Diagnosis of Diseases of the Chest

THIRD EDITION

Robert G. Fraser, M.D.
Professor Emeritus
Department of Radiology
University of Alabama at Birmingham
Birmingham, Alabama

J.A. Peter Paré, M.D.
Professor Emeritus
Department of Medicine
McGill University
Montreal, Quebec

P.D. Paré, M.D.
Professor of Medicine
University of British Columbia
Head, Respiratory Division
University of British Columbia and
    St. Paul's Hospital
Vancouver, British Columbia

Richard S. Fraser, M.D.
Associate Professor of Pathology
McGill University
Pathologist, Montreal General Hospital
Head, Department of Pathology
Montreal Chest Hospital Institute
Montreal, Quebec

George P. Genereux, M.D.
Late Professor of Radiology
University of Saskatchewan, Saskatoon
Radiologist, University of Saskatchewan Hospital
Saskatoon, Saskatchewan

1991
W.B. SAUNDERS COMPANY
Harcourt Brace Jovanovich, Inc.
Philadelphia London Toronto Montreal Sydney Tokyo

W. B. SAUNDERS COMPANY
Harcourt Brace Jovanovich, Inc.

The Curtis Center
Independence Square West
Philadelphia, PA 19106

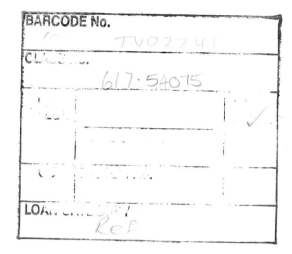

Library of Congress Cataloging-in-Publication Data
(Revised for vol. 4)

Diagnosis of diseases of the chest.

Rev. ed. of: Diagnosis of diseases of the chest /
Robert G. Fraser, J. A. Peter Paré. 2nd ed. 1977–
Includes bibliographies and indexes.

1. Chest—Disease—Diagnosis—Collected works.
2. Thoracic Diseases—diagnosis.   3. Thoracic Radiology.
1. Fraser, Robert G.

RC941.D52   1991   87–4678

ISBN 0–7216–3879–1 (set)

ISBN 0–7216–3870–8 (v. 1)

ISBN 0–7216–3871–6 (v. 2)

ISBN 0–7216–3872–4 (v. 3)

ISBN 0–7216–3873–2 (v. 4)

Listed here is the latest translated edition of this book together with the language of the translation and the publisher.

Spanish (1st edition)—Salvat Editores S.A., Muntaner 262, 08021 Barcelona, Spain

German (2nd edition)—Schattauer (F.K.) Verlag GmbH, Lenzhalde 3, Postfach 2945, 7 Stuttgart 1, Germany

Portuguese (2nd edition)—Editora Manole Ltda., Rua Conselheiro Ramalho 516, CEP 01325, São Paulo, Brazil

Editor: Lisette Bralow
Designer: W. B. Saunders Staff
Production Manager: Peter Faber
Manuscript Editor: Terry Belanger
Illustration Coordinator: Walt Verbitski
Indexer: Julie Figures
Indexer of Names: Kathy Garcia

Volume   I ISBN   0–7216–3870–8
Volume II ISBN   0–7216–3871–6
Volume III ISBN   0–7216–3872–4
Volume IV ISBN   0–7216–3873–2
Set ISBN   0–7216–3879–1

Diagnosis of Diseases of the Chest, Third Edition

Printed in the United States of America.

Last digit is the print number: 9   8   7   6   5   4   3   2   1

Diagnosis of Diseases of the Chest

THIRD EDITION

Robert G. Fraser, M.D.
Professor Emeritus
Department of Radiology
University of Alabama at Birmingham
Birmingham, Alabama

J.A. Peter Paré, M.D.
Professor Emeritus
Department of Medicine
McGill University
Montreal, Quebec

P.D. Paré, M.D.
Professor of Medicine
University of British Columbia
Head, Respiratory Division
University of British Columbia and
    St. Paul's Hospital
Vancouver, British Columbia

Richard S. Fraser, M.D.
Associate Professor of Pathology
McGill University
Pathologist, Montreal General Hospital
Head, Department of Pathology
Montreal Chest Hospital Institute
Montreal, Quebec

George P. Genereux, M.D.
Late Professor of Radiology
University of Saskatchewan, Saskatoon
Radiologist, University of Saskatchewan Hospital
Saskatoon, Saskatchewan

1991
W.B. SAUNDERS COMPANY
Harcourt Brace Jovanovich, Inc.
Philadelphia London Toronto Montreal Sydney Tokyo

W. B. SAUNDERS COMPANY
Harcourt Brace Jovanovich, Inc.

The Curtis Center
Independence Square West
Philadelphia, PA 19106

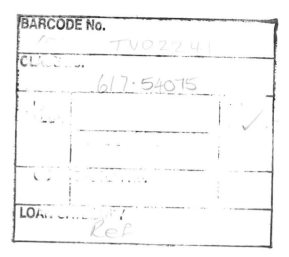

Library of Congress Cataloging-in-Publication Data
(Revised for vol. 4)

Diagnosis of diseases of the chest.

Rev. ed. of: Diagnosis of diseases of the chest /
Robert G. Fraser, J. A. Peter Paré. 2nd ed. 1977–
Includes bibliographies and indexes.

1. Chest—Disease—Diagnosis—Collected works.
2. Thoracic Diseases—diagnosis.   3. Thoracic Radiology.
1. Fraser, Robert G.

RC941.D52   1991   87–4678

ISBN 0–7216–3879–1 (set)

ISBN 0–7216–3870–8 (v. 1)

ISBN 0–7216–3871–6 (v. 2)

ISBN 0–7216–3872–4 (v. 3)

ISBN 0–7216–3873–2 (v. 4)

Listed here is the latest translated edition of this book together with the language of the translation and the publisher.

Spanish (1st edition)—Salvat Editores S.A., Muntaner 262, 08021 Barcelona, Spain

German (2nd edition)—Schattauer (F.K.) Verlag GmbH, Lenzhalde 3, Postfach 2945, 7 Stuttgart 1, Germany

Portuguese (2nd edition)—Editora Manole Ltda., Rua Conselheiro Ramalho 516, CEP 01325, São Paulo, Brazil

Editor: Lisette Bralow
Designer: W. B. Saunders Staff
Production Manager: Peter Faber
Manuscript Editor: Terry Belanger
Illustration Coordinator: Walt Verbitski
Indexer: Julie Figures
Indexer of Names: Kathy Garcia

Volume   I ISBN   0–7216–3870–8
Volume   II ISBN   0–7216–3871–6
Volume III ISBN   0–7216–3872–4
Volume IV ISBN   0–7216–3873–2
Set ISBN   0–7216–3879–1

Diagnosis of Diseases of the Chest, Third Edition

Printed in the United States of America.

Last digit is the print number: 9   8   7   6   5   4   3   2   1

DEDICATION

This volume is dedicated to our wives—
Joanne, Anne, Lisa, and Marie-Claire.

PREFACE TO
THE THIRD EDITION

—vanity of vanities; all is vanity.
What profit hath a man of all his labour which
he taketh under the sun?
One generation passeth away, and another
generation cometh.

—ECCLESIASTES 1:2

It has been 20 years since the two senior authors began writing the first edition of this book, and during the preliminary stages of planning for the third edition, we grudgingly acknowledged a mild but inescapable attrition in the motivation and initiative we possessed formerly. More importantly, we recognized the need to prepare to hand over the reins for the writing of future editions to dependable and tested hands. As a result, we felt obliged to augment the authorship of this edition with young, fertile minds, and we didn't have far to look: our two sons, RSF and PP, were devoting much of their professional lives to the pathologic and physiologic manifestations of chest disease, respectively, and it was logical that they should take up the cudgel to prevent their fathers from wallowing in their own misconceptions. We also felt the need for the addition of a third creative mind, this time a radiologist, to bring about renewed vigor and enthusiasm to the description and illustration of roentgenologic pathology; again we had to look no further than our own back yard to find GG, an internationally renowned radiologist with a vast clinical experience in chest disease. As the first volume of this third edition has evolved, it has become abundantly clear that we possessed much wisdom in seeking the collaboration of these three. The new authors have reorganized many chapters and have greatly improved the text by preparing a much more accurate description and illustration of the pathologic manifestations of thoracic disease, a more thorough discussion of normal and pathologic physiology, and fresh new material on the roentgenologic manifestations of many conditions.

It was stated in the Preface to the First Edition that the book was written with the aim of emphasizing the value of the roentgenogram as the *first* rather than the *major* step in the diagnosis of chest disease. In the subsequent 15 year interval, we have not seen cause to alter this opinion. However, despite the usefulness of this approach from a practical day-to-day viewpoint, we have come to realize more fully that the ultimate foundation upon which diagnosis must be based is a knowledge of chest disease itself. In addition to a thorough familiarity with normal structure and function, this includes a detailed knowledge of physiologic and pathologic alterations as well as the etiologies and pathogenetic mechanisms behind them. Although intimated in the first two editions, this belief has reached full fruition in the present text in which all aspects of the normal and diseased chest have been given roughly equal coverage. Whatever emphasis was formerly placed on roentgenology is now of necessity less evident. This should not be interpreted as a diminution in our belief of the importance of the roentgenogram in diagnosis but rather as an extension of the previously unstated but implied importance of the broader view. This approach has necessarily involved the inclusion of a vast amount of new information and has resulted unavoidably in a comprehensive reference work rather than a textbook. The scope of the text is such that it will find its greatest use in the hands of specialists such as respirologists, thoracic surgeons, and radiologists and pathologists whose particular interest lies in diseases of the chest. However, those with a more general outlook, such as internists and house officers, will also find the book useful as an occasional reference source.

What will the reader find new? In addition to the more extensive coverage of pathology and physiology and the addition of new knowledge that has appeared in the literature over the 7 or 8 year span, fresh material has appeared on the control of breathing, the respiratory muscles in health and disease, breathing during sleep, the development of the lung, host defense mechanisms, opportunistic infections, pulmonary vasculitides, the acquired immunodeficiency syndrome, the lung in transplantation, and drug-induced pulmonary disease. In addition, there is a complete reorganization of the chapter on neoplasms based on the 1982 WHO classification, and there are extensive additions to the discussion of the obstructive airway diseases, particularly with regard to pathophysiology and bronchial reactivity. A number of illustrations have been replaced and many new ones added, with emphasis on computed tomography and, to a lesser extent, magnetic resonance imaging. Virtually all illustrations of gross and microscopic pathology are new, and it is hoped that they will provide new insights into pathologic/radiologic correlation.

Since the publication of the Second Edition, a spectacular expansion of knowledge has occurred concerning the structure and function of the lung in health and disease; as a result, it has proved impossible to carry out a simple revision, and in most areas the book has been almost completely rewritten. However, all attempts have been made not to increase its length: the addition of new material, particularly in sections dealing with pathology and pathophysiology, has been balanced by the removal of out-of-date-text. To achieve a roughly equal size of the new volumes, it has been necessary to alter the order of chapters somewhat from that in the first two editions. The tables of differential diagnosis and decision trees have been incorporated into Volume IV rather than occupying a separate volume as in the second edition. The rapidity with which new knowledge is appearing has also made it necessary to publish the four volumes sequentially rather than simultaneously. We regret the necessity for this, but were we to await completion of the later volumes, the first volume would be long out of date, requiring thorough revision; the inevitable result would be a vicious cycle whereby none of the volumes would ever be published!

As anticipated, the writing style of each of the five authors has varied considerably, requiring considerable subediting in an attempt to unify syntax and nomenclature. In this regard, we and others have been concerned with the variable terminology employed by physicians in the description of the normal and diseased thorax. In an attempt to obviate this variability, in 1975 a joint committee of the American College of Chest Physicians and the American Thoracic Society published a glossary of pulmonary terms and symbols pertinent to the medical and physiologic aspects of the normal and diseased chest (Chest 67:538, 1975). At about the same time, the Fleischner Society formed a committee on nomenclature that designed and subsequently published a glossary of words and terms that they recommended for roentgenologic terminology (AJR 143:509, 1984). Since several of the terms recommended by the ACCP/ATS Committee for use in the classification of diseases, in physical examination, and in respiratory therapy are at variance with those used in this book, we have chosen to include only the terms and symbols used in respiratory physiology and pathophysiology. Both the modified ACCP/ATS and the Fleischner glossaries are printed at the beginning of each volume, and the reader is urged to review them and use them regularly.

The burgeoning knowledge in the field of chest disease continues unabated. The 20-odd journals that the two senior authors reviewed in the preparation of the first and second editions have been expanded not only by the proliferation of new biomedical publications and the inclusion of a number of recognized journals in other specialized clinical disciplines, but also by the many physiology and pathology journals that were not included in the original review. As a consequence, the near-10,000 references cited in the second edition will certainly be exceeded in the third. Bibliographies have been placed at the end of each chapter and their position indicated by a black slash on page edges, thus facilitating their identification.

Once again, we invite our readers to inform us of differences of opinion they may have with the contents of this book or to offer their advice as to how future editions may be improved. It is only through such interchange of information and opinion that we can hope to establish on a firm basis the knowledge necessary for a full understanding of respiratory disease.

RGF
JAPP
PDP
RSF
GPG

ACKNOWLEDGMENTS

Coordination of the contributions of two authors in the preparation of the first two editions of this book proved to be a formidable undertaking, but in fact was relatively simple compared with the enormous problems created by attempts to assimilate material from five separate sources in this third edition. The writing of the manuscript and the choice and preparation of new illustrations were the most formidable parts of the undertaking, but the many steps necessary to the final product required the unselfish and enthusiastic contributions of many hands and minds, and the support and encouragement we received from many of our friends are greatly appreciated and duly acknowledged.

It is not possible to overstate our gratitude to our secretaries, who handled magnificently the tedious and necessarily exacting task of listing and filing references, transcribing manuscript from tape, typing the several drafts up to and including the final one, and cheerfully coping with the innumerable problems encountered. Anne Paré of Val Morin, Quebec; Peggy Stewart of St. Paul's Hospital, Vancouver; Donna O'Connor of the Montreal General Hospital; and Marianne Constantine of the Montreal Chest Hospital exhibited exemplary patience and devotion in accomplishing these thorny chores. Although these individuals have earned our heartfelt thanks, the efforts by Lynn Hogan and Susan Ullery-Lynch of the Hospital of the University of Alabama at Birmingham deserve special praise, since it was their lot to type not only the contributions from their boss but also the edited manuscript from the other four authors. Joanne Fraser carried out the tedious job of recording, filing, and checking the innumerable references, an extremely frustrating chore that she performed with meticulous accuracy. The devotion and diligence with which all these people carried out their tasks are deeply appreciated.

The majority of the case histories and roentgenograms reproduced here are of patients of staff members of the Royal Victoria Hospital, the Montreal General Hospital, the Montreal Chest Hospital Institute, the Hospital of the University of Alabama at Birmingham, and the Medical Center of the University of Saskatchewan. All illustrations of pathology are derived from patients in the Montreal General Hospital and the Montreal Chest Hospital Institute. Our indebtedness to our colleagues who were caring for these patients cannot be overemphasized, not only for their generosity in permitting us to publish these case reports but also for the benefit of their experience and guidance over the years.

The superb photographic work throughout these volumes was the accomplishment of the Department of Visual Aids of the Royal Victoria Hospital; Susie Gray and Tony Zagar of the Department of Radiology, the University of Alabama at Birmingham; David Mandeville of the University of Saskatchewan Hospital; and Joseph Donohue and Anthony Graham of Montreal. Their craftsmanship and rich experience in photography are readily apparent in these pages. Caroline Luty, Adriana Torrisi, and Maria Masluck provided expert assistance in the preparation of the pathologic material. We would also like to thank Dr. Jack Fulmer for his review of the section on sarcoidosis and for his suggestions for revision, and Dr. Nestor Müller for providing us with several high resolution CT images.

Throughout our labors, we received much support and cooperation from the publishers, notably Lisette Bralow, who effectively and sympathetically minimized the many obstacles we encountered.

Finally, and with immense gratitude, we recall the patience and understanding displayed by our wives and children throughout our labors. Without their continuous encouragement, this book surely would not have been completed, and we acknowledge their many virtues with much love.

RGF
JAPP
PDP
RSF
GPG

PREFACE TO
THE FIRST EDITION

This book was written with the aim of defining an approach to the diagnosis of diseases of the chest based on the abnormal roentgenogram. Experience over the years has led the authors to the conclusion that the chest roentgenogram represents the focal point or sheet anchor in the diagnosis of the majority of pulmonary diseases, many patients presenting with either no symptoms and signs or entirely nonspecific ones. This emphasis on the roentgenogram as the first step in reaching a diagnosis does not represent an attempt to relegate history and physical examination to a position of no importance, but merely an effort to place them in proper perspective. In no other medical field is diagnosis so dependent upon the intelligent integration of information from roentgenologic, clinical, laboratory, and pathologic sources as in diseases of the chest. We submit that the roentgenogram is the starting point in this investigation; the knowledge of structural change thus obtained, when integrated with pertinent clinical findings and results of pulmonary function tests and other ancillary diagnostic procedures, enables one to arrive at a confident diagnosis. Some patients manifest symptoms and signs that themselves are virtually diagnostic of some chest disorders, but even in such cases the confirmation of diagnosis requires the presence of an appropriate roentgenographic pattern.

A glance through the pages will reveal an abundance of roentgenographic illustrations that might create the illusion that this book is written primarily for the roentgenologist, but this is not our intention. In fact, the clinical, morphologic, and laboratory aspects of many diseases are described at greater length than the roentgenologic, a fact pointing up the broad interest we hope the book will engender among internists, surgeons, and family practitioners interested in chest disease. The numerous illustrations reflect the aim of the book—to emphasize the value of the roentgenogram as the *first* rather than the *major* step in diagnosis.

During the writing of the book, our original plan was considerably modified as the format unfolded and we became even more aware of the complexities of design and organization. Originally, our approach to differential diagnosis suggested a division of chapters on the basis of specific roentgenographic patterns. It soon became apparent, however, that since many diseases give rise to various different roentgenographic patterns, this method of presentation would require tedious repetition of clinical and laboratory details in several chapters. To obviate this, we planned tables of differential diagnosis, listing etiologic classifications of diseases that produce specific roentgenographic patterns and describing briefly the clinical and laboratory characteristics of each disease, thus facilitating recognition of disease states. The tables are designed to be used with the text in the following manner. When a specific pattern of disease is recognized, the appropriate table should be scanned and those conditions selected that correspond most closely with the clinical picture presented by the patient. Additional information about the likeliest diagnostic possibilities can be obtained by referring to the detailed discussions in the relevant sections of the text (page numbers are cited after each diagnosis). The tables relate to 17 basic patterns of bronchopulmonary, pleural, and mediastinal disease; they are grouped together in Chapter 5 in Volume I and may be located with ease from the black marks found on the upper corners of their pages. Each table is preceded by a detailed description and representative illustrations of the specific roentgenographic pattern. An attempt has been made to indicate the relative incidence of the diseases.

Although our original plan called for a one volume presentation, it soon became apparent that the length of the text and the number and size of illustrations necessary for full coverage of the subject required two volumes. Volume I includes descriptions of the normal chest, methods and techniques of investigation, clinical features, and roentgenologic signs of chest diseases, the tables of differential diagnosis, and chapters devoted to diseases of developmental origin and the infectious diseases; in Volume II appear detailed discussions of the morphologic, roentgenologic, and clinical aspects of all other diseases of the thorax arranged in chapters according to etiology.

The roentgenograms have been reproduced by two different techniques, the majority in Volume I by the logEtronic method and those in Volume II by direct photography. The publishers have been generous in allotting sufficient space for the reproduction of the roentgenograms in a size adequate for good detail recognition.

Much of the material in the book has been based on our personal experience gained in the past almost two decades, during which we have had a predominant interest in pulmonary disease. Obviously, this experience has been greatly enhanced by the extensive literature that has accumulated during these years, and we are mindful of the tremendous help we have received from the contributions of others. Our free use of the literature is reflected in the extensive bibliography.

Certain differences from the contents of other books on respiratory disease will be noted. First, this text contains no reference to treatment. Since drug therapies and surgical techniques are constantly changing, any attempt to include them would make the book out of date almost before it was published. Second, we have intentionally made only passing reference to pulmonary disease peculiar to children, a full description of which would require a complete separate text.

The relative incidence of respiratory diseases has changed considerably over the last quarter century. In some diseases, such as tuberculosis and bronchiectasis, a decreased frequency reflects improved public health measures and therapeutic innovations; in others, man's therapeutic triumphs have proved a mixed blessing, enabling patients with disabling chronic respiratory disease to live longer despite formerly fatal pneumonias. Perhaps even more important, man himself is responsible for varying the spectrum of respiratory disease as a result of his irresponsible insistence upon increasing the amount and variety of atmospheric pollutants. Inhaled contaminated air not only is regarded as the major etiologic factor in chronic obstructive pulmonary disease and the inorganic dust pneumoconioses, but also has been incriminated in the etiology of several hypersensitivity diseases of the lungs. This last group comprises the "extrinsic" form of allergic alveolitis. The number of conditions involved, when added to the better known "intrinsic" counterpart—the collagen diseases—is largely responsible for the length of the chapter devoted to immunologic diseases. Other changes that have contributed to the "new face" of pulmonary disease include increasing knowledge of the hormonal effects of neoplasms; the discovery that various immunologic defects may reduce host resistance to infection; and finally the appearance in the western world of parasitic infestations and bacterial infections formerly considered so rare in those areas as to warrant little consideration in differential diagnosis, but now of some importance because of the modern day ease of intercontinental travel. Although the novelty of these recent changes may have led the authors to consider them in greater detail and length than is their due, the emphasis may serve to bring them into proper perspective.

Finally, we recognize our fallibility. It is inevitable that some observations in a text of this magnitude will prove erroneous in time or will find disagreement among our knowledgeable readers. This we expect and accept. We sincerely hope that such differences of opinion will be made known to us, so that they may be weighed and, where appropriate, introduced into subsequent editions or revisions. It is only through such interchange of information and opinion that we can hope to establish on a firm basis the knowledge necessary to a full understanding of respiratory disease.

R.G.F.
J.A.P.P.

CONTENTS

VOLUME IV

Glossary of Words, Terms and Symbols in Chest Medicine and Roentgenology

"Then you should say what you mean," the March Hare went on.
"I do," Alice hastily replied; "at least—at least, I mean what I say—that's the same thing, you know."
"Not the same thing a bit!" said the Hatter. "Why, you might just as well say that 'I see what I eat' is the same thing as 'I eat what I see!'"

This well-known excerpt from Lewis Carroll's *Alice's Adventures in Wonderland* points out a problem that confronts many physicians in today's constantly expanding scientific literature—the use of words and terms that mean different things to different people. The frequency with which imprecise or frankly erroneous words are employed to describe roentgenographic images (for example) is astonishing; common usage has created a jargon that has led to confusion if not to actual communication breakdown. In 1975, a joint committee of the American College of Chest Physicians and the American Thoracic Society published a glossary of pulmonary terms and symbols* pertinent to the medical and physiologic aspects of chest disease, but it omitted words that specifically related to chest roentgenology. As a consequence, the Fleischner Society formed a Committee on Nomenclature several years ago to draw up a glossary of roentgenologic words and terms and this task now has been completed and the glossary published.† We list herewith a number of words, terms, and symbols selected from the two publications that we hope our readers will refer to and use. The precise definition of some words has been altered slightly to coincide with usage in this book.

---

*Pulmonary Terms and Symbols; A report of the ACCP/ATS Joints Committee on Pulmonary Nomenclature. Chest *67*:583, 1975.
†Glossary of Terms for Thoracic Radiology: Recommendations of the Nomenclature Committee of the Fleischner Society. Am J Roentgenol *143*:509, 1984.

WORDS OR TERMS USED IN ROENTGENOLOGY

Word or Term	Comments
abscess *n., pl.* -es. 1. (pathol.) An inflammatory mass, the central part of which has undergone purulent liquefaction necrosis. It may communicate with the bronchial tree. 2. (radiol.) Within the lung, a mass presumed to be caused by infection. The presence of gas within the mass, with or without a fluid level, represents a cavity (q.v.) and implies a communication with the bronchial tree. Otherwise, a pulmonary mass can be considered to represent an abscess in the morphlogic sense only by inference. *Qualifiers:* Expressing clinical course: acute, chronic. Expressing etiology: bacterial, fungal, etc. Expressing site of involvement: lung, mediastinum, etc.	Should be used only with reference to masses of presumed infectious etiology. The word is not synonymous with cavity (*q.v.*).

WORDS OR TERMS USED IN ROENTGENOLOGY *Continued*

Word or Term	Comments
acinar pattern *n.* (radiol.) A collection of round or elliptic, ill-defined, discrete or partly confluent opacities in the lung, each measuring 4 to 8 mm in diameter and together producing an extended, inhomogeneous shadow. *Synonyms:* Rosette pattern; acinonodose pattern (used specifically with reference to endobronchial spread of tuberculosis); alveolar pattern.	An inferred conclusion usually used as a descriptor. An acceptable term, preferred to cited synonyms (especially "alveolar pattern," which is an inaccurate descriptor).
acinar shadow *n.* (radiol.) A round or slightly elliptic pulmonary opacity 4 to 8 mm in diameter presumed to represent an anatomic acinus rendered opaque by consolidation. Usually employed in the presence of many such opacities (*see* acinar pattern).	An inferred conclusion sometimes applicable as a roentgenologic descriptor.
acinus *n.* (anat.) The portion of lung parenchyma distal to the terminal bronchiole and consisting of respiratory bronchioles, alveolar ducts, alveolar sacs, and alveoli (*see* acinar shadow, acinar pattern).	A specific feature of pulmonary anatomy.
aeration *n.* (physiol./radiol.) 1. The state of containing air. 2. The state or process of being filled or inflated with air. *Qualifiers:* overaeration (preferred) or hyperaeration; underaeration (preferred) or hypoaeration. *Synonym:* Inflation.	An acceptable term with reference to the inspiratory phase of respiration. Inflation is preferred in sense 2.
air, *n.* (radiol.) Inspired atmospheric gas. The word is sometimes used to describe gas within the body regardless of its composition or site.	With reference to pneumothorax, subcutaneous emphysema, or the content of the stomach, colon, etc., gas is the more accurate term and is preferred.
air bronchiologram *n.* (radiol.) The equivalent of air bronchogram but in airways assumed to be bronchioles because of their peripheral location and diameter.	An acceptable term.
air bronchogram *n.* (radiol.) The roentgenographic shadow of an air-containing bronchus peripheral to the hilum and surrounded by airless lung (whether by virtue of absorption of air, replacement of air, or both), a finding generally regarded as evidence of the patency of the more proximal airway. Hence, any bandlike tapering and/or branching lucency within opacified lung corresponding in size and distribution to a bronchus or bronchi and presumed to represent an air-containing segment of the bronchial tree.	A specific feature of roentgenologic anatomy whose identify is often inferred. A useful and recommended term.
air-fluid level *n.* (radiol.) A local collection of gas and liquid that, when traversed by a horizontal x-ray beam, creates a shadow characterized by a sharp horizontal interface between gas density above and liquid density below.	A useful roentgenologic descriptor. Since with rare exception (*e.g.*, fat-fluid level) the upper of the two absorbant media is "air" (gas), it is sufficient to describe such an appearance as a "fluid level."
air space *n.* (*adj.* air-space) (anat./radiol.) The gas-containing portion of lung parenchyma, including the acini and excluding the interstitium and purely conductive portions of the lung. *Synonyms:* Acinar consolidation, alveolar consolidation (when used as an adjective in relation to air-space consolidation).	An inferred conclusion usually used as a roentgenologic descriptor. An acceptable term whose use as an adjective is also appropriate.

WORDS OR TERMS USED IN ROENTGENOLOGY *Continued*

Word or Term	Comments
air-trapping *n.* (pathophysiol./radiol.) The retention of excess gas in all or part of the lung at any stage of expiration.	A specific roentgenologic sign to be employed only if excess air retention is demonstrated by a dynamic study, *e.g.,* inspiration-expiration roentgenography or fluoroscopy. *Not* to be used with reference to overinflation of the lung at full inspiration (total lung capacity).
airway *n., adj.* (anat./radiol.) A collective term for the air-conducting passages from the larynx to and including the respiratory bronchioles. *Synonyms:* Conducting airway; tracheobronchial tree.	A useful anatomic term. May be used as an adjective in relation to disease or abnormality. Note that the respiratory bronchioles are both conducting and gas-exchanging airways and thus constitute the transitory zone.
alveolarization *n.* (radiol.) The opacification of groups of alveoli by a contrast medium.	A misnomer whose use is to be deplored. Excessive filling of peripheral lung structure by contrast media usually employed for bronchography may opacify respiratory bronchioles but not alveoli. Thus, the correct term is "bronchiolar filling or opacification."
anterior junction line *n.* (radiol.) A vertically oriented linear or curvilinear opacity approximately 1 to 2 mm wide, commonly projected on the tracheal air shadow. It is produced by the shadows of the right and left pleurae in intimate contact between the aerated lungs anterior to the great vessels (and sometimes the heart); hence, it never extends above the suprasternal notch (*cf.* posterior junction line). *Synonyms:* Anterior mediastinal septum, line, or stripe.	A specific feature of roentgenologic anatomy; to be preferred to cited synonyms.
aortopulmonary window *n.* 1. (anat.) A mediastinal space bounded anteriorly by the posterior surface of the ascending aorta; posteriorly by the anterior surface of the descending aorta; superiorly by the inferior surface of the aortic arch; inferiorly by the superior surface of the left pulmonary artery; medially by the left side of the trachea, left main bronchus, and esophagus; and laterally by the left lung. Within it are situated fat, the ductus ligament, the left recurrent laryngeal nerve, and lymph nodes. 2. (radiol.) A zone of relative lucency in the mediastinal shadow that is seen to best advantage in the left anterior oblique or lateral projection and that corresponds to the anatomic space defined above. On a posteroanterior roentgenogram of the chest, the lateral margin of the space constitutes the aortopulmonary window interface. *Synonym:* Aortic-pulmonic window.	A specific feature of roentgenologic anatomy.
atelectasis *n.* (pathophysiol./radiol.) Less than normal inflation of all or a portion of the lung with corresponding diminution in volume. *Qualifiers* may be employed to indicate severity (mild, moderate, severe), mechanism (resorption, relaxation, cicatrization, adhesive), or distribution (*e.g.,* lobar, platelike [*q.v.*], discoid). *Synonyms:* Collapse, loss of volume, anectasis.	Generally this term is preferable to "collapse" in describing loss of volume. The word "collapse" connotes total atelectasis in which lung tissue has been reduced to its smallest volume. Anectasis is usually used in reference to failure of lung expansion in the neonate.

WORDS OR TERMS USED IN ROENTGENOLOGY *Continued*

Word or Term	Comments
azygoesophageal recess *n.* 1. (anat.) A space or recess in the right side of the mediastinum into which the medial edge of the right lower lobe (crista pulmonis) extends. It is limited superiorly by the arch of the azygos vein, inferiorly by the diaphragm, posteriorly by the azygos vein in front of the vertebral column, and medially by the esophagus and its adjacent structures. (The exact relationship between the medial edge of the lung and the mediastinal structures is variable.) 2. (radiol.) In a frontal chest roentgenogram, a vertically oriented interface between air in the right lower lobe and the adjacent mediastinum that represents the medial limit of the anatomic azygoesophageal recess. *Synonyms:* Infraazygos recess; right pleuroesophageal line or stripe; right paraesophageal line or stripe.	A specific feature of roentgenologic anatomy. The use of the term "recess" to identify an interface is inappropriate; thus, azygoesophageal recess interface is preferred.
bat's-wing distribution *n.* (radiol.) A spatial arrangement of roentgenographic opacities in a frontal roentgenogram that bears a vague resemblance to the shape of a bat in flight; said of coalescent, ill-defined opacities that are approximately bilaterally symmetric and that are confined to the medulla of the lungs (*q.v.*). *Synonym:* Butterfly distribution.	A roentgenologic descriptor of limited usefulness.
bleb *n.* 1. (pathol.) A gas-containing space within or contiguous to the visceral pleura of the lung. 2. (radiol.) A local, thin-walled lucency contiguous with the pleura, usually at the lung apex. *Synonyms:* Type I bulla (pathol.); bulla; a form of pulmonary air cyst (radiol.)	An inferred conclusion seldom justifiable by roentgenogram alone. Bulla or air cyst is preferred.
bronchiole *n.* (anat./radiol.) An airway that contains no cartilage in its wall. A bronchiole may be purely conducting (up to and including the terminal bronchiole) or transitory (the respiratory bronchioles that carry out both conduction and gas exchange).	A specific feature of pulmonary anatomy.
bronchocele *n. See* mucoid impaction.	
bronchus *n.* (anat./radiol.) A conducting airway distal to the tracheal bifurcation that contains cartilage in its wall.	A specific feature of pulmonary anatomy.
bulla *n., pl.* -lae. 1. (pathol.) A sharply demarcated region of emphysema; a gas-containing space that may contain nothing but gas or may contain overdistended and ruptured alveolar septa and blood vessels. 2. (radiol.) Sharply demarcated hyperlucent area of avascularity within the lung, measuring 1 cm or more in diameter and possessing a wall less than 1 mm in thickness. *Qualifiers:* small, medium, large.	The preferred term to describe all thin-walled air-containing spaces in the lung with the exception of pneumatocele (*q.v.*).
butterfly distribution *n.* (radiol.) *See* bat's-wing distribution.	To be distinguished from the use of this term in general medicine to describe the distribution of certain cutaneous lesions.

WORDS OR TERMS USED IN ROENTGENOLOGY *Continued*

Word or Term	**Comments**

calcification *n.* 1. (pathophysiol.) (a) The process by which one or more deposits of calcium salts are formed within lung tissue or within a pulmonary lesion. (b) Such a deposit of calcium salts. 2. (radiol.) A calcific opacity within the lung that may be organized (*e.g.*, concentric lamination), but which does not display the trabecular organization of true bone. *Qualifiers:* "eggshell," "popcorn," target, laminated, flocculent, nodular, etc.

An explicit conclusion; may be used as a descriptor. To be distinguished from ossification (*q.v.*).

carina *n.* (anat./radiol.) The keel-shaped ridge that separates the right and left main bronchi at the tracheal bifurcation.

A specific feature of pulmonary anatomy.

carinal angle *n.* (anat./radiol.) The angle formed by the right and left main bronchi at the tracheal bifurcation.

Synonyms: Bifurcation angle; angle of tracheal bifurcation.

A definitive anatomic and roentgenologic measurement.

cavity *n.* 1. (pathol.) A mass within lung parenchyma, the central portion of which has undergone liquefaction necrosis and has been expelled via the bronchial tree, leaving a gas-containing space, with or without associated fluid. 2. (radiol.) A gas-containing space within the lung surrounded by a wall whose thickness is greater than 1 mm and usually irregular in contour.

A useful descriptor without etiologic connotation. The word must not be used interchangeably with abscess (*q.v.*), which may exist without bronchial communication and therefore without cavitation.

circumscribed *adj.* (radiol.) Possessing a complete or nearly complete visible border.

An acceptable descriptor.

clot *n.* (pathol.) A semisolidified mass of blood elements.

Cf. thrombus.

coalescence *n.* (radiol.) The joining together of a number of opacities into a single opacity; confluence (*q.v.*).

An acceptable descriptor.

coin lesion *n.* (radiol.) A sharply defined, circular opacity within the lung suggestive of the appearance of a coin and usually representing a spherical or nodular lesion.

Synonyms: Pulmonary nodule, pulmonary mass.

A roentgenologic descriptor, the use of which is to be condemned. The term "coin" may be descriptive of the shadow, but certainly not of the lesion producing it.

collapse *n.* (radiol.) A state in which lung tissue has undergone complete atelectasis.

The term is acceptable when employed strictly as defined, but "atelectasis" is preferred, since the degree of loss of lung volume can be qualified by mild, moderate, or severe.

collateral ventilation *n.* (physiol./radiol.) The process by which gas passes from one lung unit (acinus, lobule, segment, or lobe) to a contiguous unit via alveolar pores (pores of Kohn), canals of Lambert, or direct airway anastomoses.

Synonym: Collateral air drift.

An inferred conclusion usually based on fairly reliable signs. A useful term. The channels of peripheral airway communication also function as a mechanism for transmission of liquid from one unit to another (*e.g.*, in acute airspace pneumonia).

confluence *n.* (radiol.) The nature of opacities that are contiguous with or adjacent to one another.

Antonym: Discrete (*q.v.*).

A useful descriptor; confluence is to be distinguished from coalescence (*q.v.*), which is the act of becoming confluent.

WORDS OR TERMS USED IN ROENTGENOLOGY *Continued*

Word or Term	Comments
consolidation *n.* 1. (pathophysiol.) The process by which air in the lung is replaced by the products of disease, rendering the lung solid (as in pneumonia). 2. (radiol.) An essentially homogeneous opacity in the lung characterized by little or no loss of volume, by effacement of pulmonary blood vessels, and sometimes by the presence of an air bronchogram (*q.v.*).	An inferred conclusion, applicable only in an appropriate clinical setting when the opacity can with reasonable certainty be attributed to replacement of alveolar air by exudate, transudate, or tissue. Not to be used with reference to all homogeneous opacities.
corona radiata *n.* (radiol.) A circumferential pattern of fine linear spicules, approximately 5 mm long, extending outward from the margin of a solitary pulmonary nodule through a zone of relative lucency.	A sign of limited usefulness in the differentiation of benign and malignant nodules.
cor pulmonale *n.* 1. (pathol./clin.) Right ventricular hypertrophy and/or dilatation occurring as a result of an abnormality of lung structure or function. 2. (radiol.) The combination of pulmonary arterial hypertension and chronic lung disease, with or without evidence of enlargement of right heart chambers. *Qualifiers:* acute, chronic.	An inferred roentgenologic conclusion based on usually reliable signs. An acceptable descriptor. Despite the pathologic definition, roentgenologic evidence of cardiomegaly need not be present.
cortex *n.* (radiol.) The peripheral 2 to 3 cm of lung parenchyma adjacent to the visceral pleura, either over the convexity of the thorax or in the interlobar fissures. (*See* medulla and hilum.)	The peripheral part of an arbitrary subdivision of the lung into three zones from the hilum to the visceral pleura. Of limited usefulness.
CT number *n.* (radiol./physics) In computed tomography, a quantitative numerical statement of the relative attenuation of the x-ray beam at a specified point; loosely, the relative attenuation of a specified tissue absorber, usually expressed in Hounsfield units (HU).	
cyst *n.* 1. (pathol.) A circumscribed space whose contents may be liquid or gaseous and whose wall is generally thin and well defined and lined by epithelium. 2. (radiol.) A gas-containing space of any size possessing a thin wall. *Qualifiers:* foregut (bronchogenic, esophageal duplication); postinfectious.	This term is entirely nonspecific and should not possess inferred conclusion as to etiology. It is the preferred term to describe any thin-walled gas-containing space in the lung possessing a wall thickness greater than 1 mm.
defined *adj.* (radiol.) The character of the border of a shadow. *Qualifiers:* well, sharply, poorly, distinctly.	An acceptable descriptor.
demarcated *adj.* (radiol.) Distinct from adjacent structures. *Qualifiers:* well, sharply, poorly.	An acceptable descriptor. (*Cf.* defined.)
dense *adj.* (radiol.) Possessing density (*q.v.*). Usually used in describing or comparing roentgenographic shadows with respect to their light transmission.	A recommended term in the context defined. Should not be used in referring to the opacity of an absorber of x-radiation. (*See* opaque, opacity.)
density *n.* 1. (physics) The mass of a substance per unit volume. 2. (photometry/radiol.) The opacity of a roentgenographic shadow to visible light; film blackening. 3. (radiol.) The shadow of an absorber more opaque to x-rays than its surround; an opacity or radiopacity. 4. The degree of opacity of an absorber to x-rays, usually expressed in terms of the nature of the absorber (*e.g.*, bone, water, or fat density).	In sense 2, the term refers to a fundamental characteristic of the roentgenogram, and its use is recommended. In senses 3 and 4, it refers to the character of the absorber and has an exactly opposite connotation with respect to film blackening. Because of this potential confusion, the term should *never* be used to mean an "opacity" or "radiopacity."

WORDS OR TERMS USED IN ROENTGENOLOGY *Continued*

Word or Term	Comments
diffuse *adj.* 1. (pathophysiol.) Widely distributed through an organ or type of tissue. 2. (radiol.) Widespread and continuous (said of shadows and by inference of the states or processes producing them). *Synonyms:* Disseminated, generalized, systemic, widespread.	A useful and acceptable term. In the context of chest radiology, "diffuse" connotes widespread, anatomically continuous but not necessarily complete involvement of the lung or other thoracic structure or tissue; "disseminated" connotes widespread but anatomically discontinuous involvement; and "generalized" connotes complete or nearly complete involvement whereas "systemic" connotes involvement of a thoracic structure or tissue as part of a process involving the entire body.
discrete *adj.* (radiol.) Separate, individually distinct; hence, with respect to opacities, usually circumscribed. *Antonyms:* Confluent, coalescent.	An acceptable descriptor.
disseminated *adj.* 1. (pathophysiol.) Widely but discontinuously distributed through an organ or type of tissue. 2. (radiol.) Widespread but anatomically discontinuous (said of shadows and by inference of the states or processes producing them). *Synonyms:* Diffuse (*q.v.*), generalized, systemic.	A useful and acceptable term.
doubling time *n.* (radiol.) The time span over which a pulmonary nodule or mass doubles in volume (increases its diameter by a factor of 1.25).	An acceptable term. The concept should be used with caution as a criterion for distinguishing benign from malignant nodules.
embolus *n.* 1. (pathol.) A clot or mass of foreign material that has been carried by the bloodstream to occlude partly or completely the lumen of a blood vessel. 2. (radiol.) (a) A lucent defect or obstruction within an opacified blood vessel presumed to represent an embolus in the pathologic sense. (b) An acutely dilated pulmonary artery persumed to represent the presence of blood clot or other embolic material. *Qualifiers:* acute, chronic; air, fat, amniotic fluid, parasitic, neoplastic, tissue, foreign material (*e.g.*, iodized oil, mercury, talc); septic, therapeutic, paradoxic.	In sense 2(a), an inferred conclusion based on reliable evidence (arteriography); in sense 2(b), based on highly suggestive evidence (conventional roentgenography) in the appropriate clinical setting. A useful descriptor, particularly in arteriography.
emphysema *n.* 1. (pathol.) (a) A morbid condition of the lung characterized by abnormally expanded air spaces distal to the terminal bronchiole, with or without destruction of the air-space walls (per Ciba Conference, 1959). (b) As above, but "with destruction of the walls of involved air spaces" specified (per World Health Organization, 1961, and American Thoracic Society, 1962). 2. (radiol.) Overinflation of all or a portion of one or both lungs, with or without associated oligemia (*q.v.*), presumed to represent morphologic emphysema.	In radiology, an inferred conclusion based on usually reliable signs (if the disease is moderate or advanced). Applicable only in an appropriate clinical setting and, in the sense of the ATS definition, not applicable to spasmodic asthma or compensatory overinflation.
fibrocalcific *adj.* (radiol.) Of or pertaining to sharply defined, linear, and/or nodular opacities containing calcification(s) (*q.v.*), usually occurring in the upper lobes and presumed to represent old granulomatous lesions.	A widely used and acceptable roentgenologic descriptor.

WORDS OR TERMS USED IN ROENTGENOLOGY *Continued*

Word or Term

Comments

fibronodular *adj.* (radiol.) Of or pertaining to sharply defined, approximately circular opacities occurring singly or in clusters, usually in the upper lobes, and associated with linear opacities and distortion (retraction) of adjacent structures. A finding usually presumed to represent old granulomatous disease.

An inferred conclusion usually employed as a roentgenologic descriptor. Its use is not recommended.

fibrosis *n.* 1. (pathol.) (a) Cellular fibrous tissue or dense acellular collagenous tissue. (b) The process of proliferation of fibroblasts leading to the formation of fibrous or collagenous tissue. 2. (radiol.) Any opacity presumed to represent fibrous or collagenous tissue; applicable to linear, nodular, or stellate opacities that are sharply defined, that are associated with evidence of loss of volume in the affected portion of the lung and/or with deformity of adjacent structures, and that show no change over a period of months or years. Also applicable with caution to a diffuse pattern of opacity if there is evidence of progressive loss of lung volume or if the pattern of opacity is unchanged over time.

In radiology, an inferred conclusion often used as a descriptor. An acceptable term if used in strict accordance with the criteria cited.

fissure *n.* 1. (anat.) The infolding of visceral pleura that separates one lobe or a portion of a lobe from another. 2. (radiol.) A linear opacity normally 1 mm or less in width that corresponds in position and extent to the anatomic separation of pulmonary lobes or portions of lobes. *Qualifiers:* minor, major, horizontal, oblique, accessory, anomalous, azygos, inferior accessory.

Synonym: Interlobar septum.

A specific feature of anatomy.

Fleischner's line(s) *n.* (radiol.) A straight, curved, or irregular linear opacity that is visible in multiple projections; is usually situated in the lower half of the lung; is usually approximately horizontal but may be oriented in any direction; and may or may not appear to extend to the pleural surface. Such lines vary markedly in length and width; their exact pathologic significance is unknown.

An acceptable term. However, the term "linear opacity," properly qualified with respect to location, dimensions, and orientation, is preferred. There are no synonyms ("platelike," "discoid," and "platter" atelectasis should *not* be employed as synonyms; in the absence of clear histologic evidence of the significance of Fleischner's lines, the inferred identification of such lines with a form of atelectasis is unwarranted).

fluffy *adj.* (radiol.) In describing opacities: ill-defined, lacking clear-cut margins; resembling down.

Synonyms: Shaggy, poorly defined.

An imprecise descriptor of limited usefulness.

ground-glass pattern *n.* (radiol.) Any extended, finely granular pattern of pulmonary opacity within which normal anatomic details are partly obscured. Term derived from a fancied resemblance to etched or abraded glass.

Synonym: Granular pattern.

A nonspecific roentgenologic descriptor of limited usefulness; the synonym is preferred.

hernia *n.* (clin./morphol./radiol.) The protrusion of all or part of an organ or tissue through an abnormal opening.

An inferred conclusion to be used only within the precise terms of the definition. Thus, in the thorax the word is appropriate in relation to the diaphragm but should not be used with reference to pulmonary overinflation and mediastinal displacement.

WORDS OR TERMS USED IN ROENTGENOLOGY *Continued*

Word or Term	Comments
hilum, *n., pl.* -la. 1. (anat.) A depression or pit in that part of an organ where the vessels and nerves enter. 2. (radiol.) The composite shadow at the root of each lung composed of bronchi, pulmonary arteries and veins, lymph nodes, nerves, bronchial vessels, and associated areolar tissue. *Synonyms:* Lung root; hilus (hili).	A specific element of pulmonary anatomy. Hilum (hila) is preferred to hilus (hili).
homogeneous *adj.* (radiol.) Of uniform opacity or texture throughout. *Antonyms:* Inhomogeneous, nonhomogeneous, heterogeneous.	A useful roentgenologic descriptor. Inhomogeneous is the preferred antonym.
honeycomb pattern *n.* 1. (pathol.) A multitude of irregular cystic spaces in pulmonary tissue that are generally lined with bronchiolar epithelium and have markedly thickened walls composed of dense fibrous tissue, with or without associated chronic inflammation. 2. (radiol.) A number of closely approximated ring shadows representing air spaces 5 to 10 mm in diameter with walls 2 to 3 mm thick that resemble a true honeycomb; a finding whose occurrence implies "end-stage" lung.	It is recommended that the term be used strictly in accordance with the dimensional limits cited, in which case it possesses specific connotation.
hyperemia *n.* 1. (pathol./physiol.) An excess of blood in a part of the body; engorgement. 2. (radiol.) Increased blood flow. *Synonym:* Pleonemia (*q.v.*).	While semantically correct, this word has come through common usage to mean the increased blood flow that is part of the inflammatory response. We recommend that it be used as a descriptor only in arteriography. The synonym is preferred when indicating increased blood flow to the lungs.
hypertension *n.* (clin./radiol.) Elevation above normal levels of systolic and/or diastolic pressure within the systemic or pulmonary vascular bed. Generally accepted empiric levels of pressure for systemic arterial hypertension are 140 systolic, 90 diastolic; systemic venous hypertension, 12 mm Hg; pulmonary arterial hypertension, 30 mm Hg systolic; 15 diastolic; pulmonary venous hypertension, 12 mm Hg. *Synonym:* High blood pressure.	With the exception of systemic arterial hypertension, roentgenologic assessment of hypertension in each of the four vascular compartments constitutes an inferred conclusion, although based on usually reliable signs.
infarct *n.* (Literally, a portion of tissue stuffed with extravasated blood or serum.) 1. (pathol.) A zone of ischemic necrosis surrounded by hyperemic lung resulting from occlusion of the region's feeding vessel, usually by an embolus. 2. (radiol.) A pulmonary opacity that, by virtue of its temporal development and in the appropriate clinical setting, is considered to result from thromboembolic occlusion of a feeding vessel. The opacity is commonly but not exclusively hump-shaped and pleura-based when viewed in profile and poorly defined and round when viewed *en face*.	An inferred roentgenologic conclusion acceptable in the proper clinical setting and with appropriate signs. Subsequent events may establish that the opacity was the result of either hemorrhage or tissue necrosis. The word should not be used in the absence of an opacity (*e.g.,* with oligemia).

WORDS OR TERMS USED IN ROENTGENOLOGY *Continued*

Word or Term	Comments
infiltrate *n.* 1. (pathophysiol.) Any substance or type of cell that occurs within or spreads through the interstices (interstitium and/or alveoli) of the lung, which is foreign to the lung or which accumulates in greater than normal quantity within it. 2. (radiol.) (a) An ill-defined opacity in the lung that neither destroys nor displaces the gross morphology of the lung and is presumed to represent an infiltrate in the pathophysiologic sense. (b) Any ill-defined opacity in the lung.	An inferred and often unwarranted conclusion used as a descriptor. The term is almost invariably used in sense 2(b), in which it serves no useful purpose, and, lacking a specific connotation, is so variably used as to cause great confusion. The term's use as a descriptor is to be condemned. The preferred word is "opacity," properly qualified with respect to location, dimensions, and definition.
inflation *n.* (physiol./radiol.) The state or process of being expanded or filled with gas; used specifically with reference to the expansion of the lungs with air. *Qualifiers:* overinflation (preferred) or hyperinflation; underinflation (preferred) or hypoinflation. *Synonyms:* Aeration, inhalation, inspiration.	"Inflation" connotes expansion with gas or air. "Aeration" connotes the admission of air, exposure to air. "Inhalation" refers specifically to the act of drawing air into the lungs in the process of breathing (as opposed to exhalation); "inspiration," with reference to breathing, is similar in connotation. The word "inflation" is the preferred term, since it avoids the confusion that surrounds the meaning of aeration as a result of common misusage.
interface *n.* (radiol.) The common boundary between the shadows of two juxtaposed structures or tissues of different texture or opacity (*e.g.,* lung and heart). *Synonyms:* Edge, border.	A useful roentgenologic descriptor.
interstitium *n.* (anat./radiol.) A continuum of loose connective tissue throughout the lung consisting of three subdivisions: (a) bronchoarterial (axial), surrounding the bronchoarterial bundles from the hila to the point at which bronchiolar walls become intimately related to lung parenchyma; (b) parenchymal (acinar), situated between alveolar and capillary basement membranes; and (c) subpleural, situated between the pleura and lung parenchyma and continuous with the interlobular septa and perivenous interstitial space that extends from the lung periphery to the hila. *Synonym:* Interstitial space.	A useful anatomic term. The interstitium of the lung is not normally visible roentgenographically and only becomes visible when disease (*e.g.,* edema) increases its volume and attenuation.
Kerley line *n.* (radiol.) A linear opacity, which, depending on its location, extent, and orientation, may be further classified as follows: Kerley A line—an essentially straight linear opacity 2 to 6 cm in length and 1 to 3 mm in width, usually situated in an upper lung zone, that points toward the hilum centrally and is directed toward but does not extend to the pleural surface peripherally. Kerley B line—a straight linear opacity 1.5 to 2 cm in length and 1 to 2 mm in width, usually situated at the lung base, and oriented at right angles to the pleural surface with which it is usually in contact. Kerley C lines—a group of branching, linear opacities producing the appearance of a fine net, situated at the lung base and representing Kerley B lines seen *en face*. *Synonym:* Septal line(s).	A specific feature of pathologic/roentgenologic anatomy. Except when it is essential to distinguish A, B, and C lines, the term "septal line" is preferred. "Lymphatic line" is anatomically inaccurate and should never be used.

WORDS OR TERMS USED IN ROENTGENOLOGY *Continued*

Word or Term	Comments
line *n.* (radiol.) A longitudinal opacity no greater than 2 mm in width (*cf.* stripe).	A useful word appropriately employed in the description of roentgenographic shadows within the mediastinum (*e.g.,* anterior junction line) or lung (interlobar fissures).
linear opacity *n.* (radiol.) A shadow resembling a line; hence, any elongated opacity of approximately uniform width. *Synonyms:* Line, line shadow, linear shadow, band shadow.	A generic roentgenologic descriptor of great usefulness. "Band shadow" and "line shadow" have been employed by some to identify elongated shadows more than 2 mm wide and less than 2 mm wide, respectively; "linear opacity," qualified by a statement of specific dimensions, is the preferred term. The length, width, anatomic location, and orientation of such a shadow should be specified.
lobe *n.* (anat./radiol.) One of the principal divisions of the lungs (usually three on the right, two on the left), each of which is enveloped by the visceral pleura except at the hilum and in areas of developmental deficiency where fissures are incomplete. The lobes are separated in whole or in part by pleural fissures.	A specific feature of pulmonary anatomy.
lobule *n.* (anat./radiol.) A unit of lung structure. A subdivision of lung parenchyma that is of two types: (a) primary, arising from the last respiratory bronchiole and consisting of a series of alveolar ducts, atria, alveolar sacs, and alveoli, together with their accompanying blood vessels and nerves; (b) secondary, composed of a variable number of acini (usually 3 to 5) and bounded in most cases by connective tissue septa.	Acinus is the preferred anatomic/physiologic unit of lung structure. Since a primary lobule is not visible roentgenographically, the use of the term has been largely abandoned. When unmodified, the word "lobule" refers to a secondary lobule. A secondary pulmonary lobule occasionally becomes visible when it is either selectively consolidated or its surrounding connective tissue septa become visible from a process such as edema.
lucency *n.* (radiol.) The shadow of an absorber that attenuates the primary x-ray beam less effectively than do surrounding absorbers. Hence, in a roentgenogram, any circumscribed area that appears more nearly black (of greater photometric density) than its surround. Usually applied to local shadows of air density whose attenuation is less than that of surrounding lung (*e.g.,* a bulla) or of fat density when surrounded by a more effective absorber such as muscle. *Synonyms:* Radiolucency, translucency, transradiancy.	This term employed by analogy with "opacity," is acceptable in American usage, although it is etymologically indefensible. In British usage, "transradiancy" is preferred.
lymphadenopathy *n.* (clin./pathol./radiol.) Any abnormality of lymph nodes; by common usage usually restricted to enlargement of lymph nodes. *Synonym:* Lymph node enlargement.	Since "adeno-" specifically relates to a glandular structure and since lymph nodes are not glands, the term is a misnomer and its use is to be condemned in favor of its synonym.
marking(s) *n.* (radiol.) A descriptor variously used with reference to the shadows produced by a combination of normal pulmonary structures (blood vessels, bronchi, etc.). Usually used in the plural and following "lung" or "bronchovascular." *Synonym:* Linear opacity.	When used alone, a vague descriptor of little value and not recommended. With proper qualification, the term is acceptable.

WORDS OR TERMS USED IN ROENTGENOLOGY *Continued*

Word or Term

Comments

mass *n.* (radiol.) Any pulmonary or pleural lesion represented in a roentgenogram by a discrete opacity greater than 30 mm in diameter (without regard to contour, border characteristics, or homogeneity), but explicitly shown or presumed to be extended in all three dimensions.

Synonym: Tumor (*q.v.*).

A useful and recommended descriptor. Should always be qualified with respect to size, location, contour, definition, homogeneity, opacity, and number. Its use as a qualifier of "lesion" is to be deplored.

medulla *n.* (radiol.) That portion of the lung situated between the hilum and cortex (*q.v.*).

A term and concept of limited usefulness.

miliary pattern *n.* (radiol.) A collection of tiny discrete opacities in the lungs, each measuring 2 mm or less in diameter, and generally uniform in size and widespread in distribution.

Synonym: Micronodular pattern.

An acceptable descriptor without etiologic connotation.

mucoid impaction *n.* (radiol.) A broad I-, Y-, or V-shaped roentgenographic opacity caused by the presence within a proximal airway (lobar, segmental, or subsegmental bronchus) of thick, tenacious mucus, usually associated with airway dilatation. The shape of the opacity depends upon the branching pattern of airway involved.

Synonym: Bronchocele (*q.v.*).

An inferred conclusion based on usually reliable signs. A useful descriptor preferred to its synonym.

Mueller maneuver *n.* (physiol.) Inspiration against a closed glottis, usually but not necessarily from a position of residual volume.

A useful technique for producing transient decrease in intrathoracic pressure.

nodular pattern *n.* (radiol.) A collection of innumerable, small discrete opacities ranging in diameter from 2 to 10 mm, generally uniform in size and widespread in distribution, and without marginal spiculation (*cf.* reticulonodular pattern).

An acceptable roentgenologic discriptor without specific pathologic or etiologic implications. The size of the nodules should be specified, either as a range or as an average.

nodule *n.* (radiol.) Any pulmonary or pleural lesion represented in a roentgenogram by a sharply defined, discrete, approximately circular opacity 2 to 30 mm in diameter (*cf.* mass).

Synonym: Coin lesion (*q.v.*).

A useful and recommended descriptor to be used in preference to its synonym, which is a colloquial abomination. Should always be qualified with respect to size, location, border characteristics, number, and opacity.

oligemia *n.* 1. (pathol./physiol.) Reduced blood flow to the lungs or a portion thereof. 2. (radiol.) General or local decrease in the apparent width of visible pulmonary vessels, suggesting less than normal blood flow. *Qualifiers:* acute, chronic; local, general.

Synonym: Reduced blood flow.

An inferred conclusion usually used as descriptor and appropriately based on reliable signs. An acceptable term.

opacity *n.* (radiol.) The shadow of an absorber that attenuates the x-ray beam more effectively than do surrounding absorbers. Hence, in a roentgenogram, any circumscribed area that appears more nearly white (of lesser photometric density) than its surround. Usually applied to the shadows of nonspecific pulmonary collections of fluid, tissue, etc., whose attenuation exceeds that of the surrounding aerated lung.

Synonym: Radiopacity (*cf.* density).

An essential and recommended roentgenologic descriptor. In the context of roentgenologic reporting, "radiopaque" is acceptable but seems redundant; however, it is preferred in British usage. "Density" (*q.v.*) should *never* be used in this context.

WORDS OR TERMS USED IN ROENTGENOLOGY *Continued*

Word or Term	Comments
opaque *adj.* (radiol.) Impervious to x-rays. *Synonym:* Radiopaque.	Opaque and radiopaque are both acceptable terms, although the former is preferred (*see* opacity).
ossification *n.* (radiol.) Calcific opacities within the lung that represent trabecular bone; applicable to calcific opacities that either display morphologic characteristics of trabecular bone (trabeculation and a defined cortex) or occur in association with a lesion known histologically to produce trabecular bone within lung (*e.g.,* mitral stenosis). *Synonyms:* Ossific nodulation, ossific nodule(s).	A useful roentgenologic term, although usually an inferred conclusion. To be distinguished from "calcification" (*q.v.*).
paraspinal line *n.* (radiol.) A vertically oriented interface usually seen in a frontal chest roentgenogram to the left (rarely to the right) of the thoracic vertebral column. It extends from the aortic arch to the diaphragm and represents contact between aerated lower lobe and adjacent mediastinal tissues. The anatomic interface is situated posterior to the descending aorta and is seen between the left lateral margin of the aorta and the spine. *Synonyms:* Left paraspinal pleural reflection; left paraspinal interface.	A specific feature of roentgenologic anatomy. Either of the synonyms cited is preferred inasmuch as the shadow represents an interface, not a line.
parenchyma *n.* 1. (anat.) The gas-exchanging portion of the lung consisting of the alveoli and their capillaries, estimated to comprise approximately 90 per cent of total lung volume. 2. (radiol.) All lung tissue exclusive of visible pulmonary vessels and airways.	A useful anatomic concept and an acceptable roentgenologic descriptor.
perfusion *n.* (physiol./radiol.) The passage of blood into and out of the lung. *Synonym:* Pulmonary blood flow.	A useful and recommended term.
phantom tumor *n.* (radiol.) A shadow produced by a local collection of fluid in one of the interlobar fissures (most often the minor fissure), usually possessing an elliptic configuration in one roentgenographic projection and a rounded configuration in the other, thus resembling a tumor. It is commonly caused by cardiac decompensation and usually disappears with appropriate therapy. *Synonyms:* Vanishing tumor, pseudotumor.	An explicit diagnostic conclusion from serial roentgenograms but only an inferred conclusion from a single examination. An acceptable descriptor.
platelike atelectasis *n.* (radiol.) A linear or planar opacity presumed to represent diminished volume in a portion of the lung; usually situated in lower lung zones. *Synonyms:* Platter, linear, or discoid atelectasis.	An inferred conclusion usually not subject to proof and often unwarranted. Its use as a descriptor is not recommended. "Linear opacity" is preferred.
pleonemia *n.* (pathol./physiol./radiol.) Increased blood flow to the lungs or a portion thereof, manifested roentgenologically by a general or local increase in the width of visible pulmonary vessels. *Synonyms:* Increased blood flow, hyperemia.	An inferred conclusion often used as a descriptor and based on usually reliable signs. An acceptable term preferrable to hyperemia (*q.v.*).
pneumatocele *n.* (pathol./radiol.) A thin-walled, gas-filled space within the lung usually occurring in association with acute pneumonia (most commonly of staphylococcal etiology) and almost invariably transient.	An inferred conclusion. An acceptable descriptor if used in accordance with the precise definition.

WORDS OR TERMS USED IN ROENTGENOLOGY *Continued*

Word or Term	Comments
pneumomediastinum *n.* (pathol./radiol.) A state characterized by the presence of gas in mediastinal tissues outside the esophagus, tracheobronchial tree, or pericardium. *Qualifiers:* spontaneous, traumatic, diagnostic. *Synonym:* Mediastinal emphysema.	An appropriate descriptor based on roentgenologic signs alone; preferred to its synonym.
pneumonia *n.* (pathol./radiol.) Infection (or noninfectious inflammation) of the air spaces and/or interstitium of the lung. *Qualifiers* may be employed to indicate temporal course (acute, chronic), predominant anatomic involvement (air-space or lobar, interstitial, bronchial), or etiology (bacterial, viral, fungal). *Synonym:* Pneumonitis.	An inferred conclusion, based on usually reliable signs. Generally preferred to its synonym, although the latter is sometimes used to designate infection caused by viruses or *Mycoplasma pneumoniae.*
pneumothorax *n.* (pathol./radiol.) A state characterized by the presence of gas within the pleural space. *Qualifiers:* spontaneous, traumatic, diagnostic, tension (*q.v.*).	A diagnostic conclusion appropriately based on roentgenologic evidence alone.
popcorn calcification *n.* (radiol.) A cluster of sharply defined, irregularly lobulated, calcific opacities, usually within a pulmonary nodule, suggesting the appearance of popcorn.	An acceptable descriptor.
posterior junction line *n.* (radiol.) A vertically oriented, linear or curvilinear opacity approximately 2 mm wide, commonly projected on the tracheal air shadow, and usually slightly concave to the right. It is produced by the shadows of the right and left pleurae in intimate contact between the aerated lungs. It represents the plane of contact between the lungs posterior to the trachea and esophagus and anterior to the spine; hence, in contrast to the anterior junction line, it may project both above and below the suprasternal notch. *Synonyms:* Posterior mediastinal septum; posterior mediastinal line; supraaortic posterior junction line or stripe; mesentery of the esophagus.	A specific feature of roentgenologic anatomy; to be preferred to cited synonyms.
posterior tracheal stripe *n.* (radiol.) A vertically oriented linear opacity ranging in width from 2 to 5 mm, extending from the thoracic inlet to the bifurcation of the trachea, and visible only on lateral roentgenograms of the chest. It is situated between the air shadow of the trachea and the right lung and is formed by the posterior tracheal wall and contiguous mediastinal interstitial tissue. *Synonym:* Posterior tracheal band.	A specific feature of radiologic anatomy; to be preferred to its synonym.
primary complex *n.* 1. (pathol.) The combination of a focus of pneumonia due to a primary infection (*e.g.,* tuberculosis or histoplasmosis) with granulomas in the draining hilar or mediastinal lymph nodes. 2. (radiol.) (a) One or more irregular opacities of variable extent and location assumed to represent consolidation of lung parenchyma, associated with enlargement of hilar or mediastinal lymph nodes, an appearance presumed to represent active infection. (b) One or more small, sharply defined parenchymal opacities (often calcified) associated with calcification of hilar or mediastinal lymph nodes, an appearance usually regarded as evidence of an inactive process.	A useful inferred conclusion. "Primary complex" is to be preferred to "Ranke complex," which is acceptable but rarely used. "Ghon complex" represents an inappropriate use of the eponym and is unacceptable (Ghon described the pulmonary abnormality alone, which thus becomes a Ghon focus or Ghon lesion).

WORDS OR TERMS USED IN ROENTGENOLOGY *Continued*

Word or Term	Comments

profusion *n.* (radiol.) The number of small opacities per unit area or zone of lung. In the ILO classification of radiographs of the pneumoconioses, the qualifiers 0 through 3 subdivide the profusion into 4 categories. The profusion categories may be further subdivided by employing a 12-point scale.

A useful word to describe the number of opacities in any diffuse disease, including the pneumoconioses.

pseudocavity *n.* (radiol.) A state in which a pulmonary nodule or mass possesses a central portion that is more lucent than its periphery (thus suggesting cavitation) but in which subsequent computed tomography or pathologic examination reveals only the presence of necrotic tissue high in lipid content, with no true cavity.

Synonym: Simulated cavity.

An inferred conclusion sometimes used as a descriptor. The term is without etiologic connotation.

pulmonary edema *n.* 1. (pathophysiol.) The accumulation of liquid in the interstitial compartment of the lung with or without associated alveolar filling. Specifically, the accumulation of water, protein, and solutes (transudate), usually due to one or a combination of the following: (a) increased pressure in the microvascular bed, (b) increased microvascular permeability, or (c) impaired lymphatic drainage. Also, the accumulation of water, protein, solutes, and inflammatory cells (exudate) in response to inflammation of any type (*e.g.,* infection, allergy, trauma, or circulating toxins). 2. (radiol.) A pattern of opacity (usually bilaterally symmetrical) believed to represent interstitial thickening or alveolar filling when associated findings and/or history suggest one of the processes enumerated above. *Qualifiers:* interstitial, air-space, alveolar.

Synonyms: Wet, boggy, or moist lung.

An inferred conclusion often employed as a descriptor, based on usually reliable signs. A useful and acceptable term when used in an appropriate clinical setting. The synonyms are colloquialisms to be avoided.

respiratory failure *n.* (physiol.) A state characterized by an arterial Po_2 below 60 mm Hg or an arterial Pco_2 above 49 mm Hg, at rest at sea level, resulting from impaired respiratory function.

Synonym: Pulmonary insufficiency.

A useful term that should be restricted to clinical and physiologic usage. It is preferred to its synonym.

reticular pattern *n.* (radiol.) A collection of innumerable small linear opacities that together produce an appearance resembling a net. *Qualifiers:* fine, medium, coarse.

Synonym: Small irregular opacities (in the ILO classification of radiographs of the pneumoconioses).

A recommended descriptor that usually indicates predominant abnormality of the pulmonary interstitium. The synonym should be restricted to the roentgenographic characterization of pneumoconiosis.

reticulonodular pattern *n.* (radiol.) A collection of innumerable small, linear, and nodular opacities that together produce a composite appearance resembling a net with small superimposed nodules. In common usage, the reticular and nodular elements are dimensionally of similar magnitude. *Qualifiers:* fine, medium, coarse.

An acceptable roentgenologic descriptor that usually indicates predominant abnormality of the pulmonary interstitium.

right tracheal stripe *n.* (radiol.) A vertically oriented linear opacity approximately 2 to 3 mm wide extending from the thoracic inlet to the right tracheobronchial angle. It is situated between the air shadow of the trachea and the right lung and is formed by the right tracheal wall and contiguous mediastinal interstitial tissue and pleura.

Synonym: Right paratracheal stripe or band.

A specific feature of radiologic anatomy; to be preferred to the cited synonym since the opacity is caused chiefly by the tracheal wall itself.

WORDS OR TERMS USED IN ROENTGENOLOGY *Continued*

Word or Term	Comments
segment *n.* (anat./radiol.) One of the principal anatomic subdivisions of the pulmonary lobes served by a major branch of a lobar bronchus. *Qualifier:* bronchopulmonary.	A useful anatomic and roentgenologic descriptor.
septal line(s) *n.* (radiol.) Usually used in the plural, a generic term for linear opacities of varied distribution produced when the interstitium between pulmonary lobules is thickened (*e.g.*, by fluid, dust deposition, cellular material). *Synonym:* Kerley line (*q.v.*).	A specific feature of roentgenologic pathology, sometimes inferred. A recommended term. "Kerley line" is acceptable, particularly when seeking to identify a particular type of septal line (*e.g.*, Kerley B line).
shadow *n.* (radiol.) In clinical roentgenography, any perceptible discontinuity in film blackening (or fluoroscopic image or CRT display) attributed to the attenuation of the x-ray beam by a specific anatomic absorber or lesion on or within the body of the patient; an opacity or lucency. The word should always be qualified as precisely as possible with respect to size, contour, location, opacity, lucency, and so on.	A useful and recommended descriptor to be employed only when more specific identification is not possible.
silhouette sign *n.* (radiol.) 1. The effacement of an anatomic soft tissue border by either a normal anatomic structure (*e.g.*, the inferior border of the heart and left hemidiaphragm) or a pathologic state such as airlessness of adjacent lung or accumulation of fluid in the contiguous pleural space. 2. A sign of conformity, and hence, of the probable adjacency of a pathologic opacity to a known structure.	Useful in detecting and localizing an opacity along the axis of the x-ray beam. Although the physical basis underlying the production of this sign is contentious, the term is a widely accepted and useful descriptor. Despite the fact that the definition implies *loss* of silhouette, the term has acquired such common popularity that its continued use is recommended.
small irregular opacities *n.* (radiol.) A collection of innumerable small linear opacities that together produce an appearance resembling a net. In the ILO/1980 classification of radiographs of the pneumoconioses, the qualifiers s, t, and u subdivide the dimensions of the opacities into three diameter ranges—up to 1.5 mm, 1.5 to 3 mm, and 3 to 10 mm, respectively. *Synonym:* Reticular pattern (*q.v.*).	A term to be employed specifically to describe roentgenographic manifestations of the pneumoconioses; the synonym is preferred for nonpneumoconiotic disease.
small rounded opacities *n.* (radiol.) A collection of innumerable pulmonary nodules ranging in diameter from bare visibility up to 10 mm, usually widespread in distribution. In the ILO/1980 classification of radiographs of the pneumoconioses, the qualifiers p, q, and r subdivide the dimensions of the opacities into three diameter ranges—up to 1.5 mm, 1.5 to 3 mm, and 3 to 10 mm, respectively. *Synonym:* Nodular pattern (*q.v.*).	A term to be employed specifically to describe roentgenographic manifestations of the pneumoconioses; the synonym is preferred for nonpneumoconiotic disease.

WORDS OR TERMS USED IN ROENTGENOLOGY *Continued*

Word or Term	Comments
stripe *n.* (radiol.) A longitudinal composite opacity measuring 2 to 5 mm in width (*cf.* line).	An acceptable descriptor when limited to anatomic structures within the mediastinum (*e.g.,* right tracheal stripe).
subsegment *n.* (anat./radiol.) A unit of pulmonary tissue supplied by a bronchus of lesser order than a segmental bronchus.	A useful anatomic and roentgenologic descriptor.
tension *adj.* 1. (physiol./clin.) When used with reference to pneumo- or hydrothorax, a state characterized by cardiorespiratory functional impairment. 2. (radiol.) The accumulation of gas or fluid in a pleural space in an amount sufficient to cause airlessness of the ipsilateral lung, marked depression of the ipsilateral hemidiaphragm, and displacement of the mediastinum to the opposite side.	An inferred conclusion to be used only in the presence of clinical cardiorespiratory embarrassment. In fact, "tension" in relation to pneumothorax exists only during the expiratory phase of the respiratory cycle, since pleural pressure on inspiration is usually subatmospheric. The word should not be employed as in the term "tension cyst," which does not satisfy the criteria cited.
thromboembolism *n.* (pathol./clin./radiol.) Partial or complete occlusion of the lumen of a blood vessel by a thrombus (*q.v.*).	An inferred conclusion sometimes based on reliable signs (in conventional roentgenography) or a diagnostic conclusion based on roentgenologic evidence alone (in angiography).
thrombosis *n.* (pathol./radiol.) The state or process of thrombus formation within a blood vessel or heart chamber.	*Cf.* clot.
thrombus *n.* (pathol./radiol.) A mass of semisolidified blood, composed chiefly of platelets and fibrin with entrapped cellular elements, at the site of its formation in a blood vessel or heart chamber.	A useful descriptor to be employed only in the precise sense of the definition. (*Cf.* embolus.)
tramline shadow *n.* (radiol.) Parallel or slightly convergent linear opacities that suggest the planar projection of tubular structures and that correspond in location and orientation to elements of the bronchial tree. They are generally assumed to represent thickened bronchial walls. *Synonyms:* Thickened bronchial wall, tubular shadow (*q.v.*).	A roentgenologic descriptor which is not recommended in deference to either of the synonyms. Such shadows are of possible pathologic significance only when they occur outside the limits of the hilar shadows where bronchial walls may be seen normally.
tubular shadow *n.* (radiol.) 1. Paired, parallel, or slightly convergent linear opacities presumed to represent the walls of a tubular structure seen *en face* (*e.g.,* a bronchus). 2. An approximately circular opacity presumed to represent the wall of a tubular structure seen end-on. *Synonyms:* Tramline shadow (*q.v.*), thickened bronchial wall.	Acceptable if the anatomic nature of a shadow is obscure; otherwise the more precise "thickened bronchial wall" is to be preferred.
tumor *n.* 1. (general) A swelling or morbid enlargement. 2. (pathol./radiol.) Literally, a mass (*q.v.*), not differentiated as to its neoplastic or non-neoplastic nature. *Synonym:* Mass.	A useful descriptor, although "mass" is preferred. The use of the word as a synonym for neoplasm is to be condemned.

WORDS OR TERMS USED IN ROENTGENOLOGY *Continued*

Word or Term	Comments
Valsalva maneuver *n.* (physiol.) Forced expiration against a closed glottis, usually but not necessarily from a position of total lung capacity.	A useful technique to produce transient increase in intrathoracic pressure.
vasoconstriction *n.* 1. (physiol.) Narrowing of muscular blood vessels by contraction of their muscle layer. 2. (radiol.) Local or general reduction in the caliber of visible pulmonary vessels (oligemia [*q.v.*]), presumed to result from decreased flow occasioned by contraction of muscular pulmonary arteries. *Qualifiers:* hypoxic, reflex.	An inferred conclusion based on usually reliable signs. The word is not synonymous with oligemia; although the latter is a *sign* of vasoconstriction, it may also occur when vessel narrowing is organic (as in emphysema) rather than functional and potentially reversible.
vasodilation *n.* (radiol.) The local or general increase in the width of visible pulmonary vessels resulting from increased pulmonary blood flow. *Synonym:* Vasodilatation.	An inferred conclusion based on usually reliable signs.
ventilation *n.* (physiol./radiol.) The movement of air into and out of the lungs; inspiration and expiration. *Qualifiers:* hyperventilation (preferred), or overventilation; hypoventilation (preferred), or underventilation.	The term always implies a biphasic dynamic process of admission and expulsion; hence, it cannot be assessed from a single static image (*see* inflation).

TERMS AND SYMBOLS USED IN RESPIRATORY PHYSIOLOGY AND PATHOPHYSIOLOGY

GENERAL SYMBOLS

P	Pressure, blood, or gas
$\dot{X}$	A time derivative indicated by a dot above the symbol (rate). This symbol is used for both instantaneous flow and volume per unit time
%X	Per cent sign *preceding* a symbol indicates percentage of the predicted normal value
X/Y%	Per cent sign *following* a symbol indicates a ratio function with the ratio expressed as a percentage. Both components of the ratio must be designated; e.g., $FEV_1/FVC\% = 100 \times FEV_1/FVC$
X_A or Xa	A small capital letter or lower case letter on the same line following a primary symbol is a qualifier to further define the primary symbol. When small capital letters are not available on typewriters or to printers, large capital letters may be used as subscripts; e.g., $X_A = XA$

GAS PHASE SYMBOLS

PRIMARY SYMBOLS (LARGE CAPITAL LETTERS)

V	Gas volume. The particular gas as well as its pressure, water vapor conditions, and other special conditions must be specified in text or indicated by appropriate qualifying symbols
F	Fractional concentration of gas

COMMON QUALIFYING SYMBOLS

I	Inspired
E	Expired
A	Alveolar
T	Tidal
D	Dead space or wasted ventilation
B	Barometric
L	Lung
STPD	Standard conditions: Temperature 0 degrees Centigrade, pressure 760 mm Hg, and dry (0 water vapor)
BTPS	Body conditions: Body temperature, ambient pressure, and saturated with water vapor at these conditions

ATPD	Ambient temperature and pressure, dry
ATPS	Ambient temperature and pressure, saturated with water vapor at these conditions
an	Anatomic
p	Physiologic
rb	Rebreathing
f	Respiratory frequency per minute
max	Maximal
t	Time

BLOOD PHASE SYMBOLS

PRIMARY SYMBOLS (LARGE CAPITAL LETTERS)

Q	Blood volume
$\dot{Q}$	Blood flow, volume units and time must be specified
C	Concentration in the blood phase
S	Saturation in the blood phase

QUALIFYING SYMBOLS (LOWER CASE LETTERS)

b	Blood in general
a	Arterial
c	Capillary
ć	Pulmonary end-capillary
v	Venous
$\bar{v}$	Mixed venous

VENTILATION AND LUNG MECHANICS TESTS AND SYMBOLS

LUNG VOLUME COMPARTMENTS*

RV	Residual volume; that volume of air remaining in the lungs after maximal exhalation. The method of measurement should be indicated in the text or, when necessary, by appropriate qualifying symbols
ERV	Expiratory reserve volume; the maximal volume of air exhaled from the end-expiratory level

---

*Primary components are designated as volumes. When volumes are combined they are designated as capacities. All are considered to be at BTPS unless otherwise specified.

V_T Tidal volume; that volume of air inhaled or exhaled with each breath during quiet breathing, used only to indicate a subdivision of lung volume

IRV   Inspiratory reserve volume; the maximal volume of air inhaled from the end-inspiratory level

IC   Inspiratory capacity; the sum of IRV and V_T

IVC   Inspiratory vital capacity; the maximal volume of air inhaled from the point of maximal expiration

VC   Vital capacity; the maximal volume of air exhaled from the point of maximal inspiration

FRC   Functional residual capacity; the sum of RV and ERV (the volume of air remaining in the lungs at the end-expiratory position). The method of measurement should be indicated, as with RV

TLC   Total lung capacity; the sum of all volume compartments or the volume of air in the lungs after maximal inspiration. The method of measurement should be indicated, as with RV

RV / TLC%   Residual volume to total lung capacity ratio, expressed as a per cent

CV   Closing volume; the volume exhaled after the expired gas concentration is inflected from an alveolar plateau during a controlled breathing maneuver. Since the value obtained is dependent on the specific test technique, the method used must be designated in the text and, when necessary, specified by a qualifying symbol. Closing volume is often expressed as a ratio of the VC, i.e., (CV/VC%)

CC   Closing capacity; closing volume plus residual volume, often expressed as a ratio of TLC, i.e., (CC/TLC%)

VL   Actual volume of the lung, including the volume of the conducting airways

V_A Alveolar gas volume

FORCED SPIROMETRY MEASUREMENTS*

FVC   Forced vital capacity; vital capacity performed with a maximally forced expiratory effort

FIVC   Forced inspiratory vital capacity; the maximal volume of air inspired with a maximally forced effort from a position of maximal expiration

FEVt   Forced expiratory volume (timed). The volume of air exhaled in the specified time during the performance of the forced vital capacity; e.g., FEV_1 for the volume of air exhaled during the first second of the FVC

FEVt / FVC%   Forced expiratory volume (timed) to forced vital capacity ratio, expressed as a percentage

FEF25–75%   Mean forced expiratory flow during the middle of the FVC (formerly called the maximal mid-expiratory flow rate)

PEF   The highest forced expiratory flow measured with a peak flow meter

$\dot{V}maxX$ Forced expiratory flow, related to the total lung capacity or the vital capacity of the lung at which the measurement is made. *Modifiers refer to the amount of lung volume remaining when the measurement is made.* For example: $\dot{V}max75\%$ = Instantaneous forced expiratory flow when the lung is at 75% of its TLC

$\dot{V}max50$ Instantaneous forced expiratory flow when 50% of the vital capacity remains to be exhaled

$\dot{V}maxXp$ Forced expiratory flow at "X" percentage of vital capacity on a partial flow volume curve, initiated from a volume below TLC

MVVx   Maximal voluntary ventilation. The volume of air expired in a specified period during repetitive maximal respiratory effort

MEASUREMENTS OF VENTILATION

$\dot{V}_E$ Expired volume per minute (BTPS)

$\dot{V}_I$ Inspired volume per minute (BTPS)

$\dot{V}_{CO_2}$ Carbon dioxide production per minute (STPD)

$\dot{V}_{O_2}$ Oxygen consumption per minute (STPD)

$\dot{V}_A$ Alveolar ventilation per minute (BTPS)

V_D The physiologic dead space volume defined as V_D/f

$\dot{V}_D$ Ventilation per minute of the physiologic dead space (wasted ventilation), BTPS, defined by the following equation:
$$\dot{V}_D = \dot{V}_E(Pa_{CO_2} - P_{ECO_2})/Pa_{CO_2}$$

V_{DAN} Volume of the anatomic dead space (BTPS)

$\dot{V}_{DAN}$ Ventilation per minute of the anatomic dead space, that portion of conducting airway in which no significant gas exchange occurs (BTPS)

---

*All values are BTPS unless otherwise specified.

V_DA The alveolar dead space volume defined as V_DA/f

$\dot{V}_DA$ Ventilation of the alveolar dead space (BTPS), defined by the following equation: $V_DA = V_D - V_{DAN}$

MEASUREMENTS OF MECHANICS OF BREATHING*

PRESSURE TERMS

Paw   Pressure in the airway, level to be specified

Pao   Pressure at the airway opening

Ppl   Intrapleural pressure

P_A Alveolar pressure

P_L Transpulmonary pressure

Pbs   Pressure at the body surface

P(A-ao)   Pressure gradient from alveolus to airway opening

Pw   Transthoracic pressure

Ptm   Transmural pressure pertaining to an airway or blood vessel

Pes   Esophageal pressure used to estimate Ppl

Pga   Gastric pressure; used to estimate abdominal pressure

Pdi   Transdiaphragmatic pressure; used to estimate the tension across the diaphragm

Pdi Max   Maximal transdiaphragmatic pressure; used to measure the strength of diaphragmatic muscle contraction

PI Max (also MIP)   Maximal inspiratory pressure; measured at the mouth, used to assess the strength of inspiratory muscles

PE Max (also MEP)   Maximal expiratory pressure; measured at the mouth, used to assess the strength of the expiratory muscles

FLOW-PRESSURE RELATIONSHIPS†

R   A general symbol for resistance, pressure per unit flow

Raw   Airway resistance

Rti   Tissue resistance

R_L Total pulmonary resistance, measured by relating flow-dependent transpulmonary pressure to airflow at the mouth

Rus   Resistance of the airways on the alveolar side (upstream) of the point in the airways where intraluminal pressure equals Ppl, measured under conditions of maximal expiratory flow

Rds   Resistance of the airways on the oral side (downstream) of the point in the airways where intraluminal pressure equals Ppl, measured under conditions of maximal expiratory flow

Gaw   Airway conductance, the reciprocal of Raw

Gaw/V_L Specific conductance, expressed per liter of lung volume at which G is measured (also SGaw)

VOLUME-PRESSURE RELATIONSHIPS

C   A general symbol for compliance, volume change per unit of applied pressure

Cdyn   Dynamic compliance, compliance measured at points of zero gas flow at the mouth during active breathing. The respiratory frequency should be designated; e.g., Cdyn40

Cst   Static compliance, compliance determined from measurements made during conditions of interruption of air flow

C/V_L Specific compliance

E   Elastance, pressure per unit of volume change, the reciprocal of compliance

Pst   Static transpulmonary pressure at a specified lung volume; e.g., PstTLC is static recoil pressure measured at TLC (maximal recoil pressure)

PstTLC/ TLC   Coefficient of lung reaction expressed per liter of TLC

W   A general symbol for mechanical work of breathing, which requires use of appropriate qualifying symbols and description of specific conditions

BREATHING PATTERN

TI   Inspiratory time

TE   Expiratory time

T_{Tot} Total respiratory cycle time

T_I/T_{Tot} Ratio of inspiratory to total respiratory cycle time—Duty cycle

V_T Tidal volume

---

*All pressures are expressed relative to ambient pressure and gases are at BTPS unless otherwise specified.

†Unless otherwise specified, the lung volume at which all resistance measurements are made is assumed to be FRC.

V_T/T_I Mean inspiratory flow

V_T/T_E Mean expiratory flow

V_E $\dfrac{V_t \times T_i}{T_i \times T_{Tot}}$

$P(A\text{-}a)O_2$ Alveolar-arterial oxygen pressure difference. The previously used symbol, $A\text{-}aDO_2$ is not recommended.

$C(a\text{-}\bar{v})O_2$ Arteriovenous oxygen content difference

DIFFUSING CAPACITY TESTS AND SYMBOLS

Dx Diffusing capacity of the lung expressed as volume (STPD) of gas (x) uptake per unit alveolar-capillary pressure difference for the gas used. Unless otherwise stated, carbon monoxide is assumed to be the test gas: i.e., D is D_{CO}. A modifier can be used to designate the technique: e.g., Dsb is single breath carbon monoxide diffusing capacity and Dss is steady state CO diffusing capacity

D_M Diffusing capacity of the alveolar capillary membrane (STPD)

θx Reaction rate coefficient for red cells; the volume STPD of gas (x) which will combine per minute with 1 unit volume of blood per unit gas tension. If the specific gas is not stated, θ is assumed to refer to CO and is a function of existing O_2 tension

Qc Capillary blood volume (usually expressed as Vc in the literature, a symbol inconsistent with those recommended for blood volumes). When determined from the following equation, Qc represents the effective pulmonary capillary blood volume, i.e., capillary blood volume in intimate association with alveolar gas:

$$\frac{1}{D} = \frac{1}{D_M} + \frac{1}{\theta \cdot Qc}$$

D/V_A Diffusion per unit of alveolar volume with D expressed STPD and V_A expressed as liters BTPS. This method is preferred to the occasional practice of expressing both values STPD

BLOOD GAS MEASUREMENTS*

$PaCO_2$ Arterial carbon dioxide tension

SaO_2 Arterial oxygen saturation

$C\acute{c}O_2$ Oxygen content of pulmonary end-capillary blood

---

*Symbols for these measurements are readily composed by combining the general symbols recommended earlier.

PULMONARY SHUNTS

$\dot{Q}sp$ Physiologic shunt flow (total venous admixture) defined by the following equation when gas and blood gas data are collected during ambient air breathing:

$$\dot{Q}sp = \frac{C\acute{c}O_2 - CaO_2}{C\acute{c}O_2 - C\bar{v}O_2} \cdot \dot{Q}$$

$\dot{Q}san$ A special case of $\dot{Q}sp$ (often called anatomic shunt flow) defined by the above equation when blood and gas data are collected after sufficiently prolonged breathing of 100% O_2 to assure an alveolar N_2 less than 1%

$\dot{Q}s/\dot{Q}t$ The ratio $\dot{Q}sp$ or $\dot{Q}_{SAN}$ to total cardiac output

BRONCHIAL REACTIVITY

PC_{20} Provocative concentration of an inhaled agonist producing a 20% decrease in FEV_1

PD_{20} Provocative dose of an inhaled agonist producing a 20% decrease in FEV_1

$PD_{40}SGaw$ Provocative dose of an inhaled agonist producing a 40% decrease in SGaw

Isocapnic hyperventilation (eucapnic hyperventilation) = "hyperventilation" with addition of CO_2 to the inspired air to keep end tidal PCO_2 constant (Iso) and/or normal (Eu-). Used to assess bronchoconstrictive response to cold and/or dry air

SLEEP STUDIES

Polysom-nography   The evaluation during sleep of vital functions and a quantitative evaluation of sleep parameters overnight

NREM   Nonrapid eye movement sleep

REM   Rapid eye movement sleep

Apnea   Cessation of air flow for greater than 10 seconds

Sleep apnea   The presence of 30 or greater apneas in an overnight, 7 hour sleep study. (Apnea frequency >4/hr)

Obstructive apnea — Apnea with respiratory effort

Central apnea — Apnea without respiratory effort

Mixed apnea — Apnea initially without, but later with, respiratory effort

Hypopnea — Reduced respiratory effort with associated decrease in arterial saturation

Apnea index — Number of apneas divided by the total sleep time in hours

Arousal — Short neurologic awakening

PULMONARY DYSFUNCTION

TERMS RELATED TO ALTERED BREATHING

Many terms are in use, such as tachypnea, hyperpnea, hypopnea, and so on. Simple descriptive terms, such as rapid, deep, or shallow breathing, should be used instead.

Dyspnea — A subjective sensation of difficult or labored breathing

Overventila- — A general term indicating excessive ventilation. When unqualified, it refers to *alveolar overventilation*, excessive ventilation of the gas-exchanging areas of the lung manifested by a fall in arterial CO_2 tension. The term *total overventilation* may be used when the minute volume is increased regardless of the alveolar ventilation. (When there is increased wasted ventilation, total overventilation may occur when alveolar ventilation is normal or decreased)

Underventila-tion — A general term indicating reduced ventilation. When otherwise unqualified, it refers to alveolar underventilation, decreased effective alveolar ventilation manifested by an increase in arterial CO_2 tension. (Over- and underventilation are recommended in place of hyper- and hypoventilation to avoid confusion when the words are spoken)

TERMS DESCRIBING BLOOD GAS FINDINGS

Hypoxia — A term for reduced oxygenation

Hypoxemia — A reduced blood oxygen content or tension

Hypocarbia — (hypocapnia) A reduced arterial carbon dioxide tension

Hypercarbia — (hypercapnia) An increased arterial carbon dioxide tension

TERMS DESCRIBING ACID-BASE FINDINGS

Acidemia — A pH less than normal; the value should always be given

Alkalemia — A pH greater than normal; the value should always be given

Hypobasemia — Blood bicarbonate level below normal

Hyperbasemia — Blood bicarbonate level above normal

Acidosis — A clinical term indicating a disturbance that can lead to acidemia. It usually is indicated by hypobasemia when metabolic (nonrespiratory) in origin and by hypercarbia when respiratory in origin. There may or may not be accompanying acidemia. The term should always be qualified as metabolic (nonrespiratory) or respiratory

Alkalosis — A clinical term indicating a disturbance that can lead to alkalemia. It usually is indicated by hyperbasemia when metabolic (nonrespiratory) in origin and by hypocarbia when respiratory in origin. There may or may not be accompanying alkalemia. The term should always be qualified as metabolic (nonrespiratory) or respiratory

OTHER TERMS

Pulmonary insufficiency — Altered function of the lungs that produces clinical symptoms, usually including dyspnea

Acute respiratory failure — Rapidly occurring hypoxemia or hypercarbia due to a disorder of the respiratory system. The duration of the illness and the values of arterial oxygen tension and arterial carbon dioxide tension used as criteria for this term should be given. The term *acute ventilatory failure* should be used only when the arterial carbon dioxide tension is increased. The term *pulmonary failure* has been used to indicate respiratory failure due specifically to disorders of the lungs

Chronic respiratory failure — Chronic hypoxemia or hypercarbia due to a disorder of the respiratory system. The duration of the condition and the values of arterial oxygen tension and arterial carbon dioxide tension used as criteria for this term should be given

Obstructive pattern — (Obstructive ventilatory defect) Slowing of air flow during forced ventilatory maneuvers

Restrictive pattern
(Restrictive ventilatory defect) Reduction of vital capacity not explainable by airways obstruction

Impairment
A measurable degree of anatomic or functional abnormality which may or may not have clinical significance. *Permanent impairment* is that which persists after maximal medical rehabilitation has been achieved

Disability
A legally determined state in which a patient's ability to engage in a specific activity under a particular circumstance is reduced or absent because of physical or mental impairment. *Permanent disability* exists when no substantial improvement of the patient's ability to engage in the specific activity can be expected

14

CHAPTER

Drug- and Poison-Induced Pulmonary Disease

DRUG-INDUCED PULMONARY DISEASE

The seriousness of disease resulting from drug therapy is revealed by the estimate that approximately 5 per cent of all patients admitted to hospitals suffer adverse drug reactions of sufficient severity to cause marked morbidity, prolonged hospitalization, permanent sequelae, or a contribution to a fatal outcome.[1] The vast majority of such

2417

disease is iatrogenic; however, children[2] and, to a lesser extent, adults occasionally develop severe pulmonary disease following an overdose of drugs in accidental or suicidal poisoning. Pulmonary disease induced by medication is a growing problem, largely as a result of the increased use of cytotoxic drugs in the treatment of both benign and malignant disease. Several excellent reviews on this subject have been published;[3-12] of particular note is a recent "state of the art" article.[13, 14]

Drug reactions within the lungs can be divided into six fairly well-defined categories (the first three are described elsewhere in this book): (1) bronchospasm (see page 2052), (2) systemic lupus erythematosus-like syndrome (see page 1191), (3) intravenous abuse of oral medications (see page 1794), (4) transitory pulmonary opacities presumed to represent eosinophilic pneumonia, (5) interstitial or airspace pneumonitis, and (6) permeability pulmonary edema (use of the word "permeability" by itself to refer to noncardiogenic pulmonary edema is clearly erroneous, since it should be prefaced by "increased"; however, its use is deeply ingrained in current medical parlance, and it is employed without the adjective throughout this book). In this section we discuss the latter three categories, especially those reactions characterized by reparable or irreparable damage to the alveolocapillary membrane. Other drug-induced thoracic disorders involving the pleura, the mediastinum, and the neuromuscular control of breathing are considered in the appropriate sections of the text.

Reactions within the lungs to a variety of drugs can cause irreparable damage, disability, and even death or can have transitory clinical and roentgenographic manifestations with eventual total clinical remission. Even in the latter group, however, follow-up sometimes reveals residual derangement of pulmonary function despite the fact that patients feel well and have normal chest roentgenograms.

Mechanisms of drug-induced lung damage are not completely understood but appear to be either immunologic (usually associated with a favorable outcome) or cytotoxic (in most cases accompanied by irreparable damage and fibrosis).[13] The toxicity of specific drugs varies, some being dose-related and others not. Some authors[4] consider that individual susceptibility plays a major role in the severity of a drug reaction, even with those agents known to cause cumulative, dose-related pulmonary damage. In many cases, the simultaneous use of multiple drugs, sometimes in association with irradiation, high concentrations of oxygen, or the presence of pulmonary disease unrelated to drugs can make identification of the responsible agent difficult.

There are no specific clinical, functional, or roentgenographic findings in drug-induced pulmonary disease; in the majority of cases, even pathologic examination of tissue serves only to confirm a clinical suspicion and is not itself diagnostic. In most instances, the diagnosis is suspected because of the insidious onset of dyspnea and cough in a patient receiving a drug (or drugs) recognized as being potentially damaging to the lungs. Onset with fever is common and diffuse rales are often audible. Drugs that initiate capillary leakage or bronchospasm tend to be associated with a more abrupt clinical presentation, and physical examination usually reveals profuse rales or rhonchi, respectively. Some patients may be asymptomatic, the presence of a drug reaction being suggested by the appearance of a diffuse reticulonodular pattern on the chest roentgenogram or by a significant reduction in diffusing capacity. Since the disease process can extend from the interstitium into the alveoli, the roentgenographic pattern may be mixed, or, in the case of those drugs that cause noncardiogenic pulmonary edema, predominantly airspace. Pulmonary dysfunction may be barely detectable or may be severe and require positive pressure ventilation to maintain life; although generally restrictive in type with a low DL_{CO}, the pattern may be mixed. In fact, in some patients in whom the sensitivity to drugs has an immunologic pathogenesis, the insufficiency is predominantly obstructive.

As with clinical and roentgenographic findings, histologic changes tend to be relatively nonspecific and take three general forms: (1) alveolar/interstitial inflammation, usually caused by lymphocytes, with a variable degree of fibrosis; (2) alveolar/interstitial or airspace inflammation (or both) accompanied by significant tissue eosinophilia but little or no fibrosis; or (3) alveolar/interstitial and airspace edema associated with hyaline membranes and relatively few inflammatory cells (diffuse alveolar damage). None of these histologic patterns is in any way specific or diagnostic, but as indicated above they can support a diagnosis of drug toxicity in the presence of an appropriate history. The differential diagnosis of drug-induced pulmonary disease includes the underlying illness being treated (usually a malignancy) and superimposed infection, often opportunistic in nature.

The mechanism of lung injury, pathologic characteristics, roentgenographic manifestations, clinical features, and pulmonary function abnormalities of drug reactions are summarized in Table 14–1.

CHEMOTHERAPEUTIC AND IMMUNOSUPPRESSIVE AGENTS

Cytotoxic Antibiotics

BLEOMYCIN

Bleomycin is isolated from a strain of Streptomyces verticillus and is used primarily in the treatment of lymphoma, squamous cell carcinoma, and testicular neoplasms.[15] The present therapeutic trend is to combine this agent with a variety of other cytotoxic drugs, particularly cyclophosphamide; although it is believed that there may be some

Text continued on page 2424

Table 14–1. Drug-Induced Disease of the Thorax

DRUG	MECHANISM OF LUNG INJURY	PATHOLOGIC ABNORMALITIES	ROENTGENOGRAPHIC FEATURES	CLINICAL FEATURES	PULMONARY FUNCTION ABNORMALITIES
Cytotoxic Antibiotics					
Bleomycin	Hypersensitivity in a minority; direct toxicity in most (oxidants)	Diffuse alveolar damage progressing to fibrosis; eosinophilic pneumonia in a minority	Combined coarse reticulation and airspace opacities (predominantly lower zonal)	Toxicity in 1–2%; usually progressive dyspnea, rarely acute pulmonary insufficiency; oxygen and radiation have synergistic toxicity	Reduction in vital capacity and diffusing capacity, especially capillary blood volume component
Mitomycin	Direct pulmonary toxicity, exact mechanism unknown	Diffuse alveolar damage	Same as bleomycin	Toxicity in 3–5%; usually slowly progressive dyspnea and cough, rarely acute; possible synergism with other drugs; 50% mortality	Restrictive lung disease and reduced DL_{CO}
Pepleomycin	Same as bleomycin	Same as bleomycin	Same as bleomycin	Toxicity in 6%; same as bleomycin	Same as bleomycin
Neocarzinostatin	—	—	—	Vasculitis	—
Alkylating Agents					
Busulfan	Exact mechanism unknown, probably oxidants	Large, bizarre, atypical mononuclear cells (altered type II cells); alveolitis, increased fibroblasts and collagen, type II cell hyperplasia	Bibasilar reticulonodular and less frequently airspace opacities	Toxicity in 4%; usually slowly progressive dyspnea, cough, fever, and weakness; usually long-term therapy (average 3–4 years); synergistic toxicity with other cytotoxic drugs and radiation; poor prognosis	Restrictive lung disease; reduced DL_{CO}
Cyclophosphamide	Same as busulfan	Similar to busulfan	Similar to busulfan	Toxicity in 1%; acute or subacute onset of dyspnea, cough, and fever a variable time after onset of therapy; synergistic with oxygen and radiation	Similar to busulfan
Chlorambucil	Same as busulfan	Similar to busulfan	Similar to busulfan	Rare cause of pulmonary toxicity; subacute onset of dyspnea, cough, fever, and anorexia; 50% mortality	Similar to busulfan
Melphalan	Same as busulfan	Similar to busulfan	Similar to busulfan	Rare cause of pulmonary toxicity; similar symptoms to other alkylating agents	Similar to busulfan
Nitrosoureas (BCNU)	Same as busulfan	Similar to busulfan	Similar to busulfan	Similar to other alkylating agents	Similar to busulfan

Table continued on following page

Table 14–1. Drug-Induced Disease of the Thorax *Continued*

DRUG	MECHANISM OF LUNG INJURY	PATHOLOGIC ABNORMALITIES	ROENTGENOGRAPHIC FEATURES	CLINICAL FEATURES	PULMONARY FUNCTION ABNORMALITIES
Antimetabolites					
Methotrexate and azathioprine	Cellular immune response	Alveolitis ± eosinophilia ± granuloma formation; fibrosis 10%	Combined interstitial + airspace; rarely hilar nodes	Toxicity in 5%; no clear dose response; may be concurrent skin and liver involvement; 1% mortality	Restrictive; hypoxemia
Antiarrhythmics					
Amiodarone	Induction of lysosomal storage disease (phospholipidosis); ? immunologic	Alveolitis + type II cell hyperplasia; lysosomal inclusions on electron microscopy	Diffuse reticular and patchy airspace disease	Toxicity in 1–6%; insidious onset of dyspnea, weakness, weight loss. Dx on BAL by lysosomal inclusions in macrophages; usually reversible	Restrictive; decreased DL_{CO}
Lidocaine	—	—	Airspace opacities	ARDS picture (rare)	—
Tocainide	—	Alveolitis or fibrosis	Interstitial disease	Gradual onset; reversible	Restrictive; decreased DL_{CO}
Antimicrobials					
Nitrofurantoin	Acute: immunologic hypersensitivity reaction	Acute: interstitial and alveolar eosinophilic infiltration; chronic: fibrosis ±	Diffuse reticular pattern; occasionally pleural effusion	Acute: hours to days after ingestion; blood eosinophilia + + +, fever, cough, dyspnea, chest pain, and skin rash	Restrictive; decreased DL_{CO}
	Chronic: oxidant damage	Eosinophils		Chronic: insidious course; eosinophilia +	
Sulfasalazine (salazosulfa-pyridine)	Immunologic hypersensitivity reaction	Bronchiolitis obliterans with organizing pneumonia; tissue eosinophilia and eosinophils in BAL fluid	Patchy airspace consolidation	Dry cough, fever, dyspnea; often skin rash and eosinophilia 1–6 months after starting therapy	Restrictive or obstructive pattern
Sulfonamides, penicillin, para-aminosalicylic acid, and tetracycline	Similar to sulfasalazine	Similar to sulfasalazine	Similar to sulfasalazine	Similar to sulfasalazine	Similar to sulfasalazine
Neomycin, streptomycin, dihydrostrepto-mycin, viomycin, kanamycin, and polymixin B and E	Competitive or noncompetitive blockade at neuromuscular junction	—	Small lungs; atelectasis	Ventilatory respiratory failure secondary to muscle weakness; patients with myasthenia and renal failure especially susceptible; can follow intraperitoneal administration of drugs	Decreased lung volumes and inspiratory and expiratory pressures

Table 14–1. Drug-Induced Disease of the Thorax *Continued*

DRUG	MECHANISM OF LUNG INJURY	PATHOLOGIC ABNORMALITIES	ROENTGENOGRAPHIC FEATURES	CLINICAL FEATURES	PULMONARY FUNCTION ABNORMALITIES
Anticonvulsants					
Diphenylhydantoin (phenytoin)	Immunologic hypersensitivity reaction	Lymphocytic alveolitis; necrotizing vasculitis	Diffuse reticulonodular pattern; mediastinal lymph node enlargement	Fever, dry cough, and dyspnea 3 to 6 weeks after starting therapy; generalized lymph node enlargement; blood eosinophilia; lymphocytes in BAL fluid; hepatitis; resolution of acute symptoms in 2 weeks	Restriction and gas exchange impairment; residual gas exchange impairment is possible
Carbamazepine (Tegretol)	Similar to phenytoin	Similar to phenytoin	Similar to phenytoin	Similar to phenytoin	Similar to phenytoin
Analgesics					
Acetylsalicylic acid (aspirin) (ASA)	Increased pulmonary microvascular permeability secondary to either increased intracranial pressure or altered prostaglandin metabolism	Few reports; high protein edema; occasionally a picture simulating desquamative interstitial pneumonia	Airspace pulmonary edema	Usually history of large-dose, chronic ASA ingestion; dyspnea, lethargy, and confusion; rapidly reversible with decreased blood ASA levels	Impairment of gas exchange
Naproxen	? Same as ASA but associated with eosinophilia	?	Airspace pulmonary edema	Only four cases reported; cough, fever, and blood eosinophilia; rapid resolution	Impairment of gas exchange
Antirheumatics					
Penicillamine	Type I immunologic reaction for eosinophilic syndrome, type III for renal-pulmonary hemorrhage	No biopsies in eosinophilic syndrome; interrupted IgG and complement in basement membrane in renal-pulmonary hemorrhage; bronchiolitis obliterans	Three patterns: (1) reticulonodular with some airspace opacities, (2) diffuse airspace opacity (hemorrhage), and (3) hyperinflation in bronchiolitis obliterans	Toxicity rare and dose-related; at least four clinical syndromes: (1) eosinophilic syndrome, (2) hemoptysis and hematuria (Goodpasture-like), (3) bronchiolitis obliterans (in rheumatoid arthritis), and (4) myasthenia-like syndrome; dyspnea insidious or abrupt, poor prognosis in pulmonary-renal and bronchiolitis syndromes	Restrictive or obstructive

Table continued on following page

Table 14–1. Drug-Induced Disease of the Thorax *Continued*

DRUG	MECHANISM OF LUNG INJURY	PATHOLOGIC ABNORMALITIES	ROENTGENOGRAPHIC FEATURES	CLINICAL FEATURES	PULMONARY FUNCTION ABNORMALITIES
Gold	Probable hypersensitivity reaction, cell-mediated	Lymphocytic and plasma cell alveolitis ± fibrosis; type II cell hyperplasia	Diffuse interstitial and airspace opacities	Lung toxicity in 1% of patients; one third of patients have blood eosinophilia; presentation can be acute or subacute; fever, cough, and dyspnea; usually prompt resolution	Lung restriction and gas exchange impairment; may be residual impairment
Sympathomimetics Terbutaline, ritodrine, isoxsuprine	? Acute increase in microvascular permeability or pressure, or both	?	Airspace pulmonary edema	Used for tocolytic therapy to delay preterm labor; rarely acute pulmonary edema; rapid recovery	Severe hypoxemia
Narcotics and Sedatives Heroin, methadone, Darvon, naloxone Librium, Placidyl, paraldehyde, and codeine	Increased pulmonary microvascular permeability; ? immunologic; ? neurologic	High protein edema	Diffuse airspace pulmonary edema with normal heart size	Accompanies narcotic or sedative overdose; patients are comatose; rapid resolution	Severe hypoxemia; reversible lung restriction
Antidepressants and antipsychotics Imipramine, trimipramine, and chlorpromazine	Immunologic hypersensitivity reaction; occasionally increased pulmonary microvascular permeability	?	Patchy airspace consolidation	Cough and dyspnea; acute pulmonary edema associated with the neuroleptic malignant syndrome	?
Miscellaneous Hydrochlorothiazide	Possible hypersensitivity reaction	?	Diffuse interstitial and airspace edema	Rare; rapid onset of cough, dyspnea, and cyanosis; associated dermatitis and hepatitis; rapid recovery	Severe hypoxemia
Beclomethasone diproprionate	Possible hypersensitivity to 10% oleic acid dispensing agent	?	Airspace consolidation	Eosinophilia and "pneumonia" on switching from oral to inhaled steroid; rapid resolution	?
ACE inhibitors (captopril and enalapril)	Neutral endopeptidase inhibition; enhanced neuropeptide action	?	None	Cough and bronchospasm	Occasionally exacerbation of airway obstruction in asthmatics; increased bronchial hyper-responsiveness

Table 14–1. Drug-Induced Disease of the Thorax *Continued*

DRUG	MECHANISM OF LUNG INJURY	PATHOLOGIC ABNORMALITIES	ROENTGENOGRAPHIC FEATURES	CLINICAL FEATURES	PULMONARY FUNCTION ABNORMALITIES
Silicone	Increased pulmonary microvascular permeability	Diffuse alveolar damage	Interstitial and airspace pulmonary edema	Following subcutaneous injection in transsexual men; fever, chest pain, and dyspnea; ARDS	Gas exchange impairment
Cocaine	?	Rarely pulmonary granuloma; one case of bronchiolitis	?	Rarely implicated in pulmonary toxicity	?
Practolol (beta-adrenergic blocking agent)	?	Sclerosing peritonitis and pleuropulmonary fibrosis	?	Now withdrawn from market; caused fatal respiratory failure in some patients	Lung restriction
Propranolol and other β-blockers	β-adrenergic blockade removing protective effect of chronic β-stimulation in patients with asthma and COPD	—	Worsening hyperinflation	Worsening dyspnea, cough, and airway obstruction in patients with pre-existing asthma and COPD	Worsening airway obstruction; increased airway hyper-responsiveness
Contrast media (ethiodized oil, sodium iothalamate, and diatrizoate meglumine [Gastrografin])	Ethiodized oil causes fatty acid embolism; water-soluble media cause damage because of hypertonicity	Alveolar inflammation and high-protein edema	Diffuse airspace edema	Acute or subacute pulmonary edema; water-soluble media predispose to pulmonary edema in patients with heart disease	Hypoxemia; impaired diffusing capacity
Talc	?	?	Diffuse airspace edema	10 g talc injected intrapleurally led to ARDS over a 3-day period	Hypoxemia
Disodium chromoglycate	Allergic hypersensitivity reaction	?	Patchy airspace consolidation	Rarely, this inhaled drug used to treat allergic disease causes pulmonary eosinophilia	Hypoxemia
Penicillin, cephalosporins, phenylglycine acid chloride, piperazine hydrochloride, psyllium, methyldopa, spiramycin, amprolium hydrochloride, tetracycline, sulfone chloramides	Allergic or nonallergic airway narrowing	—	Hyperinflation	Bronchospasm in a patient with or without pre-existing asthma	Airflow obstruction

synergistic toxic effect from the combined therapy and despite the acknowledged toxicity of cyclophosphamide, it is generally concluded that the major source of lung damage in this combination is bleomycin.[13] Pulmonary disease caused by bleomycin has been recognized for many years[16] and possesses an incidence that ranges from as low as 3 per cent in most series[4, 9] to as high as 40 per cent in others.[10]

The mechanism of pulmonary injury in bleomycin toxicity is unclear. In a minority of patients, it appears to be primarily immunologic and to consist of reversible eosinophilic pneumonia.[17, 18] The majority of patients, however, manifest rapidlyprogressive interstitial pneumonitis that is associated with a mortality rate as high as 50 per cent.[19–21] The drug is concentrated in lung and skin, organs that are relatively deficient in the hydrolase enzyme that inactivates the drug; once within its target cells, the drug has the ability to cleave DNA, possibly by generating certain oxygen radicals.[22] It has been speculated that the production of such radicals is responsible for cell death and eventually interstitial fibrosis. Reactive oxygen metabolites are generally accepted as the agents of lung damage associated with radiation therapy or the administration of high concentrations of oxygen; the synergistic effect when bleomycin is combined with these forms of therapy, either simultaneously or sequentially,[7, 9, 10, 13, 19, 20] thus supports the hypothesis of oxygen radical-induced bleomycin toxicity. Berend[23] has demonstrated a protective effect of hypoxia on bleomycin lung toxicity in the rat, which supports the concept of oxidant damage. Experimental[24] and clinical[13, 25] studies have indicated an increase in severity and incidence of pulmonary fibrosis in animals and patients receiving concurrent bleomycin and high inspired concentrations of oxygen. As a consequence, supplemental oxygen administered to any patient with a history of bleomycin treatment should be at the lowest possible level;[13] in addition, when surgery is undertaken, continuous intraoperative and postoperative monitoring of arterial oxygen tension has been recommended.[26]

Despite this evidence in favor of oxygen radical-induced lung damage, some experimental findings suggest that other factors may be important in the pathogenesis of bleomycin lung toxicity.[22] For example, it has been postulated that polymorphonuclear leukocytes or lymphocytes also may play a role in the pathogenesis.[13, 27, 28] Bronchoalveolar lavage in animals administered bleomycin reveals an increased percentage of polymorphonuclear leukocytes,[28, 29] and it is conceivable that these cells could cause a release of toxic substances such as oxidants and proteases. Polymorphonuclear leukocytes also produce collagenase. In a study of hamsters depleted of neutrophils with rabbit antineutrophilic serum, Clark and Kuhn[30] found increased levels of lung collagen in the animals compared with nondepleted controls, and they attributed this increase

to a lack of collagenase enzyme. There is also experimental evidence for a contributory role of complement in the development of bleomycin-induced fibrosis.[31]

The development of bleomycin-induced pulmonary disease is dose-related,[4, 9, 10] with the overall incidence of 3 to 5 per cent rising to 35 per cent when the cumulative dose is over 450 units.[21] However, pulmonary disease can develop with total doses lower than this[20, 32, 33] and, in fact, has been reported following administration of as little as 100 units.[20] In animal studies, very low doses of bleomycin have been shown to result in some degree of interstitial fibrosis.[9, 34, 35] Risk is increased in patients receiving combined cytotoxic drug therapy, high inspired oxygen, and radiation therapy. Some evidence has been presented that continuous intravenous infusion of the drug is less likely than biweekly administration to result in pulmonary disease,[10] but further studies are required to confirm this apparent advantage.[13]

Pathologic findings in the lungs of patients[36] and experimental animals[37] administered bleomycin have been extensively reported. The earliest changes are related to endothelial cell damage and consist of edema, intra-alveolar fibrin, and hemorrhage.[13, 37] This histologic stage may be reflected in physiologic evidence of a substantial decrease in the pulmonary capillary blood volume component (V_C) of the DL_{CO}[38] and in biochemical evidence of a reduction in serum angiotensin-converting enzyme.[39] The initial endothelial cell damage is followed by destruction of type I pneumocytes,[13] hyperplasia of type II pneumocytes, and metaplasia of airway and alveolar epithelium;[4, 37] the latter is often squamous in type and may be caused by a direct effect of bleomycin on differentiated type II cells.[40] In the final stage, collagen production within alveolar walls and airspaces results in interstitial fibrosis.[37] Cytologically atypical pneumocytes with hyperchromatic and irregularly shaped nuclei that are sometimes apparent after the administration of alkylating agents are not a common feature of bleomycin toxicity.[7]

Roentgenographic abnormalities consist of a reticular pattern that tends to progress to patchy or massive airspace consolidation (Fig. 14–1).[20] In a study of 20 patients with pulmonary complications associated with combination chemotherapy regimens containing bleomycin, Balikian and his associates[41] found that the pulmonary disease showed a striking basal predominance, in several cases being localized to the costophrenic regions. These abnormalities may develop prior to, synchronous with, or following the appearance of clinical symptoms of cough and shortness of breath on exertion, both of which suggest pulmonary toxicity.[19] An unusual manifestation of bleomycin toxicity is the development of multiple pulmonary nodules that can simulate metastases but that tend to disappear on drug withdrawal.[42–45]

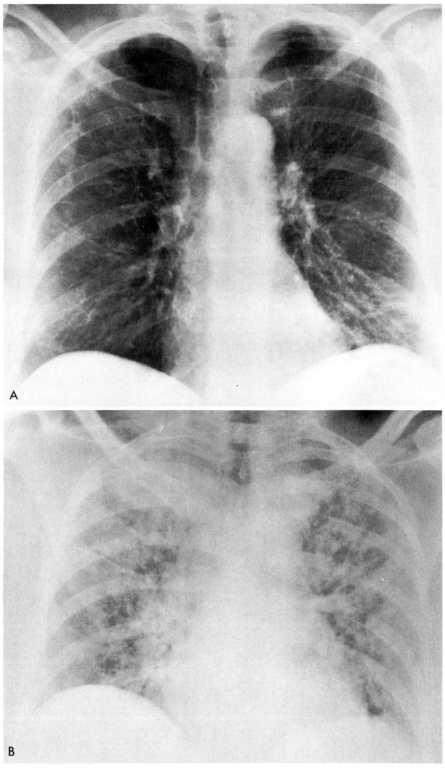

Figure 14–1. Acute Pulmonary Reaction to Bleomycin. Four months prior to the roentgenograms illustrated, large cell lymphoma was discovered in the left clavicle of this 55-year-old woman. Shortly thereafter, a 6-week course of chemotherapy was instituted that included a total of 198 units of bleomycin, 10.6 mg of vincristine, and 65 mg daily of prednisone. At the end of the 6-week course, she was begun on maintenance therapy with cyclophosphamide, 100 mg daily. Shortly thereafter, she noted the onset of weakness, dry cough, and a stuffy nose. She had a fever of 103° F, severe leukopenia (total white blood count 700 per cu mm), and was found to be anergic. At this time, a posteroanterior roentgenogram *(A)* showed an almost normal appearance of the lungs apart from some prominence of vascular markings. Five days later *(B)* extensive disease had developed throughout both lungs, the pattern of which suggests diffuse interstitial and airspace involvement of the parenchyma. An open lung biopsy was performed that day, sections being taken from the lingula and left lower lobe. Pathologic examination showed extensive interstitial pneumonitis. Shortly thereafter, the patient developed acute respiratory failure from which recovery was prolonged.

Symptoms include fever, cough, and dyspnea on exertion and occur in both the acute hypersensitivity reaction and the more insidiously progressive diffuse interstitial fibrosis.[7, 13, 19] Rales may be detected, particularly at the lung bases. In some patients, the disease can progress rapidly to fatal pulmonary insufficiency.[20] The tendency for deposition of the drug in the skin can cause hyperpigmentation and swelling of the fingers, palms, and soles of the feet.[34]

Pulmonary function tests, particularly vital capacity and diffusing capacity, have been used to monitor patients receiving bleomycin and have been reported to detect lung involvement at an early stage when the chest roentgenogram is still normal.[21, 32] Since patients receiving this drug are often weakened or anemic as a result of their underlying malignancy, and since progressive reduction in V_C and DL_{CO} may be caused by these conditions alone, the results of the tests must be interpreted with caution.[46] Pulmonary capillary blood volume (V_C), a component of DL_{CO}, is reduced in anemic patients, and it is necessary to apply a correction factor before estimating diffusing capacity. In fact, the authors of two separate studies concluded that the DL_{CO} is not a useful predictor of which patients will develop interstitial fibrosis.[46, 47] Determination of V_C, after correcting for hemoglobin concentration, has been reported to reflect pulmonary endothelial damage;[38] however, Van Barneveld and colleagues[48] found that a decrease in V_C protects patients against bleomycin-induced pneumonitis, probably by an associated reduction in the quantity of bleomycin within the lungs. In a study of 39 patients with disseminated testicular nonseminomatous neoplasm treated with a combination chemotherapy containing bleomycin, vinblastine, and the nephrotoxic agent cis-diamine-dichloro platinum (CDDP),[48] these same investigators measured DL_{CO} and its component parts (the alveolocapillary membrane and pulmonary capillary blood volume components), alveolar volume, and vital capacity. Eight of the 39 patients (20.5 per cent) developed bleomycin-induced pneumonitis. The investigators found that the combination of a low normal creatinine clearance and a decrease in vital capacity and alveolar volume unassociated with a decrease in V_C pointed to an increased risk; they concluded that it is worthwhile to monitor these parameters and, if necessary, to modify the chemotherapy of a patient at risk. That a reduction in renal function is a major risk factor for the development of bleomycin-induced pneumonitis was borne out by another study[47] in which 2 of 15 patients treated with bleomycin for malignancy died as a result of pulmonary toxicity; both had evidence of sustained nephrotoxicity during chemotherapy.

Only 1 to 2 per cent of patients receiving bleomycin therapy die of pulmonary toxicity.[49] Death usually follows a prolonged period of increasing dyspnea but can be associated in an occasional patient with rapidly progressive respiratory insufficiency.[20] For example, two patients treated for carcinoma of the tonsil without concomitant radiotherapy died 45 and 52 days, respectively, after the onset of therapy.[50] Complete clinical and roentgenologic recovery can be associated with a persistent reduction in DL_{CO} and the presence of residual fibrosis pathologically.[33] However, in one long-term follow-up of eight patients,[51] previously documented pulmonary dysfunction eventually reverted to normal. Although the role played by corticosteroids in resolving pulmonary pneumonitis is controversial, animal studies[52] have supported a beneficial action.

MITOMYCIN

Mitomycin is an alkylating antibiotic that is derived from Streptomyces caespitous and is used mainly in the treatment of patients with gastrointestinal and, occasionally, breast and cervical malignancies;[10, 13] it is usually combined with vincristine or vindesine and 5-fluorouracil, drugs not generally regarded as being toxic to the lungs.[13, 53] In two series, pulmonary toxicity occurred in 6 of 200 (3 per cent)[54] and 6 of 116 (5 per cent)[55] patients. In a review of the literature in 1986,[13] it was estimated that over 30 cases of this form of drug-induced pulmonary disease had been reported. Although a few cases have occurred with the sole use of mitomycin,[56] most have been in patients who received it in combination with other cytotoxic drugs assumed not to induce pulmonary damage; nevertheless, the possibility of a synergistic effect cannot be excluded. Long-term treatment is not required to produce pulmonary damage;[10, 13] one report indicated that 3 patients had developed interstitial pneumonitis 3 to 6 months after initiation of therapy.[56] The total dose required to induce damage also varies considerably; these 3 patients received cumulative doses of 60, 102, and 156 mg,[56] whereas in 6 patients in another report, the total dosage ranged from 20 mg up to 100 mg/m^2.[55]

The mechanism by which mitomycin induces damage has not been elucidated, but since the drug possesses alkylating properties its mode of action may be similar to that of cyclophosphamide and other alkylating agents. There is some evidence that O_2 administration and radiation therapy enhance the risk of the development of mitomycin-induced pulmonary disease.[10, 13]

Pathologic characteristics are similar to those associated with other cytotoxic drugs and include endothelial damage, necrosis of type I pneumocytes, proliferation of type II cells, and collagen deposition.[57] One group of investigators[58] has described a syndrome consisting of noncardiogenic pulmonary edema, microangiopathic hemolytic anemia, and renal failure, accompanied by immunofluorescent evidence of vascular changes and fibrinogen-fibrin deposits. A hypersensitivity form of eosinophilic pneumonitis has not been reported.

In the few descriptions of roentgenographic manifestations of mitomycin-induced pulmonary damage, the pattern has consisted of coarse reticular and airspace opacities with lower zonal predominance; it has been likened to the pattern observed in bronchiolitis obliterans and organizing pneumonia.[13, 55, 56] Pleural effusion has been described in a number of cases and appears to be a more common feature of mitomycin toxicity than of other cytotoxic drug reactions.[13]

Mitomycin toxicity is usually suspected when the patient develops a dry cough and progressive dyspnea, symptoms that may subside with cessation of therapy.[55] Most patients remain afebrile.[13, 55] Other side effects include nausea, vomiting, alopecia, and renal and cardiac toxicity.[55] Symptoms can occur in the absence of roentgenographic abnormality. In the rare patient who presents with capillary leakage, the onset of dyspnea is abrupt and the roentgenographic pattern consists of widespread edema.

In a limited number of reports, pulmonary function tests have shown a restrictive defect and decreased DL_{CO}.[13] We are not aware of pulmonary function tests being performed prospectively to monitor the potential development of pulmonary disease.

The mortality rate of mitomycin-induced toxicity is said to be about 50 per cent; some reports suggest that cure is possible when the drug is withdrawn and corticosteroids administered.[13]

OTHER CYTOTOXIC ANTIBIOTICS

Of 113 patients in one report of the use of *pepleomycin*, a derivative of bleomycin,[59] definite pulmonary toxicity occurred in 7 patients (6.2 per cent); 6 of the 7 died of pulmonary fibrosis despite prednisone therapy. Clinical, roentgenographic, and histopathologic manifestations were identical to those of bleomycin pulmonary toxicity. There is a single report of a patient who developed vasculitis following an unusually large dose of *neocarzinostatin*;[60] circulating antibodies to the agent were identified.

Alkylating Agents

BUSULFAN

This chemotherapeutic agent was the first drug to be incriminated as a cause of diffuse interstitial fibrosis.[61, 62] It is used in the treatment of myeloproliferative disorders, particularly chronic myelogenous leukemia. Although clinically recognized pulmonary toxicity occurs in only about 4 per cent of patients,[49, 63, 64] Heard and Cooke[63] performed a pathologic study of the lungs of 14 patients who had received busulfan therapy and found 6 (46 per cent) to have alveolar fibrosis associated with large, cytologically atypical alveolar mononuclear cells. The mechanism of damage is unknown, but the primary target appears to be epithelial cells.[13] Clinically apparent pulmonary toxicity tends to occur only with long-term use, ranging from 8 months to 10 years in several studies (average, 3 to 4 years).[49, 61, 62, 65] Prior use of other cytotoxic drugs or radiation therapy increases the risk.[66] Although toxicity does not appear to be directly dose-dependent, no patient treated with a total dose less than 500 mg has developed pulmonary disease in the absence of other potentially toxic influences such as radiation therapy or other chemotherapeutic agents.[13, 49]

The pathologic finding most characteristic of busulfan-induced pulmonary disease is the presence of large, cytologically atypical mononuclear cells (Fig. 14–2)[63, 64, 67] that have been identified on electron microscopy as being altered type II pneumocytes.[68] Although atypical pneumocytes are also found in pulmonary disease induced by other drugs, the extent and severity of atypia are generally greater with busulfan. The finding of cytologic atypia in tissues other than the lung (such as the pancreas)[69] suggests that the abnormality is not simply the result of a reparative or inflammatory process but is a direct effect of the drug itself. Other pathologic manifestations include an increase in fibroblasts associated with collagen deposition in both interstitium and airspaces, an infiltration of mononuclear cells, and, in the early stage, fibrinous edema and hyaline membrane formation (Fig. 14–2).[63, 69] Interstitial calcification[61, 67] and ossification[70] are occasionally seen in association with pulmonary fibrosis. Two reports have appeared of patients with chronic myelogenous leukemia being treated with busulfan who developed pulmonary alveolar proteinosis,[71, 72] an association attributed to the relationship between the two diseases rather than to the therapy (*see* page 1558).

The chest roentgenogram usually shows a diffuse reticulonodular pattern, sometimes with lower zonal predominance (Fig. 14–3); airspace opacities also can be present and probably occur more often with busulfan than with other drugs.[13] Pleural effusion has been reported in two cases.[73]

The onset of disease clinically is usually insidious, the major complaints being dry cough, fever, weakness, weight loss, and dyspnea.[61, 74] Many patients are severely disabled by shortness of breath.[75] By removing an inhibitor of tyrosinase, busulfan accelerates the formation of melanin from tyrosine and thus results in hyperpigmentation of the skin; as a result, some patients resemble those with Addison's disease.[74]

No data have appeared in the literature to support the prospective use of pulmonary function tests in following patients on long-term busulfan therapy. Once disease has become evident, lung volumes and diffusing capacity are usually reduced.[64, 65, 76]

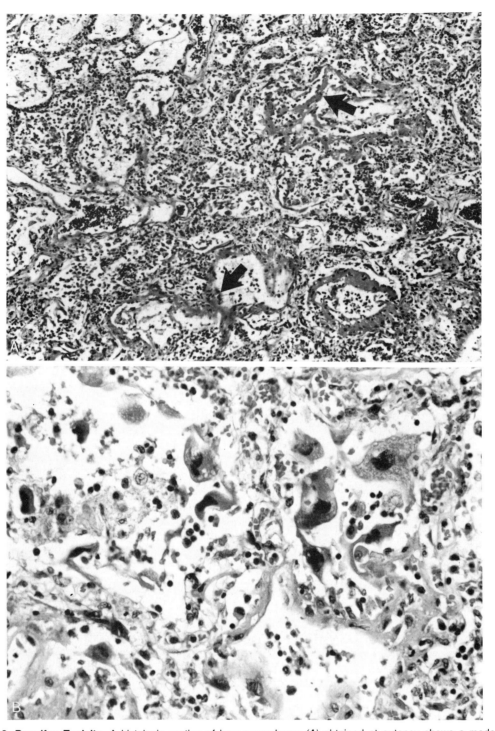

Figure 14–2. Busulfan Toxicity. A histologic section of lung parenchyma *(A)* obtained at autopsy shows a moderate degree of interstitial thickening by lymphocytes, extensive airspace filling by macrophages and other mononuclear inflammatory cells, and multifocal hyaline membranes *(arrows)*. A magnified view of three alveoli *(B)* shows type II pneumocytes to be greatly increased in size and to contain irregularly shaped and cytologically atypical nuclei. The patient was taking 3 mg of busulfan daily for therapy of acute myelogenous leukemia. (*A* × 80; *B* × 275.)

The diagnosis of busulfan-induced pulmonary disease may be suggested by the finding of the atypical pneumocytes in expectorated or lavaged material,[9] but, as with other drugs, an open lung biopsy is usually required to exclude other causes for the roentgenographic abnormalities. The prognosis is bad;[4, 7] the mean survival time after diagnosis of pulmonary fibrosis is 5 months.[49, 75, 77]

Prognosis may be improved by early detection, cessation of drug therapy, and possibly the initiation of corticosteroid therapy.

CYCLOPHOSPHAMIDE

This alkylating cytotoxic drug is used widely in the treatment of malignancies and autoimmune

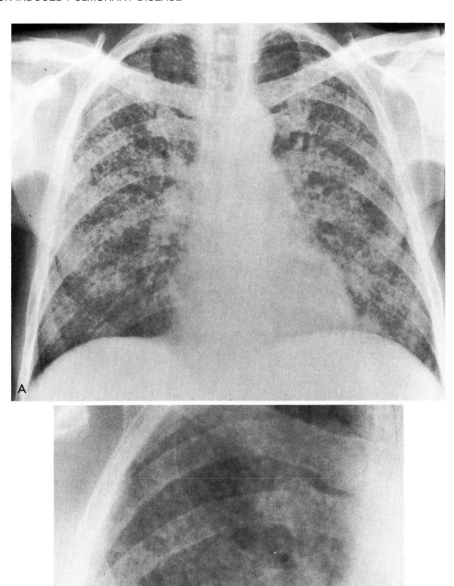

Figure 14–3. Busulfan Toxicity. This 61-year-old woman was being treated for chronic myeloid leukemia with busulfan in a dose of 2 mg three times a day. At the time of this roentgenogram, she was complaining of severe exertional dyspnea and showed signs of congestive heart failure. The posteroanterior roentgenogram *(A)* and magnified view of the right upper zone *(B)* reveal a widespread coarse reticulonodular pattern throughout both lungs without anatomic predominance. The pattern suggests a predominant interstitial abnormality. The major functional abnormality was a reduction in diffusing capacity to less than half of that predicted. The patient died approximately 1 year later, and at necropsy there was observed generalized fibrous thickening of the alveolar walls with preservation of lung architecture.

connective tissue disease. It is often combined with other chemotherapeutic agents, particularly vinca alkaloids; this creates the potential for confusion as to which agent is responsible for the pulmonary disease or for doubt as to whether the toxicity may be the result of a synergistic effect. There is also evidence that pneumonitis can develop with a variety of cytotoxic drugs in patients who have previ-

ously received a course of cyclophosphamide therapy.[7] However, there is no doubt that the drug can cause significant pulmonary damage in experimental animals when it is administered alone.[78]

Cyclophosphamide is a widely used cytotoxic agent and the incidence of pulmonary toxicity must be very low, probably less than 1 per cent.[13] The development of interstitial fibrosis has been re-

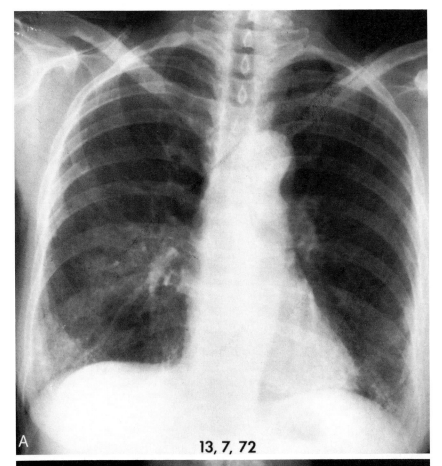

13, 7, 72

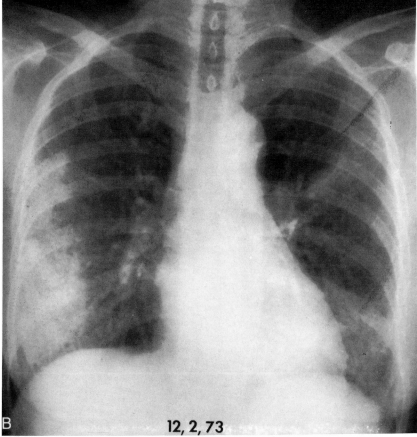

12, 2, 73

Figure 14–4. Cyclophosphamide-Induced Pulmonary Disease. A posteroanterior roentgenogram *(A)* reveals ill-defined opacities in the midportion of the right lung and at both lung bases. The appearance suggested a combination of interstitial and airspace abnormality. Seven months later *(B)*, the opacities had become largely airspace in character and, on the right side at least, showed considerable peripheral dominance.

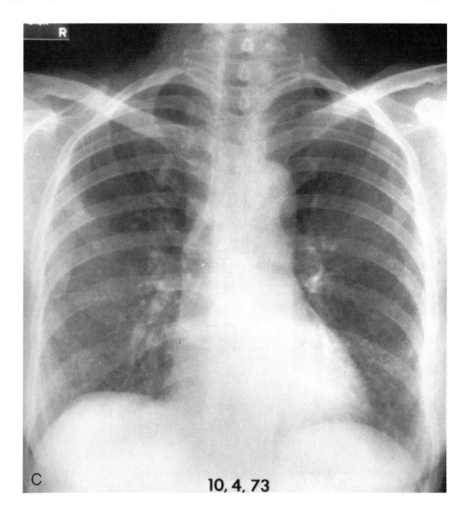

Figure 14–4 *Continued* Two months later following withdrawal of the medication *(C)*, the appearance of the chest was almost normal. This middle-aged woman was being treated with cyclophosphamide for lymphoma.

10, 4, 73

ported following administration of as little as 150 mg of the drug,[49] although the risk of serious toxicity appears to increase with higher doses. For example, in one series,[7] all but one patient who recovered had received less than a 10 g total dose whereas most of those who died had received approximately 40 g.[13, 79] In mice, oxygen administration has been reported to have a synergistic effect with cyclophosphamide in the production of toxicity, although synergism does not exist with radiation.[80] In humans, limited studies[13] have suggested that the risk of pulmonary damage is increased when cyclophosphamide is combined with oxygen; in addition, very high-dose cyclophosphamide[81] appears to sensitize the lung to radiation damage.

The pathologic findings in cyclophosphamide-induced pulmonary disease are said to be similar to those of busulfan toxicity[7] and consist of organizing intra-alveolar exudates, fibrosis, and the presence of cytologically atypical alveolar epithelial cells.[82]

The chest roentgenogram reveals changes similar to those of other drug-induced pulmonary diseases—a diffuse reticulonodular pattern with basal predominance, sometimes with an airspace component (Fig. 14–4). In one patient who developed the abrupt onset of dyspnea, the roentgenogram revealed airspace pulmonary edema.[79] Children re-

ceiving cyclophosphamide therapy have been reported to have reduced anteroposterior chest diameter, presumably resulting from loss of lung volume secondary to drug effect during their adolescent growth spurt.[83]

The clinical onset of pulmonary disease is acute or subacute more often than chronic, although the time interval between initiation of therapy and development of symptoms varies markedly;[7, 84] symptoms can develop within months in some patients[84] but take years to become apparent in others. In one patient who had been receiving 50 to 100 mg of the drug daily for malignant lymphoma, biopsy-proved interstitial fibrosis was detected after 13 years.[85] Two children who had received daily oral cyclophosphamide for 3 to 4 years developed serious pulmonary fibrosis 4 and 6 years later.[83] Cough and dyspnea are major complaints, and fever occurs in more than 50 per cent of patients.[7, 82, 86] Pulmonary function tests show a restrictive ventilatory defect and a reduced diffusing capacity.[7, 86]

The prognosis for patients who develop pulmonary toxicity as a result of cyclophosphamide therapy depends on how early it is recognized and perhaps on whether corticosteroid therapy has been instituted; approximately 60 per cent of patients recover. It is probable that patients who receive prednisone along with cyclophosphamide are protected from developing toxicity.[7] Cessation of cyclophosphamide therapy can be followed by resolution of the pulmonary disease,[86] usually in association with corticosteroid administration.[84, 87]

CHLORAMBUCIL

This alkylating agent is used chiefly in the treatment of hematologic malignancies and is a rare cause of pulmonary toxicity; only 10 cases had been reported by 1986.[13] Two patients who developed interstitial fibrosis had received total doses of 2.5 g[88] and 4.1 g.[89] There is no information in the literature to suggest a synergistic effect with other oxidants.

The pathology is similar to that of busulfan and cyclophosphamide toxicity;[89] in one description of an open lung biopsy specimen,[90] the findings consisted of perivascular and interstitial fibrosis, hyperplasia and atypia of alveolar lining cells, and alveolar filling by mononuclear cells and exudate.

The chest roentgenogram reveals a diffuse, predominantly bibasilar, reticulonodular pattern,[13] on occasion said to be coarse.[89] In one patient, the interstitial disease was reported to be confined to the upper lobes.[91]

Onset of clinical symptoms ranges from 6 months to 3 years after the beginning of therapy.[13] Symptoms tend to be subacute in nature and include anorexia, weight loss, fatigue, fever, cough, and dyspnea.[89] One patient has been reported in whom recurrent attacks of respiratory distress developed 9 to 12 days after each treatment;[92] despite a normal chest roentgenogram, an open lung biopsy specimen revealed findings compatible with drug-induced pulmonary disease. Finger clubbing[91] and rales[89] have been found on physical examination. Pulmonary function tests show a restrictive pattern and a decrease in DL_{CO}.[89, 90] Five of the 10 reported patients died.[13] Cessation of drug therapy and administration of steroids can result in resolution of the pulmonary disease.[89]

MELPHALAN

Melphalan, a phenylalanine derivative of nitrogen mustard, is used chiefly in the treatment of multiple myeloma. Since only seven documented cases of pulmonary toxicity have been reported, the incidence of toxicity is obviously low.[13, 93] However, despite this infrequent occurrence of clinically detected pulmonary disease, one retrospective autopsy study[94] revealed evidence of histopathologic abnormality in 5 of 10 patients exposed to this drug.

The pathology does not differ from that described with other alkylating agents—interstitial pulmonary fibrosis associated with proliferation and atypia of alveolar epithelial cells.[95, 96]

The chest roentgenogram has been reported to show a reticular pattern,[13] although a predomi-

nantly nodular pattern also has been described.[97] Pleural effusion was identified in one patient.[93]

Symptoms and signs tend to appear within 1 to 4 months of the initiation of therapy,[13] and are identical to those of chlorambucil, as are pulmonary function test abnormalities.[96] Five of the seven reported patients died of respiratory failure;[13] one of the other two patients showed clearing of the roentgenographic abnormalities but persistence of symptoms and reduced diffusing capacity.[96]

NITROSOUREAS

The pharmacologic action of the nitrosoureas is similar to that of other alkylating agents and consists of interference with DNA synthesis and impedance of DNA repair.[98] These drugs are used chiefly in the treatment of intracranial neoplasms, melanoma, gastrointestinal malignancies, and lymphoma.[10, 13] Following their increased use in the late 1960s and early 1970s, the number of reported cases of pulmonary damage increased. In a 1986 review, the number of cases was estimated at 70;[13] most of these were caused by BCNU (carmustine [1,3-bis (2-chloroethyl)-1-nitrosourea]).

Although many of the reported cases of pulmonary toxicity caused by BCNU occurred in patients receiving this drug alone, some have developed in combination with other cytotoxic agents, particularly cyclophosphamide. Because the dose of BCNU in these cases was lower than that generally recognized as producing interstitial fibrosis, a synergistic effect has been suggested.[4, 99] The incidence of pulmonary toxicity from BCNU therapy ranges from 1 to 20 per cent in different series.[4, 99–102] Such a large range in incidence reflects the total dose administered and the length of survival from the primary disease—the larger the dose and the longer the survival, the greater chance of a patient's developing pulmonary damage. An increased risk associated with a total dose of 1 g or more has been well documented.[4, 103] For example, in a series of 93 patients being treated for malignant glioma, Aronin and associates[102] found that 50 per cent of those who received 1.5 g or more developed interstitial fibrosis. In a more recent study in which BCNU was the only chemotherapeutic agent employed in the treatment of 318 patients with malignant glioma,[104] no clinical evidence of pulmonary damage was identified in patients who received a total dose less than 902 mg/m², whereas 10 of 107 patients who received more than this dose developed detectable pulmonary toxicity. In one series,[99] 4 patients who developed pulmonary toxicity from BCNU therapy had received prior mediastinal irradiation; this possibly indicates a synergistic effect.

The pathologic findings are similar to those of other forms of cytotoxic pulmonary damage:[13] interstitial fibrosis; hypertrophy and atypia of alveolar lining cells; and desquamated pneumocytes, histiocytes, and proteinaceous material filling alveolar spaces.[105, 106] Similarly nonspecific roentgenographic manifestations consist of a reticulonodular pattern with basal predominance. Cases of pathologically proved interstitial fibrosis have been reported in which chest roentgenograms have been normal.[13, 100]

Clinical evidence of pulmonary damage usually appears from a month to a year after the institution of therapy;[4] however, one patient developed symptoms 2½ years after cessation of treatment.[98] Symptoms include dry cough, fatigue, and dyspnea.[98, 103, 105] The DL_{CO}, PaO_2, and VC are reduced.[4, 10, 13]

The course of the disease is usually insidious over a period of months,[13] although pulmonary toxicity can be rapidly progressive and fatal.[106, 107] Since most patients treated with BCNU also receive prednisone to lessen cerebral edema, it is difficult to assess the role that corticosteroids play in the prevention or treatment of BCNU-induced pulmonary damage.

Nitrosoureas other than BCNU rarely cause pulmonary toxicity. Lomustine (CCNU)[108, 109] and semustine (methyl CCNU)[110] have been reported to induce pulmonary damage in three patients and one patient, respectively; the findings were identical to those described for BCNU.

OTHER CHEMOTHERAPEUTIC AGENTS

A number of other drugs used in the treatment of malignancy are suspect in cases of pulmonary toxicity, but they are usually administered in combination with other medications known to be hazardous so their roles in causing pulmonary damage are difficult to assess.[111, 112] For example, the vinca alkaloids, *vinblastine* and *vindesine*, are almost invariably used in combination with other drugs, particularly mitomycin. This combination of drugs has been reported to cause interstitial lung disease;[113] however, in two patients who developed fatal acute pulmonary edema while receiving vinblastine and mitomycin,[113] it is probable that the toxicity was caused by the latter drug. Vindesine, however, appears to be capable of inducing a temporary acute bronchospastic reaction. In one patient it was associated with objective evidence of obstruction on pulmonary function testing.[114] Vindesine also may play at least some role in the development of progressive interstitial fibrosis.[114, 115] *Procarbazine*, although often used in combination with other drugs,[13, 116] also has been associated with an acute allergic reaction, in one case characterized by eosinophilia, urticaria, and arthralgia.[116, 117] A challenge with procarbazine alone reproduced the reaction in this patient.[117]

In a study of 42 patients on whom computed tomography (CT) was performed both before and after treatment with *cis*-platinum, vinblastine, and bleomycin (CVB) for metastatic testicular carcinoma, 21 patients (3 symptomatic, 18 asymptomatic) were shown to develop reversible subpleural reticular and airspace opacities.[118]

ANTIMETABOLITES

METHOTREXATE

In contrast to the medications discussed above, methotrexate usually causes pulmonary disease that is reversible and that can result from hypersensitivity rather than from direct toxic damage to the alveolocapillary membrane;[119–122] however, chronic interstitial fibrosis develops in some patients.[119, 123–125] Methotrexate is used in the treatment of malignancy[13] and a variety of nonmalignant diseases such as psoriasis, pemphigus,[120, 121, 123, 126–128] and rheumatoid arthritis.[129–133] Regardless of the method of administration—oral, intravenous, or intrathecal—methotrexate has been associated with pulmonary toxicity. In 1986,[13] it was estimated that over 50 cases had been reported since the condition was first described almost 20 years previously,[119, 134] an admittedly low number considering the frequency with which the drug is administered; an incidence of approximately 5 per cent is probably realistic.[130] In one report,[134] an incidence of 41 per cent toxicity in a group of children receiving maintenance methotrexate therapy was not confirmed by pathologic examination and was undoubtedly an overestimation. We consider that this series must have included some patients with complicating infection or pulmonary dissemination of the disease being treated.

Methotrexate is a folic acid analogue that inhibits cellular reproduction by causing an acute intracellular deficiency of folate coenzymes.[13] It is probable that the mechanism causing lung damage is related to this deficiency. However, other factors may be important; in a recent study, it was shown that peripheral blood leukocytes elaborate a leukocyte inhibitory factor and that bronchoalveolar lavage fluid contains an inverted lymphocyte-subset ratio. This study provides evidence that the mechanism of pulmonary toxicity may consist of a cellular immune response to the drug. Specific risk factors have not been identified and a clear-cut dose relationship has not been shown. The frequency of dosage and duration of therapy may be important, since patients who receive daily or weekly therapy for prolonged periods are more likely to manifest toxicity.[4, 13] Although it has been said that lung damage seldom occurs on a dose less than 20 mg/wk,[4, 7] five reports have appeared recently of patients with rheumatoid arthritis who developed clinical and roentgenographic evidence of interstitial disease on a dose ranging from 5 to 15 mg/wk.[129–132, 135] All but one of these patients recovered completely on withdrawal of the drug, with or without corticosteroid therapy.

The rapidly reversible nature of interstitial pneumonitis in many patients receiving low-dose methotrexate does not justify open lung biopsy to confirm the diagnosis. It is suspected that these are patients whose tissue shows an extensive mononuclear inflammatory component, with or without granuloma formation and tissue eosinophilia, as reported in a number of cases.[4, 9, 49, 136, 137] In approximately 10 per cent of patients who develop pulmonary toxicity, interstitial fibrosis is either proven pathologically or is assumed to be present because of persistent roentgenographic abnormality.[124, 125, 137] Diffuse pulmonary edema with hyaline membrane formation has been seen in patients who have received methotrexate intrathecally.[13]

The roentgenographic changes are fairly characteristic and should suggest the diagnosis in the proper clinical setting. Initially, the chest roentgenogram reveals a diffuse reticular pattern indicating widespread interstitial disease (Fig. 14–5). This progresses rapidly to patchy acinar consolidation (Fig. 14–6), which, in time, reverts once again to an interstitial pattern followed by complete resolution.[119, 122, 136, 138, 139] Multiple nodules[137] and, in at least two patients, hilar lymph node enlargement also have been reported.[121, 137] Pleural effusion has been described.[105] Roentgenographically, demonstrable disease may be present for periods ranging from a few days[122] to a year or longer.[119]

The duration of maintenance methotrexate therapy before symptoms and signs of toxicity become clinically apparent ranges from 1 month to 5 years;[7, 120] in one patient the duration was 18 years.[126] In the majority of cases the onset is acute-to-subacute and is characterized by fever, cough, dyspnea, and headache; pleuritic pain is unusual.[13, 31] There are usually no abnormal findings on physical examination of the chest.[119, 122, 139] Digital clubbing has been described,[126] and skin eruptions have been noted in 17 per cent of cases.[137] Liver disease, including cirrhosis, is a recognized complication of prolonged therapy.[121, 140–143] A moderate blood eosinophilia is common,[119, 120, 139] variously cited as occurring in 41 per cent[13] to over 65 per cent of cases.[9] Pulmonary function tests show a restrictive pattern.[13] A surprising finding in our experience and that of others is a very low PaO_2.[119, 129]

As indicated above, patients on low-dose maintenance methotrexate therapy usually show a rapid clearing of symptoms and of roentgenographic abnormality following withdrawal of the medication.[129–132, 144] The mortality rate has been estimated at 1 per cent.[49, 137] Cases have been reported in which clearing has occurred despite continuation or reinstitution of therapy.[49, 137]

OTHER ANTIMETABOLITES

Azathioprine (Imuran), a drug commonly used to suppress rejection in patients who have received organ transplants, has been implicated as a cause of interstitial pneumonitis and fibrosis.[13, 145–147] However, it must be considered an uncommon cause of pulmonary toxicity in view of its widespread use. A recent report of renal allograft recipients on whom open lung biopsy was performed has suggested a dose-related effect, with pathologic changes including diffuse alveolar damage and interstitial pneumonitis and fibrosis; four of the five patients with fibrosis died of respiratory insufficiency.[147] Some patients with these pathologic findings recover, possibly reflecting drug dosage or early recognition of toxicity.[145, 147]

Pulmonary toxicity to *cytosine arabinoside* has been reported in individual patients[148] and in 22 per cent of 72 patients who were treated with this drug for acute leukemia.[149] Symptoms and roentgenographic abnormalities were detected a median of 6 days after the initiation of high-dose intravenous therapy. A high incidence of pulmonary disease was also reported in a retrospective autopsy study of 93 patients.[150]

In one series of 29 patients who were receiving *cyclosporin A* to prevent graft-versus-host disease following bone marrow transplantation for leukemia and aplastic anemia, 5 patients developed adult respiratory distress syndrome 8 to 18 days after the initiation of this therapy;[151] whether this was truly an effect of the drug or was simply a complication of transplantation is unclear.

ANTIMICROBIAL AGENTS

NITROFURANTOIN (FURADANTIN)

The incidence of pulmonary toxicity related to the use of nitrofurantoin (Furadantin), an oral medication commonly used in the treatment of urinary tract infections, is difficult to estimate. Almost 1,000 cases have been reported,[14, 133, 152–164] including 447 cases among 921 adverse reactions to the drug identified in Sweden over a 10-year period.[160] Despite a decrease in usage of the drug during the 1980s, the incidence of toxic manifestations increased, a paradox interpreted by the authors of the Swedish study as an indication of sensitization of the Swedish population. The incidence of adverse reactions in the United Kingdom is considerably lower than that in Sweden,[164] an observation that has been attributed either to differences in reporting or to dosages prescribed in the two countries. The higher incidence in women and the elderly is probably a reflection of the patient population receiving this medication.[156, 160]

Two distinct presentations are seen in nitrofurantoin-induced lung disease: (1) acute, developing hours to days after the onset of treatment; and (2) chronic and insidious, becoming manifest after weeks to years of continuous therapy. In the Swedish series, 87 per cent of cases were of the acute

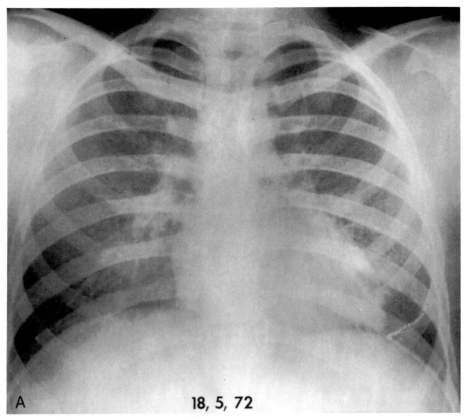

18, 5, 72

Figure 14–5. Methotrexate-Induced Pulmonary Disease. A posteroanterior roentgenogram *(A)* and a magnified view of the left upper zone *(B)* reveal a fine reticular pattern indicating diffuse interstitial lung disease. Lung volume is reduced. This middle-aged man complained of mild dyspnea on effort. He was receiving methotrexate therapy for psoriasis.

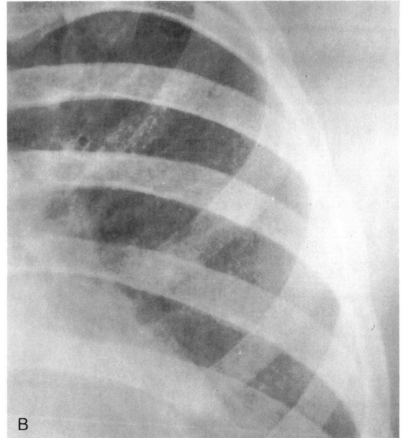

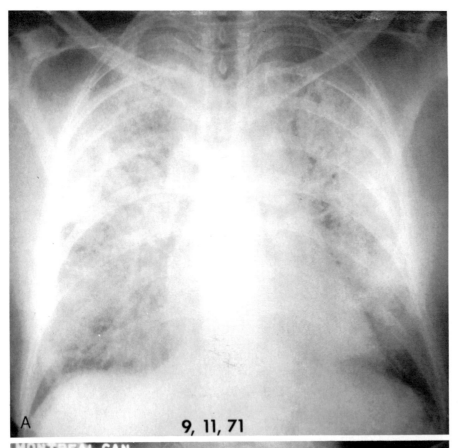

9, 11, 71

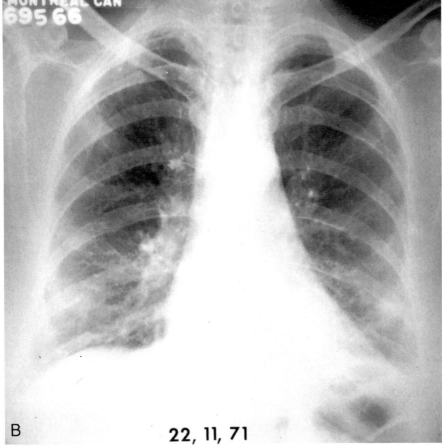

MONTREAL CAN
695 66

22, 11, 71

Figure 14–6. Methotrexate-Induced Pulmonary Disease. A posteroanterior roentgenogram *(A)* reveals massive bilateral airspace consolidation containing a well-defined air bronchogram. Heart size is within normal limits. This appearance is highly suggestive of diffuse airspace pulmonary edema, specifically of increased permeability type. Almost 2 weeks later, following withdrawal of methotrexate therapy for rheumatoid arthritis *(B)*, the massive edema had cleared almost completely.

variety.[160] This form of toxicity almost certainly constitutes a hypersensitivity reaction, a conclusion based on several factors, including its abrupt onset, its reversibility with cessation of therapy, the presence of eosinophilia, the results of *in vitro* and *in vivo* studies of lymphocytes from patients with reactions and from animal experiments,[14] and the presence of interstitial and alveolar mononuclear and polymorphonuclear inflammation with varying degrees of eosinophilia on lung biopsy. Granuloma formation, sometimes with an appearance resembling allergic alveolitis,[165] also has been described.[156, 159]

The chronic form of disease probably represents direct toxic damage due to tissue destruction from oxidants, a conclusion based on experimental studies in animals that have shown hyperoxic enhancement and antioxidant suppression of pulmonary damage.[14] Although some patients with the chronic form of drug damage are found pathologically to have inflammatory changes characteristic of the acute form, most show interstitial pneumonitis and fibrosis indistinguishable from idiopathic fibrosing alveolitis;[155, 158, 163] sometimes the pattern of desquamative or giant cell interstitial pneumonitis is present.[157]

In both the acute and chronic forms of nitrofurantoin-induced lung disease, the chest roentgenogram characteristically reveals a diffuse reticular pattern with some basilar predominance.[153, 154, 167-171] The pattern resembles interstitial pulmonary edema, and, in fact, the rapid clearing that occurs when the drug is withdrawn suggests that edema plays a considerable role in the production of the roentgenographic opacities.[172] In two patients, septal lines have been recognized,[172] and in one patient widespread acinar shadows were detected and were assumed to be caused by diffuse capillary leakage. One patient has been reported in whom all the clinical and roentgenographic features of adult respiratory distress syndrome (ARDS) developed after two weeks of therapy.[162] Pleural effusion may be present[167, 168] and in the acute form may be an isolated finding.[133, 156] Clinical and physiologic evidence of pulmonary toxicity occasionally can become manifest in the absence of roentgenographic abnormality.[154, 160, 169]

In the acute form of the disease, the patient becomes febrile and dyspneic and develops a nonproductive cough within a few days of continuous medication; approximately 25 per cent of patients complain of chest pain. A skin rash and arthralgia occur in 10 to 20 per cent.[153, 154, 156, 160, 168, 169, 173, 174] As implied above, sensitization appears to play a role in acute disease, since symptoms develop more rapidly in patients who have received the drug previously. The chronic form of disease has a more insidious onset; after months to years of nitrofurantoin medication, dry cough and gradually increasing shortness of breath on exertion develop.[155-158, 163, 173] Rales may be heard at the lung bases; in a minority of patients, pleural effusion[154, 157] and clubbing[163] may develop. In the Swedish series,[160] peripheral blood eosinophilia of 5 per cent or more was present in 83 per cent of patients with the acute form and in 40 per cent of those with chronic disease; pleural fluid eosinophilia also has been reported.[133] Profound lymphopenia caused by depletion of T cells has been described in five patients with acute nitrofurantoin pleuropulmonary reactions.[133] In both acute and chronic varieties, a restrictive pattern is found on physiologic assessment.[156, 160, 174] The diffusing capacity and the PaO$_2$ may be very low, particularly in the acute form.[133, 159, 163]

The prognosis is excellent in the acute variety, all evidence of disease usually disappearing within 4 to 8 weeks.[159] However, death can occur as a result of respiratory failure,[161] as in 2 of 398 cases in the Swedish series.[160] In the latter study, 10 per cent of patients with chronic disease died, although complete clearing occasionally occurred in this group on cessation of therapy.[158, 175] A fatal case of massive pulmonary hemorrhage, occurring 24 hours after re-exposure to nitrofurantoin, has been reported in an alcoholic with cirrhosis and esophageal varices.[161] Improvement in function can occur following drug withdrawal despite persistence of roentgenographic abnormalities;[155, 157] by contrast, complete roentgenographic resolution can occur in the presence of residual impairment in the diffusing capacity.[163]

Clinical and roentgenographic changes similar to those associated with nitrofurantoin toxicity accompany therapy with *furazolidone*, a compound chemically related to nitrofurantoin.[176]

SULFASALAZINE

When used in the treatment of inflammatory bowel disease, sulfasalazine (also known as salazosulfapyridine, salicylazosulfapyridine, salazopyrin, and Azulfidine) is broken down into sulfapyridine and 5-aminosalicylate. Pulmonary toxicity has been reported in 12 patients,[14, 177-183] in the majority of whom the presentation consisted of acute transitory pulmonary disease accompanied by peripheral blood eosinophilia, criteria for the diagnosis of Löffler's syndrome. Two patients were known to be allergic to salicylates and one to sulfonamides. Biopsy specimens have revealed interstitial fibrosis and bronchiolitis obliterans with organizing pneumonia;[14, 178, 179, 183] tissue eosinophilia was present in one patient.[178] Bronchoalveolar lavage fluid in one patient contained a significant number of eosinophils.[184]

Descriptions of chest roentgenograms in published cases are somewhat vague, consisting of ill-defined infiltrates (sic). A chest roentgenogram reproduced in one article revealed nonsegmental peripheral airspace consolidation characteristic of eosinophilic pneumonia.[77] In the one patient we have seen with this drug-induced disease, the chest roentgenogram showed patchy airspace opacities confined to the upper lobes; the blood eosinophilia and roentgenographic resolution following withdrawal of therapy simulated Löffler's syndrome.

The clinical presentation varies little from patient to patient[177–181] and consists of dry cough, progressive dyspnea, and fever, often associated with a skin rash and blood eosinophilia; these findings become manifest 1 to 6 months after initiation of treatment. In at least two instances,[177, 179] patients were challenged after cessation of therapy and positive responses were obtained. Both restrictive[14, 183] and obstructive[14, 178] changes have been found on pulmonary function testing. Follow-up studies usually reveal a complete return to normal, although rare examples of residual bronchiolitis obliterans or interstitial fibrosis have been reported.[14, 178, 183]

OTHER ANTIMICROBIAL AGENTS

A number of other antibiotics have been associated with a hypersensitivity lung reaction similar to that seen with sulfasalazine.[4, 14, 185] These include *sulfonamides*, administered either orally or as vaginal creams;[9, 188–190] *penicillin*;[191] *para-aminosalicylic acid*;[192] *cephalosporin*;[194] and *tetracycline*.[195] In two patients, tetracycline was responsible for severe reactions characterized by reversible lower lobe interstitial and airspace opacities, peripheral blood eosinophilia, and PaO_2 values of 44 and 46;[195] neither patient was challenged. An interaction between *amphotericin B* and leukocyte transfusions was originally reported to cause diffuse interstitial disease and alveolar hemorrhage,[196] but this was not confirmed in two subsequent studies.[197, 198]

ANTIARRHYTHMIC DRUGS

AMIODARONE

Amiodarone hydrochloride is an iodinated benzofuran derivative used in the treatment of cardiac arrhythmias. It was originally believed that this drug lacked deleterious side effects, possibly because of the relatively low dosage employed in Europe; however, recent reports indicate that it is an important cause of drug-induced pulmonary damage,[199] with the incidence of toxicity ranging from 1 to 6 per cent.[14, 199–201] Higher maintenance doses employed in the United States may be responsible for the observed increase in incidence.[14, 202] In the English language literature, a conservative estimate of the number of clinically and roentgenographically diagnosed cases is over 100.[199–227] A small number of presumed cases of toxicity based on prospective studies that have shown transitory impairment of pulmonary function were not included in this estimate.[212, 221]

The mechanism of lung damage has not been determined, although on the basis of light and electron microscopic findings, most authorities support a disturbance of metabolism. Marchlinski and associates[199] consider amiodarone to be one of a group of compounds whose chemical structure includes a nonpolar ring system and a hydrophilic cationic side chain capable of inducing the lysosomal storage disease, phospholipidosis, a pathogenetic concept that has been supported by others.[201, 202, 209, 224] A few investigators have found evidence for cell-mediated immunologic disturbance;[213, 220] the report of an inverted ratio of helper/suppressor T lymphocytes[220] has not been confirmed in a more recent study.[211] In one study, complement was found to be deposited in alveolar septa.[203]

Although a clear-cut relationship between dose and toxicity has not been demonstrated, most cases reported in the literature have received 400 mg/day or more prior to the appearance of pulmonary disease.[199, 200, 202, 203, 207, 219] However, several authors[206, 221, 225] have recorded the development of interstitial pulmonary disease with maintenance doses of less than 400 mg/day. In two prospective studies in which pulmonary function has been monitored, a distinct correlation has been found between dose and the detection of decreased lung volumes and diffusing capacity.[211, 212] Rotmensch and colleagues[226] have shown that the risk of developing adverse reactions is related to the concentration of amiodarone in the serum: they found that adverse reactions were common in patients with serum values exceeding 2.5 mg/liter, although pulmonary complications occurred at lower levels as well. It is possible that an additional factor of idiosyncrasy determines which patients will show amiodarone-induced pulmonary toxicity.[211]

Lung damage has its onset months after the initiation of amiodarone therapy.[14, 199, 207, 208] The drug is deposited in various organs and tissues throughout the body but particularly in the lungs where the concentration has been found to be four to seven times higher than in other organs.[225] The drug is eliminated slowly, which may explain the interval of 1 or more months after the cessation of therapy before complete roentgenographic and clinical resolution occurs.

Light microscopy of the lung in amiodarone toxicity typically reveals inflammation and fibrosis of the alveolar septa,[212, 216] hyperplasia of type II pneumocytes,[216] and the accumulation of intra-alveolar macrophages (Fig. 14–7).[212, 214, 216] These macrophages and, to a lesser extent type II pneumocytes, have a distinctive clear, foamy cytoplasm that can be seen ultrastructurally to contain numerous, often enlarged lysosomal inclusions (Fig. 14–7).[199, 202, 212, 214, 216] These are characteristic in appearance, one or more clusters of thin osmiophilic lamellae being surrounded by an amorphous electron-dense rim. The inclusions are also seen in pulmonary endothelial and interstitial cells and have been shown by dispersive x-ray analysis to contain iodine, a constituent of the amiodarone molecule.[212] Similar membrane-bound lamellar inclusions have been described in skin, Schwann cells, muscle fibers, and corneal epithelial cells.[212, 214, 216] The inclusion-bearing macrophages can be identified in BAL specimens, supporting a diagnosis of amiodarone toxicity.[211, 213] It is important to note, however, that inclusions can also be seen in patients without evidence of disease,[216] and their mere presence is not diagnostic of drug-related tissue damage. In addition to the typical histologic appearance described

above, there also have been reports of diffuse alveolar damage,[201, 216] necrotizing pneumonia (in a patient who also had hyperglycemia),[217] and necrotizing bronchiolitis associated with an infiltration of eosinophils.[224]

Chest roentgenograms are almost invariably described as showing a diffuse reticular and patchy airspace pattern,[199–201, 203, 204, 206, 207] the airspace opacities sometimes being predominant in the upper lobes.[199, 200, 207] Gefter and associates[200] found the

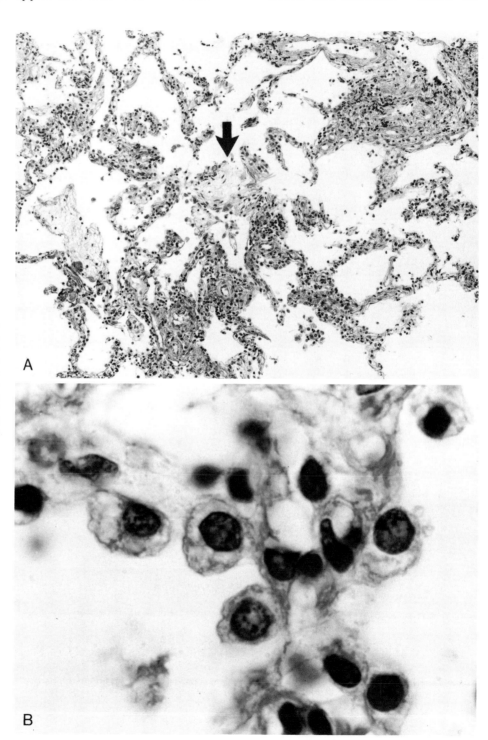

Figure 14–7. Amiodarone Toxicity: Interstitial Pneumonitis. A histologic section of lung parenchyma *(A)* shows a moderate degree of interstitial fibrosis and lymphocytic infiltration; focally, apparently active fibrosis is present *(arrow).* A magnified view of one alveolar wall *(B)* shows several type II pneumocytes with coarsely vacuolated cytoplasm.

Illustration continued on following page

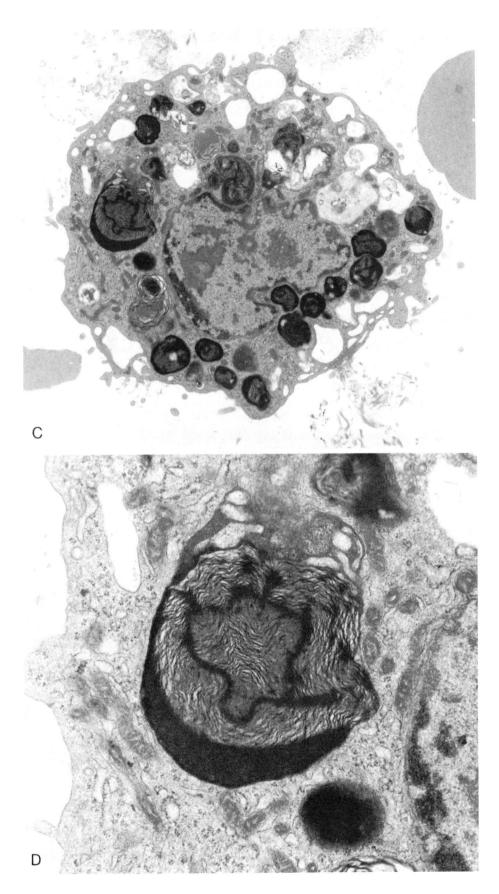

C

D

Figure 14–7 *Continued* Ultrastructural examination of an alveolar macrophage within an alveolar space *(C)* shows the cytoplasm to contain numerous phagosomes, some of which are enlarged and many of which contain densely osmiophilic material. A magnified view of one phagosome *(D)* shows a laminated inclusion organized in geographic segments with a crescent-shaped zone of amorphous electron-dense material at the periphery. This lung biopsy is from a 63-year-old man who had been taking 200 mg of amiodarone daily for 2 months. (*A* × 110, *B* × 1500, *C* × 7720 and *D* × 28,370.)

peripheral areas of consolidation to resemble those of chronic eosinophilic pneumonia, and two of the four roentgenograms reproduced by Marchlinski and colleagues[199] clearly have this appearance. Pleural thickening has been described;[199] one patient presented with bilateral exudative pleural effusions associated with toxic involvement of other organs.[228]

The clinical presentation is usually that of the insidious onset of dyspnea on exertion accompanied by a dry cough, weight loss, and weakness.[199–202, 206, 214] Fever and chest pain are rare.[199, 200, 202] In a few patients, the onset is acute, suggesting an infectious process.[201] The white cell count is usually normal or slightly elevated; marked leukocytosis is rare.[199, 202]

Nonpulmonary complications of amiodarone therapy are frequent and include blue-gray skin discoloration and photodermatitis, thyroid dysfunction (both hypo- and hyperthyroidism), corneal microdeposits, skin rashes, gastrointestinal symptoms, neurotoxicity (manifested by muscle weakness, peripheral neuropathy, and extrapyramidal symptoms), hepatic dysfunction, and bradycardia.[14, 199, 208]

In the presence of established disease, pulmonary function tests show restrictive impairment[199, 206, 211] and a severe reduction in gas transfer.[204, 206] In one study designed to determine the use of pulmonary function tests in assessing early pulmonary toxicity,[202] it was concluded that they were of little or no value; however, more recent prospective analyses[212, 221] have clearly shown that such surveillance is valid and that it can identify patients whose disease could progress to more serious and perhaps irreversible pulmonary damage.

The prognosis following withdrawal of medication and initiation of corticosteroid therapy is excellent, and very few cases of irreversible damage have been reported. However, the long half-life of the drug, estimated at 30 days,[14] creates considerable difficulty in assessing the value of corticosteroid therapy.[202, 204–207, 210, 212, 218, 219, 221–223, 225] Monitoring serum amiodarone concentration may well be a valid means of assuring the drug's efficacy and of avoiding its toxicity.[226] The possibility has been raised of the development of ARDS as a complication in patients with previous amiodarone pulmonary toxicity who undergo cardiothoracic surgical procedures.[215]

OTHER ANTIARRHYTHMIC DRUGS

Although not recognized as an antiarrhythmic that causes pulmonary toxicity, *lidocaine* used as a local anesthetic has been reported to cause acute capillary leakage on two separate occasions in the same patient.[229] *Tocainide*, an investigational antiarrhythmic drug that possesses chemical and pharmacologic properties similar to those of lidocaine, has been responsible for interstitial pneumonitis in four patients.[14, 230] Clinical and roentgenographic evidence of toxicity became apparent months after the onset of therapy[230] and resolved following withdrawal of the drug; however, two of the patients manifested some residual impairment of diffusing capacity.[14]

ANTICONVULSANT DRUGS

DIPHENYLHYDANTOIN

Diphenylhydantoin, also known as phenytoin, is used principally to control seizures and is believed to act through stabilization of neuronal membranes.[14] It was originally thought that toxicity could be manifested by both an acute hypersensitivity reaction[231, 232] and a more chronic and insidious form of interstitial pneumonitis,[233] but the occurrence of the latter syndrome was not substantiated by two subsequent prospective studies.[234, 235] The manifestations of the acute variety include blood eosinophilia and a diffuse reticulonodular pattern on the chest roentgenogram, both of which resolve within 2 weeks following drug withdrawal.[231, 236] Bronchoalveolar lavage in patients with acute reversible interstitial pneumonitis has suggested a predominantly lymphocytic type of alveolitis.[232, 237] Mediastinal node enlargement simulating lymphoma also has been reported.[238, 239]

Pathologic reports are scarce; transbronchial biopsy specimens in some patients have revealed an infiltrate of lymphocytes within alveolar septa.[232, 236, 237] Necrotizing granulomatous vasculitis has been described in several patients who manifested fever, dermatitis, and peripheral eosinophilia;[240, 241] interstitial fibrosis was identified in the lower lobes of one patient.[240]

Chest roentgenograms show a diffuse reticulonodular pattern, in some cases with mediastinal node enlargement.[14, 236, 238, 239] Clinical findings include fever, dyspnea, and a nonproductive cough that appears within 3 to 6 weeks after the onset of treatment; most patients have manifestations of systemic involvement, including generalized node enlargement, dermatitis, and clinical and laboratory evidence of hepatitis.[14, 231, 236, 242] Acute pulmonary toxicity can result in severe impairment of gas exchange:[236] in a long-term study of pulmonary function in 50 patients who had taken phenytoin for two or more years, abnormalities of gas exchange consisting of impaired diffusing capacity, low levels of PaO_2, and increased $P(A-a)O_2$ were found in 45 per cent.[243] Unfortunately, in this study there is no reference to chest roentgenograms or to any change in function following cessation of therapy.

CARBAMAZEPINE

Carbamazepine, also known as Tegretol, is used chiefly in the control of neuralgia. As with diphenylhydantoin, the onset of toxicity is acute and consists of diffuse interstitial pneumonia, eosinophilia, and a skin rash. In one affected patient, a lymphocyte-stimulation test with carbamazepine was strongly positive, whereas there was no reaction in healthy controls or in patients receiving carbamazepine therapy without adverse effects.[244] Four patients with this drug-induced disease have been described.[244–247] One report is suspect[247] in that the chest roentgenogram showed a segmental lesion and the patient was an asthmatic, features suggesting mucoid impaction; nevertheless, clearing occurred with withdrawal of the medication.

ANALGESIC DRUGS

ACETYLSALICYLIC ACID (ASPIRIN)

Aspirin is a cause of permeability pulmonary edema, particularly in middle-aged and elderly individuals who become habituated as a result of ingesting large doses to alleviate pain. In contrast, a younger group of patients is admitted to hospitals because of intentional overdoses; they may become comatose but rarely manifest overt pulmonary edema.[248–251] However, fatal salicylate-induced pulmonary edema can occur even in children and has been correlated with high serum salicylate levels and anion gaps.[252]

Studies of sheep, in which pulmonary edema has been induced by salicylate ingestion, have confirmed the clinical impression that the edema results from increased capillary permeability.[253] Pulmonary artery wedge pressure has been found to be normal in several studies,[249, 254, 255] and the constituents of airway fluid have been identical to those in plasma.[14, 256] The mechanism of increased permeability is unknown, but two possibilities have been suggested:[14, 249] (1) increased intracranial pressure causes neurogenic pulmonary edema as a result of deposition of the drug in brain tissue, and (2) inhibition of prostaglandin production results in vasodilatation and increased permeability. In some cases hypoproteinemia may play a role in the capillary leakage.[256] Serum salicylate levels are usually 30 mg/ml or more; however, there is not a clear dose relationship, since many patients with similar blood levels do not develop edema.[249, 251, 252, 255, 256] In two separate studies,[249, 251] cigarette smoking was identified as a risk factor.

Chest roentgenograms reveal the typical diffuse airspace pattern of pulmonary edema.[249, 251, 255] Patients are dyspneic, lethargic, and confused; they tend to have proteinuria, perhaps reflecting increased capillary permeability in the systemic circulation. A history of chronic acetylsalicylic acid ingestion, usually in large quantities, is invariable.[255–257] Patients tend to be dehydrated, and it is possible that treatment of the hypovolemia with crystalloidal fluids can sometimes contribute to the

development of edema.[256] Since the pulmonary edema responds well to measures that decrease serum salicylate levels, the prognosis is good.[249]

NAPROXEN

Four patients have been described who developed acute pulmonary airspace opacities (presumably edema) while taking naproxen.[258, 259] In all cases the onset was acute and consisted of weakness, fatigue, cough, low-grade fever, and blood eosinophilia. All findings resolved within days to weeks after withdrawal of the drug. One patient was subsequently challenged and showed a similar reaction.[258]

ANTIRHEUMATIC DRUGS

PENICILLAMINE

A derivative of penicillin, penicillamine is a chelator of lead, copper, zinc, and mercury. The drug is used to treat lead poisoning, Wilson's disease, cysteinuria, and connective tissue diseases, particularly rheumatoid arthritis. It is probable that the variety of pulmonary complications caused by this drug is greater than with any other drug that causes lung toxicity. In addition to rare examples of lupus-like[260] and myasthenia-like diseases,[261] a number of cases of presumed drug-induced alveolitis,[262–265] bronchiolitis obliterans,[266–270] and a Goodpasture-like syndrome[271–274] have been reported. The association of penicillamine therapy with the hemorrhagic pulmonary-renal syndrome and hypersensitivity pneumonitis appears to be valid. However, since rheumatoid disease is a well-recognized cause of bronchiolitis and since all published cases of penicillamine-induced bronchiolitis have occurred in patients with rheumatoid arthritis, it is possible that in some, if not all, cases, the bronchiolitis obliterans was a feature of the underlying disease rather than being caused by the drug. Similarly, patients with rheumatoid arthritis who are being treated with penicillamine and who develop roentgenographic evidence of a diffuse reticulonodular pattern that does not respond to withdrawal of the medication may have a complication of the disease process itself rather than a reaction to the drug.

The incidence of penicillamine-induced pulmonary toxicity must be extremely low. Risk of toxicity is not dose-related.[14] The mechanism of acute reversible pulmonary disease, usually accompanied by eosinophilia,[263–265, 270] is very likely a type I immunologic reaction, whereas limited pathologic findings suggest that the pulmonary-renal syndrome is type III.

To the best of our knowledge, no patients with the acute pulmonary eosinophilic syndrome have been biopsied. Biopsy specimens of two patients with persistent interstitial disease revealed all the changes characteristically associated with drug cytotoxicity.[14, 270] Gross and histologic findings in patients with the pulmonary-renal syndrome have been those of Goodpasture's syndrome;[271] however, in two patients immunofluorescent studies showed an interrupted pattern of staining with IgG and complement rather than the linear reaction typical of anti-glomerular basement membrane antibody in classic Goodpasture's syndrome.[271, 273]

Roentgenographic manifestations are of three types: (1) a reticulonodular pattern, with or without limited airspace opacities, indicating the presence of interstitial disease;[263] (2) overinflation unaccompanied by parenchymal abnormality, associated with advanced bronchiolitis obliterans; and (3) diffuse opacities characteristic of airspace consolidation, typically seen in patients with a Goodpasture-like syndrome.[14]

Patients with penicillamine-induced pulmonary disease present with cough and dyspnea that usually develop insidiously over a period of weeks; however, the onset of dyspnea is typically abrupt in patients with pulmonary hemorrhage.[14] Rales, and in some cases rhonchi, may be heard at the lung bases.[14, 263] Other manifestations include stomatitis, dermatitis,[14] and rarely cholestatic hepatitis.[264] In patients with bronchiolitis, pulmonary function tests can reveal evidence of severe obstruction, even when the chest roentgenogram is within normal limits.[14]

The prognosis of patients with the acute hypersensitivity syndrome is excellent. The clinical and roentgenographic abnormalities resolve rapidly following withdrawal of medication, usually with the help of steroid therapy.[262, 263] Many patients with the pulmonary-renal and bronchiolitis obliterans syndromes die.[14, 271]

GOLD

Chrysotherapy employing sodium aurothiomalate is effective in inflammatory arthritis. Side effects of its use are frequent and usually involve the skin or mucous membranes. Lung toxicity has been estimated to occur in less than 1 per cent of patients receiving this drug,[14] although over 65 cases have been reported in the literature.[14, 276–290] Cooke and Bamji[741] failed to find adverse effects of gold therapy on pulmonary function in 110 cases of rheumatoid arthritis; 96 cases were studied retrospectively and 14 prospectively.

The mechanism of pulmonary damage is thought to be a hypersensitivity reaction, with approximately one third of patients showing peripheral eosinophilia.[279, 287] There is also evidence for a cell-mediated immune reaction. For example, two groups of workers have reported that in vitro exposure to gold causes blastogenesis of lymphocytes.[14, 277] Although this observation was not confirmed by McCormick and associates,[285] these investigators did find elaboration of lymphokines (migration inhibiting factor and macrophage chemotactic factor) by peripheral lymphocytes of patients with pulmonary toxicity after incubation with gold salts; normal controls and patients receiving gold therapy without pulmonary toxicity did not manifest this effect. A genetic susceptibility may exist as revealed by a strong association between toxicity and the presence of certain major histocompatibility antigens.[290] Risk of toxicity does not appear to be dose-related.

Histologic examination reveals hyperplasia of type II pneumocytes[281] and lymphocyte and plasma cell infiltration of alveolar septa accompanied by varying degrees of fibrosis.[276, 277] Gold can be identified within lysosomes of macrophages and pulmonary capillary endothelial cells;[292] however, as with amiodarone, it has not been established whether this represents a marker of drug administration or is related to the pathogenesis of disease. There are two reports of patients developing bronchiolitis obliterans while receiving gold therapy;[266, 293] as with penicillamine, however, it is probable that this complication was the result of underlying rheumatoid disease rather than the therapy.

The chest roentgenogram has been described as showing diffuse interstitial and patchy airspace opacities;[278, 279, 281, 294] in one report,[281] the diffuse patchy (presumably airspace) opacities observed initially were subsequently replaced by a reticulonodular pattern.

Pulmonary hypersensitivity to gold salts usually presents acutely or subacutely, thereby aiding in the differentiation from interstitial fibrosis associated with rheumatoid disease whose onset is insidious.[287, 294] Patients often are febrile and complain of progressive shortness of breath on exertion and a dry cough;[278, 281, 287] almost half have an associated dermatitis.[14] Physical examination may reveal rales.[278, 281] A restrictive pattern and hypoxemia are found on physiologic assessment.[277, 281, 287, 288] Challenging with the drug may confirm the clinical association.[276, 277, 279]

The response to cessation of therapy is good; we are aware of only one reported death from pulmonary damage.[279] Steroids are usually administered and probably hasten recovery. Some residual restriction on pulmonary function testing or reticulonodularity on chest roentgenograms may be observed.[279, 283, 287, 288, 294]

SYMPATHOMIMETIC DRUGS

The tocolytic betamimetics, *terbutaline, ritodrine,* and *isoxsuprine,* used in the treatment of preterm labor, have been implicated in the development of permeability pulmonary edema.[14, 295–298] The complication has a very low incidence. Only 7 of 2,557 patients in one study[295] and 7 of 1,407 in another were affected.[296] The clinical situation is clouded somewhat in such patients by the potential for thromboembolism, amniotic fluid embolism, fluid overload, anemia and the necessity for transfusions, and the administration of other drugs, particularly corticosteroids;[295, 299] one or more of these could conceivably play a major role or at least contribute to the development of the edema. Hemodynamic data in such patients support the mechanism of edema formation as being noncardiogenic in type.[295]

The chest roentgenogram reveals classic signs of airspace edema.[14] Symptoms and clinical findings develop within 2 to 3 days of the initiation of therapy and can be associated with extreme hypoxemia. However, the prognosis is excellent; the discontinuation of therapy and the administration of oxygen and of diuretics, with or without digoxin, are successful in reversing the process in most cases.[14, 296]

NARCOTIC AND SEDATIVE DRUGS

Opiates and related drugs have been recognized as causes of pulmonary edema since the original description by Osler in 1880.[300] Most patients are heroin addicts who have taken an overdose; the incidence of permeability pulmonary edema in such circumstances ranges from 48 to 75 per cent.[301, 302] Of 149 patients with heroin overdose reported from New York City,[302] 71 developed pulmonary edema and 6 died. Pulmonary edema also has been reported as a result of overdosage of *methadone*,[303–308] *propoxyphene* (Darvon),[309] *chlordiazepoxide* (Librium),[310] *ethchlorvynol* (Placidyl),[311] *paraldehyde*,[312] *codeine*,[313] *bromocarbamide*,[314] *febarbamate*,[315] and *naloxone*.[316, 317]

The hallmark of increased capillary permeability[318]—a high protein content of pulmonary edema fluid—has been well documented in patients with heroin overdose.[319] The precise mechanism that causes capillary leakage has not been elucidated, although it is probable that the hypoxemia and acidosis that accompany severe respiratory center depression cause endothelial damage. Based on findings of reduced levels in the serum and deposition in the lungs of IgM and complement components, some investigators[320, 321] have proposed an immunologic mechanism. Theoretically, pulmonary edema in narcotic overdose also could have a neurogenic origin; in fact, opiate receptors have been discovered near the medullary respiratory center,[322] and the application of drugs in this area has produced edema in dogs.[14] Such a mechanism could explain the paradoxical development of edema following the administration of the opiate antagonist, naloxone.[316, 317]

The pathologic[323] and roentgenographic[291, 301, 324, 325] manifestations of pulmonary edema resulting from narcotic overdose are indistinguishable from those of other etiology (Fig. 14–8). The pattern is usually bilateral and symmetric. Heart size is normal. Roentgenographic resolution characteristically occurs in as brief a time as 24 to 48 hours.[325–327] The appearance of pulmonary edema may be delayed after admission to the hospital, sometimes for as long as 6 to 10 hours.[326, 328] Pulmonary edema caused by methadone overdose is roentgenographically similar to that caused by heroin and other toxic drugs[302] except that it is somewhat slower to resolve (2 to 4 days).[303, 304, 329] Prolonged absorption of methadone from the gastrointestinal tract has been suggested as the likeliest explanation of this delayed clearance.

The drug abuser with pulmonary edema is usually admitted in coma, often with frothy, pink edema fluid oozing from nostrils and mouth. A white blood count may show leukocytosis or occasionally leukopenia.[326, 330] Hypoxemia is severe and is accompanied by a mixed acidosis.[304, 306, 307, 326] By the time the first arterial blood gas is drawn, hypoxemia is probably the result of a combination of alveolar hypoventilation from depression of the respiratory center, shunt, and ventilation-perfusion inequality from airspace edema. Patients who manifest hypocapnia have presumably recovered from central nervous system depression; persisting hypoxemia and acidosis then reflect the severe pulmonary edema and hypoperfusion of tissues. Lung function studies performed shortly after recovery from the edema show a severe restrictive ventilatory defect with reduced vital capacity and total lung capacity; the impairment disappears over a period of a few days.[331, 332]

ANTIDEPRESSANT AND ANTIPSYCHOTIC DRUGS

Imipramine,[333, 334] *trimipramine*,[335] and *chlorpromazine*[326] have been associated with an acute and transient febrile pulmonary disease associated with eosinophilia. Two patients have been described who developed severe bronchiolitis and interstitial pneumonitis while receiving the tricyclic antidepressant, *amitriptyline*.[337, 338] Five patients have been described who developed ARDS from an overdose of tricyclic antidepressants.[339]

A rare manifestation of toxicity to major tranquilizers consists of permeability pulmonary edema that occurs as one of the features of the malignant neuroleptic syndrome,[340] an acute febrile disease characterized by severe muscle rigidity, neurologic changes, and autonomic dysfunction.[14]

CONTRAST MEDIA

Reference was made previously to the pulmonary toxicity that is associated with embolization of ethiodized oil used for lymphangiography (*see* page 1803). This somewhat subacute form of ARDS possesses many features that resemble fatty acid em-

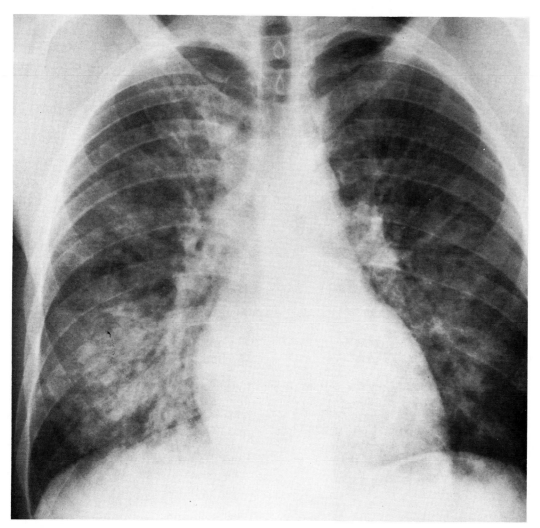

Figure 14–8. Acute Pulmonary Edema Caused by Drug Abuse. A posteroanterior roentgenogram reveals widespread, patchy airspace consolidation typical of acute pulmonary edema of any etiology. Several hours previously, this 19-year-old man had injected intravenously a high dose of Demerol and methadone. He had an uneventful recovery.

bolism and may have a similar pathogenesis. Silvestri and associates[341] reproduced this complication of lymphangiography in rabbits and showed the onset of hypoxemia 24 hours after injection; impairment of gas exchange and alveolar and interstitial inflammation, hemorrhage, and edema peaked on the fourth day. In humans, a significant drop in diffusing capacity has been recorded, being maximal in 48 hours and returning to normal in 1 month.[342–346] These observations coincide well with animal studies in which complete restoration of normal pulmonary function and morphology has been shown to occur in 6 weeks.[341]

Water-soluble contrast media occasionally have been reported to cause pulmonary edema.[347–352] Although this may represent an idiosyncratic reaction, it is more likely the consequence of the osmolarity of the solutions employed, particularly *sodium iothalamate* and *diatrizoate meglumine* (Gastrografin) whose osmolarity is five to ten times that of plasma.[350] In 1964, Harris and associates[353] instilled Gastrografin into the intestines of dogs and dem-

onstrated an influx of fluid from the plasma into the bowel lumen, with a consequent decrease in the animals' circulating plasma volume. Similar experiments were carried out by Reich on the lungs of Long-Evans rats:[348] water and normal saline were absorbed rapidly and completely and caused no complications, but both Gastrografin and 76 per cent *Renografin* resulted in flooding of the alveoli with edema fluid and rapid death. Since a 10 per cent solution of oral Hypaque (sodium diatrizoate) in water is isotonic, it is clear that the solutions most frequently used clinically are hypertonic (20 to 42 per cent) and are capable of producing an osmotic gradient across a membrane in relation to normal plasma. Some patients in whom pulmonary edema develops following intravenous administration of iodinated contrast media[350–352] are otherwise healthy and the presence of a normal wedge pressure and a high protein content of the edema fluid indicates a permeability pathogenesis.[351, 352] In a few patients with underlying heart disease,[350, 354] hyperosmolality created by the contrast media causes an overloading of the circulation which undoubtedly plays a role in the pathogenesis.

Some patients undergoing upper gastrointestinal examination with water-soluble contrast media[347-349] for suspected disease of the esophagus and stomach develop acute pulmonary edema following aspiration of this liquid; affected patients usually have chronic pulmonary disease.

MISCELLANEOUS DRUGS

Hydrochlorothiazide has been implicated as a cause of permeability pulmonary edema in eight patients.[14, 355-358] The first report appeared in 1968[356] and the most recent in 1981;[357] strangely, we have been unable to find any reports written since then. Two of these patients developed the edema after an initial ingestion of thiazides; the others had received the drug previously,[14] one following treatment with a closely related drug, bendroflumethazide.[358]

The mechanism of edema formation is unknown, but the acute reaction, the association with other clinical manifestations such as dermatitis and hepatitis,[14] the development of a similar reaction on a second dose of the drug,[355, 357] and the rapid clinical and roentgenographic resolution on withdrawal of the drug all point to a hypersensitivity response. In one study,[357] pulmonary wedge pressures were normal, confirming the permeability nature of the edema.

Cough, dyspnea, cyanosis, and rales at the lung bases developed 20 to 60 minutes after the ingestion of hydrochlorothiazide in all cases. Chest roentgenograms showed a combined interstitial and airspace pattern compatible with pulmonary edema, and complete recovery occurred with cessation of therapy.[14]

There are four reports[359] of patients who developed eosinophilia and airspace "pneumonia" after switching from oral corticosteroids to an aerosol of *beclomethasone diproprionate*. The reaction could have represented an acute hypersensitivity response to the 10 per cent oleic acid used as a dispersing agent or to the hydrocarbon propellant. Following reinstitution of the drug, one patient developed ARDS. The diagnosis of bronchopulmonary aspergillosis was considered in all cases, but aspergilli and mucous plugs were not found. Clearing was prompt when the patients were restarted on oral corticosteroids.

The angiotensin-converting enzyme (ACE) inhibitors *captopril* and *enalapril maleate* used in the treatment of hypertension can cause severe coughing; some patients also develop bronchospasm accompanied by a decrease in expiratory flow rates.[360, 361] These side effects of ACE inhibitors imply a role for ACE in the cough reflex, possibly by metabolism of substrates other than angiotensin I.[362]

Pulmonary disease has been reported in four transsexual men following subcutaneous injections of *silicone*.[363, 364] Three patients developed fever, chest pain, dyspnea, and roentgenographic evidence of acute interstitial and patchy airspace disease 24 hours after injection; silicone was identified in bronchoalveolar lavage fluid. The fourth patient[364] developed ARDS and died; at autopsy, silicone was found in various organs of the body, particularly the lungs.

Cocaine, a widely abused drug, has been implicated only occasionally as a cause of pulmonary toxicity. Pulmonary edema has been reported as a complication of cocaine[365] or "crack"[366] smoking, although pneumomediastinum and pneumothorax have been the most common roentgenographic abnormalities reported in the literature. Persistent reduction in diffusing capacity with otherwise normal pulmonary function has been described in long-term inhalers.[367, 368] In one patient who had been inhaling free-base cocaine,[369] an open lung biopsy revealed bronchiolitis obliterans with organizing pneumonia; following a very stormy clinical course requiring positive end-expiratory pressure (PEEP), the patient was found to have residual obstructive disease and air trapping. Granulomas have been identified in the lungs of a cocaine sniffer who denied intravenous injection of talc-based drugs;[370] they were considered to be related to the cellulose content of the cocaine mixture. Eight young people inhaled *strychnine* by mistake, believing it was cocaine. Most of them suffered convulsions and required artificial ventilation; one died.[371]

Beta-adrenergic blocking agents (β-blockers) can produce a systemic lupus erythematosus-like syndrome and can also precipitate acute bronchospasm. *Practolol*, a β-blocker that has been withdrawn from the market, has been reported to cause severe sclerosing peritonitis and pleuropulmonary fibrosis that became manifest months after treatment had ended; several patients died of respiratory failure.[372, 373] *Propranolol* has initiated cardiogenic edema in patients with a pheochromocytoma,[374, 375] presumably by inducing β₁ and β₂ blockade that resulted in unopposed alpha effects and sudden elevation of afterload.

Adult respiratory distress syndrome developed in three patients in whom *talc* was instilled intrapleurally for treatment of malignant effusion.[376] Fever, increasing dyspnea, and finally ARDS developed over a 72-hour period following the injection of 10 g of talc in 250 ml of saline. The mixture was retained for 2 hours and then drained; one patient died. All three patients had normal pulmonary artery wedge pressures.

In one patient taking *anabolic steroids*, multiple foci of ectatic pulmonary vessels ("pulmonary peliosis") similar to those encountered in the liver in peliosis of that organ have been described.[377]

The use of *perfluorochemicals* as artificial blood has been reported to be associated with the presence of foamy macrophages throughout the reticuloendothelial system and the lungs in humans[378] and in experimental animals.[379]

Although most strongly associated with pleural disease, *ergotamine* and its derivative *bromocriptine* have been reported to cause pulmonary fibrosis.[380, 381]

Interleukin-2 has been shown to cause pulmonary edema, cardiac arrhythmias, and unstable angina. Of eight patients who underwent intravenous bolus therapy with recombinant interleukin-2 for metastatic melanoma or renal cell carcinoma, Conant and her colleagues[382] found that five developed pulmonary edema.

POISON-INDUCED PULMONARY DISEASE

In contrast to drug-induced pulmonary disease, which in most cases represents a side effect of medication used as treatment for a symptom or clinical disorder, poison-induced pulmonary toxicity almost always occurs as a result of accidental exposure or suicidal intent. The great majority of the involved toxic substances are inhaled as noxious gases or soluble aerosols, often in an occupational setting, but with increasing frequency they are originating from environmental pollution in the vicinity of production sites or in association with vehicular accidents during transport. A minority of poisons, including insecticides, herbicides, various aromatic hydrocarbons, and the toxin responsible for the Spanish toxic-allergic syndrome, can reach the pulmonary alveolocapillary membrane by absorption through the skin or as a result of ingestion or even intravenous injection.

INSECTICIDES AND HERBICIDES

There appears to be a strong conviction that a variety of pesticides are toxic to the lungs and that every effort should be made to avoid inhalation of these chemicals when they are used as sprays. In a study from Denmark,[383] a questionnaire was sent out to fruit growers and farmers during the spraying season: 41 per cent of the 181 respondents stated that they had developed symptoms during the period of exposure. Subsequent examination showed a decrease in peak flow rates in 19 per cent and abnormal chest roentgenograms in 24 per cent of individuals studied. The roentgenographic pattern was predominantly interstitial, although some cases of airspace consolidation were also observed, sometimes with cavitation. Difficulty in identifying the specific chemicals responsible for the pulmonary toxicity is caused by the great variety of available insecticides and the multiple ingredients that they contain. The organophosphates constitute one group of chemicals that has been positively incrim-

inated; the major examples of this group are parathion and malathion. These chemicals can be absorbed through the skin or from the respiratory tract, gastrointestinal tract, or conjunctiva; they can also cause pulmonary injury when injected intravenously.

In addition to the acute toxic effects caused by these and other insecticides, there is evidence that some (particularly insecticides containing arsenic) have a pathogenetic role in the development of pulmonary carcinoma (*see* page 1336).

Organophosphate Poisoning

Poisoning with these substances occurs most commonly in agricultural workers during or shortly after the spraying of crops and less often in industrial workers during manufacture and transport; it also occurs accidentally in children and intentionally in suicide attempts.[384] The condition is serious: in a group of 157 patients treated for organophosphate insecticide poisoning in South Africa, 41 patients were admitted to an intensive care unit and 12 died.[385] Parathion is the major cause of fatal poisoning, with more than 50 deaths being reported during a 6-month period in Florida.[386]

Parathion and *malathion* are converted to paraxon and malaoxon in the liver. The toxicity of these latter substances is worse than that of their parents. They exert their effect by inhibiting acetylcholinesterase at nerve endings.[387] Symptoms and signs are attributable mainly to the accumulation of acetylcholine at cholinergic synapses, resulting in an initial stimulation and later inhibition of synaptic transmission. Miosis, diaphoresis, increased salivation, bronchorrhea, bronchoconstriction, bradycardia, and hyperperistalsis develop. At automatic ganglia and neuromuscular junctions, nicotinic action, both sympathetic and motor, is manifested by muscular fasciculations, particularly of the diaphragm,[740] followed by fatiguability and eventual paralysis of skeletal muscle. Stimulation of cholinergic receptors in the central nervous system, followed by subsequent depression, results in coma. Depending on the route and the amount of poison taken, the time interval between exposure and the onset of symptoms ranges from 5 minutes (after a massive dose) to 24 hours. Death can result from central nervous system depression or from diaphragmatic paralysis, the effects of the latter being compounded by bronchoconstriction and hypersecretion of airway mucus.[384]

Li and associates[388] collected 13 cases of organophosphate insecticide poisoning over a period of 10 years in Beijing, China; 10 of the 13 patients developed pulmonary edema which resolved completely within 2 to 5 days following institution of appropriate therapy. Since the pathophysiologic consequences of organophosphate poisoning result from excessive cholinergic activity, the antidote is continuous atropine and, in some cases, positive pressure ventilation.[385]

Other Insecticides

Proproxur (Baygon), a member of the carbamylester family, possesses pharmacologic action—the binding of acetylcholinesterase—similar to that of the organophosphates. Pulmonary edema, coma, bronchorrhea, and miosis have been described in patients who have attempted suicide with this poison.[389]

Toxaphene, a chlorinated camphene, is an amber, waxy, solid material containing about 68 per cent chlorine. Its inhalation has been said to result in extensive bilateral "allergic bronchopneumonia."[390] The roentgenographic pattern varies with the severity of exposure from "simple bronchopneumonia" of mid- and lower-lung zones to extensive "miliary" disease.[390] Hilar lymph nodes may be enlarged. In the few reported cases, resolution usually took about 3 weeks. Pulmonary function tests reveal an obstructive pattern. Blood eosinophilia and elevation of serum globulin levels can be seen.

Thallium, a drug formerly recognized as a rodenticide and insecticide, is now used industrially in the production of optic lenses, low-temperature thermometers, semiconductors, pigments, and scintillation counters. Although it is more commonly associated with central nervous system and gastrointestinal toxicity, it has been reported to be responsible for ARDS in four patients, two of whom died;[391] autopsy revealed pulmonary edema and fibrosis.

Paraquat

A bipyridylium herbicide, paraquat has been available in the United Kingdom since 1962 as a 20 per cent concentrate (Gramoxone) and as a 5 per cent solid form (Weedol). It was introduced into North America in 1964 in the form of three solutions containing 29 per cent (Orthoparaquat), 42 per cent (Orthodualparaquat), and 0.44 per cent (Ortho-spot) herbicide. Poisoning results from ingestion of the drug either by mistake or, in most cases, for suicidal purposes. In addition, there are well-documented cases of respiratory failure and death resulting from absorption of the poison through the skin.[392–394] It generally has been assumed that inhalation toxicity could not occur because of the particle size;[395] however, a patient has been described in whom chest tightness and dyspnea developed following the spraying of an adjacent field with paraquat. That the paraquat may have been responsible was lent some support by the fact that the patient's garden was subsequently defoliated, revealing a number of dead mice and moles.[396]

Paraquat poisoning, although relatively uncommon, is a very serious disorder, because 33 to 55 per cent of affected individuals die.[397, 398] During a 13-year period since the first fatal cases were reported in 1964, more than 560 poisoning deaths were reported to the manufacturers.[399] Some patients who survive manifest residual pulmonary dysfunction;[398, 400] the concentration of herbicide ingested in these individuals is almost invariably small. The ingestion of 200 ml or more in an attempt to commit suicide results in death in 24 hours or less, whereas accidental poisoning, which usually occurs from imbibing a mouthful of concentrated solution of paraquat (15 or 20 ml, commonly from an unlabeled container),[401] causes irreversible respiratory failure in 5 to 10 days. The form of poisoning that occurs in individuals who absorb paraquat through the skin is less acute than that which follows ingestion, perhaps reflecting a smaller dosage, but the poison is still often fatal.[392, 394]

Pathogenesis

It is believed that paraquat acts like other oxidants (oxygen, ozone, irradiation therapy, and cytotoxic drugs) in damaging lung tissue. It participates readily in electron transfer reactions, during which it oxidizes a substrate by accepting electrons.[402] These biochemical reactions result in the production of superoxide ions that cause peroxidation of lipid cellular membranes,[401, 403, 404] a metabolic process that is reflected in an increase in serum malondialdehyde levels.[405] Experimental studies in which low doses of ozone and paraquat have been administered to rats have shown similar histologic and biochemical manifestations.[406] This concept of an oxidant-like mechanism has been supported by studies in which poisoned rats administered oxygen died much more rapidly than those breathing ambient air.[402] It has even been postulated that paraquat exerts its toxic action by sensitizing the lungs to oxygen at atmospheric pressure.[407]

Pathologic Characteristics

Large doses of paraquat cause severe acute pulmonary edema and hemorrhage, resulting in rapid death. Ultrastructural studies of rats administered paraquat intravenously have shown type I alveolar epithelial cell damage, with little evidence of endothelial cell injury.[403] In individuals who survive for several days, hyaline membranes and an intra-alveolar fibrinous exudate are also often present (histologically identical to the exudative phase of diffuse alveolar damage seen with numerous other pulmonary injuries; *see* Fig. 10–61, page 1934). Loose fibroblastic connective tissue subsequently appears (representing the proliferative phase of diffuse alveolar damage *see* Fig. 10–62, page 1936) and is eventually converted into mature fibrous tissue, usually associated with microcyst formation. Collagen has been shown to increase in amount at about the 20th day of intoxication,[408] and it is probable that fibrosis is progressive once a threshold tissue concentration of the poison has been reached. Although there is some experimental evidence that fibrosis occurs predominantly within the airspaces, observations in humans at autopsy indicate that the process occurs in both the interstitium and airspaces.[403, 407] Whether this discrepancy is due to a true species difference in reaction or to the effects of different concentrations or routes of entry of the poison is not clear. Since patients with paraquat intoxication usually receive oxygen, sometimes in high concentration, it is possible that this therapy may be partly responsible for the observed pathologic changes.

One study from Capetown, South Africa,[393] has produced strong evidence that pathologic changes can occur as a result of prolonged absorption of low concentrations of paraquat through the skin. The authors describe a case of a vineyard sprayer who developed skin lesions from paraquat leaking from a defective spraying apparatus and who died after a subacute course of respiratory failure. Of nine coworkers, the diffusing capacity was reduced in six, and in the two on whom lung biopsy was performed, the pulmonary arteries showed evidence of medial hypertrophy and fresh and organized thrombi. These same investigators[393] applied low concentrations of paraquat to the skin of rats and produced similar medial hypertrophy of pulmonary vessels. These morphologic findings may provide support for biologic experimental investigations in which mice injected intraperitoneally with paraquat showed a linear dose-response increase in serum levels of angiotensin-converting enzyme,[409] a substance present in large quantity in pulmonary endothelial cells.

In addition to the lung, the main target organs in paraquat toxicity include the kidney (tubular necrosis), the liver (midzone necrosis), the heart (myocarditis),[410] and the adrenals (cortical necrosis).

ROENTGENOGRAPHIC MANIFESTATIONS

Roentgenographic changes in the lungs of individuals who die within hours of paraquat ingestion show diffuse bilateral airspace consolidation. In those who survive, the chest roentgenogram shows fine, discrete, and confluent granular opacities that appear 3 to 7 days after poison ingestion. In one patient who developed this roentgenographic pattern 7 days after imbibing paraquat, the lung was removed prior to transplantation; histologic examination of the resected lung revealed thickening of alveolar walls by an infiltration of inflammatory cells and fibroblasts.[411] Roentgenographic changes characteristically progress rapidly to a pattern resembling severe pulmonary edema (Fig. 14–9).[412] Although chances of survival seem relatively small once roentgenographic abnormalities have developed in the lungs, a case has been reported of a middle-aged man who survived after drinking two mouthfuls of paraquat.[400] His chest roentgenogram 18 months later revealed thickened bronchial walls and peripheral linear shadowing (sic) consistent with the presence of mild, diffuse interstitial pulmonary fibrosis; his chest roentgenogram prior to the insult was perfectly normal.

CLINICAL MANIFESTATIONS

In most cases a history of accidental paraquat ingestion or suicidal attempt will be diagnostic of poisoning. The drug is absorbed through the skin of fruit growers and farmers and often causes cutaneous lesions.[392–394] Cases have been described from Papua, New Guinea, in which poisoning followed the cutaneous application of paraquat in attempts to treat scabies and body lice.[394] Suicidal attempts with paraquat are almost invariably successful; the patient presents with vomiting, abdominal pain, and burning of the mouth and throat. Death occurs within hours to a few days from pulmonary edema and renal and hepatic failure.[398] An oropharyngeal membrane has been described that closely resembles that of diphtheria, except that it is situated predominantly on the tongue rather than the pharynx.[413] Some patients show a brief period of apparent recovery[397] before developing respiratory failure 5 to 10 days after admission. Eighteen per cent methemoglobinemia has been reported in an alcoholic patient who imbibed paraquat and survived; his methemoglobinemia responded to methylene blue therapy.[414]

PROGNOSIS

The prognosis is largely dependent on the dose ingested. Once there is clinical or roentgenographic evidence of pulmonary involvement, death is usual.[398, 400, 415] Prompt treatment, including gastric lavage, purgatives, instillation of betonite or fuller's earth into the stomach, administration of mannitol to increase urinary flow, and hemoperfusion using activated extruded charcoal or cation exchange resin, may be of benefit. If at all possible, oxygen therapy should be avoided.[401, 404, 415–417] Theoretically, antioxidants such as superoxide dismutase and vitamin E should be useful;[404, 405] however, in one experiment in which mice received dismutase before and after intraperitoneal injection of paraquat, no protection was detected.[418] Blood and urine levels of paraquat may prove to be of value, not only in diagnosis but also to establish prognosis.[397, 398, 405] In one patient,[419] however, the herbicide was absent in multiple urine and blood specimens and yet was detected in high concentration in all major organs at autopsy. Lung transplantation has been performed in patients with paraquat poisoning,[410, 411] but we are unaware of any long-term success. The Toronto Lung Transplant group[410] has experienced the consequences of transplantation before com-

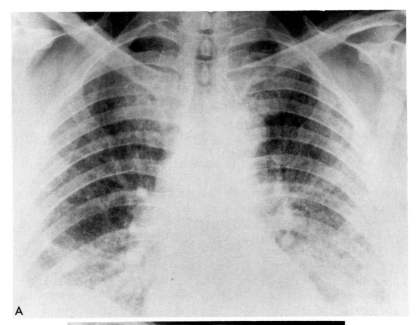

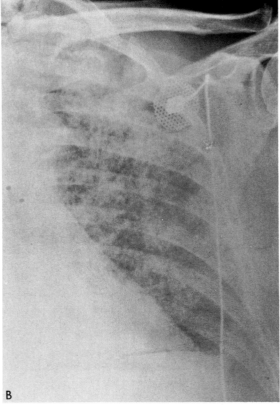

Figure 14–9. Paraquat Poisoning. During the major flood suffered by Brisbane, Australia, in 1974, this 64-year-old man added to his rum the contents of a Coke bottle that was washed up by the floods. Unfortunately, the bottle contained paraquat. On admission to the hospital, a posteroanterior roentgenogram *(A)* revealed an extensive fine granular reticulation throughout both lungs, with a suggestion of patchy airspace consolidation in both bases. Three days later *(B),* the consolidation had extended considerably and now appeared to affect both interstitium and airspaces in a rather uniform manner. The patient died a few days later. (Courtesy of Dr. Peter Goy and Dr. Sid Moro, Royal Brisbane Hospital, Brisbane, Australia.)

pletely ridding the body of this poison: one patient received a lung transplant for paraquat-induced pulmonary damage some weeks after ingestion of the poison and subsequently developed paraquat toxicity in the transplanted lung as a result of poison released from tissue stores.

SPANISH TOXIC-OIL SYNDROME

In the summer of 1981, a previously unrecognized pneumonic-paralytic-eosinophilic syndrome occurred in Spain in epidemic form.[420–422] Epidemiologic studies strongly indicated that the agent responsible for this disease was rapeseed oil that was denatured by the addition of 2 per cent aniline and was illegally marketed as a cooking oil. During an 8-month period, over 13,000 persons who had imbibed this oil were hospitalized; 277 died, the mortality rate being estimated at 1 to 2 per cent.[421, 423] The incidence of the syndrome decreased dramatically in early June of 1981 when the Spanish government removed all suspected oil from the market.

To date the specific toxin responsible has not been identified.[421–423] The suggestion that the poison may have been a fatty-acid anilide[420] has not been generally accepted, because oleoanilides are not regarded as sufficiently toxic to induce such morbidity and mortality.[424] Root-Bernstein and Westall[425] suggested that the epidemic might have a dual etiology: *Mycoplasma pneumoniae* infection appeared to be rampant at the time of the epidemic, and the question was raised as to whether the infection may have acted synergistically with the contaminated oil to cause the disorder.

Pathologic changes in the early stages of the syndrome are those of pulmonary edema accompanied by a scanty, largely mononuclear inflammatory infiltrate. Ultrastructural studies at this time show degenerative changes in both type I and type II pneumocytes.[427] Individuals who survive the acute event may show pulmonary vascular changes consistent with hypertension; in some, a lymphocytic vasculitis is also present.[166] In one clinicopathologic study of individuals who died of pulmonary hypertension,[429] pathologic abnormalities included plexiform lesions, thrombosis and severe intimal fibrosis of veins.

The initial clinical and roentgenographic presentation consisted of an "atypical" pneumonia, usually accompanied by fever, rash, myalgia, and marked eosinophilia. In some patients a period of respiratory failure terminated in death. About 20 per cent of those who survived developed a syndrome of neuromuscular disease, sicca syndrome, and scleroderma-like changes in the skin;[423, 428] some patients developed ventilatory failure as a result of respiratory muscle dysfunction. Other residual manifestations included eosinophilia (at a somewhat lower range), abnormal liver function tests, and a reduced diffusing capacity suggesting persistent interstitial lung disease.[422, 423] The most recent follow-up of patients 5 years after the epidemic[428] revealed notable persistence of scleroderma-like features; other late findings included musculoskeletal pain, cramps, livedo reticularis, carpal tunnel syndrome, and digital tuft changes. Pulmonary arterial hypertension also has been recognized as a significant sequela, although in the majority of patients it resolved spontaneously. However, a subset of patients has been recognized in whom pulmonary hypertension showed a malignant course leading rapidly to death.

FLUOROCARBON AND HYDROCARBON POISONING

Hydrocarbon poisoning can take several forms, depending on the toxic substance involved, the mode of contamination (whether inhaled, ingested, or absorbed through the skin), and the dose/time relationship of exposure. Three major clinical presentations are recognized: (1) the consequences of ingestion by young children of halogenated aromatic hydrocarbons (petroleum products), (2) the acute clinical manifestations of inhalation by adolescents and adults of chlorinated volatile hydrocarbons, and (3) the sequelae of chronic exposure to aliphatic and aromatic hydrocarbons in the addicted and in those occupationally exposed.

Ingestion

It has been estimated that 5[430] to 25 per cent[431] of all poisonings in children result from the ingestion of petroleum products, the most common of which is kerosene.[432, 433] Other liquids ingested include gasoline,[434] furniture polish,[435] lighter fluid, cleaning fluid, insecticides, and other household materials. Although poisoning is important in terms of the number of individuals affected, the resulting disease, fortunately, is of relatively mild severity. For example, in one survey of 950 children under 5 years of age who were suspected of having ingested products containing hydrocarbons,[430] 800 were asymptomatic at the time of initial evaluation and remained so during a 6- to 8-hour period of observation. The remaining 150 children had abnormal chest roentgenograms, although 71 were symptom-free. Complications occurred only in the 79 children who had both symptoms and abnormal chest roentgenograms; of these, 2 died and 5 developed progressive pulmonary disease.

Considerable controversy has raged over the pathogenesis of this form of poison-induced pulmonary disease. One hypothesis supports absorption from the intestinal tract with subsequent transportation to the pulmonary endothelium, and another invokes emesis and aspiration of vomitus with direct alveolocapillary damage. Experimental studies in animals have produced conflicting results. There is no doubt that intratracheal injection of aromatic hydrocarbons into animals produces hemorrhagic edema, suppuration, and necrosis.[432, 436–439] However, the instillation of hydrocarbons into the peritoneal cavity or stomach of animals (unaccompanied by esophageal regurgitation) has resulted in the development of pulmonary disease in some studies[440] but not in others.[436, 441] These somewhat contradictory results perhaps can be explained by varying toxicity and dosage of the hydrocarbon used; for example, in one study,[442] it was estimated that the dose instilled into a dog's stomach had to be 140 times that instilled into the trachea in order to produce a chemical pneumonitis.

There have been two reports[442, 443] of intravenous injection of small quantities of hydrocarbons into humans with resulting fever, pleural and abdominal pain, and hemoptysis; chest roentgenograms showed bilateral patchy airspace opacities that cleared completely in 3 days and in 1 week.

In other series, the percentage of children who developed roentgenographic changes varied considerably and undoubtedly depended on the selection of patients. For example, in one study[432] the incidence of abnormal chest roentgenograms was estimated to be 70 to 90 per cent,[432] whereas in the study previously cited of 950 children who were believed to have swallowed petroleum distillates, only 150 (15 per cent) developed roentgenographic changes.[430] The authors of the latter article conceded that their low incidence may have reflected the inclusion of some children who either did not actually swallow the poison or who ingested such small amounts that they would have been excluded from other series.

The chest roentgenogram is usually found to be abnormal within an hour of the ingestion of kerosene,[432, 433] but abnormality appears somewhat later following furniture polish ingestion.[435] The severity of the pulmonary abnormality varies with the amount ingested.[432] The typical roentgenographic pattern is one of patchy airspace consolidation characteristic of pulmonary edema and involves predominantly the basal portions of the lungs, usually bilaterally symmetric.[431–433, 435] Sometimes the hila are indistinct and hazy as a result of contiguous pulmonary disease, a finding that can occur alone but is more often associated with basal changes of acute aspiration edema. Roentgenographic resolution tends to be slow (up to 2 weeks)[432, 433] and usually lags well behind clinical improvement. Pneumatoceles may develop:[444–446] of 338 children with hydrocarbon ingestion studied by Harris and Brown,[446] 134 (40 per cent) developed acute pneumonia; of these, 14 demonstrated pneumatocele formation during resolution of the pneumonia. The pneumatoceles were often large, septate, and irregular, and sometimes contained fluid levels.

In the absence of witnesses to the incident, the diagnosis may be suspected from the odor of the offending agent on the child's breath. Vomiting follows shortly after ingestion and presumably is associated with aspiration. Symptoms usually are mild, but there is correlation between the amount of hydrocarbon ingested, the severity of clinical findings, and the extent of roentgenographic abnormalities.[432] A follow-up study of 14 asymptomatic children 10 years after an episode of kerosene ingestion showed subclinical functional impairment of small airways that seemed to be related to the severity of the acute insult; 4 of the 8 children who had had abnormal chest roentgenograms at the time of the incident continued to show changes.[396]

Inhalation

The practice of inhaling fluorocarbons and hydrocarbons for "kicks" originated on the West Coast of the United States in the early 1950s and subsequently developed into a small epidemic that resulted in 110[447] to 140[448] deaths, most of which occurred in the late 1960s. More recent reports of 80 deaths per year from solvent abuse in the United

Kingdom[449] and the arrest of 237 adults for solvent sniffing in Denver, Colorado, in 1979[450] clearly attest to a perpetuation of this habit. Hydrocarbons abused include various cements, glues, lacquers, paints, fingernail polish remover, lighter and cleaning fluids, gasoline, and antifreeze. Fluorocarbons (freons) are used as propellants in a great variety of commercial products packaged in aerosol cans and are usually inhaled from plastic bags. When inhaled in high concentrations, volatile hydrocarbons induce euphoria and hallucinations, with subsequent central nervous system (CNS) depression.

Rare cases of presumed permeability pulmonary edema have been described following the inhalation of toluene,[451] trichloroethylene, and tetrachloroethylene,[452] and two attacks of respiratory arrest have been documented in a punk rocker with a 6-year history of solvent abuse.[453] However, the major health hazard of inhaled hydrocarbons lies in their action on the myocardium.[454] Not only may conduction be impaired, but cardiac muscle becomes sensitive to sympathomimetic amines, resulting in arrhythmias. This sensitization may be intensified by hypoxemia, hypercapnia, stress, or physical activity.[447, 448, 455, 456] Animal studies have shown a spectrum of toxic cardiovascular effects of freons, of which arrhythmia is only one.[448] Since catecholamines are recognized inducers of cardiac arrhythmias, the combination of volatile hydrocarbons and bronchodilators is likely to be particularly hazardous. Some authors[448, 455] believe that the increased mortality of young asthmatics in England in the 1960s may have been caused, at least in part, by myocardial sensitization from fluorocarbons used as propellants in aerosol bronchodilators; however, studies in volunteers have revealed the concentration of alveolar fluorocarbon associated with aerosol catecholamine use to be at a level generally considered innocuous.[457] Inhalation of hydrocarbons, particularly trichloroethyelene, trichloroethane,[458] and toluene (a main constituent of paint)[450] can also result in liver, kidney, and CNS damage.

In addition to the arrhythmias and sudden death occasioned by sniffing of volatile hydrocarbons, repeated abuse can have chronic pathologic, roentgenographic, and clinical manifestations. A lung biopsy specimen of a chronic paint sniffer has been described as showing alveolitis and the intraalveolar and lymph node accumulation of particleladen macrophages.[459] Paint sniffers can develop muscle weakness, gastrointestinal symptoms (including pain and bleeding), and a variety of neuropsychiatric disorders.[450] Severe electrolyte disturbances also occur occasionally, rhabdomyolysis presumably being caused by hypophosphatemia.[450] Peripheral neuropathy has been reported in two young individuals who intentionally and repeatedly inhaled naphtha fumes (mixtures of aliphatic hydrocarbons containing n-hexane).[460] There are two reports of a chronic diffuse nodular pattern on chest roentgenograms from repeated "fire breathing," a process requiring the ignition of a rapidly exhaled mouthful of a volatile hydrocarbon.[461, 462]

Occupational exposure to inhaled hydrocarbons can also cause disease. When a heavy concentration is inhaled, the result can be sudden death, presumably from cardiac arrhythmia,[463] but there is also evidence that inhalation of a low concentration of hydrocarbons over a long period of time can cause damage. A controlled study of 25 cable plant workers exposed to mist and vapors of mineral oils and kerosene over a period ranging from 5 to 35 years has shown an increased incidence of impaired pulmonary function and roentgenographic evidence of reticulonodularity at the lung bases; in one worker, the presence of pulmonary fibrosis was confirmed at autopsy.[464] Unidentified saturated and unsaturated aliphatic hydrocarbons have been reported to cause respiratory allergy or irritation in cooks who broil food over mesquite wood rather than charcoal.[465]

Polychlorinated biphenyls (PCB) are chlorinated aromatic hydrocarbon compounds that can exert deleterious effects on the lungs either by inhalation or through skin absorption; there is laboratory evidence that they can also damage the liver.[466] Workers exposed to PCB in power capacitor manufacturing develop irritation of the mucous membranes; conjunctivitis, cough, and expectoration correlate with blood levels of PCB that are many times greater than those in the general population.[466–468] In one study of pulmonary function of 243 workers exposed to PCB during a mean length of employment of more than 15 years, 34 workers (14 per cent) showed a reduced forced vital capacity (FVC) of less than 80 per cent of predicted; of 326 workers who had chest roentgenograms, 6 (2 per cent) showed ILO s-opacities of 1/0 or greater (*see* page 2281).[468]

INHALED TOXIC GASES AND AEROSOLS

Several gases and liquids in a finely dispersed state can cause acute (and sometimes chronic) damage to the pulmonary airways and parenchyma. The reaction depends to some extent on the chemical composition of the gas or aerosol. Some of these substances, particularly those that are highly soluble such as sulfur dioxide, ammonia, and chloride, are so irritating to the mucous membranes of the nose that, on exposure, individuals may stop breathing and try to run away. Less soluble gases, including phosgene, nitrogen dioxide, ozone, and highly concentrated oxygen, may be inhaled deeply into the lungs before the irritating effect is perceived. Other gases, particularly when in low concentration, produce acute bronchitis or bronchiolitis that subsides spontaneously without the chemical exposure being recognized. Despite these generalizations, it is important to remember that the *concentration* of the gas and the *duration* of the exposure are the chief factors that determine clinical presentation and pulmonary pathology. Under appropriate circumstances, any one of these toxic gases can cause immediate or delayed pulmonary edema[469–471] and airway or alveolar epithelial damage.

The form of pulmonary disease that results from inhalation of such toxic substances is variable. In many instances, the inhaled toxin leads to extensive alveolocapillary damage with resultant permeability pulmonary edema. In other cases, the chemical injury appears to affect predominantly the airways,[470, 471] resulting in fulminating bronchitis and bronchiolitis, sometimes complicated by atelectasis and bacterial pneumonia. Patients who survive the acute insult may feel relatively well for about 3 weeks and then suffer abrupt clinical deterioration, with cough, shortness of breath, and fever. This delayed development is reflected pathologically by bronchiolitis obliterans.[472–474] Histologically, this is similar to the bronchiolitis obliterans caused by other etiologies (*see* page 2221): small bronchi and bronchioles are plugged with cellular fibrinous exudate that subsequently undergoes organization by ingrowth of fibroblasts from the bronchiolar walls, resulting in partial or complete airway occlusion. This complication can also occur in individuals with diffuse pulmonary edema who survive the acute event. In addition to these abnormalities, it is probable that repeated exposure to a low concentration of certain gases or aerosols can cause a more insidious irritation of the airways, with the development of chronic bronchitis (*see* page 2092).

Oxidants

In addition to inhaled gases such as oxygen, ozone, and nitrogen dioxide, the herbicide paraquat (*see* page 2448), irradiation therapy (*see* Chapter 15), and some cytotoxic drugs used as chemotherapeutic agents (*see* page 2418) have the potential to damage tissue by producing highly reactive metabolic products of oxygen that can inactivate protective enzymes in the cell, damage DNA, and destroy lipid membranes.[475–478] These agents of oxidant tissue damage are products of normal oxidation-reduction processes and include hydrogen peroxide, superoxide radical, hydroxyl radical, and singlet excited oxygen.[477, 479]

Under hyperoxic conditions and in the presence of certain poisons, intracellular production of these oxygen-free radicals increases markedly, resulting in chain reactions involving oxygen radicals. These radicals then cause a number of effects, including peroxidation of polyunsaturated lipids situated within the cell or on the cell membrane, depolymerization of mucopolysaccharides, protein sulfhydryl oxidation and cross-linking (resulting in enzyme inactivation), and nucleic acid damage.[477, 479–481] It has been shown that radioactive substances administered parenterally to animals escape into lung alveolar fluid following exposure to relatively low concentrations of ozone[482] and nitrogen dioxide,[483] thus paralleling the early biochemical changes. It also has been postulated that some of the increased lipid peroxidation associated with cell damage may be the effect rather than the cause of cell damage.[484]

An additional source of oxygen radicals may be the large number of neutrophils that appear in pulmonary tissue as a result of oxidant injury; it has been suggested that hyperoxia damages alveolar macrophages, resulting in the release of chemotactic factors that attract neutrophils to the lung.[485] To support this theory, experiments have been conducted with rats in which they were treated with 95 per cent oxygen for 6 hours. The chemoattractant activity of BAL fluid increased ten-fold, an increase that correlated with the number of neutrophils in the lavage fluid.[486]

In the presence of hyperoxia, structural abnormalities appear in as short a time as 24 hours.[475] These can occur along the whole length of the respiratory tract, although involvement may be uneven and vary from animal to animal.[487] Animals exposed to a low concentration of ozone[487] or to one atmosphere of oxygen[488] show similar histologic changes: ciliated cells become vacuolated and their mitochondria become condensed with abnormal cristae configuration. Type I alveolar epithelial cells become swollen and may desquamate; type II cells may appear normal[487] but usually undergo proliferation, resulting in a more or less continuous cuboidal epithelium lining the alveoli.[488] Endothelial cells are also affected,[489] possibly as a result of lipid peroxidation of erythrocyte membranes. Although alveolar macrophages may be somewhat more resistant to oxidizing substances than other cells of the respiratory tract, metabolic abnormalities can be found in these cells in animals after exposure to 100 per cent oxygen for 48 to 72 hours[490] and to nitrogen dioxide or ozone following a period of hyperoxia.[491] More prolonged administration of oxygen or ozone (5 ppm) results in structural alteration and impairment of macrophage function and in intrapulmonary antibacterial defense mechanisms.[492]

As may be judged from the above comments, the free radical theory of oxidant toxicity is largely dependent on animal experimentation. Such studies also demonstrate a remarkable struggle by the lung to produce a variety of antioxidant defense systems to prevent damage from these cytotoxic oxygen metabolites.[477, 478] The enzymes generally assumed to be responsible for maintaining low levels of oxygen radicals and thus protecting against oxidants include superoxide dismutase (SOD), catalase, glutathione and the glutathione enzymes, glutathione reductase, and glucose-6-phosphate dehydrogenase (G6PD). SOD increases the dismutation rate of the superoxide radical and thus accomplishes its removal before it can react directly with cellular components.[477] Catalase serves to eliminate hydrogen

peroxide and thus avoid lipid peroxidation by hydroxyl radicals.[477, 478] High concentrations of reduced glutathione (GSH) and low levels of the oxidized form (GSSG) are necessary for the survival of animals. Glutathione in its reduced form is a substrate that is preferred to protein sulfhydryls for oxidants, thus preventing protein sulfhydryl oxidation. Maintenance of high GSH and low GSSG levels is important because GSSG can react with protein sulfhydryls to form mixed glutathione-protein sulfides that can inactivate proteins; the optimal GSH–GSSG ratio is accomplished by the enzymes glutathione reductase and G6PD.[477, 478]

Prior exposure to inhaled oxidants, intermittently or in low concentration, exerts a protective effect in some species of animals, an effect that correlates with the production of antioxidants in lung tissue.[477–480, 488, 493, 494] Almost all adult rats die within 3 days if exposed to 100 per cent oxygen;[493–495] however, if initially they are exposed to sublethal concentrations of oxygen (in the range of 70 to 85 per cent) for one week or to low concentrations of ozone (0.1 to 0.5 ppm), they can subsequently survive for long periods in 100 per cent oxygen or in ordinarily lethal edemogenic concentrations of ozone.[477–479, 493–495] Since sublethal exposure to ozone and oxygen is associated with a proliferation of type II pneumocytes, it has been suggested that these cells are responsible for production of SOD.[494] This hypothesis would also explain the increased tolerance to oxygen observed in rabbits whose lungs have been injured previously by the intravenous injection of oleic acid;[496] these animals develop a proliferation of type II pneumocytes and simultaneously become resistant to ordinarily lethal hyperoxia. Despite good evidence that a pre-exposure to 70 to 85 per cent oxygen increases resistance to lung toxicity from 100 per cent oxygen,[477, 478, 494] two experimental studies on animals have indicated that exposure to 40 to 60 per cent oxygen may have the opposite effect.[497, 498] The explanation for this apparent paradox has not been established.

One group of workers[499] has shown that immunosuppressed mice do not have this adaptive tolerance to oxidants and has proposed that an underlying immunologic mechanism is responsible. In addition to the protective role of endogenous superoxidase dismutase, it has been suggested on the basis of animal studies[478] that exogenous SOD and vitamin E can exert a beneficial effect if administered in close chronologic proximity to exposure to oxidants.

OXYGEN

Physicians have become aware only during the past 30 years or so that oxygen therapy for respiratory disease can itself produce pathologic changes in the lungs that are of clinical and physiologic importance.[500–508] Studies directed at the assessment of clinical, physiologic, and anatomic alterations in the lungs of patients exposed to high concentrations of oxygen are complicated by the knowledge that some of the changes observed may be caused by the underlying disease, concurrent drug therapy, or artificial ventilation.[509] For example, in one review of the clinical and pathologic findings in 22 patients who had undergone prolonged mechanical ventilation with high concentrations of oxygen,[510] the authors concluded that oxygen could have been a contributory cause of pulmonary injury in 1 of the 6 patients who died and in 3 of the 13 survivors who showed abnormal pulmonary function 1 year later. This dilemma is perhaps most evident in newborn infants with hyaline membrane disease.[501, 504] In this clinical setting, Northway and his colleagues[501] have described a pathologic and roentgenographic evolution from a classic picture of infantile respiratory distress syndrome to one of exudation and necrosis accompanied by a roentgenographic appearance of almost complete opacification of the lungs; this then progresses to diffuse atelectasis and emphysema, creating a "spongy" pattern both roentgenographically and morphologically (bronchopulmonary dysplasia). Similar pathologic changes have been described in adults with varying underlying diseases and a requirement for prolonged oxygen therapy.[510]

Pratt[502] was the first to associate the development of interstitial fibrosis with such an exposure to oxygen. In a study of 70 patients receiving oxygen therapy by artificial ventilation, Nash and associates[500] described two histologic phases, the exudative and the proliferative, both of which were identical to diffuse alveolar damage of other etiology. The exudative phase was characterized by capillary congestion, proteinaceous material and hemorrhage within alveoli, and well-defined hyaline membranes lining all portions of the acinar airspaces. In the proliferative phase, alveolar and interlobular septal fibroblastic proliferation and hyperplasia of alveolar lining cells were observed. These two distinct phases of oxygen toxicity in humans resemble the reaction seen in animals after exposure to a high concentration of oxygen—an early acute edematous reaction followed by fibroblastic and proliferative changes that appear after the animal has developed tolerance to hyperoxia.[493, 511]

For obvious reasons there is a paucity of studies of the effects of hyperoxia on humans with healthy lungs. In one report, normal volunteers who inhaled one atmosphere of pure oxygen for 6 to 12 hours failed to show hemodynamic or gas exchange defects.[512] In another prospective study of patients after open heart surgery, one group was administered pure oxygen and a second group oxygen in limited concentration for periods up to 48 hours. The clinical course of the two groups was similar, and no differences were found in intrapulmonary shunting, effective compliance, or in the ratio of

dead space to tidal volume (V_D/V_T). On the other hand, in a study of patients with irreversible brain damage, the patients who breathed pure oxygen had significant changes in pulmonary function compared with those who breathed air; after a period of 40 hours of breathing 100 per cent oxygen, the former group showed an increase in wasted ventilation and intrapulmonary shunting. Small decreases in static and dynamic compliance and diffusing capacity have been detected in normal subjects breathing one atmosphere of oxygen for 30 to 48 hours.[513, 514] Sackner and associates[515] ventilated anesthetized dogs with both air and supplemental oxygen; in the latter group, tracheal irritation was observed and mucous velocity fell 45 per cent from baseline values after inhalation of 100 per cent oxygen for 2 hours and 51 per cent after inhalation of 50 per cent oxygen for 30 hours. This dysfunction is related to the toxic effect on macrophages[492] and may permit increased susceptibility to bronchopulmonary infection with prolonged use of high concentrations of oxygen.

Although the toxic level of oxygen has yet to be precisely defined, there appears to be ample clinical evidence that man can tolerate an FIO_2 of 50 per cent for prolonged periods of time without developing irreversible pulmonary damage.[516] The potential deleterious effects of a combination of oxidants should be borne in mind, however, and unless death from hypoxia appears imminent, high concentrations of oxygen should be avoided in patients with pulmonary disease caused by cytotoxic drugs, paraquat poisoning, or radiation pneumonitis.

OZONE

Unlike most other gases described in this section, ozone has not produced serious acute pulmonary disease in humans to the best of our knowledge. Nevertheless, there is abundant evidence that chronic inhalation of even low concentrations can cause structural changes in animal lungs and functional changes in both animal and human lungs. Ozone constitutes 90 per cent of the measured oxidant in photochemical smog,[479] and in certain urban areas the concentration of ozone in the atmosphere in parts per million (ppm) is equal to that known to cause structural and physiologic changes. High concentrations of ozone are also found within airplanes at altitudes above 30,000 feet, in proximity to high-tension electrical discharges from welding in both air and oxygen, and in various industries in which this gas is used as an oxidizing agent.[517]

Studies of the acute effects of ozone on the lungs of a variety of animals have clearly demonstrated that the gas can induce both structural[487, 518–521] and functional[522] changes. Although the details of the pathologic abnormalities vary somewhat, presumably reflecting differences in animal species, experimental techniques, and ozone concentrations, injury has been generally shown to be most prominent in the respiratory and distal membranous bronchioles. Depending on the stage at which the tissue is examined, this injury may take the form of either epithelial necrosis or regeneration. Damage to the tracheobronchial epithelium[519, 520] and alveolar capillary endothelium[521] also has been noted by some investigators. Functional changes in acute ozone exposure have been less extensively investigated. In one study, they were found in only a minority of cats exposed to 0.26 ppm but were present in almost all animals exposed to 1.0 and 0.5 ppm.[522] These changes consisted primarily of an increase in pulmonary resistance; diffusing capacity remained within normal limits. The increased pulmonary resistance resulted from damage to conducting airways that was felt to be consistent with the structural changes found after exposure to ozone levels insufficient to induce pulmonary edema.

Morphologic changes in rat lungs exposed to low concentrations of ozone and the protective effects of vitamin E have been reported by two groups of investigators.[480, 523] Sato and associates[523] used scanning electron microscopy to detect the earliest changes in rat airways and alveoli to exposure of 0.3 ppm ozone. The major change occurred in the cilia, which were seen to be swollen and matted together; in addition, the surface of alveolar ducts and alveoli throughout the parenchyma showed scattered areas of cytoplasmic swelling and attachment of round bodies. Damage to epithelial cells occurred earlier and was more severe in rats that were deficient in vitamin E, but even these animals appeared to acquire a tolerance to repeated ozone exposure, presumably as a result of superoxide dismutase production. In the studies carried out by Roehm and associates,[480] all rats exposed to 1.0 ppm ozone succumbed from pulmonary edema within 22 days. LD50 was 8.2 days for vitamin E-depleted animals and 18.5 days for those receiving vitamin E. In another study,[524] rats exposed to 0.8 to 1.5 ppm for 7 days were compared with a control group breathing filtered air: analysis of lung minces showed that the net rate of collagen synthesis in the group treated with ozone was increased several-fold, in a dose-dependent manner, compared with rats breathing air; this increased synthesis could be prevented by methylprednisolone. Activity of proline hydroxylase (an enzyme that can be regarded as a marker of collagen biosynthesis) and of hydroxyproline (the product of its reaction) has been measured in rat lungs exposed to low concentrations of ozone.[525] A negligible effect was observed at a level of 0.2 ppm, whereas at the end of a 7-day exposure to 0.5 and 0.8 ppm, enzyme activity was found to increase approximately 150 and 200 per cent, respectively. A tolerance once again appeared to be manifested by a fall-off in enzyme activity after 30 days and its return to normal within 60 days despite continued ozone exposure.

Pathologic and functional abnormalities also have been studied in several animal species after *prolonged* ozone exposure.[526–528] In some studies,[526, 527] the pathologic changes have been localized predominantly about respiratory bronchioles and have consisted of epithelial hyperplasia and hypertrophy associated with small aggregates of macrophages in adjacent alveoli. It was observed with some interest that these abnormalities appeared to be less severe after prolonged exposure compared with acute exposure, thus suggesting an adaptive reaction. In one investigation in rats,[528] abnormalities (accumulation of macrophages and fibroblasts) were found to be most marked in alveolar ducts and adjacent alveoli; in this study, findings diminished dramatically following a 24-week "recovery period" in clean air. Functional abnormalities in the animals in this last investigation[528] were mild but statistically significant, and included an increase in functional residual capacity (FRC) and residual volume (RV) and a decrease in DL_{CO}; these findings disappeared following a 3-month recovery period.

Although these metabolic and morphologic changes have been identified only in experimental animals, it is possible that they may be highly pertinent to ozone toxicity in humans, since the concentrations of ozone in most animal studies are roughly equivalent to levels detected in smog over heavily polluted urban areas. A number of investigators[529–533] have shown that acute exposure of normal volunteers to low concentrations of ozone (0.5 to 0.9 ppm) results in dry cough, chest discomfort, and impaired pulmonary function. Considerable variation is observed among individuals in their symptomatic and functional responses, probably explained on the basis of hyper-reactivity of airways, smoking habits, tolerance developed from prolonged exposure, and the degree of exercise attained.[529, 531–535] The functional derangement that follows ozone exposure is invariably obstructive in pattern and can be demonstrated by a variety of pulmonary function tests.[531–536]

In the earlier discussion in this section dealing with the pathogenesis of lung damage resulting from oxidants, certain experiments were described in which pre-exposure to low concentrations of oxidants was shown to result in adaptation or tolerance that presumably reflected protective enzyme production, particularly of superoxide dismutase. The same phenomenon occurs with ozone; for example, one study[529] has shown that "healthy" Los Angeles volunteers are more resistant to physiologic change when exposed to concentrations of ozone capable of producing symptoms than urban dwellers from less polluted areas. A number of experiments in healthy volunteers[537–539] and in patients with chronic bronchitis[540] have confirmed this phenomenon of adaptation; it develops within 2 to 5 days of exposure but is relatively short-lived, lasting from 4 days to 3 weeks after cessation of exposure.[539] The duration of adaptation is shortest in subjects who are most sensitive to ozone.

NITROGEN DIOXIDE

Nitrogen dioxide (NO_2), like ozone, is a component of photochemical smog. Although its concentration is insufficient to cause serious concern,[541] it possesses an effect identical to that of ozone on pulmonary parenchymal cells and thus represents a potential hazard to humans. Considerable experimental work has been performed on animals in which the toxic effects on the lungs of relatively low concentrations of NO_2 have been documented; in addition, an abundance of clinical experience has accumulated in which the dire consequences of exposure to a heavy concentration of this gas by humans has been demonstrated. Rarely, other oxides of nitrogen (e.g., dinitrogen tetroxide) also have been implicated in human disease.[542]

Animal experiments have shown that short-term exposure to NO_2 in a concentration less than 17 ppm will result in changes in bronchopulmonary epithelial and capillary endothelial cells.[543–546] As with oxygen (O_2) and ozone (O_3), tolerance develops with repeated exposure coincident with regeneration of type II alveolar epithelial cells.[545] Continued exposure of rats to a low concentration of NO_2 results in increased production of collagen fibrils in the pulmonary interstitium,[547] particularly around respiratory bronchioles. In a study of BAL fluid of adult hamsters administered 30 ppm NO_2 for 30 days, Kleinerman and his coworkers have shown a significant increase in the number of macrophages and in elastase activity.[548] In an additional study of the blotchy mouse exposed to 20 ppm NO_2 for 28 days, Ranga and Kleinerman observed a marked progression of the inherited emphysema that has been described in these animals.[549] The additive toxic effect of various oxidants on pulmonary cells of animals is exemplified by the deleterious consequences of adding O_2 to the NO_2 administered to mice.[550]

Experimental studies of the effects of low concentrations of NO_2 in man have revealed few abnormalities. Nonsmoking human volunteers have been subjected to an atmosphere containing 0.62 ppm NO_2 while exercising for 15 to 60 minutes, and no evidence of cardiopulmonary dysfunction could be detected.[551] Twenty-two volunteers with chronic obstructive pulmonary disease (COPD) were exercised for 1 hour in a controlled environmental chamber containing NO_2 in concentrations ranging from 0.0 to 2.0 ppm; subsequent complete pulmonary function testing failed to reveal any impairment.[551] Despite these negative results, one group of workers found a significant increase in blood levels of glutathione in 19 subjects after 2 hours' exposure to 0.2 ppm NO_2;[743] this substance is recognized as an important antioxidant.

The dangers of exposure to a high, in contrast to a low, concentration of oxides of nitrogen are appreciable. They were first described by Desgranges in 1804,[552] an account translated into English 170 years later.[553] This hazard has been recognized for many years in industry,[554] in which bronchopulmonary disease occurs following exposure to fuming nitric acid[555, 556] or to fumes from the burning of shoe polish[557] or during mining operations in association with the use of explosives.[555, 558] A rather freak exposure involved the Apollo astronauts during their descent from space following the Apollo-Soyuz training program in 1975;[542] at approximately 23,000 feet the spacecraft cabin was filled with a yellow-brown gas consisting of monomethylhydrazine and dinitrogen tetroxide, the principal toxic irritants in rocket fuels. The pulmonary reaction was similar to that described below.

Although the occupational settings mentioned above are interesting and important in their own right, little doubt exists that, from the point of view of the number of cases, the most important condition resulting from NO_2 inhalation is silo-filler's disease.[559–561] For 3 to 10 days after a silo has been filled, the fresh silage produces nitric oxide which, on contact with the air, oxidizes to form nitrogen dioxide and its polymer, nitrogen tetroxide.[562, 563] These two gases, being heavier than air, remain just above the silage and are apparent as a brownish-yellow "cloud." Anyone who enters the silo during this period will inhale NO_2 with resultant bronchopulmonary irritation; the severity of toxicity is in proportion to the duration and level of exposure. Mild exposure results in inflammation of the bronchial and bronchiolar mucosa, whereas intensive exposure can cause fatal pulmonary edema.

Following moderate to severe exposure, the course is triphasic:

First Phase. An immediate reaction occurs within the lungs that consists of acute, severe bronchiolitis and peribronchiolitis, sometimes accompanied by denuding of the epithelium; diffuse alveolar damage also has been documented in some patients.[561] The clinical picture is characterized by the abrupt onset of cough, dyspnea, weakness, and a choking feeling that usually persist. Pulmonary edema can develop within 4 to 24 hours (Fig. 14–10)[553] but usually clears completely if the patient survives.

Second Phase. Symptoms abate during this period, which lasts from 2 to 5 weeks, although cough, malaise, and shortness of breath of lesser severity may persist; weakness may worsen. The chest roentgenogram is normal.

Third Phase. This phase becomes manifest up to 5 weeks after the initial exposure[563–565] and is characterized pathologically by bronchiolitis obliterans. Roentgenographically, there is "miliary nodulation" whose appearance tends to lag somewhat behind the recurrence of symptoms. Multiple discrete nodular opacities of varying size are scattered diffusely throughout the lungs (to a point of confluence in the more severe cases).[472, 566] The nodules may disappear as the clinical course progresses to a stage of chronic pulmonary insufficiency, although

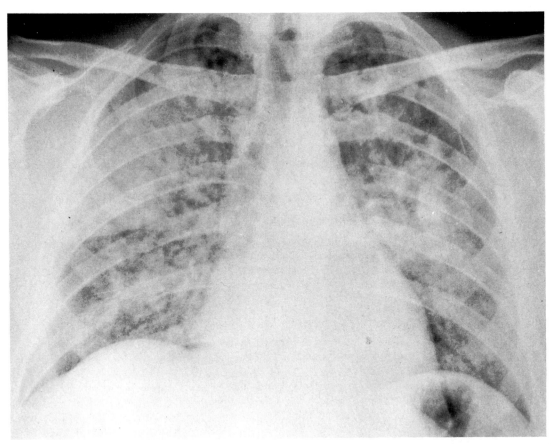

Figure 14–10. Acute Pulmonary Edema Secondary to Nitrogen Dioxide Inhalation. This 40-year-old man had spent 6 hours with several other men in an enclosed space on board ship attempting to remove a propeller with cutting torches. Such a procedure is known to be associated with accumulation of nitrogen dioxide. Toward the end of the 6 hours, the patient noted the onset of nausea, vomiting, headache, and productive cough. This posteroanterior roentgenogram reveals extensive involvement of both lungs by a process characteristic of airspace consolidation. The chest roentgenogram had returned to normal 4 days later so that the process clearly was one of edema. Two months after this roentgenogram, pulmonary function tests were normal with the exception of slight decrease in FRC, and the patient had slight residual shortness of breath on exertion.

they usually persist for a considerable time after the acute symptoms have subsided.[566] Clinically, this stage is characterized by fever, chills, progressive shortness of breath, cough, and cyanosis. Moist rales and rhonchi may be heard on auscultation. A neutrophilic leukocytosis develops in most cases, and the $PaCO_2$ may be elevated.[472] The patient may die of pulmonary insufficiency or may recover more or less completely during this stage. In some patients, a degree of obstructive impairment of pulmonary function remains.[566–569]

Horvath and associates[559] have described their experience with 23 patients exposed to NO_2 in agriculture and industry; 18 developed no more than a transient upper respiratory tract syndrome and only 5 developed pulmonary edema or bronchiolitis obliterans. From their own experience and a review of the literature, these authors concluded that NO_2 toxicity is more common than is generally appreciated and that the majority of affected individuals recover completely; however, they estimated the case fatality rate to be 29 per cent for patients with silo-filler's disease. In addition, patients who survived often had residual functional defects. Like

Becklake and her associates,[555] they found that steroids were effective in treating high concentration NO_2 pulmonary toxicity.

Sulfur Dioxide

Sulfur dioxide (SO_2) is a highly soluble gas whose major importance in pulmonary disease is as an atmospheric pollutant; continuous exposure to low concentrations in an urban environment may play a role in the pathogenesis of COPD (*see* page 2092). On contact with moist epithelial surfaces, SO_2 is hydrated and subsequently oxidized to form sulfuric acid (H_2SO_4) which causes mucosal injury; the acid may be partly neutralized, and the damage thereby diminished, by combination with endogenous ammonia within the respiratory tract.[570] Accidental exposure to high concentrations can occur in pulp and paper factories, refrigeration plants, and oil-refining and fruit-preserving industries.[571] H_2SO_4 itself is also used in photographic developing and is capable of causing reversible obstructive disease of small airways in photographers.[572, 573]

It is probable that the inhalation of SO_2 produces the same triphasic picture as does NO_2. We have seen a pulp mill worker, accidentally exposed to fumes rising from a vat of concentrated H_2SO_4, who suffered acute pulmonary edema that resolved within a few days. Three months later he manifested evidence of severe obstructive pulmonary disease caused by extensive bronchiolitis obliterans and generalized bronchiectasis (Fig. 14–11). Woodford and associates[574] have described a patient with an identical history whose course was characterized initially by acute pulmonary edema, followed by a silent period, and ending with severe irreversible obstruc-

tive disease. In reported acute accidents, the likelihood of death or residual pulmonary damage varies considerably from victim to victim; this undoubtedly reflects the severity and concentration of SO_2 exposure. For example, of 13 men exposed to burning SO_2 in the hold of a ship, only 1 died.[575] In another report of 5 men exposed in a paper mill,[576] 2 men died immediately, 1 developed severe obstructive airway disease, and 2 were asymptomatic in follow-up (although 1 of these had abnormal pulmonary function). The pulmonary function of 7 men accidentally exposed to SO_2 in a pyrite dust explosion

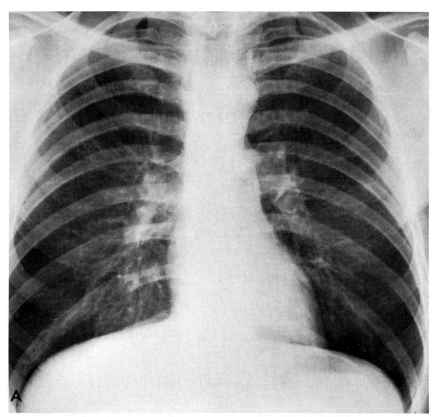

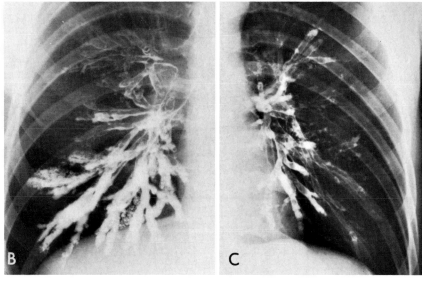

Figure 14–11. Bronchiolitis Obliterans and Bronchiectasis Secondary to Sulfur Dioxide Inhalation. Three months prior to these roentgenographic studies, this 33-year-old man was exposed to high concentrations of sulfur dioxide fumes rising from a sulfuric acid vat. Immediately following this exposure he was said to have developed acute pulmonary edema, which gradually resolved over a period of days (this acute episode was not documented locally). Three months later, a posteroanterior roentgenogram (A) was essentially normal, although close examination revealed numerous "tram lines" in the central and medullary portions of both lungs. The lungs were somewhat overinflated. Bilateral bronchography (B and C) demonstrated severe cylindrical and varicose bronchiectasis of all segmental bronchi of both lungs, the dilated bronchi terminating abruptly in squared or rounded extremities. There was an almost total absence of peripheral filling. These findings are felt to be consistent with extensive bronchiolitis obliterans in addition to bronchiectasis.

was followed for 7 years: the greatest decrease in FVC and FEV_1 and maximal midexpiratory flow was observed 1 week after the accident; after about 3 months no further decrement occurred. Four years after the accident, 3 men still manifested reversible airway obstruction, and 4 reacted positively to the histamine challenge test.[577]

Hydrogen Sulfide

Hydrogen sulfide (H_2S) produces a characteristic "rotten egg" odor at 0.2 ppm and paralyzes the sense of smell at levels of 150 ppm. Levels of 250 ppm cause irritation of mucous membranes with resultant keratoconjunctivitis, bronchitis, and pulmonary edema. Higher concentrations affect the central nervous system and cause sudden death.[578] Like cyanide, sulfide ions act as direct cytotoxins, selectively binding to cytochrome oxidase within the mitochondria and thereby disrupting the electron transport chain.

Usual sources of exposure to H_2S are the petroleum and chemical industries[579] and decaying organic matter.[578, 580] In the latter situation, production of H_2S depends on incomplete oxidation and degradation of sulfur compounds.[579] An example of acute inhalation of such waste products can be found in the dramatic description by Osbern and Crapo of "Dung Lung":[578] a cow kicked the lid of a large underground liquid manure storage tank into the tank and a farmer attempted to recover it; two other individuals tried to rescue him and all three died. This incident illustrates the danger of exposure to toxic gases released from decaying organic matter. Risk from such a source was also evident on examination of U.S. Coast Guard records of deaths at sea among fishermen over a 10-year period:[580] in 11 incidents, 32 men died from breathing a polluted atmosphere attributed to anaerobic decay of insufficiently refrigerated fish stored in an unventilated hold. Particularly in warm weather, decaying organic matter releases a variety of toxic gases, including hydrogen sulfide, ammonia, methane, carbon dioxide, and carbon monoxide; hydrogen sulfide is the most likely of these agents to cause death.

Burnett and associates[579] reviewed 5 years' experience with hydrogen sulfide poisoning in the Alberta oil fields. There were 221 cases of recognized exposure to H_2S, with an overall mortality of 6 per cent; 5 per cent of victims were dead on arrival at a hospital. Acute problems consisted of coma, dysequilibrium, and respiratory insufficiency as a result of pulmonary edema. Although 74 per cent of patients lost consciousness at the accident site, neurologic and respiratory sequelae were uncommon.

Ammonia

This toxic, highly soluble alkaline gas may play a role along with H_2S in causing bronchopulmonary disease on exposure to decaying organic matter.[578, 580] However, it is better known as a cause of lung damage in industry and farming, usually as a result of sudden rupture of or leakage from tanks of concentrated ammonia.[581–584] Vehicular accidents involving tank transportation of this gas can result in inhalation of high concentrations by those involved, often with serious consequences.[585] For example, during World War II, 47 persons were exposed to high concentrations when an ammonia container was damaged during an air raid;[586] 13 died of pulmonary edema and purulent bronchitis. Even household-strength ammonia, which has a pH of less than 12 and contains only 5 to 10 per cent of ammonia products, can cause esophageal necrosis and ARDS when ingested in large quantity for suicidal purposes.[587]

Inhalation of a large quantity of ammonia (NH_3)[586, 588] results in the production of copious serosanguineous and purulent tracheobronchial secretions; extreme inflammation and desquamation of the mucosa of the central bronchial tree can be seen bronchoscopically.[589] Postmortem examination of individuals who die shows severe bronchiectasis, with[582, 583] or without[590] obliterative bronchiolitis. Conventional chest roentgenograms of patients who survive severe exposure can be virtually normal and bronchography may be necessary to detect the bronchiectasis.[591] In one accident at sea in which a leak developed in the refrigeration system,[744] 14 fishermen had transient exposure to NH_3 lasting seconds to minutes; clinical findings consisted of inflammation of the pharynx and conjunctiva and a few rales and rhonchi on auscultation of the lungs. Although only one man showed a small patch of lung consolidation roentgenographically, the mean PaO_2 for the group was only 64 mm Hg.

Chlorine

Heavy exposure to this irritating gas can occur in industrial accidents or when the gas escapes from broken pipes or tank containers; occupational settings at particular risk are plastic and textile industries and plants for water purification.[742] Acute exposure to a high concentration of chlorine results in pulmonary edema, fever, severe acute bronchitis, conjunctivitis, nausea and vomiting, stupor, shock, and hemoptysis.[592, 593] Sudden death can occur from pulmonary edema.[594] Lesser exposure results in cough and dyspnea and sometimes roentgenographic evidence of mild interstitial edema. Postmortem examination of individuals who die from acute chlorine poisoning shows airspace edema and hemorrhage and extensive bronchial and bronchiolar epithelial necrosis;[595] evidence of epithelial damage can also be seen cytologically in bronchial brush specimens taken during life.[742] Pulmonary function tests show an obstructive pattern,[596, 597] although a number of studies have documented complete return to normal function in a few weeks;[594, 596–598] in

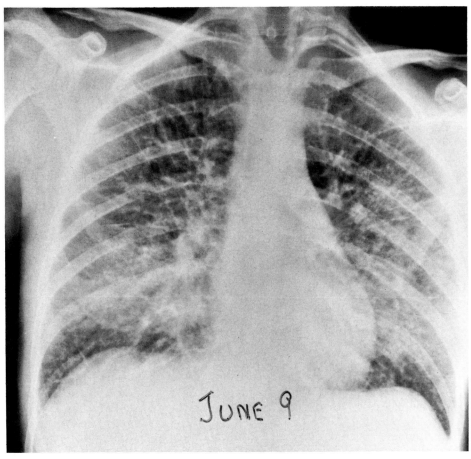

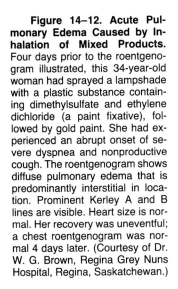

Figure 14–12. Acute Pulmonary Edema Caused by Inhalation of Mixed Products. Four days prior to the roentgenogram illustrated, this 34-year-old woman had sprayed a lampshade with a plastic substance containing dimethylsulfate and ethylene dichloride (a paint fixative), followed by gold paint. She had experienced an abrupt onset of severe dyspnea and nonproductive cough. The roentgenogram shows diffuse pulmonary edema that is predominantly interstitial in location. Prominent Kerley A and B lines are visible. Heart size is normal. Her recovery was uneventful; a chest roentgenogram was normal 4 days later. (Courtesy of Dr. W. G. Brown, Regina Grey Nuns Hospital, Regina, Saskatchewan.)

fact, pulmonary function assessment over a period of several years strongly suggests that this toxic gas does not cause irreparable lung damage.[594] Of two sisters who appeared to inhale a roughly equal quantity of chlorine, the one who was treated with corticosteroids showed stable pulmonary function whereas the untreated sister developed abnormalities that persisted for many months.[599]

A bizarre case has been reported of a patient who was addicted to inhaling chlorine gas:[600] on each of three occasions when he was admitted to the hospital after indulging, he was found to have severe, partly reversible obstructive pulmonary disease, hypoxemia, cor pulmonale, and right heart failure.

Pulmonary edema can also occur after the inhalation of other compounds containing chlorine (Fig. 14–12).

Phosgene

Although phosgene is known chiefly as a highly poisonous gas used in warfare, it is also an occasional hazard in industry. Cases of poisoning have been described following accidental inhalation of carbon tetrachloride from a fire extinguisher[598] and inhalation within small, enclosed, stove-heated spaces of chemical paint removers containing meth-

ylene chloride.[601, 602] Acute pulmonary disease also has been reported in 25 of 106 workers heavily exposed at a uranium processing plant.[603] Phosgene is the common name of a heavy, colorless gas, carbon oxychloride ($COCl_2$). When inhaled, it is hydrolyzed to hydrochloric acid and carbon dioxide. Probably as a result of the action of the former substance, sloughing of the bronchiolar mucosa, interstitial and alveolar edema, and patchy lobular emphysema occur.[598, 604] As with NO_2 there is a delay of several hours before the onset of dyspnea. Acute pulmonary edema can cause death, usually within 24 hours of exposure. If the patient survives the initial acute episode, recovery appears to be complete.[598, 602]

Mercury

Mercury poisoning can occur from exposure to either the vaporized or metallic form. Inhalation of *vaporized mercury* usually occurs in industry when an individual is exposed in a confined space such as a tank or boiler;[571] it has also been reported in a worker making fishing weights (sinkers) in a confined, nonventilated space.[605] Accidental exposure can occur in the home when metallic mercury is allowed to burn on a stove.[606–608]

Symptoms and signs tend to develop 3 to 4

hours after exposure and include gingivostomatitis, crampy abdominal pain, and diarrhea; severe tracheitis, bronchitis, bronchiolitis, and pneumonitis can be present.[606–610] The condition is particularly serious in infants in whom the bronchiolitis may be fatal; it is sometimes complicated by pneumothorax. Central nervous system symptoms are very common and can develop in the absence of pulmonary disease.[610] Other manifestations include paronychia, erosion of the nails, and a metallic taste in the mouth.[609, 610] Lung biopsy specimens can reveal minimal degrees of interstitial fibrosis.[606] Pulmonary function tests performed 2 days after exposure have shown a combination of obstructive and restrictive disease and a lowered diffusing capacity.[608]

Metallic mercury can reach the lungs by aspiration, by injection into soft tissues in suicidal attempts,[611] by accidental intravascular injection from syringes sampling venous blood, or by intentional intravascular injection by drug addicts (*see* Fig. 9–47, page 1805). Absorption into the bloodstream from deposits in the lung can cause kidney disease and death[611] or can prove innocuous.[612]

Zinc Chloride

The fumes of zinc chloride, a substance used in smoke bombs,[613] are extremely caustic to the mucous membranes and when inhaled can cause severe damage to both the tracheobronchial tree and lung parenchyma. Acute tracheobronchitis can cause death within hours.[614] Evans[614] described a catastrophe involving 70 people exposed to burning smoke generators in a tunnel: 10 of the 70 died. The major effect on the lung parenchyma is a rapidly developing diffuse interstitial fibrosis[613] manifested roentgenographically by a diffuse reticular pattern.

Manganese

Manganese oxide (pyrolusite) is employed in the smelting of manganese, in the dry-cell battery industry, and in the manufacture of coloring for glass bleaching. Individuals exposed to this substance are said to be particularly susceptible to pneumonia.[616] The results of experimental studies in mice[616, 617] and the development of upper respiratory irritation and tracheobronchitis in exposed humans suggest a chemical origin of the pneumonia. Symptoms include dry cough and fever.

Cadmium

Inhalation of cadmium fumes can cause acute or chronic disease of both the lungs and kidneys. This toxic metal is present in many foods and in cigarette tobacco. After ingestion or inhalation, it accumulates in the liver and kidneys.[618, 619] Acute exposure to a high concentration, usually of cadmium oxide which is evolved during the heating of

cadmium-coated metal with an oxyacetylene torch, results in metal fume fever (*see* page 2463) or in delayed acute pulmonary edema. Kidney stones[620] and renal glomerular and tubular damage also develop and may be fatal.[621, 622]

Cadmium workers tend to acquire physiologic and pathologic abnormalities resembling those of emphysema; it is not known whether they result from exposure to fumes or from coincidental cigarette smoking.[621] The lungs of patients with emphysema are reported to contain a significantly higher content of cadmium than unaffected lungs,[623] but since the patients with emphysema in a study by Hirst and associates included many heavy smokers and since cigarette smoke contains cadmium,[624] a cause-and-effect relationship has not been proved. However, experiments in which animals have been exposed to aerosols of cadmium alone have established beyond doubt that this metal is toxic. In one study of rats,[625] cellular injury and proliferation closely resembled the findings seen in ozone, nitrogen dioxide, and oxygen poisoning. In another study, Snider and his coworkers[626] produced bronchiolar lesions in rats by repeated exposure to cadmium chloride aerosol. Thurlbeck and Foley[627] instilled high concentrations of cadmium into the trachea of guinea pigs and produced "scar emphysema." However, despite some evidence that prolonged heavy inhalation of this metal in humans results in impairment of ventilatory function,[628–631] we find it difficult to accept that the acute lesions produced in these animal experiments are necessarily analagous to those of human emphysema.

The deleterious effects of cadmium may become manifest even after cessation of exposure. Bonnell[632] conducted a two-part study of men who worked for several years in a cadmium smelting plant. In 1953 he found a high incidence of pulmonary function impairment; a follow-up study of 100 of the men in 1959 uncovered 24 new cases of cadmium poisoning despite removal of the hazard after the original findings.[628] Of the 24 new cases, only 6 had evidence of pulmonary disease, 18 showing proteinuria only. Not all investigators have found evidence of emphysema: in one survey of 17 heavily exposed cadmium workers, Smith and associates[633] found a restrictive rather than an obstructive pulmonary function pattern; 5 of the 17 subjects showed evidence of pulmonary fibrosis roentgenographically. Other investigators have described similar physiologic and roentgenographic abnormalities.[634] Another survey of coppersmiths in Scotland who had been exposed to cadmium fumes revealed an incidence of restrictive disease greater than that observed in a control group: there was no evidence of fibrosis roentgenographically.[620] Pulmonary damage is not inevitable, even after substantial exposure to cadmium; Edling and associates[622] measured pulmonary function in cadmium workers exposed to a relatively high concentration (sufficient to cause kidney toxicity in 42 per cent) and found no evidence of pulmonary dysfunction in comparison with a control group.

Epoxides and Trimellitic Anhydride

The first description of respiratory tract disease caused by epoxy resins was by Do Pico and colleagues in 1975.[635] They described 210 rubber tire workers who developed conjunctivitis and bronchopulmonary disease that characteristically resolved while the affected individuals were on sick leave but recurred when they returned to work. Roughly one fourth of the patients revealed patchy pneumonitis and occasionally increased vascular markings, chiefly in the lower lobes. Over one third of the workers who were tested showed abnormal bronchial flow rates and diffusing capacity. Subsequent reports have described a syndrome consisting of hemoptysis, anemia,[636-639] and roentgenographic evidence of patchy airspace opacities resembling diffuse pulmonary edema. In one study,[638] diffusing capacity was increased, perhaps reflecting uptake of carbon monoxide by erythrocytes sequestered in alveoli.

Largely as a result of research emanating from Northwestern University Medical School, Chicago,[639-644] it now appears that the culpable agent is trimellitic anhydride (TMA), a low–molecular-weight reactive chemical widely used in the manufacture of plastics, epoxy resin coatings, and paints. Workers from this institution have described four syndromes induced by the inhalation of trimellitic anhydride dust or fumes: (1) an immediate-type airway response (asthma-rhinitis) that is mediated by IgE antibody directed against trimellityl-conjugated human respiratory tract proteins; (2) a late respiratory syndrome, characterized by cough, wheezing, dyspnea, myalgias, and arthralgias, that develops 4 to 12 hours after exposure (in this syndrome TMA reacts covalently with protein to form a hapten-protein complex that results in the induction of antibody, mostly IgG); (3) the TMA hemoptysis-anemia syndrome that develops following high-dose exposure to fumes when materials containing TMA are sprayed on heated metal surfaces (high levels of antibodies to trimellityl-human proteins and erythrocytes have been found in these patients); and (4) an occupational bronchitis resulting from direct irritant properties of TMA.[639-642]

The first three syndromes have a latent period between initial exposure and the onset of symptoms and there is good evidence, including the results of some experimental studies in animals, that they are immunologically mediated. Liu and associates[645] have described a system of protecting mice against TMA exposure by administering synthetic random copolymers of d-glutamic acid and d-lysine to which appropriate hapten is linked to produce antibodies. Similarly, Leach and coworkers[643] showed that the administration of cyclophosphamide protected rats from developing bronchopulmonary disease. It has been postulated[643] that a TMA antigen-antibody response within the lung activates complement, attracting polymorphonuclear leukocytes and macrophages that, in turn, induce pulmonary damage through the production of superoxide radicals. Biopsy specimens in two patients with the TMA hemoptysis-anemia syndrome showed alveolar hemorrhage and nonspecific damage of alveolar lining cells.[638, 641] In rats exposed to TMA and sacrificed at intervals,[644] BAL fluid and serum showed no evidence of lung injury or antibody response by day 2. There was evidence of minimal lung injury and low levels of antibody by day 6; by day 10, there was marked intra-alveolar hemorrhage, accumulation of inflammatory cells in alveolar septa, abundant alveolar macrophages, and evidence of endothelial and epithelial cell injury. Antibody levels in BAL fluid and serum were highly correlated with lung injury.

Limited information indicates that removal from exposure results in rapid disappearance of symptoms and a decrease in the levels of serum antibodies.[638, 642] Hypoxemia, which may be severe, and the restrictive functional defect revert to normal in patients with the hemoptysis-anemia syndrome.[638]

Fume Fevers

Metal fume fever results from inhalation of minute particles of the oxides of various metals formed during welding of galvanized iron or during cleaning of zinc-coated water tanks with a buffing machine.[646] Finely dispersed particles less than 1 micron in diameter develop when zinc, copper, magnesium, iron, cadmium, nickel, and various other metals are heated to 93° C or higher. Inhalation of the fumes results in an acute transitory illness characterized by sudden onset of thirst, a metallic taste in the mouth, irritation of the throat, substernal tightness, malaise, headache, muscle cramps, chills, and fever. Symptoms usually appear within 12 hours of exposure and subside within 24 hours without complications or sequelae. This illness has been reproduced in volunteers and in a patient with the clinical history of recurring zinc fume fever who underwent an experimental welding exposure.[647] Repeated exposure can result in increased tolerance, although re-exposure on Mondays after off-duty weekends is usually associated with a more severe episode. Moist rales and rhonchi may be heard on auscultation, and there is leukocytosis (20,000 or more leukocytes per cu mm) with neutrophilia. The chest roentgenogram either is normal or shows increased prominence of bronchovascular markings.

Polymer fume fever (synonym: polytetrafluoroethylene poisoning) is caused by inhalation of fumes that evolve as degradation products when polytetrafluoroethylene (Fluon, Teflon) is heated to high temperatures (above 250° C); the pyrolytic products of this plastic material have not been identified. Symptoms are similar to those of metal fume fever and include tightness in the chest, headache, shivering, fever, aching, weakness, and occasionally shortness of breath.[648] Two cases of pulmonary edema have been reported.[649, 650] In most reported cases in humans, fume inhalation has been associated with cigarette smoking;[648, 651] the high temperatures generated by the burning (879° C) are sufficient to produce pyrolysis products. In an influenza-like outbreak in a Massachusetts textile mill,[648] 7 of 13 employees exposed to fluorocarbon polymer developed symptoms; all were cigarette smokers. A case has been reported of a worker who had 40 episodes of fume fever before the cause was recognized.[651] In this instance and in the cases originating in the textile mill, episodes of fume fever disappeared after workers washed their hands thoroughly before they smoked cigarettes.

Formaldehyde

Increasing production and use of urea formaldehyde resins as adhesives in wood products (principally particleboard, fiberboard, and hardwood plywood) and as foam insulation in housing have made formaldehyde gas toxicity a subject of concern, perhaps more in the lay press than in the medical literature.[652, 653] Occupational exposure occurs in the manufacture of these substances, in carpentry shops,[654] and in those exposed to formalin in pathology departments[655] and mortician establishments.[656] In one study of 103 medical students exposed to low concentrations of formaldehyde during a 7-month anatomy course, no abnormalities of pulmonary function could be demonstrated, even in the 12 students who had pre-existing asthma.[657] Nonoccupational exposure occurs in buildings that contain furniture treated with urea formaldehyde foam insulation (UFFI).[658–660] The occupational health standard of 3 ppm[653] has been exceeded in mobile homes in which particleboard is used extensively.[661] Symptoms have been produced in atopic subjects exposed to 2 ppm of formaldehyde for 40 minutes in an environmental chamber.[662]

Formaldehyde is considered by some[653] to be an allergic (immunologically mediated) skin sensitizer that can also cause or exacerbate respiratory distress in individuals with pre-existing or formaldehyde-induced bronchial hyper-reactivity. Long-term studies over a period of 2 years have shown that rats and mice exposed to somewhat higher concentrations than the occupational standard of 3 ppm develop squamous cell carcinoma of the nasal passages;[663] however, a follow-up study of 136 formaldehyde plant workers employed for 1 month or more between 1950 and 1976 failed to reveal an increased incidence of nasal carcinoma or of excess deaths compared with controls.[664]

It is now generally accepted that exposure to formaldehyde can cause eye irritation, rhinitis, skin rash, and upper respiratory symptoms.[658, 659, 661] One author[652] has referred to the occasional case of acute pulmonary edema, and it is perhaps not surprising that such an occurrence might follow an acute high-level exposure. Only one study[654] has suggested any long-term pulmonary dysfunction from the inhalation of formaldehyde fumes, and several other studies have found no evidence of either acute or chronic impairment of pulmonary function.[652, 653, 656, 658–660, 662, 664] Nevertheless, we concur with the concern over possible long-term effects, particularly in people living in homes insulated with urea-formaldehyde foam.

Bronchopulmonary Disease Associated with Burns

Burns caused by fire are a major cause of morbidity and mortality in our society. Although the most significant pathophysiologic abnormalities that result are related to skin damage, secondary shock, and infection, pulmonary disease is also a common and important factor. The mechanisms of tracheal and bronchopulmonary damage are threefold, and assessment of the relative contribution of each can be extremely difficult in an individual patient.

(1) The inhalation of smoke and the variety of toxic chemicals it contains is a particularly important mechanism, especially within confined spaces. Smoke consists of gases and a suspension of small particles in hot air; the particles are composed of carbon that is coated with combustible products such as organic acids and aldehydes. The gaseous fraction has a highly variable composition depending on the material that is burning. Although most products of inhaled smoke are unidentified, carbon monoxide and carbon dioxide are the main constituents and are always present. A list of toxic combustion products of common materials has been published,[665] but only two are discussed here. *Cyanide* is a product of fires involving material such as nylon, asphalt, wool, silk, and polyurethane;[666] high carboxyhemoglobin levels correlate with high cyanide levels in the blood of fire survivors. *Polyvinyl chloride* (PVC), a plastic solid widely used as a rubber substitute for covering electric and telephone wire and cable and in many manufactured products,[667] has been implicated as a major cause of bronchopulmonary damage because of the release of hydrogen chloride gas when it burns. PVC degrades and releases hydrochloric acid at temperatures over 225° C. The effect of the acid in the gas phase is largely restricted to irritability and chiefly involves the upper respiratory tract. In a PVC fabricating plant, however, in which an extruding machine was overheated, exposed workers developed headache, nausea, and fainting; pulmonary function tests revealed restrictive impairment.[668] Loosely bound hydrochloric acid can condense on soot aerosol and thereby gain access to the lung parenchyma.

(2) Direct trauma due to heat can itself cause severe tissue damage, particularly to the mucous membranes of the upper respiratory tract. Although its relative contribution can be difficult to determine in patients injured in fires, damage can occur in situations in which there is no fire. For example, in an autopsy study of 27 individuals who died following the explosion of a steam tube in a ship's boiler room, Brinkman and Puschel[669] found that airway abnormalities extended from the trachea to the transitional airways and consisted of vacuolar swelling of epithelial cells and "coagulative" changes of the subepithelial connective tissue. The lung parenchyma showed capillary congestion and airspace hemorrhage and edema. Another example of heat-related damage to the tracheobronchial tree was reported by Jung and Gottlieb:[670] a drugged semicomatose patient aspirated hot coffee when his friends tried to revive him. Subsequent examination revealed roentgenographic evidence of pulmonary edema and burning of the mucosa distal to the trachea.

(3) In addition to the damage caused by heat and by the inhalation of smoke, pulmonary disease can be caused by the presence of coexistent shock, sepsis, renal failure, and the consequences of therapy, including overhydration.[671, 672]

The histopathologic changes observed in patients who have died within 48 hours of a fire include pulmonary congestion, edema, intravascular fibrin thrombi, and intra-alveolar hemorrhage.[673, 674] Ultrastructural studies have shown intracellular edema with focal bleb and vesicle formation in type I cells.[674] In both experimental animals and humans, smoke inhalation results in necrosis of tracheal and proximal bronchial epithelium;[675] although this change is probably diffuse in most cases, the injury occasionally results in the formation of localized endobronchial polyps composed of granulation tissue.[676] Carbon particles may be seen on the airway surface and provide a marker of inhalation. Atypical squamous cells, representing the result of reparative changes in the healing phase, can be identified in the sputum of many individuals.[677]

Pulmonary complications occur in 20 to 30 per cent of burn victims admitted to a hospital; of these, 70 to 75 per cent die.[678–681] The incidence correlates with the severity of the burn and with a history of being in an enclosed space.[679, 681, 682] During the first 24 hours, complications result from upper airway edema caused by direct heat injury or toxic products, usually in patients with head and neck burns.[683] After a latent period of 12 to 48 hours, symptoms and roentgenographic evidence of lower respiratory tract involvement develop.[684, 685] Complications that become evident 2 to 5 days after the burn consist of atelectasis, pulmonary edema, and pneumonia; the latter occurs much more frequently in the presence of inhalation injury. In a review of the records of 1,058 burn patients treated at a single institution over a 5-year period,[686] 373 (35 per cent) suffered inhalation injury diagnosed by bronchoscopy or ventilation/perfusion scintigraphy or both; 141 of these patients (38 per cent) subsequently developed pneumonia. Among the 685 patients without inhalation injury, pneumonia occurred in only 60 (8.8 per cent). Atelectasis can be caused by mucous plugging of large bronchi, presumably as a result of excessive smoke inhalation.[687] Complications that arise after 5 days include pulmonary embolism[688] and ARDS.[689] Peters[682] has stated that when tracheobronchitis occurs in patients with serious cutaneous burns, the mortality is exceedingly high, ranging from 48 to 86 per cent; a patient's condition usually follows a staged progression that is proportional to the extent and severity of the tracheobronchitis.

Putman and his colleagues[690] have described the roentgenographic findings in victims of acute smoke inhalation unassociated with skin burns; in 6 of 21 patients, chest roentgenograms obtained 4 to 24 hours after the incident revealed focal opacities that were interpreted as atelectasis and that usually cleared within 3 days. These authors[691] emphasized that the conventional chest roentgenogram is an insensitive means of determining pulmonary injury by smoke inhalation; from their study of 21 patients, they concluded that determination of blood carboxyhemoglobin and arterial blood gas levels is a more important parameter in clinical evaluation. However, Teixidor and colleagues[685] reviewed the chest roentgenograms of 62 patients who required admission to a hospital following smoke inhalation; 35 patients (62.5 per cent) developed pulmonary edema that, in most cases, appeared within 24 hours after the injury (Fig. 14–13).

Transient hypoxemia in firemen overcome by smoke inhalation is a common finding.[692] It might be expected that fire fighters who are repeatedly exposed to smoke will show cumulative lung damage. An initial follow-up of over 1,000 Boston fire fighters has demonstrated both clinical and physiologic evidence of impaired airway conductance (in addition to the effects ascribed to cigarette smoking).[693–695] However, a subsequent follow-up of this cohort of fire fighters at 3 years[696] failed to confirm the original impression: the annual decline was less than that observed over 1 year and could not be related to the number of fires fought or to other indices of acute fire exposure. In a separate study of lung function in retired fire fighters,[697] no evidence of severe impairment of respiratory function was identified over a 5-year follow-up period, although observed values were significantly lower than predicted. In addition, it was evident that subjects with respiratory complaints and impaired ventilatory capacity tended to be selectively removed from active fire fighting duty prior to retirement. Several other controlled studies,[698–702] in which pulmonary function has been assessed in fire fighters,

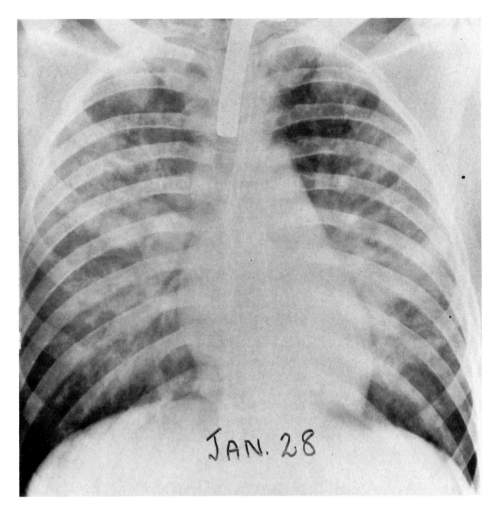

Figure 14–13. Acute Smoke Inhalation. This 30-year-old man was involved in a fire and inhaled large quantities of smoke before being rescued. He was brought to the emergency room in severe respiratory distress and a tracheostomy was required. An anteroposterior roentgenogram reveals massive consolidation of both lungs in a pattern characteristic of acute pulmonary edema. The patient had an uneventful recovery.

have failed to show short-term deterioration in function,[692] although they support the conclusion that a long-term risk of obstructive pulmonary disease exists in this occupation over and above that caused by cigarette smoking. An analysis of causes of death among 2,470 Boston fire fighters employed during the period 1915 to 1975 failed to reveal an association between occupation and cause-specific mortality.[703] By contrast, a determination of mortality by cause among 1,113 stationary engineers and firemen revealed an excess of deaths from cancer of the buccal cavity, pharynx, rectum, and lung; in the same study, no evidence for an increase in the frequency of deaths from nonmalignant respiratory disease was detected.[704]

Vinyl Chloride and Polyvinyl Chloride

Vinyl chloride (VC) and polyvinyl chloride (PVC) have been reported to cause pulmonary interstitial fibrosis and granulomatosis. The chief symptom is dyspnea, and pulmonary function tests have shown restrictive impairment.[705, 706] The roentgenographic pattern has been described as nodular or reticulonodular; in 20 (1.6 per cent) of 1,216 workers[707] and in 10 (1.2 per cent) of 818 workers[708]

exposed to PVC, profusion of opacities was described as 1/0 or greater, mostly of category p or s. Individuals who showed roentgenographic abnormalities had a history of greater exposure, of at least 5 years' duration in one report.[707] One study[709] of 509 workers exposed to PVC revealed no impairment of pulmonary function that could not be explained on the basis of cigarette consumption. Other investigators[705, 707, 708] have shown evidence of mild restrictive functional impairment.

Vinyl chloride is carcinogenic:[710] prolonged exposure to low concentrations has been shown to cause angiosarcoma of the liver,[711–713] and its monomer has been associated with an incidence of lung cancer that is higher than expected.[706, 710] An immunologically determined multisystem disorder manifested by Raynaud's phenomenon, acro-osteolysis, thrombocytopenia, portal fibrosis, and hepatic and pulmonary dysfunction also has been ascribed to PVC and VC (*see* page 2368).[714–716]

Carbon Monoxide

Carbon monoxide is an odorless gas formed by incomplete combustion of carbon-containing matter. It is produced in high concentration in fires, and inhalation of the gas is probably the most common cause of death in these circumstances. Other sources of carbon monoxide (CO) include faulty heaters, exhaust from automobiles, tobacco smoke, and mine explosions. More recently recognized sources are paint removers that contain methylene chloride (a solvent metabolized to carbon monoxide)[717] and briquets used in hibachis;[718] several fatalities have been reported following the burning of charcoal briquets within confined spaces such as trailers, station wagons, and cellars. A report from New York City[719] indicates that despite the increase in total gasoline use, the concentration of CO in large cities has remained stable and has possibly decreased since the turn of the century. This has resulted from improvements in the efficiency of internal combustion engines, changes in the types of fuel used for space heating and electrical generation, and the replacement of manufactured gas by natural gas.

The deleterious effects of carbon monoxide in humans appear to be attributable to two factors: (1) tissue hypoxia resulting from the formation of carboxyhemoglobin (COHb), which reduces the oxygen transport capacity of the blood and causes a shift of the oxyhemoglobin dissociation curve to the left, thus curtailing the amount of oxygen available to the tissues; and (2) a direct cytotoxic effect. Characteristically, clinical symptoms develop when carboxyhemoglobin saturation reaches 20 per cent; unconsciousness occurs at about 60 per cent and death at about 80 per cent. If acute carbon monoxide poisoning does not end fatally, follow-up studies have demonstrated neurologic damage characterized by personality deterioration and memory impairment.[720]

Of possibly even greater significance than acute carbon monoxide poisoning is the morbidity associated with long-term exposure to low concentrations of this gas. The blood carboxyhemoglobin level of healthy nonsmoking individuals is roughly 0.5 per cent, a figure that rises to about 3 per cent with increased hemolysis.[721] By contrast, the average COHb of a smoker who smokes one pack a day is 5.9 per cent,[722] a figure that may rise to between 10 and 20 per cent with heavy smoking.[721, 723] It is obvious that such individuals will develop significant hypoxia, particularly if they live at high altitudes. The percentage of inspired carbon monoxide may be increased in heavy traffic, since car exhausts contain between 1 and 7 per cent CO,[724] and it may also rise in closed breathing circuits such as during anesthesia or in closed air systems such as submarines.[722] It has been shown that blood levels of COHb less than 2 per cent may result in interference with time-duration discrimination, and that automobile drivers involved in accidents have higher levels of COHb than controls.[722] Experimental studies in animals[721] suggest that carbon monoxide may play a role in the formation of atheroma, and investigations in humans have shown that low

levels of CO increase myocardial ischemia and induce angina after less cardiac work than is required by control patients breathing room air.[725, 726]

In acute carbon monoxide poisoning, abnormalities may be detected on the chest roentgenogram. In a study of 62 patients observed over a 2-year period, Sone and associates[727] observed abnormalities in 18 (30 per cent). The age range of the 14 males and 48 females was 1 to 84 years (mean, 30.8 ± 4.2 years). The most common roentgenographic abnormality, observed in 11 of the 18 cases, was a ground-glass opacity of homogeneous density occurring predominantly in the peripheral zones of the lungs. An air bronchogram was not identified nor was there evidence of pulmonary venous hypertension. This change was attributed by the authors to parenchymal interstitial edema, probably caused by a combination of tissue hypoxia and a direct toxic effect of carbon monoxide on the alveolocapillary membrane. The second most common change, observed in six cases, was a parahilar haze and peribronchial and perivascular cuffing caused by interstitial edema. In these cases, there was usually an associated cardiac enlargement suggesting the presence of myocardial damage secondary to carbon monoxide toxicity. In some cases, the ground-glass appearance, parahilar haze, vascular cuffing, and cardiac enlargement coexisted in various combinations. Intra-alveolar edema was identified in three patients, all of whom had convincing evidence of cardiac enlargement. In this series, hyperbaric oxygen therapy, at a pressure of 2 absolute atmospheres, was administered to all patients immediately after admission. Roentgenographic abnormalities cleared in most patients by 3 days and in all by 5 days; however, the presence of parahilar haze or intra-alveolar edema signified a poor overall prognosis despite roentgenographic resolution. Cases of acute pulmonary edema following carbon monoxide intoxication have also been reported by others.[728, 729]

A patient has been described who became comatose and developed pulmonary edema following exposure to CO;[729] the wedge pressure was normal and protein-rich edema fluid was aspirated from his trachea, establishing the edema as permeability in type. These authors exposed rabbits to CO and caused capillary leakage. Electron microscopic examination revealed swelling of epithelial and endothelial cells, interstitial edema, and depletion of lamellar bodies in alveolar type II cells.

Thesaurosis

In its broad connotation, this term designates storage in the body of unusual amounts of normal or foreign material. However, since the original descriptions of thesaurosis by Bergmann and associates in 1958 and 1962,[730, 731] the term has become restricted to pulmonary disease resulting from the inhalation of hair spray and characterized by a granulomatous pulmonary infiltration resembling sarcoidosis.

There has been some dispute about the existence of this condition, some authors having speculated that it simply represents sarcoidosis in an individual who happens to use hair spray.[732] The basis for this dispute is related in part to the following four points:

(1) Intracutaneous injection of hair spray into experimental animals results in the local accumulation of macrophages.[733] In addition, examination of macrophages inoculated with hair spray in cell culture has shown morphologic evidence of ingestion of the substance and of macrophage activation.[733, 734] Despite these observations that suggest a cellular reaction to hair spray, inhalation studies in dogs,[426] rats, and guinea pigs[735] have failed to show evidence of significant pulmonary disease.

(2) Some roentgenologic studies have found evidence for an increased prevalence of pulmonary disease in beauticians; for example, in one follow-up study of these individuals, Gowdy and Wagstaff[736] found that 21 per cent had abnormal chest roentgenograms when first seen and that 40 per cent showed abnormalities 4 years later.

(3) The roentgenographic pattern in some individuals with supposed thesaurosis consists of a diffuse fine micronodularity simulating the pattern seen in alveolar microlithiasis and talcosis of intravenous drug abuse;[737] such an appearance is unusual (but not unknown) in sarcoidosis, especially in the presence of cough and dyspnea which most reported patients with thesaurosis have. In addition, the original patients described by Bergmann and his colleagues[738, 739] manifested roentgenographic changes identical to those of sarcoidosis.

(4) Roentgenographic clearing and symptomatic improvement tend to occur fairly rapidly following discontinuance of exposure to hair spray, and the number of reported cases in which this has occurred suggests a causal relationship.[737] However, it has been argued that again this might be a coincidental phenomenon,[732] since in many cases sarcoidosis is associated with spontaneous remission in the absence of therapy.

Considering these points, it seems reasonable to conclude that hair spray-induced pulmonary disease may exist and should be considered in an individual with appropriate roentgenographic and pathologic abnormalities and a history of excessive exposure to the substance. It must be remembered, however, that sarcoidosis is a relatively common disease and that despite the widespread use of hair spray, only a small number of cases of possible thesaurosis have been reported. The possibility of sarcoidosis developing in an individual who happens to use hair spray, therefore, should be carefully excluded before a diagnosis of thesaurosis is accepted.

Histologically, cases reported as thesaurosis have shown interstitial inflammation predominantly in a peribronchial location but also to some extent in the parenchyma. The inflammatory infiltrate consists of lymphocytes and numerous multinucleated giant cells, the latter frequently containing PAS-positive material; granulomas are also described and in some instances are indistinguishable from those seen in sarcoidosis.

Schraufnagel and his colleagues[737] have reported a radiologic/pathologic correlative study of two patients who admitted using an inordinate quantity of hair spray. Pathologically, both patients manifested interstitial granulomas indistinguishable from sarcoidosis. Roentgenographically, the pattern was similar in the two patients; it consisted of a fine micronodularity distributed widely throughout both lungs. In a review of 31 cases in the literature, these authors found that 8 cases manifested a micronodular pattern roentgenographically similar to their own two patients. Roentgenographic clearing tends to occur fairly rapidly following discontinuance of exposure; a favorable response also has been observed with corticosteroid therapy.[737]

REFERENCES

1. Brettner A, Heitzman ER, Woodin WG: Pulmonary complications of drug therapy. Radiology 96:31, 1970.
2. Fazen LE III, Lovejoy FH Jr, Crone RK: Acute poisoning in a children's hospital: A 2-year experience. Pediatrics 77:144, 1986.
3. Rosenow EC III: The spectrum of drug-induced pulmonary disease. Ann Intern Med 77:977, 1972.
4. Demeter SL, Ahmad M, Tomashefski JF: Drug-induced pulmonary disease. Part I. Patterns of response. Part II. Categories of drugs. Part III. Agents used to treat neoplasms or alter the immune system including a brief review of radiation therapy. Clev Clin Q 46:89, 1979.
5. Seltzer SE, Herman PG: Drug-induced pulmonary reactions associated with abnormal chest radiograph. JCE Radiol 1:25, 1979.
6. Sostman HD, Putman CE, Gamsu G: Diagnosis of chemotherapy lung. Am J Roentgenol 136:33, 1981.
7. Batist G, Andrews JL Jr: Pulmonary toxicity of antineoplastic drugs. JAMA 246:1449, 1981.
8. Morrison DA, Goldman AL: Radiographic patterns of drug-induced lung disease. Radiology 131:299, 1979.
9. Lippman M: Pulmonary reactions to drugs. Med Clin North Am 61:1353, 1977.
10. Weiss RB, Muggia FM: Cytotoxic drug-induced pulmonary disease: Update 1980. Am J Med 68:259, 1980.
11. Filipek WJ: Drug-induced pulmonary disease. Postgrad Med 65:131, 139, 1979.
12. Whitcomb ME, Domby WR: Drug-induced lung disease. Primary Care 5:411, 1978.
13. Cooper JAD Jr, White DA, Matthay RA: Drug-induced pulmonary disease. Part 1: Cytotoxic drugs. Am Rev Respir Dis 133:321, 1986.
14. Cooper JAD Jr, White DA, Matthay RA: Drug-induced pulmonary disease. Part 2: Noncytotoxic drugs. Am Rev Respir Dis 133:488, 1986.
15. Bennett JM, Reich SD: Bleomycin. Ann Intern Med 90:945, 1979.
16. Yagoda A, Mukherji B, Young C, et al: Bleomycin. An antitumor antibiotic: Clinical experience in 274 patients. Ann Intern Med 77:861, 1972.
17. Holoye PY, Luna MA, MacKay B, et al: Bleomycin hypersensitivity pneumonitis. Ann Intern Med 88:47, 1978.
18. Yousem SA, Lifson JD, Colby TV: Chemotherapy-induced eosinophilic pneumonia: Relation to bleomycin. Chest 88:103, 1985.
19. Samuels ML, Johnson DE, Holoye PY, et al: Large-dose bleomycin therapy and pulmonary toxicity: A possible role of prior radiotherapy. JAMA 235:1117, 1976.
20. Iacovino JR, Leitner J, Abbas AK, et al: Fatal pulmonary reaction from low doses of bleomycin. An idiosyncratic tissue response. JAMA 235:1253, 1976.
21. Pascual RS, Mosher MB, Sikand RS, et al: Effects of bleomycin on pulmonary function in man. Am Rev Respir Dis 108:211, 1973.
22. Phan SH, Fantone JC: Inhibition of bleomycin-induced pulmonary fibrosis by lipopolysaccharide. Lab Invest 50:587, 1984.
23. Berend N: Protective effect of hypoxia on bleomycin lung toxicity in the rat. Am Rev Respir Dis 130:307, 1984.
24. Tryka AF, Skornik WA, Godleski JJ, et al: Potentiation of bleomycin-induced lung injury by exposure to 70% oxygen. Am Rev Respir Dis 126:1074, 1982.
25. Goldiner PL, Carlon GC, Cvitkovic E, et al: Factors influencing postoperative morbidity and mortality in patients treated with bleomycin. Br Med J 1:1664, 1978.
26. Oxorn DC, Chung DC, Lam AM: Continuous in-vivo monitoring of arterial oxygen tension in a patient treated with bleomycin. Can Anaesth Soc J 31:200, 1984.
27. Moseley PL, Shasby DM, Brady M, et al: Lung parenchymal injury induced by bleomycin. Am Rev Respir Dis 130:1082, 1984.
28. Thrall RS, Barton RW, D'Amato DA, et al: Differential cellular analysis of bronchoalveolar lavage fluid obtained at various stages during the development of bleomycin-induced pulmonary fibrosis in the rat. Am Rev Respir Dis 126:488, 1982.
29. Fahey PJ, Utell MJ, Mayewski RJ, et al: Early diagnosis of bleomycin pulmonary toxicity using bronchoalveolar lavage in dogs. Am Rev Respir Dis 126:126, 1982.
30. Clark JG, Kuhn C III: Bleomycin-induced pulmonary fibrosis in hamsters: Effect of neutrophil depletion on lung collagen synthesis. Am Rev Respir Dis 126:737, 1982.
31. Phan SH, Thrall RS: Inhibition of bleomycin-induced pulmonary fibrosis by cobra venom factor. Am J Pathol 107:25, 1982.
32. Perez-Guerra F, Harkleroad LE, Walsh RE, et al: Acute bleomycin lung. Am Rev Respir Dis 106:909, 1972.
33. Brown WG, Hasan FM, Barbee RA: Reversibility of severe bleomycin-induced pneumonitis. JAMA 239:2012, 1978.
34. Fleischman RW, Baker JR, Thompson BR, et al: Bleomycin-induced interstitial pneumonia in dogs. Thorax 26:675, 1971.
35. Collins JF, McCullough B, Coalson JJ, et al: Bleomycin-induced diffuse interstitial pulmonary fibrosis in baboons: II. Further studies on connective tissue changes. Am Rev Respir Dis 123:305, 1981.
36. Luna MA, Bedrossian CWM, Lichtiger B, et al: Interstitial pneumonitis associated with bleomycin therapy. Am J Clin Pathol 58:501, 1972.
37. Jones AW: Bleomycin lung damage: The pathology and nature of the lesion. Br J Dis Chest 72:321, 1978.
38. Luursema PB, Star-Kroesen MA, van der Mark TW, et al: Bleomycin-induced changes in the carbon monoxide transfer factor of the lungs and its components. Am Rev Respir Dis 128:880, 1983.
39. Sorensen PG, Romer FK, Cortes D: Angiotensin-converting enzyme: An indicator of bleomycin-induced pulmonary toxicity in humans. Eur J Cancer Clin Oncol 20:1405, 1984.
40. Adamson IYR, Bowden DH: Bleomycin-induced injury and metaplasia of alveolar type 2 cells. Relationship of cellular responses to drug presence in the lung. Am J Pathol 96:531, 1979.
41. Balikian JP, Jochelson MS, Bauer KA, et al: Pulmonary complications of chemotherapy regimens containing bleomycin. Am J Roentgenol 139:455, 1982.
42. Glasier CM, Siegel MJ: Multiple pulmonary nodules: Unusual manifestation of bleomycin toxicity. Am J Roentgenol 137:155, 1981.
43. McCrea ES, Diaconis JN, Wade JC, et al: Bleomycin toxicity simulating metastatic nodules to the lungs. Cancer 48:1096, 1981.
44. Glasier CM, Siegel MJ: Multiple pulmonary nodules: Unusual manifestation of bleomycin toxicity. Am J Roentgenol 137:155, 1981.
45. Dineen MK, Englander LS, Huben RP: Bleomycin-induced nodular pulmonary fibrosis masquerading as metastatic testicular cancer. J Urol 136:473, 1986.
46. Lewis BM, Izbicki R: Routine pulmonary function tests during bleomycin therapy: Tests may be ineffective and potentially misleading. JAMA 243:347, 1980.
47. Bell MR, Meredith DJ, Gill PG: Role of carbon monoxide diffusing capacity in the early detection of major bleomycin-induced pulmonary toxicity. Aust NZ J Med 15:235, 1985.
48. Van Barneveld PWC, van der Mark TW, Sleijfer DT, et al: Predictive factors for bleomycin-induced pneumonitis. Am Rev Respir Dis 130:1078, 1984.
49. Ginsberg SJ, Comis RL: The pulmonary toxicity of antineoplastic agents. Semin Oncol 9:34, 1982.
50. Dee GJ, Austin JH, Mutter GL: Bleomycin-associated pulmonary fibrosis: Rapidly fatal progression without chest radiotherapy. J Surg Oncol 35:135, 1987.
51. Van Barneveld PWC, Sleijfer DT, van der Mark TW, et al: Natural course of bleomycin-induced pneumonitis: A follow-up study. Am Rev Respir Dis 135:48, 1987.
52. Phan SH, Thrall RS, Williams C: Bleomycin-induced pulmonary fibrosis: Effects of steroid on lung collagen metabolism. Am Rev Respir Dis 124:428, 1981.
53. Fielding JWL, Stockley RA, Brookes VS: Interstitial lung disease in a patient treated with 5-fluorouracil and mitomycin C. Br Med J 2:602, 1978.
54. Gunstream SR, Seidenfeld JJ, Sobonya RE, et al: Mitomycin-associated lung disease. Cancer Treat Rep 67:301, 1983.
55. Budzar AU, Legha SS, Luna MA, et al: Pulmonary toxicity of mitomycin. Cancer 45:236, 1980.
56. Orwoll ES, Kiessling PJ, Patterson JR: Interstitial pneumonia from mitomycin. Ann Intern Med 89:352, 1978.
57. Budzar AU, Legha SS, Luna MA, et al: Pulmonary toxicity of mitomycin. Cancer 45:236, 1980.
58. Jolivet J, Giroux L, Laurin S, et al: Microangiopathic hemolytic anemia, renal failure, and noncardiogenic pulmonary edema: A chemotherapy-induced syndrome. Cancer Treat Rep 67:429, 1983.
59. Shinkai T, Saijo N, Tominaga K, et al: Pulmonary toxicity induced by pepleomycin 3-[(S)-1-phenylethylaminol propylamino-bleomycin. Jpn J Clin Oncol 13:395, 1983.
60. Selzer SE, Griffin T, D'Orsi C, et al: Pulmonary reaction associated with neocarzinostatin therapy. Cancer Treat Rep 62:1271, 1978.
61. Oliner H, Schwartz R, Rubio F, et al: Interstitial pulmonary fibrosis following busulfan therapy. Am J Med 31:134, 1961.

62. Leake E, Smith WG, Woodliff HJ: Diffuse interstitial pulmonary fibrosis after busulphan therapy. Lancet 2:432, 1963.

63. Heard BE, Cooke RA: Busulphan lung. Thorax 23:187, 1968.

64. Burns WA, McFarland W, Matthews MJ: Busulphan-induced pulmonary disease. Report of a case and review of the literature. Am Rev Respir Dis 101:408, 1970.

65. Bates DV, Macklem PT, Christie RV: Respiratory Function in Disease; An Introduction to the Integrated Study of the Lung. 2nd ed. Philadelphia, WB Saunders Co, 1971.

66. Soble AR, Perry H: Fatal radiation pneumonia following subclinical busulfan injury. Am J Roentgenol 128:15, 1977.

67. Koss LG, Melamed MR, Mayer K: The effect of busulfan on human epithelia. Am J Clin Pathol 44:385, 1965.

68. Littler WA, Kay JM, Hastleton PS, et al: Busulphan lung. Thorax 24:639, 1969.

69. Kirschner RH, Esterly JR: Pulmonary lesions associated with busulfan therapy of chronic myelogenous leukemia. Cancer 27:1074, 1971.

70. Kuplic JB, Higley CS, Niewoehner DE: Pulmonary ossification associated with long-term busulfan therapy in chronic myeloid leukemia. Case report. Am Rev Respir Dis 106:759, 1972.

71. Miyashita T, Ojima A, Tuji T, et al: Varied pulmonary lesions with intra-alveolar large lamellar bodies in an autopsy case with busulfan therapy. Acta Pathol Jpn 27:239, 1977.

72. Aymard J-P, Gyger M, Lavallee R, et al: A case of pulmonary alveolar proteinosis complicating chronic myelogenous leukemia: A peculiar pathologic aspect of busulfan lung? Cancer 53:954, 1984.

73. Smalley RV, Wall RL: Two cases of busulfan toxicity. Ann Intern Med 64:154, 1966.

74. Harrold BP: Syndrome resembling Addison's disease following prolonged treatment with busulphan. Br Med J 1:463, 1966.

75. Podoll LN, Winkler SS: Busulfan lung. Report of two cases and review of the literature. Am J Roentgenol 120:151, 1974.

76. Littler WA, Ogilvie C: Lung function in patients receiving busulphan. Br Med J 4:530, 1970.

77. Collis CH: Lung damage from cytotoxic drugs. Cancer Chemother Pharmacol 4:17, 1980.

78. Gould VE, Miller J: Sclerosing alveolitis induced by cyclophosphamide. Ultrastructural observations on alveolar injury and repair. Am J Pathol 81:513, 1975.

79. Maxwell I: Reversible pulmonary edema following cyclophosphamide treatment. JAMA 229:137, 1974.

80. Hakkinen PJ, Whiteley JW, Witschi HR: Hyperoxia, but not thoracic x-irradiation, potentiates bleomycin and cyclophosphamide-induced lung damage in mice. Am Rev Respir Dis 126:281, 1982.

81. Trask CW, Joannides T, Harper PG, et al: Radiation-induced lung fibrosis after treatment of small cell carcinoma of the lung with very high-dose cyclophosphamide. Cancer 55:47, 1985.

82. Burke DA, Stoddart JC, Ward MK, et al: Fatal pulmonary fibrosis occurring during treatment with cyclophosphamide. Br Med J 285:696, 1982.

83. Alvarado CS, Boat TF, Newman AJ: Late-onset pulmonary fibrosis and chest deformity in two children treated with cyclophosphamide. J Pediatr 92:443, 1978.

84. Spector JI, Zimbler H, Ross JS: Early-onset cyclophosphamide-induced interstitial pneumonitis. JAMA 242:2852, 1979.

85. Abdel Karim FW, Ayash RE, Allam C, et al: Pulmonary fibrosis after prolonged treatment with low-dose cyclophosphamide: A case report. Oncology 40:174, 1983.

86. Mark GJ, Lehimgar-Zadeh A, Ragsdale BD: Cyclophosphamide pneumonitis. Thorax 33:89, 1978.

87. Spector JI, Zimbler H, Ross JS: Cyclophosphamide and interstitial pneumonitis. JAMA 243:1131, 1980.

88. Refvem O: Fatal intra-alveolar and interstitial lung fibrosis in chlorambucil-treated chronic lymphocytic leukemia. Mt Sinai J Med NY 44:847, 1977.

89. Cole SR, Myers TJ, Klatsky AU: Pulmonary disease with chlorambucil therapy. Cancer 41:455, 1978.

90. Godard P, Marty JP, Michel FB: Interstitial pneumonia and chlorambucil. Chest 76:471, 1979.

91. Clinicopathological conference. Two cases of drug-induced disease. Demonstration at the Royal College of Physicians of London. Br Med J 2:1405, 1978.

92. Lane SD, Besa EC, Justh G, et al: Fatal interstitial pneumonitis following high-dose intermittent chlorambucil therapy for chronic lymphocytic leukemia. Cancer 47:32, 1981.

93. Major PP, Laurin S, Bettez P: Pulmonary fibrosis following therapy with melphalan: Report of two cases. Can Med Assoc J 123:197, 1980.

94. Taetle R, Dickman PS, Feldman PS, et al: Pulmonary histopathologic changes associated with melphalan therapy. Cancer 42:1239, 1978.

95. Codling BW, Chakera TM: Pulmonary fibrosis following therapy with melphalan for multiple myeloma. J Clin Pathol 25:668, 1972.

96. Goucher G, Rowland V, Hawkins J: Melphalan-induced pulmonary interstitial fibrosis. Chest 77:805, 1980.

97. Westerfield BT, Michalski JP, McCombs C, et al: Reversible melphalan-induced lung damage. Am J Med 68:767, 1980.

98. Ryan BR, Walters TR: Pulmonary fibrosis: A complication of 1,3-bis(2-chloroethyl)-1-nitrosourea (BCNU) therapy. Cancer 48:909, 1981.

99. Durant JR, Norgard, MJ, Murad TM, et al: Pulmonary toxicity associated with bischloroethylnitrosourea (BCNU). Ann Intern Med 90:191, 1979.

100. Selker RG, Jacobs SA, Moore PB: BCNU (1,3-bis(2-chloroethyl)-1-nitrosourea) induced pulmonary fibrosis. Neurosurgery 7:560, 1980.

101. Wolff SN, Phillips GL, Herzig GP: High-dose carmustine with autologous bone marrow transplantation for the adjuvant treatment of high-grade gliomas of the central nervous system. Cancer Treat Rep 71:183, 1987.

102. Aronin PA, Mahalev MS Jr, Rudnick SA, et al: Prediction of BCNU pulmonary toxicity in patients with malignant gliomas: An assessment of risk factors. N Engl J Med 303:83, 1980.

103. Melato M, Tuveri G: Pulmonary fibrosis following low-dose 1,3-bis(2-chloroethyl)-1-nitrosourea (BCNU) therapy. Cancer 45:1311, 1980.

104. Weinstein AS, Diener-West M, Nelson DF, et al: Pulmonary toxicity of carmustine in patients treated for malignant glioma. Cancer Treat Rep 70:943, 1986.

105. Bellot PA, Valdiserri RO: Multiple pulmonary lesions in a patient treated with BCNU (1,3-bis(2-chloroethyl)-1-nitrosourea) for glioblastoma multiforme. Cancer 43:46, 1979.

106. Patten GA, Billi JE, Rotman HH: Rapidly progressive fatal pulmonary fibrosis induced by carmustine. JAMA 244:687, 1980.

107. Mitsudo SM, Greenwald ES, Banerji B, et al: BCNU (1,3-bis(2-chloroethyl)-1-nitrosourea) lung: Drug-induced pulmonary changes. Cancer 54:751, 1984.

108. Cordonnier C, Vernant J-P, Mital P, et al: Pulmonary fibrosis subsequent to high doses of CCNU for chronic myeloid leukemia. Cancer 51:1814, 1983.

109. Dent RG: Fatal pulmonary toxic effects of lomustine. Thorax 37:627, 1982.

110. Lee W, Moore RP, Wampler GL: Interstitial pulmonary fibrosis as a complication of prolonged methyl-CCNU therapy. Cancer Treat Rep 62:1355, 1978.

111. Zimmerman MS, Ruckdeschel JC, Hussain M: Chemotherapy-induced interstitial pneumonitis during treatment of small cell anaplastic lung cancer. J Clin Oncol 2:396, 1984.

112. White DA, Orenstein M, Godwin TA, et al: Chemotherapy-associated pulmonary toxic reactions during treatment for breast cancer. Arch Intern Med 144:953, 1984.

113. Rao SX, Ramaswamy G, Levin M, et al: Fatal acute respiratory failure after vinblastine-mitomycin therapy in lung carcinoma. Arch Intern Med 145:1905, 1985.

114. Luedke D, McLaughlin TT, Daughaday C, et al: Mitomycin C and vindesine associated pulmonary toxicity with variable clinical expression. Cancer 55:542, 1985.

115. Bott SJ, Stewart FM, Prince-Fiocco MA: Interstitial lung disease associated with vindesine and radiation therapy for carcinoma of the lung. South Med J 79:894, 1986.

116. Cersosimo RJ, Licciardello JT, Matthews SJ, et al: Acute pneumonitis associated with MOPP chemotherapy of Hodgkin's disease. Drug Intell Clin Pharm 18:609, 1984.

117. Ecker MD, Jay B, Keohane MF: Procarbazine lung. Am J Roentgenol 131:527, 1978.

118. Lien HH, Brodahl U, Telhaug R, et al: Pulmonary changes at computed tomography in patients with testicular carcinoma treated with cis-platinum, vinblastine and bleomycin. Acta Radiol (Diagn) 26:507, 1985.

119. Clarysse AM, Cathey WJ, Cartwright GE, et al: Pulmonary disease complicating intermittent therapy with methotrexate. JAMA 209:1861, 1969.

120. Whitcomb ME, Schwarz MI, Tormey DC: Methotrexate pneumonitis: Case report and review of the literature. Thorax 27:636, 1972.

121. Filip DJ, Logue GL, Harle TS, et al: Pulmonary and hepatic complications of methotrexate therapy of psoriasis. JAMA 216:881, 1971.

122. Schwartz IR, Kajani MK: Methotrexate therapy and pulmonary disease. JAMA 210:1924, 1969.

123. Goldman GC, Moschella SL: Severe pneumonitis occurring during methotrexate therapy. Report of two cases. Arch Dermatol 103:194, 1971.

124. Henderson J, Paré JAP: Unpublished data, 1976.

125. Bedrossian CWM, Miller WC, Luna MA: Methotrexate-induced diffuse interstitial pulmonary fibrosis. South Med J 72:313, 1979.

126. Kaplan RL, Waite DH: Progressive interstitial lung disease from prolonged methotrexate therapy. Arch Dermatol 114:1800, 1978.

127. Phillips TJ, Wallis PJ, Jones DH, et al: Pulmonary function in patients on long-term, low-dose methotrexate. Br J Dermatol 115:657, 1986.

128. Phillips TJ, Jones DH, Baker H: Pulmonary complications following methotrexate therapy. J Am Acad Dermatol 16(2 Pt 1):373, 1987.

129. St Clair EW, Rice JR, Snyderman R: Pneumonitis complicating low-dose methotrexate therapy in rheumatoid arthritis. Arch Intern Med 145:2035, 1985.

130. Carson CW, Cannon GW, Egger MJ, et al: Pulmonary disease during the treatment of rheumatoid arthritis with low-dose pulse methotrexate. Semin Arthritis Rheum 16:186, 1987.

131. Cannon GW, Ward JR, Clegg DO, et al: Acute lung disease associated with low-dose pulse methotrexate therapy in patients with rheumatoid arthritis. Arthritis Rheum 26:1269, 1983.

132. Engelbrecht JA, Calhoon SL, Scherrer JJ: Methotrexate pneumonitis after low-dose therapy for rheumatoid arthritis. Arthritis Rheum 26:1275, 1983.

133. Geller M, Flaherty DK, Dickie HA, et al: Lymphopenia in acute nitrofurantoin pleuropulmonary reactions. J Allergy Clin Immunol 59:445, 1977.

134. Cooperative study: Acute lymphocytic leukemia in children. Maintenance therapy with methotrexate administered intermittently. Acute leukemia group B. JAMA 207:923, 1969.

135. Ridley MG, Wolfe CS, Mathews JA: Life-threatening acute pneumonitis during low-dose methotrexate treatment for rheumatoid arthritis: A case report and review of the literature. Ann Rheum Dis 47:784, 1988.

136. Everts CS, Westcott JL, Bragg DG: Methotrexate therapy and pulmonary disease. Radiology 107:539, 1973.

137. Sostman HD, Matthay RA, Putman CE, et al: Methotrexate-induced pneumonitis. Medicine 55:371, 1976.

138. Lisbona A, Schwartz J, Lachance C, et al: Methotrexate-induced pulmonary disease. J Can Assoc Radiol 24:215, 1973.

139. Robertson HH: Medical memoranda. Pneumonia and methotrexate. Br Med J 2:156, 1970.

140. Colsky J, Greenspan EM, Warren TN: Hepatic fibrosis in children with acute leukemia after therapy with folic acid antagonists. Arch Pathol 59:198, 1955.

141. Muller SA, Farrow GM, Martalock DL: Clinical studies. Cirrhosis caused by methotrexate in the treatment of psoriasis. Arch Dermatol 100:523, 1969.

142. Epstein EH Jr, Croft JD Jr: Cirrhosis following methotrexate administration for psoriasis. Arch Dermatol 100:531, 1969.

143. Coe RO, Bull FE: Cirrhosis associated with methotrexate treatment of psoriasis. JAMA 206:1515, 1968.

144. Manni JJ, Van den Broek P: Pulmonary complications of methotrexate therapy. Clin Otolaryngol 2:131, 1977.

145. Weisenburger DD: Interstitial pneumonia associated with azathioprine therapy. J Clin Pathol 69:181, 1978.

146. Krowka MJ, Breuer RI, Kehoe TJ: Azathioprine-associated pulmonary dysfunction. Chest 83:696, 1983.

147. Bedrossian CWM, Sussman J, Conklin RH, et al: Azathioprine-associated interstitial pneumonitis. Am J Clin Pathol 82:148, 1984.

148. Hewlett RI, Wilson AF: Adult respiratory distress syndrome (ARDS) following aggressive management of extensive acute lymphoblastic leukemia. Cancer 39:2422, 1977.

149. Andersson BS, Cogan BM, Keating MJ, et al: Subacute pulmonary failure complicating therapy with high-dose ara-C in acute leukemia. Cancer 56:2181, 1985.

150. Haupt HM, Hutchins GM, Moore GW: Ara-C lung: Noncardiogenic pulmonary edema complicating cytosine arabinoside therapy of leukemia. Am J Med 70:256, 1981.

151. Bacigalupo A, Frassoni F, van Lint MT, et al: Cyclosporin A in marrow transplantation for leukemia and aplastic anemia. Exp Hematol 13:244, 1985.

152. Koch-Weser J, Sidel VW, Dexter M, et al: Adverse reactions to sulfisoxazole, sulfamethoxazole and nitrofurantoin, manifestations and specific reaction rates during 2,118 courses of therapy. Arch Intern Med 128:399, 1971.

153. Muir DCF, Stanton JA: Allergic pulmonary infiltration due to nitrofurantoin. Br Med J 1:1072, 1963.

154. Murray MJ, Kronenberg R: Pulmonary reactions simulating cardiac pulmonary edema caused by nitrofurantoin. N Engl J Med 273:1185, 1965.

155. Rosenow EC 3rd, DeRemee RA, Dines DE: Chronic nitrofurantoin pulmonary reaction. Report of five cases. N Engl J Med 279:1258, 1968.

156. Hailey FJ, Glascock HW Jr, Hewitt WF: Pleuropneumonic reactions to nitrofurantoin. N Engl J Med 281:1087, 1969.

157. Bone RC, Wolfe J, Sobonyar RE, et al: Desquamative interstitial pneumonia following chronic nitrofurantoin therapy. Chest 69(Suppl):296, 1976.

158. Simonian SJ, Kroeker EJ, Boyd DP: Chronic interstitial pneumonitis with fibrosis after long-term therapy with nitrofurantoin. Ann Thorac Surg 24:284, 1977.

159. Taskinen E, Tukiainen P, Sovijarvi AR: Nitrofurantoin-induced alterations in pulmonary tissue: A report on five patients with acute or subacute reactions. Acta Pathol Microbiol Scand (A) 85:713, 1977.

160. Holmberg L, Boman G, Bottiger LE, et al: Adverse reactions to nitrofurantoin: Analysis of 921 reports. Am J Med 69:733, 1980.

161. Averbuch SD, Yungbluth P: Fatal pulmonary hemorrhage due to nitrofurantoin. Arch Intern Med 140:271, 1980.

162. Israel RH, Gross RA, Bomba PA: Adult respiratory distress syndrome associated with acute nitrofurantoin toxicity: Successful treatment with continuous positive airway pressure. Respiration 39:318, 1980.

163. Willcox PA, Maze SS, Sandler M, et al: Pulmonary fibrosis following long-term nitrofurantoin therapy. S Afr Med J 61:714, 1982.

164. Penn RG, Griffin JP: Adverse reactions to nitrofurantoin in the United Kingdom, Sweden, and Holland. Br Med J 284:1440, 1982.

165. Magee F, Wright JL, Chan N, et al: Two unusual pathological reactions to nitrofurantoin: Case reports. Histopathology 10:701, 1986.

166. Fernández-Segoviano P, Esteban A, Martínez-Cabruja R: Pulmonary vascular lesions in the toxic oil syndrome in Spain. Thorax 38:724, 1983.

167. Bahk YW: Pulmonary paragonimiasis as a cause of Loeffler's syndrome. Radiology 78:598, 1962.

168. Robinson BR: Pleuropulmonary reaction to nitrofurantoin. JAMA 189:239, 1964.

169. Strauss WG, Griffin LM: Nitrofurantoin pneumonia. JAMA 199:765, 1967.

170. Demasi CJ: Allergic pulmonary infiltrates probably due to nitrofurantoin. Arch Intern Med 120:631, 1967.

171. Nicklaus TM, Snyder AB: Nitrofurantoin pulmonary reaction. A unique syndrome. Arch Intern Med 121:151, 1968.

172. Ngan H, Millard RJ, Lant AF, et al: Nitrofurantoin lung. Br J Radiol 44:21, 1971.

173. Sollaccio PA, Ribaudo CA, Grace WJ: Subacute pulmonary infiltration due to nitrofurantoin. Ann Intern Med 65:1284, 1966.

174. Pinerua RF, Hartnett BJS: Acute pulmonary reaction to nitrofurantoin. Thorax 29:599, 1974.

175. Robinson BW: Nitrofurantoin-induced interstitial pulmonary fibrosis: Presentation and outcome. Med J Aust 22:72, 1983.

176. Cortez LM, Pankey GA: Acute pulmonary hypersensitivity to furazolidone. Am Rev Respir Dis 105:823, 1972.

177. Berliner S, Neeman A, Shoenfeld Y, et al: Salazopyrin-induced eosinophilic pneumonia. Respiration 39:119, 1980.

178. Williams T, Eidus L, Thomas P: Fibrosing alveolitis, bronchiolitis obliterans, and sulfasalazine therapy. Chest 81:766, 1982.

179. Sigvaldason A, Sorenson S: Interstitial pneumonia due to sulfasalazine. Eur J Respir Dis 64:229, 1983.

180. Averbuch M, Halpern Z, Hallak A, et al: Sulfasalazine pneumonitis. Am J Gastroenterol 80:343, 1985.

181. Yaffe BH, Korelitz BI: Sulfasalazine pneumonitis. Am J Gastroenterol 78:493, 1983.

182. Cazzadori A, Braggio P, Bontempini L: Salazopyrin-induced eosinophilic pneumonia. Respiration 47:158, 1985.

183. Teague WG, Sutphen JL, Fechner RE: Desquamative interstitial pneumonitis complicating inflammatory bowel disease of childhood. J Pediatr Gastroenterol Nutr 4:663, 1985.

184. Valcke Y, Pauwels R, Van der Straeten M: Bronchoalveolar lavage in acute hypersensitivity pneumonitis caused by sulfasalazine. Chest 92:572, 1987.

185. Sheffer AL, Pennoyer DS: Management of adverse drug reactions. J Allergy Clin Immunol 74(2 Pt 2):580, 1984.

186. Ellis RV, McKinlay CA: Allergic pneumonia. J Lab Clin Med 26:1427, 1941.

187. Contratto AW: So-called "atypical pneumonia" among college students. N Engl J Med 229:229, 1943.

188. Fiegenberg DS, Weiss H, Kirshman H: Migratory pneumonia with eosinophilia associated with sulfonamide administration. Arch Intern Med 120:85, 1967.

189. Klinghoffer JF: Loeffler's syndrome following use of vaginal cream. Ann Intern Med 40:343, 1954.

190. Donlan CJ, Scutero JV: Transient eosinophilic pneumonia secondary to use of a vaginal cream. Chest 67:232, 1975.

191. Reichlin S, Loveless MH, Kane EG: Loeffler's syndrome following penicillin therapy. Ann Intern Med 38:113, 1953.

192. Wold DE, Zahn DW: Allergic (Löffler's) pneumonitis occurring during antituberculous chemotherapy. Report of three cases. Am Rev Tuberc 74:445, 1956.

193. Cullinan SA, Bower GC: Acute pulmonary hypersensitivity to carbamazepine. Chest 68(Suppl):580, 1975.

194. Dreis DF, Winterbauer RH, Van Norman GA, et al: Cephalosporin-induced interstitial pneumonitis. Chest 86:138, 1984.

195. Ho D, Tashkin DP, Bein ME, et al: Pulmonary infiltrates with eosinophilia associated with tetracycline. Chest 76:33, 1979.

196. Ampel NM, Ruben FL, Norden CW: Cutaneous abscess caused by Legionella micdadei in an immunosuppressed patient. Ann Intern Med 102:630, 1985.

197. Wong KH, Moss CW, Hochstein DH, et al: "Endotoxicity" of the Legionnaires' disease bacterium. Ann Intern Med 90:624, 1979.

198. Dana BW, Durie BGM, White RF, et al: Concomitant administration of granulocyte transfusions and amphotericin B in neutropenic patients: Absence of significant pulmonary toxicity. Blood 57:90, 1981.
199. Marchlinski FE, Gansler TS, Waxman HL, et al: Amiodarone pulmonary toxicity. Ann Intern Med 97:839, 1982.
200. Gefter WB, Epstein DM, Pietra GG, et al: Lung disease caused by amiodarone, a new antiarrhythmia agent. Radiology 147:339, 1983.
201. Dean PJ, Groshart KD, Porterfield JG, et al: Amiodarone-associated pulmonary toxicity: A clinical and pathologic study of eleven cases. J Clin Pathol 87:7, 1987.
202. Rakita L, Sobol SM, Mostow N, et al: Amiodarone pulmonary toxicity. Am Heart J 106(4 Pt 2):906, 1983.
203. Suarez LD, Poderoso JJ, Elsner B, et al: Subacute pneumopathy during amiodarone therapy. Chest 83:566, 1983.
204. Riley SA, Williams SE, Cooke NJ: Alveolitis after treatment with amiodarone. Br Med J 284:161, 1982.
205. Zaher C, Hamer A, Peter T, et al: Low-dose steroid therapy for prophylaxis of amiodarone-induced pulmonary infiltrates (letter). N Engl J Med 308:779, 1983.
206. Cazzadori A, Braggio P, Barbieri E, et al: Amiodarone-induced pulmonary toxicity. Respiration 49:157, 1986.
207. Pesola A, Consentino G, Vercillo C, et al: Lung disease associated with amiodarone treatment. C Ital Cardiol 15:552, 1985.
208. Raeder EA, Podrid PJ, Lown B: Side effects and complications of amiodarone therapy. Am Heart J 109(5 Pt 1):975, 1985.
209. Dake MD, Madison JM, Montgomery CK, et al: Electron microscopic demonstration of lysosomal inclusion bodies in lung, liver, lymph nodes, and blood leukocytes of patients with amiodarone pulmonary toxicity. Am J Med 78:506, 1985.
210. Pozzi E, Sada E, Luisetti M, et al: Interstitial pneumopathy and low-dosage amiodarone. Eur J Respir Dis 65:620, 1984.
211. Liu FL, Cohen RD, Downar E, et al: Amiodarone pulmonary toxicity: Functional and ultrastructural evaluation. Thorax 41:100, 1986.
212. Adams PC, Gibson GJ, Morley AR, et al: Amiodarone pulmonary toxicity: Clinical and subclinical features. Q J Med 59:449, 1986.
213. Israel-Biet D, Venet A, Caubarrere I, et al: Bronchoalveolar lavage in amiodarone pneumonitis: Cellular abnormalities and their relevance to pathogenesis. Chest 91:214, 1987.
214. Kennedy JI, Myers JL, Plumb VJ: Amiodarone pulmonary toxicity: Clinical, radiologic, and pathologic correlations. Arch Intern Med 147:50, 1987.
215. Nalos PC, Kass RM, Gang ES, et al: Life-threatening postoperative pulmonary complications in patients with previous amiodarone pulmonary toxicity undergoing cardiothoracic operations. J Thorac Cardiovasc Surg 93:904, 1987.
216. Myers JL, Kennedy JI, Plumb VJ: Amiodarone lung: Pathologic findings in clinically toxic patients. Hum Pathol 18:349, 1987.
217. Pollak PT, Sami M: Acute necrotizing pneumonitis and hyperglycemia after amiodarone therapy: Case report and review of amiodarone-associated pulmonary disease. Am J Med 76:935, 1984.
218. Farmakis M, Litos G, Melissinos C, et al: Diffuse interstitial pulmonary disease during amiodarone treatment. Arzneimittelforsch 34:223, 1984.
219. Jirik FR, Henning H, Huckell VF: Diffuse alveolar damage syndrome associated with amiodarone therapy. Can Med Assoc J 128:1192, 1983.
220. Akoun GM, Gauthier-Rahman S, Milleron BJ, et al: Amiodarone-induced hypersensitivity pneumonitis: Evidence of an immunological cell-mediated mechanism. Chest 85:133, 1984.
221. Kudenchuk PJ, Pierson DJ, Greene HL, et al: Prospective evaluation of amiodarone pulmonary toxicity. Chest 86:541, 1984.
222. Quyyumi AA, Ormerod LP, Clarke SW, et al: Pulmonary fibrosis: A serious side-effect of amiodarone therapy. Eur Heart J 4:521, 1983.
223. Koslin DB, Chapman P, Youker JE, et al: Amiodarone-induced pulmonary toxicity. J Can Assoc Radiol 35:195, 1984.
224. Costa-Jussa FR, Corrin B, Jacobs JM: Amiodarone lung toxicity: A human and experimental study. J Pathol 144:73, 1984.
225. Darmanata JI, van Zandwijk N, Düren DR, et al: Amiodarone pneumonitis: Three further cases with a review of published reports. Thorax 39:57, 1984.
226. Rotmensch HH, Belhassen B, Swanson BN, et al: Steady-state serum amiodarone concentrations: Relationships with antiarrhythmic efficacy and toxicity. Ann Intern Med 101:462, 1984.
227. Wright AJ, Brackenridge RG: Pulmonary infiltration and bone marrow depression complicating treatment with amiodarone. Br Med J 284:1303, 1982.
228. Gonzalez-Rothi RJ, Hannan SE, Hood CI, et al: Amiodarone pulmonary toxicity presenting as bilateral exudative pleural effusions. Chest 92:179, 1987.
229. Howard JJ, Mohsenifar Z, Simons SM: Adult respiratory distress syndrome following administration of lidocaine. Chest 81:644, 1982.
230. Perlow GM, Jain BP, Pauker SG, et al: Tocainide-associated interstitial pneumonitis. Ann Intern Med 94:489, 1981.
231. Fruchter L, Laptook A: Diphenylhydantoin hypersensitivity reaction associated with interstitial pulmonary infiltrates and hypereosinophilia. Ann Allergy 47:453, 1981.
232. Chamberlain DW, Hyland RH, Ross DJ: Diphenylhydantoin-induced lymphocytic interstitial pneumonia. Chest 90:458, 1986.
233. Moore MT: Pulmonary changes in hydantoin therapy. JAMA 171:1328, 1959.
234. Low NL, Yahr MD: The lack of pulmonary fibrosis in patients receiving diphenylhydantoin. JAMA 174:1201, 1960.
235. Livingston S, Whitehouse D, Pauli LL: Study of the effects of diphenylhydantoin sodium on the lungs. N Engl J Med 264:648, 1961.
236. Michael JR, Rudin ML: Acute pulmonary disease caused by phenytoin. Ann Intern Med 95:452, 1981.
237. Munn NJ, Baughman RP, Ploysongsang Y, et al: Bronchoalveolar lavage in acute drug-hypersensitivity pneumonitis probably caused by phenytoin. South Med J 77:1594, 1984.
238. Saltzstein SL, Ackerman LV: Lymphadenopathy induced by anticonvulsant drugs and mimicking clinically and pathologically malignant lymphomas. Cancer 12:164, 1959.
239. Heitzman ER: Lymphadenopathy related to anticonvulsant therapy: Roentgen findings simulating lymphoma. Radiology 89:311, 1967.
240. Yermakov VM, Hitti IF, Sutton AL: Necrotizing vasculitis associated with diphenylhydantoin: Two fatal cases. Hum Pathol 14:182, 1983.
241. Gaffey CM, Chun B, Harvey JC, et al: Phenytoin-induced systemic granulomatous vasculitis. Arch Pathol Lab Med 110:131, 1986.
242. Haruda F: Phenytoin hypersensitivity: 38 cases. Neurology 29:1480, 1979.
243. Hazlett DR, Ward GW, Madison DS: Pulmonary function loss in diphenylhydantoin therapy. Chest 66:660, 1974.
244. De Swert LF, Ceuppens JL, Teuwen D, et al: Acute interstitial pneumonitis and carbamazepine therapy. Acta Paediatr Scand 73:285, 1984.
245. Cullinan SA, Bower GC: Acute pulmonary hypersensitivity to carbamazepine. Chest 68:580, 1975.
246. Stephan WC, Parks RD, Tempest B: Acute hypersensitivity pneumonitis associated with carbamazepine therapy. Chest 74:463, 1978.
247. Lee T, Cochrane GM, Amlot P: Pulmonary eosinophilia and asthma associated with carbamazepine. Br Med J 282:440, 1981.
248. Gaensler EA, Weisel RD: The risks in abdominal and thoracic surgery in COPD. Postgrad Med 54:183, 1973.
249. Heffner JE, Sahn SA: Salicylate-induced pulmonary edema. Clinical features and prognosis. Ann Intern Med 95:405, 1981.
250. Leatherman JW, Drage CW: Adult respiratory distress syndrome due to salicylate intoxication. Minn Med 65:677, 1982.
251. Walters JS, Woodring JH, Stelling CB, et al: Salicylate-induced pulmonary edema. Radiology 146:289, 1983.
252. Fisher CJ Jr, Albertson TE, Foulke GE: Salicylate-induced pulmonary edema: Clinical characteristics in children. Am J Emerg Med 3:33, 1985.
253. Bowers RE, Brigham KL, Owen PJ: Salicylate pulmonary edema: The mechanism in sheep and review of the clinical literature. Am Rev Respir Dis 115:261, 1977.
254. Heffner J, Starkey T, Anthony P: Salicylate-induced noncardiogenic pulmonary edema. West J Med 130:263, 1979.
255. Liebman RM, Katz HM: Pulmonary edema in a 52-year-old woman ingesting large amounts of aspirin. JAMA 246:2227, 1981.
256. Hormaechea E, Carlson RW, Rogove H, et al: Hypovolemia, pulmonary edema and protein changes in severe salicylate poisoning. Am J Med 66:1046, 1979.
257. Andersen R, Refstad S: Adult respiratory distress syndrome precipitated by massive salicylate poisoning. Intensive Care Med 4:211, 1978.
258. Nader DA, Schillaci RF: Pulmonary infiltrates with eosinophilia due to naproxen. Chest 83:280, 1983.
259. Buscaglia AJ, Cowden FE, Brill H: Pulmonary infiltrates associated with naproxen. JAMA 251:65, 1984.
260. Gould DM, Daves ML: A review of roentgen findings in systemic lupus erythematosus (SLE). Am J Med Sci 235:596, 1958.
261. Bocanegra T, Espinoza LR, Vasey FB, et al: Myasthenia gravis and penicillamine therapy of rheumatoid arthritis. JAMA 244:1822, 1980.
262. Eastmond CJ: Diffuse alveolitis as complication of penicillamine treatment for rheumatoid arthritis. Br Med J 1:1506, 1976.
263. Davies D, Jones JKL: Pulmonary eosinophilia caused by penicillamine. Thorax 35:957, 1980.
264. Kumar A, Bhat A, Gupta DK, et al: D-penicillamine-induced acute hypersensitivity pneumonitis and cholestatic hepatitis in a patient with rheumatoid arthritis. Clin Exp Rheumatol 3:337, 1985.
265. Petersen J, Moller I: Miliary pulmonary infiltrates and penicillamine. Br J Radiol 51:915, 1978.
266. Estes D, Christian CL: The natural history of systemic lupus erythematosus by prospective analysis. Medicine 50:85, 1971.

267. Fessel WJ: Systemic lupus erythematosus in the community. Arch Intern Med 134:1027, 1974.
268. Wallace SL, Diamond H, Kaplan D: Recent advances in rheumatoid diseases: The connective tissue diseases other than rheumatoid arthritis—1970 and 1971. Ann Intern Med 77:455, 1972.
269. Cohen AS, Reynolds WE, Franklin EC, et al: Preliminary criteria for the classification of systemic lupus erythematosus. Bull Rheum Dis 21:643, 1971.
270. Camus P, Degat OR, Justrabo E, et al: D-penicillamine–induced severe pneumonitis. Chest 81:376, 1982.
271. Fuleihan FJD, Abboud RT, Hubaytar R: Idiopathic pulmonary hemosiderosis. Case report with pulmonary function tests and review of the literature. Am Rev Respir Dis 98:93, 1968.
272. Ewan PW, Jones HA, Rhodes CG, et al: Detection of intrapulmonary hemorrhage with carbon monoxide uptake: Application in Goodpasture's syndrome. N Engl J Med 295:1391, 1976.
273. Clinical Pathologic Conference: Pulmonary hemorrhage and renal failure. Am J Med 60:397, 1976.
274. Robboy SJ, Minna JD, Coleman RW, et al: Pulmonary hemorrhage syndrome as a manifestation of disseminated intravascular coagulation: Analysis of ten cases. Chest 63:718, 1973.
275. Barber KA, Jackson R: Neonatal lupus erythematosus: Five new cases with HLA typing. Can Med Assoc J 129:139, 1983.
276. Winterbauer RH, Wilske KR, Wheelis RF: Diffuse pulmonary injury associated with gold treatment. N Engl J Med 294:919, 1976.
277. Geddes DM, Brostoff J: Pulmonary fibrosis associated with hypersensitivity to gold salts. Br Med J 1:1444, 1976.
278. Scharf J, Nahir M, Kleinhaus U, et al: Diffuse pulmonary injury associated with gold therapy. JAMA 237:2412, 1977.
279. Gould PW, McCormack PL, Palmer DG: Pulmonary damage associated with sodium aurothiomalate therapy. J Rheumatol 4:252, 1977.
280. Sepuya SM, Grzybowski S, Burton JD, et al: Diffuse lung changes associated with gold therapy. Can Med Assoc J 118:816, 1978.
281. James DW, Whimeter WF, Hamilton EBD: Gold lung. Br Med J 1:1523, 1978.
282. Weaver LT, Law JS: Lung changes after gold salts. Br J Dis Chest 72:247, 1978.
283. Tala E, Jalava S, Nurmela T, et al: Pulmonary infiltrates associated with gold therapy: Report of a case. Scand J Rheumatol 8:97, 1979.
284. Terho EO, Torkko M, Vaita R: Pulmonary damage associated with gold therapy: A report of two cases. Scand J Respir Dis 60:345, 1979.
285. McCormick J, Cole S, Lahirir B, et al: Pneumonitis caused by gold salt therapy: Evidence for the role of cell-mediated immunity in its pathogenesis. Am Rev Respir Dis 122:145, 1980.
286. Ettensohn DB, Roberts NJ Jr, Condemi JJ: Bronchoalveolar lavage in gold lung. Chest 85:569, 1984.
287. Morley TF, Komansky HJ, Adelizzi RA, et al: Pulmonary gold toxicity. Eur J Respir Dis 65:627, 1984.
288. Schapira D, Nahir M, Scharf Y: Pulmonary injury induced by gold salts treatment. Med Interne 23:259, 1985.
289. Gortenuti G, Parrinello A, Vicentini D: Diffuse pulmonary changes caused by gold salt therapy: Report of a case. Diagn Imag Clin Med 54:298, 1985.
290. Partanen J, van Assendelft AH, Koskimies S, et al: Patients with rheumatoid arthritis and gold-induced pneumonitis express two high-risk major histocompatibility complex patterns. Chest 92:277, 1987.
291. Morrison WJ, Wetherill S, Zyroff J: The acute pulmonary edema of heroin intoxication. Radiology 97:347, 1970.
292. Nickels J, van Assendelft AHW, Tukiainen P: Diffuse pulmonary injury associated with gold treatment. Acta Path Microbiol Immunol Scand Sect A 91:265, 1983.
293. Rabhan NB, Minkin W: Criteria for classification of systemic lupus erythematosus. JAMA 231:846, 1973.
294. Evans RB, Ettensohn DB, Fawaz-Estrup F, et al: Gold lung: Recent developments in pathogenesis, diagnosis, and therapy. Semin Arthritis Rheum 16:196, 1987.
295. Mabie WC, Pernoll ML, Witty JB, et al: Pulmonary edema induced by betamimetic drugs. South Med J 76:1354, 1983.
296. Nimrod C, Rambihar V, Fallen E, et al: Pulmonary edema associated with isoxsuprine therapy. Am J Obstet Gynecol 148:625, 1984.
297. Pisani RJ, Rosenow EC 3rd: Pulmonary edema associated with tocolytic therapy. Ann Intern Med 110:714, 1989.
298. Gupta RC, Foster S, Romano PM, et al: Acute pulmonary edema associated with the use of oral ritodrine for premature labor. Chest 95:479, 1989.
299. Evron S, Samueloff A, Mor-Yosef S, et al: Pulmonary edema occurring after isoxsuprine and dexamethasone treatment for preterm labor: Case report. J Perinat Med 11:272, 1983.
300. Osler W: Oedema of left lung-morphia poisoning. In Published Memoirs and Communications. Pathological Report of the Montreal General Hospital, No 2, p 39. Montreal, The Gazette Printing Co., 1880.
301. Wilen SB, Ulreich S, Rabinowitz JG: Roentgenographic manifestations of methadone-induced pulmonary edema. Radiology 114:51, 1975.
302. Duberstein JL, Kaufman DM: A clinical study of an epidemic of heroin intoxication and heroin-induced pulmonary edema. Am J Med 51:704, 1971.
303. Frand UI, Shim CS, Williams MH Jr: Methadone-induced pulmonary edema. Ann Intern Med 76:975, 1972.
304. Schaaf JT, Spivack ML, Rath GS, et al: Pulmonary edema and adult respiratory distress syndrome following methadone abuse. Am Rev Respir Dis 107:1047, 1973.
305. Gardner R: Methadone misuse and death by overdosage. Br J Addict 65:113, 1970.
306. Kjeldgaard JM, Hahn GW, Heckenlively JR, et al: Methadone-induced pulmonary edema. JAMA 218:882, 1971.
307. Fraser DW: Methadone overdose. Illicit use of pharmaceutically prepared parenteral narcotics. JAMA 217:1387, 1971.
308. Presant S, Knight L, Klassen GA: Methadone-induced pulmonary edema. Can Med Assoc J 113(Suppl):966, 1975.
309. Bogartz LJ, Miller WC: Pulmonary edema associated with propoxyphene intoxication. JAMA 215:259, 1971.
310. Richman S, Harris RD: Acute pulmonary edema associated with Librium abuse. A case report. Radiology 103:57, 1972.
311. Glauser FL, Smith WR, Caldwell J, et al: Ethchlorvynol (Placidyl)-induced pulmonary edema. Ann Intern Med 84:46, 1976.
312. Mountain R, Ferguson S, Fowler A, et al: Noncardiac pulmonary edema following administration of parenteral paraldehyde. Chest 82:371, 1982.
313. Sklar J, Timms RM: Codeine-induced pulmonary edema. Chest 72:230, 1977.
314. Sugihara H, Hagedorn M, Böttcher D, et al: Interstitial pulmonary edema following bromocarbamide intoxication. Am J Pathol 75:457, 1974.
315. Gali JM, Vilanova JL, Mayos M, et al: Febarbamate-induced pulmonary eosinophilia: A case report. Respiration 49:231, 1986.
316. Flacke JW, Flacke WE, Williams GD: Acute pulmonary edema following naloxone reversal of high-dose morphine anesthesia. Anesthesiology 47:376, 1977.
317. Taff RH: Pulmonary edema following naloxone administration in a patient without heart disease. Anesthesiology 59:576, 1983.
318. Staub NC: "State of the art" review. Pathogenesis of pulmonary edema. Am Rev Respir Dis 109:358, 1974.
319. Katz S, Aberman A, Frand UI, et al: Heroin pulmonary edema. Evidence for increased pulmonary capillary permeability. Am Rev Respir Dis 106:472, 1972.
320. Smith WR, Wells ID, Glauser FL, et al: Immunologic abnormalities in heroin lung. Chest 68:651, 1975.
321. Smith WR, Glauser FL, Dearden LC, et al: Deposits of immunoglobulin in the pulmonary tissue of patients with "heroin lung." Chest 73:471, 1978.
322. Snyder SH: Opiate receptors in the brain. N Engl J Med 296:266, 1977.
323. Helpern M, Rho Y-M: Deaths from narcotism in New York City. Incidence, circumstances, and postmortem findings. NY J Med 66:2391, 1966.
324. Jaffe RB, Koschmann EB: Intravenous drug abuse: Pulmonary, cardiac, and vascular complications. Am J Roentgenol 109:107, 1970.
325. Light RW, Dunham TR: Severe slowly resolving heroin-induced pulmonary edema. Chest 67:61, 1975.
326. Steinberg AD, Karliner JS: The clinical spectrum of heroin pulmonary edema. Arch Intern Med 122:122, 1968.
327. Master K: Heroin pulmonary edema. Chest 64:147, 1973.
328. Saba GP II, James AE Jr, Johnson BA, et al: Pulmonary complications of narcotic abuse. Am J Roentgenol 122:733, 1974.
329. Zyroff J, Slovis TL, Nagler J: Pulmonary edema induced by oral methadone. Radiology 112:567, 1974.
330. Alexander M: Surveillance of heroin-induced deaths in Atlanta 1971 to 1973. JAMA 229:677, 1974.
331. Karliner JS, Steinberg AD, Williams MH Jr: Lung function after pulmonary edema associated with heroin overdoses. Arch Intern Med 124:350, 1969.
332. Frand UI, Shim CS, Williams MH Jr: Heroin-induced pulmonary edema: Sequential studies of pulmonary function. Ann Intern Med 77:29, 1972.
333. Wilson IC, Gambill JM, Sandifer MG: Loeffler's syndrome occurring during imipramine therapy. Am J Psychiatry 119:892, 1963.
334. Joynt RJ, Clancy J: Extreme eosinophilia during imipramine therapy. Am J Psychiatry 118:170, 1961.
335. Paré JAP: Unpublished data, 1975.
336. Shear MK: Chlorpromazine-induced PIE syndrome. Am J Psychiatry 135:492, 1978.
337. Marshall A, Moore K: Pulmonary disease after amitriptyline overdosage. Br Med J 1:716, 1973.
338. Sunshine P, Yaffe SJ: Amitriptyline poisoning. Clinical and pathological findings in a fatal case. Am J Dis Child 106:501, 1963.

339. Varnell RM, Godwin JD, Richardson ML, et al: Adult respiratory distress syndrome from overdose of tricyclic antidepressants. Radiology 170:667, 1989.
340. Smego RA, Durack DT: The neuroleptic malignant syndrome. Arch Intern Med 142:1183, 1982.
341. Silvestri RC, Huseby JS, Rughani I, et al: Respiratory distress syndrome from lymphangiography contrast medium. Am Rev Respir Dis 122:543, 1980.
342. Fraimow W, Wallace S, Lewis P, et al: Changes in pulmonary function due to lymphangiography. Radiology 85:231, 1965.
343. Fallat RJ, Powell MR, Youker JE, et al: Pulmonary deposition and clearance of 131I-labeled oil after lymphography in man: Correlation with lung function. Radiology 97:511, 1970.
344. Weg JG, Harkleroad LE: Aberrations in pulmonary function due to lymphangiography. Dis Chest 53:534, 1968.
345. Gold WM, Youker J, Anderson S, et al: Pulmonary-function abnormalities after lymphangiography. N Engl J Med 273:519, 1965.
346. White RJ, Webb JAW, Tucker AK, et al: Pulmonary function after lymphography. Br Med J 4:775, 1973.
347. Ansell G: A national survey of radiological complications: Interim report. Clin Radiol 19:175, 1968.
348. Reich SB: Production of pulmonary edema by aspiration of water-soluble nonabsorbable contrast media. Radiology 92:367, 1969.
349. Chiu CL, Gambach RR: Hypaque pulmonary edema: A case report. Radiology 111:91, 1974.
350. Malins AF: Pulmonary oedema after radiological investigation of peripheral occlusive vascular disease: Adverse reaction to contrast media. Lancet 1:413, 1978.
351. Greganti MA, Flowers WM Jr: Acute pulmonary edema after the intravenous administration of contrast media. Radiology 132:583, 1979.
352. Chamberlin WH, Stockman GD, Wray NP: Shock and noncardiogenic pulmonary edema following meglumine diatrizoate for intravenous pyelography. Am J Med 67:684, 1979.
353. Harris PD, Neuhauser EBD, Gerth R: The osmotic effect of water soluble contrast media on circulating plasma volume. Am J Roentgenol 91:694, 1964.
354. Cameron JD: Pulmonary edema following drip-infusion urography. Radiology 111:89, 1974.
355. Beaudry C, Laplante L: Severe allergic pneumonitis from hydrochlorothiazide. Ann Intern Med 78:251, 1973.
356. Steinberg AD: Pulmonary edema following ingestion of hydrochlorothiazide. JAMA 204:825, 1968.
357. Dorn MR, Walker BK: Noncardiogenic pulmonary edema associated with hydrochlorothiazide therapy. Chest 79:482, 1981.
358. Bell RT, Lippmann M: Hydrochlorothiazide-induced pulmonary edema: Report of a case and review of the literature. Arch Intern Med 139:817, 1979.
359. Mollura JL, Bernstein R, Fine SR, et al: Pulmonary eosinophilia in a patient receiving beclomethasone diproprionate aerosol. Ann Allergy 42:326, 1979.
360. Carruthers SG: Severe coughing during captopril and enalapril therapy. Can Med Assoc J 135:217, 1986.
361. Popa V: Captopril-related (and induced?) asthma. Am Rev Respir Dis 136:999, 1987.
362. Morice AH, Lowry R, Brown MJ, et al: Angiotensin-converting enzyme and the cough reflex. Lancet 2:1116, 1987.
363. Chastre J, Basset F, Viau F, et al: Acute pneumonitis after subcutaneous injections of silicone in transsexual men. N Engl J Med 308:764, 1983.
364. Coulaud JM, Labrousse J, Carli P, et al: Adult respiratory distress syndrome and silicone injection. Toxicol Eur Res 5:171, 1983.
365. Hoffman CK, Goodman PC: Pulmonary edema in cocaine smokers. Radiology 172:463, 1989.
366. Eurman DW, Potash HI, Eyler WR, et al: Chest pain and dyspnea related to "crack" cocaine smoking: Value of chest radiography. Radiology 172:459, 1989.
367. Weiss RD, Goldenheim PD, Mirin SM, et al: Pulmonary dysfunction in cocaine smokers. Am J Psychiatry 138:1110, 1981.
368. Itkonen J, Schnoll S, Glassroth J: Pulmonary dysfunction in "free base" cocaine users. Arch Intern Med 144:2195, 1984.
369. Patel RC, Dutta D, Schonfeld SA: Free-base cocaine use associated with bronchiolitis obliterans organizing pneumonia. Ann Intern Med 107:186, 1987.
370. Cooper CB, Bai TR, Heyderman E, et al: Cellulose granuloma in the lungs of a cocaine sniffer. Br Med J 286:2021, 1983.
371. O'Callaghan WG, Joyce N, Counihan HE, et al: Unusual strychnine poisoning and its treatment: Report of eight cases. Br Med J 285:478, 1982.
372. Marshall AJ, Eltringham WK, Barritt DW, et al: Respiratory disease associated with practolol therapy. Lancet 2:1254, 1977.
373. Hall DR, Morrison JB, Edwards FR: Pleural fibrosis after practolol therapy. Thorax 33:822, 1978.
374. Wark JD, Larkins RG: Pulmonary oedema after propranolol therapy in two cases of phaeochromocytoma. Br Med J 1:1395, 1978.
375. Sloand EM, Thompson BT: Propranolol-induced pulmonary edema and shock in a patient with pheochromocytoma. Arch Intern Med 144:173, 1984.
376. Rinaldo JE, Owens GR, Rogers RM: Adult respiratory distress syndrome following intrapleural instillation of talc. J Thorac Cardiovasc Surg 85:523, 1983.
377. Lie JT: Pulmonary peliosis. Arch Pathol Lab Med 109:878, 1985.
378. Ohnishi Y, Kitazawa M: Application of perfluorochemicals in human beings—A morphological report of a human autopsy case with some experimental studies using rabbit. Acta Pathol Jpn 30(3):489, 1980.
379. Kitazawa M, Ohnishi Y: Long-term experiment of perfluorochemicals using rabbits. Virchows Arch Pathol Anat 398:1, 1982.
380. Wiggins J, Skinner C: Bromocriptine-induced pleuropulmonary fibrosis. Thorax 41:328, 1986.
381. Taal BG, Spierings ELH, Hilvering C: Pleuropulmonary fibrosis associated with chronic and excessive intake of ergotamine. Thorax 38:396, 1983.
382. Conant EF, Fox KR, Miller WT: Pulmonary edema as a complication of Interleukin-2 therapy. Am J Roentgenol 152:749, 1989.
383. Lings S: Pesticide lung: A pilot investigation of fruit-growers and farmers during the spraying season. Br J Ind Med 39:370, 1982.
384. Namba T, Nolte CT, Jackrel J, et al: Poisoning due to organophosphate insecticides. Acute and chronic manifestations. Am J Med 50:475, 1971.
385. Du Toit PW, Muller FO, Van Tonder WM, et al: Experience with the intensive care management of organophosphate insecticide poisoning. S Afr Med J 60:227, 1981.
386. Bledsoe FH, Seymour EQ: Acute pulmonary edema associated with parathion poisoning. Radiology 103:53, 1972.
387. Neal EA: Enzymic mechanism of metabolism of the phosphorothionate insecticides. Arch Intern Med 128:118, 1971.
388. Li C, Miller WT, Jiang J: Pulmonary edema due to ingestion of organophosphate insecticide. Am J Roentgenol 152:265, 1989.
389. Salisburg BD, Tate CF, Davies JE: Baygon-induced pulmonary edema. Chest 65:455, 1974.
390. Warraki S: Respiratory hazards of chlorinated camphene. Arch Environ Health 7:253, 1963.
391. Roby DS, Fein AM, Bennett RH, et al: Cardiopulmonary effects of acute thallium poisoning. Chest 85:236, 1984.
392. Newhouse M, McEvoy D, Rosenthal D: Percutaneous paraquat absorption: An association with cutaneous lesions and respiratory failure. Arch Dermatol 114:1516, 1978.
393. Levin PJ, Klaff LJ, Rose AG, et al: Pulmonary effects of contact exposure to paraquat: A clinical and experimental study. Thorax 34:150, 1979.
394. Wohlfahrt DJ: Fatal paraquat poisonings after skin absorption. Med J Aust 1:512, 1982.
395. Kimbrough RD: Toxic effects of the herbicide paraquat. Chest 65(Suppl):65S, 1974.
396. George M, Hedworth-Whitty RB: Non-fatal lung disease due to inhalation of nebulised paraquat. Br Med J 280:902, 1980.
397. Editorial: Paraquat poisoning. Lancet 2:1018, 1971.
398. Higenbottam T, Crome P, Parkinson C, et al: Further clinical observations on the pulmonary effects of paraquat ingestion. Thorax 34:161, 1979.
399. Harley JB, Grinspan S, Root RK: Paraquat suicide in a young woman: Results of therapy directed against the superoxide radical. Yale J Biol Med 50:481, 1977.
400. Anderson CG: Paraquat and the lung. Australas Radiol 14:409, 1970.
401. Fairshter RD, Wilson AF: Paraquat poisoning. Manifestations and therapy. Am J Med 59:751, 1975.
402. Fisher HK, Clements JA, Wright RR: Enhancement of oxygen toxicity by the herbicide paraquat. Am Rev Respir Dis 107:246, 1973.
403. Thurlbeck WM, Thurlbeck SM: Pulmonary effects of paraquat poisoning. Chest 69(Suppl):276, 1976.
404. Fairshter RD: Paraquat toxicity and lipid peroxidation. Arch Intern Med 141:1121, 1981.
405. Yasaka T, Ohya I, Matsumoto J, et al: Acceleration of lipid peroxidation in human paraquat poisoning. Arch Intern Med 141:1169, 1981.
406. Montgomery MR, Casey PJ, Valls AA, et al: Biochemical and morphological correlation of oxidant-induced pulmonary injury: Low dose exposure to paraquat, oxygen, and ozone. Arch Environ Health 34:396, 1979.
407. Rebello G, Mason JK: Pulmonary histological appearances in fatal paraquat poisoning. Histopathology 2:53, 1978.
408. Yamaguchi M, Takahashi T, Togashi H, et al: The corrected collagen content in paraquat lungs. Chest 90:251, 1986.
409. Hollinger MA, Patwell SW, Zuckerman JE, et al: Effect of paraquat on serum angiotensin-converting enzyme. Amer Rev Respir Dis 121:795, 1980.
410. The Toronto Lung Transplant Group: Sequential bilateral lung

transplantation for paraquat poisoning: A case report. J Thorac Cardiovasc Surg 89:734, 1985.

411. Matthew H, Logan A, Woodruff MFA, et al: Paraquat poisoning—lung transplantation. Br Med J 3:759, 1968.

412. Davidson JK, MacPherson P: Pulmonary changes in paraquat poisoning. Clin Radiol 23:18, 1972.

413. Stephens DS, Walker DH, Schaffner W, et al: Pseudodiphtheria: Prominent pharyngeal membrane associated with fatal paraquat ingestion. Ann Intern Med 94:202, 1981.

414. Ng LL, Naik RB, Polak A: Paraquat ingestion with methaemoglobinaemia treated with methylene blue. Br Med J 284:1445, 1982.

415. Fisher HK, Humphries M, Bails R: Paraquat poisoning. Recovery from renal and pulmonary damage. Ann Intern Med 75:731, 1971.

416. Smith LL, Wright A, Wyatt I, et al: Effective treatment for paraquat poisoning in rats and its relevance in treatment of paraquat poisoning in man. Br Med J 4:569, 1974.

417. Maini R, Winchester JP: Removal of paraquat from blood by haemoperfusion over sorbent materials. Br Med J 3:281, 1975.

418. Giri SN, Hollinger MA, Schiedt MJ: The effects of paraquat and superoxide dismutase on pulmonary vascular permeability and edema in mice. Arch Environ Health 36:149, 1981.

419. Conradi SE, Olanoff LS, Dawson WT Jr: Fatality due to paraquat intoxication: Confirmation by postmortem tissue analysis. J Clin Pathol 80:771, 1983.

420. Tabuenca JM: Toxic-allergic syndrome caused by ingestion of rapeseed oil denatured with aniline. Lancet 2:567, 1981.

421. Rigau-Pérez JG, Pérez-Alvarez L, Duēnas-Castro S, et al: Epidemiologic investigation of an oil-associated pneumonic paralytic eosinophilic syndrome in Spain. Am J Epidemiol 119:250, 1984.

422. De la Cruz JL, Oteo LA, López C, et al: Toxic-oil syndrome: Gallium-67 scanning and bronchoalveolar lavage studies in patients with abnormal lung function. Chest 88:398, 1985.

423. Follow-up on epidemic pneumonia with progression to neuromuscular illness—Spain. MMWR 31:93, 1982.

424. Gordon RS: Oleoanilides and Spanish oil poisoning. Lancet 2:1171, 1981.

425. Root-Bernstein RS, Westall FC: Mycoplasma pneumoniae and a dual etiology for Spanish oil syndrome. Nature 301:178, 1983.

426. Giovacchini RP, Becker GH, Brunner MJ, et al: Pulmonary disease and hair-spray polymers. Effects of long-term exposure of dogs. JAMA 193:298, 1965.

427. Martinez-Tello FJ, Navas-Palacios JJ, Ricoy JR, et al: Pathology of a new toxic syndrome caused by ingestion of adulterated oil in Spain. Virchows Arch (Pathol Anat) 397:261, 1982.

428. Alonso-Ruiz A, Zea-Mendoza AC, Salazar-Vallinas JM, et al: Toxic oil syndrome: A syndrome with features overlapping those of various forms of scleroderma. Semin Arthritis Rheum 15:200, 1986.

429. Gómez-Sánchez MA, Mestre de Juan MJ, Gómez-Pajuelo C, et al: Pulmonary hypertension due to toxic oil syndrome. A clinicopathologic study. Chest 95:325, 1989.

430. Anas N, Namasonthi V, Ginsburg CM: Criteria for hospitalizing children who have ingested products containing hydrocarbons. JAMA 246:840, 1981.

431. Bonte FJ, Reynolds J: Hydrocarbon pneumonitis. Radiology 71:391, 1958.

432. Reynolds J, Bonte FJ: Kerosene pneumonitis. Tex Med 56:34, 1960.

433. Brünner S, Rovsing H, Wulf H: Roentgenographic changes in the lungs of children with kerosene poisoning. Am Rev Respir Dis 89:250, 1964.

434. Nome O, Ditlefsen EML: Acute gasoline poisoning. Four cases. Nord 61:140, 1959.

435. Jimenez JP, Lester RG: Pulmonary complications following furniture polish ingestion. A report of 21 cases. Am J Roentgenol 98:323, 1966.

436. Wolfe BM, Brodeur AE, Shields JB: The role of gastrointestinal absorption of kerosene in producing pneumonitis in dogs. J Pediatr 76:867, 1970.

437. Gross P, McNerney JM, Babyak MA: Kerosene pneumonitis: An experimental study with small doses. Am Rev Respir Dis 88:656, 1963.

438. Steele RW, Conklin RH, Mark HM: Corticosteroids and antibiotics for the treatment of fulminant hydrocarbon aspiration. JAMA 219:1434, 1972.

439. Scharf SM, Heimer D, Goldstein J: Pathologic and physiologic effects of aspiration of hydrocarbons in the rat. Am Rev Respir Dis 124:625, 1981.

440. Thurlbeck WM: Conference summary. Chest 66(Suppl):40, 1974.

441. Heinisch HM, Levejohann R: The pathogenesis of radiological changes in the lungs after ingestion of petroleum distillates: An experimental study in rabbits and extrapolation of the results to children. Ann Radiol 16:263, 1973.

442. Neeld EM, Limacher MC: Chemical pneumonitis after the intravenous injection of hydrocarbon. Radiology 129:36, 1978.

443. Vaziri ND, Jeeminson-Smith P, Wilson AF: Hemorrhagic pneumo-

nitis after intravenous injection of charcoal lighter fluid. Ann Intern Med 90:794, 1979.

444. Baghdassarian OM, Weiner S: Pneumatocele formation complicating hydrocarbon pneumonitis. Am J Roentgenol 95:104, 1965.

445. Campbell JB: Pneumatocele formation following hydrocarbon ingestion. Am Rev Respir Dis 101:414, 1970.

446. Harris VJ, Brown R: Pneumatoceles as a complication of chemical pneumonia after hydrocarbon ingestion. Am J Roentgenol 125:531, 1975.

447. Bass M: Sudden sniffing death. JAMA 212:2075, 1970.

448. Harris WS: Toxic effects of aerosol propellants on the heart. Arch Intern Med 131:162, 1973.

449. Anderson HR, MacNair RS, Ramsey JD: Deaths from abuse of volatile substances: A national epidemiological study. Br Med J 290:304, 1985.

450. Streicher HZ, Gabon PA, Moss AH, et al: Syndromes of toluene sniffing in adults. Ann Intern Med 94:758, 1981.

451. Cane RD, Buchanan N, Miller M: Pulmonary oedema associated with hydrocarbon inhalation. Intensive Care Med 3:31, 1977.

452. Patel R, Janakiraman N, Towne WD: Pulmonary edema due to tetrachloroethylene. Environ Health Perspect 21:247, 1977.

453. Cronk SL, Barkley DEH, Farrell MF: Respiratory arrest after solvent abuse. Br Med J 290:897, 1985.

454. Macdougall IC, Isles C, Oliver JS, et al: Fatal outcome following inhalation of Tipp-Ex. Scott Med J 32:55, 1987.

455. Frank R: Are aerosol sprays hazardous? Am Rev Respir Dis 112:485, 1975.

456. The Medical Letter, 15: No. 21, p 86 (Issue 385), 1973. Published by The Medical Letter, Inc., 56 Harrison Street, New Rochelle, NY 10801.

457. Draffan GH, Dollery CT, Williams FM, et al: Alveolar gas concentrations of fluorocarbons 11 and 12 in man after use of pressurized aerosols. Thorax 29:95, 1974.

458. Litt IF, Cohen MI: "Danger—Vapor harmful": Spot-remover sniffing. N Engl J Med 281:543, 1969.

459. Engstrand DA, England DM, Huntington RW III: Pathology of paint sniffers' lung. Am J Forensic Med Pathol 7:232, 1986.

460. Tenenbein M, de Groot W, Rajani KR: Peripheral neuropathy following intentional inhalation of naphtha fumes. Can Med Assoc J 131:1077, 1984.

461. Buchanan DR, Lamb D, Seaton A: Punk rocker's lung: Pulmonary fibrosis in a drug-snorting fire-eater. Br Med J 283:1661, 1981.

462. Cartwright TR, Brown ED, Brashear RE: Pulmonary infiltrates following butane "fire-breathing." Arch Intern Med 143:2007, 1983.

463. Jones RD, Winter DP: Two case reports of deaths on industrial premises attributed to 1,1,1-trichloroethane. Arch Environ Health 38:59, 1983.

464. Skyberg K, Ronneberg A, Kamoy JI, et al: Pulmonary fibrosis in cable plant workers exposed to mist and vapor of petroleum distillates. Environ Res 40:261, 1986.

465. Johns RE Jr, Lee JS, Agahian B, et al: Respiratory effects of mesquite broiling. J Occup Med 28:1181, 1986.

466. Smith AB, Schloemer J, Lowry LK, et al: Metabolic and health consequences of occupational exposure to polychlorinated biphenyls. Br J Ind Med 39:361, 1982.

467. Shigematsu N, Ishimaru S, Saito R, et al: Respiratory involvement in polychlorinated biphenyls poisoning. Environ Res 16:92, 1978.

468. Warshaw R, Fischbein A, Thornton J, et al: Decrease in vital capacity in PCB-exposed workers in a capacitor manufacturing facility. Ann NY Acad Sci 320:277, 1979.

469. Kleinfeld M, Messite J, Giel CP: Pulmonary edema of noncardiac origin. Am J Med Sci 235:660, 1958.

470. Kleinfeld M: Acute pulmonary edema of chemical origin. Arch Environ Health 10:942, 1965.

471. Conner E, Dubois A, Comroe J: Acute chemical injury of the airway and lungs. Anesthesiology 23:538, 1962.

472. Lowry T, Schuman LM: "Silo-filler's disease"—A syndrome caused by nitrogen dioxide. JAMA 162:153, 1956.

473. McAdams AJ, Jr: Bronchiolitis obliterans. Am J Med 19:314, 1955.

474. Baar HS, Galindo J: Bronchiolitis fibrosa obliterans. Thorax 21:209, 1966.

475. Currie WD, Pratt PC, Sanders AP: Hyperoxia and lung metabolism. Chest 66:19S, 1974.

476. Hueter FG, Fritzhand M: Oxidants and lung biochemistry. A brief review. Arch Intern Med 128:48, 1971.

477. Deneke SM, Fanburg BL: Normobaric oxygen toxicity of the lung. N Engl J Med 303:76, 1980.

478. Frank L, Massaro D: Oxygen toxicity. Am J Med 69:117, 1980.

479. Cross CE, DeLucia AJ, Reddy AK, et al: Ozone interactions with lung tissue. Biochemical approaches. Am J Med 60:929, 1976.

480. Roehm JN, Hadley JH, Menzel DB: Antioxidants vs. lung disease. Arch Intern Med 128:88, 1971.

481. Mustafa MG, DeLucia AJ, Cross CE, et al: Effect of ozone exposure on lung mitochondrial oxidative metabolism. Chest 66(Suppl):16S, 1974.

482. Alpert SM, Schwartz BB, Lee SD, et al: Alveolar protein accumulation. A sensitive indicator of low level oxidant toxicity. Arch Intern Med 128:69, 1971.
483. Sherwin RP, Richters V: Lung capillary permeability. Nitrogen dioxide exposure and leakage of tritiated serum. Arch Intern Med 128:61, 1971.
484. Halliwell B, Gutteridge JMC: Lipid peroxidation, oxygen radicals, cell damage, and antioxidant therapy. Lancet 1:1396, 1984.
485. Harada RN, Bowman CM, Fox RB, et al: Alveolar macrophage secretions: Initiators of inflammation in pulmonary oxygen toxicity. Chest 81(Suppl):S52, 1982.
486. Fox RB, Hoidal JR, Brown DM, et al: Pulmonary inflammation due to oxygen toxicity: Involvement of chemotactic factors and polymorphonuclear leukocytes. Am Rev Respir Dis 123:521, 1981.
487. Boatman ES, Sato S, Frank R: Acute effects of ozone on cat lungs. II. Structural. Am Rev Respir Dis 110:157, 1974.
488. Weibel ER: Oxygen effect on lung cells. Arch Intern Med 128:54, 1971.
489. Clark JM, Lambertsen CJ: Pulmonary oxygen toxicity: A review. Pharmacol Rev 23:37, 1971.
490. Fisher AB, Diamond S, Mallen S, et al: Effect of 48- and 72-hour oxygen exposure on the rabbit alveolar macrophage. Chest 66(Suppl):4S, 1974.
491. Simons JR, Theodore J, Robin ED: Common oxidant lesion of mitochondrial redox state produced by nitrogen dioxide, ozone and high oxygen in alveolar macrophages. Chest 66(Suppl):9S, 1974.
492. Huber GL, Mason RJ, LaForce M, et al: Alterations in the lung following the administration of ozone. Arch Intern Med 128:81, 1971.
493. Paegle RD, Spain D, Davis S: Pulmonary morphology of chronic phase of oxygen toxicity in adult rats. Chest 66(Suppl):7S, 1974.
494. Crapo JD, Barry BE, Foscue HA, et al: Structural and biochemical changes in rat lungs occurring during exposure to lethal and adaptive doses of oxygen. Am Rev Respir Dis 122:123, 1980.
495. Crapo JD: Superoxide dismutase and tolerance to pulmonary oxygen toxicity. Chest 67(Suppl):39S, 1975.
496. Winter PM, Smith G, Wheelis RF: The effect of prior pulmonary injury on the rate of development of fatal oxygen toxicity. Chest 66(Suppl):1S, 1974.
497. Hayatdavoudi G, Crapo JD, Foscue HA, et al: Evidence of the toxicity of 60 per cent oxygen on rat lungs. Am Rev Respir Dis 117(Suppl):346, 1978.
498. Frank L, Massaro D: Accelerated O₂ toxicity in 100 per cent O₂ after pre-exposure to lower FiO₂. Protection with endotoxin treatment (abstract). Clin Res 28:425A, 1980.
499. Farad R, Simmons G, Feldman N, et al: Impairment of adaptive tolerance to oxygen toxicity by systemic immunosuppression. Chest 67(Suppl):42S, 1975.
500. Nash G, Blennerhassett JB, Pontoppidan H: Pulmonary lesions associated with oxygen therapy and artificial ventilation. N Engl J Med 276:368, 1967.
501. Northway WH Jr, Rosan RC, Porter DY: Pulmonary disease following respirator therapy of hyaline-membrane disease. Bronchopulmonary dysplasia. N Engl J Med 276:357, 1967.
502. Pratt PC: Pulmonary capillary proliferation induced by oxygen inhalation. Am J Pathol 34:1033, 1958.
503. Bruns PD, Shields LV: The pathogenesis and relationship of the hyaline-like pulmonary membrane to premature neonatal mortality. Am J Obstet Gynecol 61:953, 1951.
504. Hawker JM, Reynolds EOR, Taghizadeh A: Pulmonary surface tension and pathological changes in infants dying after respirator treatment for severe hyaline membrane disease. Lancet 2:75, 1967.
505. Shanklin DR, Wolfson SL: Therapeutic oxygen as a possible cause of pulmonary hemorrhage in premature infants. N Engl J Med 277:833, 1967.
506. Balentine JD: Pathologic effects of exposure to high oxygen tensions. A review. N Engl J Med 275:1038, 1966.
507. Roberton NRC, Gupta JM, Dahlenburg GW, et al: Oxygen therapy in the newborn. Lancet 1:1323, 1968.
508. Pontoppidan H, Berry PR: Regulation of the inspired oxygen concentration during artificial ventilation. JAMA 201:11, 1967.
509. Kapanci Y, Tosco R, Eggerman J, et al: Oxygen pneumonitis in man: Light- and electron-microscopic morphometric studies. Chest 62:162, 1972.
510. Gillbe CE, Salt JC, Branthwaite MA: Pulmonary function after prolonged mechanical ventilation with high concentrations of oxygen. Thorax 35:907, 1980.
511. Pratt PC, Sanders AP, Currie WD: Oxygen toxicity and gas mixtures: Morphology. Chest 66(Suppl):8S, 1974.
512. Van DeWater JM, Kagey KS, Miller IT, et al: Oxygen response of the lung to six to twelve hours of 100 per cent inhalation in normal man. N Engl J Med 283:621, 1970.
513. Burger EJ Jr, Mead J: Static properties of lungs after oxygen exposure. J Appl Physiol 27:191, 1969.
514. Caldwell PR, Lee WL Jr, Schildkraut HS, et al: Changes in lung volume, diffusing capacity, and blood gases in men breathing oxygen. J Appl Physiol 21:1477, 1966.
515. Sackner MA, Hirsch JA, Epstein S, et al: Effect of oxygen in graded concentrations upon tracheal mucous velocity. A study in anesthetized dogs. Chest 69:164, 1976.
516. Jackson RM: Pulmonary oxygen toxicity. Chest 88:900, 1985.
517. Editorial: Ozone in smog. Lancet 2:1077, 1975.
518. Castleman WL, Dungworth DL, Schwartz LW, et al: Acute respiratory bronchiolitis. An ultrastructural and autoradiographic study of epithelial cell injury and renewal in rhesus monkeys exposed to ozone. Am J Pathol 98:811, 1980.
519. Wilson DW, Plopper CG, Dungworth DL: The response of the Macaque tracheobronchial epithelium to acute ozone injury. Am J Pathol 116:193, 1984.
520. Mellick PW, Dungworth DL, Schwartz LW, et al: Short-term morphologic effects of high ambient levels of ozone on lungs of Rhesus monkeys. Lab Invest 36:82, 1977.
521. Plopper CG, Dungworth DL, Tyler WS: Pulmonary lesions in rats exposed to ozone. A correlated light and electron microscopic study. Am J Pathol 71:375, 1973.
522. Watanabe S, Frank R, Yokoyama E: Acute effects of ozone on lungs of cats. I. Functional. Am Rev Respir Dis 108:1141, 1973.
523. Sato S, Kawakami N, Maeda S, et al: Scanning electron microscopy of the lungs of vitamin E-deficient rats exposed to a low concentration of ozone. Am Rev Respir Dis 113:809, 1976.
524. Hesterberg TW, Last JA: Ozone-induced acute pulmonary fibrosis in rats: Prevention of increased rates of collagen synthesis by methylprednisolone. Am Rev Respir Dis 123:47, 1981.
525. Hussain MZ, Mustafa MG, Chow CK, et al: Ozone-induced increase of lung proline hydroxylase activity and hydroxyproline content. Chest 69(Suppl):273, 1976.
526. Boorman GA, Schwartz LW, Dungworth DL: Pulmonary effects of prolonged ozone insult in rats. Morphometric evaluation of the central acinus. Lab Invest 43:108, 1980.
527. Eustis SL, Schwartz LW, Kosch PC, et al: Chronic bronchiolitis in nonhuman primates after prolonged ozone exposure. Am J Pathol 105:121, 1981.
528. Gross KB, White HJ: Functional and pathologic consequences of a 52-week exposure to 0.5 ppm ozone followed by a clean air recovery period. Lung 165:283, 1987.
529. Hackney JD, Linn WS, Mohler JG, et al: Experimental studies on human health effects of air pollutants. II. Four-hour exposure to ozone alone and in combinations with other pollutant gases. Arch Environ Health 30:379, 1975.
530. Bates DV, Ball GM, Burnham CD, et al: Short-term effects of ozone on the lung. J Appl Physiol 32:176, 1972.
531. Kagawa J, Toyama T: Effects of ozone and brief exercise on specific airway conductance in man. Arch Environ Health 30:36, 1975.
532. Kagawa J: Respiratory effects of two-hour exposure with intermittent exercise to ozone, sulfur dioxide and nitrogen dioxide alone and in combination in normal subjects. Am Ind Hyg Assoc J 44:14, 1983.
533. Kagawa J: Exposure-effect relationship of selected pulmonary function measurements in subjects exposed to ozone. Int Arch Occup Environ Health 53:345, 1984.
534. Hackney JD, Linn WS, Buckley RD, et al: Scientific communications. Experimental studies on human health effects of air pollutants. I. Design considerations. Arch Environ Health 30:373, 1975.
535. Kerr HD, Kulle TJ, McIlhany ML, et al: Effects of ozone on pulmonary function in normal subjects. An environmental-chamber study. Am Rev Respir Dis 111:763, 1975.
536. Hazucha M, Silverman F, Parent C, et al: Pulmonary function in a man after short-term exposure to ozone. Arch Environ Health 27:183, 1973.
537. Linn WS, Medway DA, Anzar UT, et al: Persistence of adaptation to ozone in volunteers exposed repeatedly for 6 weeks. Am Rev Respir Dis 125:491, 1982.
538. Bromberg PA, Hazucha MJ: Is "adaptation" to ozone protective? Am Rev Respir Dis 125:489, 1982.
539. Horvath SM, Gliner JA, Folinsbee LJ: Adaptation to ozone: Duration of effect. Am Rev Respir Dis 123:496, 1981.
540. Kulle TJ, Milman JH, Sauder LR, et al: Pulmonary function adaptation to ozone in subjects with chronic bronchitis. Environ Res 34:55, 1984.
541. Editorial: Ozone in smog. Lancet 2:1077, 1975.
542. DeJournette RL: Rocket propellant inhalation in the Apollo-Soyuz astronauts. Radiology 125:21, 1977.
543. Dowell AR, Kilburn KH, Pratt PC: Short-term exposure to nitrogen dioxide. Effects on pulmonary ultrastructure, compliance, and the surfactant system. Arch Intern Med 128:74, 1971.
544. Williams RA, Rhoades RA, Adams WS: The response of lung tissue and surfactant to nitrogen dioxide exposure. Arch Intern Med 128:101, 1971.

545. Evans MJ, Stephens RJ, Freeman G: Effects of nitrogen dioxide on cell renewal in the rat lung. Arch Intern Med 128:57, 1971.
546. Evans MJ, Cabral LC, Stephens RJ, et al: Acute kinetic response and renewal of the alveolar epithelium following injury by nitrogen dioxide. Chest 65(Suppl):62S, 1974.
547. Stephens RJ, Freeman G, Evans MJ: Ultrastructural changes in connective tissue in lungs of rats exposed to NO_2. Arch Intern Med 127:873, 1971.
548. Kleinerman J, Ip MPC, Sorensen J: Nitrogen dioxide exposure and alveolar macrophage elastase in hamsters. Am Rev Respir Dis 125:203, 1982.
549. Ranga V, Kleinerman J: Lung injury and repair in the blotchy mouse: Effects of nitrogen dioxide inhalation. Am Rev Respir Dis 123:90, 1981.
550. Pelled B, Shechter Y, Alroy G, et al: Deleterious effects of oxygen at ambient and hyperbaric pressure in the treatment of nitrogen dioxide-poisoned mice. Am Rev Respir Dis 108:1152, 1973.
551. Folinsbee LJ, Horvath SM, Bedi JF, et al: Effect of 0.62 ppm NO_2 on cardiopulmonary function in young male nonsmokers. Environ Res 15:199, 1978.
552. Desgranges JB: Sur une morte prompte occasionné par le gaz nitreux. J Med Chir Pharmacol 8:487, 1804.
553. Ramirez FJ: The first death from nitrogen dioxide fumes. The story of a man and his dog. JAMA 229:1181, 1974.
554. Gailitis J, Burns LE, Nally JB: Silo-filler's disease. Report of a case. N Engl J Med 258:543, 1958.
555. Becklake MR, Goldman HI, Bosman AR, et al: The long-term effects of exposure to nitrous fumes. Am Rev Tuberc 76:398, 1957.
556. Pfitzer EA, Yevich PP, Greene EA, et al: Acute toxicity of red fuming nitric acid-hydrofluoric acid vapor mixture. AMA Arch Ind Health 18:218, 1958.
557. LaFleche LR, Boivin C, Leonard C: Nitrogen dioxide—A respiratory irritant. Can Med Assoc J 84:1438, 1961.
558. Delaney LT Jr, Schmidt HW, Stroebel CF: Silo-filler's disease. Mayo Clin Proc 31:189, 1956.
559. Horvath EP, doPico GA, Barbee RA, et al: Nitrogen dioxide-induced pulmonary disease: Five new cases and a review of the literature. JOM 20:103, 1978.
560. Fleetham JA, Munt PW, Tunnicliffe BW: Silo-filler's disease. Can Med Assoc J 119:482, 1978.
561. Douglas WW, Hepper NG, Colby TV: Silo-filler's disease. Mayo Clin Proc 64:291, 1989.
562. Scott EG, Hunt WB Jr: Silo-filler's disease. Chest 63:701, 1973.
563. Ramirez J, Dowell AR: Silo-filler's disease: Nitrogen dioxide-induced lung injury. Long-term follow-up and review of the literature. Ann Intern Med 74:569, 1971.
564. Tse RL, Bockman AA: Nitrogen dioxide toxicity. Report of four cases in firemen. JAMA 212:1341, 1970.
565. Jones GR, Proudfoot AT, Hall JI: Pulmonary effects of acute exposure to nitrous fumes. Thorax 28:61, 1973.
566. Cornelius EA, Betlach EH: Silo-filler's disease. Radiology 74:232, 1960.
567. Leib GMP, Davis WN, Brown T, et al: Chronic pulmonary insufficiency secondary to silo-filler's disease. Am J Med 24:471, 1958.
568. Moskowitz RL, Lyons HA, Cottle HR: Silo-filler's disease. Clinical, physiologic and pathologic study of a patient. Am J Med 36:457, 1964.
569. Fleming GM, Chester EH, Montenegro HD: Dysfunction of small airways following pulmonary injury due to nitrogen dioxide. Chest 75:720, 1979.
570. Larson TV, Frank R, Covert DS, et al: Measurements of respiratory ammonia and the chemical neutralization of inhaled sulfuric acid aerosol in anesthetized dogs. Am Rev Respir Dis 125:502, 1982.
571. Morgan WKC, Seaton A: Occupational Lung Disease. Philadelphia, WB Saunders, 1975, p 241.
572. Kipen HM, Lerman Y: Respiratory abnormalities among photographic developers: A report of three cases. Am J Ind Med 9:341, 1986.
573. Hodgson MJ, Parkinson DK: Respiratory disease in a photographer. Am J Ind Med 9:349, 1986.
574. Woodford DM, Coutu RE, Gaensler EA: Obstructive lung disease from acute sulfur dioxide exposure. Respiration 38:238, 1979.
575. Hamilton A, Hardy HL: Industrial Toxicology. 3rd ed. Acton, Mass, Publishing Sciences Group, Inc, 1974, p 210.
576. Charan NB, Myers CG, Lakshminarayan S, et al: Pulmonary injuries associated with acute sulfur dioxide inhalation. Am Rev Respir Dis 119:555, 1979.
577. Harkonen H, Nordman H, Korhonen O, et al: Long-term effects of exposure to sulfur dioxide: Lung function four years after a pyrite dust explosion. Am Rev Respir Dis 128:890, 1983.
578. Osbern LN, Crapo RO: Dung lung: A report of toxic exposure to liquid manure. Ann Intern Med 95:312, 1981.
579. Burnett WW, King EG, Grace M, et al: Hydrogen sulfide poisoning: Review of 5 years experience. Can Med Assoc J 117:1277, 1977.

580. Glass RI, Ford R, Allegra DT, et al: Deaths from asphyxia among fishermen. JAMA 244:2193, 1980.
581. Meuret G, Fueter R, Gloor F: Early stage of fulminant idiopathic pulmonary fibrosis cured by intense combination therapy using cyclophosphamide, vincristine and prednisone. Respiration 36:228, 1978.
582. Price SK, Hughes JE, Morrison SC, et al: Fatal ammonia inhalation: A case report with autopsy findings. S Afr Med J 64:952, 1983.
583. Sobonya R: Fatal anhydrous ammonia inhalation. Hum Pathol 8:293, 1977.
584. Arwood R, Hammond J, Ward GG: Ammonia inhalation. J Trauma 25:444, 1985.
585. Hatton DV, Leach CS, Beaudet AL, et al: Collagen breakdown and ammonia inhalation. Arch Environ Health 34:83, 1979.
586. Caplin M: Ammonia gas-poisoning. Forty-seven cases in a London shelter. Lancet 241:95, 1941.
587. Klein J, Olson KR, McKinney HE: Caustic injury from household ammonia. Am J Emerg Med 3:320, 1985.
588. Slot CMJ: Ammonia gas burns. An account of six cases. Lancet 235:1356, 1938.
589. Flury KE, Dines DE, Rodarte JR, et al: Airway obstruction due to inhalation of ammonia. Mayo Clin Proc 58:389, 1983.
590. Hoeffler HB, Schweppe HI, Greenberg SD: Bronchiectasis following pulmonary ammonia burn. Arch Pathol Lab Med 106:686, 1982.
591. Kass I, Zamel N, Dobry CA, et al: Bronchiectasis following ammonia burns of the respiratory tract. A review of two cases. Chest 62:282, 1972.
592. Weill H, George R, Schwarz M, et al: Late evaluation of pulmonary function after acute exposure to chlorine gas. Am Rev Respir Dis 99:374, 1969.
593. Chester EH, Gillespie DG, Krause FD: The prevalence of chronic obstructive pulmonary disease in chlorine gas workers. Am Rev Respir Dis 99:365, 1969.
594. Jones RN, Hughes JM, Glindmeyer H, et al: Lung function after acute chlorine exposure. Am Rev Respir Dis 134:1190, 1986.
595. Adelson L, Kaufman J: Fatal chlorine poisoning: Report of two cases with clinicopathologic correlation. Am J Clin Pathol 56:430, 1971.
596. Rosenthal T, Baum GL, Frand U, et al: Poisoning caused by inhalation of hydrogen chloride, phosphorus oxychloride, phosphorus pentachloride, oxalyl chloride, and oxalic acid. Chest 73:623, 1978.
597. Hasan FM, Gehshan A, Fuleihan FJ: Resolution of pulmonary dysfunction following acute chlorine exposure. Arch Environ Health 38:76, 1983.
598. Seidelin R: The inhalation of phosgene in a fire extinguisher accident. Thorax 16:91, 1961.
599. Chester EH, Kaimal J, Payne CB Jr, et al: Pulmonary injury following exposure to chlorine gas: Possible beneficial effects of steroid treatment. Chest 72:247, 1977.
600. Rafferty P: Voluntary chlorine inhalation: A new form of self-abuse? Br Med J 281:1178, 1980.
601. Gerritsen WB, Buschmann CH: Phosgene poisoning caused by the use of chemical paint removers containing methylene chloride in ill-ventilated rooms heated by kerosene stoves. Br J Ind Med 17:187, 1960.
602. English JM: A case of probable phosgene poisoning. Br Med J 1:38, 1964.
603. Polednak, AP: Mortality among men occupationally exposed to phosgene in 1943–1945. Environ Res 22:357, 1980.
604. Everett ED, Overholt EL: Phosgene poisoning. JAMA 205:243, 1968.
605. Gore I Jr, Harding SM: Sinker lung: Acute metallic mercury poisoning associated with the making of fish weights. Ala J Med Sci 24:267, 1987.
606. Hallee TJ: Diffuse lung disease caused by inhalation of mercury vapor. Am Rev Respir Dis 99:430, 1969.
607. Natelson EA, Blumenthal BJ, Fred HL: Acute mercury vapor poisoning in the home. Chest 59:677, 1971.
608. Lien DC, Todoruk DN, Rajani HR, et al: Accidental inhalation of mercury vapour: Respiratory and toxicologic consequences. Can Med Assoc J 129:591, 1983.
609. Haddad JK, Stenberg E Jr: Bronchitis due to acute mercury inhalation. Report of two cases. Am Rev Respir Dis 88:543, 1963.
610. Tamir M, Bronstein B, Behar M, et al: Mercury poisoning from an unsuspected source. Br J Ind Med 21:299, 1964.
611. Johnson HRM, Koumides O: Unusual case of mercury poisoning. Br Med J 1:340, 1967.
612. Wallach L: Aspiration of elemental mercury—Evidence of absorption without toxicity. N Engl J Med 287:178, 1972.
613. Milliken JA, Waugh D, Kadish ME: Acute interstitial pulmonary fibrosis caused by a smoke bomb. Can Med Assoc J 88:36, 1963.
614. Evans EH: Casualties following exposure to zinc chloride smoke. Lancet 2:368, 1945.

615. Riddervold J, Halvasen K: Bacteriological investigations on pneumonia and pneumococcus carriers in Sauda, an isolated industrial community in Norway. Acta Pathol Microbiol Scand 20:272, 1943.
616. Davies TAL: Manganese pneumonitis. Br J Ind Med 3:111, 1946.
617. Davies TAL, Harding HK: Manganese pneumonitis. Further clinical and experimental observations. Br J Ind Med 6:82, 1949.
618. Lewis GP, Coughlin LL, Jusko WJ, et al: Contribution of cigarette smoking to cadmium accumulation in man. Lancet 1:291, 1972.
619. Editorial: Cadmium and the lung. Lancet 2:1134, 1973.
620. Scott R, Paterson PJ, McKirdy A, et al: Clinical and biochemical abnormalities in coppersmiths. Lancet 2:396, 1976.
621. Beton DC, Andrews GS, Davies HJ, et al: Acute cadmium fume poisoning. Five cases with one death from renal necrosis. Br J Ind Med 23:292, 1966.
622. Edling C, Elinder CG, Randma E: Lung function in workers using cadmium containing solders. Br J Ind Med 43:657, 1986.
623. Hirst RN, Perry HM, Cruz MG, et al: Elevated cadmium concentration in emphysematous lungs. Am Rev Respir Dis 108:30, 1973.
624. Lewis GP, Lyle H, Miller S: Association between elevated hepatic water-soluble protein-bound cadmium levels and chronic bronchitis and/or emphysema. Lancet 2:1330, 1969.
625. Palmer KC, Snider GL, Hayes JA: Cellular proliferation induced in the lung by cadmium aerosol. Am Rev Respir Dis 112:173, 1975.
626. Snider GL, Hayes JA, Korthy AL, et al: Centrilobular emphysema experimentally induced by cadmium chloride aerosol. Am Rev Respir Dis 108:40, 1973.
627. Thurlbeck WM, Foley FD: Experimental pulmonary emphysema: The effect of intratracheal injection of cadmium chloride solution in the guinea pig. Am J Pathol 42:431, 1963.
628. Bonnell JA, Kazantzis G, King E: A follow-up study of men exposed to cadmium oxide fume. Br J Ind Med 16:135, 1959.
629. Kazantzis G, Flynn FV, Spowage JS, et al: Renal tubular malfunction and pulmonary emphysema in cadmium pigment workers. Q J Med 32:165, 1963.
630. DeSilva PE, Donnan MB: Chronic cadmium poisoning in a pigment manufacturing plant. Br J Ind Med 38:76, 1981.
631. Lauwerys RR, Roels HA, Buchet J-P, et al: Investigations on the lung and kidney function in workers exposed to cadmium. Environ Health Perspect 28:137, 1979.
632. Bonnell JA: Emphysema and proteinuria in men casting copper-cadmium alloys. Br J Ind Med 12:181, 1955.
633. Smith TJ, Petty TL, Reading JC, et al: Pulmonary effects of chronic exposure to airborne cadmium. Am Rev Respir Dis 114:161, 1976.
634. Anthony JS, Zamel N, Aberman A: Abnormalities in pulmonary function after brief exposure to toxic metal fumes. Can Med Assoc J 119:586, 1978.
635. doPico GA, Rankin J, Chosy LW, et al: Respiratory tract disease from thermo-setting resins. Study of an outbreak in rubber tire workers. Ann Intern Med 83:177, 1975.
636. Herbert FA, Orford R: Pulmonary hemorrhage and edema due to inhalation of resins containing trimellitic anhydride. Chest 75:546, 1979.
637. Patterson R, Addington W, Banner AS, et al: Antihapten antibodies in workers exposed to trimellitic anhydride fumes: A potential immunopathogenetic mechanism for the trimellitic anhydride pulmonary disease-anemia syndrome. Am Rev Respir Dis 120:1259, 1979.
638. Rice DL, Jenkins DE, Gray JM, et al: Chemical pneumonitis secondary to inhalation of epoxy pipe coating. Arch Environ Health 32:173, 1977.
639. Ahmad D, Morgan WK, Patterson R, et al: Pulmonary haemorrhage and haemolytic anaemia due to trimellitic anhydride. Lancet 2:328, 1979.
640. Patterson R, Addington W, Banner AS, et al: Antihapten antibodies in workers exposed to trimellitic anhydride fumes: A potential immunopathogenetic mechanism for the trimellitic anhydride pulmonary disease-anemia syndrome. Am Rev Respir Dis 120:1259, 1979.
641. Rivera M, Nicotra B, Byron GE, et al: Trimellitic anhydride toxicity: A cause of acute multisystem failure. Arch Intern Med 141:1071, 1981.
642. Zeiss CR, Wolkonsky P, Chacon R, et al: Syndromes in workers exposed to trimellitic anhydride: A longitudinal clinical and immunologic study. Ann Intern Med 98:8, 1983.
643. Leach CL, Hatoum NS, Ratajczak HV, et al: Evidence of immunologic control of lung injury induced by trimellitic anhydride. Am Rev Respir Dis 137:186, 1988.
644. Zeiss CR, Leach CL, Smith LJ, et al: A serial immunologic and histopathologic study of lung injury induced by trimellitic anhydride. Am Rev Respir Dis 137:191, 1988.
645. Liu F-T, Bargatze RF, Katz DH: Induction of immunologic tolerance to the trimellitate haptenic group in mice: Model for a therapeutic approach to trimellitic anhydride-induced hypersensitivity syndromes in humans? J Allergy Clin Immunol 66:322, 1980.

646. Rohrs LC: Metal-fume fever from inhaling zinc oxide. AMA Arch Intern Med 100:44, 1957.
647. Vogelmeier C, Konig G, Bencze K, et al: Pulmonary involvement in zinc fume fever. Chest 92:946, 1987.
648. Wegman DH, Peters JM: Polymer fume fever and cigarette smoking. Ann Intern Med 81:55, 1974.
649. Robbins JJ, Ware RL: Pulmonary edema from Teflon fumes. N Engl J Med 271:360, 1964.
650. Evans EA: Pulmonary edema after inhalation of fumes from polytetrafluoroethylene (PTFE). J Occup Med 15:599, 1973.
651. Williams N, Smith K: Polymer fume fever, an elusive diagnosis. JAMA 219:1587, 1972.
652. Yodaiken RE: The uncertain consequences of formaldehyde toxicity. JAMA 246:1677, 1981.
653. Bernstein RS, Stayner LT, Elliot LJ, et al: Inhalation exposure to formaldehyde: An overview of its toxicology, epidemiology, monitoring, and control. Am Ind Hyg Assoc J 45:778, 1984.
654. Alexandersson R, Kolmodin-Hedman B, Hedenstierna G: Exposure to formaldehyde: Effects on pulmonary function. Arch Environ Health 37:279, 1982.
655. Kwong F, Kraske G, Nelson AM, et al: Acute symptoms secondary to formaldehyde exposure in a pathology resident. Ann Allergy 50:326, 1983.
656. Levine RJ, DalCorso RD, Blunden PD, et al: The effects of occupational exposure on the respiratory health of West Virginia morticians. J Occup Med 26:91, 1984.
657. Uba G, Pachorek D, Bernstein J, et al: Prospective study of respiratory effects of formaldehyde among healthy and asthmatic medical students. Am J Ind Med 15:91, 1989.
658. Harris JC, Rumack BH, Aldrich FD: Toxicology of urea formaldehyde and polyurethane foam insulation. JAMA 245:243, 1981.
659. Day JH, Lees REM, Clark RH, et al: Respiratory response to formaldehyde and off-gas of urea formaldehyde foam insulation. Can Med Assoc J 131:1061, 1984.
660. Norman GR, Pengelly LD, Kerigan AT, et al: Respiratory function of children in homes insulated with urea formaldehyde foam insulation. Can Med Assoc J 134:1135, 1986.
661. Dally KA, Hanrahan LP, Woodbury MA, et al: Formaldehyde exposure in nonoccupational environments. Arch Environ Health 36:277, 1981.
662. Witek TJ Jr, Schachter EN, Tosun T, et al: An evaluation of respiratory effects following exposure to 2.0 ppm formaldehyde in asthmatics: Lung function, symptoms, and airway reactivity. Arch Environ Health 42:230, 1987.
663. Campbell JS, Harrison JR: Current status of urea-formaldehyde foam insulation. Can Med Assoc J 125:329, 1981.
664. Marsh GM: Proportional mortality patterns among chemical plant workers exposed to formaldehyde. Br J Ind Med 39:313, 1982.
665. Done AK: The toxic emergency: Where there's smoke, there may be more than fire. Emerg Med 13:111, 1981.
666. Clark CJ, Campbell D, Reid WH: Blood carboxyhaemoglobin and cyanide levels in fire survivors. Lancet 1:1332, 1981.
667. Dyer RF, Esch VH: Polyvinyl chloride toxicity in fires, hydrogen chloride toxicity in fire fighters. JAMA 235:393, 1976.
668. Froneberg B, Johnson PL, Landrigan PJ: Respiratory illness caused by overheating of polyvinyl chloride. Br J Ind Med 39:239, 1982.
669. Brinkmann B, Püschel K: Heat injuries to the respiratory system. Virchows Arch A Pathol Anat Histol 379:299, 1978.
670. Jung RC, Gottlieb LS: Respiratory tract burns after aspiration of hot coffee. Chest 72:125, 1977.
671. Editorial: The lung in burns. Lancet 2:673, 1981.
672. Moylan JA, Chan C-K: Inhalation injury: An increasing problem. Ann Surg 188:34, 1978.
673. Hasleton PS, McWilliam L, Haboubi NY: The lung parenchyma in burns. Histopathology 7:333, 1983.
674. Burns TR, Greenberg SD, Cartwright J, et al: Smoke inhalation: An ultrastructural study of reaction to injury in the human alveolar wall. Environ Res 41:447, 1986.
675. Thorning DR, Howard ML, Hudson LD, et al: Morphologic changes in rabbits exposed to pine wood smoke. Hum Pathol 13:355, 1982.
676. Williams DO, Vanecko RM, Glassroth J: Endobronchial polyposis following smoke inhalation. Chest 84:774, 1983.
677. Cooney W, Dzuira B, Harper R, et al: The cytology of sputum from thermally injured patients. Acta Cytol 16:433, 1972.
678. Phillips AW, Tanner JW, Cope O: Burn therapy. IV. Respiratory tract damage (an account of the clinical, x-ray and postmortem findings) and the meaning of restlessness. Ann Surg 158:799, 1963.
679. Achauer BM, Allyn PA, Furnas DW, et al: Pulmonary complications of burns: The major threat to the burn patient. Ann Surg 177:311, 1973.
680. Whitener DR, Whitener LM, Robertson KJ, et al: Pulmonary function measurements in patients with thermal injury and smoke inhalation. Am Rev Respir Dis 122:731, 1980.
681. Teixidor HS, Novick G, Rubin E: Pulmonary complications in burn patients. J Can Assoc Radiol 34:264, 1983.

682. Peters WJ: Inhalation injury caused by the products of combustion. Can Med Assoc J 125:249, 1981.
683. Raman TK, Dobbins JR, Berte JB: Respiratory burns during oxygen therapy. Chest 57:485, 1970.
684. Crapo RO: Smoke-inhalation injuries. JAMA 246:1694, 1981.
685. Teixidor HS, Rubin E, Novick GS, et al: Smoke inhalation: Radiologic manifestations. Radiology 149:383, 1983.
686. Shirani KZ, Pruitt BA Jr, Mason AD Jr: The influence of inhalation injury and pneumonia on burn mortality. Ann Surg 205:82, 1987.
687. Pietak SP, Delahaye DJ: Airway obstruction following smoke inhalation. Can Med Assoc J 115:329, 1976.
688. Achauer BM, Allyn PA, Furnas DW, et al: Pulmonary complications of burns: The major threat to the burn patient. Ann Surg 177:311, 1973.
689. Beachley MC, Ghahremani GG: The radiographic spectrum of pulmonary complications in burn victims. Am J Roentgenol 128:441, 1977.
690. Putman CE, Loke J, Matthay RA, et al: Radiographic manifestations of acute smoke inhalation. Am J Roentgenol 129:865, 1977.
691. Putman CE, Loke J, Matthay RA, et al: Radiographic manifestations of acute smoke inhalation. Am J Roentgenol 129:865, 1977.
692. Tashkin DP, Genovesi MG, Chopra S, et al: Respiratory status of Los Angeles firemen: One-month follow-up after inhalation of dense smoke. Chest 71:445, 1977.
693. Sidor R, Peters JM: Prevalence rates of chronic non-specific respiratory disease in fire fighters. Am Rev Respir Dis 109:255, 1974.
694. Peters JM, Theriault GP, Fine LJ, et al: Chronic effect of fire fighting on pulmonary function. N Engl J Med 291:1320, 1974.
695. Sidor R, Peters JM: Fire fighting and pulmonary function. An epidemiologic study. Am Rev Respir Dis 109:249, 1974.
696. Musk AW, Peters JM, Wegman DH: Lung function in fire fighters, I: A three year follow-up of active subjects. Am J Public Health 67:626, 1977.
697. Musk AW, Peters JM, Wegman DH: Lung function in fire fighters, II: A five year follow-up of retirees. Am J Public Health 67:630, 1977.
698. Unger KM, Snow RM, Mestas JM, et al: Smoke inhalation in firemen. Thorax 35:838, 1980.
699. Loke J, Farmer W, Matthay RA, et al: Acute and chronic effects of fire fighting on pulmonary function. Chest 77:369, 1980.
700. Genovesi MG: Effects of smoke inhalation. Chest 77:335, 1980.
701. Young I, Jackson J, West S: Chronic respiratory disease and respiratory function in a group of fire fighters. Med J Aust 1:654, 1980.
702. Sparrow D, Bosse R, Rosner B, et al: The effect of occupational exposure on pulmonary function: A longitudinal evaluation of fire fighters and nonfire fighters. Am Rev Respir Dis 125:319, 1982.
703. Musk AW, Monson RR, Peters JM, et al: Mortality among Boston firefighters, 1915–1975. Br J Ind Med 35:104, 1978.
704. Decoufle P, Lloyd JW, Salvin LG: Mortality by cause among stationary engineers and stationary firemen. JOM 19:679, 1977.
705. Cordasco EM, Demeter SL, Kerkay J, et al: Pulmonary manifestations of vinyl and polyvinyl chloride (interstitial lung disease); newer aspects. Chest 78:828, 1980.
706. Lilis R: Vinyl chloride and polyvinyl chloride exposure and occupational lung disease. Chest 78:826, 1980.
707. Mastrangelo G, Manno M, Marcer G, et al: Polyvinyl chloride pneumoconiosis: Epidemiological study of exposed workers. JOM 21:540, 1979.
708. Boutar CA, Copland LH, Thornley PE, et al: Epidemiological study of respiratory disease in workers exposed to polyvinylchloride dust. Thorax 35:644, 1980.
709. Chivers CP, Lawrence-Jones C, Paddle GM: Lung function in workers exposed to polyvinyl chloride dust. Br J Ind Med 37:147, 1980.
710. Buffler PA, Wood S, Eifler C, et al: Mortality experience of workers in a vinyl chloride monomer production plant. JOM 21:195, 1979.
711. Wegman DH, Peters JM, Jaeger RJ, et al: Vinyl chloride: Can the worker be protected? N Engl J Med 294:653, 1976.
712. Anderson H, Miller A, Selikoff IJ: Pulmonary changes among vinyl chloride polymerization workers. Chest 69(Suppl):299, 1976.
713. Dannaher CL, Tamburro CH, Yam LT: Occupational carcinogenesis: The Louisville experience with vinyl chloride-associated hepatic angiosarcoma. Am J Med 70:279, 1981.
714. Ward AM, Udnoon S, Watkins J, et al: Immunological mechanisms in the pathogenesis of vinyl chloride disease. Br Med J 1:936, 1976.

715. Suciu I, Prodan L, Ilea E, et al: Clinical manifestations in vinyl chloride poisoning. Ann NY Acad Sci 246:53, 1975.
716. Martseller HJ, Lelbach WK: Unusual splenomegalic liver disease as evidenced by peritoneoscopy and guided liver biopsy among polyvinyl chloride production workers. Ann NY Acad Sci 246:95, 1975.
717. Stewart RD, Hake CL: Paint-remover hazard. JAMA 235:398, 1976.
718. Wilson EF, Rich TH, Messman HC: The hazardous hibachi. Carbon monoxide poisoning following use of charcoal. JAMA 221:405, 1972.
719. Morandi M, Eisenbud M: Carbon monoxide exposure in New York City: A historical overview. Bull NY Acad Med 56:817, 1980.
720. Smith JS, Brandon S: Morbidity from acute carbon monoxide poisoning. A three-year follow-up. Br Med J 1:318, 1973.
721. Astrup P: Some physiological and pathological effects of moderate carbon monoxide exposure. Br Med J 4:447, 1972.
722. Goldsmith JR, Landaw SA: Carbon monoxide in human health. Science 162:1352, 1968.
723. Cowie J, Sillett EW, Ball KP: Carbon-monoxide absorption by cigarette smokers who change to smoking cigars. Lancet 1:1033, 1973.
724. Editorial: Carbon monoxide poisoning—A timely warning. N Engl J Med 278:849, 1968.
725. Aronow WS, Isbell MW: Carbon monoxide effect on exercise-induced angina pectoris. Ann Intern Med 79:392, 1973.
726. Anderson EW, Adelman RJ, Strauch JM, et al: Effect of low-level carbon monoxide exposure on onset and duration of angina pectoris. A study in ten patients with ischemic heart disease. Ann Intern Med 79:46, 1973.
727. Sone S, Higashihara T, Kotake T, et al: Pulmonary manifestations in acute carbon monoxide poisoning. Am J Roentgenol 120:865, 1974.
728. Kittredge RD: Pulmonary edema in acute carbon monoxide poisoning. Am J Roentgenol 113:680, 1971.
729. Fein A, Grossman RF, Jones JG, et al: Carbon monoxide effect on alveolar epithelial permeability. Chest 78:726, 1980.
730. Bergmann M, Flance IJ, Blumenthal HT: Thesaurosis following inhalation of hair spray: A clinical and experimental study. N Engl J Med 258:471, 1958.
731. Bergmann M, Flance IJ, Cruz PT, et al: Thesaurosis due to inhalation of hair spray. Report of twelve new cases, including three autopsies. N Engl J Med 266:750, 1962.
732. Herrero EU, Feigelson HH, Becker A: Sarcoidosis in a beautician. Am Rev Respir Dis 92:280, 1965.
733. Gebbers J-O, Tetzner C, Burkhardt A: Alveolitis due to hair-spray. Virchows Arch A Pathol Anat Histol 382:323, 1979.
734. Wright JL, Cockcroft DW: Lung disease due to abuse of hairspray. Arch Pathol Lab Med 105:363, 1981.
735. Brunner MJ, Giovacchini RP, Wyatt JP, et al: Pulmonary disease and hair-spray polymers: A disputed relationship. JAMA 184:851, 1963.
736. Gowdy JM, Wagstaff MJ: Pulmonary infiltration due to aerosol thesaurosis. A survey of hairdressers. Arch Environ Health 25:101, 1972.
737. Schraufnagel DE, Paré JAP, Wang NS: Micronodular pulmonary pattern: Association with inhaled aerosol. Am J Roentgenol 137:57, 1981.
738. Bergmann M, Flance IJ, Blumenthal HT: Thesaurosis following inhalation of hair spray: A clinical and experimental study. N Engl J Med 258:471, 1958.
739. Bergmann M, Flance IJ, Cruz PT, et al: Thesaurosis due to inhalation of hair spray. Report of twelve new cases, including three autopsies. N Engl J Med 266:750, 1962.
740. Hunter D: Devices for the protection of the worker against injury and disease. Part II. Br Med J 1:506, 1950.
741. Cooke NT, Bamji AN: Gold and pulmonary function in rheumatoid arthritis. Br J Rheumatol 22:18, 1983.
742. Shroff CP, Khade MV, Srinivasan M: Respiratory cytopathology in chlorine gas toxicity: A study in 28 subjects. Diagn Cytopathol 4:28, 1988.
743. Chaney S, Blomquist D, DeWitt P, et al: Biochemical changes in humans upon exposure to nitrogen dioxide while at rest. Arch Environ Health 36:53, 1981.
744. Montague TJ, MacNeil AR: Mass ammonia inhalation. Chest 77:496, 1980.

15

Diseases of the Thorax Caused by External Physical Agents

Trauma to the thorax can result in a wide variety of effects on the chest wall, diaphragm, mediastinum, trachea, and lungs. The results may be direct (for example, fractures of the ribs, spine, or shoulder girdles; diaphragmatic hernia; esophageal rupture; and pulmonary contusion or laceration) or indirect (such as air embolism resulting from the escape of air into pulmonary veins subsequent to parenchymal laceration). Because the manifestations of such trauma are dissimilar in different sites, each is considered separately. As might be anticipated, however, a great deal of overlap occurs. Also, the effects of penetrating and nonpenetrating trauma may be quite different and thus require separate consideration. "Trauma" is used here in its broad sense to indicate all affections of the thorax resulting from external physical agents (with the exception of certain inhalation and embolic diseases); thus, irradiation injury is included in this category. It is also appropriate to include in this chapter the consequences of surgery, both thoracic and nonthoracic, and complications caused by various diagnostic, therapeutic, and monitoring procedures including intubation.

Pre-existing or coincidental pulmonary disease can make the lung more susceptible to traumatic damage or can be ascribed in error to the traumatic episode. An example of the former situation is rupture of a bulla secondary to rib fracture and development of pneumothorax. Mistakenly ascribing pulmonary damage to trauma might be exemplified by the discovery, after a traumatic episode, of a pleural effusion that on subsequent investigation proved to be of tuberculous etiology;[1] in fact, in certain circumstances it is possible that underlying disease such as tuberculosis may be activated by chest trauma.[2]

Although diagnosis of the majority of traumatic abnormalities of the thorax can be established with reasonable confidence by conventional roentgenographic methods, certain conditions (for example, laceration of the aorta) require special diagnostic procedures, including computed tomography (CT) and aortography, to confirm the injury and establish its extent. Toombs and his colleagues[3] have emphasized the importance of CT in the study of patients following acute chest trauma; in their series of 20 patients, many abnormalities were discovered on CT that were not apparent on conventional roentgenograms. In another study of 85 consecutive patients with chest trauma, Wagner and his colleagues[33] found 151 abnormalities (excluding rib fractures) on roentgenograms and 423 on CT scans; further, 99 lacerations were identified on CT and only 5 on roentgenograms. The value of CT in blunt chest trauma has recently been reviewed.[477]

EFFECTS ON THE LUNGS OF NONPENETRATING TRAUMA

PULMONARY PARENCHYMAL CONTUSION

Pulmonary contusion consists of the exudation of edema fluid and blood into the parenchyma of the lung in both its airspace and interstitial components[4–9] unaccompanied by substantial tissue disruption; it is the most common pulmonary complication of blunt chest trauma. In nonpenetrating injuries it occurs more often than rib fracture[5, 6] and, indeed, rib fractures are frequently absent.[10,11] The severity of the injury necessary to produce contusion varies from a trivial glancing blow to major trauma resulting from motor vehicle or aircraft accidents.[10] Nonmilitary blast injuries account for a small percentage of cases.[11, 12] Pulmonary contusion has been reported following extracorporeal shock-wave lithotripsy.[13]

Roentgenographically, the pattern varies from irregular, patchy areas of airspace consolidation to diffuse and extensive homogeneous consolidation (Fig. 15–1). As might be expected, the distribution of the contused areas does not conform to lobes or segments.[4, 5, 7] Although the major change is usually in the lung directly deep to the traumatized areas, damage may occur also, or even predominantly, on the opposite side as a result of a contrecoup effect.[9, 14] In blast injuries the contusion is typically bilateral,[9] although again the major change occurs in the thoracic area that faced the blast. Increase in the size and loss of definition of the vascular markings extending out from the hila indicate the presence of hemorrhage and edema in the peribronchovascular interstitial space.[5, 7]

The time between the trauma and the detection of roentgenographic abnormality is important, particularly in the differentiation from traumatic fat embolism. In contusion, changes are apparent roentgenographically soon after trauma (almost invariably within 6 hours),[7, 10] whereas in traumatic fat embolism they usually become manifest only 1 to 2 days or more after injury. Resolution of lung contusion typically occurs rapidly, improvement being noted within 24 to 48 hours[6, 15] and clearing being complete within 3 to 10 days (Fig. 15–2).[4–7, 16, 17] Shaw[18] has described a somewhat atypical type of pulmonary "contusion" resulting from the impact of rubber bullets; parenchymal opacification develops immediately and persists for weeks to months (the protracted time course suggests that these opacities represented hematomas rather than simple contusion).

Clinically, the findings are seldom striking; in fact, symptoms may be entirely absent[7, 19] or may be masked by the many other injuries the patient has.[20] Pain is not a prominent feature except from other aspects of the trauma. Hemoptysis is said to occur in 50 per cent of cases, and there may be mild fever; shortness of breath may develop in the presence of severe contusion.[7, 10] Pulmonary contusion can be the site of secondary infection.[21]

PULMONARY PARENCHYMAL LACERATION, TRAUMATIC LUNG CYST, AND HEMATOMA

Rather uncommonly, closed chest trauma results in the development of one or more cystic spaces within the lung that can remain air-filled or that can fill partly or completely with blood. The

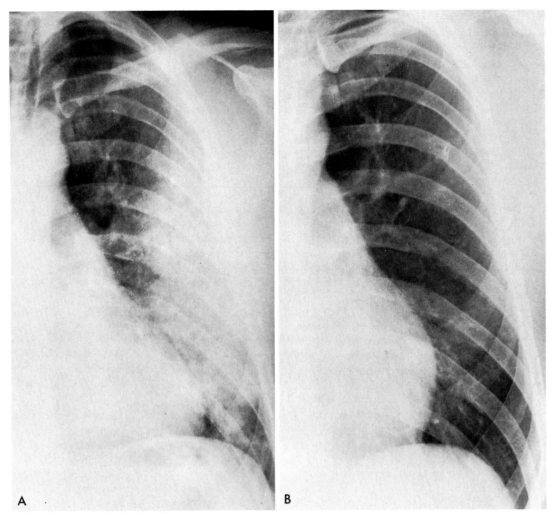

Figure 15–1. Pulmonary Contusion. Six hours before the roentgenographic examination illustrated in *(A)*, this 33-year-old man was involved in a car accident in which he suffered severe trauma to the posterior portion of his left chest. A view of the left hemithorax from an anteroposterior roentgenogram reveals homogeneous consolidation of the posterolateral portion of the left lung in nonsegmental distribution. The margins of the consolidation are very indistinctly defined and there is no air bronchogram. No ribs were fractured. The right lung was clear. Six days later *(B)*, complete clearing had occurred.

trauma usually is blunt and often severe, as in automobile accidents. Children and young adults seem to be particularly prone, probably because of the greater flexibility of their thoracic walls; in fact, in young patients, the trauma can be relatively minor and still result in rather large parenchymal lacerations.[22]

Three mechanisms have been suggested to explain the development of traumatic lung cysts: (1) The physical force ruptures alveolar tissue, and the inherently elastic lung parenchyma recoils from the ruptured area, leaving a spherical cystic lesion.[23, 24] (2) Sudden compression of an area of lung closes off a segment of the peripheral bronchial tree and creates within it a bursting, explosive pressure that is expended in the rupture of alveolar walls within the lobules supplied by the occluded bronchus.[25] (3) The propagation of a concussion wave creates shearing stresses that tear the substance of the lung.[5]

These lesions may be apparent roentgenographically immediately after trauma but more commonly are not seen until a few hours or even several days later.[26, 27] Regardless of the mechanism of their production, it is logical to assume that they develop coincident with the trauma. The fact that they are not identified immediately could be ascribed to two circumstances: (1) In the absence of hemorrhage, their paper-thin margins and lack of contrast with contiguous parenchyma render them invisible. (2) Their presence may be masked by surrounding pulmonary contusion (Fig. 15–3).[9]

Pathologically, the features of traumatic lung cysts have been infrequently described.[28] The occasional excised specimen has shown the "cyst" wall to be composed of fibrous or granulation tissue; since there is no epithelial lining, the use of the term cyst is thus, strictly speaking, incorrect and some authors designate the lesion a pseudocyst.[28] A parenchymal hematoma consists of a collection of blood of variable size that compresses adjacent lung tissue (Fig. 15–4); an acute inflammatory reaction is occasionally present at the periphery.

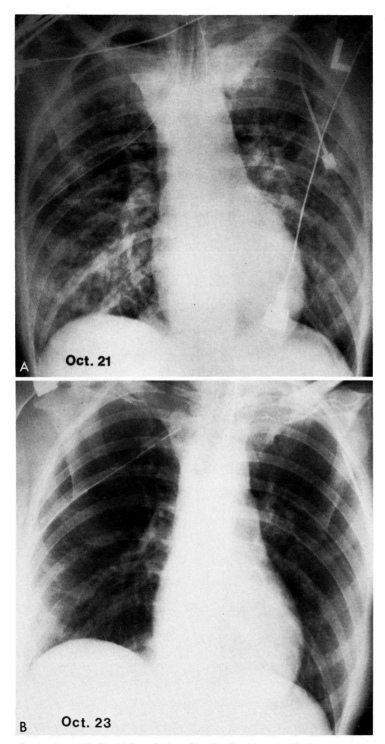

Figure 15–2. Pulmonary Contusion with Rapid Resolution. Shortly after his arrival in the emergency room following an automobile accident, this 22-year-old man showed roentgenographic evidence of poorly defined patchy airspace consolidation throughout both lungs *(A)*. The appearance is one of pulmonary edema of any cause, although the history and normal cardiac size obviously favor traumatic contusion. Complete clearing had occurred 48 hours later *(B)*.

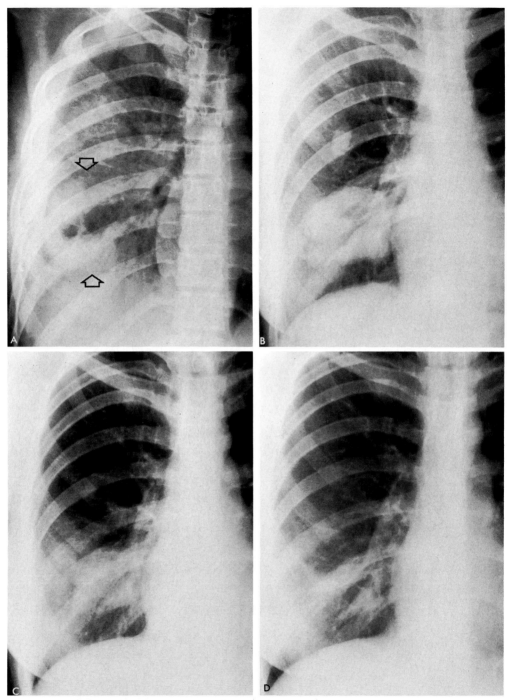

Figure 15–3. Pulmonary Contusion and Hematoma. This 15-year-old girl suffered a severe blow to the right side of her chest in a car accident. Three hours after the accident, an anteroposterior roentgenogram *(A)* demonstrates extensive consolidation of the parenchyma of the right lung due to pulmonary contusion (the left lung was clear). In addition to the diffuse opacity, an indistinctly defined shadow of greater density is present in the right base *(arrows)*, containing a central radiolucency; there is a large hemothorax. Three weeks later *(B)*, the general opacity caused by contusion has completely cleared, as has the hemothorax. However, there remains a large, sharply circumscribed, lobulated shadow that represents the hematoma vaguely visible in *(A)*. A much smaller hematoma can be identified in the lung directly above the major lesion. Approximately 1 month later *(C)*, the mass has undergone considerable decrease in size and is not as sharply defined. One month later *(D)*, the hematoma is still present in the form of an elliptical shadow. Complete clearing did not occur until 6 months later. (Courtesy of Dr. J. G. Monks, Rosetown Union Hospital, Rosetown, Saskatchewan.)

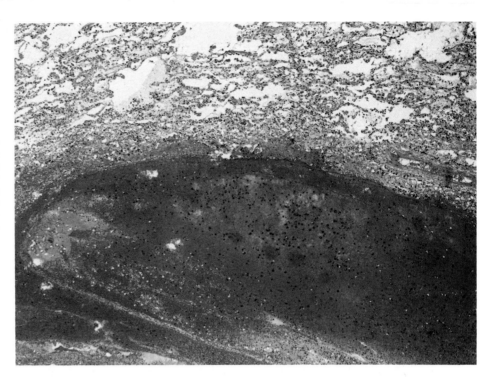

Figure 15–4. Pulmonary Hematoma. A histologic section of lung taken from the lower lobe of an individual involved in a motor vehicle accident 24 hours prior to death shows a well-defined focus of hemorrhage somewhat compressing adjacent lung parenchyma. (× 40.)

Roentgenographically, traumatic cysts appear as single or multiple lesions,[14, 29] unilocular or multilocular,[27] ranging from oval to spherical and from 2 cm to 14 cm in diameter (Fig. 15–5).[25] Usually they are located subpleurally in peripheral areas of the lung.[10, 27] In the majority of cases they develop under the point of maximal injury, but in some they occur in a remote location as a result of a contrecoup effect. Their appearance depends in large measure on whether hemorrhage has occurred into them. Approximately half the lesions present as thin-walled, air-filled spaces with or without fluid levels (Fig. 15–6),[30] and the remainder as homogeneous, well-circumscribed masses of water density—pulmonary hematomas (Fig. 15–7). Pneumothorax occurs occasionally.[25]

A characteristic of these lesions is their tendency to persist for a long time, frequently up to 4 months (Fig. 15–7).[8, 31] However, they generally decrease in size progressively; if this is not apparent within 6 weeks, the possibility must be considered that trauma may have been purely coincidental to a solitary nodule of other etiology.[10, 23] The frequent designation of these masses as "vanishing lung tumor"[14] should not be confused with similar terminology applied to encysted interlobar effusion in cases of congestive heart failure. The development of a cystic lesion at the base of the left lung following trauma has been confused with a ruptured diaphragm;[32] however, visibility of an outline of the diaphragm should make such a misdiagnosis unlikely.

CT has been shown to be much more sensitive than conventional roentgenography in the identification of pulmonary abnormalities following trauma. In a study of 85 consecutive patients with chest trauma, Wagner and his colleagues[33] found 151 abnormalities (excluding rib fractures) on roentgenograms and 423 on CT scans; further, 99 lacerations were identified on CT and only 5 on roentgenograms. CT can be particularly useful in the demonstration of paramediastinal traumatic cysts.[29]

In the majority of patients, there are no symptoms attributable to this lesion. Hemoptysis occurs rarely and is probably attributable to the emptying of a pulmonary hematoma.[30] A traumatic lung cyst occasionally has been reported as becoming infected.[34] Pulmonary hematomas indistinguishable from those caused by closed chest trauma sometimes develop following segmental or wedge resection of the lung.[14, 35] In addition, bleeding into bullae of patients with advanced chronic obstructive pulmonary disease (COPD) during mechanical ventilation has been reported; the resulting shadows simulate traumatic lung cysts.[36]

FRACTURES OF THE TRACHEA AND BRONCHI

Fractures (*synonyms:* rupture, transection) of the tracheobronchial tree usually result from blunt trauma to the anterior chest in vehicular accidents; occasionally they occur as a result of overdistention of the cuff of an endotracheal tube.[37] The incidence is highest in males under 40 years of age. It has been stated that in adults particularly the trauma is severe enough to result in fractures of the first three ribs, but the incidence of this abnormality varies widely in different series. For example, such fractures were observed in 53 per cent of cases in

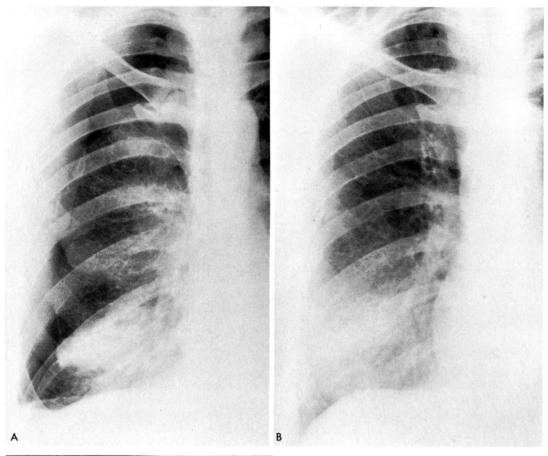

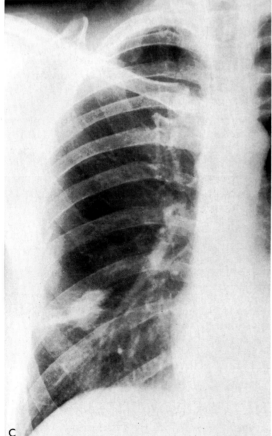

Figure 15–5. Traumatic Pulmonary Contusion, Hematoma, and Pneumothorax. This 38-year-old man suffered a severe blow to the right side of the chest in a car accident. Two hours later, a posteroanterior roentgenogram *(A)* revealed a hydropneumothorax with approximately 50 per cent collapse of the right lung (the left lung was normal); ribs 6 and 7 were fractured in the posterior axillary line. A poorly defined shadow of inhomogeneous density is present in the lower portion of the right lower lobe. Three days later *(B)*, the pneumothorax has disappeared following closed tube drainage, and the shadow in the right lower lobe is still poorly defined because of surrounding contusion. Three weeks later *(C)*, the shadow has undergone considerable decrease in size; it did not disappear completely until 2 months later.

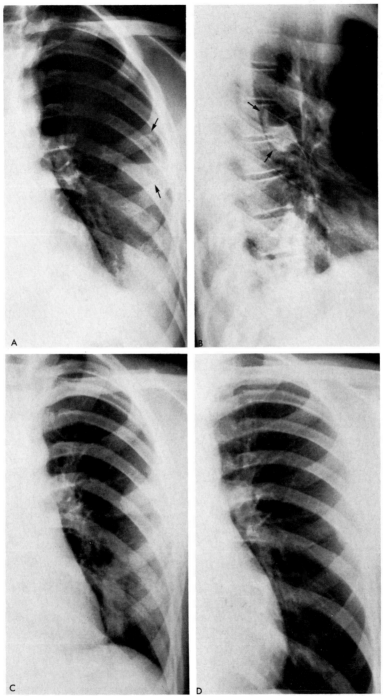

Figure 15–6. Traumatic Pulmonary Contusion, Laceration, and Hematoma. This 18-year-old man suffered a severe blow to the left side of his chest in a car accident 4 days previously. Views of the left hemithorax from posteroanterior *(A)* and lateral *(B)* roentgenograms reveal inhomogeneous, nonsegmental consolidation of the lower portion of the left lung caused by pulmonary contusion. In the midportion of the left lung is a thin-walled cystic space containing a prominent air-fluid level *(arrows* in both projections); this space represents a pulmonary laceration into which hemorrhage has occurred. Eight days later *(C),* most of the contusion in the lung base has cleared, and the shadow caused by the pulmonary laceration is a little smaller. Four months later *(D),* a small shadow measuring about 1 cm in diameter is still present as a residuum of the hematoma. (Courtesy of Dr. J. G. Monks, St. Paul's Hospital, Saskatoon, Saskatchewan.)

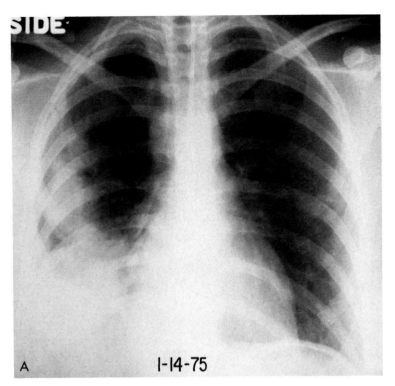

Figure 15–7. Multiple Unilateral Pulmonary Hematomas. This 17-year-old girl was involved in a two-car collision in which she sustained fractures of her right scapula and humerus. The day after admission, an anteroposterior roentgenogram *(A)* revealed extensive parenchymal consolidation in the lower two-thirds of the right lung in nonsegmental distribution; the left lung was clear. There was some widening of the superior mediastinum, undoubtedly from venous hemorrhage.

one series,[38] in an astonishing 91 per cent of patients in another,[39] but in only 1 of 50 patients in a more recent study.[40] In children, rib fractures are seldom seen, presumably owing to the resiliency of the chest wall.

Although the precise mechanism of tracheobronchial transection is not clear, it probably consists of a sudden crushing compression of air against a closed glottis and a shearing action of the vertebral column against the airway.[41] It is possible that the lateral widening of the thorax and lungs that occurs during the deceleration can also play a role, with the degree of lateral traction exceeding bronchial elasticity and with a tear resulting at or just distal to the carina.[42]

Fractures of the bronchi, more common than those of the trachea, constitute about 80 per cent of all tracheobronchial injuries.[16] They are usually parallel to the cartilage rings and involve the mainstem bronchi 1 to 2 cm distal to the carina.[6, 16, 43, 44] The right side is affected more often than the left; pulmonary vessels are rarely damaged.[45] Fractures of the intrathoracic trachea are horizontal and usually occur just above the carina.[6, 16, 43, 44, 46] Occasionally, the proximal trachea ruptures as a result of blunt trauma to the throat, and in such circumstances other cervical structures are usually involved;[46] the tracheal tear tends to be vertical in the membranous portion and can be associated with vascular damage.[16, 47]

Roentgenologically, the most common finding is pneumothorax,[43, 48] although this is not present in 30 per cent of cases,[49] probably because in some cases fracture affects the bronchi within the me-

diastinum and the mediastinal parietal pleura remains intact. Certain combinations of roentgenographic findings are considered to be highly suggestive of tracheobronchial fracture: (1) a large pneumothorax that does not respond to chest tube drainage because of the free communication between the fractured airway and the pleural space;[44, 50–52] (2) pneumothorax and pneumomediastinum in the absence of pleural effusion;[53] and (3) mediastinal and deep cervical emphysema in a trauma patient who is not receiving positive pressure ventilation.[54] Following bronchial rupture, a small amount of air can escape from the airway and remain localized to the surrounding connective tissues where it can be demonstrated roentgenographically.[6] Displacement of fracture ends can cause bronchial obstruction and atelectasis of an entire lung (Fig. 15–8);[5, 6, 43, 48, 53] it is important to recognize that atelectasis may be a late development, and the discovery of such a change some time after an accident should strongly suggest the diagnosis. Fractures of one or more of the first three ribs may provide additional supportive evidence.[38, 55] Rollins and Tocino[56] have drawn attention to the importance of recognizing an overdistended endotracheal balloon cuff as a sign of tracheal rupture; the overdistention results from herniation of the balloon through the tracheal tear into the mediastinum. The "fallen lung sign"—collapse of a lung toward the lateral chest wall—has recently been touted by Unger and her colleagues[478] as a reliable indicator of airway injury.

In approximately 10 per cent of patients, tracheobronchial fracture is unassociated with any

Text continued on page 2493

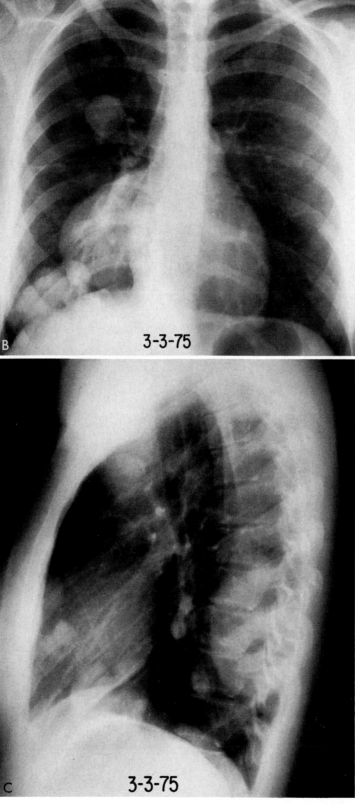

Figure 15–7 *Continued* Two months later, roentgenograms in posteroanterior *(B)* and lateral *(C)* projections revealed multiple, sharply circumscribed homogeneous nodules in the right lung ranging from 1 to 6 cm in diameter (12 discrete nodules can be identified). No cavitation was present and the left lung remained clear.

Illustration continued on following page

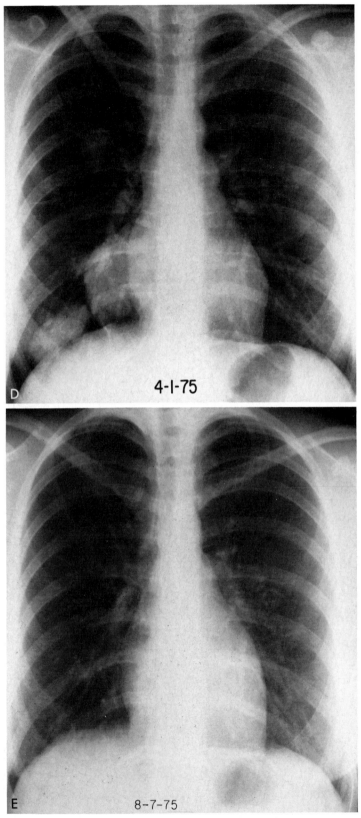

Figure 15–7 *Continued* Approximately 1 month later *(D)*, the nodules had diminished considerably in size, and several had disappeared altogether. Seven months after the injury, all signs of disease had disappeared and the chest roentgenogram *(E)* was perfectly normal. (Courtesy of Dr. John D. Armstrong, Jr., University of Utah College of Medicine and Valley West Hospital, Salt Lake City, Utah.)

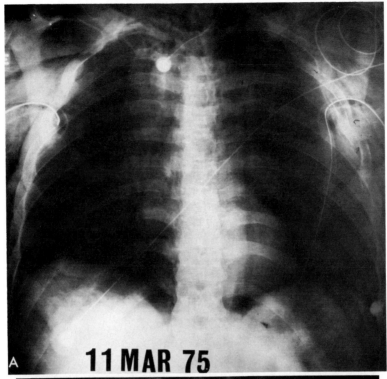

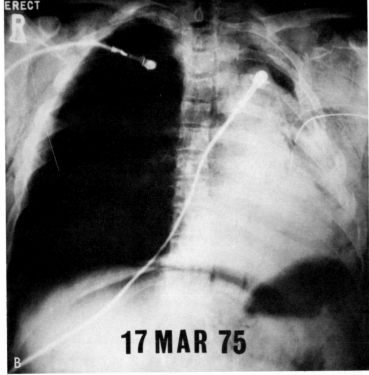

Figure 15–8. Fracture of the Left Main Bronchus. On admission to the hospital following a crushing injury to his chest, this 33-year-old man showed roentgenographic evidence *(A)* of severe subcutaneous and mediastinal emphysema and fractures of multiple left ribs, including the first, second, and third (not visible on the illustration). Bilateral pneumothorax had been treated in the emergency room by intubation. At this time, both lungs were well expanded. Six days later *(B),* there had occurred almost total collapse of the left lung. Bronchoscopy revealed an obstruction in the midportion of the left main bronchus. The obstructing material resembled a blood clot, although in some areas the bronchoscopist thought he was looking at the edge of a cartilaginous ring.

Illustration continued on following page

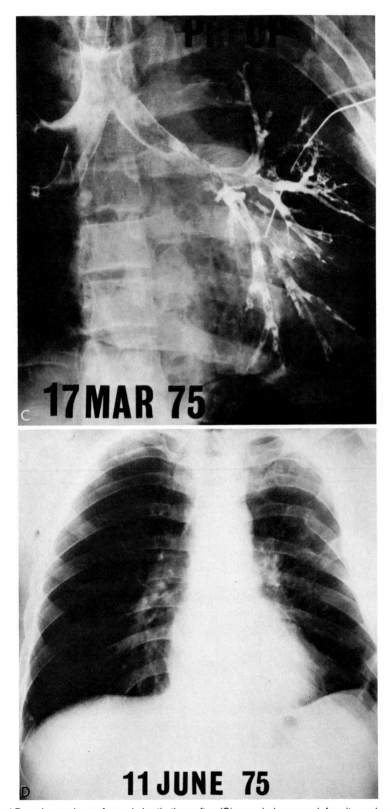

Figure 15–8 *Continued* Bronchography performed shortly thereafter *(C)* revealed severe deformity and narrowing of the distal end of the left main bronchus just before its bifurcation. At thoracotomy, the left main bronchus was found to be completely disrupted just proximal to its bifurcation and this was repaired by end-to-end anastomosis. Three months later *(D),* the left lung was well expanded, the only residual roentgenographic changes being those usually anticipated following severe trauma.

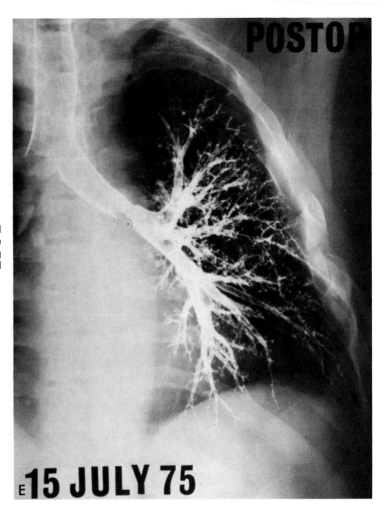

Figure 15–8 *Continued* Both bronchoscopy and bronchography *(E)* at this time revealed a stricture of the left main bronchus at the site of anastomosis, reducing its lumen by approximately half. (Courtesy of Dr. Harold Stolberg, Hamilton Civic Hospitals, Hamilton, Ontario.)

roentgenographically demonstrable abnormality or with much in the way of symptoms or signs.[16] It is probable that in such cases the peribronchial connective tissue is preserved, preventing passage of air into the mediastinum or pleura. Thus, the consequence of the trauma may not become evident until the patient presents with atelectasis of a lobe or lung as a result of bronchial stenosis.[57] A review of 90 such cases showed that in one third of the patients the condition was not diagnosed until 1 month to 19 years after the traumatic episode,[48] a finding that underlines the need for a high index of suspicion and early bronchoscopy to establish the diagnosis. Bronchoscopy is superior to bronchography in the early stages of the injury,[58] although the latter procedure may be of value in the assessment of bronchial deformity in later, more chronic stages (Fig. 15–8). In either stage, tomography may be of help in revealing large defects in the trachea or major bronchi.

Traumatic tracheobronchial fracture is very uncommon, its rarity probably contributing to the infrequency with which it is recognized early. In the series described by Burke,[39] 68 per cent of cases were not diagnosed until obstructive pneumonitis had developed in the lung distal to the fracture.

Symptoms and signs include cyanosis, hemoptysis, shock, and cough; rarely, there is pain caused by hemorrhage into the pleural space.[48] Air usually is identifiable in the subcutaneous tissues, initially involving the neck and upper thorax and later becoming generalized.[44]

The overall mortality of patients who suffer tracheobronchial fracture resulting from blunt trauma is approximately 30 per cent; over half of these patients die within 1 hour of injury.[38] Approximately 10 per cent of patients who reach the hospital alive subsequently die.[39] Early diagnosis is extremely important, since primary surgical repair results in anatomic and functional restoration.[42, 59, 60] If the presence of tracheobronchial fracture goes unrecognized, the eventual development of stenosis and stricture can result in destruction of distal parenchyma. In such circumstances, resectional rather than reparative surgery is usually indicated,[46] although successful late repair has been reported.[61] Traumatic rupture of a bronchus can cause severe $\dot{V}/\dot{Q}$ inequality as a result of persistent perfusion of unventilated lung.[62] However, in a follow-up study of seven patients in whom a transected main bronchus had been repaired 2 to 14 (average, 7½) years previously, all showed normal $\dot{V}/\dot{Q}$ scans and normal flow-volume curves while breathing air and an air-helium mixture.[63]

LUNG TORSION

Torsion of a lung or lobe has been described under three sets of circumstances:[64] (1) spontaneously, usually in association with some other pulmonary or diaphragmatic abnormality such as pneumonia,[65, 66] accessory pulmonary lobe, or diaphragmatic hernia; (2) following trauma; and (3) as a complication of thoracic surgery, usually following lobectomy.[67–69, 252] As a complication of trauma, torsion of a whole lung occurs most commonly in children, presumably because of the easy compressibility of a child's thoracic cage. The trauma usually is severe, such as when a child is run over by a vehicle, and torsion occurs most often when the major force is applied to the compressible lower thorax. The lung is twisted through 180 degrees so that its base comes to lie at the apex of the hemithorax and its apex at the base. The diagnosis should be obvious from the roentgenographic appearance of the chest. The pattern of pulmonary vascular markings is altered in a predictable manner, with the interlobar artery sweeping upward toward the apex and the lower lung vessels being comparatively diminutive. If the torsion is not relieved, vascular supply can be compromised and the lung can become roentgenographically opaque as a result of exudation of edema fluid and blood into the airspaces.[6, 70, 71] The resultant density has been described as "ground-glass" in appearance.[71]

In an analysis of nine cases of pulmonary torsion associated with a variety of intrathoracic abnormalities (not necessarily trauma), Felson[64] found the following roentgenographic manifestations: (1) a collapsed or consolidated lobe that is situated in an unusual location on a conventional roentgenogram, on conventional or computed tomograms, or on an angiogram or bronchogram; (2) hilar displacement in a direction inappropriate for that lobe; (3) alteration in the normal position and sweep of the pulmonary vasculature; (4) rapid opacification of an ipsilateral lobe following trauma or thoracic surgery; (5) marked change in position of an opacified lobe on sequential roentgenograms; and (6) a bronchial "cutoff" with no evidence of a mass.

ATELECTASIS

Posttraumatic collapse of a lobe—or very occasionally of a whole lung—is not common, but when present constitutes a cause of significant intrapulmonary shunting and hypoxemia at a time when a patient's clinical status may be critical. The cause of the atelectasis is not always clear, although it is probable that most cases result from bronchial obstruction from blood clots[5] or mucous plugs. In such circumstances, bronchoscopy will readily reveal the cause and permit prompt relief of the obstruction. In an occasional patient, however, total collapse of a lobe or even a lung occurs without apparent reason, and bronchoscopy reveals no evidence of bronchial fracture or occlusion.[72] Whether or not the atelectasis in such cases is related to surfactant deficit (adhesive atelectasis) or some other cause is unknown, but the affected parenchyma usually re-expands spontaneously without roentgenographic or functional residua.[72]

There is also evidence that mechanical percussion or hand clapping of the chest wall during physiotherapy can result in focal atelectasis. Studies of gas exchange in patients undergoing these procedures have shown variable results; some studies have found a decrease in arterial Pao_2[467, 468] and others an increase.[469] Experiments on dogs have shown small foci of subpleural atelectasis adjacent to the region of clapping or percussion.[470] Although the pathogenesis of this process is unclear, Zidulka and his colleagues[470] have suggested that differences in the amount of atelectasis may underlie the variation in the results of gas exchange studies noted clinically.

ADULT RESPIRATORY DISTRESS SYNDROME

One of the most ominous consequences of prolonged shock in the immediate posttraumatic period is the adult respiratory distress syndrome (Fig. 15–9). It is thoroughly described in Chapter 10 (see page 1927).

EFFECTS ON THE PLEURA OF NONPENETRATING TRAUMA

Hemothorax and pneumothorax are common manifestations of nonpenetrating trauma, and each may develop from a variety of causes. For example, blood can enter the pleural space from injury to vessels of the chest wall, diaphragm, lung, or mediastinum. Although pneumothorax most commonly develops as a consequence of pulmonary interstitial emphysema (see farther on), it may result from two other mechanisms, tracheobronchial fracture and esophageal rupture; both carry potentially grave consequences. Those conditions in which hydrothorax has resulted from trauma to mediastinal structures (rupture of the aorta, the thoracic duct, or the esophagus) are considered in the section on mediastinal trauma. Similarly, pneumothorax caused by tracheobronchial fracture has been dealt with in the previous section and that caused by esophageal rupture is discussed in the section on the mediastinum that follows. We are concerned here with hemothorax and pneumothorax devel-

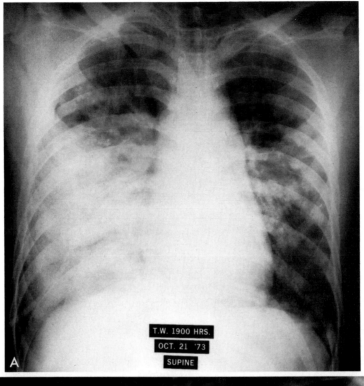

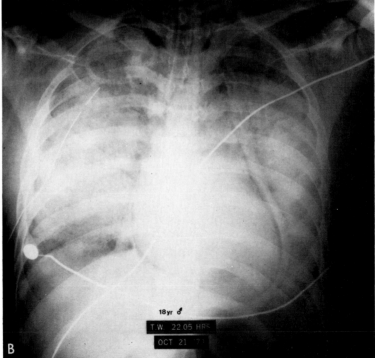

Figure 15–9. Traumatic Pulmonary Contusion, Pneumomediastinum, Pneumopericardium, Pneumothorax, and Adult Respiratory Distress Syndrome (ARDS). Following admission to the hospital of this 18-year-old man after a severe motor vehicle accident, a chest roentgenogram in the supine position *(A)* revealed massive patchy consolidation of both lungs consistent with severe pulmonary contusion. Three hours later *(B)*, both lungs were uniformly consolidated and a pneumopericardium had developed; a tube had been introduced into the right pleural space to drain a pneumothorax.

Illustration continued on following page

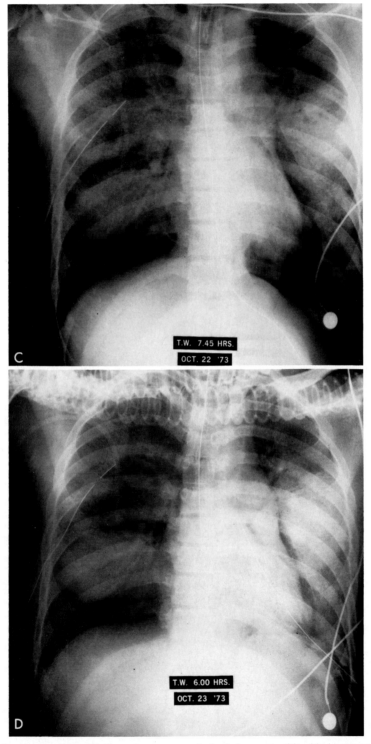

Figure 15–9 *Continued* By 12 hours later *(C)*, the pulmonary opacity had shown considerable improvement; the pneumopericardium had disappeared but there was now evidence of a large left pneumothorax. The next day *(D)*, a tube was introduced into the left pleural space for drainage of the pneumothorax. A well-defined opacity was now evident in the lower portion of the right lung—a pulmonary hematoma.

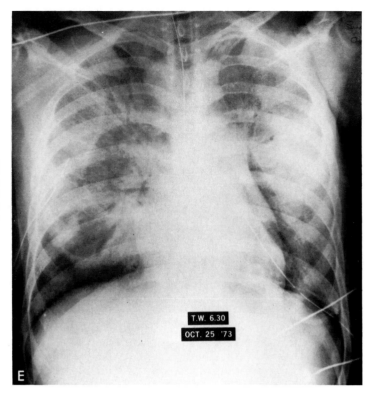

Figure 15–9 *Continued* Four days after admission *(E),* the lungs were still massively consolidated. Persistence of such opacity for this length of time is inconsistent with pulmonary contusion alone and it is necessary to invoke the diagnosis of ARDS. The outcome was fatal. (Courtesy of Dr. John Clement, Vancouver General Hospital, Vancouver, British Columbia.)

oping as a consequence of direct damage to the pleura.

HEMOTHORAX

Although hemorrhage may result from laceration of the parietal or visceral pleura by fractured ribs, hemothorax or pneumothorax (or both) may occur in closed chest trauma without evidence of fracture. When blood enters the pleural space it coagulates rapidly, but, presumably as a result of physical agitation produced by movement of the heart and lungs, the clot may be defibrinated and leave fluid indistinguishable roentgenologically from effusion from any other cause.[6, 73] When a solid clot does remain it may prove a hindrance to adequate thoracentesis, a procedure that should be carried out thoroughly to prevent later troublesome fibrothorax. As in empyema, loculation tends to occur early in hemothorax and increases still further the difficulty of achieving needle drainage. Reynolds and Davis[6] emphasized the importance of the site of hemorrhage in relation to the quantity of hemothorax. When bleeding is from a vessel in the chest wall, diaphragm, or mediastinum, the hemothorax tends to increase despite the quantity of blood present. By contrast, when the blood comes from the pulmonary vasculature the expanding hemothorax compresses the lung, with resultant pulmonary vascular tamponade that may produce hemostasis.

The roentgenographic demonstration of small quantities of blood requires examination of the patient in the lateral decubitus position.[16, 17] Although an accumulation of pleural fluid following trauma is usually owing to hemorrhage, very occasionally it results from other causes, such as traumatic subarachnoid pleural fistula[74] or rupture of the esophagus (*see* farther on). Similarly, widening of the pleural line, particularly over the apex, may be produced by faulty placement of a central venous catheter, with resultant hemorrhage from a subclavian vein or the instillation of fluid through the catheter.[17] Traumatic hemothorax may be associated with pneumothorax, thereby producing hemopneumothorax.

The blood in traumatic hemothorax may contain a large number of eosinophils,[75] a finding that is rarely accompanied by blood eosinophilia.[76, 77]

PNEUMOTHORAX

Pneumothorax-complicating trauma may occur without roentgenographic evidence of rib fracture; for example, in one series of 15 survivors of attempted suicide who jumped into water from a considerable height (50 M), 10 patients developed a pneumothorax within 12 hours and in only 4 of these was there an associated rib fracture.[78] When fracture is present the likely mechanism is laceration of the visceral pleura by rib fragments, and in such circumstances hemothorax may be expected as a concomitant finding. When no fractures are visible the mechanism is variable; it is possible that rupture occurs through an area of pre-existing blebs or bullae, although Williams and Bonte[73] feel that pulmonary emphysema plays little if any role. We are of a similar opinion and suggest the alternative mechanism of pulmonary *interstitial* emphysema secondary to pulmonary trauma and parenchymal laceration. This explanation also provides adequate reason for the occurrence of pneumomediastinum and subcutaneous emphysema without rib fracture. In this regard it is noteworthy that subcutaneous emphysema may result from closed chest trauma without associated pneumothorax (in 13 of 166 patients in one report[79]). This finding may be logically explained on the basis of pulmonary interstitial emphysema with subsequent tracking of air to the mediastinum and out through the thoracic inlet into the neck and lateral chest wall (Fig. 15–10).

Traumatic pneumothorax sometimes develops on the undamaged side, presumably as a result of contrecoup transmission of forces.[73]

When a pneumothorax is small and the visceral pleural line is poorly visualized, roentgenography at full expiration may reveal the partially collapsed lung to better advantage. When a patient's condition does not warrant roentgenography in the erect position, examination in the lateral decubitus position permits identification of very small quantities of air in the pleural space.[17]

EFFECTS ON THE MEDIASTINUM OF NONPENETRATING TRAUMA

The abnormalities with which we are primarily concerned in nonpenetrating trauma to the mediastinum include pneumomediastinum, hemorrhage, rupture of the aorta and major vessels, perforation of the esophagus, and rupture of the thoracic duct. Traumatic abnormalities of the heart and pericardium are not within the scope of this book.

PNEUMOMEDIASTINUM

Traumatic pneumomediastinum may develop after closed chest trauma, and in such circumstances it is probably produced by the same mechanism as spontaneous pneumomediastinum—the rupture of alveoli into the perivascular sheath as a result of an abrupt increase in pressure or sheer stress. Pneumomediastinum may also follow traumatic rupture of the esophagus or fracture of the tracheobronchial tree; in either case, the mediastinal emphysema may be associated with acute mediastinitis. Sometimes perforation of the esophagus or the tracheobronchial tree occurs during or following diagnostic instrumentation. It may be due directly to the

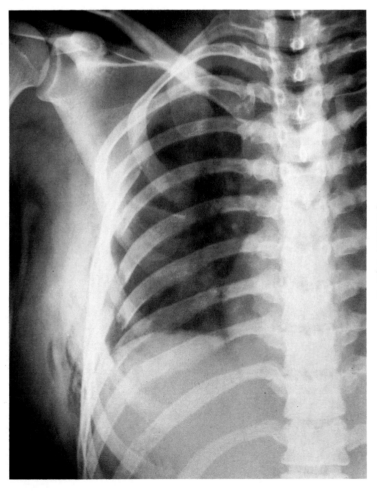

Figure 15–10. Subcutaneous Emphysema Associated with Multiple Fractured Ribs in the Absence of Pneumothorax. An anteroposterior roentgenogram in the supine position reveals multiple grossly displaced fractures of the right rib cage in the posterior axillary line. There is considerable subcutaneous emphysema in adjacent soft tissues but no pneumothorax. (However, a small pneumothorax might not be visible on this roentgenogram exposed with the patient supine.)

trauma or could conceivably result from the paroxysmal coughing engendered by these procedures.[80,81] Air may also enter the mediastinum along deep fascial planes as a result of trauma or surgical procedures to the neck or in association with zygomaticomaxillary fractures.[82]

The roentgenographic signs are identical to those of pneumomediastinum from any cause (see Chapter 19).

MEDIASTINAL HEMORRHAGE

The majority of cases of mediastinal hemorrhage result from trauma, usually of a severe nature, such as that associated with an automobile accident and chest cage compression.[83, 84] The trauma is often iatrogenic, usually from faulty placement of a central venous line in a subclavian vein. Less common causes include rupture of an aortic aneurysm[85, 86] and extension of blood from the retropharyngeal soft tissues secondary to trauma or to spontaneous hemorrhage associated with coagulation disorders. Undoubtedly the majority of cases of mediastinal hemorrhage go unrecognized, the amount of bleeding being insufficient to produce symptoms and signs.

Roentgenologically, hemorrhage typically results in uniform, symmetrical widening of the mediastinum in any of its compartments (Fig. 15–11). Local accumulation of blood in the form of a hematoma is manifested by a homogeneous mass that may project to one or both sides of the mediastinum and may be situated in any compartment.[86–88]

Radionuclide imaging with ^{131}I macroaggregated albumin has been advocated as a method of demonstrating venous rupture in patients in whom increasing mediastinal widening causes concern.[90] However, since rupture of the thoracic aorta or one of its major branches must be considered a distinct possibility in any patient with progressive mediastinal widening, either CT or aortography must remain the most definitive diagnostic procedure in such cases.[91]

Symptoms and signs of mediastinal hemorrhage seldom are striking. Suspicion may be aroused when retrosternal pain that radiates into the back develops in a patient who suffered chest trauma recently. A hematoma of sufficient size and appropriate location may compress the superior vena cava.[83, 85]

RUPTURE OF THE THORACIC AORTA AND ITS BRANCHES

Rupture of the aorta is a well-recognized sequela of closed chest injury; approximately 70 per cent of cases follow severe automobile accidents.[92] Because of the variable mobility of different portions of the aorta, sudden deceleration produces shearing stresses, the more mobile anterior portion of the aortic arch being "whipped" on the more fixed posterior arch and paraspinal aorta.[93] Thus, approximately 95 per cent of all aortic ruptures occur in the region of the aortic isthmus at the site of the ligamentum arteriosum;[93] the remaining 5 per cent are immediately above the aortic valve. Immediate death is the usual result. Only 10 to 20 per cent of all patients with this injury live longer than 1 hour,[93] and less than 5 per cent survive long enough for a chronic traumatic aneurysm to develop.

Pathologically, the tear usually begins in the intima and proceeds outward. The most minimal lesion is a transverse intimal tear; the more severe lesions involve the media and adventitia.

ROENTGENOGRAPHIC MANIFESTATIONS

A wide variety of signs have been described over the years as being useful in the diagnosis of aortic rupture. Some of these have stood the test of time, while others have fallen into disrepute as the result of demonstrated low sensitivity and specificity. Since aortography remains the definitive method of establishing the diagnosis, an attempt is made at the end of the following descriptions to indicate which abnormalities should be regarded as the most reliable indications for that procedure.

Widening of the Upper Half of the Mediastinum. Plain roentenograms of the chest almost invariably reveal widening of the superior mediastinum as a result of hemorrhage (Fig. 15–12), although the hemorrhage eventually may prove to be of venous origin due to either direct trauma or iatrogenic causes such as malpositioning of a central venous line.[94] From a study of 158 patients with a widened vascular pedicle, Milne and his coworkers[95] found that extravascular hemorrhage resulting from aortic injury tended to cause the pedicle to widen predominantly to the left of the midline while, at the same time, causing disappearance of the shadow of the tracheal stripe and the azygos vein. They emphasize that this combination of changes contrasts with the situation pertaining in the presence of an increase in systemic blood volume (or the supine position), in which the vascular pedicle widens predominantly to the right and the azygos vein dilates concomitantly; these differences can assist in distinguishing physiologic from pathologic widening of the pedicle.

Loss of Contour of the Aortic Knob. The aortic knob is generally invisible, an important sign that should alert the roentgenologist to the possibility of aortic rupture (Fig. 15–12). However, it must be emphasized that in some cases the shadow of the aortic knuckle is preserved and this must not be construed as evidence to exclude the diagnosis.[96]

Deviation of the Trachea and Left Main Bronchus. As the hematoma enlarges, the left main bronchus may be deviated anteriorly, inferiorly, and

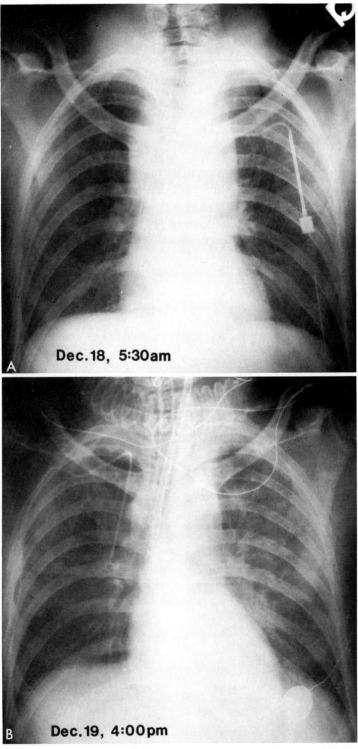

Figure 15–11. Traumatic Mediastinal Hemorrhage. A roentgenogram of the chest in anteroposterior projection, supine position *(A)* of this young man following severe closed chest trauma reveals moderate widening of the upper half of the mediastinum, roughly symmetric on both sides. The lungs are unremarkable. Approximately 36 hours later *(B)*, the widening had diminished considerably. There is now evidence of a uniform opacity over both lungs which, in a supine view, is good evidence for bilateral pleural effusion, in this case hemothorax.

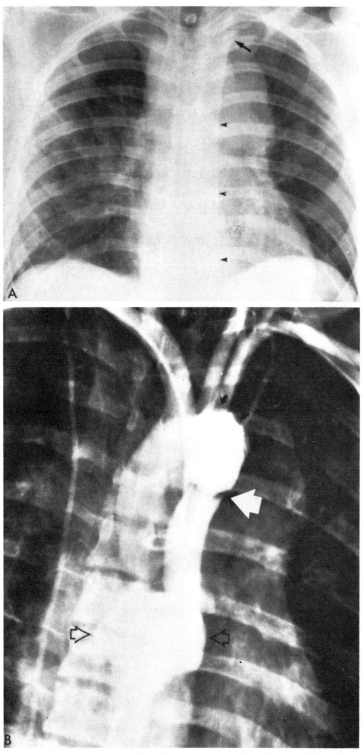

Figure 15–12. Traumatic Aneurysm and Rupture of the Thoracic Aorta. This 16-year-old boy crashed into a telephone pole in an automobile traveling at 85 mph. Shortly after his arrival in the emergency room, a chest roentgenogram in anteroposterior projection *(A)* revealed marked widening of the upper mediastinum and loss of visualization of the aortic knob. A wide paravertebral opacity *(arrowheads)* extends up to the apex, creating an extrapleural apical cap *(arrow)*. The suspicion of aortic rupture was confirmed by aortography *(B)*. The site of primary aortic laceration is indicated by a *thick arrow,* the irregular bulge immediately above *(small arrows)* representing dissection proximally. Several cm distally is a large, well-circumscribed collection of contrast medium *(open arrows),* which represents an extra-aortic hematoma from a second rupture. The patient exsanguinated following section of the mediastinal pleura at thoracotomy.

to the right, and the trachea may be displaced to the right. These signs are said to be present in about 75 per cent of patients.[97] However, one of the authors has reviewed the conventional roentgenograms of several confirmed cases examined at the University of Alabama at Birmingham and found convincing evidence of tracheal displacement in none.

Displacement of a Nasogastric Tube. Some studies[98, 99] have emphasized the importance of identifying displacement of a nasogastric tube to the right; for example, Gerlock and associates[99] found that when both the trachea and nasogastric tube were shifted to the right, the patient had a 96 per cent probability of having an acute rupture of the thoracic aorta. By contrast, however, a more recent postmortem study of eight victims of fatal motor vehicle accidents with documented aortic rupture showed that five had nasogastric tube deviation to the right and three to the left,[100] suggesting that rightward nasogastric tube deviation is not as sensitive as has been suggested.

Displacement of the Right Paraspinous Interface. This sign has been found by some workers to be highly reliable (Fig. 15–12): in a retrospective review of the roentgenographic findings in 14 patients with proven acute traumatic rupture of the aorta, Peters and Gamsu[101] found displacement of the right paraspinous interface in 8 patients; the sign was not seen roentgenographically in any patient who did not have evidence of rupture on thoracic aortography.

Widening of the Right Tracheal Stripe. Another sign that has been suggested as a possible indicator of aortic tear is widening of the right tracheal stripe to a diameter greater than 5 mm (Fig. 15–12);[102] in a study of 102 consecutive patients with blunt chest trauma, Woodring and his associates found that all patients with a right paratracheal stripe less than 5 mm in width had a normal aortogram, whereas in those patients whose right tracheal stripe measured 5 mm or greater, aortography revealed major arterial injury in 23 per cent.

The Left Apical Cap. A potential space exists between the isthmus of the aorta and the parietal pleura of the left lung. Provided that the parietal pleura is intact, extravasated blood can track cephalad along the course of the left subclavian artery between the parietal pleura and the extrapleural soft tissues, with a resulting homogeneous opacity over the apex of the left hemithorax—the extrapleural apical cap (Fig. 15–12).[103] In a recent prospective and retrospective study of 45 patients with traumatic rupture of the aorta in which the value of the left apical cap was assessed, Simeone and his colleagues[104] found that in 7 patients a left apical cap was the only clearly visible abnormality. In 11 patients, a cap was present together with a poorly defined aortic knob, while in 13 patients there was the additional finding of mediastinal widening. All of the classic signs of aortic rupture were present

in 14 patients, except for an apical cap. In the same series, 12 of the 32 angiograms were performed solely because of the presence of an apical cap: 2 were positive for aortic rupture and 10 were negative. These findings suggest that left apical cap *by itself* constitutes an unreliable sign of acute aortic rupture.

Left Hemothorax. Hemothorax complicating traumatic rupture of the aorta is common and is almost invariably left-sided.[105] It should not be attributed erroneously to left-sided rib fractures.

Fracture of the First and Second Ribs. Formerly considered a potential indicator of aortic/bracheocephalic trauma, fractures of the first and second ribs are now thought to represent unreliable signs on the strength of several well-documented studies.[106–108]

Mediastinal Width/Chest Width Ratio. In 1981, Seltzer and his colleagues published the results of a study of plain roentgenograms of 20 patients with proven traumatic aortic rupture conducted specifically to test the accuracy of the ratio of mediastinal width to chest width.[109] They found that if they defined a ratio of 0.25 or larger at the level of the aortic arch as being abnormal, 95 per cent of cases with ruptured aortas would be identified, and 25 per cent false-positive studies would result; if the ratio were increased to 0.28 or greater, the sensitivity would be decreased to 85 per cent but the specificity increased to 100 per cent. However, in a reappraisal of this sign in 1984, Marnocha and his associates[110] found that the ratio was of insufficient sensitivity and specificity to be clinically useful in confirming or excluding aortic rupture.

Occasionally, mediastinal hemorrhage following severe chest trauma can result from damage to one of the great vessels arising from the aortic arch. In fact, avulsion of the innominate artery from the arch has been stated to be the second most common type of aortic injury in which the patient survives long enough for diagnostic evaluation.[111] The plain roentgenographic findings are similar to those of rupture of the aortic isthmus, with the possible exception that the outline of the descending aorta may be preserved.[111] The angiographic findings are diagnostic. Traumatic aneurysms may be multiple: a case has been reported[112] of a 15-year-old girl who was involved in an automobile accident that resulted in general mediastinal widening caused by traumatic aneurysms of the innominate and left common carotid arteries and of the inferior wall of the transverse arch of the aorta. Repeat aortography 15 months later revealed no change in the size or configuration of the three aneurysms (one might wonder why she had not been operated upon).

According to Lundell and her colleagues,[113] traumatic laceration of the ascending aorta represents only about 5 per cent of all thoracic aortic injuries seen clinically; however, the incidence of this injury at autopsy is much higher (approximately 20 per cent). The authors point out that this disparity is caused by the frequent association of severe and often fatal cardiac injury that occurs in roughly 80 per cent of cases (compared with 25 per cent when the laceration is at the isthmus). Although these injuries are rarely recognized during life, the fact that cases are occasionally reported[113] emphasizes the importance of opacifying the entire aorta from the aortic valve to the diaphragm in any patient in whom the possibility of aortic laceration is entertained.

Dennis and Rogers[464] have recently emphasized the difficulty of distinguishing the signs of fractures of the upper thoracic spine from those of aortic rupture. In a retrospective analysis of the frontal chest roentgenograms of 54 patients with traumatic fractures of at least one vertebral body from C-6 to T-8, they found 37 patients (69 per cent) with signs generally considered to be consistent with aortic laceration—upper mediastinal widening equal to or greater than 8 cm, left apical cap, widened tracheal stripe to 5 mm or more, and deviation of a nasogastric tube to the right of the T-4 spinous process. The spinal fracture could be identified on the initial roentgenogram in approximately half of the 37 patients.

Early recognition of aortic rupture is imperative in view of the poor survival rates of undiagnosed patients with this type of injury.[115] Approx-imately 20 per cent of patients with aortic rupture survive the initial trauma, although the majority of survivors develop a thin-walled aneurysm which, if untreated, will rupture within 2 weeks in approximately 60 per cent of these patients and within 10 weeks in 90 per cent.[116] Despite these dismal statistics, some aneurysms of traumatic origin are unrecognized at the time and may remain so for many years until a screening chest roentgenogram of an asymptomatic patient reveals the abnormality.[117-121] Rarely, a patient presents with symptoms and signs of rupture of an aortic aneurysm that was caused by severe trauma many years previously but was not recognized (Fig. 15–13).

VALIDITY OF ROENTGENOGRAPHIC SIGNS AND INDICATIONS FOR AORTOGRAPHY

Since 1982 a number of papers have been published in which an attempt has been made to assess the relative value of the many signs described above in the diagnosis of traumatic rupture of the thoracic aorta.[122-126, 465] The majority opinion recorded in these studies included the following: no single roentgenographic sign is highly specific for vascular injury, and the most reliable signs of aortic disruption are mediastinal widening and an abnormal aortic outline. However, to illustrate how dis-

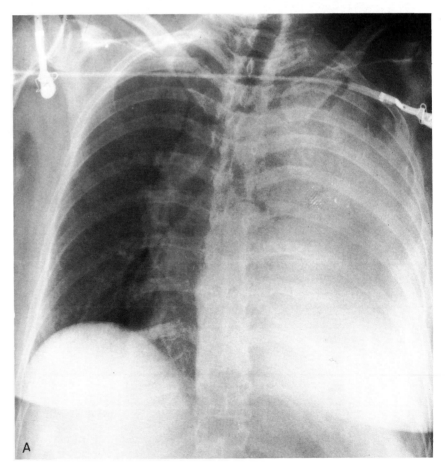

Figure 15–13. Traumatic Aneurysm of the Aorta: Delayed Rupture 20 Years After Trauma. This 53-year-old woman was admitted to the hospital approximately 24 hours after the abrupt onset of severe chest pain and worsening dyspnea. A roentgenogram of the chest in anteroposterior projection, supine position *(A)* discloses a massive left pleural effusion which, on thoracentesis, proved to be blood.

Illustration continued on following page

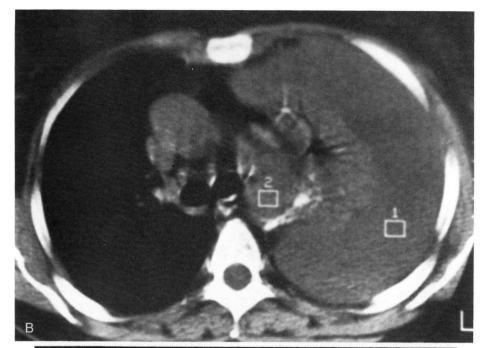

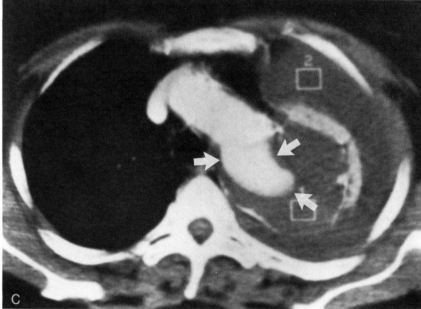

Figure 15–13 *Continued* A computed tomographic (CT) scan at the level of the tracheal bifurcation *(B)* shows the left pleural space to be filled with fluid, the density of which is identical to that of the blood in the descending thoracic aorta. Marked calcification of the wall of the aorta can be identified on this scan. A CT scan at the level of the aortic arch following a bolus injection of contrast medium *(C)* reveals a large saccular aneurysm extending off the left side of the arch *(arrows).*

parate the experiences of various investigators can be, we record the results of two fairly recent studies in which the reliability of roentgenographic signs in aortic rupture was assessed:

(1) From a study of 86 consecutive patients with blunt chest trauma and possible aortic rupture on whom supine chest roentgenograms were available for review, Marnocha and Maglinte[125] analyzed 16 radiographic signs both independently and in combination. Only 2 of these signs were found to be statistically significant—deviation of a nasogastric tube to the right at the T-4 level and depression of the left mainstem bronchus greater than 40 degrees from the horizontal. In 4 consecutive years of experience, these authors did not encounter a single case of aortic rupture if the aortic knob and contour appeared normal and the trachea and nasogastric tube were not deviated.

(2) In a retrospective review of the chest roentgenograms of 205 patients with blunt chest trauma who underwent aortography, Mirvis and his colleagues[126] found 41 confirmed cases of aortic rupture. Discriminant analysis of 16 radiographic signs indicated that the most reliable signs were loss of the aortopulmonary window, abnormality of the contour of the aortic arch, shift of the trachea to the right, and widening of the left paraspinal line (unassociated with spinal fracture). These authors found that no single roentgenographic sign, or combination of signs, demonstrated sufficient sen-

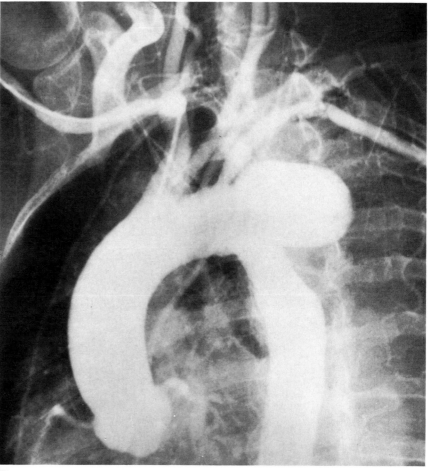

Figure 15–13 *Continued* An aortogram in left anterior oblique projection *(D)* demonstrates a large saccular aneurysm arising from the aorta just distal to the takeoff of the left subclavian artery. The only previous trauma that the patient could recall was an automobile accident approximately 20 years previously in which she suffered a severe injury to her thorax against a steering wheel. She had not been investigated for possible thoracic injury at that time.

D

sitivity to identify all cases of traumatic aortic rupture from conventional chest roentgenograms without the performance of a large number of negative aortographic studies.

Also of considerable interest was the observation by Gundry and his colleagues[124] that of 25 patients with traumatic rupture of the aorta, *all* of those under the age of 65 years had a widened mediastinum; in fact, this was the only finding that taken alone correlated significantly with aortic rupture (P = 0.001). By contrast, only 2 of 6 patients over the age of 65 years had a widened mediastinum. This led the authors to conclude that all elderly persons with severe truncal trauma probably should have aortography even in the absence of mediastinal widening.

Although aortography remains the definitive method of establishing the diagnosis of acute aortic rupture and of defining its anatomic extent, CT also has been reported to be of diagnostic value (Fig. 15–14): in a CT study of 10 patients suspected of having thoracic aortic injury following acute multiple trauma, Heiberg and her colleagues[127] made a diagnosis of aortic transection in 4 patients; there were no false-negative or false-positive examinations. The CT findings included (1) false aneurysm, (2) linear lucency within the opacified

aortic lumen caused by the torn edge of the aortic wall, (3) marginal irregularity of the opacified aortic lumen, (4) periaortic or intramural aortic hematoma, and (5) dissection. Interestingly, in this series the extent of associated mediastinal hemorrhage and the amount of blood in the pleural space were not useful as indicators of aortic injury; similarly, shift of the trachea and esophagus to the right or the absence thereof was not discriminatory.

On the basis of the many studies that we have reviewed, we believe that the following three conclusions are warranted: (1) In any patient who has suffered severe chest trauma on whom conventional chest roentgenograms reveal upper mediastinal widening and loss of configuration of the aortic knob, CT or aortography or both should be performed to establish the diagnosis and reveal the anatomic extent of the rupture. (2) Patients over the age of 65 years probably should have at least a CT whether or not there is roentgenographic evidence of mediastinal widening. (3) Considered individually, it is doubtful whether the other signs described above should constitute sufficient indication for aortography; however, even in the absence of mediastinal widening, any combination of three of the described signs should raise one's index of suspicion to a high level and should probably war-

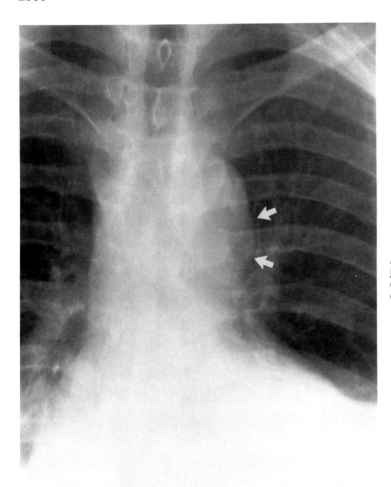

Figure 15–14. Traumatic Laceration of the Aorta.
A detail view of the mediastinum in posteroanterior projection *(A)* reveals a small bulge on the descending arch of the aorta *(arrows);* there is also a left pleural effusion of moderate size.

A   16 ⋅⋅ 4 ⋅⋅ 80

rant at least CT and possibly aortography (Fig. 15–14).

CLINICAL MANIFESTATIONS

Clinical findings that suggest the presence of traumatic rupture of the aorta include the following: (1) a systolic murmur over the precordium or medial to the left scapula; (2) hoarseness (caused by pressure of the hematoma on the left recurrent laryngeal nerve); and (3) hypertension in the upper extremities and hypotension or weak pulses in the lower extremities.[21] In a review of the literature, Finkelmeier and associates[128] found 413 cases of chronic traumatic aneurysm of the thoracic aorta reported from 1950 to 1980. Signs or symptoms of aneurysm expansion developed within 5 years of injury in 42 per cent of the patients and within 20 years in 85 per cent (*see* Fig. 15–13). The most common symptom was pain, usually accompanied by roentgenographic evidence of progressive enlargement of the aortic shadow. A follow-up of the 60 patients who did not undergo surgery showed that 20 had died of their aortic lesions, most of them in the absence of symptoms. Of the 300 patients who had surgery, only 4.6 per cent died, most of them as a result of hemorrhage.

PERFORATION OF THE ESOPHAGUS

Rupture of the esophagus from closed chest trauma is rare and results in changes localized to the mediastinum and pleura.[73, 129, 130] Of considerably greater frequency is the rupture that occurs as a complication of esophagoscopy or gastroscopy,[131] overzealous dilatation of a stricture or achalasia, disruption of the suture line following esophageal resection and anastomosis, or, as in two reported cases,[132] passage of an esophageal obturator airway used by paramedical personnel during cardiopulmonary resuscitation.

The usual result of esophageal rupture is acute mediastinitis manifested roentgenographically by mediastinal widening, usually more evident superiorly and typically possessing a smooth, sharply defined margin (*see* Fig. 11–1, page 1973). Air may be visible within the mediastinal compartments as well as in the soft tissues of the neck.[80, 81, 133] If the mediastinal pleura is ruptured, there is early development of hydrothorax or hydropneumothorax.

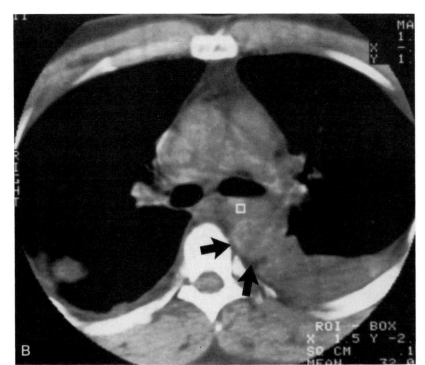

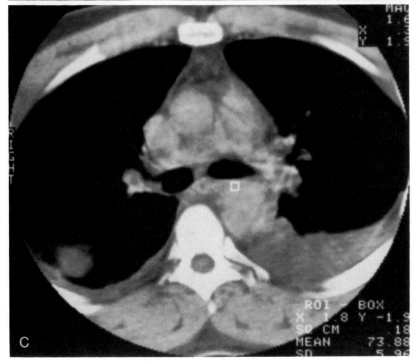

Figure 15–14 *Continued* Because of concern over the possibility of an aortic laceration, a CT scan was performed: the scan just below the level of the carina before the injection of contrast medium *(B)* shows a loss of definition of the aorta except along its medial and posteromedial borders *(arrows)*; following the injection of contrast medium *(C)*, the density within the box anterior to the aorta showed an increase from 32 to 73 Hounsfield units, indicating a leakage of blood into the mediastinum. The left pleural effusion did not show a corresponding increase in density; the cause of the right lower lobe opacity was not established.

Illustration continued on following page

Identification of ingested material (such as milk) in pleural fluid is diagnostic. If the pleural integrity is maintained, mediastinal changes develop rapidly and pleural effusion develops late.[134] In the majority of cases the site of rupture can be identified precisely—although sometimes with considerable difficulty—only by roentgenographic evidence of extravasation of ingested contrast material. The type of contrast medium that should be employed in such a study is still somewhat controversial. In an experimental study in which various combinations of contrast media and flora were instilled into the mediastinum of 30 domestic cats, Vessal and his colleagues[135] found that water-soluble contrast media caused no significant histologic reaction. Barium resulted in granuloma formation but had no additional deleterious effect when mixed with varying concentrations of normal human bacterial flora of the mouth. These authors recommended that because of its superior physical properties, barium

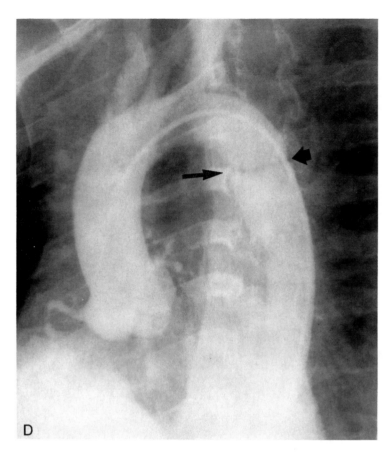

D

Figure 15–14 *Continued* An aortogram in right posterior oblique projection *(D)* reveals a lucent defect in the descending arch *(arrows)*, representing the tear in the aortic wall.

appears to be the contrast agent of choice in difficult clinical problems relating to esophageal rupture or perforation.

Chills and high fever are common, and effects of obstruction of the superior vena cava may be apparent. Vomitus may contain blood.[130] Physical examination usually reveals subcutaneous emphysema in the soft tissues of the neck or Hamman's sign on auscultation over the apex of the heart. When the diagnosis is not suspected initially and treatment is not instituted promptly, the inflammation may progress to abscess formation, with subsequent perforation of the abscess into a bronchus or the pleural cavity. The resultant esophagobronchial or esophagopleural fistulae usually can be identified by contrast roentgenographic examination or, with esophagopleural fistula, by microscopic examination of pleural fluid.[136] The pleural fluid also contains a concentration of amylase that is higher than that of the blood as a result of contamination by saliva.

It has been established that morbidity and mortality increase considerably with delay in treatment.[134] In one series,[138] mortality increased threefold when surgery was delayed beyond 24 hours.

RUPTURE OF THE THORACIC DUCT

Rupture of the thoracic duct, resulting in chylothorax, may develop from surgical procedures, nonpenetrating injuries, or penetrating wounds from a bullet or knife.[6, 73] The anatomic course of the thoracic duct and the site of damage establish on which side the chylothorax develops. As it enters the thorax the duct lies slightly to the right of the midline, so that rupture in its lower third—an unusual site in crushing injuries—leads to right-sided chylothorax. The duct crosses the midline to the left in the midthorax, so that its disruption above this point as a result of crushing injury or, more commonly, surgical trauma, tends to produce left-sided chylothorax. Chylothorax resulting from nonpenetrating thoracic trauma may be bilateral;[139] 5 of 28 cases reported by Shackelford and Fisher[140] were so situated.

Several days may elapse between the time of chest trauma and the development of roentgenographically demonstrable pleural fluid,[6, 73] a time lag that should strongly suggest this entity. The reason offered by Reynolds and Davis[6] is that initially the extravasated chyle is confined to the mediastinal space and ruptures into the pleural space only when the accumulation has acquired sufficient pressure. Rea[141] states that the average latent period is 12 days, and Thorne[142] reported a case in which the interval was 11 months. In this latter patient, a mediastinal opacity representing a "chyloma" was identified roentgenologically 3 months before rupture into the pleural cavity. A case recently has been reported in which a traumatic "lymphocele" was demonstrated by lymphoscintigraphy with modified ^{99m}Tc sulfur colloid.[143]

The rupture of large quantities of chyle from the mediastinum into the pleural space may give rise to the abrupt onset of respiratory difficulty. Thoracentesis yielding milky fluid of high fat content confirms the diagnosis, and the precise site of rupture may be established by lymphangiography.

EFFECTS ON THE DIAPHRAGM OF NONPENETRATING TRAUMA

The only abnormality of the diaphragm occurring as a result of trauma is rupture or tear. This may be caused by direct penetrating injury or blunt nonpenetrating trauma to the abdomen or thorax; the number of cases attributable to each type of trauma is roughly equal.[144, 145] The most common causal trauma is an automobile accident or falling from a height. In some cases rupture follows a bout of hyperemesis[145–148] or, more rarely, repair of a hiatus hernia by the Allison technique.[149, 150] It may follow a seemingly insignificant blow to the chest or abdomen. In some cases herniation of abdominal contents through the site of rupture occurs at the time of the accident, but its presence is masked by injuries to other organs. In other cases, major herniation of abdominal contents may occur into the thorax without associated signs or symptoms and be detected months or years later on a screening chest roentgenogram. The latter situation is probably not uncommon; it has been estimated that 9 out of 10 traumatic diaphragmatic hernias are overlooked at the time of injury.[151]

Traumatic hernias account for only a small percentage of all diaphragmatic hernias—for example, only 11 (5 per cent) of 260 cases reviewed by Marchand.[152] By contrast, 90 per cent of strangulated diaphragmatic hernias are of traumatic origin.[16, 150] According to the older literature, the left hemidiaphragm is affected in 90 to 98 per cent of cases,[144, 145, 147, 151, 153, 154] possibly because the right hemidiaphragm is protected by the liver, which dissipates the force of indirect trauma and helps to prevent laceration. Despite this generally accepted view of left-sided predominance, it is clear that right diaphragmatic hernias are more likely to be overlooked than those of the left side, and it is almost certain that the incidence of right-sided hernias is considerably higher than is generally appreciated. Laws and Waldschmidt,[155] in fact, found the incidence of right and left hemidiaphragmatic hernias to be identical. (In a letter to the editor of the Journal of the American Medical Association, they additionally cited two references of series showing a 2-to-1 and a 3-to-1 predominance of left to right.) Further, in a recent analysis of 42 cases of diaphragmatic rupture secondary to blunt trauma, it was found that the left hemidiaphragm was affected in 24 cases (57 per cent), the right in 15 cases (36 per cent), and both in 3 cases (7 per cent).[156] The central and posterior portions of the left hemidiaphragm are most commonly involved. The hernial contents depend on the size and position of the rupture and can include omentum, stomach, small and large intestines, spleen, kidney, and even pancreas. As might be anticipated, there is no peritoneal sac.

Roentgenographically, the left hemidiaphragm cannot be traced and abnormal shadows are visible

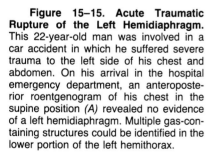

Figure 15–15. Acute Traumatic Rupture of the Left Hemidiaphragm. This 22-year-old man was involved in a car accident in which he suffered severe trauma to the left side of his chest and abdomen. On his arrival in the hospital emergency department, an anteroposterior roentgenogram of his chest in the supine position (A) revealed no evidence of a left hemidiaphragm. Multiple gas-containing structures could be identified in the lower portion of the left hemithorax.

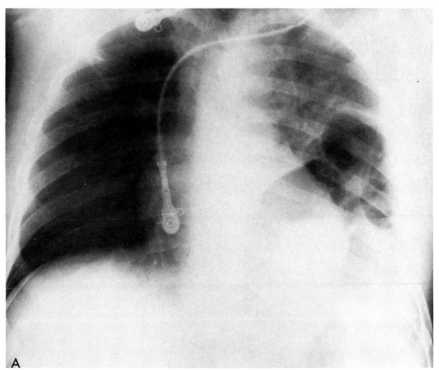

A

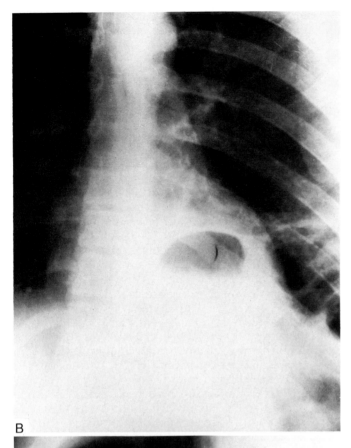

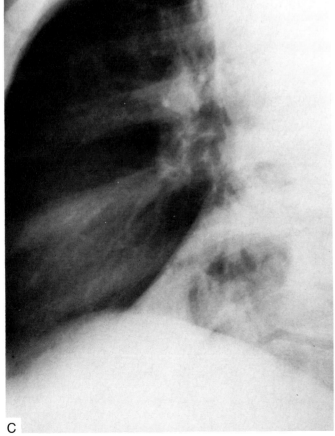

Figure 15–15 *Continued* Later the same day, anteroposterior *(B)* and lateral *(C)* roentgenograms in the erect position revealed a gas-containing structure in the medial portion of the left hemithorax posteriorly, showing a prominent air-fluid level in the erect position; this is the stomach. In addition, there is almost total airlessness of the left lower lobe owing to atelectasis. A large left diaphragmatic laceration was satisfactorily repaired.

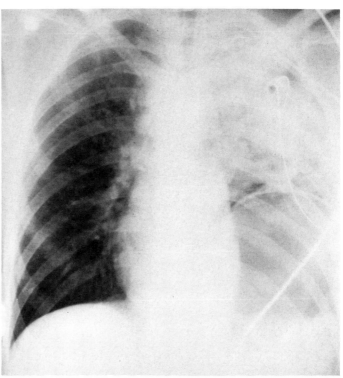

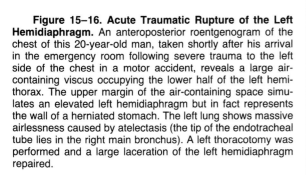

Figure 15–16. Acute Traumatic Rupture of the Left Hemidiaphragm. An anteroposterior roentgenogram of the chest of this 20-year-old man, taken shortly after his arrival in the emergency room following severe trauma to the left side of the chest in a motor accident, reveals a large air-containing viscus occupying the lower half of the left hemithorax. The upper margin of the air-containing space simulates an elevated left hemidiaphragm but in fact represents the wall of a herniated stomach. The left lung shows massive airlessness caused by atelectasis (the tip of the endotracheal tube lies in the right main bronchus). A left thoracotomy was performed and a large laceration of the left hemidiaphragm repaired.

in the left hemithorax (Fig. 15–15). These shadows depend on the nature of hernial contents and are commonly inhomogeneous owing to the presence of air-containing bowel, usually with fluid levels. In contrast to Bochdalek hernias, a portion of the stomach is often present (Fig. 15–16). The roentgenographic appearance can simulate eventration or diaphragmatic paralysis, and differentiation may be possible only with barium examination of the gastrointestinal tract, computed tomography, or real-time sonography.[157] Of major differential importance is the fact that with hernia afferent and efferent loops of bowel are constricted as they traverse the orifice in the diaphragm (Fig. 15–17), whereas in eventration or paralysis the loops tend to be widely separated.

Traumatic diaphragmatic hernia is usually suspected on roentgenographic examination following injury, although it is surprising how often an unsuspected diaphragmatic tear is found at thoracotomy or laparotomy performed for some other purpose.[144] Minagi and associates[164] have stressed the importance of recognizing minor alteration of diaphragmatic contour as an early sign of diaphragmatic rupture. Although relatively nonspecific in nature, local elevation or irregularity of configuration should suggest the possibility of tear in the appropriate clinical setting, as was the case in four of the nine patients described by these authors.

The association of fractured ribs, particularly the lower ones, is also of obvious importance in suggesting the diagnosis of traumatic rupture. Strangulation of hernial contents occurs in some

cases; in fact, 90 per cent of all strangulated diaphragmatic hernias are traumatic in origin.[150] Unilateral pleural effusion, hemothorax, and pneumothorax are also important roentgenographic signs suggesting this complication:[158, 471, 472] when strangulation is absent fluid seldom collects in the affected pleural space, since any fluid that forms as a result of irritation can pass into the abdomen through the rent in the diaphragm.

When rupture occurs in the right hemidiaphragm, a portion of the liver may herniate through the rent and create a mushroom-like mass within the right hemithorax, the herniated liver being constricted by the tear. In such circumstances, herniation may be suspected by the high position of the lower border of the liver as indicated by the position of the hepatic flexure.[155, 159]

Diaphragmatic rupture can be associated with several unusual complications. Rarely, a tear in the left hemidiaphragm involves the pericardial sac and allows passage of various organs into this space;[165] such a case has been reported in which the diagnosis was verified by CT.[160] Exceptionally, rupture of the left hemidiaphragm results in bronchopancreatic fistula, an abnormality that occurs more frequently following acute pancreatitis;[161, 162] a suspected diagnosis can be confirmed by finding a high level of amylase in the sputum.[162] A thoracobiliary fistula can also develop. Oparah and Mandal[163] have described 4 such cases and found 12 cases reported in the literature; all patients had suffered injuries to both the diaphragm and the liver. The chest roentgenogram usually revealed an elevated right

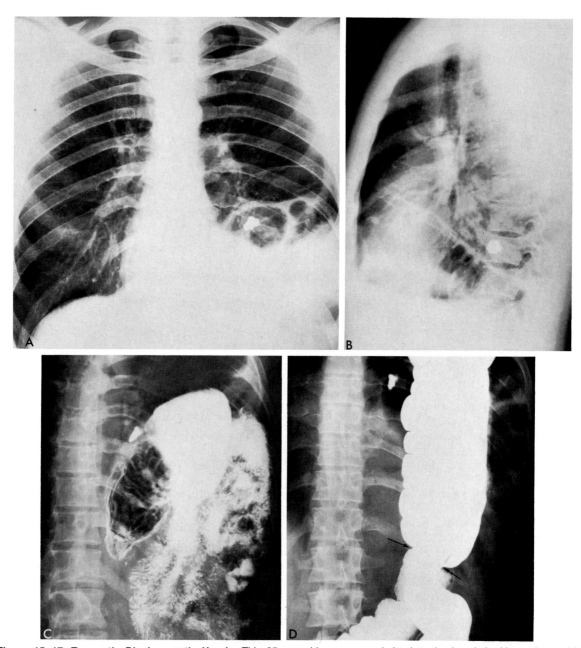

Figure 15–17. Traumatic Diaphragmatic Hernia. This 25-year-old man was admitted to the hospital with a 12-year history of discomfort in the left chest and upper abdomen, a symptom that had been present more or less continuously since he was wounded in 1944 by a piece of shrapnel that entered the left side of his chest between the eighth and ninth ribs. On admission, posteroanterior *(A)* and lateral *(B)* roentgenograms revealed numerous air-containing viscera within the lower portion of the left hemithorax. The left hemidiaphragm could not be identified clearly along any of its surface. The metallic foreign body was readily visualized. Barium examination of the upper gastrointestinal tract *(C)* showed much of the stomach and several loops of small bowel within the left hemithorax. Barium opacification of the colon *(D)* demonstrated a long segment of splenic flexure within the left hemithorax, the point at which the colon passed through the rent in the diaphragm being indicated by *arrows*. At thoracotomy, a large defect measuring 3 inches in diameter was found in the left hemidiaphragm; most of the stomach, part of the large bowel, and a considerable amount of small bowel were situated within the left hemithorax. Successful repair was performed.

hemidiaphragm and pleural effusion. Seven of the 16 patients had biloptysis and two thirds developed bile empyema.

The majority of hernias give rise to symptoms, although they may not be noted for months or even years after the traumatic episode.[147, 148, 166] Immediate symptoms consist of severe substernal pain, vomiting, shock, and dyspnea resulting from lung compression. Associated injuries are common; in one series of 42 cases, they occurred in 38 patients and usually numbered two or more in each patient.[156] The most frequent injuries are rupture of the spleen, perforation of a hollow abdominal viscus, and fractured ribs. Intestinal obstruction as a result of strangulation occurs most commonly in cases of long-standing hernia.[144] Following blunt trauma, an extremely scaphoid anterior abdominal wall should make one suspicious of a diaphragmatic hernia (Gibson's sign).[21]

EFFECTS ON THE CHEST WALL OF NONPENETRATING TRAUMA

FRACTURES OF THE RIBS

Fractures of the rib cage as a result of blunt trauma most commonly involve the fourth to tenth ribs. Fracture of the first rib is uncommon and in many cases is of the "fatigue" (stress) type, commonly in asymptomatic active young women.[167] Traumatic fracture of the first and second ribs can result from direct or indirect violence and when it affects the middle third may fail to unite.[167] The severity of the trauma required to fracture these ribs may result in serious intrathoracic damage, including torsion of the lung and tracheobronchial fracture. Albers and associates[168] divided 75 patients with 90 first-rib fractures into two groups. Group I consisted of 13 patients with a fracture of one or both first ribs only, and group II (62 patients) had multiple rib fractures that included the first rib. In group I, intrathoracic injuries were mild and included none involving major vessels, whereas in group II many of the patients sustained severe intrathoracic injury, 58 per cent involving the aorta. The lack of an association between isolated first-rib fractures and tracheobronchial or aortic rupture likely is attributable to the nature of the trauma, which is frequently accompanied by maxillofacial or neurologic injuries.[106] Fractures of the ninth, tenth, or eleventh ribs are apt to be associated with splenic or hepatic injury and sometimes with serious intra-abdominal hemorrhage.[21]

The possibility of hemothorax, pneumothorax, or hemopneumothorax complicating severe rib fracture renders it desirable—if not necessary—to perform chest roentgenography several hours after trauma.[79] The fracture of multiple ribs may result in a "flail" chest, which may lead rapidly to severe respiratory failure, a complication usually apparent clinically in paradoxical movement of the chest wall. Blood gas analysis is imperative to assess the presence and course of respiratory failure in these cases.

Cough fractures of the ribs occur more often in women than in men[169, 170] and almost invariably involve the sixth to ninth ribs, most often the seventh and usually in the posterior axillary line.[169, 170] Unless special care is taken to obtain roentgenograms of superior quality detailing the involved ribs, cough fractures may go undetected until evidenced by callus formation some time later.

The diagnosis of fractured ribs may be suggested clinically by the abrupt onset of chest pain after blunt trauma or a severe bout of coughing. The pain is accentuated by breathing; in some cases, a sensation of "something snapping" is noted by the patient.

Severe sudden compression of the thorax, regardless of whether it is associated with rib fractures, can result in a dramatic clinical picture of ecchymosis and edema of the face known as "traumatic asphyxia."[171] This complication is believed to be the result of reflux of blood from the right side of the heart into the great veins of the head and neck. Ninety per cent of patients who present with this clinical picture as the sole manifestation of trauma and who survive the first few hours after injury will recover, survival rate being inversely proportional to the extent and severity of associated injuries.[171]

Patients who survive severe crush injuries to the chest usually show little residual defect. In a follow-up study of 54 patients who had required tracheostomy and intermittent positive pressure ventilation (IPPV) following severe injury, Davidson and associates[172] found that only 1 in 5 patients was left with evidence of chest wall deformity, and in none was this severe. The authors attributed this excellent outcome to the efficiency of IPPV in preventing paradoxical chest movement. Although chest roentgenograms on these patients frequently demonstrated localized areas of pleural thickening, there was no instance of the subsequent development of significant fibrothorax. Mean values for forced vital capacity (FVC) and forced expiratory volume per second (FEV_1) showed surprisingly small reductions for the group as a whole. However, it was thought that many patients suffered from cough, sputum production, and dyspnea of greater severity than was indicated by objective tests. Another study of the late respiratory sequelae of blunt chest trauma[173] resulted in similar findings: in an assessment of 86 survivors of such trauma for respiratory symptoms, the incidence of cough, wheezing, and dyspnea was found to be high despite a mean FEV_1 and FVC within the normal range.

DISLOCATION OF THE CLAVICLE

Potential serious morbidity and even death associated with posterior dislocation of the clavicle at the sternoclavicular joint have been noted.[174] Although retrosternal dislocation of the clavicle is rare—of 63 sternoclavicular dislocations recorded at the Mayo Clinic over a 50-year period[175] only 3 were retrosternal—the displaced clavicle may produce serious morbidity by impinging on the trachea, the esophagus, or the great vessels or major nerves in the superior mediastinum. Prompt diagnosis is important, not only because of the serious consequences of compression of major structures but because closed reduction can usually be achieved if treatment is instituted within 24 to 48 hours of the injury. Open surgical reduction is required if diagnosis is delayed.[174]

FRACTURES OF THE SPINE

Fractures of thoracic vertebral bodies may result in extraosseous hemorrhage and the development of unilateral or bilateral paraspinal masses (Fig. 15–18). Although the fracture is usually evident roentgenographically, the major evidence of its presence may be deformity of the contiguous paraspinal soft tissues. When pleural effusion develops in association with signs of spinal cord injury at the thoracic level, the possibility of subarachnoid-pleural fistula should be considered and can be confirmed by myelography.[74]

POSTTRAUMATIC HERNIA OF THE LUNG

Protrusion of a portion of lung through an abnormal aperture of the thoracic cage may be congenital or traumatic in origin and may be cervical, thoracic, or diaphragmatic in position. The protrusion is covered by both parietal and visceral pleura. Congenital hernias occur most frequently in the supraclavicular fossa, less often at the costo-chondral junction. Traumatic hernias may follow chest trauma or surgery,[176] and in a small percentage of cases the weakened area is the result of inflammatory or neoplastic damage to the thoracic cage.[177]

The most common location of posttraumatic herniation is the parasternal region just medial to the costochondral junction, where the intercostal musculature is thinnest. The patient usually complains of a bulge appearing during coughing and straining, and, in most cases, the diagnosis is evidenced by the clinical finding of a soft crepitant mass that develops under these conditions and disappears during expiration or rest. In one patient with multiple rib fractures and a flail chest, positive end-expiratory pressure (PEEP) was considered to play a role in herniation; lung parenchyma herniated through pectoral and intercostal muscles, internal thoracic fascia, and ruptured parietal pleura.[178] Chest roentgenograms will reveal pulmonary parenchymal tissue herniating through an obvious defect in the rib cage (Fig. 15–19)[179] or through a supraclavicular fossa. Optimal visualization requires the Valsalva maneuver, with or with-

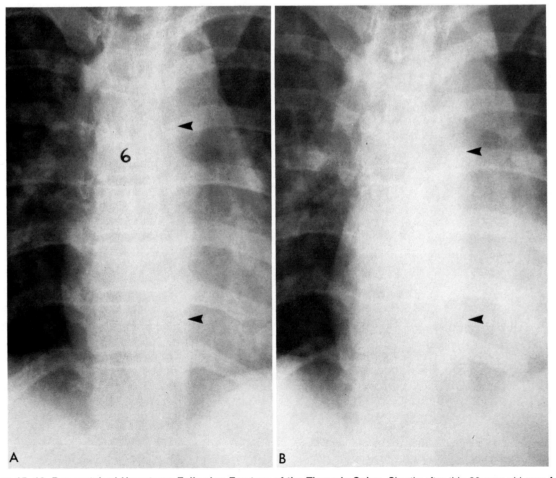

Figure 15–18. Paravertebral Hematoma Following Fracture of the Thoracic Spine. Shortly after this 20-year-old man fell from a moderate height, an anteroposterior view of the thoracic spine *(A)* revealed a slight reduction in the vertical diameter of the sixth thoracic vertebral body. The paraspinal soft tissues showed no abnormality *(arrowheads)*. Three days later *(B)*, there has occurred a moderate lateral displacement of the paraspinal line *(arrowheads)* owing to hemorrhage.

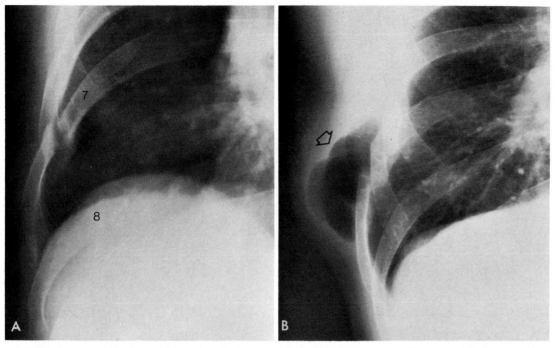

Figure 15–19. Hernia of the Lung. Approximately 1 year prior to the roentgenograms illustrated, this 46-year-old man suffered comminuted fractures of the axillary portions of ribs 6, 7, and 8 on the right in a crush injury to his chest. Healing of the rib fractures had occurred such that there was considerable separation between ribs 7 and 8 *(A)*. The patient noted a soft, fluctuant bulge in the axillary region of his chest on coughing and straining. Roentgenography of the chest in full inspiration during the Valsalva maneuver *(B)* demonstrated herniation of a sizable portion of lung through the defect in the rib cage into the contiguous soft tissues of the axilla *(arrow)*. The roentgenogram illustrated in *(A)* was exposed at full expiration and shows no evidence of lung herniation. The defect was successfully repaired surgically.

out tangential roentgenographic projection, or CT.[479]

A rare consequence of blunt trauma has been described[180] in a patient in whom a pocket of air collected in the chest wall at the site of the injury; it was postulated that air had replaced the blood in a hematoma.

PULMONARY EFFECTS OF NONTHORACIC TRAUMA

A number of pleuropulmonary abnormalities occur as a consequence of trauma in which the pathogenesis is unrelated to direct injury to the thorax (although chest injury may have occurred as well). Some of these effects are specific to trauma, including traumatic fat embolism, traumatic air embolism, and the hypoxemia associated with severe head trauma, while others are nonspecific, such as pulmonary thromboembolism and adult respiratory distress syndrome. In a prospective study of 119 patients with multiple fractures or with fractures of long bones or hip, Cole[181] found that 42 patients (35 per cent) had PaO_2 values of less than 79 mm Hg on the first day. The lowest PaO_2 levels were observed in patients with multiple fractures. Only 11 patients had abnormal chest roentgenograms; in one patient with a PaO_2 of 47 mm Hg, the chest roentgenogram was considered normal. In most

patients, PaO_2 had returned to normal by the sixth day and all patients survived. It is to be assumed that such cases represent increased capillary leakage resulting from the presence of fat, associated hypotension, or perhaps an (as yet) undetermined cause. The hypoxemia that sometimes follows isolated severe head injury is equally complex; in some patients, it is the result of pulmonary edema (*see* page 1926), whereas in others it has been clearly shown to be caused by ventilation/perfusion mismatching.[182, 183] The latter could result from both bronchiolar constriction and a failure of the homeostatic mechanism that attenuates perfusion to hypoventilated areas.

If there is reason to believe that the chest was also injured, the only other condition that need be considered in the differential diagnosis of a roentgenographic pattern of diffuse opacification following trauma is severe pulmonary contusion. Sometimes this distinction can be difficult, although contusion tends to be less diffuse and to clear more rapidly.

EFFECTS ON THE THORAX OF PENETRATING TRAUMA

The usual roentgenographic appearance of the path of a bullet through lung parenchyma is a rather poorly defined homogeneous shadow which,

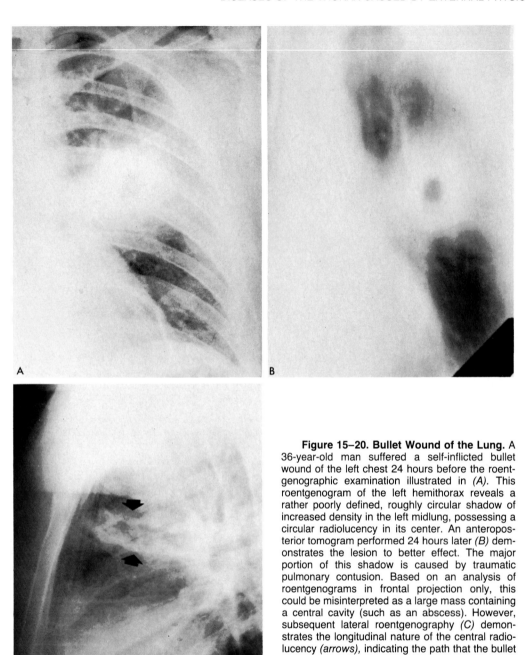

Figure 15–20. Bullet Wound of the Lung. A 36-year-old man suffered a self-inflicted bullet wound of the left chest 24 hours before the roentgenographic examination illustrated in *(A)*. This roentgenogram of the left hemithorax reveals a rather poorly defined, roughly circular shadow of increased density in the left midlung, possessing a circular radiolucency in its center. An anteroposterior tomogram performed 24 hours later *(B)* demonstrates the lesion to better effect. The major portion of this shadow is caused by traumatic pulmonary contusion. Based on an analysis of roentgenograms in frontal projection only, this could be misinterpreted as a large mass containing a central cavity (such as an abscess). However, subsequent lateral roentgenography *(C)* demonstrates the longitudinal nature of the central radiolucency *(arrows)*, indicating the path that the bullet took in its passage through the lung. The only residuum of this process was a small linear scar.

as might be expected, is more or less circular when viewed in the direction in which the bullet passed and longitudinal when viewed in perpendicular projection. The indistinct definition is caused by hemorrhage and edema into the parenchyma surrounding the bullet track. The hemorrhage usually clears in a few days, leaving a "longitudinal" hematoma that may not resolve for several weeks or months. Resolution usually is complete and without residua, although we have seen patients in whom a longitudinal scar remained.[184] In a small percentage of cases, a central radiolucency may be apparent along the bullet's course and reveal communication between the central core of blood and the bronchial tree (Fig. 15–20).[185] In such circumstances, a history of hemoptysis can be elicited in most cases. In one patient with this manifestation, Hodson[186] was able to demonstrate by Lipiodol bronchography the communication between missile track and bronchus. In one remarkable case, the tract persisted for many

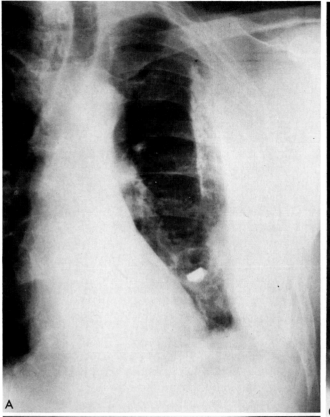

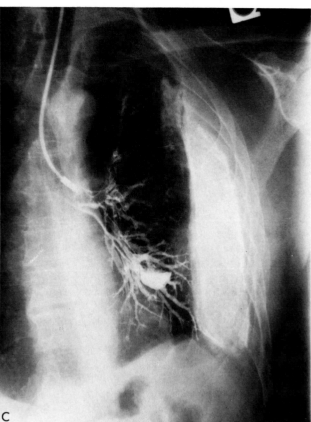

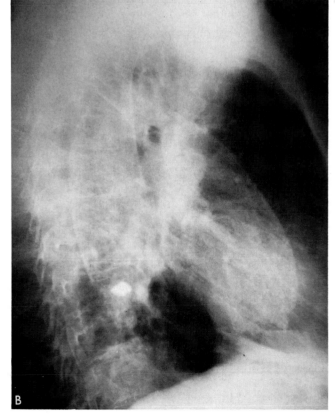

Figure 15–21. Long-Term Follow-up of Shrapnel Wound of the Left Lower Lobe and Pleura. Posteroanterior *(A)* and lateral *(B)* roentgenograms reveal moderate loss of volume of the left hemithorax associated with marked thickening of the pleura over the whole of the left lung (fibrothorax). A thick calcific plaque covers the axillary portion of the lung. A metallic foreign body is situated in the midportion of the left lower lobe, associated with a poorly defined cystic space. In view of a history of chronic productive cough, a bronchogram was performed *(C)*. Contrast medium entered the cystic space and completely obscured the metallic foreign body, thus confirming the suspicion that the fragment of shrapnel lay within the cystic space. The calcific fibrothorax was the result of traumatic hemothorax.

years, its dense fibromuscular wall lined by and presumably derived from bronchial epithelium.[184]

Penetrating wounds of the thorax from a knife or bullet may induce traumatic pneumothorax, although the searing effect of a bullet as it passes through the pleura may cauterize the tissues sufficiently to prevent escape of air into the pleural space. In one series of 250 consecutive cases of gunshot wounds involving the thorax, 90 per cent presented with hemothorax or hemopneumothorax and only 3 per cent with pneumothorax alone.[187] Hemothorax sometimes results in calcific fibrothorax (Fig. 15–21). Occasionally, a foreign body may find its way into the pleural cavity, where it may cause chronic empyema. The foreign body may have been left in the vicinity of the pleura at the time of surgery[188] or may be the direct result of a gunshot or shrapnel wound.[189] When the foreign body is metallic or otherwise opaque, it should be easily identifiable roentgenographically. The history and the scar on the skin of the chest wall provide suggestive evidence. Rarely, a knife or bullet will traverse a pulmonary artery and vein lying in close proximity and lead to the formation of an arteriovenous fistula.[190, 191]

Very occasionally, the bullet from a gunshot wound of the chest will enter the aorta and be carried distally to produce peripheral arterial embolism.[192] The younger patient appears to have a better chance of survival after bullet perforation of the aorta, possibly because greater elasticity permits the defect in the vessel to close without exsanguination and death. Whenever a patient with a gunshot wound of entry and no wound of exit shows no roentgenographic evidence of the projectile in the thorax, embolization should be suspected. Similarly, a bullet or its fragments may enter a vein and be carried to the lung, where its presence will be readily apparent.

Intrapulmonary migration of metallic foreign bodies used to stabilize the vertebrae or shoulder joint also has been reported;[193, 194] this occurs most often across the pleural space into lung parenchyma, but has also been reported to occur via the trachea, with the foreign body eventually residing in the bronchi.[193] This complication can develop during the postoperative period immediately following insertion of the pin[193] or many years later.[194] The roentgenographic appearance and clinical history should be diagnostic.

Bullets, shrapnel, and other metallic fragments that have penetrated lung parenchyma occasionally may cause intrathoracic complications many years later. Hemoptysis is the most common complication,[195–197] but others include bronchial obstruction with atelectasis,[195] abscess formation, and (as discussed previously) empyema.[189] The factors that govern the onset of disease, usually after many years of quiescence, are not precisely known but are presumably related to a slowly developing change in the position of the metallic fragments

and their erosion through significant structures, such as bronchi, vessels, or pleura. These changes in position may be noted roentgenologically, providing a diagnostic clue.[189, 196] Another uncommon, but well-documented, long-term complication is the development of carcinoma in relation to scarring associated with a metallic fragment.[184, 198–200] In this case, the carcinoma can arise either in relation to the metallic fragment itself or in the fibrous tract linking the fragment with the pleura.[200]

A final rare complication of abdominal and thoracic bullet wounds of the abdomen and thorax is intrathoracic splenosis.[201] A bullet that enters the abdomen and ruptures the spleen may traverse the diaphragm into the thorax and transport splenic cells with it. Four cases have been recorded in the literature of the subsequent development of nodules within the thorax that resembled small spleens and were proved to represent splenic implants subsequent to penetrating trauma.[201]

Despite the complications described above, penetrating injuries of the lung have surprisingly good prognoses, and the incidence of such complications is low. For example, in one series of 373 patients seen over a period of 1 year,[202] 282 were treated with intercostal thoracostomy tube only; 91 patients required thoracotomy, and there were 29 deaths. It should be remembered, however, that associated intra-abdominal injuries are common in patients with penetrating thoracic trauma. In one series of 250 consecutive cases of gunshot wounds of the thorax, 20 per cent of the patients also had injuries involving the diaphragm or one or more abdominal viscera.[187] The diaphragm can be damaged without evidence of visceral injury and with negative roentgenographic findings.[203] Such patients usually complain of abdominal pain, and examination reveals tenderness and rigidity of the abdominal wall.

THE POSTOPERATIVE CHEST

ROENTGENOGRAPHIC MANIFESTATIONS

The number of requests for roentgenographic examination of the chest with mobile apparatus at a patient's bedside has increased enormously in recent years, partly because of a remarkable growth of intensive care units and partly because of the introduction of complex cardiovascular surgical procedures that require close surveillance postoperatively. Radiologists who are required to see large numbers of such examinations recognize the necessity for a different set of guidelines in interpretation than are employed for standard roentgenograms of the chest in erect subjects, the chief reason being a tendency to over-read.[204] Abnormalities that would cause concern on standard roentgenograms are frequently of no importance in the postoperative period and, in fact, should be considered "normal" or expected findings. We have frequently been impressed by the dreadful appearance of a patient's roentgenogram 24 hours postoperatively, only to be informed by the surgeon that the patient is doing well and there is no cause for alarm. For these reasons, perhaps more than elsewhere in the interpretation of chest roentgenograms, a close correlation of clinical and roentgenographic findings is vitally important. Although daily reporting sessions in consultation with those responsible for the care of all patients in a hospital are an excellent practice, they are particularly valuable for patients in the surgical recovery room and the medical and surgical intensive care units. Such consultation sessions not only tend to prevent potentially harmful over-reading but serve to bring to the early attention of the attending physician or surgeon abnormalities that may be of clinical importance.

Unfortunately, bedside roentgenograms are almost always technically inferior to those obtained in the standard manner in a radiology department. However, we have found that use of the special techniques described in Chapter 2 (see page 323) permit better assessment of these difficult problems than is possible from conventional chest roentgenograms.

The roentgenographic abnormalities with which we are primarily concerned in the immediate postoperative period are those following thoracotomy, a subject that has been excellently reviewed by Goodman.[205] However, thoracic complications of nonthoracic surgery are also of major clinical importance, and these are considered in the next section. The majority of complications occur in the immediate postoperative period (up to the 10th day), although certain manifestations may not become apparent for several weeks or even months postoperatively (e.g., following pneumonectomy).

We find it convenient to divide postoperative roentgenograms into three broad groups, depending on the nature of observed abnormalities and the requirement for early or immediate clinical attention. This rather simplified approach has proved to be of some value in determining the course to take in any given situation.

(1) Changes are present that are ordinarily anticipated following thoracotomy, for example, subcutaneous emphysema, the accumulation of a minimal amount of pleural fluid, and no major pulmonary abnormality. In such cases, we employ the designation "satisfactory postoperative appearance" without going into any detail as to the changes observed.

(2) Abnormalities are identified that may or may not be of importance in patient care, but whose nature requires that follow-up studies be performed, for example, a pneumothorax or hydrothorax greater in amount than ordinarily anticipated, a large hematoma following wedge resection, or mediastinal widening following mediastinotomy.

(3) Abnormalities are present that require immediate attention and are sufficiently urgent to require a telephone call to the attending physician or surgeon, for example, acute atelectasis, a large pneumothorax or hydrothorax, malposition of an endotracheal tube, or pulmonary thromboembolism.

Although roentgenographic changes observed in the soft tissues of the chest wall, the thoracic cage, the pleura, the mediastinum, the diaphragm, and the lungs are in many ways interdependent and therefore should be considered together in interpretation, it serves a useful purpose to deal with them separately.

Soft Tissues of the Chest Wall

Soft tissue swelling caused by hemorrhage and edema in the vicinity of the incision is common but seldom leads to difficulty in roentgenologic interpretation and often is not roentgenographically apparent. Subcutaneous emphysema, manifested by linear streaks of gas density along the lateral chest wall and frequently in the neck, is almost invariably apparent for 2 or 3 days postoperatively. It need cause concern only when it is present in exceptionally large quantities, in which circumstance the gas may be coming from the mediastinum as a result of pulmonary interstitial and mediastinal emphysema. Such occasions are rare.

Thoracic Cage

The absence of a rib, usually the fifth or sixth, is frequently but not invariably a finding following thoracotomy. Nowadays the ribs often are spread rather than resected in both pulmonary and cardiac procedures, so that an intact rib cage is quite compatible with prior thoracotomy; ribs that have been spread may be fractured. Sternotomy is evidenced only by the presence of wire sutures.

The major abnormality to be detected in the rib cage relates to the size of one hemithorax in comparison with the other—approximation of ribs and a smaller hemithorax in the presence of atelectasis and separation of ribs and a larger hemithorax in the presence of pneumothorax. As discussed farther on, enlargement of one hemithorax may be the only sign of pneumothorax in a patient whose roentgenogram was exposed in the supine position. In such circumstances, when the pneumothorax is small a pleural line may not be visible.

Median sternotomy has become the principal surgical approach to the heart and great vessels and to a variety of mediastinal abnormalities. As pointed out by Goodman and his colleagues,[206] the incidence of complications following median sternotomy is low (less than 5 per cent), but the overall mortality rate of three of the major complications (sternal dehiscence, mediastinitis, and osteomyelitis) exceeds 50 per cent. The complications that may occur following sternotomy usually become manifest between 1 and 2 weeks postoperatively and consist of six different presentations:[466] (1) serosanguineous discharge with a stable sternum, (2) unstable sternum with or without a serosanguineous discharge, (3) sternal dehiscence without mediastinitis, (4) superficial wound infection without mediastinitis, (5) subcutaneous infection with retrosternal extension and an unstable sternum, and (6) mediastinitis with or without sternal separation. In the study by Serry and associates,[466] all patients in groups 1 and 2 survived with appropriate therapy, patients in groups 3 and 4 had a 24 per cent mortality, and in patients with deep wound infections (groups 5 and 6), the mortality rate exceeded an astonishing 70 per cent. Goodman and his colleagues[206] have emphasized the limited role that conventional roentgenography and tomography can play in the evaluation of these conditions. In a CT study of 32 patients in the immediate poststernotomy period, these authors found focal edema, focal hematomas, and minor sternal irregularities common in the 20 patients who suffered no clinical problems; by contrast, among the 12 patients with obvious postoperative problems, CT was able to distinguish the 6 patients with no significant infection from the 6 with major infection. In addition, among the latter group CT was of great value in establishing whether the infection was limited to the presternal tissues or whether it involved the anterior mediastinum.

The so-called midsternal stripe, formerly thought to represent radiographic evidence of sternal dehiscence, can be recognized in 30 to 60 per cent of patients sometime during the postoperative period and is now known to be of no diagnostic or prognostic significance.[205] Of much greater importance in establishing sternal separation is a change in the relationship of wires to their neighbors.

Curtis and his colleagues[207] have called attention to fracture of the first rib as a complication of midline sternotomy; in a review of 50 randomly selected cases, first-rib fractures were identified in 3 patients (6 per cent).

Pleura

The most common roentgenographic abnormality in the postoperative period is pleural effusion. During the 2 or 3 days after thoracotomy little or no fluid is evident, since the pleural space is effectively drained. Following removal of the drainage tube, however, a small amount of fluid often appears, only to disappear quite quickly during

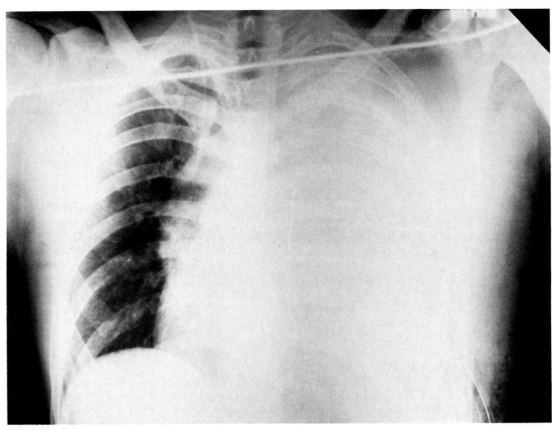

Figure 15–22. Massive Hemothorax Complicating Thoracotomy. Twenty-four hours prior to the roentgenogram illustrated, this 20-year-old man was subjected to left thoracotomy for repair of a coarctation of the aorta (minimal rib notching was apparent). The roentgenogram illustrates a massive effusion in the left pleural space with considerable shift of the mediastinum to the right. This represents a massive hemothorax caused by bleeding into the pleural space from an intercostal artery. The unusually severe hemorrhage was related to hypertrophy of the intercostal circulation secondary to coarctation.

convalescence. Minimal residual pleural thickening may remain, particularly over the lung base.

The accumulation of fluid in larger than expected amounts may result from a variety of causes, including poor positioning of the drainage tube, hemorrhage from an intercostal vessel (Fig. 15–22), or infection (empyema). In the presence of pleural adhesions, fluid may loculate in areas that are not in communication with the drainage tube, a finding that is particularly common following pleural decortication. In such circumstances, absorption of the fluid may be prolonged, sometimes requiring several weeks. Such local intrapleural collections may be simulated by an extrapleural hematoma

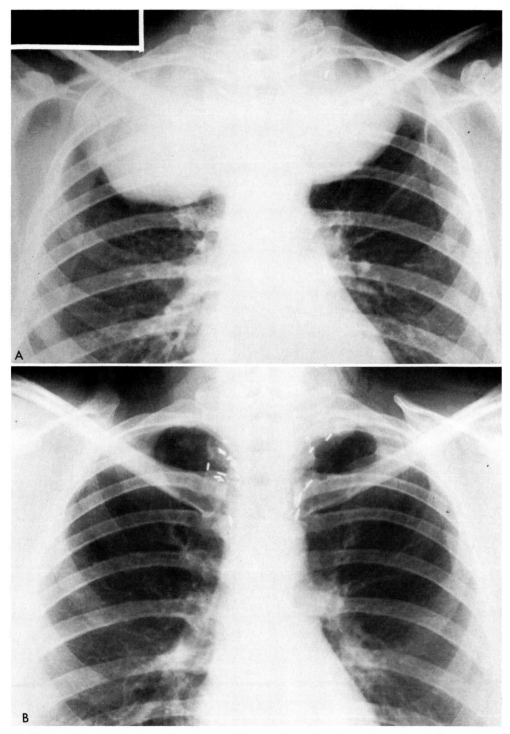

Figure 15–23. Bilateral Apical Extrapleural Hematomas Following Sympathectomy. Several days following bilateral upper thoracic sympathectomy, a roentgenogram *(A)* reveals sharply defined homogeneous masses occupying the apical portion of both hemithoraces (a preoperative roentgenogram was normal). Three months later *(B)*, the hematomas had completely resolved.

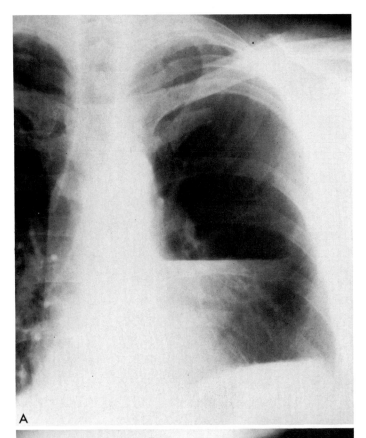

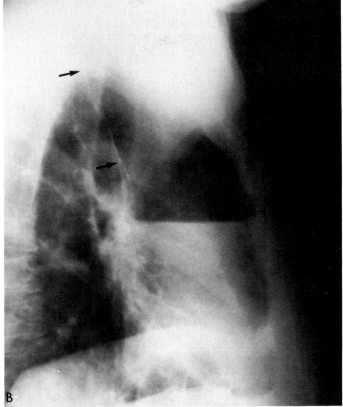

Figure 15–24. Loculated Hydropneumothorax Following Lobectomy. Posteroanterior *(A)* and lateral *(B)* roentgenograms reveal a large loculated collection of gas and fluid in the anterior portion of the left hemithorax (the upper half of the lower lobe major fissure is indicated by *arrows* in *B*). These films were made approximately 2 weeks following left upper lobectomy, the persistence of pneumothorax being caused by air leak from lower lobe parenchyma. It required several weeks for spontaneous absorption.

secondary to the thoracotomy incision, but in either event the finding is not of major importance unless the accumulation is very large or infected. Extrapleural hematomas are particularly common following surgery over the lung apex and sometimes create a rather ominous-looking shadow (Fig. 15–23), which actually is of little or no clinical significance.

In contrast to the small amount of fluid that often accumulates, gas is seldom visible in the pleural space following removal of the drainage tube, even on roentgenograms exposed with the patient erect. A word of caution regarding the assessment of possible pneumothorax: in the immediate postoperative period, roentgenograms are often exposed with the patient supine, in which position any intrapleural gas tends to be situated at the base of the hemithorax anteriorly where it may not be in communication with the drainage tube. Even a small pneumothorax in this location is usually of sufficient size to permit identification of the visceral pleural line at the base of the lung. If the line is not visible, however, suspicion of pneumothorax still should be raised by the presence of enlargement of the ipsilateral hemithorax owing to a loss of the inward retractile force of the elastic recoil of the lung. A pneumothorax of such small size should not cause symptoms, but when clinical concern is registered roentgenography should be performed in the lateral decubitus or erect position to confirm or deny the presence of pneumothorax. One should be particularly aware of the possibility of pneumothorax in circumstances in which it is unexpected, for example, following mediastinotomy for cardiac surgery, during which the mediastinal pleura may have been accidentally nicked.

Pneumothorax postoperatively may be due to a variety of causes. Lack of communication with the drainage tube is probably the most common, particularly if the gas is loculated or the tube is incorrectly positioned (e.g., in the major fissure). Other causes include leakage into the pleural space from a blown bronchial stump (bronchopleural fistula) or from a bare area of lung following wedge or segmental resection of lung (Fig. 15–24). In the presence of pleural adhesions, a loculated collection of gas may remain for a considerable period of time because of lack of communication with the drainage tube. This may be associated with a collection of fluid in the form of hydropneumothorax.

The incidence of bronchopleural fistula as a complication of pulmonary resection is approximately 2 per cent[208] and the mortality rate ranges from 16 to 22 per cent.[208, 209] It occurs as a result of necrosis of the bronchial stump or dehiscence of sutures and formerly was seen most often after pneumonectomy for tuberculosis. It is most common after right pneumonectomy and occurs rarely after lower lobectomy on either side. Characteristically, it is heralded by the sudden onset of dyspnea and expectoration of bloody fluid during the first 10 days postoperatively. The chest roentgenogram reveals an unexpected disappearance of fluid as a reflection of emptying of the pleural space by way of the tracheobronchial tree.[210] Roentgenographic evaluation of this complication can be facilitated by CT.[211] With the introduction of a modern stapling machine to effect closure of the bronchus, fistulas are becoming much less frequent.[212]

Mediastinum

The two major abnormalities of the mediastinum that occur in the postoperative period are enlargement and displacement. Enlargement results from the accumulation of either gas (pneumomediastinum is a frequent finding following mediastinotomy and should not occasion alarm) or fluid (widening of the superior mediastinum owing to venous hemorrhage and edema is also a common finding after mediastinotomy and should not be considered serious unless it is excessive or increasing). Persistence of pneumomediastinum in the absence of any other potential cause (such as tracheostomy) should raise the suspicion of interstitial pulmonary emphysema associated with some form of pulmonary disease.[213]

Position of the mediastinum is one of the most important indicators of pulmonary abnormality during the postoperative period. Displacement may occur toward or away from the side of the thoracotomy. Ipsilateral displacement is an expected finding following lobectomy or pneumonectomy. Following removal of part of a lung, mediastinal displacement is temporary; the normal midline position is regained as the remainder of the lung undergoes compensatory overinflation. Excessive displacement toward the operated side may be a sign of atelectasis in the ipsilateral lung. In the case of pneumonectomy, ipsilateral mediastinal displacement is progressive and permanent (see farther on). Mediastinal displacement *away* from the operated side may occur as a result of atelectasis in the contralateral lung or an accumulation of excessive fluid or gas in the ipsilateral pleural space.

The changes in the chest roentgenogram following pneumonectomy have been clarified by Hanson and his colleagues on the basis of a review of 110 cases.[214] Within 24 hours of pneumonectomy, the ipsilateral pleural space is air-containing, the mediastinum is shifted slightly to the ipsilateral side, and the hemidiaphragm is slightly elevated (Fig. 15–25). The postpneumonectomy space then begins to fill with serosanguineous fluid in a progressive and normally predictable manner at a rate of approximately two rib spaces a day. The majority of the 110 cases studied by Hanson and his colleagues showed 80 to 90 per cent obliteration of the space at the end of 2 weeks and complete obliteration by 2 to 4 months. Obliteration of the space occurs not only as a result of fluid accumulation but by progressive ipsilateral displacement of the mediastinum

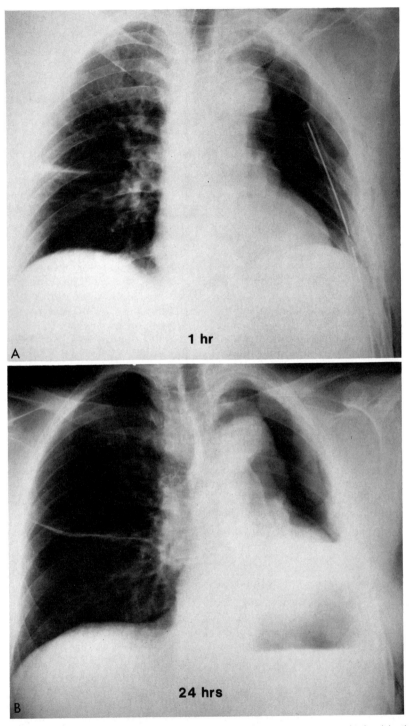

Figure 15–25. Postpneumonectomy Course, Normal. An anteroposterior roentgenogram obtained in the supine position at the bedside 1 hour following left pneumonectomy *(A)* reveals a slight reduction in the volume of the left hemithorax. The space is air-filled and the mediastinum is in the midline. At 24 hours, a roentgenogram in the erect position *(B)* shows moderate elevation of the left hemidiaphragm (as indicated by the gastric air bubble), a moderate shift of the mediastinum to the left, and a prominent air-fluid level in the plane of the third interspace anteriorly.

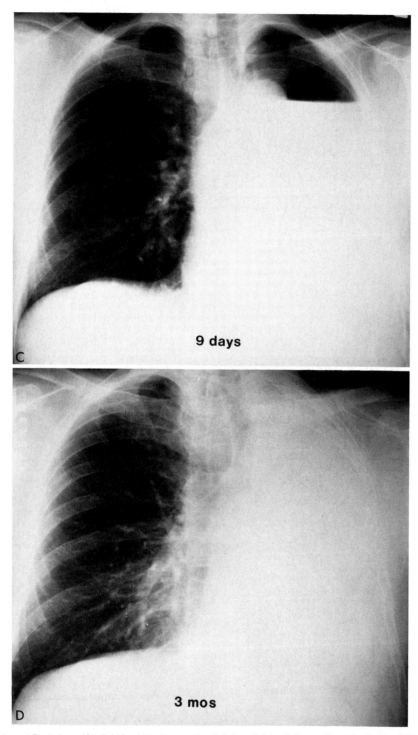

Figure 15–25 *Continued* By 9 days *(C)*, fluid had filled approximately two-thirds of the cavity of the left hemithorax but the mediastinum was still displaced to the left (note the curvature of the tracheal air column). By 3 months *(D)*, the left hemithorax had become completely airless. Note the persistent shift of the mediastinum to the left and the prominent curve of the air column of the trachea.

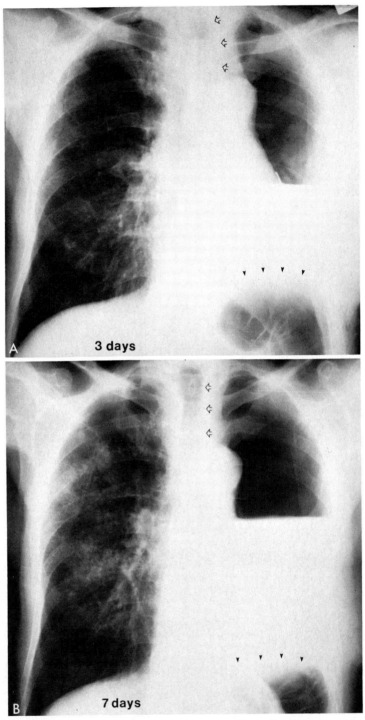

Figure 15–26. Postpneumonectomy Course Complicated by Empyema. Three days following left pneumonectomy *(A)*, the amount of fluid that has accumulated, the position of the left hemidiaphragm *(arrowheads),* and the shift of the tracheal air column to the left *(open arrows)* are all consistent with a normal postoperative course (compare with Figure 15–25). At 7 days *(B)*, however, the left hemidiaphragm *(arrowheads)* has undergone some depression and the tracheal air column *(open arrows)* has returned to the midline. Such a change should suggest empyema, bronchopleural fistula, pleural hemorrhage, or conceivably chylothorax.

and elevation of the hemidiaphragm. Mediastinal displacement is an almost invariable finding and constitutes the most reliable indicator of a normal postoperative course. It generally requires 6 to 8 months to reach its maximum. Failure of the mediastinum to shift in the postoperative period almost always indicates an abnormality in the postpneumonectomy space regardless of the character or level of the air-fluid interface.

In the series of cases studied by Hanson and associates,[214] the postpneumonectomy space filled more rapidly on the left than on the right and also when the pneumonectomy was extrapleural, that is, when it included the parietal pleura, usually in cases of infectious lung disease such as tuberculous bronchiectasis and lung abscess. The character of the fluid level was found to have little or no diagnostic or prognostic significance; the contour of the air-fluid interface was less important than the appearance of bubbles or a drop in the level of fluid by more than 2 cm. Hanson and coworkers found that the hallmark of a normal course of events following pneumonectomy was progressive shift of the mediastinum to the operative side, associated with compensatory overinflation of the contralateral lung (Fig. 15–25). The absence of such a shift in the immediate postoperative period indicated the presence of bronchopleural fistula, empyema (Fig. 15–26), hemorrhage, or occasionally chylothorax. The most sensitive indicator of *late* complications was found to be a return to the midline of a previously shifted mediastinum, particularly the tracheal air column. This indicated the presence within the postpneumonectomy space of an expanding process such as recurrent neoplasm (Fig. 15–27), bronchopleural fistula, hemorrhage, chylothorax, or empyema (Fig. 15–28). In some patients with recurrent carcinoma following pneumonectomy, conventional roentgenograms of the thorax do not manifest signs of such an expanding process within the ipsilateral hemithorax. In these cases, CT can be of great value in documenting tumor recurrence, either as enlarged mediastinal lymph nodes or as a soft tissue mass projecting into the near–water-density postpneumonectomy space.[215]

A rare event, but one of potentially catastrophic magnitude, is herniation of the heart through a pericardial defect following radical pneumonectomy in which partial pericardiectomy has been carried out or in which intrapericardial ligation of pulmonary vessels has been performed.[216, 217] This herniation may occur on either side and is frequently associated clinically with the abrupt onset of circulatory collapse or superior vena cava obstruction. Roentgenologically, the appearance varies with the side on which the pneumonectomy has been formed: if on the right, the heart is dextrorotated into the right hemithorax with production of an unmistakable appearance;[218, 219] when on the left, the heart may rotate posteriorly or laterally and herniation is usually less evident, particularly if there is a sizable accumulation of pleural fluid. On the left side, an indentation or notch may become apparent between the great vessels and the heart, simulating the appearance of congenital absence of the left side of the pericardium (*see* page 761). Hidvegi and his colleagues[220] have described a case in which herniation of the heart following left

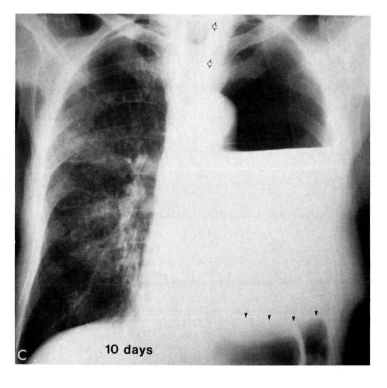

Figure 15–26 *Continued* By 10 days *(C)*, the left hemidiaphragm *(arrowheads)* had become concave superiorly and the mediastinum and tracheal air column *(open arrows)* had shifted further to the right. This was proved left-sided empyema.

10 days

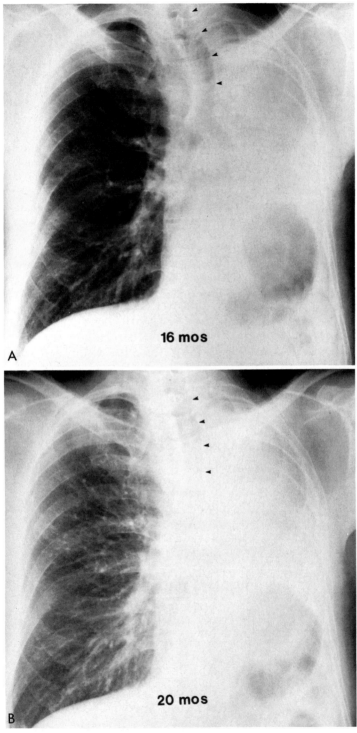

Figure 15–27. Postpneumonectomy Course: Recurrence of Neoplasm. Sixteen months following left pneumonectomy for bronchogenic carcinoma, a posteroanterior roentgenogram *(A)* reveals a normal appearance (compare with Figure 15–25). The left hemidiaphragm is markedly elevated and the heart and tracheal air column *(arrowheads)* are shifted into the left hemithorax. By 20 months *(B)*, the left side of the tracheal air column is beginning to flatten out *(arrowheads)*, suggesting the presence of an expanding process in the left hemithorax.

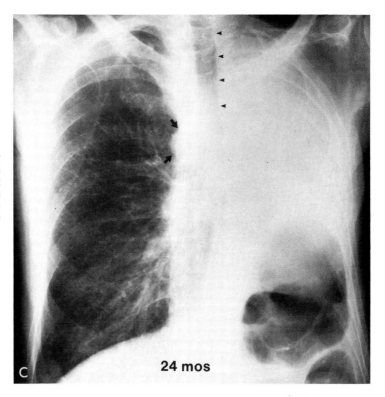

Figure 15–27 *Continued* By 24 months *(C)*, not only is the trachea in the midline *(arrowheads)* but there has developed a soft tissue mass in the region of the right tracheobronchial angle *(arrows)*, indicating a metastasis to the azygos lymph node. Recurrence of neoplasm in the pleural space and contralateral node metastasis were subsequently proved pathologically.

pneumonectomy resulted in displacement of the left chest tube, constituting the initial evidence that something was amiss. In the correct clinical setting, this grave complication should be readily recognizable radiologically, leading to life-saving thoracotomy.[221] The diagnosis can be confirmed by thoracoscopy.[222]

Another rare complication of right pneumonectomy that tends to occur a considerable time after surgery (often less than 1 year but occasionally as long as 37 years[223]) is the so-called right pneumonectomy syndrome. This condition is usually seen in children and adolescents, although in one report it was identified in a patient 50 years of age.[223] Roentgenographic manifestations include marked rightward and posterior displacement of the mediastinum, clockwise rotation of the heart and great vessels, and marked displacement of the overinflated left lung into the anterior portion of the right hemithorax. As a result of the marked rotation of the heart and great vessels, the distal trachea and left main bronchus become compressed between the aorta and pulmonary artery, with resulting dyspnea and recurrent left-sided pneumonia. CT has been shown to facilitate identification of this potentially serious complication.[223]

Diaphragm

The value of diaphragmatic position in the assessment of the postoperative chest roentgenogram depends largely on the position of the patient at the time of roentgenography. In the supine position, the normally higher position of the right hemidiaphragm is accentuated, presumably owing to the mass of the liver, and this must not be mistaken for evidence of intrathoracic abnormality. With the patient erect, the usual rules regarding diaphragmatic position pertain.

Following pneumonectomy or lobectomy, the ipsilateral hemidiaphragm is almost invariably elevated during the first few postoperative days. Following pneumonectomy, this elevation persists along with ipsilateral mediastinal shift, despite accumulation of fluid in the pleural space. Following lobectomy, diaphragmatic elevation and mediastinal displacement disappear over a period of several days or weeks as the remainder of the ipsilateral lung undergoes compensatory overinflation.

Marked elevation of a hemidiaphragm can result from injury to the phrenic nerve sustained during surgery. Elevation can also be caused by a number of pathologic states within the lungs, including atelectasis, bronchopneumonia, and thromboembolism. Differentiation of these conditions may be difficult from roentgenographic signs alone, although the time interval following surgery may be of some assistance (*see* farther on).

Depression of one hemidiaphragm is a very uncommon postoperative abnormality and is invariably caused by a massive pneumothorax or hydrothorax.

Lungs

The chest roentgenogram following thoracotomy may reveal changes to be anticipated from the nature of the surgical procedure. For example,

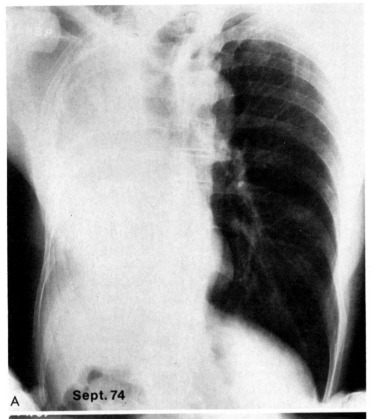

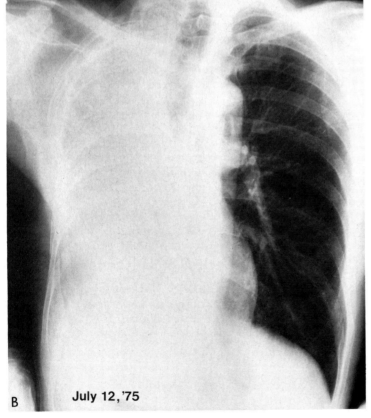

Figure 15–28. Empyema Necessitatis in a Post-pneumonectomy Space. This 53-year-old man had had a right pneumonectomy for acute lung gangrene approximately 1 year prior to the roentgenogram illustrated in *(A);* at the time of this study, he was asymptomatic. Note the marked reduction in volume of the right hemithorax, as indicated by shift of the trachea and heart to the right. On July 12, 1975 *(B),* he was admitted with fever and pain in the right side of his chest; note that both the tracheal air column and heart show less displacement to the right.

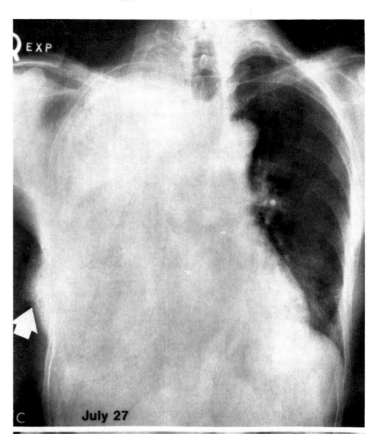

Figure 15–28 *Continued* Two weeks later *(C),* both the tracheal air column and the heart had reached a midline position owing to the presence of a large expanding process in the right postpneumonectomy space. In addition, a smooth soft tissue mass had developed in the right lateral chest wall *(arrow).* Following drainage of a large amount of pus from the right pleural space and replacement with air *(D),* a gas shadow can be seen extending outside the rib cage *(arrows)* in the identical position of the soft tissue mass previously identified. This represents extension of pus through the parietal pleura and intercostal musculature into the subcutaneous tissues of the chest wall—empyema necessitatis.

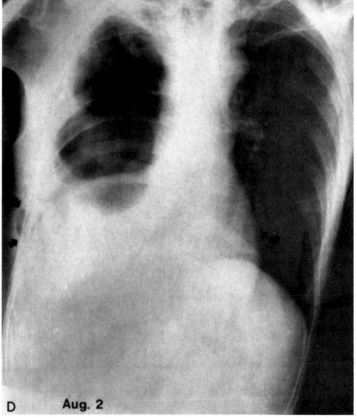

following lobectomy, rearrangement of fissures often results in displacement, which must not be misinterpreted as evidence of atelectasis. Similarly, the vascular markings become more widely spaced and lung density is reduced as a result of compensatory overinflation, signs that must not be confused with those resulting from atelectasis or from reduced perfusion due to pulmonary embolism. Hematoma formation is common following wedge or segmental resection and results from hemorrhage into the potential space at the site of excision (Fig. 15–29). Provided that the radiologist is aware of the type of surgical procedure carried out, these rather ominous-looking, yet clinically insignificant, opacities should present little difficulty in diagnosis.

Undoubtedly the most common pulmonary complication of surgical procedures is atelectasis, whether the surgery is thoracic or abdominal. In a review of the postoperative roentgenographic findings in 92 adult patients who had undergone elective cardiac surgery, Carter and his colleagues[224] found that the most common abnormality was atelectasis, although the only two postoperative complications that required decisive clinical intervention were mediastinal hemorrhage (in 7 per cent of cases) and sternal wound infection (in 3 per cent of cases). Atelectasis may vary widely in extent and may affect multiple small lobular units whose air-

lessness causes insufficient density to be appreciated roentgenologically. In such circumstances, atelectasis may be evidenced only by the demonstration on pulmonary function testing of decreased lung volume, increased venous admixture, or decreased pulmonary compliance.[225]

The mechanisms of development of postoperative atelectasis also vary considerably. The most common cause is mucous plugging from retained secretions, which occurs chiefly as a result of diminished diaphragmatic excursion caused, for example, by phrenic nerve paralysis[226] or by splinting as a result of pain.[225] Gamsu and his colleagues[227] have documented a disruption of mucociliary clearance and pooling of mucus associated with atelectasis following major surgery. During the immediate postoperative period, they insufflated powdered tantalum into the tracheobronchial tree of 18 patients who had undergone abdominal surgery and demonstrated grossly abnormal mucociliary clearance and abnormal pooling in basal bronchi in 14 patients. Although these results were obtained in patients undergoing abdominal surgery, it seems reasonable to assume that a similar mechanism exists in patients subjected to thoracotomy.

A very common, although as yet incompletely understood, abnormality that occurs postoperatively in patients who have undergone cardiopulmonary

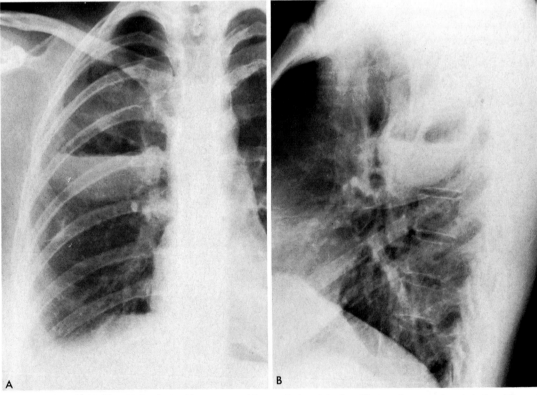

Figure 15–29. Postoperative Pulmonary Hematoma. Views of the right hemithorax from posteroanterior (A) and lateral (B) roentgenograms reveal a large, well-defined circular shadow in the upper portion of the right lung, possessing a prominent air-fluid level within it. It is very thin-walled. These roentgenograms were made approximately 3 days following wedge resection of a bulla of the right upper lobe. The shadow represents an accumulation of blood elements and gas in the bare area following resection. Over a period of 4 weeks, it underwent slow but progressive resolution and left no significant residuum. The patient was a 39-year-old woman.

bypass for open heart surgical procedures is a relatively homogeneous opacity that develops usually in the left lower lobe behind the heart. An air bronchogram is invariably associated. Although these air-containing bronchi sometimes appear crowded, there are no other convincing signs of atelectasis (Fig. 15–30); similarly, there are seldom clinical signs of pneumonia. Although the etiology remains obscure, it appears most logical to ascribe this opacity to adhesive atelectasis resulting from surfactant loss.[228] However, Benjamin and his colleagues[229] have offered an alternative explanation: in retrospective and prospective analyses of chest roentgenograms of patients following coronary artery bypass surgery, they found that a left lower lobe opacity developed in 13 of 40 patients

(32.5 per cent) who were operated on without topical cooling of the heart with ice and in a total of 111 of 162 patients (70 per cent) who were operated on with topical cooling of the heart with ice. The authors explain this difference, at least partly, on the effect of ice cooling on the phrenic nerve—the production of paralysis or paresis of the left hemidiaphragm with subsequent left lower lobe atelectasis. However, since external cooling by ice is not performed in institutions that still have a very high incidence of lower lobe opacities, it seems most unlikely that this is the only factor responsible for the atelectasis. In addition, in a study of 57 patients in whom phrenic nerve function was investigated using transcutaneous stimulation, Wilcox and colleagues[230] concluded that although phrenic pa-

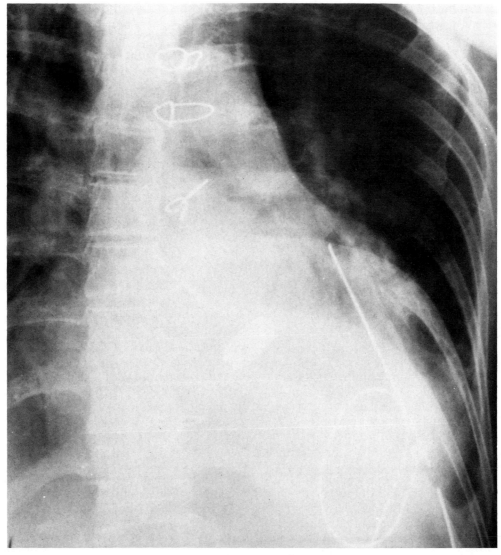

Figure 15–30. Adhesive Atelectasis of the Left Lower Lobe Following Open Heart Surgery and Extracorporeal Circulation. A view of the left lung from an anteroposterior roentgenogram exposed at the patient's bedside reveals airlessness of much of the left lower lobe associated with a prominent air bronchogram. The patient's clinical status was satisfactory, there being no fever or other signs of pneumonia. Such an appearance is so common following open heart surgery that it represents an expected finding, apparently of little clinical consequence.

resis can occur after bypass surgery and topical cold cardioplegia (5 of the 57 patients), other factors must be invoked to explain the atelectasis found in the majority of patients. Unilateral phrenic nerve paralysis has been reported to occur after surgery in 32 (1.7 per cent) of 1,891 consecutive cardiac surgical procedures on infants and children.[231]

Regardless of the nature of this left lower lobe abnormality, it appears to occasion little clinical disability and is considered by some investigators to be such a frequent finding following bypass surgery that it can be regarded as an expected part of a "satisfactory postoperative appearance."

Perhaps the most common roentgenographic abnormalities in the lungs following either thoracic or abdominal surgery take the form of broad linear opacities oriented in an oblique or horizontal plane in the lower half of either lung, often associated with an elevated hemidiaphragm. As discussed in Chapter 4 (see page 633), these "Fleischner's lines" were shown by Westcott and Cole[476] to be caused by peripheral subpleural linear collapse combined with invagination of overlying pleura. Our experience suggests that in the majority of patients who manifest these opacities, there is little clinical evidence of serious trouble; however, it should be noted that their physiologic consequences may be of some importance.

During the postoperative period, there are some patients in whom blood is shunted from pulmonary artery to pulmonary vein and yet whose chest roentgenograms reveal nothing noteworthy. A relatively common cause of hypoxemia immediately after operation is hypoventilation resulting from respiratory center depression caused by medication given during and after surgery.[232] When hypoxemia persists for several days after operation, impairment of ventilation-perfusion ratios may be demonstrated.[233, 234] Diament and Palmer's study of 23 subjects whose arterial blood gases were measured while they breathed 100 per cent oxygen before and after surgery showed a mean true shunt of 12 per cent during the postoperative period.[235] These workers correlated the degree of shunting with the roentgenographic appearances postoperatively. Shunting averaged 7 per cent in the 12 patients whose chest roentgenograms were normal, 13 per cent in the 5 patients whose chest roentgenograms showed "plate atelectasis," and 19 per cent in the 6 patients whose roentgenograms revealed segmental collapse. The authors[235] ascribed these findings to true pulmonary venoarterial shunting caused by inability of the patient to breathe deeply in the immediate postoperative period. They considered that this inability had resulted in loss of surfactant and collapse of acinar units. In another study of serial PaO$_2$ levels following upper abdominal surgery,[236] it was found that 3 of 8 patients did not regain preoperative levels by postoperative day 7. Postoperative PaO$_2$ levels appear to relate to the presence or absence of complications: in a study of

40 patients following elective cholecystectomy, Hansen and associates[237] found that in 30 patients a PaO$_2$ below 70 mm Hg correlated with abnormal stethoscopic or chest roentgenographic findings; none of the 10 patients with normal chest examinations had a PaO$_2$ below this figure. Similar findings have been reported following left thoracotomy for benign esophageal disease in 14 patients in whom no lung tissue was resected:[238] in all patients a fall in PaO$_2$ was observed postoperatively, with a mean reduction of 31 per cent. This hypoxemia was at its worst during the first 2 days, after which levels gradually returned to preoperative values.

To attribute an opacity in the lungs on a postoperative roentgenogram to residual atelectasis resulting from compression by a retractor or the surgeon's hand during the surgical procedure is tenuous; to the best of our knowledge, such effects have never been documented. Any local pulmonary opacity identified in the postoperative period must be regarded as one of the big four—atelectasis, pneumonia, infarction, or edema. The manifestations of these complications are no different from those that develop in a nonsurgical setting. As might be anticipated, diffuse pulmonary edema is much more common in patients who have undergone cardiac surgery.

An excellent systematic review of the changes that occur in pulmonary and extrapulmonary anatomy as the result of lobar collapse or resection has been recently written by Holbert and his coworkers.[239]

CLINICAL MANIFESTATIONS

Numerous factors can determine morbidity and mortality after thoracotomy and resectional surgery. Among these are (1) the general health of the patient, (2) preoperative evaluation, including assessment of lung function, (3) management by the anesthesiologist, (4) the extent of the surgery, (5) the technical ability of the surgeon, and (6) postoperative care.

The general health of the patient undoubtedly plays a role in the successful outcome of the operation. Not infrequently the requirement for surgery is urgent, if not emergent, and permits incomplete, if any, correction of existing disorders. If a reasonable interval exists between the decision for surgery and the operation itself, there is little doubt that the prognosis can be improved with proper preparation, at least in patients with either COPD or obesity. Since it has been shown that the majority of patients with pulmonary carcinoma (the most common indication for pulmonary resectional surgery) have coincident chronic obstructive pulmonary disease,[240] it is imperative that these patients be encouraged to discontinue cigarette smoking some days prior to surgery.

A fundamental aspect of preoperative preparation is a clinical and physiologic assessment of the patient's breathing reserve, both to determine the likelihood of survival after resectional surgery and to avoid creating a respiratory cripple. An experienced physician or surgeon may feel confident in making such a judgment on the basis of history and by observing the patient as he or she walks through corridors and up stairs. However, most physicians feel more comfortable with an objective determination of pulmonary function (see farther on). In patients who are considered to be operable but have clinical evidence of acute bronchitis or COPD, bronchodilators and antibiotics should be administered before surgery is undertaken. Some observers believe that preoperative instruction in breathing and coughing diminishes the frequency of postoperative complications,[241] but this assertion has been questioned by others.[242]

The anesthesiologist and the anesthetic employed can exert a significant influence over the incidence of postoperative complications. In a review of disturbances in gas exchange during anesthesia, Rehder and associates[244] found that functional residual capacity (FRC) decreases and that chest wall mechanics are altered; both oxygenation and carbon dioxide (CO_2) elimination are impaired, and both venous admixture and alveolar dead space are increased. In a more recent study,[243] it was concluded that the development of shunt during anesthesia is related to the presence of atelectasis in dependent lung regions, a conclusion that is consistent with the hypothesis that the atelectasis is caused by changes in chest wall mechanics. Serious hypoxia can result if artificial ventilation is discontinued while the respiratory center is still depressed by anesthetics or narcotics.

It is probable that the extent of surgical resection exerts considerable influence on outcome. For example, mortality is higher following pneumonectomy than lobectomy, but this may be simply a reflection of the area of gas exchange available to a patient whose remaining lung tissue is probably affected by COPD. The surgical approach is also important. For example, it has been demonstrated that when the pleura is opened, airway resistance increases abruptly, whereas if entry is by way of the mediastinum by splitting the sternum, airway conductance is not disturbed.[245]

Pulmonary dysfunction is an invariable accompaniment of thoracic and upper abdominal surgery. A decrease occurs in all lung volumes and in compliance. Perfusion of nonventilated alveoli is reflected in hypoxemia. These changes become maximal 48 to 72 hours after surgery and usually clear completely within 7 days without clinical evidence of their presence.[241] They probably result from persistent shallow breathing initiated by pain, narcotic drugs, and general anesthesia. Normal spontaneous periodic sighing ceases and must be replaced by either positive pressure inflation or voluntary maximal inspiration. Expiratory maneu-

vers, including blow bottles, serve no purpose in the postoperative period, nor does CO_2 breathing or intermittent positive pressure breathing (IPPB) with a pressure cycled machine, since the reduction in compliance causes a rapid rise in pressure and prevents filling of the lung to total lung capacity (TLC).

Pain inhibits coughing and prevents effective expectoration in addition to reducing lung volume. In a study of 24 adult male patients undergoing thoracotomy, cough pressures in the immediate postoperative period were found to be reduced to 29 per cent of their preoperative values.[246] One week following surgery, cough pressures still averaged only 50 per cent of control values, but there was a slow return to normal over the ensuing 3 weeks. The major preventive measure to overcome this physiologic dysfunction is encouragement of the patient by the physician, nurse, or therapist to cough and to inspire deeply in order to renew surfactant and to clear the airways. In a study in which a balloon catheter was inserted in the ipsilateral pleural space close to the apex, it was shown that more effective pressure on coughing can be obtained in the sitting position and that this can be further increased by manually assisted compression of the chest wall.[247] Some workers believe that assistance may be provided by properly functioning ultrasonic nebulizers.[246] Although nursing of the patient in the head-down position may facilitate drainage of secretions from the trachea, in an obese patient it may interfere considerably with gas exchange and can increase the work of breathing.[248]

Patients with pulmonary carcinoma tolerate pneumonectomy surprisingly well, considering that the majority have associated COPD.[249–251] Perfusion of the tumor-bearing lung is usually greatly reduced, to as low as 25 per cent of the total pulmonary blood flow in some cases.[250, 251] Following pneumonectomy, PaO_2 values usually improve, presumably as a result of better matching of ventilation and perfusion.[249, 253] Regional pulmonary function studies using ^{133}Xe have shown little change in distribution of ventilation and perfusion in the remaining lung after surgery, even in patients with a history of bronchitis.[249–251] The results of such studies must reflect the exclusion from resectional surgery of patients with moderate or advanced COPD, since a rise in pulmonary arterial pressure and loss of the gravity effect on perfusion are to be expected when a significant degree of emphysema is present in the remaining lung.

An unusual complication of pneumonectomy has been described in a patient with an atrial septal defect whose postoperative PaO_2 while breathing room air was 55 mm Hg in the supine position and 34 mm Hg in the erect position. It was obvious that the patient had developed pulmonary hypertension in the remaining lung, and the author[254] considered that the detrimental effect of the erect position on cardiac output and mixed venous oxygen saturation resulted in increased hypoxemia (orthodeoxia) and dyspnea (platypnea). Platypnea caused by unexplained interatrial right-to-left shunting also has been reported to occur after pneumonectomy and even lobectomy in the absence of any evidence of pulmonary hypertension.[255]

Assessment of Operative Risk

Patients with abnormal pulmonary function are more likely to get into trouble after surgery, particularly if preoperative and postoperative care is neglected.[256] Experience has shown that certain indices of pulmonary dysfunction may be more useful than others in identifying patients who are more likely to develop postoperative complications. If resectional surgery is to be confined to a lobe, such criteria may not apply, but since most lobectomies and pneumonectomies are carried out for pulmonary carcinoma, physiologic evaluation must be based on the assumption that pneumonectomy may prove necessary once the thorax is opened.[257] Pulmonary function test values that indicate a high risk for development of postoperative cardiopulmonary complications include: (1) vital capacity less than 1.0 liter; (2) FEV_1 less than 0.5 liter per second; (3) maximal midexpiratory flow less than 0.6 liter per second; (4) maximal voluntary ventilation (MVV, MBC) less than 50 per cent of predicted; (5) PaO_2 less than 55 mm Hg; and (6) elevated preoperative PCO_2.[258] Using such guidelines, it is possible to adopt a prospective approach to the selection of patients capable of undergoing pneumonectomy.[259] It has been suggested[259] that FEV_1 should be more than 50 per cent of predicted, and that the ratio of residual volume (RV) to TLC should be less than 50 per cent. Despite the foregoing, some authorities[260] are of the opinion that decisions regarding operability and extent of resection cannot be made solely on the basis of spirometric tests. Several groups[261–265, 473] employ ventilation/perfusion lung scans to assess the amount of functioning lung tissue preoperatively. In conjunction with spirometric measurements, this procedure permits calculation of the likely functional effects of pneumonectomy using the formula: postoperative FEV_1 (or FVC) equals preoperative FEV_1 (or FVC) multiplied by per cent function of regions of lung not to be resected. If the estimated postoperative FEV_1 turns out to be less than 800 ml, it has been suggested that it is advisable to carry out a further refinement of this approach to assess operability by exercising patients with a balloon inflated in the pulmonary artery of the lung to be resected: if the mean pulmonary artery pressure on exercise does not rise above 35 mm Hg and the PaO_2 does not fall below 45 mm Hg, the patient can be considered operable.[257, 259]

Several groups of investigators[266–270] have used exercise testing as a means of predicting postoperative morbidity and mortality. Although results have been somewhat conflicting, two studies[268, 269] have indicated that patients with an exercise oxygen consumption (MVO_2) greater than 20 ml/kg/min are unlikely to develop postoperative complications, whereas those with an MVO_2 less than 10 ml/kg/min can be expected to have significant morbidity and mortality. The oxygen consumption/body surface area at an arterial lactate level of 20 mg/dl ($\dot{V}O_2$/BSA at La-20) has been shown to be a useful predictor of postoperative mortality.[270] Preoperative and postoperative measurements of transdiaphragmatic pressure indicate that as a complication of pulmonary resection, respiratory failure can be caused by a reduction in diaphragmatic function.[271]

THORACIC COMPLICATIONS OF NONTHORACIC SURGERY

The major thoracic complications of abdominal surgery are atelectasis, pneumonia, thromboembolism, subphrenic abscess, cardiogenic pulmonary edema, and adult respiratory distress syndrome (ARDS).[272] This subject has been reviewed by Goodman[272] and by Harman and Lillington.[273] Atelectasis is undoubtedly the most common of these and in the majority of patients is related to retention of secretions and mucous plugging of airways. In their study of mucociliary clearance following major surgery, Gamsu and his colleagues[227] insufflated powdered tantalum into the lungs of 25 patients at the termination of surgery to outline airways from the trachea to the small bronchi. Of the 7 patients who had peripheral surgery, clearance of tantalum was progressive and usually complete within 48 hours. In contrast, 14 of 18 patients who had abdominal surgery showed grossly abnormal mucociliary clearance; at least one bronchopulmonary segment became atelectatic in all of the patients and a whole lobe or more in 6 patients. Atelectasis usually developed between 6 and 26 hours postoperatively and always occurred after pooling of mucus and tantalum was demonstrated. Tantalum was retained in the bronchi of atelectatic segments until re-expansion was evident. This study confirms in graphic fashion the importance of retention of secretions in the pathogenesis of postoperative collapse. However, given the extremely high incidence of this complication in the study group, we wonder whether the tantalum itself might have contributed to the impaired clearance and atelectasis. Retention is undoubtedly abetted by diminished diaphragmatic excursion caused by splinting as a result of pain[225] or occasionally caused by a large pneumoperitoneum following laparotomy.[274] Similar effects may follow peritoneal dialysis.[275]

In a review of the risks of abdominal and thoracic surgery in patients with chronic obstructive pulmonary disease, Gaensler and Weisel[276] pointed out that the prevalence of postoperative pulmonary complications is greater after abdominal than after thoracic surgery. Whether the same prevalence would exist in subjects without COPD is not known, but the overall incidence of complications following any form of surgery is clearly greater in patients with disturbed pulmonary function. In a study of 63 patients[277] on whom pulmonary function studies were carried out prior to various types of surgery, a striking difference was found in the prevalence of postoperative respiratory complications between the group with normal preoperative pulmonary function (3 per cent) and the group with one or more function abnormalities and a compatible clinical history (70 per cent).

Cigarette smoking and older age are risk factors for postoperative pulmonary complications;[278–280] physiologic detection of patients at risk is best accomplished by spirometry and the determination of closing capacity,[278] particularly in the supine position.[281] Routine postoperative physiotherapy may decrease the incidence of atelectasis and pulmonary infection.[282] In a series of 132 male patients over the age of 47, all of whom were cigarette smokers and lived in an industrial environment, some degree of respiratory complication developed in 85.6 per cent during the 10 days after upper abdominal surgery as judged clinically. On the second day 52.5 per cent demonstrated some roentgenographic abnormalities,[283] almost half of these being of major severity. A clinical assessment of 785 patients who underwent major surgical procedures on the lower abdomen under general anesthesia revealed a considerably lower incidence of chest complications (5 per cent).[284] However, when surgery was carried out on the upper abdomen, the complication rate rose to 10 per cent, and when surgery was performed on the gastrojejunal or biliary tracts, the incidence of complications more than doubled (21 per cent).

The roentgenographic and clinical features of acute pneumonia and pulmonary embolism are no different from those observed in other clinical settings. Subphrenic abscess, although uncommon, is almost always a complication of abdominal surgery. In a review of 1,566 abdominal operations, Sanders[285] found 15 cases of subphrenic abscess (1 per cent). Of the 13 patients on whom roentgenologic data were available, the findings were as follows: pleural effusion, 12 patients; elevated hemidiaphragm, 11; gas in an abscess, 5; and immobility of the hemidiaphragm, 3. This author stressed the importance of pleural effusion in the diagnosis of subphrenic abscess, especially when associated with an elevated hemidiaphragm. In fact, he stated that following abdominal surgery pleural effusion infrequently arises from causes other than subphrenic abscess. However, since the clinical signs (pain in the hypochondrium, limitation of respiratory motion, and fever) and roentgenographic manifestations (pleural effusion and diaphragmatic elevation) of pulmonary embolism and infarction are similar to those of subphrenic abscess, and since they both

tend to develop approximately 10 days after surgery, differentiation between the two may be difficult at times. (For additional information about subphrenic abscess, see Chapter 20).

COMPLICATIONS OF INTUBATION AND MONITORING APPARATUS

The intubation and monitoring apparatus discussed in this section includes endotracheal tubes, transtracheal catheters, chest tubes for drainage of the pleural space, abdominal drainage tubes, nasogastric tubes, venous catheters for measurement of central venous pressure (CVP) or for hyperalimentation, arterial catheters for measurement of pulmonary arterial and wedge pressures (Swan-Ganz), cardiac pacemaker leads, and the intra-aortic assist balloon. The subject of complications that arise in the introduction, maintenance, and use of devices for life support and monitoring in an intensive care unit has been completely reviewed by Ravin and colleagues.[286]

CHEST DRAINAGE TUBES

Complications of chest drainage tubes are uncommon[287, 288] and are usually readily apparent clinically. They include laceration of an intercostal artery or vein, malposition of the tube (such as in the chest wall, abdomen, or interlobar fissure), pulmonary perforation, infection (predominantly empyema), and formation of a systemic artery-pulmonary artery shunt. This subject (as well as indications and techniques for tube thoracostomy) has been reviewed by Miller and Sahn[289] and by Dalbec and Krome.[290]

Hemorrhage from a lacerated intercostal vessel can be avoided by insertion of the tube in the intercostal space as close as possible to the superior surface of a rib; intercostal vessels may be tortuous, especially in the elderly,[289] and insertion elsewhere can be dangerous. Malposition of the chest tube can occur within the pleural space, in which case the complication is one only of inadequate drainage. Such malposition can occur in several ways. For example, it should be appreciated that a tube inserted anterolaterally and directed posteriorly will drain the posterior pleural space but, with the patient lying in a supine position, will not drain a pneumothorax situated anteriorly. (For drainage of a pneumothorax, the tube is introduced anteriorly, usually through the second interspace.) Similarly, a drainage tube in any position will not drain a loculated accumulation of fluid or gas in an area not in communication with the tube's holes. The incidence of malposition of a chest tube within a major fissure probably is higher than generally believed, and in recent years a number of papers have addressed this problem.[291–293] It is important to realize that malposition often cannot be convincingly recognized on a single anteroposterior roentgenogram, although when drainage of a pneumothorax or hydrothorax is not occurring satisfactorily the abnormal position can be confirmed, if necessary, by lateral roentgenography. Although CT has been recommended for assessment of tubal malposition,[292] it would appear logical that this expensive procedure should be restricted to cases of loculated empyema in which proper tube positioning is imperative for adequate drainage.

Malposition of a chest tube can also occur outside the pleural space, within the chest wall or abdomen, in which case it should be readily apparent roentgenographically. This may be associated with serious complications, such as laceration of the diaphragm, liver, stomach, or colon.[287]

Pulmonary perforation is rarely recognized *in vivo* as a complication of tube insertion, at least in adults.[287, 288] However, in one necropsy study, three such cases were identified:[294] two of these were part of a series of 18 patients who had had chest tubes inserted and had subsequently died, indicating an incidence of perforation of 11 per cent. Such perforation is usually minimal in extent but occasionally can be substantial (Fig. 15–31). It is often associated with the use of a trocar to aid tube insertion; underlying pulmonary parenchymal consolidation or fibrous interpleural adhesions also probably increase the risk of perforation by decreasing or eliminating the possibility of the lung retracting when the pleural space is entered. Roentgenologic and clinical findings are absent in most cases; rarely, parenchymal hemorrhage can result in hemoptysis and the production of a linear opacity in the region of the chest tube.[294]

Infection of the pleural space related to the presence of a thoracostomy tube is uncommon; in one study of 1,249 trauma patients, it was documented in 30 patients (2.4 per cent).[287] Even rarer is the development of necrotizing fasciitis of the chest wall following tube insertion for empyema.[295]

In children particularly, insertion of a thoracostomy tube can cause a transitory pleural reaction with fibrin formation that may be confused roentgenographically with a bulla, pneumothorax, or atelectasis; the reaction occurs in direct proportion to the length of time the tube is left in place.[296] Chest tube tracks that remain following partial or complete removal of thoracostomy tubes can simulate normal structures or pathologic states; their incidence has been estimated to be approximately 15 per cent.[297] This subject recently has been reviewed by Panicek and his colleagues.[297]

A rare complication of closed tube thoracostomy is systemic-to-pulmonary artery vascular shunt;[296, 298, 299] in one reported case,[299] the fistula was fed by large, tortuous, intercostal artery collaterals originating from the lateral thoracic and thoracoacromial branches of the right axillary artery and anterior intercostal branches of the internal mammary artery. The plain chest roentgenogram showed an ill-defined opacity projected over the right third anterior interspace. Aids to the diagnosis of such a complication include the presence of a continuous murmur and roentgenographic evidence of unilateral rib notching.[300]

Other rare complications of chest tube insertion include Horner's syndrome[462] and entrapment and "infarction" of pulmonary tissue within one of the side holes or the end hole of the tube.[301]

ABDOMINAL DRAINAGE TUBES

Potentially serious complications can follow transgression of the pleural space during placement of interventional drainage catheters into the liver and upper abdomen.[302, 303] Two recent studies[302, 303] have emphasized the importance of not puncturing the ninth intercostal space in the midaxillary line, because in virtually all cadaver studies carried out needles inserted through this interspace have traversed pleura. Nichols and his colleagues[303] have advised a left subxiphoid approach in patients with abscesses, ascites, emphysema, undue anxiety, and, in the case of biliary drainage, benign or purely left-sided disease.

NASOGASTRIC TUBES

Since the majority of nasogastric tubes are opaque, any malposition should be readily apparent roentgenographically. The two most common misplacements are coiling within the esophagus and incomplete insertion; in each case, the function of the nasogastric tube clearly is not being served. A complication of far greater clinical importance is the faulty insertion of the nasogastric tube into the tracheobronchial tree rather than into the esophagus; the tip sometimes ends up in unusual locations such as the mediastinum (Fig. 15–32) or abdomen (Fig. 15–33); such malposition can be particularly hazardous if the tube is meant for hyperalimentation, because the injection of a large amount of fluid into the lungs or pleural cavity, rather than the stomach, can have disastrous consequences (Fig. 15–34). Even in the presence of an endotracheal tube with an inflated cuff, a nasogastric tube can be passed inadvertently into the tracheobronchial tree because of the low-pressure cuffs often used today.[304] Miller[305] has pointed out that a patient on a positive pressure breathing apparatus in whom a feeding tube has been inadvertently placed in the tracheobronchial tree close to the pleural surface is in danger of developing a large pneumothorax on removal of the tube. In this type of situation, the attending physician or surgeon should be warned that the feeding tube may be acting as a "finger in the dike" and that insertion of a thoracostomy tube into the pleural space may be advisable before the

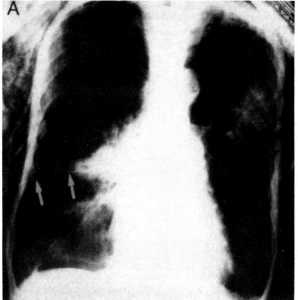

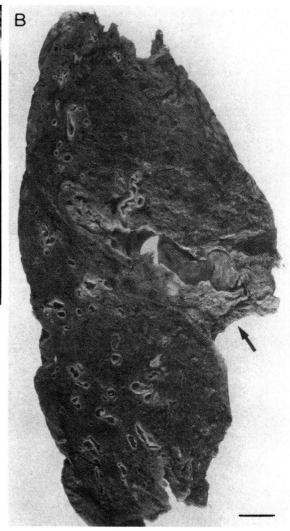

Figure 15–31. Pulmonary Perforation Secondary to Tube Thoracostomy. A chest roentgenogram *(A)* obtained the day following insertion of a thoracostomy tube (with aid of a trocar) for spontaneous pneumothorax reveals extensive subcutaneous emphysema and a triangular opacity with the base obscuring the right hilum; the position of the tube is indicated by *arrows*. The patient was a 75-year-old man who did not complain of chest pain nor did he have hemoptysis. He died 7 weeks later. A section of right lung obtained at autopsy *(B)* shows a roughly linear tract extending from the middle lobe *(arrow)* into the posterior aspect of the upper lobe. The origin of the tract in the middle lobe corresponded to the chest wall scar where the tube had been inserted (bar = 1.5 cm). (From Fraser RS: Human Pathol *19:*512, 1988.)

feeding tube is withdrawn. Inadvertent placement of feeding tubes into the tracheobronchial tree, with subsequent insertion into the pleural space, appears to be a particular complication of the use of the narrow-bore nasogastric tube with stylet,[306–308] and is most apt to occur in patients with impaired mental status or diminished gag, cough, or swallowing reflexes.[308]

Enteral nutrition in patients receiving mechanical ventilation can sometimes result in bacterial colonization of the stomach; in such cases, the gastric flora can colonize the trachea and cause nosocomial respiratory infection.[309]

ENDOTRACHEAL TUBES

During the first few days after insertion of an endotracheal tube, serious complications are infrequent and occur more often in association with emergency resuscitation than with more routine respiratory therapy.[310] The incidence in one large series of patients on inhalation therapy was 10 per cent.[311] The chief complication is large airway obstruction resulting from malpositioning of the tube too low in the trachea and major bronchi. In the vast majority of instances, the endotracheal tube enters the right main bronchus (in 27 of 28 cases in one series[310]), and the orifice of the left main bronchus is occluded by the balloon cuff of the endotracheal tube, resulting in complete obstruction and atelectasis of the left lung (*see* Fig. 11–3, page 1977). If the tube is advanced sufficiently down into the right main bronchus, the right upper lobe bronchus may be occluded, with resultant atelectasis of this lobe as well as the left lung (*see* Fig. 11–4, page 1978) or of the right middle lobe alone. The latter complication occurred in one patient in the Twigg and Buckley series of 28 patients.[310] Occasionally the tube enters the left rather than the right main-stem bronchus, leading to obstruction of the latter.

The rate at which atelectasis occurs depends on the gas content of the lung at the moment of occlusion. Total collapse requires 18 to 24 hours if the parenchyma is air-containing, but it may occur

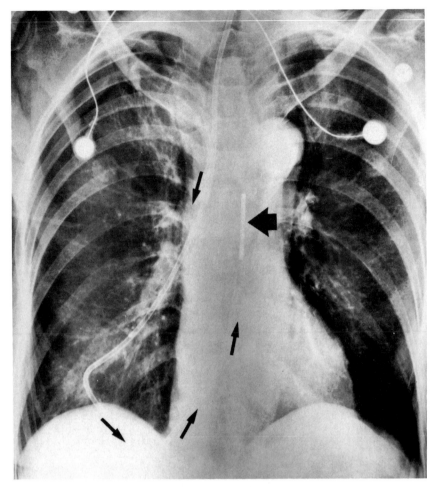

Figure 15–32. Faulty Insertion of a Dobbhoff Feeding Tube. The circuitous course taken by this Dobbhoff feeding tube can be established only partly from this anteroposterior roentgenogram. Obviously the catheter passed into the right lower lobe and then as it turned to the left it presumably penetrated the visceral pleura covering this lobe. It then passed superiorly either within the mediastinum or in the pleural space adjacent to the azygoesophageal recess to a point where its tip overlies the region of the tracheal carina *(large arrow)*. In contrast to the devastating effects of the faulty insertion illustrated in Figure 15–33, this patient suffered no ill effects following removal of the tube.

in a matter of minutes if the lung contains 100 per cent oxygen (often the case in acute respiratory emergencies). Withdrawal of the tube typically results in rapid re-expansion of the collapsed lung or lobe.

According to Twigg and Buckley,[310] the ideal location of the tip of an endotracheal tube is 3 cm distal to the vocal cords. However, since in our experience the vocal cords are infrequently visualized on bedside roentgenograms, the carina seems a much more logical point from which to establish reference. Conrardy and associates[312] recommended that with the head and neck in a neutral position, the ideal distance between the tip of the endotracheal tube and the carina is 5 ± 2 cm. These authors also showed that flexion and extension of the neck cause a 2 cm descent and ascent, respectively, of the tip of the endotracheal tube; if the position of the neck can be established from the roentgenogram (through visualization of the mandible), the ideal distance between the tip of the endotracheal tube and the carina should be 3 ± 2 cm with the neck flexed and 7 ± 2 cm with the neck extended. As pointed out by Goodman and his colleagues[313] if the carina is not visualized, it is sufficient to establish the relationship of the tip of the endotracheal tube to the fifth, sixth, or seventh thoracic vertebral bodies, this relationship pertaining in 92 of 100 patients whose bedside chest roentgenograms were studied. In infants, Todres and his associates[314] have emphasized the importance of correlating the position of the tip of the endotracheal tube with the position of the patient's head. In a study of 16 intubated newborn infants in whom chest roentgenograms were obtained with the head fully flexed and fully extended, movement of the tip of the endotracheal tube ranged from 7 to 28 mm, being closest to the carina in full flexion.

The roentgenographic findings are typical and should present no difficulty in interpretation. Clinically, the examining physician should not be misled by hearing breath sounds transmitted from the normal or overinflated contralateral lung through the collapsed lung.

Malpositioning of an endotracheal tube in the esophagus is very uncommon and is usually evident clinically. Because the trachea and esophagus are superimposed on an anteroposterior roentgenogram, such malpositioning is usually not apparent; however, Smith and colleagues[480] have recently shown that the faulty position can be accurately identified in a 25 degree right posterior oblique projection.

Complications, such as tracheal stenosis, that

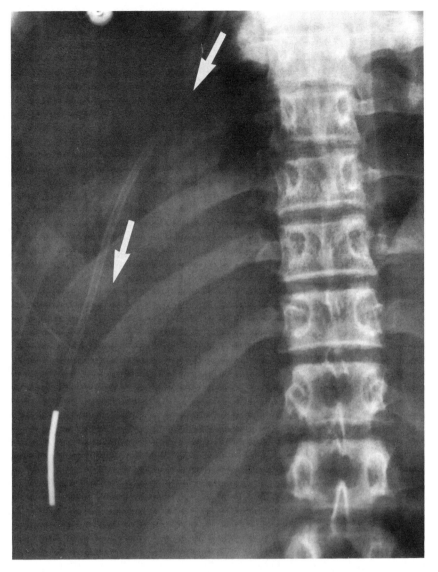

Figure 15–33. Faulty Insertion of a Dobbhoff Feeding Tube. A view of the lower portion of the right hemithorax and upper abdomen in anteroposterior projection reveals a feeding tube that has passed via the bronchi of the right lower lobe to a point projected over the lower portion of the liver and the posterolateral portion of the right tenth rib (*arrows* indicate the course of the tube). Judging from this single projection, it is almost certain that the visceral pleura has been penetrated but whether or not the tip has penetrated the diaphragm was not established. Following removal of the tube, the patient developed a right pneumothorax that required thoracostomy tube insertion; she subsequently developed a right-sided empyema that required thoracotomy for drainage.

result from prolonged inflation of the cuff of an endotracheal tube are discussed in Chapter 11 in relation to large airway obstruction (*see* page 1987).

TRANSTRACHEAL CATHETERS

The use of chronic indwelling transtracheal catheters to administer oxygen to patients with COPD has been described in several reports.[315–317] Complications of their use include subcutaneous emphysema, localized skin infection or hemorrhage, abnormal tracheal mucous production, breakage of catheter parts into the trachea, and the formation of partly occlusive mucous or mucopurulent plugs around the catheter tip.[315, 316] Fletcher and colleagues[316] described an example of the last-named complication in which a plug was adherent to the catheter and measured 2.5 × 1.8 cm; they noted that dislodgement of such a plug could result in bronchial obstruction and that further growth could seriously compromise tracheal air flow.

MONITORING APPARATUS

Percutaneous Central Venous Catheters

The increasing use of prepackaged polyethylene catheters to monitor central venous pressure and to provide a route for hyperalimentation has revealed a number of complications with which the respiratory physician and the radiologist should be thoroughly familiar. Some complications, either early or late, pertain to the catheterization procedure itself and relate to abnormalities within or around the catheterized vein. Other complications, perhaps the majority, arise from incorrect positioning of the tip of the catheter.

Several extensive reviews of the literature on complications of central venous catheterization have been published,[318–326] and the reader cannot avoid being impressed by the great variety and the serious consequences of potential complications. Central venous catheters can be inserted via an arm vein, a subclavian vein (by either an infraclavicular or supraclavicular route), or an external or internal jug-

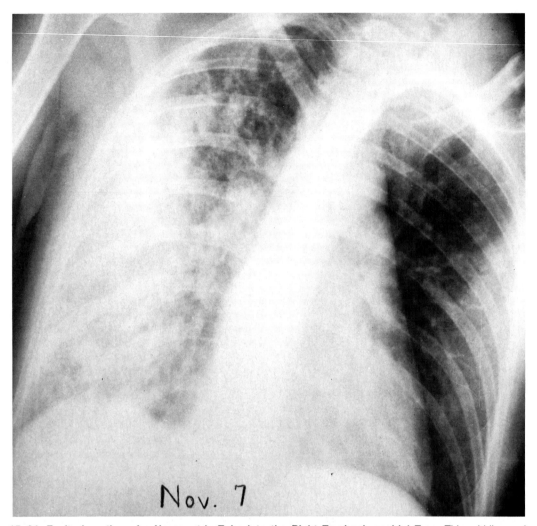

Figure 15–34. Faulty Insertion of a Nasogastric Tube into the Right Tracheobronchial Tree. This middle-aged woman was brought to the emergency department in a coma following a drug overdose. A nasogastric tube was introduced in order to lavage the stomach and 1,000 ml of saline injected. An anteroposterior roentgenogram shortly thereafter reveals massive airspace consolidation throughout the right lung; the left lung is clear. The saline had been injected into the right lung through a malpositioned tube. Complete roentgenographic clearing had occurred 3 days later.

ular vein. The majority of faulty placements occur in arm and infraclavicular subclavian approaches. From arm vein insertion, only 66 to 74 per cent of catheters reach their proper location, and the results via external jugular placement are even less satisfactory;[327] supraclavicular subclavian, or internal jugular approaches result in a relatively small percentage of improper placements. In a review of the complications of central venous catheterization, Langston[328] found that only 186 (62 per cent) of 300 central venous lines were positioned in the subclavian or innominate veins or superior vena cava at the time of the initial chest roentgenogram obtained immediately after catheterization. Of the remainder, 48 (16 per cent) were in the internal jugular vein (Fig. 15–35), 39 (13 per cent) in the right atrium or right ventricle, two in the azygos vein, one in a left-sided superior vena cava that drained into the coronary sinus, and two were coiled in the subclavian vein; 22 were in extrathoracic sites other than the internal jugular vein. In none of

these cases was the incorrect position recognized clinically. The problem with faulty placement is that pressure recorded in the jugular vein is not equivalent to central venous pressure. However, since it is often within the normal range and may show only slightly diminished dynamics, it is unlikely that the malposition of the catheter can be recognized through pressure measurements alone.

There are four major complications of central venous catheterization:

Phlebothrombosis. Although this is probably the most common complication of venous catheterization, its incidence is difficult to establish.[329] The thrombus is typically sterile and causes no symptoms; it is attributable to reaction to the foreign material of the catheter and trauma to the vessel wall rather than to the type of fluid administered. Of 240 patients studied by Walters and associates,[329] only 4 patients had symptomatic subclavian vein thrombosis. Phlebograms performed on 20 consecutive patients, however, showed four instances of

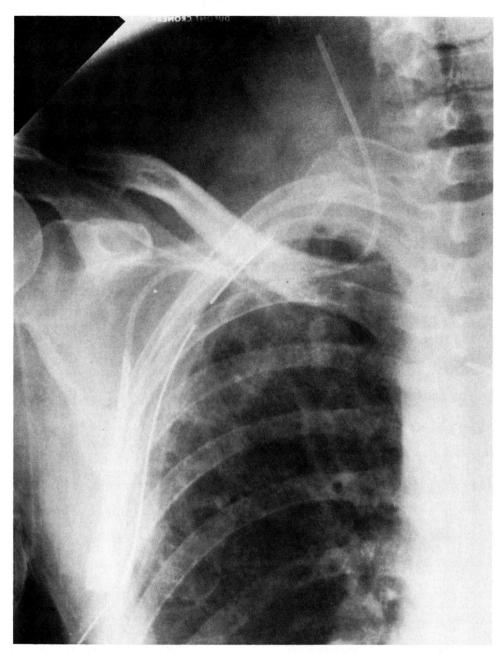

Figure 15–35. Malpositioning of a Subclavian Catheter in the Jugular Vein. The catheter occupies a correct position in the subclavian vein but then ascends the jugular vein. Such a position probably will not record true central venous pressure.

axillary vein thrombosis from which the patients suffered no symptoms. Catheters left in place for long periods of time are more likely to cause thrombosis of large veins.

Perforation of a Vein. A vein can be perforated either at the time of insertion[330–335] or some time later;[324, 336–345, 474] late perforation is caused by gradual erosion of a relatively thin-walled intrathoracic vessel by the catheter, partly as a result of cardiac and respiratory movements affecting the catheter tip.[346] Depending on the vein involved, perforation can result in pneumothorax, hemothorax, hydrothorax, mediastinal hemorrhage (Fig. 15–36), bronchopulmonary-venous fistula, or extrapleural hematoma (Fig. 15–37).[321–324, 333, 335–342, 347–349] Unilat-

eral pneumothorax is undoubtedly the most common of these. A particularly serious consequence is bilateral pneumothorax,[330] a complication that arises when an unsuspected perforation with consequent pneumothorax occurs in an unsuccessful attempt on one side followed by induction of a pneumothorax with a catheter insertion on the contralateral side. Rarely, pleural effusion also can be bilateral and massive.[330, 334, 344, 345, 350, 351] The great majority of vein perforations occur following introduction of catheters for pressure measurements and hyperalimentation; they occur less often with electrode insertion for cardiac pacing[352] and with catheter placement for providing vascular access for plasmapheresis and hemodialysis.[353] It is obvious that

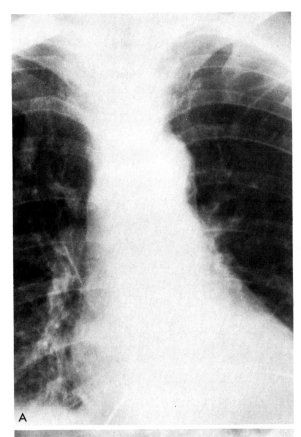

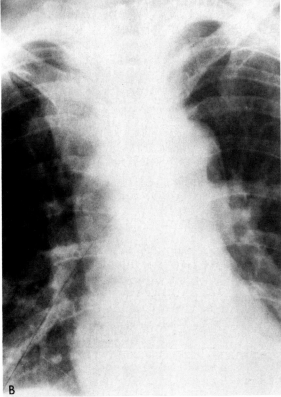

Figure 15–36. Mediastinal Hemorrhage Following Faulty Insertion of a Subclavian Catheter. The roentgenogram illustrated in (A) reveals a normal appearance of the upper mediastinum. Three days later (B), following attempted insertion of a right subclavian line, there has occurred moderate widening of the superior mediastinum as a result of venous hemorrhage secondary to perforation of a vein by the catheter.

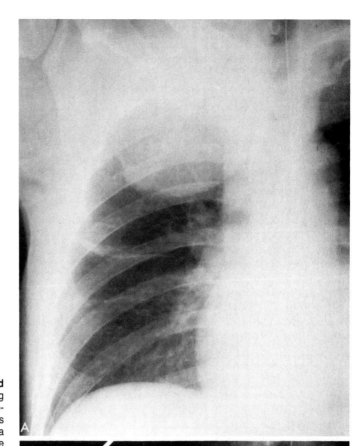

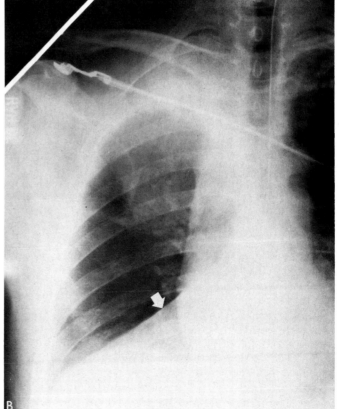

Figure 15–37. Apical Hematoma Following Attempted Insertion of a Subclavian Catheter. Several hours following attempted insertion of a right subclavian catheter, an antero-posterior roentgenogram *(A)* reveals a large homogeneous mass occupying the upper third of the right hemithorax (a previous roentgenogram was normal). One week later *(B)*, the opacity was slightly larger and less well defined. Coincidentally, there had developed complete airlessness of the right lower lobe caused by atelectasis, presumably from an obstructing mucous plug (*arrow* points to downward displaced major fissure).

when venous perforation occurs into the pleura, lung, or mediastinum, patients receiving hyperalimentation are at greater risk for serious complications (Fig. 15–38).[326, 354] "Pneumonia" has been reported following the development of a venopulmonary fistula,[355] and lung abscess has occurred after passage of a catheter through the heart and pulmonary artery.[356] Air embolism also has been reported as a complication of subclavian vein catheterization;[347, 357, 358] it can occur on either insertion or withdrawal of the catheter.

Perforation of the Myocardium. Of the 300 patients studied by Langston,[328] the tip of the central venous catheter was in the right atrium or right ventricle in 40 patients (13 per cent). This is obviously an extremely hazardous position for any patient, particularly if the catheter has a firm or sharp tip; perforation of the right atrium or ventricle may result in fatal pericardial tamponade (from either blood or infused fluid).[359] Also, such a catheter position may readily cause arrhythmias. This is well recognized by physicians who regularly perform cardiac catheterization in the laboratory.

Catheter Coiling, Knotting, and Breaking (Figs. 15–39 and 15–40). Coiled catheters traumatize the vein and are much more likely to perforate, break, and embolize. They also show a much greater tendency to twist into knots; although the knots sometimes can be manipulated free, this is not always possible, and thoracotomy is occasionally required for removal.[360]

Miscellaneous complications of central venous catheterization include sepsis,[321, 323] pulmonary embolization of fragments of catheters,[321–323] thoracic duct laceration,[321] and damage to the brachial plexus, sympathetic chain, or the phrenic, recurrent laryngeal, or 9th to 12th cranial nerves.[321, 323, 324, 475]

Indwelling Balloon-Tipped Pulmonary Arterial Catheters

Flow-directed balloon-tipped (Swan-Ganz) catheters for monitoring circulatory hemodynamics in critically ill patients have been used with increasing frequency since their first description in 1970.[361] Complications of these catheters have been reviewed[362–365] and include atrial and ventricular dysrhythmias, rupture of the balloon, knotting of the catheter, perforation of the pulmonary artery, perforation of the visceral pleura (with resultant pneumothorax or hemothorax)[365, 375, 379] false aneurysms of the pulmonary artery,[366, 367] tears of the pulmonary valve,[114] and pulmonary artery occlusion and infarction. The catheters also can act as a nidus for bacterial colonization[380] and platelet consumption,[381] with the potential of causing sepsis or contributing to hemorrhage. Such events are not rare; in one prospective study of 528 catheterizations, serious complications were considered to have occurred in 23 (4.4 per cent).[463]

Pulmonary artery occlusion, with or without infarction, is probably the most common pulmonary complication. In their series of 125 patients undergoing catheterization, Foote and his colleagues[363] identified some sort of ischemic lesion in 9 patients (7.2 per cent). Another review of 391 patients documented evidence of thromboembolism in 16 patients (4 per cent).[368] Pulmonary artery occlusion can result from one or more of four mechanisms: (1) irritation of the endothelium of the vena cava, right-sided heart chambers, or a major pulmonary artery by the catheter tip or inflated balloon that results in thrombus formation and subsequent embolization; (2) formation of thrombus around the distal end of the catheter itself that leads to subsequent embolization; (3) prolonged inflation of the balloon for recording of wedge pressure that results in peripheral ischemia and infarction; and (4) tightening of a large intracardiac loop of the catheter by hemodynamic action that can propel the tip of the catheter to a point where it occludes a small peripheral artery with resultant infarction (Fig. 15–41). As pointed out by Chun and Ellestad,[369] the last mechanism can be avoided if the technique described by Swan and associates is strictly adhered to—the balloon is inflated as soon as a large-caliber vein is encountered and the catheter is permitted to float into the pulmonary artery. The incidence of pulmonary artery occlusion rises sharply as the length of time the catheter is left *in situ* increases. In one series,[364] all 5 patients in whom the Swan-Ganz catheter was maintained in position for over 72 hours developed infarcts. Shin and Ho[370] have reported two cases in which septic infarction occurred distal to the tip of a Swan-Ganz catheter, with resultant abscess formation and the development of large cavities following expulsion of liquefied material into the tracheobronchial tree.

It has been estimated that the pulmonary artery is perforated in 0.1 to 0.2 per cent of all cases of catheter insertion,[371] although it may occur more often than those figures would indicate. For example, in one necropsy review, 4 such cases were identified in a consecutive series of 270 cases (1.5 per cent) but in only 1 case was the perforation suspected clinically.[371] The most common clinical situation associated with perforation is cardiac surgery, an observation attributed by Stone and colleagues,[372] to one or more of three factors: (1) shrinkage of heart chambers as a result of evacuation of blood with distal migration of the catheter; (2) cooling of the perfusate and cardiovascular tissue that leads to increased rigidity of the tubing and vessel walls; and (3) manipulation of the heart that causes increased movement of the catheter.

As might be expected, the usual result of pulmonary artery perforation is hemorrhage, generally into pulmonary parenchyma but on occasion predominantly into the bronchovascular interstitium[373] or pleural space. Only a few cases have been examined pathologically;[371] in many cases, the site of

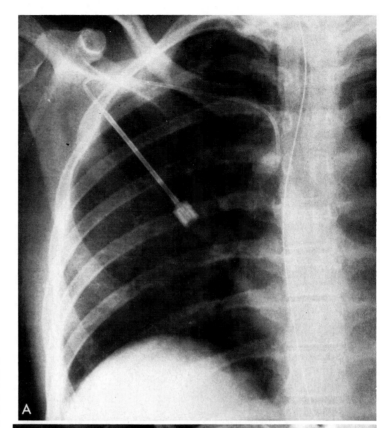

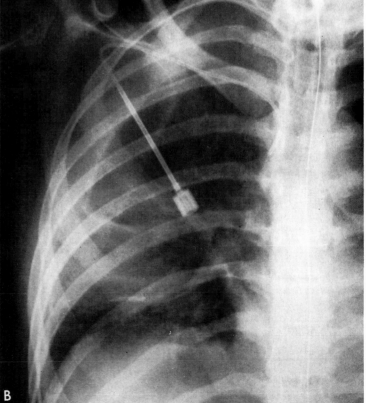

Figure 15–38. Faulty Position of Subclavian Catheter in the Pleural Space. Immediately following insertion of a right subclavian catheter, an anteroposterior roentgenogram *(A)* reveals the tip to lie in a position consistent with the superior vena cava, although it could be argued that it is more medial than usual. Following injection of several hundred ml of fluid for hyperalimentation, a second roentgenogram exposed in the supine position *(B)* reveals a large accumulation of fluid in the right pleural space, indicating that the tip of the catheter had perforated the vein and mediastinal parietal pleura.

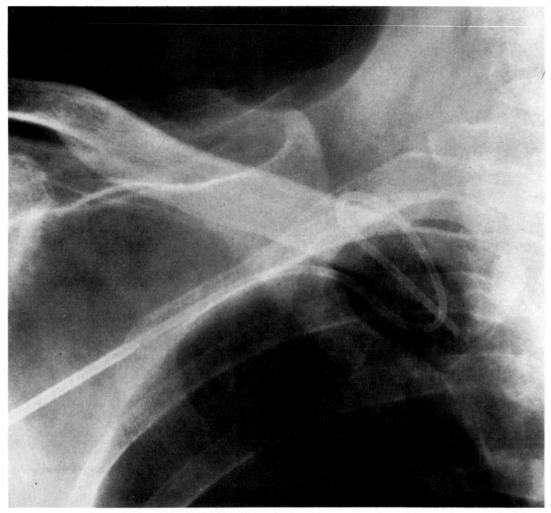

Figure 15–39. Malpositioning (Coiling) of a Subclavian Catheter. An anteroposterior roentgenogram of the apical portion of the right hemithorax reveals a subclavian catheter that has coiled through a 360-degree arc. It is almost certain that the tip of this catheter does not lie within the subclavian vein.

rupture has been undetected, whereas in others a localized intraparenchymal hematoma or nodule of intraparenchymal thrombus reveals the location (Fig. 15–42). Perforation should be suspected roentgenologically when an airspace opacity develops near the tip of the catheter. The diagnosis is virtually confirmed if there is associated hemoptysis, the main clinical manifestation,[374–376] which can be massive.[377, 378]

The prime purpose of the Swan-Ganz catheter is the determination of pressure within the pulmonary artery and within the left atrium as measured through the wedged catheter. It has been shown in both the experimental animal[382] and in humans at the time of open heart surgery[383] that when the tip of the catheter is positioned at or above the level of the left atrium, the wedge pressure measured by the catheter is not an accurate estimate of left atrial pressure when positive end-expiratory pressure (PEEP) is being administered; in such positions, the catheter consistently recorded pressures higher than left atrial pressure. In all other situations

where catheters were located below the left atrium, they were accurate at every level of PEEP tested. The admonition is obvious: when PEEP is being used, the position of a Swan-Ganz catheter should be confirmed by a lateral chest roentgenogram; when the catheter is situated above the level of the left atrium, it should be repositioned.

INTRA-AORTIC COUNTERPULSATION BALLOON

This catheter has been gaining in popularity for use in conditions characterized by low output cardiac decompensation and cardiogenic shock. The device provides augmentation of diastolic coronary artery perfusion as well as reduced impedance to ventricular ejection.[384, 385] Reported complications resulting from its use include[286, 385] damage to the aorta including dissection, laceration of the wall, and subadventitial hematoma formation; red blood cell destruction; embolic phenomena; vascular in-

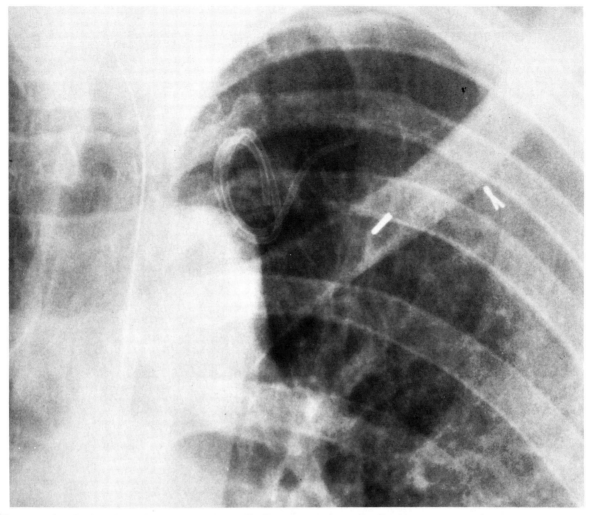

Figure 15–40. Broken Central Venous Pressure (CVP) Line. A tightly coiled CVP catheter can be identified overlying the upper portion of the left lung. The catheter had broken at its point of entry and had retracted inward to constitute a foreign body in the soft tissues of the anterior chest wall.

sufficiency of the catheterized limb; and balloon rupture with secondary gas embolism. As emphasized by Ravin and his colleagues,[286] however, the most common complication observed by radiologists is improper positioning. The ideal position of the tip is just distal to the origin of the left subclavian artery. A more proximal position can occlude the left subclavian artery, and one more distal can result in decreased effectiveness of diastolic counterpulsation.

CARDIAC PACEMAKER LEADS

The structure of all pacemaker leads is very similar—the lead itself that contains a conducting medium and insulation, a terminal pin that allows attachment to the pulse generator, and a distal electrode. One of the problems with pacemaker leads in the past has been that of dislodgement. Earlier leads relied for positioning on the force transmitted along the lead to the interface between the electrode and myocardium; as a result, these leads were placed as close as possible to the apex of the right ventricle. The radiographic aspects of positioning of cardiac pacemaker leads has been recently reviewed by Filice and coworkers.[386]

More recent leads incorporate mechanical fixation devices to maintain position, commonly either tined or screw-in electrodes that represent passive and active fixation mechanisms respectively. These serve to maintain electrode position without relying on lead forces, thus permitting the use of smaller, more flexible leads. The tines are made of radiolucent plastic and are therefore not visible radiographically; the screw-in devices are metallic and easily seen. Atrial leads commonly possess a "J" configuration that facilitates their placement in the atrial appendage where trabeculation is profuse. Tined ventricular leads are commonly positioned at or near the apex of the right ventricle where they cause minimal complications.

The impact that radiology can make in determining the cause of pacemaker malfunction and in the evaluation of lead position and integrity can be considerable; it has been the subject of a recent

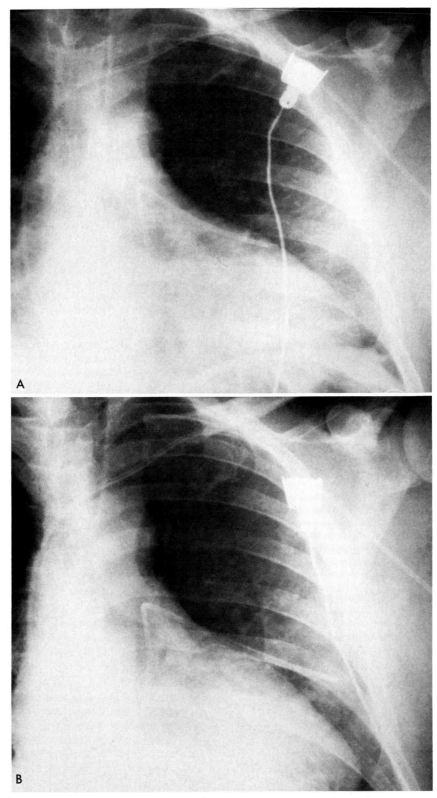

Figure 15–41. Pulmonary Infarction Associated with a Swan-Ganz Catheter. In the anteroposterior roentgenogram illustrated in *(A)*, a Swan-Ganz catheter is in position in the left lower lobe, its tip in a position consistent with a subsegmental artery. Twenty-four hours later *(B)*, the intrapulmonary extent of the catheter had increased considerably, such that its tip now lies less than 2 cm from the visceral pleural surface.

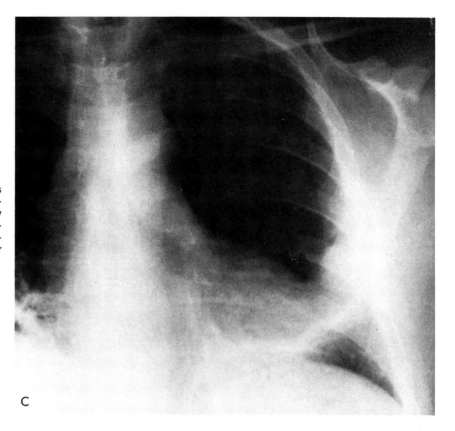

Figure 15–41 *Continued* Several days later *(C),* a wedge-shaped opacity had appeared in the left axillary lung zone highly suggestive of a pulmonary infarct; its position corresponds precisely to what was undoubtedly an impacted Swan-Ganz catheter tip.

C

review by Steiner and his colleagues.[387] Goodman and his colleagues[388] have recently described the complications to be anticipated from automatic implantable cardioverter defibrillators.

COMPLICATIONS OF DIAGNOSTIC BIOPSY PROCEDURES

Pleuropulmonary complications of diagnostic biopsy procedures, such as transbronchial biopsy, transthoracic needle aspiration, and closed chest pleural biopsy, are well-known. Because these procedures necessarily cause tissue disruption in order to obtain material for diagnosis, infiltration of air or blood into the pleural cavity, mediastinum, lung parenchyma, or bronchovascular interstitium is, to some extent, an inevitable consequence. In most instances, the extent of this infiltration is limited so that related clinical problems are minimal or nonexistent. Details of the incidence and type of complications with the different procedures are discussed at length in Chapters 2 and 3.

RADIATION INJURY OF THE LUNG

It seems reasonably safe to assume that within the therapeutic range of doses usually administered, the pulmonary parenchyma reacts to ionizing radiation in virtually 100 per cent of patients. However,

there are many variables that affect this reaction and its clinical and roentgenographic manifestations. For example, the volume of lung tissue irradiated, the radiation dose administered, the time over which it is given, and the quality of the radiation all determine in variable degrees the severity of tissue reaction.[389, 390] In addition, the lung can be affected in the absence of a demonstrable abnormality on conventional roentgenograms;[391] in these circumstances, CT[392] and pulmonary function testing may be more sensitive procedures to determine the extent of damage. Finally, it should be noted that there is some semantic confusion in the literature, the term "radiation pneumonitis" being used by some to denote a roentgenographic abnormality and by others to describe a clinical syndrome. For all these reasons, the incidence of pulmonary effects of radiation therapy varies considerably from series to series. The lungs are usually damaged by radiation aimed directly at the lungs, although they also can be injured when the beam is directed elsewhere in the thorax, such as at the mediastinum or chest wall. In only a relatively small number of patients, however—possibly no more than 5 to 15 per cent—does the latter therapy result in respiratory symptoms.[389]

In addition to the effects of roentgen therapy, radiation injury to the lungs may also follow inhalation of beta-emitting radionuclides.[407, 408] With increased use of these materials, nuclear accidents probably will become more frequent. Several such incidents have already been reported in humans.[389]

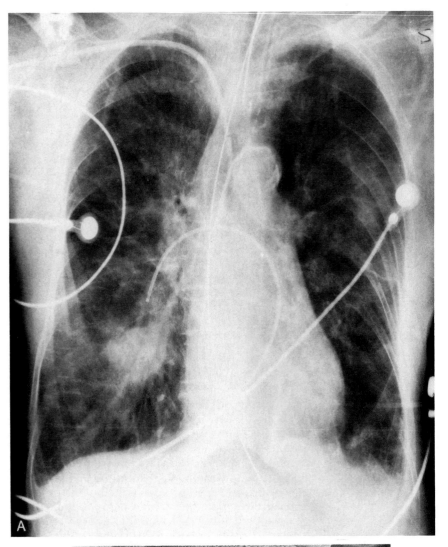

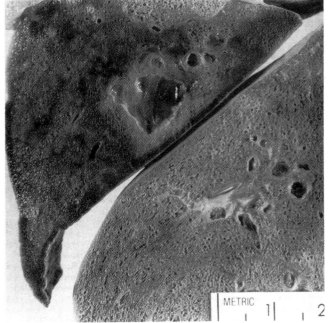

Figure 15–42. Pulmonary Artery Perforation by Swan-Ganz Catheter. A posteroanterior roentgenogram *(A)* shows the tip of a Swan-Ganz catheter in the region of the right interlobar artery. Distal to it is a fairly well-defined opacity that could be situated in either the middle or lower lobe. Shortly thereafter, this 83-year-old woman coughed up a small amount of blood and died. At autopsy, the right middle lobe *(B)* showed extensive airspace hemorrhage and a defect in a subsegmental pulmonary artery associated with an irregularly shaped intraparenchymal hematoma. (From Fraser RS: Human Pathol *18:*1246, 1987.)

In the future, in fact, inhalation likely will be the most common route by which a radionuclide enters the body. Radiation pneumonitis has been induced in beagle dogs from inhaled aerosols composed of particles of clay fused with various radionuclides,[407] a reaction that has been alleviated by bronchopulmonary lavage and intravenous chelation therapy.[409]

FACTORS THAT AFFECT THE REACTION

Volume of Lung Irradiated

This variable is considered by some investigators to be perhaps the most important factor leading to lung damage.[393, 394] For example, it has been estimated that a 30-gray total dose delivered in fractions to 25 per cent of total lung volume may not produce any symptoms, whereas an identical dose delivered in the same manner to the entire volume of both lungs would probably prove fatal.[393]

Effect of Dosage

In lungs that are normal before the administration of ionizing radiation, its effects (as measured by symptoms and signs, roentgenologic changes, and physiologic tests) probably will be proportionate to the amount of radiation delivered.[391] Radiation pneumonitis seldom occurs with a dose of less than 20 gray,[395–397] although exceptions do occur.[397, 398] Doses in excess of 60 gray given over a period of 5 to 6 weeks almost invariably lead to severe radiation pneumonitis. Despite the fact that the average dose to patients in whom roentgenographically demonstrable changes develop in the lungs is significantly higher than the average dose to those whose lungs remain normal, there are not statistically significant differences among the doses that result in minimal, moderate, or severe pulmonary changes.[397]

Time-Dose Factor

The radiation effect on the lung is related less to the total dose than to the rate at which it is delivered, since fractionation permits repair of sublethal damage between fractions.[389, 399] This biologic effect of relative equivalent therapy takes into account the total dose absorbed, the number of fractions, and the time elapsed between first and last treatments.[400, 401]

Other Factors

Other variables that influence pulmonary damage include retreatment, associated chemotherapy,[405] and corticosteroid withdrawal;[389, 390, 402–404] each of these factors apparently increases susceptibility. There is little evidence to support the clinical impression that patients with COPD are more likely to develop radiation pneumonitis than those without bronchopulmonary abnormality.[406]

PATHOGENESIS

The pathogenesis of radiation-induced pulmonary disease is complex and not completely understood.[410] It is believed that x-rays or gamma rays exert their effects by colliding with and exciting electrons which, in turn, generate ion pairs and a variety of free radicals. The latter are highly reactive and cause breakage of covalent bonds in both small and large molecules; such damage can be repaired in some instances but may be irreversible, particularly in the presence of oxygen. The resulting molecular changes can then lead to significant biochemical, structural, and functional abnormalities. These abnormalities can be considered as being caused by two classes of molecules: (1) those such as DNA that are concerned with genetic effects; and (2) a variety of nongenetic macromolecules contained in the cell cytoplasm, organelles, and membranes. Damage to the latter group can result in several immediate effects, such as leaky cell membranes or impaired transport of intracellular material; if sufficiently severe, these can lead directly to cell death. Such injury may be the mechanism of capillary endothelial and type I epithelial cell damage in early radiation pneumonitis.[410] Damage to both types of cell at this stage also may be related directly to an increase in capillary permeability and the accumulation of intra-alveolar fluid.[410]

Less obvious in its effect, at least in the early stages of radiation pneumonitis, is injury to DNA molecules. This may take several forms, including breaks that are incorrectly repaired, abnormal crosslinks, and chromosomal rearrangements. Cells containing such DNA can remain viable and apparently unharmed until they divide, at which time the progeny may die or at least show functional disturbances. This effect is most evident in cells with a rapid turnover rate and least obvious in highly differentiated cells. In the lungs, the cells most sensitive to radiation-induced chromosomal abnormalities are capillary endothelial, bronchial epithelial, and alveolar type II cells. The cytologic atypia of type II pneumocytes in radiation pneumonitis presumably reflects this genetic damage.

The precise pathogenesis of the pulmonary fibrosis that occurs in long-standing irradiated lung is unclear. Although it may be caused by a direct effect of radiation on parenchymal interstitial cells, there is experimental evidence that primary endothelial damage resulting in alteration of the normal endothelial-fibroblast interaction may be responsible.[411]

In one review,[412] it was suggested that the involvement of lung tissue outside the radiation field might indicate a delayed hypersensitivity immune reaction in response to antigen resulting from intensive irradiation. Roswit and White[412] suggest that the extraordinary latent period for the reaction, the histologic pattern, the involvement of unirradiated lung, and the beneficial response to corticosteroid therapy seem to support this hypothesis. It is also supported by the lymphocytosis that can be observed in BAL fluid and the increased gallium uptake that occurs in the contralateral lung when irradiation is confined to one hemithorax.[413]

In contrast to the evidence that irradiation of the mediastinum of dogs does not result in obstruction of lymphatic channels,[414] blockage of mediastinal lymphatics as a result of irradiation of enlarged lymph nodes in humans is believed by some investigators to result in severe bilateral pulmonary disease.[398, 415]

PATHOLOGIC CHARACTERISTICS

Our knowledge of the pathologic features of the early stages of radiation pneumonitis derives primarily from animal experiments. Although such knowledge is useful, it must be remembered that there are significant interspecies differences in the morphology of the reaction.[416, 417] In addition, some studies have employed very large doses (up to 70 gray[418]) or have exposed a whole lung rather than part of a lung to the irradiation; thus, extrapolation of experimental findings to the human condition must be made with caution.

One of the earliest and most consistent abnormalities in experimental animals is endothelial damage that is manifested initially as swelling and vacuolization of the cytoplasm, followed by necrosis and detachment from the basement membrane.[419, 420] Platelet thrombi develop and are organized by a process of either recanalization or fibrosis; this in turn can cause significant vascular narrowing and obstruction, decreased lung perfusion,[421] and pulmonary arterial hypertension.[422] Soon after irradiation, type I cells become necrotic,[419] although there is evidence that this occurs later than the damage to capillary endothelial cells.[416]

In humans, two stages of radiation damage can be recognized, an early or acute reaction (radiation pneumonitis) and a late or fibrotic stage. Many reports of pathologic changes in the early stage have been derived from autopsies of patients who died 4 to 12 weeks after completion of radiation therapy, at a time when secondary changes from superimposed infection or heart failure may have obscured or been difficult to separate from the effects of radiation. However, enough information is available from apparently uncomplicated cases and from lung biopsies to allow a reasonable description.[395, 416, 423] Typically, the reaction is characterized by a pattern of diffuse alveolar damage (Fig. 15–43) consisting of an exudate of proteinaceous material in the alveolar airspaces associated with hyaline membranes, especially in alveolar ducts and distal respiratory bronchioles. The parenchymal interstitium is thickened by congested capillaries, edema, and, with time, fibroblasts and loose connective tissue; an inflammatory cellular infiltrate is usually minimal in extent. Type II cells are hyperplastic and often have very large nuclei, sometimes bizarre in shape (Fig. 15–43). Although this latter feature can be seen in diseases of other etiology, providing the changes are sufficiently extensive and the effect of cytotoxic drugs can be excluded, it is highly suggestive of radiation damage. Evidence of epithelial injury also can be present in membranous bronchioles and bronchi, typically in the form of a loss of the normal respiratory epithelium and its replacement by a cuboidal or flattened epithelium; these epithelial cells can also show prominent nuclear atypia (Fig. 15–43).

The late or fibrotic stage of irradiation damage is characterized by parenchymal fibrosis that may be so severe that underlying architecture is difficult to identify; proliferation and fragmentation of elastic fibers are common. Although somewhat distorted by the adjacent fibrosis, airways can appear remarkably unaffected. However, bronchiolitis obliterans and (occasionally) bronchial fibrosis may be present. Arterioles and arteries often show myointimal proliferation; focal medial hyalinization and intimal foam cells also may be seen.

ROENTGENOGRAPHIC MANIFESTATIONS

Pulmonary disease is rarely, if ever, manifested either symptomatically or roentgenographically while the patient is receiving radiation therapy.[424] In fact, changes are seldom apparent roentgenographically until at least 1 month after cessation of treatment,[425] and in many cases they take as long as 4 to 6 months to appear.[424, 426] In a small series of patients followed up to 40 months after completion of irradiation, Teates and Cooper[427] found no roentgenographic evidence of changes developing later than 6 months after the cessation of therapy. By contrast, Fleming and coworkers[396] observed new changes developing up to 2 years afterward.

Acute radiation pneumonitis is manifested roentgenographically by consolidation of lung parenchyma, usually associated with considerable loss of volume (Fig. 15–44). Depending on the severity of the reaction and therefore on the dose delivered, the resultant opacity may be patchy or confluent. The volume of lung affected usually, but not always, corresponds to the area irradiated, and thus there is no tendency to segmental or lobar distribution (Fig. 15–45). The margins of affected lung, in fact, usually bear a close relationship to the position of the radiation ports.[428] Loss of volume may be severe, caused either by extensive bronchiolar plugging or more likely by a loss of surfactant (adhesive atelectasis); despite this, the major and segmental bronchi are more or less unaffected and an air bronchogram is almost invariably present (Fig. 15–46).[397, 398, 425, 426] In a prospective CT study of patients receiving radiation therapy,[429] the relatively homogeneous, nonsegmental nature of the pulmonary opacity was

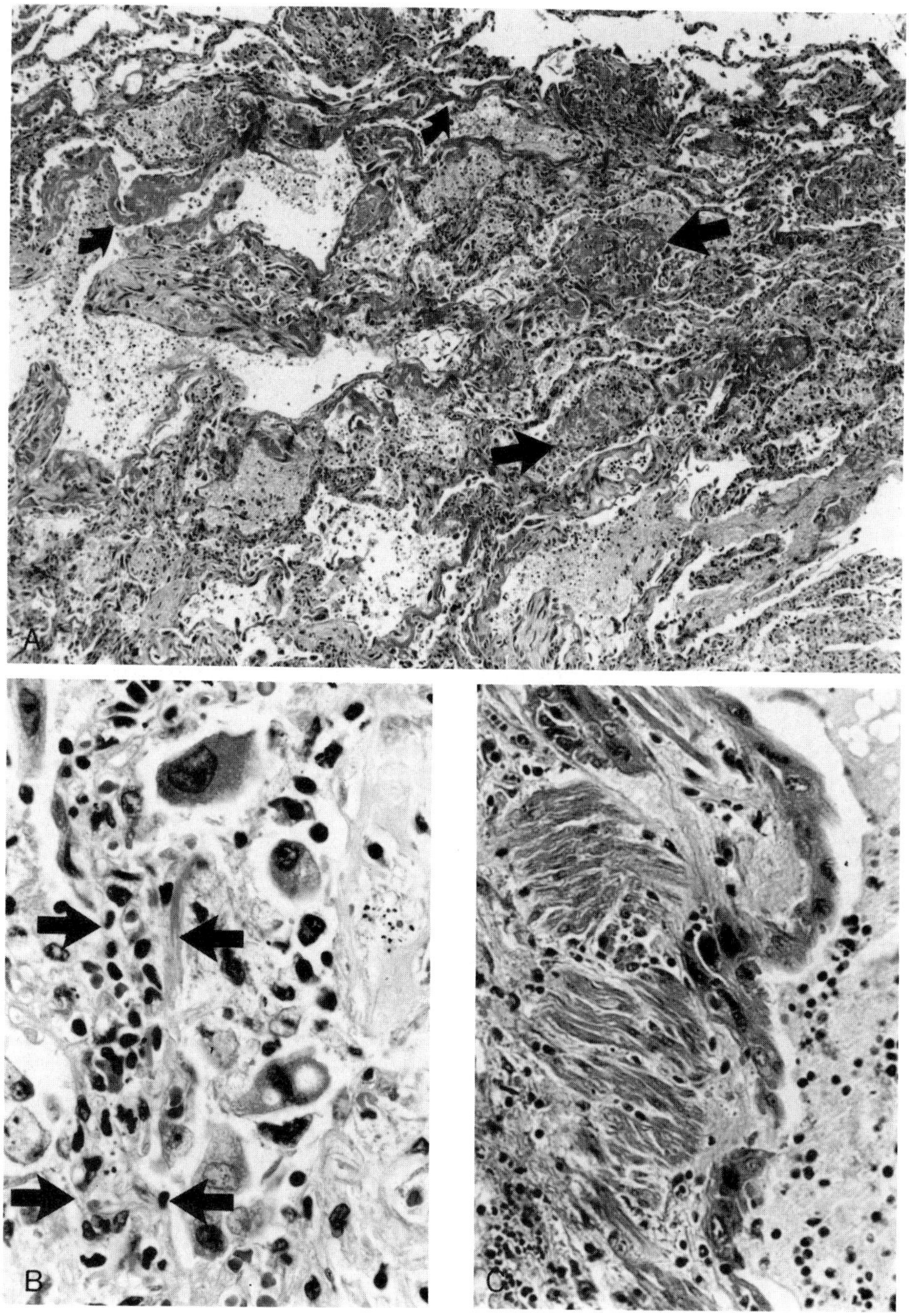

Figure 15–43. Acute Radiation Pneumonitis. A histologic section of lung parenchyma *(A)* from the upper lobe of a patient treated 3 months prior to death with radiation therapy for a left breast carcinoma reveals extensive airspace filling by a proteinaceous exudate *(straight arrows)*, mild interstitial thickening, and focal hyaline membrane formation *(curved arrows)*. A magnified view of a single alveolus *(B)* shows a mononuclear inflammatory infiltrate in the septal interstitium *(between arrows)* and several irregularly shaped type II pneumocytes with hyperchromatic and cytologically atypical nuclei. A section of bronchial wall *(C)*, also within the field of radiation, again shows a mononuclear inflammatory infiltrate as well as markedly abnormal epithelial lining cells. (A × 60; B × 400; C × 200.)

well documented, as were loss of lung volume, an air bronchogram, and restriction of the opacity to the boundaries of the radiation beam. An important exception to this rule is the obstructive atelectasis that sometimes occurs shortly after the institution of radiation therapy for an endobronchial lesion.[430] This is caused by radiation-induced edema of the bronchial wall that is already severely narrowed by the endobronchial lesion.

In contrast to the usual roentgenographic manifestations of acute radiation pneumonitis just described, rarely the appearance may be one of hyperlucent lung. Three cases of this unusual manifestation have been reported,[396, 431, 432] and we have personally seen one patient whose left lung became replaced by a multitude of large bullae following irradiation of the mediastinum for Hodgkin's disease. A lung scan pattern suggesting pulmonary embolism may result from obliterative vasculitis, as emphasized by Bateman and associates.[433] A unique sign of previous mediastinal radiation consists of bilateral superomedial hilar displacement in the absence of roentgenographic evidence of parenchymal irradiation fibrosis.[434]

The late or chronic stage of radiation damage is characterized by fibrosis (Fig. 15–47). The af-
Text continued on page 2562

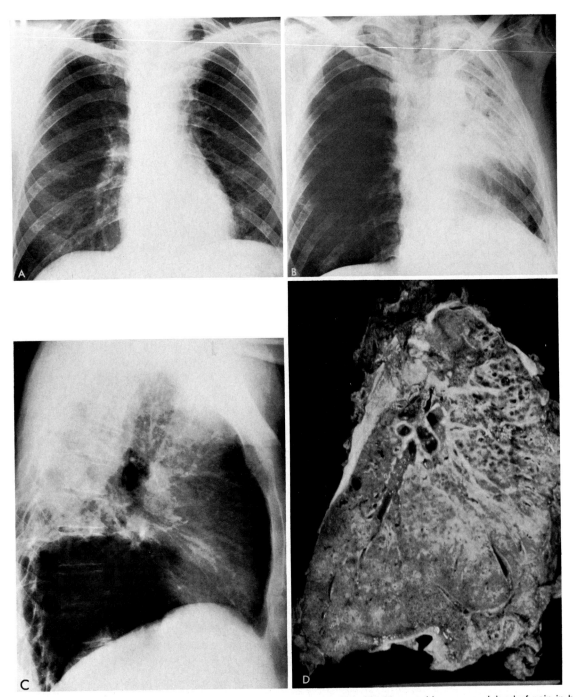

Figure 15–44. Radiation Pneumonitis. On his first admission to the hospital, this 56-year-old man complained of pain in his neck and low back, which was subsequently proved to be caused by metastases to cervical and lumbar vertebrae from a primary adenocarcinoma of the upper lobe of his left lung. A roentgenogram at that time *(A)* demonstrated moderate loss of volume of the left upper lobe as a result of the endobronchial lesion. He received cobalt teletherapy to the left upper lung and mediastinum through opposing fields. Two courses were administered, each delivering 30 gray to the left upper lung. The first course lasted 4 weeks and the second 6 weeks, the two courses being separated by approximately 1 month. Six weeks after the end of the second course of treatment, roentgenograms of the chest in posteroanterior *(B)* and lateral *(C)* projections revealed a severe loss of volume of the left lung, with marked mediastinal displacement and elevation of the hemidiaphragm. The posterior portion of the left upper lobe and the superior portion of the left lower lobe were the sites of extensive inhomogeneous consolidation and atelectasis. The patient expired 2 weeks later. At necropsy, the left upper lobe and upper third of the lower lobe were the sites of extensive fibrosis, pneumonitis, bronchiectasis, and atelectasis *(D)*. Note the sharp line of definition of affected lung parenchyma corresponding to the roentgenographic appearance in *C*.

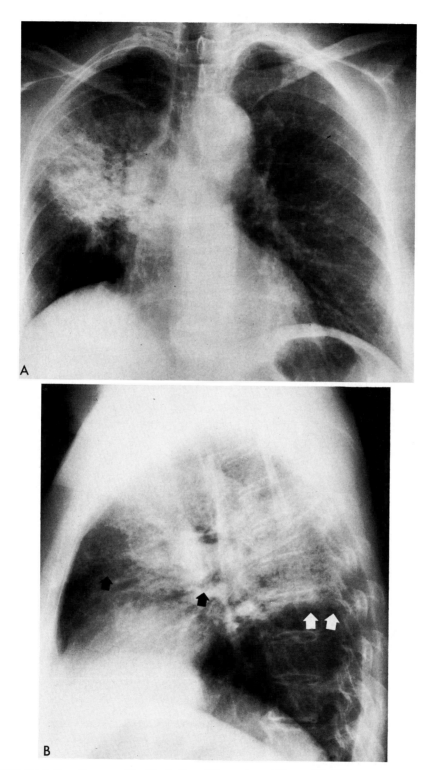

Figure 15–45. Acute Radiation Pneumonitis Illustrating "Through-and-Through" Effect. Posteroanterior *(A)* and lateral *(B)* roentgenograms reveal inhomogeneous consolidation of the upper half of the right lung associated with a prominent air bronchogram. In lateral projection *(B)*, the lower border of the consolidation is almost a straight line *(arrows)*, conforming precisely to the lower margin of the collimated beam of radiation. These films were of a 48-year-old woman approximately 3 months following an intensive course of cobalt therapy for primary bronchogenic carcinoma.

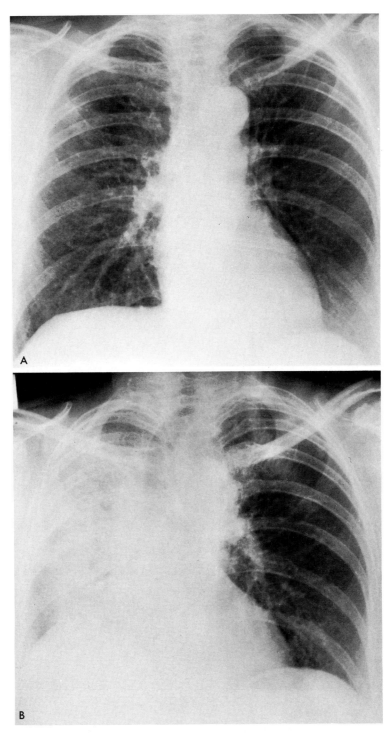

Figure 15–46. Acute Radiation Pneumonitis and Subsequent Fibrosis. This 52-year-old woman presented with a large ulcerated mass in the right breast that proved on biopsy to be carcinoma. Preoperative cobalt teletherapy was administered to the breast and mediastinum in a dosage of approximately 30 gray. The breast was then removed and over a period of 6 weeks postoperative cobalt therapy administered to the right lung in a dosage of 51 gray and to the mediastinum of 35 gray. A posteroanterior roentgenogram *(A)* at the end of the postoperative radiation therapy revealed no significant abnormalities. Three weeks later, however, a remarkable change had occurred in the appearance of the chest *(B)*, the right lung having undergone severe loss of volume as evidenced by elevation of the hemidiaphragm and shift of the mediastinum.

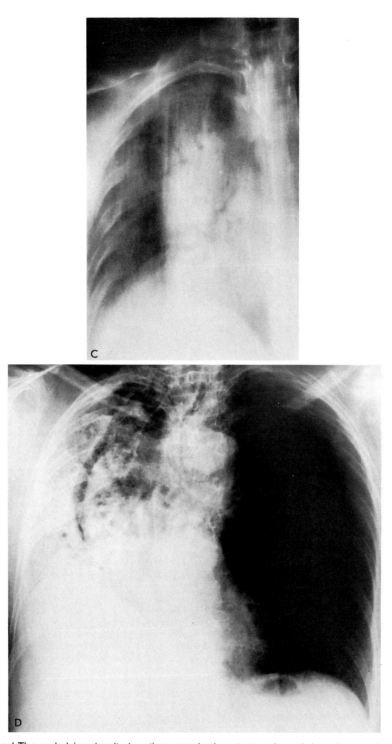

Figure 15–46 *Continued* The underlying density is rather granular in nature and an air bronchogram is identified within it (seen to better advantage in the anteroposterior tomogram of the right hemithorax illustrated in *C.*) She was treated with corticosteroids for the following month. A posteroanterior roentgenogram approximately 1 month later *(D)* revealed severe loss of volume of the right lung. The pattern observed earlier had changed to a very coarse inhomogeneous pattern in which extensive bronchiectasis was readily apparent. In subsequent years, the roentgenographic appearance of the right hemithorax underwent no further change, and the patient's only complaint was shortness of breath on climbing stairs or walking rapidly on level ground.

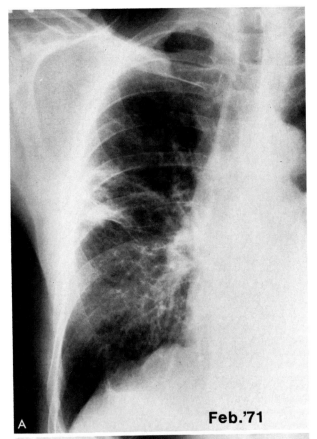

Feb.'71

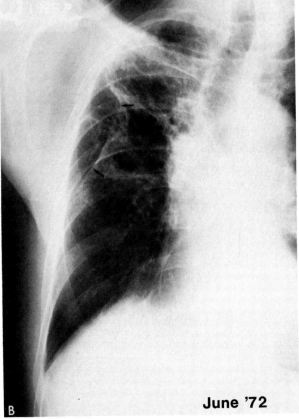

June '72

Figure 15–47. Progressive Cicatrization Atelectasis Following Irradiation Pneumonitis, Manifested by Migration of a Bulla.
Several months following completion of a course of cobalt therapy to the right hemithorax for inoperable bronchogenic carcinoma, a roentgenogram *(A)* of this 66-year-old man reveals some loss of volume of the right lung and a few patchy opacities in the axillary portion of the right upper lobe. Almost 1½ years later *(B)*, the loss of volume was more severe and there had developed a well-circumscribed cystic space in the axillary portion of the right lung *(arrows)*, representing a bulla.

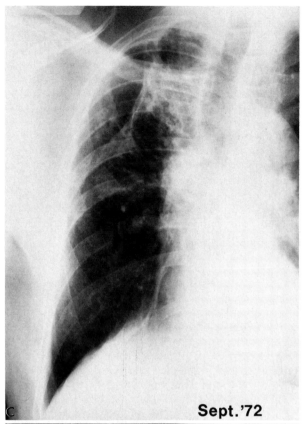

Sept.'72

Figure 15–47 *Continued* Three months later *(C)* the bulla had enlarged somewhat and had migrated superiorly in response to progressive fibrosis of the right upper lobe. A further 3 months later *(D)*, the bulla occupied the apical zone of the right hemithorax.

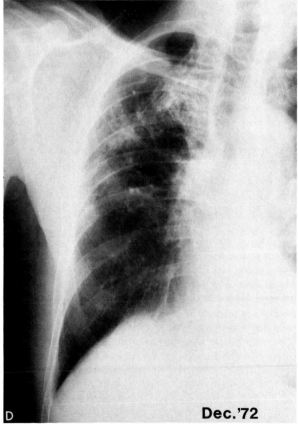

Dec.'72

fected lung shows severe loss of volume, with obliteration of all normal architectural markings (Fig. 15–48), and the peripheral parenchyma is characteristically airless and opaque as a result of replacement by fibrous tissue. It has been stated[435] that radiation fibrosis generally is well established and stable 9 to 12 months after the completion of radiation therapy. Dense fibrotic strands frequently extend from the hilum to the periphery and present an appearance suggesting severe bronchiectasis. At this stage differentiation from lymphangitic spread of carcinoma may be difficult and, in fact, may be impossible on the basis of a single roentgenographic study. However, the lack of progression with time and the roentgenographic demonstration of fairly severe changes in the absence of corresponding clinical symptoms should suggest the diagnosis of radiation fibrosis. CT has been found to permit ready differentiation of radiation-induced fibrosis from recurrent pulmonary neoplasm.[436]

Pleural effusion that can be demonstrated roentgenographically is very uncommon,[397, 437, 438] although effusions are often present at necropsy; fairly extensive thickening of the pleura may be seen both roentgenologically and pathologically (Fig. 15–48).[397, 439] The presence of pleural thickening can be established with ease on CT scans.[440] The development of pericardial effusion following radiation therapy to the mediastinum is not uncommon: in one group of 31 patients with a variety of malignancies who developed pericarditis, 10 per cent of the pericardial effusions were attributed to radiation.[441] Although this complication usually develops within a few days after initiation of therapy,[442] it can be delayed for a considerable time, even years.[442–444]

CLINICAL MANIFESTATIONS

Many patients with roentgenographic evidence of radiation damage remain asymptomatic.[397] Radiation pneumonitis rarely produces symptoms during the 1-month period after termination of therapy. When the symptoms do develop, they usually appear between 2 and 3 months, and occasionally as late as 6 months, after the completion of therapy.

Symptoms generally have an insidious onset and consist of nonproductive cough, weakness, and shortness of breath on exertion. Cough may be very troublesome and occur in spasms. The patient may have a sensation of inability to inspire to TLC and when encouraged to do so will invariably cough. Chest pain develops occasionally,[425] but hemoptysis is rare.[397, 426] Fever may be a prominent finding and is usually low-grade but sometimes high and spiking.[389] Dyspnea is generally mild and noted only on exertion but may occasion extreme respiratory distress. Death may be caused by respiratory insufficiency. Discontinuation of corticosteroids in patients receiving combined steroid and radiation therapy

can precipitate severe radiation pneumonitis.[403, 404] Tachycardia out of proportion to the fever may be observed. Crepitations at the height of inspiration are common, and there may be signs of lung consolidation in patients with severe pneumonitis. Rarely, a pleural friction rub can be heard.

Acute radiation pneumonitis may persist for up to 1 month and can either resolve completely or progress to pulmonary fibrosis. In a minority of patients, fibrosis develops insidiously without an acute phase being recognized. With the onset of fibrosis, symptoms of the acute pneumonitis gradually abate.

As previously mentioned, the institution of radiation therapy for an endobronchial neoplasm can induce edema and narrowing of the airway lumen. In our experience and that of others,[445] this effect can have disastrous consequences if the tumor is in the trachea. This complication can be prevented by preliminary treatment with corticosteroids.[446]

The development of new primary neoplasms following radiotherapy and chemotherapy is well recognized.[447, 448] Since such lesions can occur coincidentally with the malignancy under treatment or in an area outside the treatment field, they do not necessarily represent complications of therapy. Repeated small doses of radiation received either as treatment of disease or as a result of occupational exposure appear to result in an increased incidence of visceral malignancy, including that of the lung[449, 450, 453] and of the breast.[454] Even environmental pollution by low-level radiation,[451] as may be found in houses constructed over rock containing radioactive material (see page 1337), may play a significant carcinogenic role. Using data from a tri-state leukemia survey, it has been estimated that in the fetuses of mothers subjected to diagnostic radiation there is a significant risk of genetic damage resulting in subsequent leukemia.[452]

PULMONARY FUNCTION STUDIES

It is important to appreciate that in many patients receiving radiation therapy pulmonary function improves initially, presumably due to the therapeutic effect on malignant tissue within the thorax.[406, 439] The major impairment in function is restrictive in nature; vital capacity and flow rates are decreased, the former to a proportionately greater degree. Diffusing capacity is decreased when a large volume of lung is involved; it may return to normal as the acute process subsides but more commonly remains decreased as fibrosis ensues.[391, 439, 455, 456] In one report[457] that dealt with the long-term functional assessment of 36 patients irradiated for breast carcinoma, the surprising observation was made that diffusing capacity returned to normal 18 months after termination of treatment. As might be expected, the greater the amount of

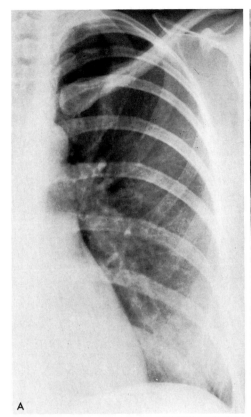

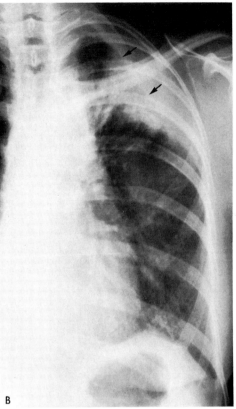

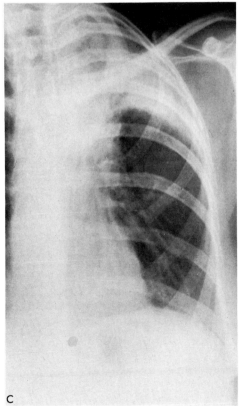

Figure 15–48. Irradiation Pneumonitis and Pleuritis. At the time of the posteroanterior roentgenogram illustrated in *(A)*, this 37-year-old woman presented with a huge carcinoma of the left breast that was considered inoperable. Over a period of 127 days, cobalt teletherapy was administered to the supraclavicular area in the amount of 61 gray and to the mediastinum in a dosage of 30 gray (an additional 80 gray were administered to the breast directly). Six months after the beginning of radiation therapy and approximately 2 months after its termination, the patient noted the onset of a dry hacking cough. A roentgenogram at that time *(B)* revealed a triangular shadow of inhomogeneous density extending upward and outward from the left hilum. A homogeneous shadow in the upper axilla (inner borders indicated by *arrows*) represents local or encapsulated pleural effusion, although there was no evidence of a free effusion in the pleural space. Several months later *(C)*, the affected lung had undergone further loss of volume and the whole apical zone of the left hemithorax had become opacified. It was now impossible to separate the parenchymal and pleural components of the radiation injury. This represents the late or fibrotic stage of irradiation pneumonitis.

lung affected the more severe the diffusion defect.[458]

In a study of the effect of unilateral thoracic irradiation on lung function in the dog, Teates[459] performed differential lung function tests for 6 months after stopping the irradiation. Measurement of the diffusing capacity by the steady-state method in the damaged lung showed reduction after 6 to 10 weeks, with simultaneous ipsilateral reduction in blood flow and ventilation, and it was concluded that hypoxemia resulted from ventilation-perfusion imbalance. In another experimental study on rats,[460] changes in expansibility of the lungs and thorax were measured after single fraction irradiation of the lungs in exposures up to 30 gray. Six weeks after irradiation, compliance (as measured by the slope of the pressure-volume curve) was found to be markedly reduced in all lungs receiving over 15 gray. The loss of compliance was apparently not related to pulmonary fibrosis, since trichrome staining revealed no increase in lung collagen.

In a physiologic-roentgenographic correlative study, Prato and his colleagues[461] performed repeated regional measurements of pulmonary blood flow and ventilation on 25 patients irradiated for breast cancer. Patients were studied before and at varying times after (16 to 407 days) the start of radiotherapy. Of all parameters measured, blood flow showed the earliest and greatest decrease. The authors state that since changes in blood flow at 60 days are predictive of changes at 300 days, it is reasonable to assume that earlier studies during the course of irradiation can be useful in predicting long-term effects. In a prospective study of patients with Hodgkin's disease in whom there was no evidence of intrathoracic involvement but who received prophylactic mantle-field radiotherapy to the chest, a 10 per cent reduction in both FVC and diffusing capacity was noted at an interval of 6 weeks to 6 months after the initiation of therapy.[392]

REFERENCES

1. Lane WZ: Lung trauma. Influence of pre-existing pulmonary disease. N Engl J Med 260:251, 1959.
2. Dubrow EL, Landis FB: Reactivation of pulmonary tuberculosis due to trauma. Chest 68:596, 1975.
3. Tombs BD, Sandler CM, Lester RG: Computed tomography of chest trauma. Radiology 140:733, 1981.
4. Williams JR, Bonte FJ: Pulmonary changes in nonpenetrating thoracic trauma. Tex Med 59:27, 1963.
5. Williams JR, Bonte FJ: Pulmonary damage in nonpenetrating chest injuries. Radiol Clin North Am 1:439, 1963.
6. Reynolds J, Davis JT: Injuries of the chest wall, pleura, pericardium, lungs, bronchi and esophagus. Radiol Clin North Am 4:383, 1966.
7. Stevens E, Templeton AW: Traumatic nonpenetrating lung contusion. Radiology 85:247, 1965.
8. Sorsdahl OA, Powell JW: Cavitary pulmonary lesions following nonpenetrating chest trauma in children. Am J Roentgenol 95:118, 1965.
9. Williams JR, Stembridge VA: Pulmonary contusion secondary to nonpenetrating chest trauma. Am J Roentgenol 91:284, 1964.
10. Errion AR, Houk VN, Kettering DL: Pulmonary hematoma due to blunt, nonpenetrating thoracic trauma. Am Rev Respir Dis 88:384, 1963.
11. Schneider M, Klein CP: Blast injury of the lungs. With report of a case occurring in peace time. Radiology 54:548, 1950.
12. Hirsch M, Bazini J: Blast injury of the chest. Clin Radiol 20:362, 1969.
13. Roth RA, Beckmann CF: Complications of extracorporeal shock-wave lithotripsy and percutaneous nephrolithotomy. Urol Clin North Am 15:155, 1988.
14. Williams JR: The vanishing lung tumor—pulmonary hematoma. Am J Roentgenol 81:296, 1959.
15. Ting YM: Pulmonary parenchymal findings in blunt trauma to the chest. Am J Roentgenol 98:343, 1966.
16. Wiot JF: The radiologic manifestations of blunt chest trauma. JAMA 231:500, 1975.
17. Paredes S, Hipona FA: The radiologic evaluation of patients with chest trauma. Med Clin North Am 59:37, 1975.
18. Shaw J: Pulmonary contusion in children due to rubber bullet injuries. Br Med J 4:764, 1972.
19. Schwartz A, Borman JB: Contusion of the lung in childhood. Arch Dis Child 36:557, 1961.
20. Hussey HH: Editorial: Pulmonary contusion. JAMA 230:264, 1974.
21. Wilson RF, Murray C, Antonenko DR: Nonpenetrating thoracic injuries. Surg Clin North Am 57:17, 1977.
22. Cochlin DL, Shaw MRP: Traumatic lung cysts following minor blunt chest trauma. Clin Radiol 29:151, 1978.
23. Joynt GHC, Jaffe F: Solitary pulmonary hematoma. J Thorac Cardiovasc Surg 43:291, 1962.
24. Milne E, Dick A: Circumscribed intrapulmonary haematoma. Br J Radiol 34:587, 1961.
25. Fagan CJ: Traumatic lung cyst. Am J Roentgenol 97:186, 1966.
26. Diller WF, Endrei E: Posttraumatische Rundherde der Lunge. (Posttraumatic coin lesions of the lungs.) Fortschr Roentgenstr 96:364, 1962.
27. Greening R, Kynette A, Hodes PJ: Unusual pulmonary changes secondary to chest trauma. Am J Roentgenol 77:1059, 1957.
28. Shirakusa T, Araki Y, Tsutsui M, et al: Traumatic lung pseudocyst. Thorax 42:516, 1987.
29. Shirakusa T, Araki Y, Tsutsui M, et al: Traumatic lung pseudocyst. Thorax 42:516, 1987.
30. Santos GH, Mahendra T: Traumatic pulmonary pseudocysts. Ann Thorac Surg 27:359, 1979.
31. Chester EH: Chest injury resulting in bullae in the lung. Report of a case. N Engl J Med 268:1068, 1963.
32. Cochlin DL, Shaw MRP: Traumatic lung cysts following minor blunt chest trauma. Clin Radiol 29:151, 1978.
33. Wagner RB, Crawford WO Jr, Schimpf PP: Classification of parenchymal injuries of the lung. Radiology 167:77, 1988.
34. Ganske JG, Dennis DL, Vanderveer JB Jr: Traumatic lung cyst: Case report and literature review. J Trauma 21:493, 1981.
35. Beumer HM, Mellema TL: Excavated haematomas after pulmonary segmental resection. Dis Chest 37:163, 1960.
36. Bonmarchand G, Lefebvre E, Lerebours-Pigeonniere G, et al: Intrapulmonary haematoma complicating mechanical ventilation in patients with chronic obstructive pulmonary disease. Intensive Care Med 14:246, 1988.
37. Roxburgh JC: Rupture of the tracheobronchial tree. Thorax 42:681, 1987.
38. Chesterman JT, Satsangi PN: Rupture of the trachea and bronchi by closed injury. Thorax 21:21, 1966.
39. Burke JF: Early diagnosis of traumatic rupture of the bronchus. JAMA 181:682, 1962.
40. Woodring JH, Fried AM, Hatfield DR, et al: Fractures of first and second ribs: Predictive value for arterial and bronchial injury. Am J Roentgenol 138:211, 1982.
41. Lynn RB, Iyengar K: Traumatic rupture of the bronchus. Chest 61:81, 1972.
42. Eastridge CE, Hughes FA Jr, Pate JW, et al: Tracheobronchial injury caused by blunt trauma. Am Rev Respir Dis 101:230, 1970.
43. Silbiger ML, Kushner LN: Tracheobronchial perforation: Its diagnosis and treatment. Radiology 85:242, 1965.
44. Larizadeh R: Rupture of the bronchus. Thorax 21:28, 1966.
45. Collins JP, Ketharanathan V, McConchie I: Rupture of major bronchi resulting from closed chest injuries. Thorax 28:371, 1973.
46. Bertelsen S, Howitz P: Injuries of the trachea and bronchi. Thorax 27:188, 1972.
47. Heceta WG, Torpoco J, Richardson RL: Extensive linear "blow-out" of the thoracic membranous trachea with innominate artery avulsion secondary to blunt chest trauma. Chest 67:247, 1975.
48. Hood RM, Sloan HE: Injuries to the trachea and major bronchi. J Thorac Cardiovasc Surg 38:458, 1959.
49. Eijgelaar A, Homan van der Heide JN: A reliable early symptom of bronchial or tracheal rupture. Thorax 25:120, 1970.
50. Haverling M: Traumatic bronchial rupture: Acute stage diagnosed by bronchography. Acta Radiol [Diagn] (Stockh) 7:72, 1968.
51. Harvey-Smith W, Bush W, Northrop C: Traumatic bronchial rupture. Am J Roentgenol 134:1189, 1980.
52. Travis SP, Layer GT: Traumatic transection of the thoracic trachea. Ann R Coll Surg Engl 65:240, 1983.
53. Döpper Th: Zur Röntgendiagnostik stumpfer Thoraxtrauman. (Roentgen diagnosis of injuries of the thorax due to blunt trauma.) Fortschr Roentgenstr 92:524, 1960.
54. Lotz PR, Martel W, Rohwedder JJ, et al: Significance of pneumomediastinum in blunt trauma to the thorax. Am J Roentgenol 132:817, 1979.
55. Hardy JD: Injuries to main-stem bronchi: Complete separation of left with successful anastomosis and instability of right due to fracture of multiple cartilages. Ann Surg 149:949, 1959.
56. Rollins RJ, Tocino I: Early radiographic signs of tracheal rupture. Am J Roentgenol 148:695, 1987.
57. Vidinel I: Displacement of the mediastinum. Chest 62:215, 1972.
58. Tyson MD, Watson TR Jr, Sibley JR: Traumatic bronchial rupture with plastic repair. N Engl J Med 258:160, 1958.
59. Streete BG, Stull FE Jr: Primary repair of fracture of the left main-stem bronchus. J Thorac Surg 36:76, 1958.
60. Weisel W, Watson RR, O'Connor TM: Long-term follow-up study of patients with bronchial anastomosis or tracheal replacement. Chest 61:141, 1972.
61. van der Schaar H, Wagenaar JPM, Swierenga J, et al: Successful late repair of a post-traumatic bronchial stricture. Thorax 27:769, 1972.
62. Lynne-Davis P, Ganguli PC, Sterns LP: Pulmonary function following traumatic rupture of the bronchus. Chest 61:400, 1972.
63. Deslauriers J, Beaulieu M, Archambault G, et al: Diagnosis and long-term follow-up of major bronchial disruptions due to nonpenetrating trauma. Ann Thorac Surg 33:32, 1982.
64. Felson B: Lung torsion: Radiographic findings in nine cases. Radiology 162:631, 1987.
65. Huang TY, Cho SR: Torsion of the lung without trauma. Radiology 132:25, 1979.
66. Shorr RM, Rodriguez A: Spontaneous pulmonary torsion. Chest 91:927, 1987.
67. Weisbrod GL: Left upper lobe torsion following left lingulectomy. J Can Assoc Radiol 38:296, 1987.
68. Kelly MV II, Kyger ER, Miller WC: Postoperative lobar torsion and gangrene. Thorax 32:501, 1977.
69. Weisbrod GL: Left upper lobe torsion following left lingulectomy. J Can Assoc Radiol 38:296, 1987.
70. Parks RE: Traumatic torsion of the lung. Case report. Radiology 67:582, 1956.
71. Daughtry DC: Traumatic torsion of the lung. N Engl J Med 256:385, 1957.

15

72. Crawford WO Jr: Pulmonary injury in thoracic and non-thoracic trauma. Radiol Clin North Am 11:527, 1973.
73. Williams JR, Bonte FJ: The Roentgenologic Aspect of Nonpenetrating Chest Injuries. Springfield, Ill, Charles C Thomas, 1961.
74. Higgins CB, Mulder DG: Traumatic subarachnoid-pleural fistula. Chest 61:189, 1972.
75. Campbell GD, Webb WR: Eosinophilic pleural effusion: A review with the presentation of seven new cases. Am Rev Respir Dis 90:194, 1964.
76. Kumar UN, Varkey B, Mathal G: Posttraumatic pleural-fluid and blood eosinophilia. JAMA 234:625, 1975.
77. Beekman JF, Bosniak S, Canter HG: Eosinophilia and elevated IgE concentration in a serous pleural effusion following trauma. Am Rev Respir Dis 110:484, 1974.
78. Robertson HT, Lakshminarayan S, Hudson LD: Lung injury following a 50-metre fall into water. Thorax 33:175, 1978.
79. Craighead CC, Glass BA: Management of nonpenetrating injuries of the chest. JAMA 172:1138, 1960.
80. Tsai SH, Cohen SS, Fenger EPK: Bronchial perforation as a complication of bronchoscopy. Am Rev Tuberc 78:106, 1958.
81. Armen RN, Morrow CS, Sewell S: Mediastinal emphysema: A complication of bronchoscopy. Ann Intern Med 48:1083, 1958.
82. Switzer P, Pitman RG, Fleming JP: Pneumomediastinum associated with zygomatico-maxillary fracture. J Can Assoc Radiol 25:316, 1974.
83. Laforet EG: Traumatic hemomediastinum. J Thorac Surg 29:597, 1955.
84. Coté J, Hodgson CH, Ellis FH Jr: Traumatic mediastinal hematoma: Report of unusual case. Proc Mayo Clin 34:264, 1959.
85. Strax TE, Ryvicker MJ, Elguezabal A: Superior vena caval syndrome due to a mediastinal hematoma secondary to a dissecting aortic aneurysm. Dis Chest 55:338, 1969.
86. Raphael MJ: Mediastinal haematoma. A description of some radiological appearances. Br J Radiol 36:921, 1963.
87. Leigh TF: Mass lesions of the mediastinum. Radiol Clin North Am 1:377, 1963.
88. Cohen G: Traumatic haemomediastinum: A case report. S Afr Med J 32:298, 1958.
89. Redding RA, Douglas WHJ, Stein M: Thyroid hormone influence upon lung surfactant metabolism. Science 175:994, 1972.
90. Bachynski JE: Rupture of a mediastinal vein detected by ^{131}I-MAA scanning. J Can Assoc Radiol 22:58, 1971.
91. Pastershank SP, Chow KC: Blunt trauma to the aorta and its major branches. J Can Assoc Radiol 25:202, 1974.
92. Fishbone G, Robbins DI, Osborn DJ, et al: Trauma to the thoracic aorta and great vessels. Radiol Clin North Am 11:543, 1973.
93. Sanborn JC, Heitzman R, Markarian B: Traumatic rupture of the thoracic aorta: Roentgen-pathological correlations. Radiology 95:293, 1970.
94. Hewes RC, Smith DC, Lavine MH: Iatrogenic hydromediastinum simulating aortic laceration. Am J Roentgenol 133:817, 1979.
95. Milne ENC, Imray TJ, Pistolesi M, et al: The vascular pedicle and the vena azygos. Part III: In trauma—The "vanishing" azygos. Radiology 153:25, 1984.
96. Sherbon KJ: Traumatic rupture of the thoracic aorta—The radiologist's responsibility. Australas Radiol 164:164, 1975.
97. Fishbone G, Robbins DI, Osborn DJ, et al: Trauma to the thoracic aorta and great vessels. Radiol Clin North Am 11:543, 1973.
98. Tisnado J, Tsai FY, Als A, et al: A new radiographic sign of acute traumatic rupture of the thoracic aorta: Displacement of the nasogastric tube to the right. Radiology 125:603, 1977.
99. Gerlock AJ Jr, Muhletaler CA, Coulam CM, et al: Traumatic aortic aneurysm: Validity of esophageal tube displacement sign. Am J Roentgenol 135:713, 1980.
100. Wales LR, Morishima MS, Reay D, et al: Nasogastric tube displacement in acute traumatic rupture of the thoracic aorta: A postmortem study. Am J Roentgenol 138:821, 1982.
101. Peters DR, Gamsu G: Displacement of the right paraspinous interface: A radiographic sign of acute traumatic rupture of the thoracic aorta. Radiology 134:599, 1980.
102. Woodring JH, Pulmano CM, Stevens RK: The right paratracheal stripe in blunt chest trauma. Radiology 143:605, 1982.
103. Simeone JF, Minagi H, Putman CE: Traumatic disruption of the thoracic aorta: Significance of the left apical extrapleural cap. Radiology 117:265, 1975.
104. Simeone JF, Deren MM, Cagle F: The value of the left apical cap in the diagnosis of aortic rupture. A prospective and retrospective study. Radiology 139:35, 1981.
105. Williams JR, Bonte FJ: The Roentgenological Aspect of Non-Penetrating Chest Injuries. Springfield, Ill, Charles C Thomas, 1961.
106. Yee ES, Thomas AN, Goodman PC: Isolated first rib fracture: Clinical significance after blunt chest trauma. Ann Thorac Surg 32:278, 1981.
107. Fisher RG, Ward RE, Ben-Menachem Y, et al: Arteriography and

108. the fractured first rib: Too much for too little? Am J Roentgenol 138:1059, 1982.
108. Woodring JH, Fried AM, Hatfield DR, et al: Fractures of first and second ribs: Predictive value for arterial and bronchial injury. Am J Roentgenol 138:211, 1982.
109. Seltzer SE, D'Orsi C, Kirshner R, et al: Traumatic aortic rupture: Plain radiographic findings. Am J Roentgenol 137:1011, 1981.
110. Marnocha KE, Maglinte DDT, Woods J, et al: Mediastinal-width/chest-width ratio in blunt chest trauma: A reappraisal. Am J Roentgenol 142:275, 1984.
111. Eller JL, Ziter FMH Jr: Avulsion of the innominate artery from the aortic arch. An evaluation of roentgenographic findings. Radiology 94:75, 1970.
112. Koury WC, Davidson KC: Multiple chronic traumatic pseudoaneurysms of the aorta and great vessels. A case report. Radiology 116:23, 1975.
113. Lundell CJ, Quinn MF, Finck EJ: Traumatic laceration of the ascending aorta: Angiographic assessment. Am J Roentgenol 145:715, 1985.
114. O'Toole JD, Wurtzbacher JJ, Wearner NE, et al: Pulmonary-valve injury and insufficiency during pulmonary-artery catheterization. N Eng J Med 301:1167, 1979.
115. Freed TA, Neal MP Jr, Vinik M: Roentgenographic findings in extracardiac injury secondary to blunt chest automobile trauma. Am J Roentgenol 104:424, 1968.
116. Parmley LF, Mattingly TW, Manion WC, et al: Nonpenetrating traumatic injury of the aorta. Circulation 17:1086, 1958.
117. Parmley LF, Mattingly TW, Manion WC, et al: Nonpenetrating traumatic injury of the aorta. Circulation 17:1086, 1958.
118. Langbein IE, Brandt PWT: Traumatic rupture of the aorta. Australas Radiol 12:102, 1968.
119. Verdant A: Chronic traumatic aneurysm of the descending thoracic aorta with compression of the tracheobronchial tree. Can J Surg 27:278, 1984.
120. Chew FS, Panicek DM, Heitzman ER: Late discovery of a posttraumatic right aortic arch aneurysm. Am J Roentgenol 145:1001, 1985.
121. Heystraten FM, Rosenbusch G, Kingma LM, et al: Chronic posttraumatic aneurysm of the thoracic aorta: Surgically correctable occult threat. Am J Roentgenol 146:303, 1986.
122. Sefcek DM, Sefczek RJ, Deeb ZL: Radiographic signs of acute traumatic rupture of the thoracic aorta. Am J Roentgenol 141:1259, 1983.
123. Barcia TC, Livoni JP: Indications for angiography in blunt thoracic trauma. Radiology 147:15, 1983.
124. Gundry SR, Williams S, Burney RE: Indications for aortography. Radiography after blunt chest trauma: A reassessment of the radiographic findings associated with traumatic rupture of the aorta. Invest Radiol 18:230, 1983.
125. Marnocha KE, Maglinte DDT: Plain-film criteria for excluding aortic rupture in blunt chest trauma. Am J Roentgenol 144:19, 1985.
126. Mirvis SE, Bidwell JK, Buddemeyer EU, et al: Value of chest radiography in excluding traumatic aortic rupture. Radiology 163:487, 1987.
127. Heiberg E, Wolverson MK, Sundaram M, et al: CT in aortic trauma. Am J Roentgenol 140:1119, 1983.
128. Finkelmeier BA, Mentzer RM Jr, Kaiser DL, et al: Chronic traumatic thoracic aneurysm: Influence of operative treatment on natural history. An analysis of reported cases, 1950–1980. J Thorac Cardiovasc Surg 84:257, 1982.
129. James OF, Moore PG: Tracheo-oesophageal fistula caused by blunt chest injury. Anaesth Intensive Care 11:59, 1983.
130. Stanbridge RDeL: Tracheo-oesophageal fistula and bilateral recurrent laryngeal nerve palsies after blunt chest trauma. Thorax 37:548, 1982.
131. Leading article: Traumatic perforation of oesophagus. Br Med J 1:524, 1972.
132. Scholl DG, Tsai SH: Esophageal perforation following the use of the esophageal obturator airway. Radiology 122:315, 1977.
133. Christoforidis A, Nelson SW: Spontaneous rupture of the esophagus with emphasis on the roentgenologic diagnosis. Am J Roentgenol 78:574, 1957.
134. Parkin GJS: The radiology of perforated oesophagus. Clin Radiol 24:324, 1973.
135. Vessal K, Montali RJ, Larson SM, et al: Evaluation of barium and Gastrografin as contrast media for the diagnosis of esophageal rupture or perforations. Am J Roentgenol 123:307, 1975.
136. Eriksen KR: Oesophageal fistula diagnosed by microscopic examination of pleural fluid. Acta Chir Scand 128:771, 1964.
137. Liebow AA, Carrington CB: The interstitial pneumonias. In Simon M, Potchen EJ, LeMay M (eds): Frontiers of Pulmonary Radiology. New York, Grune and Stratton, 1969, p 102.
138. Wichern WA: Perforation of the esophagus. Am J Surg 119:534, 1970.
139. Brook MP, Dupree DW: Bilateral traumatic chylothorax. Ann Emerg Med 17:69, 1988.

140. Shackelford RT, Fisher AM: Traumatic chylothorax. South Med J 31:766, 1938.
141. Rea D: Traumatic chylothorax in a closed chest injury. Report of a case. Br J Dis Chest 54:82, 1960.
142. Thorne PS: Traumatic chylothorax. Tubercle 39:29, 1958.
143. Ellis MC, Gordon L, Gobien RP, et al: Traumatic lymphocele: Demonstration by lymphoscintigraphy with modified ⁹⁹ᵐTc sulfur colloid. Am J Roentgenol 140:973, 1983.
144. Ebert PA, Gaertner RA, Zuidema GD: Traumatic diaphragmatic hernia. Surg Gynecol Obstet 125:59, 1967.
145. Luastela E, Tala P: Traumatic diaphragmatic hernia. Ann Chir Gynaecol Fenn 87(Suppl):1, 1959.
146. Gupta RL: Traumatic diaphragmatic hernia due to a stab wound of the chest. Br J Dis Chest 55:159, 1961.
147. Desforges G, Strieder JW, Lynch JP, et al: Traumatic rupture of the diaphragm. Clinical manifestations and surgical treatment. J Thorac Surg 34:779, 1957.
148. Efron G, Hyde I: Non-penetrating traumatic rupture of the diaphragm. Clin Radiol 18:394, 1967.
149. Allison PR: Reflux esophagitis, sliding hiatal hernia, and the anatomy of repair. Surg Gynecol Obstet 92:419, 1951.
150. Keshishian JA, Cox PA: Diagnosis and management of strangulated diaphragmatic hernias. Surg Gynecol Obstet 115:626, 1962.
151. Bernatz PE, Burnside AF Jr, Clagett OT: Problem of the ruptured diaphragm. JAMA 168:877, 1958.
152. Marchand P: Traumatic hiatus hernia. Br Med J 1:754, 1962.
153. Campbell JA: The diaphragm in roentgenology of the chest. Radiol Clin North Am 1:395, 1963.
154. Brünner A: Die sogenannte traumatische Zwerchfellhernie. (So-called traumatic diaphragmatic hernia.) Schweiz Med Wochenschr 86:1329, 1956.
155. Laws HL, Waldschmidt ML: Rupture of diaphragm (letter). JAMA 243:32, 1980.
156. Holm A, Bessey PQ, Aldrete JS: Diaphragmatic rupture due to blunt trauma: Morbidity and mortality in 42 cases. South Med J 81:956, 1988.
157. Ammann AM, Brewer WH, Maull KI, et al: Traumatic rupture of the diaphragm: Real-time sonographic diagnosis. Am J Roentgenol 140:915, 1983.
158. Harrison JF: Strangulated diaphragmatic hernia with haemothorax. Br J Dis Chest 57:59, 1963.
159. Salomon NW, Zukoski CF: Rupture of the right hemidiaphragm with eventration of the liver. JAMA 241:1929, 1979.
160. Fagan CJ, Schreiber MH, Amparo EG, et al: Traumatic diaphragmatic hernia into the pericardium: Verification of diagnosis by computed tomography. Case report. J Comput Assist Tomog 3:405, 1979.
161. Bell JW: Pancreatic-bronchial fistula. Am Rev Respir Dis 106:97, 1972.
162. Cox CL Jr, Anderson JN, Guest JL Jr: Bronchopancreatic fistula following traumatic rupture of the diaphragm. JAMA 237:1461, 1977.
163. Oparah SS, Mandal AK: Traumatic thoracobiliary (pleurobiliary and bronchobiliary) fistulas: Clinical and review study. J Trauma 18:539, 1978.
164. Minagi H, Brody WR, Laing FC: The variable roentgen appearance of traumatic diaphragmatic hernia. J Can Assoc Radiol 28:124, 1977.
165. Smith L, Lippert KM: Peritoneopericardial diaphragmatic hernia. Ann Surg 148:798, 1958.
166. Kümmerle F: Inkarzerationem von Magen und Darm nach traumatischen Zwerchfellrupturen. (Incarceration of the stomach and intestine after traumatic rupture of the diaphragm.) Deutsch Med Wochenschr 83:1544, 1958.
167. Dunbar JS: Fractures and pseudoarthrosis of the first rib. J Can Assoc Radiol 7:14, 1956.
168. Albers JE, Rath RK, Glaser RS, et al: Severity of intrathoracic injuries associated with 1st rib fractures. Ann Thorac Surg 33:614, 1982.
169. Wynn-Williams N, Young RD: Cough fracture of the ribs. Including one complicated by pneumothorax. Tubercle 40:47, 1959.
170. Pearson JEG: Cough fracture of the ribs. Br J Tuberc 51:251, 1957.
171. Moore JD, Mayer JH, Gago O: Traumatic asphyxia. Chest 62:634, 1972.
172. Davidson IA, Bargh W, Cruickshank AN, et al: Crush injuries of the chest. A follow-up study of patients treated in an artificial ventilation unit. Thorax 24:563, 1969.
173. Hanning CD, Ledingham E, Ledingham IMCA: Late respiratory sequelae of blunt chest injury: A preliminary report. Thorax 36:204, 1981.
174. Lee FA, Gwinn JL: Retrosternal dislocation of the clavicle. Radiology 110:631, 1974.
175. Nettles JL, Linscheid RL: Sternoclavicular dislocations. J Trauma 8:158, 1968.
176. Sebba L, Baigelman W: Post-surgical lung hernia. Am J Med Sci 284:40, 1982.
177. Bidstrup P, Nordentoft JM, Petersen B: Hernia of the lung. Brief survey and report of two cases. Acta Radiol [Diagn] (Stockh) 4:490, 1966.
178. Kyosola K, Reinikainen M, Siitonen P, et al: Lung hernia after blunt thoracic trauma. Acta Chir Scand 150:425, 1984.
179. Taylor DA, Jacobson HG: Posttraumatic herniation of the lung. Am J Roentgenol 87:896, 1962.
180. Banerjee A, Khanna SK, Narayanan PS: Chest wall pneumoma: A hitherto unreported clinical entity. Thorax 37:388, 1982.
181. Cole WS: Respiratory sequels to non-thoracic injury. Lancet 1:555, 1972.
182. Schumacker PT, Rhodes GR, Newell JC, et al: Ventilation-perfusion imbalance after head trauma. Am Rev Respir Dis 119:33, 1979.
183. Popp AJ, Shah DM, Berman RA, et al: Delayed pulmonary dysfunction in head-injured patients. J Neurosurg 57:784, 1982.
184. Dubeau L, Fraser RS: Long-term effects of pulmonary shrapnel injury. Report of a case with carcinoma and residual shrapnel tract. Arch Pathol Lab Med 108:407, 1984.
185. Larose JH: Cavitation of missile tracks in the lung. Radiology 90:995, 1968.
186. Hodson CJ: Four primarily radiological lesions found in traumatic chest cases. A preliminary report. Br J Radiol 17:296, 1944.
187. Oparah SS, Mandal AK: Penetrating gunshot wounds of the chest in civilian practice: Experience with 250 consecutive cases. Br J Surg 65:45, 1978.
188. Trombold JS, McCuistion AC, Harris HW: Slowly expanding intrapleural lesion due to a foreign body. Report of a case. N Engl J Med 264:172, 1961.
189. Wellington JL: The shrapnel awakes: Pyopneumothorax and chronic empyema resulting from a foreign body retained for 17 years. Can Med Assoc J 87:349, 1962.
190. Ekstrom D, Weiner M, Baier B: Pulmonary arteriovenous fistula as a complication of trauma. Am J Roentgenol 130:1178, 1978.
191. Gavant ML, Winer-Muram HT: Traumatic pulmonary artery pseudoaneurysm. J Can Assoc Radiol 37:108, 1986.
192. Klein CP: Gunshot wounds of the aorta with peripheral arterial bullet embolism: Report of 2 cases. Am J Roentgenol 119:547, 1973.
193. Richardson M, Gomes M, Tsou E: Transtracheal migration of an intravertebral Steinmann pin to the left bronchus. J Thorac Cardiovasc Surg 93:939, 1987.
194. Singh A, Singh B, Singh P: An interesting and unusual cause of hemoptysis. Chest 62:339, 1972.
195. Vogt-Moykopf I, Krumhaar D: Treatment of intrapulmonary shell fragments. Surg Gynecol Obstet 123:1233, 1966.
196. Kovnat DM, Anderson WM, Rath GS, et al: Hemoptysis secondary to retained transpulmonary foreign body. Am Rev Respir Dis 109:279, 1974.
197. Le Roux BT: Intrathoracic foreign bodies. Thorax 19:203, 1964.
198. Raeburn C, Spencer H: Lung scar cancers. Br J Tuberc 51:237, 1957.
199. Siddons AHM, MacArthur AM: Carcinomata developing at the site of foreign bodies in the lung. Br J Surg 39:542, 1952.
200. Strauss FH, Dordal E, Kappas A: The problem of pulmonary scar tumors. Arch Path 76:693, 1963.
201. Dalton ML Jr, Strange WH, Downs EA: Intrathoracic splenosis. Case report and review of the literature. Am Rev Respir Dis 103:827, 1971.
202. Graham JM, Mattox KL, Beall AC Jr: Penetrating trauma of the lung. J Trauma 19:665, 1979.
203. Sandrasagra FA: Penetrating thoracoabdominal injuries. Br J Surg 64:638, 1977.
204. Underwood GH Jr, Newell JD 2nd: Pulmonary radiology in the intensive care unit. Med Clin North Am 67:1305, 1983.
205. Goodman LR: Review: Postoperative chest radiograph. II. Alterations after major intrathoracic surgery. Am J Roentgenol 134:803, 1980.
206. Goodman LR, Kay HR, Teplick SK, et al: Complications of median sternotomy: Computed tomographic evaluation. Am J Roentgenol 141:225, 1983.
207. Curtis JA, Libshitz HI, Dalinka MK: Fracture of the first rib as a complication of midline sternotomy. Radiology 115:63, 1975.
208. Williams NS, Lewis CT: Bronchopleural fistula: A review of 86 cases. Br J Surg 63:520, 1976.
209. Malave G, Foster ED, Wilson JA, et al: Bronchopleural fistula—Present-day study of an old problem. A review of 52 cases. Ann Thorac Surg 11:1, 1971.
210. Leading article: Bronchopleural fistula. Br Med J 2:1093, 1976.
211. Heater K, Revzani L, Rubin JM: CT evaluation of empyema in the postpneumonectomy space. Am J Roentgenol 145:39, 1985.
212. Smiell J, Widmann WD: Bronchopleural fistulas after pneumonectomy. A problem with surgical stapling. Chest 92:1056, 1987.
213. Westcott JL, Cole SR: Interstitial pulmonary emphysema in children and adults: Roentgenographic features. Radiology 111:367, 1974.
214. Hanson RE, Kloiber R, Lesperance RR, et al: Unpublished data.

215. Peters JC, Desai KK: CT demonstration of postpneumonectomy tumor recurrence. Am J Roentgenol 141:259, 1983.
216. Gates GF, Sette RS, Cope JA: Acute cardiac herniation with incarceration following pneumonectomy. Radiology 94:561, 1970.
217. Tschersich HU, Skopara V Jr, Fleming WH: Acute cardiac herniation following pneumonectomy. Radiology 120:546, 1976.
218. Brady MB, Brogdon BG: Cardiac herniation and volvulus: Radiographic findings. Radiology 161:657, 1986.
219. Castillo M, Oldham S: Cardiac volvulus: Plain film recognition of an often fatal condition. Am J Roentgenol 145:271, 1985.
220. Hidvegi RS, Abdulnour EM, Wilson JAS: Herniation of the heart following left pneumonectomy. J Can Assoc Radiol 32:185, 1981.
221. Arndt RD, Frank CG, Schmitz AL, Haveson SB: Cardiac herniation with volvulus after pneumonectomy. Am J Roentgenol 130:155, 1978.
222. Rodgers BM, Moulder PV, DeLaney A: Thoracoscopy: New method of early diagnosis of cardiac herniation. J Thorac Cardiovasc Surg 78:623, 1979.
223. Shepard JO, Grillo HC, McLoud TC, et al: Right-pneumonectomy syndrome: Radiologic findings and CT correlation. Radiology 161:661, 1986.
224. Carter AR, Sostman HD, Curtis AM, et al: Thoracic alterations after cardiac surgery. Am J Roentgenol 140:475, 1983.
225. Hamilton W: Atelectasis, pneumothorax, and aspiration as postoperative complications. Anesthesiology 22:708, 1961.
226. Culiner MM, Reich SB, Abouav J: Nonobstructive consolidation atelectasis following thoracotomy. J Thorac Surg 37:371, 1959.
227. Gamsu G, Singer MM, Vincent HH, et al: Postoperative impairment of mucous transport in the lung. Am Rev Respir Dis 114:673, 1976.
228. Templeton AW, Almond CH, Seaber A, et al: Postoperative pulmonary patterns following cardiopulmonary bypass. Am J Roentgenol 96:1007, 1966.
229. Benjamin JJ, Cascade PN, Rubenfire M, et al: Left lower lobe atelectasis and consolidation following cardiac surgery: The effect of topical cooling on the phrenic nerve. Radiology 142:11, 1982.
230. Wilcox P, Baile EM, Hards J, et al: Phrenic nerve function and its relationship to atelectasis after coronary artery bypass surgery. Chest 93:693, 1988.
231. Mickell JJ, Oh KS, Siewers RD, et al: Clinical implications of postoperative unilateral phrenic nerve paralysis. J Thorac Cardiovasc Surg 76:297, 1978.
232. Hood RM, Beall AC Jr (sponsored by Gerbode FA): Hypoventilation, hypoxemia, and acidosis occurring in the acute postoperative period. J Thorac Surg 36:729, 1958.
233. Palmer KNV, Gardiner AJS, McGregor MH: Hypoxaemia after partial gastrectomy. Thorax 20:73, 1965.
234. Diament ML, Palmer KNV: Postoperative changes in gas tensions of arterial blood and in ventilatory function. Lancet 2:180, 1966.
235. Diament ML, Palmer KNV: Venous/arterial pulmonary shunting as the principal cause of postoperative hypoxaemia. Lancet 1:15, 1967.
236. Parfrey PS, Harte PJ, Quinlan JP, et al: Postoperative hypoxaemia and oxygen therapy. Br J Surg 64:390, 1977.
237. Hansen G, Drablos PA, Steinert R: Pulmonary complications, ventilation and blood gases after upper abdominal surgery. Acta Anaesthesiol Scand 21:211, 1977.
238. Bainbridge ET, Matthews HR: Hypoxaemia after left thoracotomy for benign oesophageal disease. Thorax 35:264, 1980.
239. Holbert JM, Libshitz HI, Chasen MH, et al: The postlobectomy chest: Anatomic considerations. RadioGraphics 7(5):889, 1987.
240. Legge JS, Palmer KNV: Pulmonary function in bronchial carcinoma. Thorax 28:588, 1973.
241. Bartlett RH, Gazzaniga AB, Geraghty TR: Respiratory maneuvers to prevent postoperative pulmonary complications. JAMA 224:1017, 1973.
242. Berecek KH, Janson SL: Influence of postanesthetic suggestion on the prevention of postoperative pulmonary complications. Chest 61:240, 1972.
243. Tokics L, Strandberg A, Brismar B, et al: Computerized tomography of the chest and gas exchange measurements during ketamine anaesthesia. Acta Anaesthesiol Scand 31:684, 1987.
244. Rehder K, Sessler AD, Marsh HM: General anesthesia and the lung. Am Rev Respir Dis 112:541, 1975.
245. Ghia J, Andersen NB: Pulmonary function and cardiopulmonary bypass. JAMA 212:593, 1970.
246. Byrd RB, Burns JR: Cough dynamics in post-thoracotomy state. Chest 67:654, 1975.
247. Yamazaki S, Ogawa J, Shohzu A, et al: Intrapleural cough pressure in patients after thoracotomy. J Thorac Cardiovasc Surg 80:600, 1980.
248. Marshall R: The nursing position after operation and the work of breathing. Thorax 24:330, 1969.
249. Legge JS, Palmer KNV: Effect of lung resection for bronchial carcinoma on pulmonary function in patients with and without chronic obstructive bronchitis. Thorax 30:563, 1975.
250. Hall DR: Regional lung function after pneumonectomy. Thorax 29:425, 1974.
251. Ali MK, Mountain C, Miller JM, et al: Regional pulmonary function before and after pneumonectomy using 133xenon. Chest 68:288, 1975.
252. Larsson S, Lepore V, Dernevik L, et al: Torsion of a lung lobe: Diagnosis and treatment. J Thorac Cardiovasc Surg 36:281, 1988.
253. Begin P, Deschamps C, Gauthier JJ, et al: Functional effects of pneumonectomy and bilobectomy for lung cancer. Respiration 46:8, 1984.
254. Begin R: Platypnea after pneumonectomy. N Engl J Med 293:342, 1975.
255. Springer RM, Gheorghiade M, Chakko CS, et al: Platypnea and interatrial right-to-left shunting after lobectomy. Am J Cardiol 51:1802, 1983.
256. Stein M, Cassara EL: Preoperative pulmonary evaluation and therapy in surgery. JAMA 211:787, 1970.
257. Olsen GN, Block AJ, Swenson EW, et al: Pulmonary function evaluation of the lung resection candidate: A prospective study. Am Rev Respir Dis 111:379, 1975.
258. Hodgkin JE, Dines DE, Didier EP: Preoperative evaluation of the patient with pulmonary disease. Mayo Clin Proc 48:114, 1973.
259. Block AJ, Olsen GN: Preoperative pulmonary function testing. JAMA 235:257, 1976.
260. Keagy BA, Schorlemmer GR, Murray GF, et al: Correlation of preoperative pulmonary function testing with clinical course in patients after pneumonectomy. Ann Thorac Surg 36:253, 1983.
261. Bria WF, Kanarek DJ, Kazemi H: Prediction of postoperative function following thoracic operations. Value of ventilation-perfusion scanning. J Thorac Cardiovasc Surg 86:186, 1983.
262. Loddenkemper R, Gabler A, Gobel D: Criteria of functional operability in patients with bronchial carcinoma: Preoperative assessment of risk and prediction of postoperative function. J Thorac Cardiovasc Surg 31:334, 1983.
263. Bins MC, Wever AM, Pauwels EK, et al: Krypton-81m ventilation studies as a parameter for lung capacity after lobectomy. Eur J Nucl Med 9:312, 1984.
264. Williams AJ, Cayton RM, Harding LK, et al: Quantitative lung scintigrams and lung function in the selection of patients for pneumonectomy. Br J Dis Chest 78:105, 1984.
265. Fogh J, Willie-Jorgensen P, Brynjolf I, et al: The predictive capacity of preoperative perfusion/ventilation scintigraphy, spirometry and x-ray of the lungs on postoperative pulmonary complications. A prospective study. Acta Anaesthesiol Scand 31:717, 1987.
266. Reichel J: Assessment of operative risk of pneumonectomy. Chest 62:570, 1972.
267. Colman NC, Schraufnagel DE, Rivington RN, et al: Exercise testing in evaluation of patients for lung resection. Am Rev Respir Dis 125:604, 1982.
268. Smith TP, Kinasewitz GT, Tucker WY, et al: Exercise capacity as a predictor of post-thoracotomy morbidity. Am Rev Respir Dis 129:730, 1984.
269. Bechard D, Wetstein L: Assessment of exercise oxygen consumption as preoperative criterion for lung resection. Ann Thorac Surg 44:344, 1987.
270. Miyoshi S, Nakahara K, Ohno K, et al: Exercise tolerance test in lung cancer patients: The relationship between exercise capacity and postthoracotomy hospital mortality. Ann Thorac Surg 44:487, 1987.
271. Maeda H, Nakahara K, Ohno K, et al: Diaphragm function after pulmonary resection. Relationship to postoperative respiratory failure. Am Rev Respir Dis 137:678, 1988.
272. Goodman LR: Review: Postoperative chest radiograph: I. Alterations after abdominal surgery. Am J Roentgenol 134:533, 1980.
273. Harman E, Lillington G: Pulmonary risk factors in surgery. Med Clin North Am 63:1289, 1979.
274. Bevan PG: Post-operative pneumoperitoneum and pulmonary collapse. Br Med J 2:609, 1961.
275. Berlyne GM, Lee HA, Ralston AJ, et al: Pulmonary complications of peritoneal dialysis. Lancet 2:75, 1966.
276. Gaensler EA, Weisel RD: The risks in abdominal and thoracic surgery in COPD. Postgrad Med 54:183, 1973.
277. Stein M, Koota GM, Simon M, et al: Pulmonary evaluation of surgical patients. JAMA 181:765, 1962.
278. Wiren JE, Janzon L: Respiratory complications following surgery. Improved prediction with preoperative spirometry. Acta Anaesthesiol Scand 27:476, 1983.
279. Martin LF, Asher EF, Casey JM, et al: Postoperative pneumonia. Determinants of mortality. Arch Surg 119:379, 1984.
280. Poe RH, Kallay MC, Dass T, et al: Can postoperative pulmonary complications after elective cholecystectomy be predicted? Am J Med Sci 295:29, 1988.
281. Wiren JE, Lindell SE, Hellekant C: Pre- and postoperative lung function in sitting and supine position related to postoperative chest x-ray abnormalities and arterial hypoxaemia. Clin Physiol 3:257, 1983.

282. Morran CG, Finlay IG, Mathieson M, et al: Randomized controlled trial of physiotherapy for postoperative complications. Br J Anaesth 55:1113, 1983.
283. Collins CD, Darke CS, Knowelden J: Chest complications after upper abdominal surgery: Their anticipation and prevention. Br Med J 1:401, 1968.
284. Wightman JAK: A prospective survey of the incidence of postoperative pulmonary complications. Br J Surg 55:85, 1968.
285. Sanders RC: Postoperative pleural effusions and subphrenic abscess. Clin Radiol 21:308, 1970.
286. Ravin CE, Putman CE, McLoud TC: Hazards of the intensive care unit. Am J Roentgenol 126:423, 1976.
287. Millikan JS, Moore EE, Steiner E, et al: Complications of tube thoracostomy for acute trauma. Am J Surg 140:738, 1980.
288. Daly RC, Mucha P, Pairolero PC, et al: The risk of percutaneous chest tube thoracostomy for blunt thoracic trauma. Ann Emerg Med 14:865, 1985.
289. Miller KS, Sahn SA: Chest tubes. Indications, technique, management and complications. Chest 91:258, 1987.
290. Dalbec DL, Krome RL: Thoracostomy. Emerg Med Clinics North Am 4:441, 1986.
291. Maurer JR, Friedman PJ, Wing VW: Thoracostomy tube in an interlobar fissure: Radiologic recognition of a potential problem. Am J Roentgenol 139:1155, 1982.
292. Stark DD, Federle MP, Goodman PC: CT and radiographic assessment of tube thoracostomy. Am J Roentgenol 141:253, 1983.
293. Webb WR, LaBerge JM: Radiographic recognition of chest tube malposition in the major fissure. Chest 85:81, 1984.
294. Fraser RS: Lung perforation complicating tube thoracostomy: Pathologic description of three cases. Hum Pathol 19:518, 1988.
295. Pingleton SK, Jeter J: Necrotizing fasciitis as a complication of tube thoracostomy. Chest 83:925, 1983.
296. Gilsanz V, Cleveland RH: Pleural reaction to thoracotomy tube. Chest 74:167, 1978.
297. Panicek DM, Randall PA, Witanovski LS, et al: Chest tube tracks. RadioGraphics 7(2):321, 1987.
298. Fein AB, Godwin JD, Moore AV, et al: Systemic artery-to-pulmonary vascular shunt: A complication of closed-tube thoracostomy. Am J Roentgenol 140:917, 1983.
299. Lurus AG, Cowen RL, Eckert JF: Systemic-pulmonary arteriovenous fistula following closed-tube thoracostomy. Radiology 92:1296, 1969.
300. Hirsch M, Maroko I, Gueron M, et al: Systemic-pulmonary arteriovenous fistula of traumatic origin: A case report. Cardiovasc Intervent Radiol 6:160, 1983.
301. Stahly TL, Tench WD: Lung entrapment and infarction by chest tube suction. Radiology 122:307, 1977.
302. Neff CC, Mueller PR, Ferrucci JT Jr, et al: Serious complications following transgression of the pleural space in drainage procedures. Radiology 152:335, 1984.
303. Nichols DM, Cooperberg PL, Golding RH, et al: The safe intercostal approach? Pleural complications in abdominal interventional radiology. Am J Roentgenol 141:1013, 1984.
304. Stark P: Inadvertent nasogastric tube insertion into the tracheobronchial tree. A hazard of new high-residual volume cuffs. Radiology 142:239, 1982.
305. Miller WT: Inadvertent tracheobronchial placement of feeding tubes. Letter to the editor. Radiology 167:875, 1988.
306. Hand RW, Kempster M, Levy JH, et al: Inadvertent transbronchial insertion of narrow-bore feeding tubes into the pleural space. JAMA 251:2396, 1984.
307. Grossman TW, Duncavage JA, Dennison B, et al: Complications associated with a narrow bore nasogastric tube. Ann Otol Rhinol Laryngol 93(5 Pt 1):460, 1984.
308. Woodall BH, Winfield DF, Bisset GS 3rd: Inadvertent tracheobronchial placement of feeding tubes. Radiology 165:727, 1987.
309. Pingleton SK, Hinthorn DR, Liu C: Enteral nutrition in patients receiving mechanical ventilation. Multiple sources of tracheal colonization include the stomach. Am J Med 80:827, 1986.
310. Twigg HL, Buckley CE: Complications of endotracheal intubation. Am J Roentgenol 109:452, 1970.
311. Bergström J: Intubation and tracheotomy in barbiturate poisoning. Int Anesthesiol Clin 4:323, 1966.
312. Conrardy PA, Goodman LR, Laing F, et al: Alteration of endotracheal tube position—Flexion and extension of the neck. Crit Care Med 4:7, 1976.
313. Goodman LR, Conrardy PA, Laing F, et al: Radiographic evaluation of endotracheal tube position. Am J Roentgenol 127:433, 1976.
314. Todres ID, deBros F, Kramer SS, et al: Endotracheal tube displacement in the newborn infant. J Pediatr 89:126, 1976.
315. Heimlich HJ, Carr GC: Transtracheal catheter technique for pulmonary rehabilitation. Ann Otol Rhinol Laryngol 94:502, 1985.
316. Fletcher EC, Nickeson D, Costarangos-Galarza C: Endotracheal mass resulting from a transtracheal oxygen catheter. Chest 93:438, 1988.
317. Christopher KL, Spofford BT, Brannin PK, et al: Transtracheal oxygen therapy for refractory hypoxemia. JAMA 256:494, 1986.
318. Baigrie RS, Morgan CD: Hemodynamic monitoring: Catheter insertion techniques, complications and trouble-shooting. Can Med Assoc J 121:885, 1979.
319. Mitchell SE, Clark RA: Complications of central venous catheterization. Am J Roentgenol 133:467, 1979.
320. Mitchell SE, Clark RA: Complications of central venous catheterization. Am J Roentgenol 133:467, 1979.
321. McGoon MD, Benedetto PW, Greene BM: Complications of percutaneous central venous catheterization: A report of two cases and review of the literature. Johns Hopkins Med J 145:1, 1979.
322. Weiner P, Sznajder I, Plavnick L, et al: Unusual complications of subclavian vein catheterization. Crit Care Med 12:538, 1984.
323. Kappes S, Towne J, Adams M, et al: Perforation of the superior vena cava: A complication of subclavian dialysis. JAMA 249:2232, 1983.
324. Ciment LM, Rotbart A, Galbut RN: Contralateral effusions secondary to subclavian venous catheters. Report of two cases. Chest 83:926, 1983.
325. Scott WL: Complications associated with central venous catheters. A survey. Chest 94(6):1221, 1988.
326. Fletcher JP, Little JM: Subclavian vein catheterisation for parenteral nutrition. Ann R Coll Surg Engl 70:150, 1988.
327. Dunbar RD, Mitchell R, Lavine M: Aberrant locations of central venous catheters. Lancet 1:711, 1981.
328. Langston CS: The aberrant central venous catheter and its complications. Radiology 100:55, 1971.
329. Walters MB, Stanger HAD, Rotem CE: Complications with percutaneous central venous catheters. JAMA 220:1455, 1972.
330. Maggs PR, Schwaber JR: Fatal bilateral pneumothoraces complicating subclavian vein catheterization. Chest 71:552, 1977.
331. Dronen S, Thompson B, Nowak R, et al: Subclavian vein catheterization during cardiopulmonary resuscitation. JAMA 247:3227, 1982.
332. Abraham E, Shapiro M, Podolsky S: Central venous catheterization in the emergency setting. Crit Care Med 11:515, 1983.
333. Armstrong CW, Mayhall CG: Contralateral hydrothorax following subclavian catheter replacement using a guidewire. Chest 84:231, 1983.
334. Schorlemmer GR, Khouri RK, Murray GF, et al: Bilateral pneumothoraces secondary to iatrogenic buffalo chest. An unusual complication of median sternotomy and subclavian vein catheterization. Ann Surg 199:372, 1984.
335. Shiloni E, Meretyk S, Weiss Y: Tension haemothorax: An unusual complication of central vein catheterization. Injury 16:385, 1985.
336. Holt S, Myerscough E: Pneumothorax and hydrothorax after subclavian vein cannulation. Postgrad Med J 53:226, 1977.
337. Apps MC, Clark JMF, Skeates SJ: Hydrothorax, a complication of the insertion of central venous cannulae. Intensive Care Med 3:41, 1977.
338. LaPenna R, Whinnery C: An unusual complication of subclavian vein catheterization for total parenteral nutrition. Postgrad Med 64:171, 1978.
339. Mitchell A, Steer HW: Late appearance of pneumothorax after subclavian vein catheterization: An anaesthetic hazard. Br Med J 281:1339, 1980.
340. Chute E, Cerrs FB: Late development of hydrothorax and hydromediastinum in patients with central venous catheters. Crit Care Med 10:868, 1982.
341. Ghani GA, Berry AJ: Right hydrothorax after left external jugular vein catheterization. Anesthesiology 58:93, 1983.
342. Iberti TJ, Katz LB, Reiner MA, et al: Hydrothorax as a late complication of central venous indwelling catheters. Surgery 94:842, 1983.
343. McDonnell PJ, Qualman SJ, Hutchins GM: Bilateral hydrothorax as a life-threatening complication of central venous hyperalimentation. Surg Gynecol Obstet 158:577, 1984.
344. Damtew B, Lewandowski K: Hydrothorax, hydromediastinum and pericardial effusion: A complication of intravenous alimentation. Can Med Assoc J 130:1573, 1984.
345. Molinari PS, Belani KG, Buckley JJ: Delayed hydrothorax following percutaneous central venous cannulation. Acta Anaesthesiol Scand 28:493, 1984.
346. Tocino IM, Watanabe A: Impending catheter perforation of superior vena cava: Radiographic recognition. Am J Roentgenol 146:487, 1986.
347. Paskin DL, Hoffman WS, Tuddenham WJ: A new complication of subclavian vein catheterization. Ann Surg 179:266, 1974.
348. Knight L, Tobin J Jr, L'Heureux P: Hydrothorax: A complication of hyperalimentation with radiologic manifestations. Radiology, 111:693, 1974.
349. Kotozoglou T, Mambo N: Fatal retropleural hematoma complicating internal jugular vein catheterization. A case report. Am J Forensic Med Pathol 4:125, 1983.
350. Usselman JA, Seat SG: Superior caval catheter displacement causing bilateral pleural effusions. Am J Roentgenol 133:738, 1979.

351. Hamilton S, Thompson AD, Jamieson WRE, et al: Arteriography in catheter-induced rupture of the pulmonary artery. J Can Assoc Radiol 34:326, 1983.
352. Topaz O, Sharon M, Rechavia E, et al: Traumatic internal jugular vein cannulation. Ann Emerg Med 16:1394, 1987.
353. Tapson JS, Uldall PR: Fatal hemothorax caused by a subclavian hemodialysis catheter. Thoughts on prevention. Arch Intern Med 144:1685, 1984.
354. Brennan MF, Sugarbaker PH, Moore FD: Venobronchial fistula. A rare complication of central venous catheterization for parenteral hyperalimentation. Arch Surg 106:871, 1973.
355. Demey HE, Colemont LJ, Hartoko TJ, et al: Venopulmonary fistula: A rare complication of central venous catheterization. J Parenter Enteral Nutr 11:580, 1987.
356. Norman WJ, Moule NJ, Walrond ER: Lung abscess: A complication of malposition of a central venous catheter. Br J Radiol 47:498, 1974.
357. Johnson CL, Lazarchick J, Lynn HB: Subclavian venipuncture: Preventable complications; report of two cases. Mayo Clin Proc 45:712, 1970.
358. Flanagan JP, Gradisar IA, Gross RJ, et al: Air embolus—a lethal complication of subclavian venipuncture. N Engl J Med 281:488, 1969.
359. Hunt R, Hunter TB: Cardiac tamponade and death from perforation of the right atrium by a central venous catheter. Letter to the editor. Am J Roentgenol 151:1250, 1988.
360. Rossleigh MA: Unusual complication of intravenous catheterisation. Med J Australia 1:236, 1982.
361. Swan HJC, Ganz W, Forrester J, et al: Catheterization of the heart in man with use of a flow-directed balloon-tipped catheter. N Engl J Med 283:447, 1970.
362. Goodman DJ, Rider AK, Billingham ME, et al: Thromboembolic complications with the indwelling balloon-tipped pulmonary arterial catheter. N Engl J Med 291:777, 1974.
363. Foote GA, Schabel SI, Hodges M: Pulmonary complications of the flow-directed balloon-tipped catheter. N Engl J Med 290:927, 1974.
364. McCloud TC, Putman CE: Radiology of the Swan-Ganz catheter and associated pulmonary complications. Radiology 116:19, 1975.
365. Katz JD, Cronau LH, Barash PG, et al: Pulmonary artery flow-guided catheters in the perioperative period. Indications and complications. JAMA 237:2832, 1977.
366. Dieden JD, Friloux LA III, Renner JW: Pulmonary artery false aneurysms secondary to Swan-Ganz pulmonary artery catheters. Am J Roentgenol 149:901, 1987.
367. Davis SD, Neithamer CD, Schreiber TS, et al: False pulmonary artery aneurysm induced by Swan-Ganz catheter: Diagnosis and embolotherapy. Radiology 164:741, 1987.
368. Katz JD, Cronau LH, Barash PG, et al: Pulmonary artery flow-guided catheters in the perioperative period. Indications and complications. JAMA 237:2832, 1977.
369. Chun GMH, Ellestad MH: Perforation of the pulmonary artery by a Swan-Ganz catheter. N Engl J Med 284:1041, 1971.
370. Shin MS, Ho K-J: Cavitary pulmonary lesions complicating use of flow-directed balloon-tipped catheters in two cases. Am J Roentgenol 132:650, 1979.
371. Fraser RS: Catheter-induced pulmonary artery perforation: Pathologic and pathogenic features. Hum Pathol 18:1246, 1987.
372. Stone JG, Khambatta HJ, McDaniel DD: Catheter-induced pulmonary arterial trauma: Can it always be averted? J Thorac Cardiovasc Surg 86:146, 1983.
373. Rosenblum SE, Ratliff NB, Shirey EK, et al: Pulmonary artery dissection induced by a Swan-Ganz catheter. Cleve Clin Q 51:671, 1984.
374. Forman MB, Obel IWP: Pulmonary haemorrhage following Swan-Ganz catheterization in a patient without severe pulmonary hypertension. S Afr Med J 58:329, 1980.
375. Hannan AT, Brown M, Bigman O: Pulmonary artery catheter-induced hemorrhage. Chest 85:128, 1984.
376. Pellegrini RV, Marcelli GD, DiMarco RF, et al: Swan-Ganz catheter induced pulmonary hemorrhage. J Cardiovasc Surg 28:646, 1987.
377. Rubin SA, Puckett RP: Pulmonary artery—Bronchial fistula: A new complication of Swan-Ganz catheterization. Chest 75:515, 1979.
378. Kron IL, Piepgrass W, Carabello B, et al: False aneurysm of the pulmonary artery: A complication of pulmonary artery catheterization. Ann Thorac Surg 33:629, 1982.
379. Woodcock TE, Murray S, Ledingham IM: Mixed venous oxygen saturation changes during tension pneumothorax and its treatment. Anaesthesia 39:1004, 1984.
380. Michel L, Marsh HM, McMichan JC, et al: Infection of pulmonary artery catheters in critically ill patients. JAMA 245:1032, 1981.
381. Vicente Rull JR, Loza Aquirre J, de la Puerta E: Thrombocytopenia induced by pulmonary artery flotation catheters: A prospective study. Intensive Care Med 10:29, 1984.
382. Tooker J, Huseby J, Butler J: The effect of Swan-Ganz catheter

383. Shasby DM, Dauber IM, Pfister S, et al: Swan-Ganz catheter location and left atrial pressure determine the accuracy of the wedge pressure when positive end expiratory pressure is used. Chest 80:666, 1981.
384. Brown BG, Goldfarb D, Topaz SR, et al: Diastolic augmentation by intra-aortic balloon. Circulatory hemodynamics and treatment of severe acute left ventricular failure in dogs. J Thorac Cardiovasc Surg 53:789, 1967.
385. Hyson EA, Ravin CE, Kelley MJ, et al: Intra-aortic counterpulsation balloon: Radiographic considerations. Am J Roentgenol 128:915, 1977.
386. Filice R, Hutton L, Klein G: Cardiac pacemaker leads—A radiograph perspective. J Can Assoc Radiol 35:20, 1984.
387. Steiner RM, Tegtmeyer CJ, Morse D, et al: The radiology of cardiac pacemakers. RadioGraphics 6(3):373, 1986.
388. Goodman LR, Almassi GH, Troup PJ, et al: Complications of automatic implantable cardioverter defibrillators: Radiographic CT and echocardiographic evaluation. Radiology 170:447, 1989.
389. Gross NJ: Pulmonary effects of radiation therapy. Ann Intern Med 86:81, 1977.
390. Chacko DC: Considerations in the diagnosis of radiation injury. JAMA 245:1255, 1981.
391. Cooper G Jr, Guerrant JL, Harden AG, et al: Some consequences of pulmonary irradiation. Am J Roentgenol 85:865, 1961.
392. Jones PW, Al-Hillawi A, Wakefield JM, et al: Differences in the effect of mediastinal radiotherapy on lung function and the ventilatory response to exercise. Clin Sci 67:389, 1984.
393. Rubin P, Casarett GW: Clinical Radiation Pathology. Vol. I. Philadelphia, WB Saunders, 1968.
394. Bloomer WD, Hellman S: Normal tissue responses to radiation therapy. N Engl J Med 293:80, 1975.
395. Jennings FL, Arden A: Development of radiation pneumonitis. Time and dose factors. Arch Pathol 74:351, 1962.
396. Fleming JAC, Filbee JF, Wiernik G: Sequelae to radical irradiation in carcinoma of the breast. An inquiry into the incidence of certain radiation injuries. Br J Radiol 34:713, 1961.
397. Lougheed MN, Maguire GH: Irradiation pneumonitis in the treatment of carcinoma of the breast. J Can Assoc Radiol 11:1, 1960.
398. Wiernik G: Radiation pneumonitis following a low dose of cobalt teletherapy. Br J Radiol 38:312, 1965.
399. Gish JR, Coates EO, DuSault LA, et al: Pulmonary radiation reaction: A vital-capacity and time-dose study. Radiology 73:679, 1959.
400. Ellis F: Dose, time and fractionation: A clinical hypothesis. Clin Radiol 20:1, 1969.
401. Wara WM, Phillips TL, Margolis LW, et al: Radiation pneumonitis: A new approach to the derivation of time-dose factors. Cancer 32:547, 1973.
402. Parris TM, Knight JG, Hess CE, et al: Severe radiation pneumonitis precipitated by withdrawal of corticosteroids: A diagnostic and therapeutic dilemma. Am J Roentgenol 132:284, 1979.
403. Parris TM, Knight JG, Hess CE, et al: Severe radiation pneumonitis precipitated by withdrawal of corticosteroids: A diagnostic and therapeutic dilemma. Am J Roentgenol 132:284, 1979.
404. Pezner RD, Bertrand M, Cecchi GR, et al: Steroid-withdrawal radiation pneumonitis in cancer patients. Chest 85:816, 1984.
405. Trask CWL, Joannides T, Harper PG, et al: Radiation-induced lung fibrosis after treatment of small cell carcinoma of the lung with very high-dose cyclophosphamide. Cancer 55:57, 1985.
406. Hoffbrand BI, Gillam PMS, Heaf PJD: Effect of chronic bronchitis on changes in pulmonary function caused by irradiation of the lungs. Thorax 20:303, 1965.
407. Pickrell JA, Harris DV, Mauderly JL, et al: Altered collagen metabolism in radiation-induced interstitial pulmonary fibrosis. Chest 69:311, 1976.
408. Leading article: Case of acute radiation injury. Br Med J 2:574, 1974.
409. Muggenberg BA, Mauderly JL, Boecker BB, et al: Prevention of radiation pneumonitis from inhaled cerium-144 by lung lavage in beagle dogs. Am Rev Respir Dis 111:795, 1975.
410. Gross NJ: The pathogenesis of radiation-induced lung damage. Lung 159:115, 1981.
411. Adamson IYR, Bowden DH: Endothelial injury and repair in radiation-induced pulmonary fibrosis. Am J Pathol 112:224, 1983.
412. Roswit B, White DC: Severe radiation injuries of the lung. Am J Roentgenol 129:127, 1977.
413. Gibson PG, Bryant DH, Morgan GW, et al: Radiation-induced lung injury: A hypersensitivity pneumonitis? Ann Intern Med 109:288, 1988.
414. Leeds SE, Reich S, Uhley HN, et al: The pulmonary lymph flow after irradiation of the lungs of dogs. Chest 59:203, 1971.
415. Smith JC: Radiation pneumonitis. Case report of bilateral reaction after unilateral irradiation. Am Rev Respir Dis 89:264, 1964.

height on the wedge pressure-left atrial pressure relationship in edema during positive-pressure ventilation. Am Rev Respir Dis 117:721, 1978.

416. Fajardo LF, Berthrong M: Radiation injury in surgical pathology. Am J Surg Pathol 2:159, 1978.

417. Heppleston AG, Young AE: Population and ultrastructural changes in murine alveolar cells following $^{239}PuO_2$ inhalation. J Pathol 146:155, 1985.

418. Slauson DO, Hahn FF, Chiffelle TL: The pulmonary vascular pathology of experimental radiation pneumonitis. Am J Pathol 88:635, 1977.

419. Adamson IYR, Bowden DH, Wyatt JP: A pathway to pulmonary fibrosis: An ultrastructural study of mouse and rat following radiation to the whole body and hemithorax. Am J Pathol 58:481, 1970.

420. Phillips TL: An ultrastructural study of the development of radiation injury in the lung. Radiology 87:49, 1966.

421. Teates CD: The effects of unilateral thoracic irradiation on pulmonary blood flow. Am J Roentgenol 102:875, 1968.

422. Schreiner BF Jr, Michaelson SM, Yuile CL: The effects of thoracic irradiation upon cardiopulmonary function in the dog. Am Rev Respir Dis 99:205, 1969.

423. Bennett DE, Million RR, Ackerman LV: Bilateral radiation pneumonitis: A complication of the radiotherapy of bronchogenic carcinoma. (Report and analysis of seven cases with autopsy.) Cancer 23:1001, 1969.

424. Borgström K-E, Gynning I: Roentgenographic changes in the lungs and vertebrae during intense rotation roentgen therapy of esophageal cancer. Acta Radiol 47:281, 1957.

425. Lichtenstein H: X-ray diagnosis of radiation injuries of the lung. Dis Chest 38:294, 1960.

426. Smith JC: Radiation pneumonitis. A review. Am Rev Respir Dis 87:647, 1963.

427. Teates D, Cooper G Jr: Some consequences of pulmonary irradiation. A second long-term report. Am J Roentgenol 96:612, 1966.

428. Polansky SM, Ravin CE, Prosnitz LR: Pulmonary changes after primary irradiation for early breast carcinoma. Am J Roentgenol 134:101, 1980.

429. Mah K, Poon PY, Van Dyk J, et al: Assessment of acute radiation-induced pulmonary changes using computed tomography. J Comput Assist Tomogr 10:736, 1986.

430. Goldman AL, Enquist R: Hyperacute radiation pneumonitis. Chest 67:613, 1975.

431. Farmer W, Ravin C, Schachter EN: Hyperlucent lung after radiation therapy. Am Rev Respir Dis 112:255, 1975.

432. Berdon WE, Baker DH, Boyer J: Unusual benign and malignant sequelae to childhood radiation therapy including "unilateral hyperlucent lung." Am J Roentgenol 93:545, 1965.

433. Bateman NT, Croft DN: False-positive lung scans and radiotherapy. Br Med J 1:807, 1976.

434. Harnsberger HR, Armstrong JD II: Bilateral superomedial hilar displacement: A unique sign of previous mediastinal radiation. Radiology 147:35, 1983.

435. Libshitz HI, Southard ME: Complications of radiation therapy: The thorax. Sem Roentgenol 9:41, 1974.

436. Bourgouin P, Cousineau G, Lemire P, et al: Differentiation of radiation-induced fibrosis from recurrent pulmonary neoplasm by CT. J Can Assoc Radiol 38:23, 1987.

437. Bachman AL, Macken K: Pleural effusions following supervoltage radiation for breast carcinoma. Radiology 72:699, 1959.

438. Whitcomb ME, Schwarz MI: Pleural effusion complicating intensive mediastinal radiation therapy. Am Rev Respir Dis 103:100, 1971.

439. Deeley TJ: The effects of radiation on the lungs in the treatment of carcinoma of the bronchus. Clin Radiol 11:33, 1960.

440. Srinivasan G, Kurtz DW, Lichter AS: Pleural-based changes on chest x-ray after irradiation for primary breast cancer: Correlation with findings on computerized tomography. Int J Radiat Oncol Biol Phys 9:1567, 1983.

441. Posner MR, Cohen GI, Skarin AT: Pericardial disease in patients with cancer: The differentiation of malignant from idiopathic and radiation-induced pericarditis. Am J Med 71:407, 1981.

442. Gomm SA, Stretton TB: Chronic pericardial effusion after mediastinal radiotherapy. Thorax 36:149, 1981.

443. Gomm SA, Stretton TB: Chronic pericardial effusion after mediastinal radiotherapy. Thorax 36:149, 1981.

444. Applefield MM, Cole JF, Pollock SH, et al: The late appearance of chronic pericardial disease in patients treated by radiotherapy for Hodgkin's disease. Ann Intern Med 94:338, 1981.

445. Cameron SJ, Grant IWB, Lutz W, et al: The early effect of irradiation on ventilatory function in bronchial carcinoma. Clin Radiol 20:12, 1969.

446. Cameron SJ, Grant IWB, Pearson JG, et al: Prednisolone and mustine in prevention of tumour swelling during pulmonary irradiation. Br Med J 1:535, 1972.

447. Sadove AM, Block M, Rossof AH, et al: Radiation carcinogenesis in man: New primary neoplasms in fields of prior therapeutic radiation. Cancer 48:1139, 1981.

448. Nelson DF, Cooper S, Weston MG, et al: Second malignant neo-plasms in patients treated for Hodgkin's disease with radiotherapy or radiotherapy and chemotherapy. Cancer 48:2386, 1981.

449. Doll R: Radiation hazards: 25 years of collaborative research. Br J Radiol 54:179, 1981.

450. Smith PG, Doll R: Mortality from cancer and all causes among British radiologists. Br J Radiol 4:187, 1981.

451. Kerr CB: Health consequences of environmental pollution by ionizing radiation. Med J Australia 1:685, 1981.

452. Bross IDJ, Natarajan N: Genetic damage from diagnostic radiation. JAMA 237:2399, 1977.

453. Matthay RA, Zorn SK, Mitchell MS, et al: Lung carcinoma, a complication of therapy for Hodgkin's disease? Am Rev Respir Dis 113:138, 1976.

454. Editorial: More hazards of radiation. N Engl J Med 279:714, 1968.

455. Rodman T, Karr S, Close HP: Radiation reaction in the lung. Report of a fatal case in a patient with carcinoma of the lung, with studies of pulmonary function before and during prednisone therapy. N Engl J Med 262:431, 1960.

456. Kanagami H, Baba K, Ogata K, et al: Clinical aspects of radiation fibrosis of the lung with emphasis on respiratory function. Jap J Chest Dis (Nippon Kyobu Rinsho) 21:682, 1962.

457. Cudkowicz L, Cunningham M, Haldane EV: Effects of mediastinal irradiation upon respiratory function following mastectomy for carcinoma of breast. Thorax 24:359, 1969.

458. Brady LW, Germon PA, Cander L: The effects of radiation therapy on pulmonary function in carcinoma of the lung. Radiology 85:130, 1965.

459. Teates CD: Effect of unilateral-thoracic irradiation on lung function. J Appl Physiol 20:628, 1965.

460. Shrivastava PN, Hans L, Concannon JP: Changes in pulmonary compliance and production of fibrosis in x-irradiated lungs of rats. Radiology 112:439, 1974.

461. Prato FS, Kurdyak R, Saibil EA, et al: Physiological and radiographic assessment during the development of pulmonary radiation fibrosis. Radiology 122:389, 1977.

462. Bertino RE, Wesbey GE, Johnson RJ: Horner syndrome occurring as a complication of chest tube placement. Radiology 164:745, 1987.

463. Boyd KD, Thomas SJ, Gold J, et al: A prospective study of complications of pulmonary artery catheterizations in 500 consecutive patients. Chest 84:245, 1983.

464. Dennis LN, Rogers LF: Superior mediastinal widening from spine fractures mimicking aortic rupture on chest radiographs. Am J Roentgenol 152:27, 1989.

465. Mirvis SE, Bidwell JK, Buddemeyer EU, et al: Imaging diagnosis of traumatic aortic rupture. A review and experience at a major trauma center. Invest Radiol 22:187, 1987.

466. Serry C, Bleck PC, Javid H, et al: Sternal wound complications. Management and results. J Thorac Cardiovasc Surg 80:861, 1980.

467. Connors AF, Hammon WE, Martin RJ, et al: Chest physical therapy. The immediate effect on oxygenation in acutely ill patients. Chest Physical Therapy 78:559, 1980.

468. Huseby J, Hudson L, Stark K, et al: Oxygenation during chest physiotherapy. Chest 70:430, 1976.

469. Holody B, Goldberg HS: The effect of mechanical vibration physiotherapy on arterial oxygenation in acutely ill patients with atelectasis or pneumonia. Am Rev Respir Dis 124:372, 1981.

470. Zidulka A, Chrome JF, Wight DW, et al: Clapping or percussion causes atelectasis in dogs and influences gas exchange. J Appl Physiol 66:2833, 1989.

471. Aronchick JM, Epstein DM, Gefter WB, et al: Chronic traumatic diaphragmatic hernia: The significance of pleural effusion. Radiology 168:675, 1988.

472. Radin DR, Ray MJ, Halls JM: Strangulated diaphragmatic hernia with pneumothorax due to colopleural fistula. Am J Roentgenol 146:321, 1986.

473. Markos J, Mullan BP, Hillman DR, et al: Preoperative assessment as a predictor of mortality and morbidity after lung resection. Am Rev Respir Dis 139:902, 1989.

474. Ellis LM, Vogel SB, Copeland EM 3rd: Central venous catheter vascular erosions. Diagnosis and clinical course. Ann Surg 209:475, 1989.

475. Milam MG, Sahn SA: Horner's syndrome secondary to hydromediastinum. A complication of extravascular migration of a central venous catheter. Chest 94:1093, 1988.

476. Westcott JL, Cole S: Plate atelectasis. Radiology 155:1, 1985.

477. Kerns SR, Gay SB: CT of blunt chest trauma. Am J Roentgenol 154:55, 1990.

478. Unger JM, Schuchmann GG, Grossman JE, et al: Tears of the trachea and main bronchi caused by blunt trauma: Radiologic findings. Am J Roentgenol 153:1175, 1989.

479. Bhalla M, Leitman BS, Forcade C, et al: Lung hernia: Radiographic features. Am J Roentgenol 154:51, 1990.

480. Smith GM, Reed JC, Choplin RH: Radiographic detection of esophageal malpositioning of endotracheal tubes. Am J Roentgenol 154:23, 1990.

Metabolic Pulmonary Disease

The diseases covered in this chapter, except for certain additions, were considered in the chapter, "Diseases of the Chest of Unknown Origin," in previous editions of this book. The decision to place them in a separate chapter in this edition is based on their generally accepted, or suspected, metabolic or endocrine etiology. It should be noted that many of these diseases have an inherited component.

PULMONARY ALVEOLAR PROTEINOSIS

Recognition of this rare, but fascinating, disease (also known as alveolar lipoproteinosis) has been relatively recent; it was reported for the first time by Rosen and his colleagues in 1958.[1] The disease is characterized by the deposition of a somewhat granular material high in protein and lipid content within the airspaces of the lung. The alveolar walls and interstitial tissue characteristically are normal or almost so. Although the disease occurs predominantly in patients between the ages of 20 and 50 years, very young children constitute an additional susceptible group; a number of pathologically confirmed cases have been described in infants and children.[2-5] There is a male-to-female predominance of about 2 to 1. According to Bedrossian and colleagues, approximately 260 cases had been reported by 1980.[6]

ETIOLOGY AND PATHOGENESIS

The etiology and pathogenesis of alveolar proteinosis are poorly understood. However, the bulk of evidence suggests an abnormality of the metabolism of surfactant or its clearance by alveolar macrophages. For this reason, the disease is included in this chapter, although it is possible that factors other than, or in addition to, those involved with surfactant metabolism may be important in pathogenesis.

In both humans and experimental animals, alveolar proteinosis is seen in a variety of settings. This suggests that multiple factors may be involved in the pathogenesis and that the histologic appearance characteristic of the disease may represent a final common pathway of a number of distinct pulmonary insults. These settings include the following:

(1) An immunocompromised state, especially lymphopenia, thymic aplasia, and immunoglobulin deficiency in infants and children[7] and lymphoma and leukemia in adults.[6, 8–11] Occasional cases also have been reported in patients with AIDS[12] and autoimmune connective tissue diseases.[13] Although it has been suggested that the drugs used in the therapy of some of these conditions may be responsible for the proteinosis,[11] a more attractive hypothesis is that the underlying immunodeficiency is reflected in malfunction of alveolar macrophages[6] that, in turn, leads to the accumulation of the abnormal intra-alveolar material (see farther on).

(2) Rarely, in infants and young children without evidence of underlying systemic disease.[14, 15] Some of these individuals have been siblings;[4, 16] in at least two and possibly three instances, histories of consanguinity have been obtained, strongly suggesting the possibility of a genetic factor in at least some individuals. However, in the majority of cases no family history of the disease can be elicited.

(3) In experimental animals following exposure to a variety of airborne dusts, including aluminum powder, quartz,[17–19] and fiberglass,[20] and in humans exposed to a high concentration of silicon dioxide (acute silicoproteinosis, see page 2283).[21] The early stage of the disease in animals is manifested by the presence of extruded lamellar bodies from type II pneumocytes; these are phagocytosed by alveolar macrophages that rapidly become rounded up and appear less mobile.[17] The macrophages subsequently break down and release a fine granular substance resembling that found in human alveolar proteinosis.

(4) In association with a variety of microorganisms, especially *Nocardia* sp., *Aspergillus* sp., and *Cryptococcus* sp.;[6, 16] other agents such as cytomegalovirus,[22] *Mycobacterium tuberculosis*, nontuberculous mycobacteria, *Histoplasma capsulatum*, *Candida* sp., *Mucorales* sp., and herpesvirus have been reported less frequently.[6] Although it has been suggested that the organisms themselves may be the cause of the proteinosis,[6, 22] it seems more likely that their presence is secondary and is the result of either an abnormality of macrophage function or the presence of a favorable growth environment provided by the intra-alveolar proteinaceous material (or perhaps both factors).

As the above discussion suggests, an abnormality of surfactant production, metabolism, or clearance (or a combination of these) has been strongly implicated in the pathogenesis of the disease. Many experimental investigations have attempted to confirm and elaborate upon this hypothesis. One line of study has concerned the nature of the intra-alveolar material itself. Ultrastructural investigations have shown it to consist of amorphous debris containing numerous laminated osmiophilic bodies resembling tubular myelin and the lamellar bodies of type II pneumocytes.[23–25] This suggests that at least part of the intra-alveolar material is derived from these cells and that it may represent surfactant or a component thereof. This interpretation has been supported by the immunohistochemical demonstration of a positive reaction of the intra-alveolar material to an antisurfactant antibody.[26]

In addition to these anatomic investigations, a number of studies have been directed toward determining the biochemical nature of the extracellular material obtained either by BAL or from tissue.[16, 27–33] Most authorities agree that the tissue and washings contain phospholipids, principally palmitoyl lecithin, and that the lipids and proteins are similar to those obtained in normal subjects but in increased amounts. However, some workers have described specific lipids[31] and proteins[27] in BAL fluid that are not present in normal alveolar fluid. In addition, the specific components of the fluid may not be the same in different individuals with the disease; for example, in a comparison of the BAL fluid from two patients with alveolar proteinosis, one who recovered completely and one who required repeated alveolar lavages,[29] glycoproteins were found in both patients but glycosaminoglycans only in the patient with the poor prognosis.

Thus, good evidence exists that the material accumulating within the alveoli in alveolar proteinosis is derived from type II pneumocytes and that it represents surfactant or a component thereof. There is still considerable uncertainty, however, about the cause of its accumulation. It has been suggested that an overproduction of surfactant by hyperplastic or abnormally stimulated type II pneumocytes may be responsible; however, Ramirez and Harlan[32, 33] were unable to detect any enhancement of lipid synthesis and concluded that either the removal of alveolar phospholipid is impaired or that its degradation is defective. In fact, several experiments have provided evidence of abnormal macrophage function, including impaired phagocytosis and defective antimicrobial activity.[34] The basis for the macrophage dysfunction is itself unclear. As discussed previously, Bedrossian and colleagues[6] have suggested that an underlying immunodeficiency state may be involved; however, the rarity of alveolar proteinosis compared with the relatively common occurrence of immunodeficiency states clearly indicates that other factors must be involved. It is possible that large amounts of inhaled

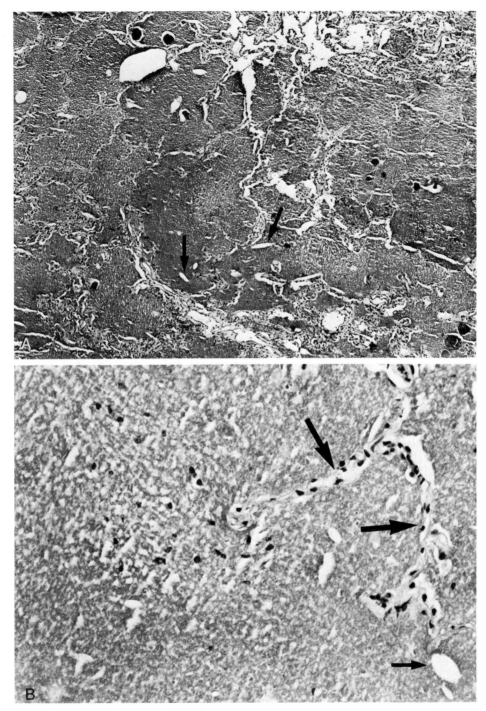

Figure 16–1. Pulmonary Alveolar Proteinosis. A histologic section of lung parenchyma *(A)* shows the alveolar airspaces to be almost completely filled by amorphous, finely granular, PAS-positive material (seen to better advantage at greater magnification in *B*). Scattered oval or elongated crystal-like spaces *(small arrows)* and mononuclear cells (lymphocytes and macrophages) are present within the material. The alveolar septa *(larger arrows in B)* are normal. (A × 50; B × 250; both PAS.)

inorganic dusts are toxic to alveolar macrophages and explain the development of alveolar proteinosis in association with silicosis. An understanding of the underlying cause of macrophage dysfunction is made more difficult by *in vitro*[35-37] and animal[17] studies in which the phagocytic function of alveolar macrophages has been shown to be suppressed by the lipoproteinaceous debris itself; this suggests that once the condition has begun a positive feedback mechanism acts to cause its continuation and possibly its worsening.

Immunologic mechanisms also may be involved in the pathogenesis of the disease.[27] For example, the production of DIP-like changes in rabbits following the intravenous injection of complete Freund's adjuvant[38] and the subsequent development of alveolar proteinosis after a second injection 2 to 4 weeks later strongly suggest some immunologic component.[39]

PATHOLOGIC CHARACTERISTICS

At autopsy, the lungs are heavy and firm; cut sections show patchy or diffuse consolidation, but the normal architecture is preserved unless there is superimposed infection. A viscous, yellowish fluid may ooze from the cut surface.[6] Microscopically, the walls of transitional airways and alveoli are usually normal or at most slightly thickened by a lymphocytic infiltrate;[40, 41] rarely, interstitial fibrosis (sometimes severe) has been described.[15, 42-44] The alveoli are filled with a finely granular, proteinaceous material that is rich in lipids and that stains eosinophilic with H&E and deep pink with para-aminosalicylic acid (PAS) (Fig. 16–1); on frozen section the material may be basophilic.[45] Acicular crystals and laminated bodies that stain with varying intensity and are believed to be cellular fragments are also seen. Intact and apparently degenerating macrophages are present within the granular material but are usually not abundant except focally at the border between normal and affected lung.

Ultrastructural investigation shows the intra-alveolar material to consist of amorphous granular debris containing numerous relatively discrete inclusions consisting of densely osmiophilic granules or moderately osmiophilic lamellar bodies, some of which resemble tubular myelin (Fig. 16–2).[23-25]

Because many patients with alveolar proteinosis recover spontaneously and their chest roentgenograms return to normal, it is thought that the intra-alveolar material is partly expectorated and partly phagocytosed and removed by the lymphatics.[46] Although enlargement of hilar lymph nodes is not apparent, either roentgenologically or pathologically, a case has been reported in which proteinaceous material was identified in a supraclavicular lymph node.[47]

ROENTGENOGRAPHIC MANIFESTATIONS

The roentgenographic pattern, with rare exceptions, is bilateral and symmetrical[48] and is identical in both distribution and character to that of pulmonary edema (Fig. 16–3). Since the process is one of airspace consolidation, the basic lesion is the acinar shadow. Confluence of acinar shadows is the rule, with the production of irregular, rather poorly defined, patchy shadows scattered widely throughout the lungs. In many cases the shadows are distributed in a "butterfly" or "bat's wing" pattern (Fig. 16–4) that is sometimes seen in pulmonary edema and commonly, but falsely, attributed to uremia.[49-51] Differentiation of the roentgenographic pattern from that of pulmonary edema of cardiac origin may be difficult, but the absence of other signs of pulmonary venous hypertension should be of considerable help: there is no tendency to cardiac enlargement, there are no signs of interstitial edema, and there is no evidence of upper lobe vessel distention. Occasionally, the roentgenographic pattern simulates diffuse interstitial lung disease despite pathologic confirmation of its predominantly alveolar location,[16, 52, 53] a paradox that also has been observed on CT scans (Fig. 16–5).[54] This may be caused by very patchy, incomplete alveolar filling wherein irregular subacinar, rather than acinar, shadows project as a reticulonodular pattern. Similarly, the development of Kerley B lines has been reported[46] and probably is related to lymphatic obstruction. These appearances render differential diagnosis even more difficult. In children, as might be expected, acinar opacities are considerably smaller than in adults, and this should be taken into consideration in pattern recognition.[2]

Resolution usually is complete roentgenographically but can occur asymmetrically and in a spotty fashion; occasionally, new foci of airspace consolidation develop in areas not previously affected.[46, 49] The formation of denser nodules and linear streaking were described by Greenspan, who suggested that these may represent pulmonary fibrosis.[49] Resolution may be associated with manifestations of bronchial obstruction, including segmental atelectasis and "obstructive overinflation."[49] In fact, one case has been described in which bullae developed, with subsequent spontaneous pneumothorax.[55] Neither lymph node enlargement nor pleural effusion occurs at any stage of the disease.

CLINICAL MANIFESTATIONS

Approximately one third of patients are asymptomatic. The remainder manifest a variety of symptoms, the most frequent being shortness of breath on exertion that is usually progressive in severity and unassociated with orthopnea. Cough is often present and usually is dry but may be associated with the expectoration of "chunky" gelatinous ma-

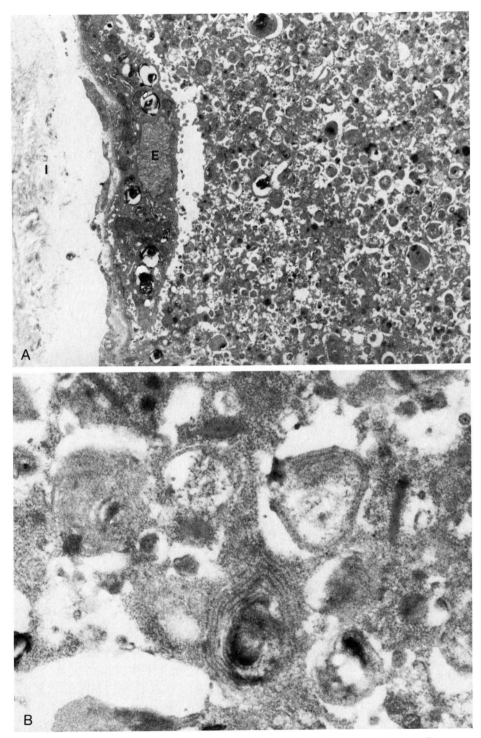

Figure 16–2. Pulmonary Alveolar Proteinosis. A transmission electron micrograph *(A)* shows a type II pneumocyte (E) overlying a somewhat fibrotic interstitium (I). The adjacent alveolar airspace is filled with numerous, variably electron-dense bodies, some of which at greater magnification *(B)* show distinct lamellations resembling those seen in the normal type II cell osmiophilic body. (A × 9,500; B × 56,000.)

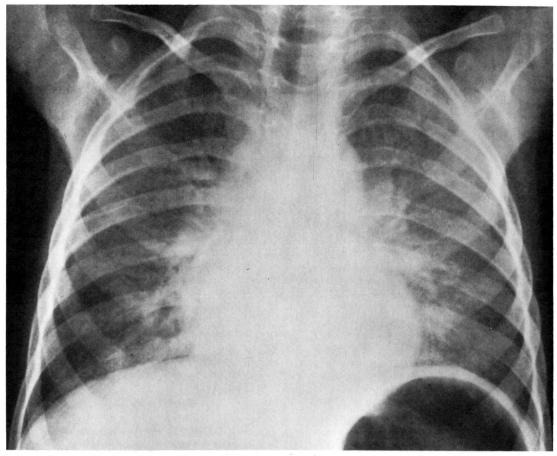

Figure 16–3. Alveolar Proteinosis in a 2-Year-Old Boy. This roentgenogram reveals extensive airspace consolidation of both lungs, uniformly distributed and associated with an air bronchogram. There is no pleural effusion or cardiomegaly. The main clinical finding was tachypnea. An open lung biopsy revealed alveolar proteinosis. On two occasions, bilateral pulmonary lavage was carried out in association with extracorporeal circulation. Despite these valiant attempts, the child died. (Courtesy of Dr. Maurice Brouillette, Brome-Mississquoi-Perkins Hospital, Cowansville, Quebec.)

terial that rarely can take the form of a bronchial cast (Fig. 16–6). Hemoptysis rarely occurs.[51] Fatigue, weight loss, and pleuritic pain may be present,[1, 46, 56–58] and a low-grade fever is said to develop at the onset of the illness in 50 per cent of patients.[1, 51] Fine or coarse rales sometimes can be heard on auscultation[46, 59] as in 12 of the 14 patients described by Rogers and his associates;[58] in the latter group the rales tended to disappear following BAL but recurred with exacerbations of the disease. Clubbing of the fingers and toes is not uncommon.[16, 57, 59–61]

Laboratory investigation reveals a normal or slightly elevated white cell count. Polycythemia is common.[60] Hyperglobulinemia is present in a minority of patients,[1, 50, 51] the increase being mainly in the alpha$_2$ and, to a lesser extent, alpha$_1$ fractions.[62] In a few patients, IgA levels have been decreased in serum,[16, 27] and IgG, IgA, and IgM levels increased in BAL fluid.[27, 28] In one case, a monoclonal serum peak in IgG was incriminated as an inhibitor of phagocytosis.[63] Hyperlipidemia and an increase in the level of serum lactate dehydrogenase (LDH) have been observed in some cases,[64] in 13 of 14 patients in one series.[58]

The diagnosis of alveolar proteinosis should be strongly suspected when a chest roentgenogram reveals a pattern consistent with pulmonary edema in a patient who does not have orthopnea. The diagnosis can be confirmed by BAL,[23, 46, 51, 65] the fluid showing the following characteristics: (1) a grossly opaque effluent, a milky effluent, or both; (2) very few alveolar macrophages; (3) large acellular eosinophilic bodies in a diffuse background of eosinophilic granules; and (4) PAS staining of the proteinaceous material with a lack of significant alcian blue staining.[66] However, in many cases the diagnosis must be confirmed by examination of tissue obtained by transbronchial[67] or open lung biopsy.

Pulmonary function studies can be completely normal or can reveal a reduction in diffusing capacity,[68, 69] vital capacity, and pulmonary compliance. Hypoxemia is caused by ventilation-perfusion inequality and intrapulmonary shunt[46, 70, 71] and may result in pulmonary hypertension that can be relieved by the breathing of oxygen.[72] The results of follow-up function studies of patients treated successfully with BAL correlate well with clinical improvement.[53, 78]

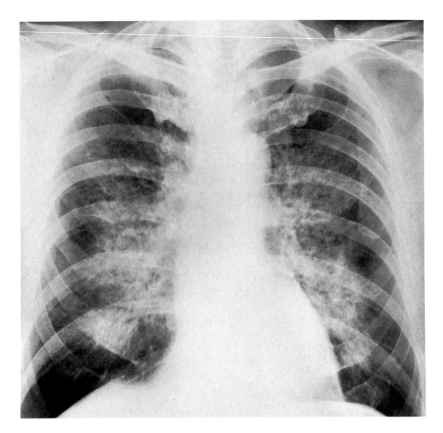

Figure 16–4. Alveolar Proteinosis. This 63-year-old man noted the onset of dyspnea and dry cough 5 months previously. A posteroanterior roentgenogram reveals involvement of the central and midzones of both lungs by patchy airspace consolidation which in many areas is confluent. The disease possesses a "butterfly" pattern of distribution, the peripheral zones of the lungs being spared. An air bronchogram is visible. Cardiac size is normal. Pulmonary function tests revealed normal values except for diffusing capacity, which was reduced by about 50 per cent.

PROGNOSIS

Although it is difficult to be precise about prognosis, several reviews of the literature suggest that the disease is fatal in about one third of cases, death resulting either from respiratory failure caused by the proteinosis or from superimposed infection.[51, 69, 74, 75] In a review of the records of 139 patients who had been followed for varying periods of time, Davidson and MacLeod[76] reported complete recovery or great improvement in 40 patients and death in 45 patients. Death was attributable to proteinosis or complicating infection in 38 of the latter group. In a prospective study of 23 patients over a period of 15 years, Kariman and associates[5] observed spontaneous remission without treatment in 24 per cent and progressive dyspnea and decrease in pulmonary function requiring BAL in 76 per cent; there were no deaths or opportunistic infections during the period of observation. Rarely, the disease is associated with interstitial fibrosis of sufficient severity to cause pulmonary insufficiency and death.[42]

Irrigation of the tracheobronchial tree by BAL is an effective therapeutic procedure that can be life-saving (Fig. 16–7); it has greatly improved the prognosis of the disease.[58, 65, 77–83] The procedure is best performed with normal saline, one side at a time, at 2- to 3-day intervals; it is important to have the assistance of a physiotherapist[84] or a mechanical chest percussor.[82] Some patients do not require more than one or two BALs,[85, 86] but a few require

whole lung lavage repeated semiannually or annually.[5, 58, 82] BAL has been performed successfully during pregnancy,[87] in a patient with one lung,[88] in patients with severe respiratory insufficiency (with the aid of hyperbaric oxygen),[89] and during cardiopulmonary bypass.[90, 91]

Spontaneous remission occurs in some patients and is usually permanent;[61] however, a patient has been described who had a relapse 18 years after the primary episode.[92] Success attributed to such oral medications as prednisolone,[62] potassium iodide,[93] enzymes,[94] and antituberculous drugs[95] may simply reflect a coincidental spontaneous remission. The same can be said for aerosolized trypsin,[61] with or without added acetylcysteine,[96] although some authorities recommend this therapy for patients who cannot tolerate BAL.

AMYLOIDOSIS

The term *amyloidosis* designates a group of diseases with numerous clinicopathologic features; all of these diseases are characterized by the extracellular deposition of an insoluble fibrillary protein traditionally termed amyloid.[97] Although originally considered to represent a single substance, it is now clear that amyloid consists of several proteins, each of which is similar physically but distinctive biochemically. The fundamental unit of this structure is a twisted array of nonbranching fibrils. The aggregation of numerous sheets of these fibrils is

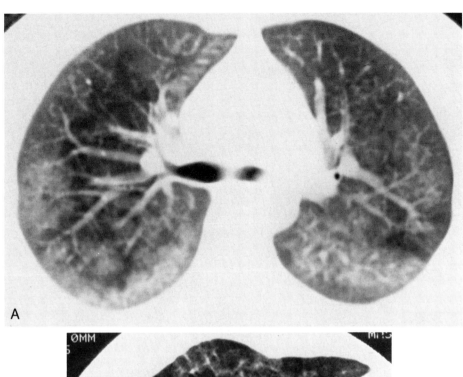

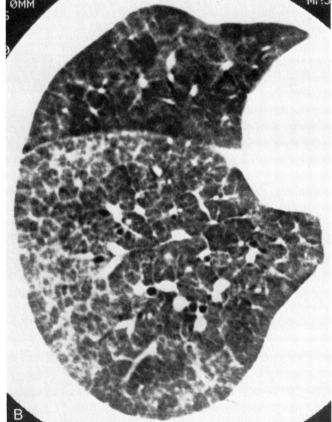

Figure 16–5. Pulmonary Alveolar Proteinosis: CT Manifestations in Two Patients. In the first patient, a 39-year-old woman, a CT scan with 10-mm collimation *(A)* reveals extensive bilateral airspace opacities with marked peripheral anatomic predominance, at least in the right lung. This appearance is consistent with virtually any diffuse airspace filling process, including alveolar proteinosis. In the second patient, a 44-year-old man, a high-resolution CT scan with 1.5-mm collimation *(B)* shows a rather coarse reticulation consistent with thickening of interlobular septa; multiple polygonal lines can be identified, creating what some would consider a honeycomb pattern. It is possible that this represents the late or fibrotic phase of the disease.

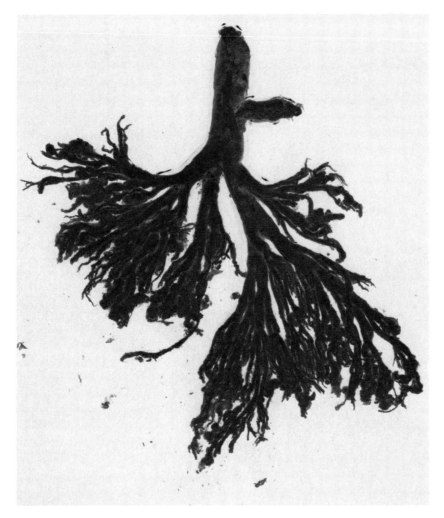

Figure 16–6. Pulmonary Alveolar Proteinosis: Bronchial Cast Formation. Illustrated is a cast of the right lower lobe bronchial tree that was expectorated by a patient with pulmonary alveolar proteinosis. The patient was a 57-year-old woman who gave a 5-year history of dyspnea and episodes of expectoration of bronchial casts similar to the one illustrated. Open lung biopsy showed the characteristic pathologic changes of pulmonary alveolar proteinosis. Despite repeated BAL, her symptoms progressed and she died of respiratory failure one year later. (Courtesy of Dr. R. Chapela and Dr. R. Sansores, National Respiratory Disease Institute of Mexico.)

responsible for the characteristic ultrastructural features and the staining and optical properties of amyloid by which it is recognized pathologically: electron microscopy reveals numerous randomly arranged, nonbranching fibrils 75 to 100 nm in diameter; light microscopy demonstrates amorphous pink staining with hematoxylin and eosin, violet-red with crystal violet (as a manifestation of metachromasia), and light red with Congo red (the latter also showing an apple-green birefringence with polarization microscopy).

Because of its great variety of clinical and pathologic manifestations, amyloidosis has been classified in several ways.[98] The traditional division has been into four major forms depending on the underlying clinical features: (1) a *primary* type, in which no associated disease is recognized or in which there is an underlying plasma cell disorder (most commonly multiple myeloma); (2) *secondary* amyloidosis, in which there is an identifiable underlying chronic abnormality such as tuberculosis, bronchiectasis, rheumatoid disease, syphilis, or certain neoplasms such as Hodgkin's disease; (3) a relatively uncommon *familial* form that can be localized to a certain tissue such as nerve; and (4) a so-called *senile* form that affects many organs and

tissues (including the lungs) and in which the majority of individuals are over 70 years of age. A subdivision of amyloidosis into localized (i.e., within a single organ or tissue) and generalized forms is also common.

Recently it has been proposed that amyloidosis could be better classified on the basis of the specific protein of which the amyloid is composed.[97] Following this concept, the most important forms are *amyloid L* (AL), associated with the deposition of immunoglobulin light chains and usually seen in association with such conditions as multiple myeloma and macroglobulinemia; and *amyloid A* (AA), associated with the deposition of a protein derived from an acute serum phase reactant (SAA) and occuring in association with chronic inflammatory diseases, certain neoplasms, and familial Mediterranean fever. A third relatively common form of amyloid is associated with the deposition of prealbumin in nerves in familial amyloidotic polyneuropathy, in the cerebral plaques of Alzheimer's disease, and in the heart and pulmonary parenchyma in "senile" amyloidosis. Serum levels of prealbumin have been found to be considerably reduced in patients with senile systemic amyloidosis and mildly reduced in those with secondary (AA) amyloidosis.[99]

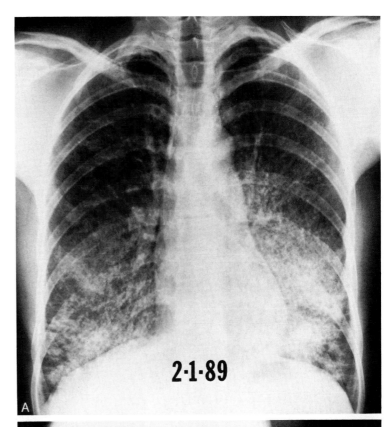

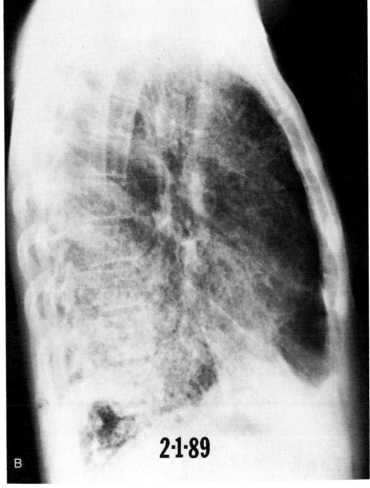

Figure 16–7. Pulmonary Alveolar Proteinosis: Response to Bronchoalveolar Lavage. Posteroanterior *(A)* and lateral *(B)* roentgenograms of the chest of this 29-year-old woman with known alveolar proteinosis reveal extensive bilateral patchy airspace opacities with middle and lower zonal predominance.

Illustration continued on following page

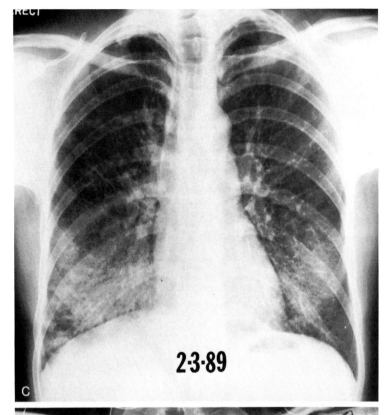

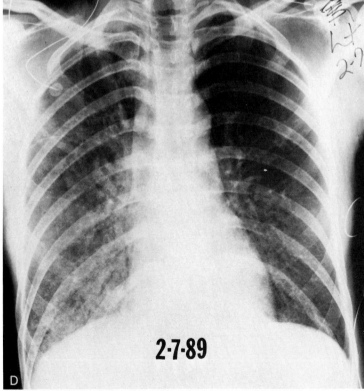

Figure 16–7 *Continued*. Approximately 1 month later, a repeat roentgenogram 24 hours following left lung lavage *(C)* shows almost complete clearing of the left-sided opacities. Four days later, a roentgenogram obtained immediately following right lung lavage *(D)* reveals marked worsening of the opacities throughout this lung, caused by the presence within lung parenchyma of lavage fluid.

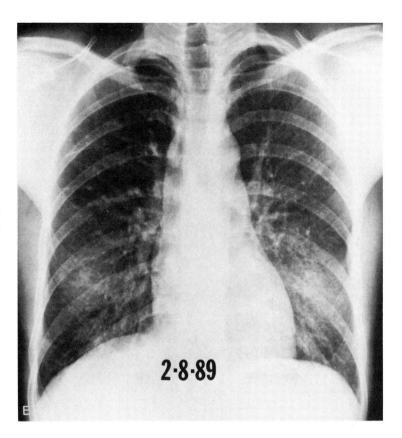

Figure 16–7 *Continued*. Twenty-four hours later *(E)*, the fluid had absorbed and the right lung was almost normal in appearance.

A fourth form of amyloid is related to local hormone deposition, such as that occurring in the pancreatic islets of patients with diabetes mellitus and in the tumor stroma of medullary thyroid carcinoma.

Wright and coworkers[100, 101] have described a simple histochemical method of identifying AA in paraffin tissue sections: when amyloid deposits stained with congo red are exposed to potassium permanganate, restaining with congo red results in a different response by different types of amyloid—AA does not restain or restains weakly, whereas AL and "senile" amyloid restain avidly. Several reports of individual cases in the literature appear to confirm the validity of this method of distinguishing the various types.[102–104]

These classifications of amyloidosis are helpful in understanding the underlying nature of the disease, but from the point of view of diagnosis and the clinical consequences of involvement of the thorax it is perhaps more useful to consider the anatomic location of disease. Three major patterns of amyloid deposition can occur within the trachea and lungs—tracheobronchial, nodular parenchymal, and diffuse parenchymal. Although these patterns can occur in combination,[105, 106] in most cases the amyloid is deposited predominantly in one pattern, thus providing some rationale for a discussion in this fashion. In addition to tracheal and pulmonary involvement, amyloidosis can also affect the pleura, pulmonary arteries, and hilar and mediastinal lymph nodes, either alone or in combination with airway or parenchymal disease (*see* farther on); rare cases also have been reported of amyloid deposition in the diaphragm (in two cases associated with respiratory failure)[107, 108] and in association with intrapulmonary neuroendocrine tumors.[98, 109]

In considering a diagnosis of thoracic amyloidosis, it must be remembered that pulmonary diseases such as chronic fibrocaseous tuberculosis, bronchiectasis,[109] lung abscess, and cystic fibrosis[102, 110–114] can themselves result in amyloidosis; although rare, this secondary phenomenon can occasionally alter the course or roentgenographic appearance of the underlying pulmonary abnormality.

PATHOGENESIS

A detailed description of the basic pathogenetic features of amyloidosis is beyond the scope of this text; the interested reader is directed to the pertinent literature for a complete discussion.[97, 100, 115] However, certain specific features related to localized pulmonary disease deserve mention. With the exception of "senile" amyloid, which appears to be composed of prealbumin,[97, 116] most localized deposits of amyloid in the lungs consist of AL.[117–119] In the great majority of these cases, there is no evidence of systemic immunologic disease (such as multiple myeloma or Waldenström's macroglobulinemia), and in the few cases that have been studied[117, 119] no serologic immunoglobulin abnormality has been demonstrated. Thus, it has been

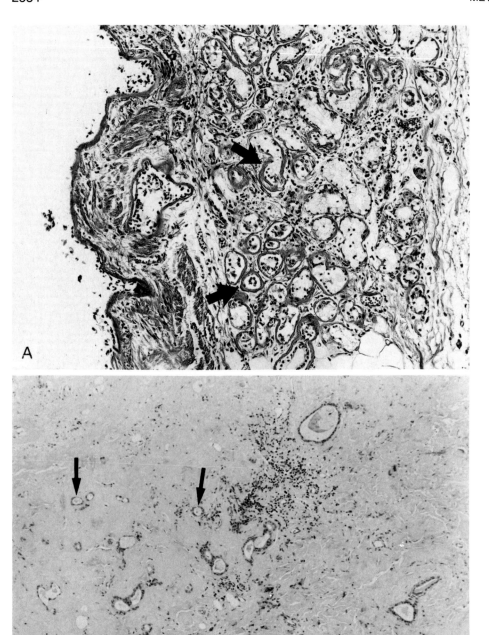

Figure 16–8. Amyloidosis: Tracheobronchial. A histologic section *(A)* shows mild amyloid deposition in relation to a bronchial gland duct and acini *(arrows)*, representing an early stage of bronchial wall amyloidosis. This was an incidental finding in a patient with familial Mediterranean fever. A histologic section *(B)* of a more advanced lesion from a grossly visible plaque in an individual with no known extrapulmonary disease shows virtual complete replacement of airway interstitial tissue by amyloid, with separation and atrophy of bronchial gland acini *(arrows)*. (A × 100; B × 60.)

speculated[119] that local immunoglobulin deposition, possibly related to either overproduction or impaired clearance secondary to a chronic inflammatory process, may be responsible for the accumulation. The presence of variable numbers of plasma cells in relation to foci of localized pulmonary or cutaneous amyloid supports this concept.[120] The cytoplasm of the plasma cells in these cases reacts with immunoglobulin light chain or Bence Jones protein antiserum (or both) whereas adjacent amyloid reacts with AL antiserum, suggesting that the plasma cells may produce and secrete immunoglob-

ulin light chains or Bence Jones protein that undergoes proteolysis to protein AL.[120]

PATHOLOGIC CHARACTERISTICS

The pathologic characteristics of the various forms of pulmonary amyloidosis have been well-described in both the older[105, 281] and more recent[117, 118, 121, 122] literature.

Airway involvement occurs most commonly in the false vocal cords,[123] trachea, and proximal bron-

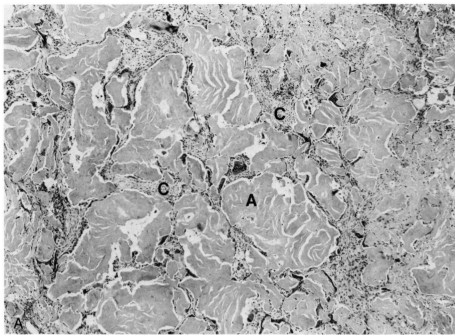

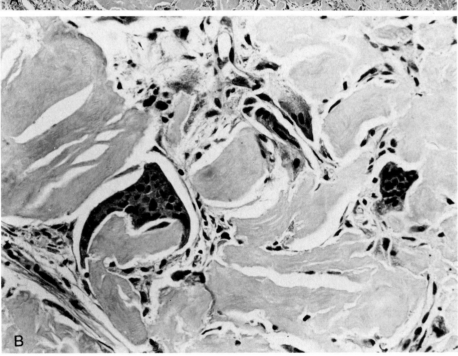

Figure 16–9. Amyloidosis: Nodular Parenchymal. A histologic section *(A)* from a well-defined 2.5-cm nodule in the right upper lobe of an asymptomatic 60-year-old man shows abundant amorphous amyloid (A) separated by a small amount of connective tissue (C) containing plasma cells, occasional lymphocytes, and rather numerous multinucleated giant cells. The latter cells are seen to better advantage in a magnified view *(B)*. (A × 40; B × 275.)

chi. Although there is overlap, it is usually manifested in one of two ways:[98, 117] a localized tumor-like growth or (more commonly) multiple discrete or confluent intramural plaques that cause distortion of the airway wall and stenosis of its lumen.[117, 119] Histologically, the amyloid is situated in the subepithelial interstitial tissue and often surrounds tracheobronchial ducts and acini, some of which may show secondary atrophy (Fig. 16–8). Calcification, ossification, and foreign body giant cell reaction may be present but are probably less common than in the nodular parenchymal form.[118] A variable number of plasma cells and lymphocytes are present between foci of amyloid deposition.

The *parenchymal nodules* of localized pulmonary amyloid can be solitary or multiple, are usually fairly well-defined, and measure 2 to 4 cm in diameter. Grossly, they have a grayish-brown, waxy appearance and may be firm or quite hard depending on the extent of associated calcification or ossification. Histologically, at the periphery of the nodule amyloid is often present in the alveolar interstitium only; however, in the central regions, normal parenchymal structure is usually lost and is replaced by a mass of amyloid, typically containing fairly numerous multinucleated giant cells and variable numbers of lymphocytes and plasma cells (Fig. 16–9). Amyloid sometimes can be identified within the

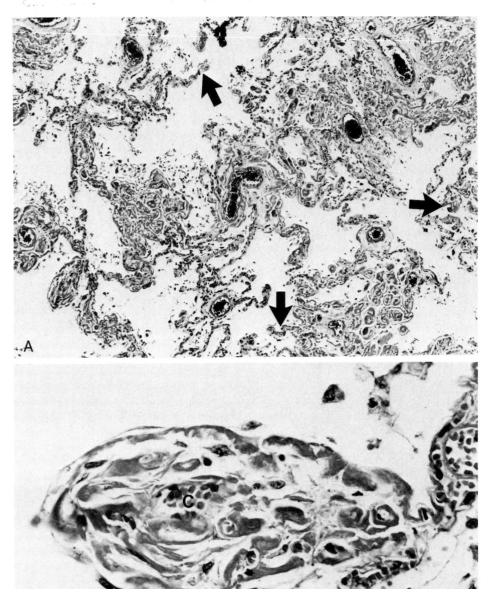

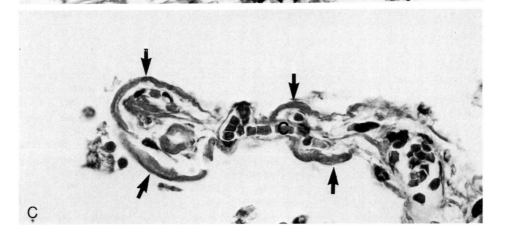

Figure 16–10. Amyloidosis: Diffuse Interstitial. A histologic section of lung parenchyma *(A)* shows amyloid deposition in the interstitium around small vessels, transitional airways, and alveolar septa *(arrows.)* Magnified views of two alveolar septa show thick *(B)* and relatively thin *(C)* deposits of amyloid situated between the capillary lumen (c) and overlying alveolar epithelium *(arrows* in *C)*. *(A* × 60, *B* × 375, *C* × 600.)

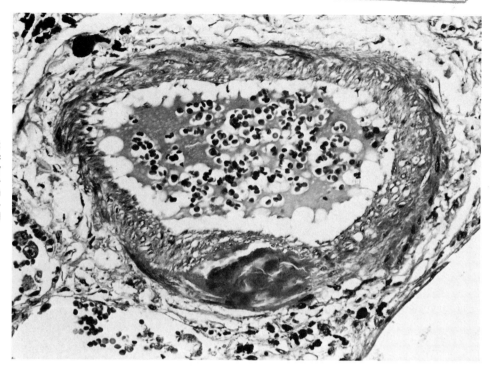

Figure 16–11. Amyloidosis: Pulmonary Arterial. A histologic section of a muscular pulmonary artery reveals focal amyloid deposition in the media. This was an incidental finding in an 87-year-old man who also had left atrial amyloidosis. ($\times$ 250.)

cytoplasm of the giant cells. Deposition of amyloid in the media of blood vessels, both within and immediately adjacent to the main mass, is common.

In *diffuse interstitial disease,* amyloid is present in the media of small (occasionally medium-sized) blood vessels and in the parenchymal interstitium (Fig. 16–10). In the latter site, it is situated in relation to endothelial and epithelial basement membranes and can appear in a uniform and more or less linear pattern or as multiple small nodules.[106] Inflammatory cells (multinucleated giant cells, plasma cells, and lymphocytes) and ossification or calcification are typically absent.

As indicated, vascular involvement is common in each of the forms of amyloidosis described above. It is also not infrequent in "senile" amyloidosis, particularly when the heart is also affected;[121] in this circumstance, the sole site of amyloid deposition is usually the vessels. In all situations, the amyloid typically accumulates in the media of small- to medium-sized pulmonary arteries (Fig. 16–11).

Amyloidosis may be confused histologically with so-called light chain deposition disease. In this abnormality, kappa or lambda light chains produced in association with a plasma cell dyscrasia are deposited in tissue but fail to polymerize into the β-pleated sheet typical of amyloid; extracellular deposits are thus formed that are histologically similar to but ultrastructurally and histochemically different from amyloid. Although most often identified in the kidneys, such deposits also have been reported in the lungs.

ROENTGENOGRAPHIC MANIFESTATIONS

In the tracheobronchial form, roentgenographic features range from general accentuation of bronchovascular markings associated with overinflation to the effects of more severe bronchial obstruction, such as atelectasis or obstructive pneumonitis. The latter may involve a segment, a lobe, or an entire lung.[124–126] The nodular parenchymal form is manifested by solitary or multiple masses (Fig. 16–12), in some cases with cavitation.[117, 126–129] Calcification or ossification may also occur,[125, 130, 131] although less commonly than is identified histologically. Computed tomography can be helpful in revealing the calcification.[132] A case has been described in which a homogeneous mass measuring several centimeters in diameter and situated at the apex of the left lung was associated with destruction of the first rib, thus simulating a Pancoast tumor;[133] conventional tomography revealed the presence of calcification within the mass, which diminished the likelihood of neoplasia. The diagnosis of amyloidosis was made pathologically from material obtained by trephine biopsy. Obstructive bronchial amyloidosis and peripheral parenchymal disease occasionally occur concomitantly.[124, 125]

Pulmonary involvement is less common in generalized *secondary* amyloidosis than in the primary or "senile" type[98–100, 117, 134] and usually takes the form of diffuse parenchymal disease that tends to be of slight or moderate severity (Fig. 16–13). Pulmonary involvement is a frequent occurrence in generalized *primary* disease;[98] 35 to 70 per cent of patients show roentgenographic evidence of deposition in the lung,[135, 136] usually in the form of diffuse parenchymal disease. The diffuse parenchymal form can be manifested by a nodular pattern that simulates miliary tuberculosis, silicosis, or sarcoidosis.[137]

Hilar[138–141] and mediastinal[142, 143] lymph nodes

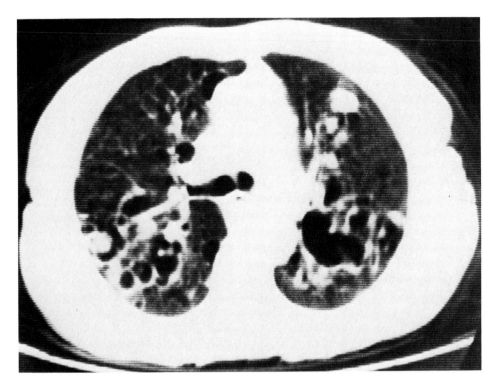

Figure 16–12. Amyloidosis: Nodular Parenchymal. A CT scan at the level of the carina reveals multiple nodular and thick, irregular linear opacities throughout both lungs. A number of air-containing "cystic" spaces probably represent bullae. The patient is an elderly woman who complained of dyspnea. (Courtesy of Dr. Michael O'Donovan, Montreal General Hospital, Montreal, Quebec.)

are occasionally affected in amyloidosis, either with or without associated pulmonary parenchymal disease. This may be apparent roentgenographically as lymph node enlargement that can be massive and associated with dense calcification. Pleural effusion is uncommon.[131, 144, 145]

CLINICAL MANIFESTATIONS

The plaque-like form of tracheobronchial amyloidosis can cause symptoms that simulate bronchial asthma;[146, 147] hemoptysis is common[125, 126, 146] as are recurrent bronchitis and pneumonia.[126, 148] Laryngeal amyloidosis is frequently associated with hoarseness,[123, 149] and macroglossia can cause obstructive sleep apnea.[150] Discrete tracheal and endobronchial papillary lesions seldom cause symptoms and are usually discovered incidentally at bronchoscopy; however, they can be large enough to cause airway obstruction, atelectasis, and bronchiectasis.[149, 151] Other symptoms and signs depend on the volume of lung affected and whether infection is present.

The nodular parenchymal form of amyloidosis usually provokes no symptoms[118, 152, 153] and is discovered on a screening chest roentgenogram; rarely, the nodules are extensive and large enough to cause respiratory symptoms and even failure.[154] A patient has been described in whom multinodular deposits of amyloid compressed small bronchi and caused bronchiectasis and fatal hemorrhage.[155] New lesions occasionally have been reported to appear following surgical excision of nodules,[154] but whether this represents the effect of inadequate

resection or the development of independent lesions is unclear.

Dyspnea and respiratory insufficiency are seen rarely in the nodular form of pulmonary amyloidosis, more commonly in tracheobronchial disease, and frequently in the diffuse alveolar septal form.[117, 118, 134, 156] Dyspnea may be secondary to heart failure; cardiac involvement is a common feature of both primary and "senile" amyloidosis.[111, 121] Repeated hemoptysis in patients with the alveolar septal form has been ascribed to medial dissection of pulmonary arteries.[157]

Amyloidosis should be considered in any patient whose chest roentgenogram reveals one of the described patterns and who has involvement of multiple tissues and organs or who has clinical findings suggesting the presence of a disease known to be associated with amyloid deposition. These include infectious diseases (e.g., lung abscess, tuberculosis, and osteomyelitis),[100, 158] diseases associated with recurrent infections (e.g., bronchiectasis, hypogammaglobulinemia, and cystic fibrosis),[102, 110–114, 145, 159] and noninfectious inflammatory diseases (e.g., rheumatoid arthritis, spondylitis, systemic lupus erythematosus, and familial Mediterranean fever).[100, 160, 161] The number of reported cases of amyloidosis associated with cystic fibrosis (CF) has risen dramatically since the original description of this association in 1977;[111] the complication probably reflects the greater longevity being achieved in patients with CF, since all reported cases have been in adolescents and young adults. In a retrospective autopsy study of 33 clinically documented patients with CF who were at least 15 years of age at the time of death, one group of investigators[114] found 11 with amyloid deposits in multiple organs.

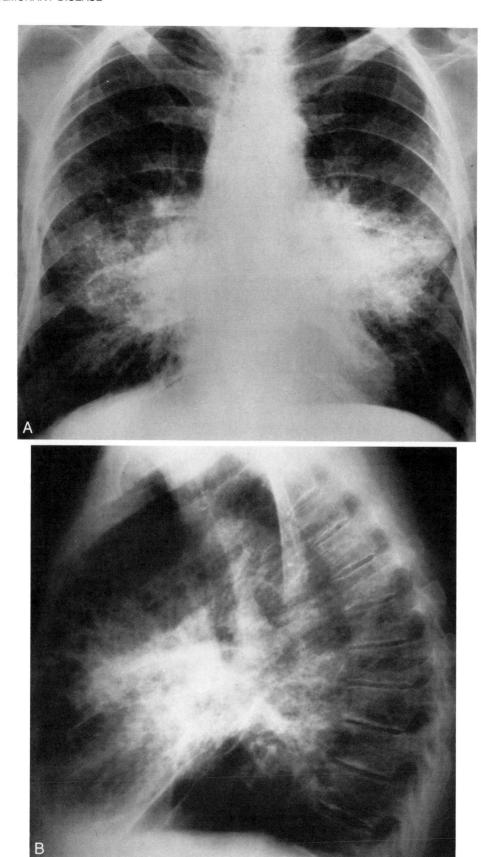

Figure 16–13. Parenchymal Amyloidosis. Posteroanterior *(A)* and lateral *(B)* roentgenograms reveal fairly large, poorly defined inhomogeneous opacities in the medial and central portions of both lungs that possess a "butterfly" distribution. The lungs are otherwise normal. Possible hilar lymph node enlargement cannot be evaluated because of contiguity of the parenchymal disease. Open lung biopsy revealed the typical features of parenchymal amyloidosis.

Strangely, this 33 per cent incidence was not duplicated in an autopsy review in Boston of 23 CF patients with long-term survival in whom no evidence of amyloidosis was found.[102]

In a minority of patients with tracheobronchopathia osteochondroplastica (*see* page 1996), amyloid is found in the airway lesions.[106, 162]

Biopsy of rectal tissue or of subcutaneous abdominal fat[163] may be required to confirm the diagnosis. When disease is localized to the lungs, transbronchial biopsy,[164] open lung biopsy, or transthoracic needle aspiration usually yields diagnostic tissue; rarely, amyloid can be identified in bronchial brushing specimens.[164] Bronchoscopy reveals irregular nodular filling defects with an intact covering mucous membrane.[125, 146, 147, 165] Pleural involvement has been diagnosed by Cope needle biopsy.[144] A fatal complication has been reported in a patient who bled excessively following transbronchial biopsy and required intubation and positive-pressure ventilation;[166] the latter procedure resulted in massive arterial air embolism.

Circulating and tissue-bound monoclonal light chains, more often lambda than kappa, are frequently present in patients with primary amyloidosis.[103, 118, 123, 129, 156, 167] In other patients, including those with secondary amyloidosis, nonspecific immunoglobulin abnormalities may be observed, with serum levels of IgA, IgG, and IgM being either increased or decreased. In the 7 per cent of patients with multiple myeloma who have amyloidosis, IgG (less commonly IgA) monoclonal gammopathy is invariable.[168, 169]

The prognosis in the nodular parenchymal type of amyloidosis is much better than in the tracheobronchial or diffuse interstitial forms; in most cases the nodules remain stationary in size or grow slowly and cause no symptoms. Spontaneous regression has been described.[170] Although considered unusual, resolution of secondary amyloidosis associated with skeletal tuberculosis has been reported following treatment of the infection.[171] Two patients with primary disease have been reported to survive as long as 7 years[172] and 14 years;[172] the latter patient had nodular lesions. Complicating renal failure in AA amyloidosis of familial Mediterranean fever usually proves fatal at an early age; it is believed to be preventable with early colchicine therapy.[161] By contrast, patients with diffuse interstitial disease[152] or with rare respiratory muscle involvement[107, 108] often die from respiratory insufficiency. The thromboembolic complications of multiple myeloma[173] are most common in patients with complicating amyloidosis.

LIPID STORAGE DISEASE

GAUCHER'S DISEASE

Gaucher's disease is an autosomal recessive abnormality characterized by a deficiency of β-glucosidase, the enzyme that catabolizes glucosylceramide.[174, 175] This deficiency results in an accumulation of this substance in reticuloendothelial cells whose appearance becomes altered to form *Gaucher cells*. These cells contain striated PAS-positive inclusions that resemble wrinkled tissue paper and that accumulate in organs of the reticuloendothelial system, particularly the liver, spleen, lymph nodes, bones, and, in the infantile form of the disease, the brain. Clinically and roentgenographically significant involvement of other tissues and organs, including the lungs, occurs sporadically.

Three varieties of the disease are recognized: (1) *neurologic* (or infantile) type that occurs in infants and is fatal before the age of 2 years; (2) *visceral* (or juvenile) type that becomes manifest between the age of 6 months and early adolescence and is associated with rapid enlargement of the liver and spleen and with death from intercurrent infection or a hemorrhagic diathesis; and (3) *osseous* (or adult) type that occurs in late adolescence or adulthood and is characterized by splenomegaly and bone involvement. Patients with the osseous type can survive for more than 40 years. The majority of patients with Gaucher's disease are female and more than 95 per cent are Jews.

Pulmonary involvement in Gaucher's disease has been described in all three forms[176] but is uncommon; in a review of the literature in 1975, Wolson[177] found only 10 cases in which pulmonary disease of any form was demonstrated. Two more recent reports describe four additional cases in children, all of whom died from respiratory insufficiency.[178, 179] Histologically, Gaucher cells are found predominantly in the alveolar interstitium and adjacent airspaces;[178–180] they can be few in number or so numerous that the underlying lung structure is difficult to appreciate. Bone marrow emboli containing Gaucher cells derived from pathologic fractures or bone infarcts occasionally can be identified in pulmonary vessels.[176]

Roentgenographic manifestations consist of a reticulonodular or miliary pattern affecting both lungs diffusely (Fig. 16–14).[180] Lytic lesions, occasionally seen in the ribs, represent foci of bone involvement.

Clinically significant pulmonary involvement is usually manifested by dyspnea and sometimes by pulmonary hypertension[176] and respiratory failure.[178, 179] Elevated levels of serum angiotensin–converting enzyme (ACE) have been described,[182] a finding that is sometimes incorrectly interpreted as suggesting a diagnosis of sarcoidosis.

NIEMANN-PICK DISEASE

Niemann-Pick disease is caused by an inherited fault in the production of sphingomyelinase. This deficiency results in the deposition of the ceramide phospholipid, sphingomyelin, in the liver, spleen,

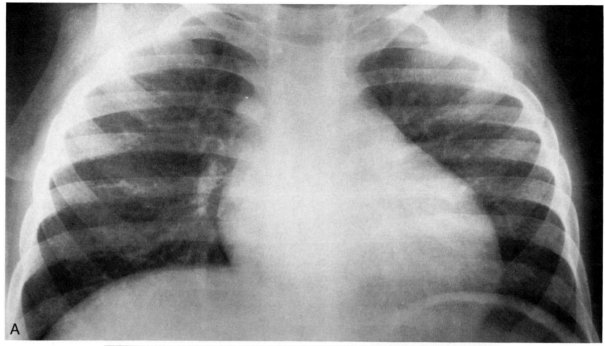

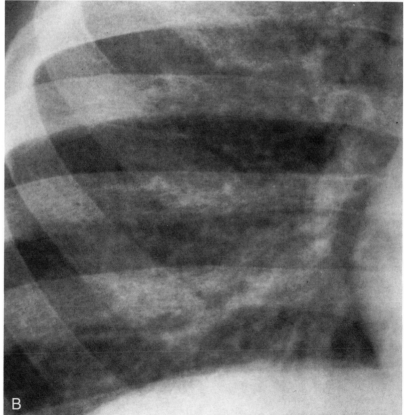

Figure 16–14. Gaucher's Disease. A posteroanterior roentgenogram *(A)* and a magnified view of the right lower zone *(B)* reveal a fine reticular pattern throughout both lungs without anatomic predominance. There are no associated abnormalities such as lymph node enlargement or pleural effusion. Lung volume is small, but this could be a technical aberration. (Courtesy of Dr. JS Dunbar.)

lung, bone marrow, and brain. Five clinical variants have been described that depend on the age of onset and predominant organs affected. Many patients die in infancy or childhood; however, some individuals survive into adulthood, occasionally presenting with the first manifestations of their disease at that time.[183]

Pathologically, aggregates of large multivacuolated "foam" cells (NP cells) are present in the parenchyma of many organs, particularly the brain, spleen, liver, lungs, bone marrow, and lymph nodes. The foaminess is caused by cytoplasmic inclusions containing regularly arranged lamellae of lipid.[184] In the lungs, NP cells appear to be most numerous in the alveoli.[185] Histiocytes containing fine and coarse granules that stain deep blue with May-Grünwald-Giemsa stain ("sea-blue histiocytes") have been detected in some patients, most often in bone marrow.[183]

Roentgenographic manifestations in the lungs consist of a diffuse reticulonodular pattern (Fig. 16–15);[183, 185, 186] the nodules measure from 1 to 2 mm in diameter and are associated with linear strands that have been said to create a honeycomb pattern.[186] Hepatomegaly and peripheral lymph node enlargement are common; pulmonary involvement can cause respiratory failure.

FABRY'S DISEASE

Fabry's disease (angiokeratoma corporis diffusum universali) is caused by an inherited deficiency of alpha-galactosidase A, the enzyme responsible for metabolizing ceramide trihexoside. The deficiency results in the accumulation of a number of glycolipids in endothelial, muscle, and mesenchymal cells in several organs and tissues including the skin, kidneys, and heart. The initial clinical presentation is usually in the form of red spots in the skin and is followed 5 to 10 years later by the development of renal and myocardial failure.

Although some authors[187] have expressed skepticism about the validity of reports of lung involvement in Fabry's disease, occasional well-documented cases[188] indicate that this does indeed occur. However, in most individuals the functional significance of such involvement is unclear. In one study of seven patients with Fabry's disease, Rosenberg and his colleagues[189] found evidence of airflow obstruction whose severity was out of proportion to the smoking history; the authors suggested that the physiologic abnormality may have been caused by airway narrowing secondary to glycolipid accumulation demonstrated in biopsy specimens of airway epithelial cells. Another report described a woman whose clinical presentation suggested multiple pulmonary emboli but whose chest roentgenogram revealed only slight accentuation of lung markings;[190] because of a history of several episodes of hemoptysis, it was thought likely that the changes

were caused by multiple angiomas in the tracheobronchial tree similar to those that were present in the skin. Arterial blood gas analysis revealed a decrease in the PaO_2 and an increase in the alveolar-arterial oxygen gradient. The patient died, but unfortunately necropsy was not performed.

GM₁ GANGLIOSIDOSIS

GM_1 gangliosidosis is caused by a deficiency of β-galactosidase and is characterized by the accumulation in various organs of histiocytes containing a monocyaloganglioside. The condition usually affects infants or young children and is manifested principally by mental retardation, sometimes with hepatosplenomegaly and skeletal abnormalities. In the occasional patient in whom pulmonary disease has been identified, aggregates of foamy macrophages similar to those of Niemann-Pick disease have been found predominantly within alveoli.[191] "Miliary shadows" have been described on chest roentgenograms, and the condition has been said to cause respiratory insufficiency.[191]

HERMANSKY-PUDLAK SYNDROME

The Hermansky-Pudlak syndrome is an autosomal recessive condition characterized by tyrosinase-positive oculocutaneous albinism, a storage pool platelet defect, and the accumulation of ceroid pigment in macrophages throughout the body.[192, 193] The disease is uncommon, approximately 200 cases having been reported by 1985,[193] and is seen most often in individuals from Puerto Rico and southern Holland.[194, 195]

Ceroid is a complex chromolipid, the origin and chemical structure of which are incompletely understood. It is recognized histologically as a finely granular brown pigment that is PAS-positive, diastase-resistant, and acid-fast and that shows brilliant yellow-orange fluorescence when viewed with ultraviolet light. Ultrastructurally,[193] the pigment is finely granular or (less commonly) whorled and is found most often in membrane-bound vacuoles. The latter finding and other observations[193, 196] suggest that the ceroid is stored within lysosomes, thus representing a possible enzymatic defect; however, the nature of such a defect is unknown.

Involvement of the pulmonary interstitium has been documented in a number of reports.[192–197] Histologically, it consists of mild to severe parenchymal and peribronchial fibrosis associated with variable numbers of ceroid-laden macrophages. The pathogenetic relationship between the macrophages and the fibrosis is unclear. In one study of pulmonary inflammatory cells obtained by BAL from patients with the syndrome,[197] superoxide production by stimulated alveolar macrophages was increased compared with normal; the authors spec-

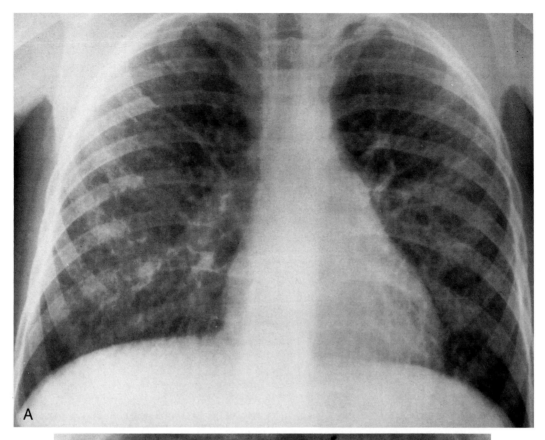

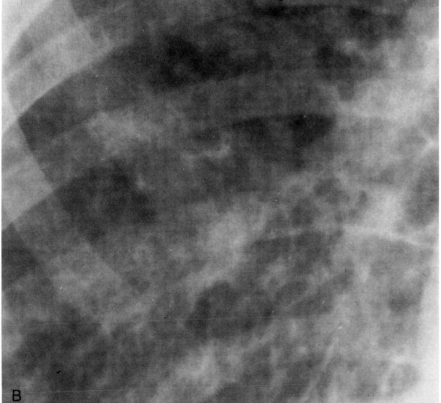

Figure 16–15. Niemann-Pick Disease. A posteroanterior roentgenogram *(A)* and a magnified view of the right lower lung zone *(B)* reveal a coarse reticular pattern throughout both lungs without anatomic predominance. The pattern indicates diffuse interstitial lung disease. There are no associated findings such as lymph node enlargement or pleural effusion. This adolescent boy had a sibling who was also affected but to a lesser degree. (Courtesy of Dr. JS Dunbar.)

ulated that ceroid-laden macrophages may be more responsive to exogenous stimuli and that subsequent release of toxic oxygen metabolites may cause the pulmonary fibrosis.

Roentgenographic manifestations of pulmonary disease in patients with the Hermansky-Pudlak syndrome consist of a reticulonodular pattern caused by interstitial fibrosis. In a description of the roentgenographic features of four patients, Leitman and his colleagues[198] found the pattern to range from a fine reticulation to a coarse reticulonodulation associated with bullae and bronchiectasis (an illustration in the article shows considerable upper zonal predominance of the latter changes).

Clinically, in addition to the abnormal skin pigmentation and ocular signs, patients complain of progressive dyspnea and appear to be susceptible to infection and a bleeding tendency. Pulmonary function studies reveal a restrictive pattern; hypoxemia at rest is characteristic. Some patients develop a nonspecific inflammatory and granulomatous involvement of the colon similar to Crohn's disease.[192, 196]

IDIOPATHIC PULMONARY CEROIDOSIS

Rare cases have been reported in which ceroid-laden macrophages have accumulated within alveolar airspaces in the absence of evidence of significant extrathoracic disease.[199, 200] The etiology, pathogenesis, and natural history of the condition are unknown. Some cases have been associated with mild interstitial fibrosis, dyspnea, and pulmonary function abnormalities.[199, 200]

GLYCOGEN STORAGE DISEASE

Involvement of thoracic structures other than the heart is only rarely detectable either clinically or roentgenographically in glycogen storage disease. However, aggregates of intra-alveolar foamy macrophages containing glycogen-like material have been noted in some cases,[201] and can cause respiratory dysfunction and roentgenographic abnormality. *Pompe's disease* (acid maltase deficiency) is a type II glycogen storage disease characterized by the accumulation of glycogen in skeletal muscle and a variety of visceral organs. Although the condition usually affects infants and is fatal, occasional cases have been reported with an onset in adulthood.[202] Involvement of the diaphragm and respiratory muscles of the chest wall in these individuals can cause dyspnea and respiratory failure;[202] this facet is considered in greater detail in Chapter 21.

MUCOPOLYSACCHARIDE STORAGE DISORDERS

Deficient activity of lysosomal enzymes involved in the catabolism of glycosaminoglycans causes disease that predominantly affects the skeletal, cardiovascular, and central nervous systems. Patients with some of these metabolic disorders die in childhood or adolescence, whereas others with conditions such as Hurler's, Hunter's, and Morquio's syndromes survive into adulthood. Respiratory complications include kyphoscoliosis, respiratory failure, susceptibility to pulmonary infection, and airway obstruction, sometimes accompanied by sleep apnea.[203]

HERITABLE DISEASES OF CONNECTIVE TISSUE

Over 100 distinct heritable disorders of connective tissue exist, each presumed to be caused by a mutation in a single gene that controls the structure or metabolism of one or more macromolecules.[204] In several of these inborn errors of metabolism, specific enzyme deficiencies have been recognized and are believed to be responsible for the clinical manifestations, including abnormalities of the thoracic cage and pleuropulmonary interstitium.[205, 206]

Lysyl oxidase is the enzyme responsible for the initial deamination of lysine and hydroxylysine, which results in the formation of compounds that produce the characteristic cross-links of elastin and collagen. Lysyl oxidase has a cupric ion as a cofactor, and animals on copper-deficient diets show changes in tissues and organs that are considered to be the result of an interference with cross-linking of collagen and elastin.[207, 208] Defective binding between collagen and elastin also occurs in animals fed on the seed of *Lathyrus odoratus*[209] and is believed to be the underlying mechanism for the inherited emphysema-like changes found in the lungs of the "blotchy mouse."[207]

Even in young individuals, advanced emphysema can develop in a variety of heritable disorders of connective tissue, including cutis laxa (generalized elastolysis),[206, 210, 211] osteogenesis imperfecta,[212] and Marfan's syndrome.[213–215] In some of these disorders, a deficiency of lysyl hydroxylase appears to play a role in pathogenesis.

MARFAN'S SYNDROME

The underlying biochemical defect of this heritable disorder is unknown; the syndrome is defined and diagnosed clinically on the strength of cardinal features in the skeletal, ocular, and cardiovascular systems.[206, 216] In one study in which the profiles of the collagen cross-linking compounds in the skin and aortic tissue of affected patients were compared with those of normal subjects,[217] it was found that the amount of chemically stable forms of intermolecular cross-links was reduced in the patients. The authors proposed that an abnormality of nonenzymatic steps involved in the maturation of collagen causes the defective collagen organization in Marfan's syndrome. Some (but not all) patients have increased levels of urinary hydroxyproline, an indication of accelerated collagen turnover.[208]

Although the predominant pulmonary abnormality is emphysema, other manifestations include bullae (usually apical), recurrent pneumothorax,[218–220] upper lobe fibrosis, frequent respiratory infections, and bronchiectasis.[220] Isolated "cystic medial necrosis" of a pulmonary artery associated with a dissecting aneurysm also has been reported, in the absence of other stigmata of Marfan's syndrome.[221] Scoliosis can be very deforming[216] and may require surgery for correction.[222] In a retrospective review of the medical records in one genetics clinic,[219] the authors found that the incidence of spontaneous pneumothorax in patients over 12 years of age with Marfan's syndrome was 4.4 per cent (11 of 249); 7 patients had recurrent or bilateral pneumothorax and 9 had apical bullae detectable on chest roentgenograms. In another series of 100 patients with Marfan's syndrome seen at the Brompton hospital,[220] 11 patients had a history of spontaneous pneumothorax, recurrent in 10 and bilateral in 6.

Cardiovascular manifestations are common and include aortic dissection, mitral valve prolapse, and aortic and mitral valve regurgitation.[216] The sudden onset of chest pain in a patient with Marfan's syndrome indicates the development of either pneumothorax or dissecting aneurysm of the aorta (more likely the latter). Dissecting aneurysm has been reported as a frequent manifestation of Marfan's syndrome during pregnancy: in a review of the literature, Pyeritz[223] found 32 reports of pregnancy in patients with Marfan's syndrome, of whom 20 developed a dissecting aneurysm; 16 of these patients died and 4 survived. By contrast, Pyeritz reported no deaths among the 26 pregnant patients with Marfan's syndrome who were followed in his clinic.

EHLERS-DANLOS SYNDROME

The Ehlers-Danlos syndrome consists of a group of inherited disorders of connective tissue divided into 11 different types on the basis of clinical, genetic, and biochemical features. In some types, specific enzyme deficiencies appear to play a role in the pathogenesis; for example, in type 4, the variety predominantly associated with fragile skin and vessel rupture, there is a deficiency of type III procollagen produced by fibroblasts.[224] Structural abnormalities of collagen tissue are the cause of the most apparent clinical findings of abnormal fragility of tissues and hyperextensibility of joints.[225, 226]

Pleuropulmonary and thoracic skeletal abnormalities, including bullae, pneumothorax, and scoliosis, are very similar to those of Marfan's syndrome.[227] Easy bruisability is a prominent feature, especially in type 4 disease, and rupture of vessels,

including those of the pulmonary circulation, can be life-threatening. Fragility of tissue manifested by rupture of vessels or of the uterus can have serious consequences in pregnancy.[228, 229] Some cases have been reported in which involvement of the bronchial tree resulted in weakness of the walls and subsequent bronchiectasis; probably of a similar nature were the multiple, transient fluid-filled pulmonary cysts described in a 12-week-old infant with Ehlers-Danlos syndrome.[230] The chest roentgenogram can be normal or can reveal changes characteristic of bronchiectasis.

Of the 400 patients with Ehler-Danlos syndrome found by Beighton in a literature review, 20 died suddenly.[231]

PSEUDOXANTHOMA ELASTICUM

Jackson and Loh[232] described a single patient with pseudoxanthoma elasticum in whom a lung biopsy showed fragmented and swollen elastic tissue in pulmonary vessels and calcification of alveolar septa and vessel walls. They considered these changes to be a manifestation of this disease in the lungs, although they noted that other histologic studies of pulmonary tissue in this condition had failed to document similar changes.

ALKAPTONURIA (OCHRONOSIS)

Alkaptonuria is a rare hereditary disorder caused by a lack of homogentisic acid oxidase. The result is secretion of homogentisic acid in the urine and its accumulation in cartilage and other connective tissues; with time, this causes abnormal connective tissue pigmentation (ochronosis) and arthritis. A characteristic slate-gray or coal-black color of the tracheobronchial cartilage rings has been described at both autopsy and bronchoscopy.[233] The pigment accumulates predominantly in the peribronchial fibrous tissue, but also can be seen in the cartilage matrix, fibrous tissue of the mucosa, and parenchymal scars.[233] The spinal column, especially in the lumbar region, shows degeneration of intervertebral disks with narrowing of disk spaces and dense calcification of remaining disk material.

HOMOCYSTINURIA

Homocystinuria is a biochemical abnormality, the most common cause of which is a deficiency of cystathionine β-synthase. Many of the clinical manifestations of this hereditary disorder, including ectopia lentis and a variety of skeletal and connective tissue abnormalities, are related to abnormal connective tissue, probably secondary to defective cross-linking of collagen. Pathologically and roentgenographically, the skeleton is osteoporotic, and the vertebrae show rarefaction of spongy bone with biconcave (codfish) compression fractures. An exceptionally high incidence of thrombosis and thromboembolism is unexplained.[234]

PULMONARY ABNORMALITIES IN SYSTEMIC ENDOCRINE DISEASE

DIABETES MELLITUS

The most common and serious pulmonary complication of diabetes mellitus is infection, a subject discussed in some detail in Chapter 6 (*see* page 885). In addition, there have been a few studies of the intrinsic pathologic abnormalities in the lungs of patients with this disease. Vracko and his colleagues[235] measured the thickness of the alveolar epithelial and capillary basal laminae in diabetic patients and age-matched controls; they found both measurements to be significantly greater in the diabetics, although the increased thickness was much less than that observed in the basal laminae of muscle and renal tubules. In an experimental study of alloxan-induced diabetes in rats, an increase in the thickness of the capillary basal lamina was also demonstrated;[236] in addition, a variety of ultrastructural changes in type II pneumocytes, including a decrease in the amount of surfactant, were observed. These changes may be reflected in the mild, duration-related reduction in lung elastic recoil, pulmonary diffusing capacity, and pulmonary capillary blood volume that are observed in patients with insulin-dependent diabetes mellitus.[237] An unusual pulmonary abnormality has been documented by Reinilä in a retrospective autopsy study of 339 diabetics.[238] He found 20 patients (5.9 per cent) with perivascular "xanthogranulomas" consisting of aggregates of multinucleated giant cells and foamy histiocytes; in a control group of 156 individuals, only 3 (1.9 per cent) were similarly affected. The pathogenesis of this change is unclear; it is of no known functional or roentgenographic significance.

Cardiac arrest occurring in diabetic patients who develop severe autonomic neuropathy following pneumonia, anesthesia, or administration of depressant drugs has been attributed to an inability of the chemoreceptors to respond to hypoxia.[239, 240] Similarly, the threshold for cough reflex response to inhaled citric acid was found to be higher in diabetics with autonomic neuropathy than in nonneuropathic control diabetic patients; this suggests impairment of the vagal innervation of the bronchial tree.[241]

HYPOPITUITARISM AND ACROMEGALY

Both experimental[242] and physiological[243] investigations suggest that growth hormone exerts an important influence on lung structure. De Troyer and his colleagues[243] have shown that patients with hypopituitarism have a restrictive type of ventilatory impairment, total lung capacity being approximately 75 per cent of normal; by contrast, despite deficiency of one or more pituitary hormones, patients with acromegaly have large lungs with a total lung capacity approximately 25 per cent greater than matched controls. Other investigators[244] have confirmed the significant increase in lung volumes in acromegalics and, in addition, have described abnormal small airway function.

HYPOTHYROIDISM

An abnormal accumulation of fluid is known to occur in the pericardial and pleural spaces in patients with myxedema in the absence of cardiovascular, renal, or other causes of fluid retention.[245, 246] Patchy airspace disease has been described as well and in one study was presumed to be edema, although there was no dyspnea or cardiomegaly; the disease cleared on treatment of myxedema.[247]

Hypoxemia can also occur in patients with myxedema, usually in association with obesity and hypoventilation and often with coma.[248–251] However, some of these patients are not obese and their blood gas values have been shown to return to normal on thyroid therapy despite little or no change in body weight.[252, 253] Naeye[254] has documented the presence of amorphous eosinophilic material in relation to pulmonary capillaries and small pulmonary veins in 4 of 14 patients with inadequately treated myxedema; he suggested that this material consists of acid and (possibly) neutral mucopolysaccharides and that its presence might explain the hypoxemia detected in some patients.

HYPERPARATHYROIDISM

Hypercalcemia associated with hyperparathyroidism can result in diffuse metastatic calcification of the lungs and the heart. Usually detectable only by histologic examination, it is sometimes severe enough to be visible roentgenographically, especially with dual-energy digital radiography (*see* page 595).[255] Parathyroid hormone undoubtedly plays a role in the ectopic calcium deposition that occurs in patients with kidney[256] and liver[257, 258] transplants and in those with chronic renal failure, especially in patients undergoing maintenance hemodialysis; such metastatic calcification frequently involves the pulmonary parenchyma.[259–261] This form of ectopic calcification is to be differentiated from the diffuse dendriform pulmonary ossification associated with bronchitis and bronchiectasis.[262, 263]

KLINEFELTER'S SYNDROME

This inherited endocrine syndrome is characterized classically by small, firm testes, azoospermia, gynecomastia, elevated urinary gonadotropins, and often eunuchoid skeletal proportions. These patients are said to be prone to bronchitis, bronchiectasis, and asthma. Huseby and Petersen[264] studied 24 patients with the disorder and found 4 with asthma, 4 with chronic cough, 2 with an obstructive defect, and 11 with reduced functional residual capacity; the last-named was attributed to chest wall abnormality, since the lungs were considered to be normal.

NON-NEOPLASTIC HEMATOLOGIC DISORDERS

ACUTE CHEST SYNDROME OF SICKLE-CELL DISEASE

"Acute chest syndrome" occurs in patients with homozygous sickle-cell anemia (SS disease) and hemoglobin sickle-cell (SC) disease and consists of episodes of abrupt onset of fever, chest pain, leukocytosis, and roentgenographic evidence of pleuropulmonary disease. It is very common and is usually attributed to pneumonia, particularly when it occurs in children. Although there is little doubt that these patients are more susceptible to pneumococcal, hemophilus, and mycoplasma pneumonia, most studies[265–270] indicate that infection is a relatively rare cause, even in children. It is now evident that most episodes are caused by sickling leading to obstruction in the pulmonary vessels, a conclusion that has been corroborated to some extent by autopsy studies.[271] It is possible that the increasing use of pneumococcal vaccination and penicillin prophylaxis has significantly reduced the number of such episodes caused by infection,[267, 269] and as a result the etiology of the acute chest syndrome has changed.

CARBONIC ANHYDRASE II DEFICIENCY SYNDROME

This autosomal recessive syndrome includes osteopetrosis, renal tubular acidosis, cerebral calcification, mental retardation, growth failure, typical facial appearance, abnormal teeth, and a deficiency of carbonic anhydrase II in erythrocytes. Restrictive lung disease has been described in two patients.[272]

THALASSEMIA MAJOR

This inherited disorder of beta globulin synthesis is manifested largely by anemia and osteoporosis.

It can be associated with a restrictive respiratory defect with low PaO_2 and reduced static compliance, findings that are explained by a decrease in the growth of airspaces relative to the vascular bed and major airways during childhood.[273]

THROMBOTIC THROMBOCYTOPENIC PURPURA

Thrombotic thrombocytopenic purpura is a syndrome characterized by microangiopathic hemolytic anemia, thrombocytopenia, neurologic abnormalities, fever, and renal dysfunction. Bone and his colleagues[274] have described six patients with this disorder who developed an ARDS-like syndrome with respiratory failure. The patients were dyspneic and hypoxemic and showed roentgenographic evidence of pulmonary parenchymal opacities; five required mechanical ventilation. Four died and at autopsy the lungs were found to be edematous and hemorrhagic with hyaline membranes and thrombi. Disseminated intravascular coagulation was ruled out by the absence of clotting defects.

MISCELLANEOUS METABOLIC ABNORMALITIES

LIPID PROTEINOSIS

This rare familial metabolic disorder originally was considered to be a disease of the skin and the mucous membranes of the oral cavity and larynx,[275] but is now recognized as a generalized abnormality that can affect many organ systems, including the central nervous system, gastrointestinal tract, urinary tract, lymph nodes, striated muscle, and lungs.[276] The disorder follows a mendelian autosomal recessive pattern of transmission, and there are many cases of consanguinity reported in the parents of affected individuals.

Pathologically, the condition is characterized by the deposition in affected tissues of an amorphous eosinophilic material that has been demonstrated by histochemical analysis to contain a lipid; this led early investigators to suspect that the disorder was a lipoidosis. More recently, biochemical and electron microscopic studies have suggested that the material is principally a glycoprotein elaborated by fibrocytes.[277]

In 1967, Caplan[278] first described visceral involvement in patients with lipid proteinosis, with pulmonary abnormality being restricted to a minor degree of infiltration in the walls of capillaries. Roentgenographic abnormalities in the respiratory tract include diffuse or nodular thickening of the vocal cords and, in the case reported by Weidner and associates,[276] a diffuse reticulonodular pattern throughout both lungs simulating diffuse interstitial pulmonary fibrosis.

Patients with lipid proteinosis characteristically are seen for the first time by either the dermatologist (with a presentation of markedly thickened eyelids) or the otolaryngologist (with a presentation of chronic hoarseness). A number of patients suffer epileptiform attacks, but visceral lesions otherwise rarely initiate symptoms.[278]

FAMILIAL RETARDATION OF GROWTH, RENAL AMINOACIDURIA, AND COR PULMONALE

One report has appeared of this strange combination of abnormalities, which was found in three of six children of asymptomatic nonconsanguineous parents.[279, 280] Only one of the three children sur-
vived to the age of 10 years. The finding of greatest interest in the two children who died was a diffuse change in the skeletal musculature, consisting of fatty infiltration, loss of cross-striation, increased collagen content, foci of flocculation, and abortive attempts at regeneration in some large and medium-sized muscle fibers. In each of the three children, the left lung was smaller than normal and was the site of atelectasis and infection involving the basilar segments; the children experienced recurrent pulmonary infections. Arterial P_{CO_2} was elevated and P_{O_2} diminished, indicative of an "alveolar hypoventilation syndrome" that was considered to be caused by deficient musculature. All three children had aminoaciduria and aminoacidemia, metabolic abnormalities that were also detected in other members of the family.

REFERENCES

1. Rosen SH, Castleman B, Liebow AA: Pulmonary alveolar proteinosis. N Engl J Med 58:1123, 1958.
2. McCook TA, Kirks DR, Merton DF, et al: Pulmonary alveolar proteinosis in children. Am J Roentgenol 137:1023, 1981.
3. Avery ME, Ohlsson A, Cumming W, et al: In Godwin JT (ed): Clinicopathologic conference. Case presentation. King Faisal Special Hosp Med J 4:33, 1984.
4. Teja K, Cooper PH, Squires JE, et al: Pulmonary alveolar proteinosis in four siblings. N Engl J Med 305:1390, 1981.
5. Kariman K, Kylstra JA, Spook A: Pulmonary alveolar proteinosis: Prospective clinical experience in 23 patients for 15 years. Lung 162:223, 1984.
6. Bedrossian CWM, Luna MA, Conklin RH, et al: Alveolar proteinosis as a consequence of immunosuppression. A hypothesis based on clinical and pathologic observations. Hum Pathol 11:527, 1980.
7. Colón AR, Lawrence RD, Mills SD, et al: Childhood pulmonary alveolar proteinosis (PAP). Am J Dis Child 121:481, 1971.
8. Green D, Dighe P, Ali NO, et al: Pulmonary alveolar proteinosis complicating chronic myelogenous leukemia. Cancer 46:1763, 1980.
9. Carnovale R, Zornoza J, Goldman AM, et al: Pulmonary alveolar proteinosis: Its association with hematologic malignancy and lymphoma. Radiology 122:303, 1977.
10. Lakshminarayan S, Schwarz MI, Stanford RE: Unsuspected pulmonary alveolar proteinosis complicating acute myelogenous leukemia. Chest 69:433, 1976.
11. Aymard J-P, Gyger M, Lavallee R, et al: A case of pulmonary alveolar proteinosis complicating chronic myelogenous leukemia. Cancer 53:954, 1984.
12. Ruben FL, Talamo TS: Secondary pulmonary alveolar proteinosis occurring in two patients with acquired immune deficiency syndrome. Am J Med 80:1187, 1986.
13. Samuels MP, Warner J: Pulmonary alveolar lipoproteinosis complicating juvenile dermatomyositis. Thorax 43:939, 1988.
14. Knight DP, Knight JA: Pulmonary alveolar proteinosis in the newborn. Arch Pathol Lab Med 109:529, 1985.
15. Teja K, Cooper PH, Squires JE, et al: Pulmonary alveolar proteinosis in four siblings. N Engl J Med 305:1390, 1981.
16. Webster JR, Battifora H, Furey C, et al: Pulmonary alveolar proteinosis in 2 siblings with decreased immunoglobulin-A. Am J Med 69:786, 1980.
17. Corrin B, King E: Pathogenesis of experimental pulmonary alveolar proteinosis. Thorax 25:230, 1970.
18. Gross P, deTreville RTP: Alveolar proteinosis. Its experimental production in rodents. Arch Pathol 86:255, 1968.
19. Heppleston AG, Wright NA, Stewart JA: Experimental alveolar lipoproteinosis following the inhalation of silica. J Pathol 101:293, 1970.
20. Lee KP, Barras CE, Griffith FD, et al: Pulmonary response to glass fiber by inhalation exposure. Lab Invest 40:123, 1979.
21. Buechner HA, Ansari A: Acute silico-proteinosis. A new pathologic variant of acute silicosis in sandblasters, characterized by histologic features resembling alveolar proteinosis. Dis Chest 55:274, 1969.
22. Ranchod M, Bissell M: Pulmonary alveolar proteinosis and cytomegalovirus infection. Arch Pathol Lab Med 103:139, 1979.
23. Costello JF, Moriarty DC, Branthwaite MA: Diagnosis and management of alveolar proteinosis: The role of electron microscopy. Thorax 30:121, 1975.
24. Heppleston AG, Young AE: Alveolar lipo-proteinosis: An ultrastructural comparison of the experimental and human forms. J Pathol 107:107, 1972.
25. Gilmore LB, Talley FA, Hook GE: Classification and morphometric quantitation of insoluble materials from the lungs of patients with alveolar proteinosis. Am J Pathol 133:252, 1988.
26. Singh G, Katyal SL: Surfactant apoprotein in nonmalignant pulmonary disorders. Am J Pathol 101:51, 1980.
27. Bell DY, Hook GER: Pulmonary alveolar proteinosis: Analysis of airway and alveolar proteins. Am Rev Respir Dis 119:979, 1979.
28. Ito M, Takeuchi N, Ogura T, et al: Pulmonary alveolar proteinosis: Analysis of pulmonary washings. Br J Dis Chest 72:313, 1978.
29. Satoh K, Arai H, Yoshida T, et al: Glycosaminoglycans and glycoproteins in bronchoalveolar lavage fluid from patients with pulmonary alveolar proteinosis. Inflammation 7:347, 1983.
30. Takemura T, Fukuda Y, Harrison M, et al: Ultrastructural, histochemical, and freeze-fracture evaluation of multilamellated structures in human pulmonary alveolar proteinosis. Am J Anat 179:258, 1987.
31. Sahu S, DiAugustine RP, Lynn WS: Lipids found in pulmonary lavage of patients with alveolar proteinosis and in rabbit lung lamellar organelles. Am Rev Respir Dis 114:177, 1976.
32. Ramirez J, Harlan WR Jr: Pulmonary alveolar proteinosis. Nature and origin of alveolar lipid. Am J Med 45:502, 1968.
33. Ramirez J: Pulmonary alveolar proteinosis. Treatment by massive bronchopulmonary lavage. Arch Intern Med 119:147, 1967.
34. Golde DW, Territo M, Finley TN, et al: Defective lung macrophages in pulmonary alveolar proteinosis. Ann Intern Med 85:304, 1976.
35. Gonzalez-Rothi RJ, Harris JO: Pulmonary alveolar proteinosis. Further evaluation of abnormal alveolar macrophages. Chest 90:656, 1986.
36. Muller-Quernheim J, Schopf RE, Benes P, et al: A macrophage-suppressing 40-kD protein in a case of pulmonary alveolar proteinosis. Klin Wochenschr 65:893, 1987.
37. Nugent KM, Pesanti EL: Macrophage function in pulmonary alveolar proteinosis. Am Rev Respir Dis 127:780, 1983.
38. Deodhar SD, Bhagwat AG: Desquamative interstitial pneumonia-like syndrome in rabbits. Arch Pathol 84:54, 1967.
39. Bhagwat AG, Wentworth P, Conen PE: Observations on the relationship of desquamative interstitial pneumonia and pulmonary alveolar proteinosis in childhood: A pathologic and experimental study. Chest 58:326, 1970.
40. Spencer H: Pathology of the Lung: Excluding Pulmonary Tuberculosis. London–New York, Pergamon Press, 1962.
41. Divertie MB, Brown AL Jr, Harrison EG Jr: Pulmonary alveolar proteinosis. Two cases studied by electron microscopy. Am J Med 40:351, 1966.
42. Hudson AR, Halprin GM, Miller JA, et al: Pulmonary interstitial fibrosis following alveolar proteinosis. Chest 65:700, 1974.
43. Kaplan AI, Sabin S: Case report: Interstitial fibrosis after uncomplicated pulmonary alveolar proteinosis. Postgrad Med 61:263, 1977.
44. Clague HW, Wallace AC, Morgan WKC: Pulmonary interstitial fibrosis associated with alveolar proteinosis. Thorax 38:865, 1983.
45. Corsello BF, Choi H: Basophilic staining in pulmonary alveolar proteinosis. Report of three cases. Arch Pathol Lab Med 108:68, 1984.
46. Ramirez J: Pulmonary alveolar proteinosis. A roentgenologic analysis. Am J Roentgenol 92:571, 1964.
47. Sieracki JC, Horn RC Jr, Kay S: Pulmonary alveolar proteinosis: Report of three cases. Ann Intern Med 51:728, 1959.
48. Mendenhall E Jr, Solu S, Easom HF: Pulmonary alveolar proteinosis. Am Rev Respir Dis 84:876, 1961.
49. Greenspan RH: Chronic disseminated alveolar diseases of the lung. Semin Roentgenol 2:77, 1967.
50. Landis FB, Rose HD, Sternlieb RO: Pulmonary alveolar proteinosis. A case report with unusual clinical features and laboratory manifestations. Am Rev Respir Dis 80:249, 1959.
51. Kroeker EJ, Korfmacher S: Pulmonary alveolar proteinosis. Report of case with application of a special sputum examination as an aid to diagnosis. Am Rev Respir Dis 87:416, 1963.
52. Miller PA, Ravin CE, Smith GJW, et al: Pulmonary alveolar proteinosis with interstitial involvement. Am J Roentgenol 137:1069, 1981.
53. Yeh SD, White DA, Stover-Pepe DE, et al: Abnormal gallium scintigraphy in pulmonary alveolar proteinosis (PAP). Clin Nucl Med 12:294, 1987.
54. Godwin JD, Müller NL, Takasugi JE: Pulmonary alveolar proteinosis: CT findings. Radiology 169:609, 1988.
55. Anton HC, Gray B: Pulmonary alveolar proteinosis presenting with pneumothorax. Clin Radiol 18:428, 1967.
56. Lull GF Jr, Beyer JC, Maier JG, et al: Pulmonary alveolar proteinosis. Report of two cases. Am J Roentgenol 82:76, 1959.
57. Jones CC: Pulmonary alveolar proteinosis with unusual complicating infections. A report of two cases. Am J Med 29:713, 1960.
58. Rogers RM, Levin DC, Gray BA, et al: Physiologic effects of bronchopulmonary lavage in alveolar proteinosis. Am Rev Respir Dis 118:255, 1978.
59. McDowell C, Williams SE, Hinds JR: Pulmonary alveolar proteinosis. Report of a case. Aust Ann Med 8:137, 1959.
60. Ray RL, Salm R: A fatal case of pulmonary alveolar proteinosis. Thorax 17:257, 1962.
61. Jay SJ: Pulmonary alveolar proteinosis: Successful treatment with aerosolized trypsin. Am J Med 66:348, 1979.
62. Lovette JB, Magovern GJ, Kent EM: Alveolar proteinosis. Arch Intern Med 108:611, 1961.

63. Mork JN, Johnson JR, Zinneman HH, et al: Pulmonary alveolar proteinosis associated with IgG monoclonal gammopathy. Arch Intern Med 121:278, 1968.
64. Ramirez J: Pulmonary alveolar proteinosis. Treatment in a case complicated by tuberculosis. Am Rev Respir Dis 95:491, 1967.
65. Ramirez-Rivera J, Liebman M, Bartone JC: Pulmonary alveolar proteinosis. Diagnostic and pathologic implications of pulmonary washings. Am J Clin Pathol 45:415, 1966.
66. Martin RJ, Coalson JJ, Rogers RM, et al: Pulmonary alveolar proteinosis: The diagnosis by segmental lavage. Am Rev Respir Dis 121:819, 1980.
67. Rubinstein I, Mullen JB, Hoffstein V: Morphologic diagnosis of idiopathic pulmonary alveolar lipoproteinosis revisited. Arch Intern Med 148:813, 1988.
68. Glay A: Pulmonary alveolar proteinosis. (Report of a case.) J Can Assoc Radiol 17:16, 1960.
69. Oka S, Shiraishi K, Ogata K, et al: The course of the first case in Japan of pulmonary alveolar proteinosis. Am Rev Respir Dis 93:608, 1966.
70. Fraimow W, Cathcart RT, Taylor RC: Physiologic and clinical aspects of pulmonary alveolar proteinosis. Ann Intern Med 52:1177, 1960.
71. Snider TH, Wilner FM, Lewis BM: Cardiopulmonary physiology in a case of pulmonary alveolar proteinosis. Ann Intern Med 52:1318, 1960.
72. Oliva PB, Vogel JHK: Reactive pulmonary hypertension in alveolar proteinosis. Chest 58:167, 1970.
73. Fraimow W, Cathcart RT, Krishner JJ et al: Pulmonary alveolar proteinosis. A correlation of pathological and physiological findings in a patient followed up with serial biopsies of the lung. Am J Med 28:458, 1960.
74. Plenk HP, Swift SA, Chambers WL, et al: Pulmonary alveolar proteinosis—A new disease? Radiology 74:928, 1960.
75. Nicholas JJ, Auchincloss JH Jr, Rudolph L: Pulmonary alveolar proteinosis. A case with improvement after a short course of endobronchial instillations of heparin. Ann Intern Med 62:358, 1965.
76. Davidson JM, MacLeod WM: Pulmonary alveolar proteinosis. Br J Dis Chest 63:13, 1969.
77. Ramirez J, Kieffer RF Jr, Ball WC Jr: Bronchopulmonary lavage in man. Ann Intern Med 63:819, 1965.
78. Ramirez J, Campbell GD: Pulmonary alveolar proteinosis. Endobronchial treatment. Ann Intern Med 63:429, 1965.
79. McLaughlin JS, Ramirez J: Pulmonary alveolar proteinosis. Treatment by pulmonary segmental flooding. Am Rev Respir Dis 89:745, 1964.
80. Wasserman K, Blank N, Fletcher G: Lung lavage (alveolar washing) in alveolar proteinosis. Am J Med 44:611, 1968.
81. Farca A, Maher G, Miller A: Pulmonary alveolar proteinosis. JAMA 224:1283, 1973.
82. Selecky PA, Wasserman K, Benfield JR, et al: The clinical and physiological effect of whole-lung lavage in pulmonary alveolar proteinosis: A ten-year experience. Ann Thorac Surg 24:451, 1977.
83. Du Bois RM, McAllister WA, Branthwaite MA: Alveolar proteinosis: Diagnosis and treatment over a 10-year period. Thorax 38:360, 1983.
84. Bracci L: Role of physical therapy in management of pulmonary alveolar proteinosis. A case report. Phys Ther 68:686, 1988.
85. Wilson JW, Rubinfeld AR, White A, et al: Alveolar proteinosis treated with a single bronchial lavage. Med J Aust 145:158, 1986.
86. Busque L: Pulmonary lavage in the treatment of alveolar proteinosis. Can Anaesth Soc J 24:380, 1977.
87. Matuschak GM, Owens GR, Rogers RM, et al: Progressive intrapartum respiratory insufficiency due to pulmonary proteinosis. Amelioration by therapeutic whole-lung bronchopulmonary lavage. Chest 86:496, 1984.
88. Heymach GJ III, Shaw RC, McDonald JA, et al: Fiberoptic bronchopulmonary lavage for alveolar proteinosis in a patient with only one lung. Chest 81:508, 1982.
89. Jansen HM, Zuurmond WW, Roos CM, et al: Whole-lung lavage under hyperbaric oxygen conditions for alveolar proteinosis with respiratory failure. Chest 91:829, 1987.
90. Zapol WM, Wilson R, Hales C, et al: Venovenous bypass with a membrane lung to support bilateral lung lavage. JAMA 251:3269, 1984.
91. Freedman AP, Pelias A, Johnston RF, et al: Alveolar proteinosis lung lavage using partial cardiopulmonary bypass. Thorax 36:543, 1981.
92. Wilson DO, Rogers RM: Prolonged spontaneous remission in a patient with untreated pulmonary alveolar proteinosis. Am J Med 82:1014, 1987.
93. Mather CL, Hamlin GB: Pulmonary alveolar proteinosis: A case followed from diagnosis to recovery. N Engl J Med 272:1156, 1965.
94. Brodsky I, Mayock RL: Pulmonary alveolar proteinosis. Remission after therapy with trypsin and chymotrypsin. N Engl J Med 265:935, 1961.
95. Ozaki T, Nakayama T, Ishimi H, et al: Glucocorticoid receptors in bronchoalveolar cells from patients with idiopathic pulmonary fibrosis. Am Rev Respir Dis 126:968, 1982.
96. Smith LJ, Ankin MG, Katzenstein A-L, et al: Management of pulmonary alveolar proteinosis: Clinical conference in pulmonary disease from Northwestern University, McGaw Medical Center, Chicago. Chest 78:765, 1980.
97. Kisilevsky R: Biology of disease. Amyloidosis: A familiar problem in the light of current pathogenetic developments. Lab Invest 49:381, 1983.
98. Editorial: Amyloid and the lower respiratory tract. Thorax 38:84, 1983.
99. Westermark P, Pitkanen P, Benson L, et al: Serum prealbumin and retinol-binding protein in the prealbumin-related senile and familial forms of systemic amyloidosis. Lab Invest 52:314, 1985.
100. Wright JR, Calkins E: Clinical-pathologic differentiation of common amyloid syndromes. Medicine 60:429, 1981.
101. Wright JR, Calkins E, Humphrey RL: Potassium permanganate reaction in amyloidosis. A histologic method to assist in differentiating forms of this disease. Lab Invest 36:274, 1977.
102. Travis WD, Castile R, Vawter G, et al: Secondary (AA) amyloidosis in cystic fibrosis. A report of three cases. Am J Clin Pathol 85:419, 1986.
103. Wakasa K, Sakurai M, Koezuka I, et al: Primary tracheobronchial amyloidosis. A case report and review of reported cases. Acta Pathol Jpn 34:145, 1984.
104. Tamura K, Nakajima N, Makino S, et al: Primary pulmonary amyloidosis with multiple nodules. Eur J Radiol 8:128, 1988.
105. Whitwell F: Localized amyloid infiltrations of the lower respiratory tract. Thorax 8:309, 1953.
106. Monreal FA: Pulmonary amyloidosis: Ultrastructural study of early alveolar septal deposits. Hum Pathol 15:388, 1984.
107. Streeten EA, de la Monte SM, Kennedy TP: Amyloid infiltration of the diaphragm as a cause of respiratory failure. Chest 89:760, 1986.
108. Santiago RM, Scharnhorst D, Ratkin G, et al: Respiratory muscle weakness and ventilatory failure in AL amyloidosis with muscular pseudohypertrophy. Am J Med 83:175, 1987.
109. Gordon HW, Miller R Jr, Mittman C: Medullary carcinoma of the lung with amyloid stroma: A counterpart of medullary carcinoma of the thyroid. Hum Pathol 4:431, 1973.
110. Biberstein M, Wolf P, Pettross B, et al: Amyloidosis complicating cystic fibrosis. Am J Clin Pathol 80:752, 1983.
111. Ristow SC, Condemi JJ, Stuard ID, et al: Systemic amyloidosis in cystic fibrosis. Am J Dis Child 131:886, 1977.
112. Prior J, Crawford AD: Systemic amyloidosis complicating cystic fibrosis. Br J Dis Chest 74:84, 1980.
113. Michalsen H, Storrøsten OT, Lindboe CF: Generalized amyloidosis in cystic fibrosis. Eur J Respir Dis 66:306, 1985.
114. McGlennen RC, Burke BA, Dehner LP: Systemic amyloidosis complicating cystic fibrosis. A retrospective pathologic study. Arch Pathol Lab Med 110:879, 1986.
115. Glenner GG: Amyloid deposits and amyloidosis. The Beta-fibrilloses. N Engl J Med 302:1283, 1333, 1980.
116. Pitkänen P, Westermark P, Cornwell GG III: Senile systemic amyloidosis. Am J Pathol 117:391, 1984.
117. Cordier JF, Loire R, Brune J: Amyloidosis of the lower respiratory tract. Clinical and pathologic features in a series of 21 patients. Chest 90:827, 1986.
118. Hui AN, Koss MN, Hochholzer L, et al: Amyloidosis presenting in the lower respiratory tract. Clinicopathologic, radiologic, immunohistochemical, and histochemical studies on 48 cases. Arch Pathol Lab Med 110:212, 1986.
119. Da Costa P, Corrin B: Amyloidosis localized to the lower respiratory tract: Probable immunoamyloid nature of the tracheobronchial and nodular pulmonary forms. Histopathology 9:703, 1985.
120. Masuda C, Mohri S, Nakajima H: Histopathological and immunohistochemical study of amyloidosis. Br J Dermatol 119:33, 1988.
121. Smith RRL, Hutchins GM, Moore GW, et al: Type and distribution of pulmonary parenchymal and vascular amyloid. Correlation with cardiac amyloidosis. Am J Med 66:96, 1979.
122. Chen KTK: Amyloidosis presenting in respiratory tract. Pathol Ann 24:253, 1989.
123. Michaels L, Hyams VJ: Amyloid in localised deposits and plasmacytomas of the respiratory tract. J Pathol 128:29, 1979.
124. Cotton RE, Jackson JW: Localized amyloid "tumours" of the lung simulating malignant neoplasms. Thorax 19:97, 1964.
125. Mosetitsch W: Amyloid "tumoren" der lungen. (Amyloid tumors of the lungs.) Fortschr Roentgenstr 94:579, 1961.
126. Rubinow A, Celli BR, Cohen AS, et al: Localized amyloidosis of the lower respiratory tract. Am Rev Respir Dis 118:603, 1978.
127. Condon RE, Pinkham RD, Hames GH: Primary isolated nodular pulmonary amyloidosis. Report of a case. J Thorac Cardiovasc Surg 48:498, 1964.
128. Vaara J, Tukiainen H, Syrjanen K, et al: Solitary amyloid tumour

of the lung: A rare complication of primary amyloidosis. Eur J Respir Dis 67:385, 1985.

129. Jimenez C, Vital C, Merlio JP, et al: Plasmacytoma and gastric amyloidosis associated with nodular pulmonary amyloidosis. Ann Pathol 8:155, 1988.

130. Fors B, Rydén L: Tumoral amyloidosis of the lung. Acta Pathol Microbiol Scand 61:1, 1964.

131. Bhate DV: Case of the spring season: Diffuse primary amyloidosis with nodular calcified lung lesions. Semin Roentgenol 14:81, 1979.

132. Savader SJ, Nokes SR, Chappel G: Case report and review: Computed tomography of multiple nodular pulmonary amyloidosis. Comput Radiol 11:111, 1987.

133. Gibney RTN, Connolly TP: Pulmonary amyloid nodule simulating Pancoast tumor. J Can Assoc Radiol 35:90, 1984.

134. Celli BR, Rubinow A, Cohen AS, et al: Patterns of pulmonary involvement in systemic amyloidosis. Chest 74:543, 1978.

135. Briggs GW: Amyloidosis. Ann Intern Med 55:943, 1961.

136. Mathews WH: Primary systemic amyloidosis. Am J Med Sci 228:317, 1954.

137. Wang CC, Robbins LL: Amyloid disease. Its roentgen manifestations. Radiology 66:489, 1956.

138. Hsiu J-G, Stitik FP, D'Amato NA, et al: Primary amyloidosis presenting as a unilateral hilar mass. Report of a case diagnosed by fine needle aspiration biopsy. Acta Cytol 30:55, 1986.

139. Thompson PJ, Jewkes J, Corrin B, et al: Primary bronchopulmonary amyloid tumour with massive hilar lymphadenopathy. Thorax 38:153, 1983.

140. Wilson SR, Sanders DE, Delarue NC: Intrathoracic manifestations of amyloid disease. Radiology 120:283, 1976.

141. Desai RA, Mahajan VK, Benjamin S, et al: Pulmonary amyloidoma and hilar adenopathy. Rare manifestations of primary amyloidosis. Chest 76:170, 1979.

142. Melato M, Antonutto G, Falconieri G, et al: Massive amyloidosis of mediastinal lymph nodes in a patient with multiple myeloma. Thorax 38:151, 1983.

143. Osnoss KL, Harrell DD: Isolated mediastinal mass in primary amyloidosis. Chest 78:786, 1980.

144. Knapp MJ, Roggli VL, Kim J, et al: Pleural amyloidosis. Arch Pathol Lab Med 112:57, 1988.

145. Simon BG, Moutsopoulos HM: Primary amyloidosis resembling sicca syndrome. Arthritis Rheum 22:932, 1979.

146. Prowse CB, Elliott RIK: Diffuse tracheo-bronchial amyloidosis: A rare variant of a protean disease. Thorax 18:326, 1963.

147. Brown J: Primary amyloidosis. Clin Radiol 15:358, 1964.

148. Hodge DS, Anderson WR, Tsai SH: Primary diffuse bronchial amyloidosis. Arch Pathol Lab Med 101:615, 1977.

149. Simpson GT 2nd, Strong MS, Skinner M, et al: Localized amyloidosis of the head and neck and upper aerodigestive and lower respiratory tracts. Ann Otol Rhinol Laryngol 93:374, 1984.

150. Carbone JE, Barker D, Stauffer JL: Sleep apnea in amyloidosis. Chest 87:401, 1985.

151. Flemming AFS, Fairfax AJ, Arnold AG, et al: Treatment of endo-bronchial amyloidosis by intermittent bronchoscopic resection. Br J Dis Chest 74:183, 1980.

152. Lee S-C, Johnson HA: Multiple nodular pulmonary amyloidosis. A case report and comparison with diffuse alveolar-septal pulmonary amyloidosis. Thorax 30:178, 1975.

153. Moldow RE, Bearman S, Edelman MH: Pulmonary amyloidosis simulating tuberculosis. Am Rev Respir Dis 105:114, 1972.

154. Laden SA, Cohen ML, Harley RA: Nodular pulmonary amyloidosis with extrapulmonary involvement. Hum Pathol 15(6):594, 1984.

155. Lee AB, Bogaars HA, Passero MA: Nodular pulmonary amyloidosis. A cause of bronchiectasis and fatal pulmonary hemorrhage. Arch Intern Med 143:603, 1983.

156. Hardy TJ, Myerowitz RL, Bender BL: Diffuse parenchymal amyloidosis of lungs and breast. Its association with diffuse plasmacytosis and kappa-chain gammopathy. Arch Pathol Lab Med 103:583, 1979.

157. Road JD, Jacques J, Sparling JB: Diffuse alveolar septal amyloidosis presenting with recurrent hemoptysis and medial dissection of pulmonary arteries. Am Rev Respir Dis 132:1368, 1985.

158. Winter JH, Milroy R, Stevenson RD, et al: Secondary amyloidosis in association with Aspergillus lung disease. Br J Dis Chest 80:400, 1986.

159. Gaffney EF, Lee JCK: Systemic amyloidosis and hypogammaglobulinemia. Arch Pathol Lab Med 102:558, 1978.

160. Nomura S, Kumagai N, Kanoh T, et al: Pulmonary amyloidosis associated with systemic lupus erythematosus. Arthritis Rheum 29:680, 1986.

161. Meyerhoff J: Familial Mediterranean fever: Report of a large family, review of the literature, and discussion of the frequency of amyloidosis. Medicine 59:66, 1980.

162. Jones AW, Chatterji AN: Primary tracheobronchial amyloidosis with tracheobronchopathia osteoplastica. Br J Dis Chest 71:268, 1977.

163. Westermark P, Stenkvist B: A new method for the diagnosis of systemic amyloidosis. Arch Intern Med 132:522, 1973.

164. Kline LR, Dise CA, Ferro TJ, et al: Diagnosis of pulmonary amyloidosis by transbronchial biopsy. Am Rev Respir Dis 132:191, 1985.

165. Kamberg S, Loitman BS, Holtz S: Amyloidosis of the tracheobronchial tree. N Engl J Med 266:587, 1962.

166. Strange C, Heffner JE, Collins BS, et al: Pulmonary hemorrhage and air embolism complicating transbronchial biopsy in pulmonary amyloidosis. Chest 92:367, 1987.

167. Cathcart ES, Ritchie RF, Cohen AS, et al: Immunoglobulins and amyloidosis. An immunologic study of sixty-two patients with biopsy-proved disease. Am J Med 52:93, 1972.

168. Kyle RA: Multiple myeloma. Review of 869 cases. Mayo Clin Proc 50:29, 1975.

169. Morgan JE, McCaul DS, Rodriquez FH, et al: Pulmonary immunologic features of alveolar septal amyloidosis associated with multiple myeloma. Chest 92:704, 1987.

170. Hof DG, Rasp FL: Spontaneous regression of diffuse tracheobronchial amyloidosis. Chest 76:237, 1979.

171. Sunga MN Jr, Reyes CV, Zvetina J, et al: Resolution of secondary amyloidosis 14 years after adequate chemotherapy for skeletal tuberculosis. South Med J 82:92, 1989.

172. Eisenberg R, Sharma OP: Primary pulmonary amyloidosis. An unusual case with 14 years' survival. Chest 89:889, 1986.

173. Catovsky D, Ikoku NB, Pitney WR, et al: Thromboembolic complications in myelomatosis. Br Med J 3:438, 1970.

174. Brady RO: The sphingolipidoses. N Engl J Med 275:312, 1966.

175. Fifer WR: Atypical primary pulmonary histiocytosis-X. Am Rev Respir Dis 87:568, 1963.

176. Smith RRL, Hutchins GM, Sack GH Jr, et al: Unusual cardiac, renal and pulmonary involvement in Gaucher's disease. Interstitial glucocerebroside accumulation, pulmonary hypertension and fatal bone marrow embolization. Am J Med 65:352, 1978.

177. Wolson AH: Pulmonary findings in Gaucher's disease. Am J Roentgenol 123:712, 1975.

178. Schneider EL, Epstein CJ, Kaback MJ, et al: Severe pulmonary involvement in adult Gaucher's disease. Report of three cases and review of the literature. Am J Med 63:475, 1977.

179. Peters SP, Lee RE, Glew RH: Gaucher's disease: A review. Medicine 56:425, 1977.

180. Jackson DC, Simon G: Unusual bone and lung changes in a case of Gaucher's disease. Br Med J 38:698, 1965.

181. Puhr L: Mikrolithiasis alveolaris pulmonum. (Pulmonary alveolar microlithiasis.) Virchows Arch (Pathol Anat) 290:156, 1933.

182. Lieberman J, Beutler E: Elevation of serum angiotensin-converting enzyme in Gaucher's disease. N Engl J Med 294:1442, 1976.

183. Long RG, Lake BD, Pettit JE, et al: Adult Niemann-Pick disease. Its relationship to the syndrome of the sea-blue histiocyte. Am J Med 62:627, 1977.

184. Skikne MI, Prinsloo I, Webster I: Electron microscopy of lung in Niemann-Pick disease. J Pathol 106:119, 1972.

185. Crocker AC, Farber S: Niemann-Pick disease: A review of eighteen patients. Medicine 37:1, 1958.

186. Lachman R, Crocker A, Schulman J, et al: Radiological findings in Niemann-Pick disease. Radiology 108:659, 1973.

187. Bartimmo EE Jr, Guisan M, Moser KM: Pulmonary involvement in Fabry's disease: A reappraisal. Follow-up of a San Diego kindred and review of the literature. Am J Med 53:755, 1972.

188. Bagdade JD, Parker F, Ways PO, et al: Fabry's disease. A correlative clinical, morphologic, and biochemical study. Lab Invest 18:681, 1968.

189. Rosenberg DM, Ferrans VJ, Fulmer JD, et al: Chronic airflow obstruction in Fabry's disease. Am J Med 68:898, 1980.

190. Parkinson JE, Sunshine A: Angiokeratoma corporis diffusum universale (Fabry) presenting as suspected myocardial infarction and pulmonary infarcts. Am J Med 31:951, 1961.

191. Matsumoto T, Matsumori H, Taki T, et al: Infantile GM$_1$-gangliosidosis with marked manifestation of lungs. Acta Path Jap 29(2):269, 1979.

192. Garay SM, Gardella JE, Fazzini EP, et al: Hermansky-Pudlak syndrome. Pulmonary manifestations of a ceroid storage disorder. Am J Med 66:737, 1979.

193. Schinella RA, Greco MA, Garay SM, et al: Hermansky-Pudlak syndrome: A clinicopathologic study. Hum Pathol 16:366, 1985.

194. DePinho RA, Kaplan KL: The Hermansky-Pudlak syndrome. Report of three cases and review of pathophysiology and management considerations. Medicine 64:192, 1985.

195. Hoste P, Willems J, Devriendt J, et al: Familial diffuse interstitial pulmonary fibrosis associated with oculocutaneous albinism. Report of two cases with a family study. Scand J Respir Dis 60:128, 1979.

196. Takahashi A, Yokoyama T: Hermansky-Pudlak syndrome with special reference to lysosomal dysfunction. A case report and review of the literature. Virchows Arch (A) 402:247, 1984.

197. Rankin JA: Hermansky-Pudlak syndrome and interstitial lung disease: Report of a case with lavage findings. Am Rev Respir Dis 130:138, 1984.

16

198. Leitman BS, Balthazar EJ, Garay SM, et al: The Hermansky-Pudlak syndrome: Radiographic features. J Can Assoc Radiol 37:41, 1986.
199. Sastre J, Renedo G, González Mangado N, et al: Pulmonary ceroidosis. Chest 91:281, 1987.
200. Takahashi K, Hakozaki H, Kojima M: Idiopathic pulmonary ceroidosis. Acta Path Jap 28(2):301, 1978.
201. Caplan H: A case of endocardial fibro-elastosis with features of glycogen-storage disease. J Pathol Bact 76:77, 1958.
202. Lightman NI, Schooley RT: Adult-onset acid maltase deficiency. Case report of an adult with severe respiratory difficulty. Chest 72(2):250, 1977.
203. Semenza GL, Pyeritz RE: Respiratory complications of mucopolysaccharide storage disorders. Medicine 67:209, 1988.
204. Prockop DJ, Kivirikko KL: Heritable diseases of collagen. N Engl J Med 311:376, 1984.
205. Pyeritz RE: Connective tissue in the lung: Lessons from the Marfan syndrome. Ann Intern Med 103:289, 1985.
206. Mainardi CL, Kang AH: Collagen disease: A new perspective. Am J Med 71:913, 1981.
207. Fisk DE, Kuhn C: Emphysema-like changes in the lungs of the blotchy mouse. Am Rev Respir Dis 113:787, 1976.
208. Pyeritz RE, McKusick VA: Basic defects in the Marfan syndrome. N Engl J Med 305:1011, 1981.
209. McKusick VA: Heritable Disorders of Connective Tissue, 4th ed. St Louis, CV Mosby, 1972, p 187.
210. Goltz RW, Hult A-M, Goldfarb M, et al: Cutis laxa. A manifestation of generalized elastolysis. Arch Dermatol 92:373, 1965.
211. McKusick VA: Heritable Disorders of Connective Tissue, 4th ed. St Louis, CV Mosby, 1972.
212. McKusick VA: Heritable Disorders of Connective Tissue, 2nd ed. St Louis, CV Mosby, 1960, p 249.
213. Bolande RP, Tucker AS: Pulmonary emphysema and other cardiorespiratory lesions as part of the Marfan abiotrophy. Pediatrics 33:356, 1964.
214. McKusick VA: Heritable Disorders of Connective Tissue, 4th ed. St Louis, CV Mosby, 1972, p 372.
215. Murdoch JL, Walker BA, Halpern BL, et al: Life expectancy and causes of death in the Marfan syndrome. N Engl J Med 286:804, 1972.
216. Pyeritz RE, McKusick VA: The Marfan syndrome: Diagnosis and management. N Engl J Med 300:772, 1979.
217. Boucek RJ, Noble NL, Gunja-Smith Z, et al: The Marfan syndrome: A deficiency in chemically stable collagen cross-links. N Engl J Med 305:988, 1981.
218. Berliner S, Dean H, Pinkhas J: Spontaneous pneumothorax in a patient with Marfan syndrome. Respiration 42:127, 1981.
219. Hall JR, Pyeritz RE, Dudgeon DL, et al: Pneumothorax in the Marfan syndrome: Prevalence and therapy. Ann Thorac Surg 37:500, 1984.
220. Wood JR, Bellamy D, Child AH, et al: Pulmonary disease in patients with Marfan syndrome. Thorax 39:780, 1984.
221. Shilkin KB, Low LP, Chen BTM: Dissecting aneurysm of the pulmonary artery. J Pathol 98:25, 1969.
222. Verghese C: Anaesthesia in Marfan's syndrome. Anaesthesia 39:917, 1984.
223. Pyeritz RE: Maternal and fetal complications of pregnancy in the Marfan syndrome. Am J Med 71:784, 1981.
224. Clark JG, Kuhn C III, Uitto J: Lung collagen in type IV Ehlers-Danlos syndrome: Ultrastructural and biochemical studies. Am Rev Respir Dis 122:971, 1980.
225. Barabas AP: Heterogeneity of the Ehlers-Danlos syndrome: Description of three clinical types and a hypothesis to explain the basic defect(s). Br Med J 2:612, 1967.
226. Robitaille GA: Ehlers-Danlos syndrome and recurrent hemoptysis. Ann Intern Med 61:716, 1964.
227. Smit J, Alberts L, Balk AG: Pneumothorax in the Ehlers-Danlos syndrome: Consequence or coincidence? Scand J Respir Dis 59:239, 1978.
228. Hammerschmidt DE, Arneson MA, Larson SL, et al: Maternal Ehlers-Danlos syndrome type X. JAMA 248:2487, 1982.
229. Rivera-Alsina ME, Kwan P, Zavisca FG, et al: Complications of the Ehlers-Danlos syndrome in pregnancy. A case report. J Reprod Med 29:757, 1984.
230. Baumer JH, Hankey S: Transient pulmonary cysts in an infant with the Ehlers-Danlos syndrome. Br J Radiol 53:598, 1980.
231. Beighton P: Lethal complications of Ehlers-Danlos syndrome. Br Med J 3:656, 1968.
232. Jackson A, Loh C-L: Pulmonary calcification and elastic tissue damage in pseudoxanthoma elasticum. Histopathol 4:607, 1980.
233. Gaines JJ Jr: The pathology of alkaptonuric ochronosis. Hum Pathol 20:40, 1989.
234. Mudd SH, Levy HL: Disorders of transsulfuration. In Stanbury JB, Wyngaarden JB, Fredrickson DS, et al (eds): The Metabolic Basis of Inherited Disease, 5th ed. New York, McGraw-Hill, 1982, p 527.
235. Vracko R, Thorning D, Huang TW: Basal lamina of alveolar epithelium and capillaries: Quantitative changes with aging and in diabetes mellitus. Am Rev Respir Dis 120:973, 1979.
236. Sugahara K, Ushijima K, Morioka T, et al: Studies of the lung in diabetes mellitus. 1. Ultrastructural studies of the lungs in alloxan-induced diabetic rats. Virchows Arch (Pathol Anat) 390:313, 1981.
237. Sandler M, Bunn AE, Stewart RI: Cross-section study of pulmonary function in patients with insulin-dependent diabetes mellitus. Am Rev Respir Dis 135:223, 1987.
238. Reinilä A: Perivascular xanthogranulomatosis in the lungs of diabetic patients. Arch Pathol Lab Med 100:542, 1976.
239. Page McB, Watkins PJ: Cardiorespiratory arrest and diabetic autonomic neuropathy. Lancet 1:14, 1978.
240. Lloyd-Mostyn RH, Watkins PJ: Defective innervation of heart in diabetic autonomic neuropathy. Br Med J 3:15, 1975.
241. Vianna LG, Gilbey SG, Barnes NC, et al: Cough threshold to citric acid in diabetic patients with and without autonomic neuropathy. Thorax 43:569, 1988.
242. Brody JS, Buhain WJ: Hormonal influence on post-pneumonectomy lung growth in the rat. Respir Physiol 19:344, 1973.
243. De Troyer A, Desir D, Copinschi G: Regression of lung size in adults with growth hormone deficiency. Q J Med (New Series 49) 195:329, 1980.
244. Siafakas NM, Sigalas J, Filaditaki B, et al: Small airway function in acromegaly. Bull Eur Physiopathol Respir 23:329, 1987.
245. Schneierson SJ, Katz M: Solitary pleural effusion due to myxedema. JAMA 168:1003, 1958.
246. Brown SD, Brashear RE, Schnute RB: Pleural effusion in a young woman with myxedema. Arch Intern Med 143:1458, 1983.
247. Sadiq MA, Davies JC: Unusual lung manifestations of myxoedema. Br J Clin Pract 31:224, 1977.
248. Forester CF: Coma in myxedema. Report of a case and review of the world literature. Arch Intern Med 111:734, 1963.
249. Menendez CE, Rivlin RS: Thyrotoxic crisis and myxedema coma. Med Clin North Am 57:1463, 1973.
250. Weg John C, Calverly JR, Johnson C: Hypothyroidism and alveolar hypoventilation. Arch Intern Med 115:302, 1965.
251. Wilson WR, Bedell GN: The pulmonary abnormalities in myxedema. J Clin Invest 39:42, 1960.
252. Massumi RA, Winnacker JJ: Severe depression of the respiratory center in myxedema. Am J Med 36:876, 1964.
253. Domm BM, Vassalo CL: Myxedema coma with respiratory failure. Am Rev Respir Dis 107:842, 1973.
254. Naeye RL: Capillary and venous lesions in myxedema. Lab Invest 12:465, 1963.
255. Sanders C, Frank MS, Rostand SG, et al: Metastatic calcification of the heart and lungs in end-stage renal disease: Detection and quantification by dual-energy digital chest radiography. Am J Roentgenol 149:881, 1987.
256. Breitz HB, Sirotta PS, Nelp WB, et al: Progressive pulmonary calcification complicating successful renal transplantation. Am Rev Respir Dis 136:1480, 1987.
257. Munoz SJ, Nagelberg SB, Green PJ, et al: Ectopic soft tissue calcium deposition following liver transplantation. Hepatology 8:476, 1988.
258. Raisis IP, Park CH, Yang SL, et al: Lung uptake of technetium-99m phosphate compounds after liver transplantation. Clin Nucl Med 13:188, 1988.
259. Bestetti-Bosisio M, Cotelli F, Schiaffino E, et al: Lung calcification in long-term dialysed patients: A light and electronmicroscopic study. Histopathology 8:69, 1984.
260. Haque AK, Rubin SA, Leveque CM: Pulmonary calcification in long-term hemodialysis: A mimic of pulmonary thromboembolism. Am J Nephrol 4:109, 1984.
261. Jolles H, Johnson AC, Ell SR: Subcutaneous calcifications masquerading as pulmonary lesions in long-term hemodialysis. Review of nodular pulmonary opacities in the population undergoing hemodialysis. Chest 88:234, 1985.
262. Ndimbie OK, Williams CR, Lee MW: Dendriform pulmonary ossification. Arch Pathol Lab Med 111:1062, 1987.
263. Kawakami Y, Abe S, Nishimura K, et al: Diffuse pulmonary ossification associated with chronic bronchitis. Jpn J Med 26:409, 1987.
264. Huseby JS, Petersen D: Pulmonary function in Klinefelter's syndrome. Chest 80:31, 1981.
265. Charache S, Scott JC, Charache P: "Acute chest syndrome" in adults with sickle cell anemia. Microbiology, treatment, and prevention. Arch Intern Med 139:67, 1979.
266. Buchanan GR, Smith SJ, Holtkamp CA, et al: Bacterial infection and splenic reticuloendothelial function in children with hemoglobin SC disease. Pediatrics 72:93, 1983.
267. Poncz M, Kane E, Gill FM: Acute chest syndrome in sickle cell disease: Etiology and clinical correlates. J Pediatr 107:861, 1985.
268. Scharf MB, Lobel JS, Caldwell E, et al: Nocturnal oxygen desaturation in patients with sickle cell anemia. JAMA 249:1753, 1983.
269. Sprinkle RH, Cole T, Smith S, et al: Acute chest syndrome in

children with sickle cell disease. A retrospective analysis of 100 hospitalized cases. Am J Pediatr Hematol Oncol 8:105, 1986.

270. Powers D, Weidman JA, Odom-Maryon T, et al: Sickle cell chronic lung disease: Prior morbidity and the risk of pulmonary infection. Medicine 67:66, 1988.

271. Haupt HM, Moore GW, Bauer TW, et al: The lung in sickle cell disease. Chest 81:332, 1982.

272. Ohlsson A, Cumming WA, Paul A, et al: Carbonic anhydrase II deficiency syndrome: Recessive osteopetrosis with renal tubular acidosis and cerebral calcification. Pediatrics 77:371, 1986.

273. Cooper DM, Mansell AL, Weiner MA, et al: Low lung capacity and hypoxemia in children with thalassemia major. Am Rev Respir Dis 121:639, 1980.

274. Bone RC, Henry JE, Petterson J, et al: Respiratory dysfunction in thrombotic thrombocytopenic purpura. Am J Med 65:262, 1978.

275. Hardcastle SW, Rosenstrauch WJ: Lipoid proteinosis. A case report. S Afr Med J 66:273, 1984.

276. Weidner WA, Wenzl JE, Swischuk LE: Roentgenographic findings in lipoid proteinosis: A case report. Am J Roentgenol 110:457, 1970.

277. Shore RN, Howard BV, Howard WJ, et al: Lipoid proteinosis, demonstration of normal lipid metabolism in cultured cells. Arch Dermatol 110:591, 1974.

278. Caplan RM: Visceral involvement in lipoid proteinosis. Arch Dermatol 95:149, 1967.

279. Rowley PT, Mueller PS, Watkin DM, et al: Familial growth retardation, renal aminoaciduria and cor pulmonale. I. Description of a new syndrome, with case reports. Am J Med 31:187, 1961.

280. Rosenberg LE, Mueller PS, Watkin DM: A new syndrome: Familial growth retardation, renal aminoaciduria and cor pulmonale. II. Investigation of renal function, amino acid metabolism and genetic transmission. Am J Med 31:205, 1961.

281. Prowse CB: Amyloidosis of the lower respiratory tract. Thorax 13:308, 1958.

16

17

Pulmonary Disease of Unknown Origin

SARCOIDOSIS

Sarcoidosis (*synonyms:* Boeck's sarcoid, Besnier-Boeck-Schaumann disease) is a disease of unknown etiology that is difficult to define in precise terms. In 1976, a subcommittee on Classification and Definition of Sarcoidosis of the New York Academy of Science proposed the following definition:[1]

Sarcoidosis is a multisystem granulomatous disorder of unknown etiology most commonly affecting young adults and presenting most frequently with bilateral lymphadenopathy, pulmonary infiltration, and skin or

eye lesions. The diagnosis is established most securely when clinicoradiographic findings are supported by histologic evidence of widespread noncaseating epithelioid cell granulomas in more than one organ or a positive Kveim-Siltzbach skin test. Immunological features are depression of delayed-type hypersensitivity suggesting T-cell anergy and raised serum immunoglobulins suggesting B-cell overactivity. There may also be hypercalciuria with or without hypercalcemia. The course and prognosis correlate with the mode of onset. An acute onset usually heralds a self-limiting course with spontaneous resolution, while an insidious onset may be followed by relentless progressive fibrosis. Corticosteroids relieve symptoms and suppress inflammation and granuloma formation.

EPIDEMIOLOGY

Precise figures regarding the incidence of sarcoidosis are difficult to obtain, partly because its presence in the majority of patients is first identified on screening chest roentgenograms of asymptomatic individuals; this implies that many cases never come to clinical attention. For example, from a comprehensive review of the world literature to 1967,[2] Scadding found that approximately 50 per cent of patients with sarcoidosis were asymptomatic when the disease was first recognized; 25 per cent presented with respiratory symptoms, usually dyspnea; and the remaining 25 per cent had extrathoracic symptoms only, often related to the skin or eyes. Our own experience has been similar. The following statistics relating to the incidence and prevalence of sarcoidosis must be considered in the light of these observations.

Sarcoidosis shows considerable variation in reported incidence in different countries and continents. Although to a large extent such geographic variation undoubtedly is related to true differences in incidence, it probably is also a reflection of local awareness and interest in the disease. As a generalization, the disease is more common in temperate than in tropical climates,[2] most large series having been reported from Scandinavia, England, and the United States.[3-9] The incidence in Sweden is 64 per 100,000 population and in Norway 26.7 per 100,000;[10] in the United States a reasonable estimate of prevalence of a roentgenographic pattern consistent with the diagnosis is about 10 per 100,000 examinations.[2, 11, 12] The disease is uncommon in Southeast Asia;[11] in Japan, for example, the incidence is 5.6 per 100,000.[10] It is especially rare among the Chinese. A mass community roentgenographic survey of 3.6 million persons in Taiwan did not uncover a single case;[13] however, four confirmed cases have been described more recently in Hong Kong Chinese,[14] and of eight patients with sarcoidosis seen over a period of 10 years in Singapore, five were Chinese.[15] In the United States, recognition of the disease in a Chinese patient justifies publication.[13, 16]

Sarcoidosis is rarely seen in African[2] or South American blacks or mulattoes[17] but is unusually common in the black population of the United States. This is particularly true in black women, in whom the incidence has been estimated to be 10 to 17 times that in Caucasians.[3, 4] A disproportionately high incidence also has been observed in Puerto Ricans living in the United States[18, 19] and in West Indians in the United Kingdom.[20] The disease appears to be more prevalent in rural areas, a distribution that has been particularly noted in the southeastern United States[21] and in Switzerland.[22] Epidemiologic studies of military personnel[23, 24] suggested that the greatest concentration of sarcoidosis in the United States is in the eastern, and particularly the southeastern, portion of the country. However, two subsequent surveys of patients from the general population failed to confirm such a geographic predominance, probably because of the fact that in these two series, females outnumbered males by three to one.[5, 6]

Sex incidence varies among series, with no predominance in some series and a definite female predominance in others;[2, 3] the clear-cut increased risk in black American women has been mentioned. Although the disease may occur at any age, it is recognized most commonly in patients between the ages of 20 and 40 years.[2, 4] In Mayock's review of 1,254 cases,[4] 50 per cent of the patients were in this age group; only 2 per cent were under the age of 10 years and only 4 per cent over the age of 60 years. A well-documented case of sarcoidosis of recent origin in an 81-year-old woman in the United Kingdom has been touted as the oldest patient reported with this disease in the world.[25] Estimates of the incidence of the disease in children may be low, since screening chest roentgenograms are less likely to be obtained in this age group.[26] This lack of screening of asymptomatic children is perhaps the explanation for reports in the American medical literature suggesting that sarcoidosis is more apt to be associated with symptoms in children than in adults;[27, 28] for example, in an analysis of the clinical and roentgenographic characteristics of pulmonary sarcoidosis in 26 children ranging in age from 2.5 to 17 years (mean 13 years), Merten and his colleagues[29] found that 25 of the children (96 per cent) were symptomatic at the time of diagnosis. By contrast, in a study in Japan where schoolchildren have yearly chest roentgenograms, of 45 children with a diagnosis of sarcoidosis, 42 were asymptomatic.[26] In very young children under the age of 4 years, the incidence of symptoms referable to the joints, skin, and eyes is unusually high, most reported patients being Caucasian.[28, 30]

ETIOLOGY AND PATHOGENESIS

The etiology of sarcoidosis is unknown, but the observation that the lungs and regional thoracic lymph nodes are the structures most often involved (in 80 to 90 per cent of cases in large series[31, 32]) suggests that the disease is caused by some agent that enters the body via the lungs, presumably by inhalation. Support for this hypothesis lies in the finding of an increased percentage of lymphocytes and activated alveolar macrophages in bronchoalveolar lavage (BAL) fluid from patients with extrathoracic sarcoidosis who show no clinical, roentgenographic,[33] or physiologic[34] evidence of pulmonary or mediastinal disease.

The most popular etiologic agents that have come under suspicion are microorganisms, particularly *Mycobacterium tuberculosis*[35] and nontuberculous mycobacteria.[36] Experimental evidence suggesting a transmissible agent such as a microorganism was reported by Mitchell and his associates who found that they could produce granulomas in the footpads or viscera of mice by inoculating homogenates of human sarcoid tissue.[37–39] In addition, the electron microscopic observation by Wang and his associates[40] (since duplicated by Dewar and colleagues[285]) of tadpole-shaped structures in granulomas from four patients with sarcoidosis suggests the possibility of an infectious agent. Tubulospherical bodies have been identified by transmission electron microscopy in vitreous leukocytes of patients with sarcoidosis and have been transmitted directly to mice, resulting in granulomatous uveitis.[962] A peculiar association between sarcoidosis and infection by the gram negative rod *Yersinia enterocolitica* has been described;[41] although this organism most often involves the gastrointestinal tract, it can cause a clinical picture that is virtually identical to sarcoidosis, including the presence of erythema nodosum and acute arthritis (*see* page 850). Despite the evidence suggesting an infectious etiology, culture of affected tissue is invariably sterile and microorganisms are not seen with special tissue stains. In addition, there is no evidence of human-to-human transmission of the disease. Other possible etiologic agents have been discussed in greater detail by Scadding[35] and by Williams.[42]

Although the pathogenesis of sarcoidosis is also poorly understood, there is abundant evidence that some abnormality of immune function is important. Much of the work documenting this connection has been related to an analysis of cells and immune mediators obtained by BAL. In normal, nonsmoking individuals, a typical BAL cell population consists of over 90 per cent macrophages, 9 per cent lymphocytes, and less than 1 per cent polymorphonuclear leukocytes. Of the lymphocytes, over 90 per cent are T cells, of which approximately 50 per cent are helper (Th) cells, 25 per cent suppressor (Ts) cells, and less than 10 per cent B cells. In cigarette smokers with no evidence of pulmonary disease, the cell differential is similar to that of normal individuals except that the neutrophil content is increased up to 5 per cent and the number of alveolar macrophages is proportionally decreased.[43] By contrast with those two groups, the BAL fluid of patients with active sarcoidosis contains approximately 60 per cent macrophages and 40 per cent lymphocytes.[43] This increase in lymphocytes is caused almost entirely by an increase in the Th subset;[44–49] in most reports, the proportion of helper to suppressor T cells ranges from about 6.5:1[49] to as high as 10.5:1.[44, 45] Proliferation of lymphocytes and an increased Th-Ts ratio also have been described in other pulmonary interstitial diseases, such as drug-induced toxicity,[50, 51] pneumoconiosis,[71] and amyloidosis;[52] however, proportions greater than 2.5:1 are seldom encountered.[53] The pathogenesis of this T-cell proliferation may be related to the production of interleukin-1, a monokine that probably originates from activated alveolar macrophages that have been shown to stimulate the recruitment and proliferation of pulmonary alveolar Th cells.[54] However, the reason for the specific expansion of activated Th cells is unclear; it does not appear to be caused by an inherent abnormality of Ts cells or of their suppressor T-cell function.[55, 56] In addition, a role has not been identified for the recently described circulating IgM anti-T cell autoantibody;[57] this antibody binds mostly to suppressor T cells but has no inhibitory effects *in vitro* on their activation or proliferative response.[58]

Although T-cell abnormalities in BAL fluid are the most obvious, the proportion and type of a variety of other cells are also abnormal. Subpopulations of alveolar macrophages in patients with active sarcoidosis differ from those of normal subjects;[59–62] many are immature, probably as a result of their recent recruitment from blood monocytes.[63] In addition, most,[64–68] but not all,[69] investigators have found the density of class II major histocompatibility complex (MHC) HLA-DR (Ia-like) antigen expression of alveolar macrophages to be increased in pulmonary sarcoidosis, a finding that appears to be linked to a combination of lymphocytosis, T-lymphocyte subtype distribution, and the production of chemical mediators. Neutrophils are rarely found in BAL fluid of nonsmoking patients with sarcoidosis,[70] although they may be present in greater proportion than normal in advanced, presumably inactive fibrotic disease.[72] BAL fluid also shows an increase in the number of killer (K) and natural killer (NK) lymphocytes,[44] HLA-DR antigen-bearing lymphocytes,[62, 73–75] and mast cells, many with evidence of accentuated mediator release.[76] Ultrastructural features of "activation" have been described in 10 to 70 per cent of these and other cells in BAL fluid from patients with sarcoidosis.[78] It is of some interest from a pathogenetic point of view that the proportion of cells present in pulmonary interstitial tissue in biopsy specimens of normal subjects and of patients with sarcoidosis is similar to that found in BAL fluid.[62, 70, 79]

In addition to the cellular abnormalities of BAL fluid in patients with sarcoidosis, a variety of immune-related mediators are present in the supernatant of BAL/activated Th cells grown in culture, mediators that are undoubtedly important in the pathogenesis of the disease (Fig. 17–1). These include monocyte chemotactic factor, migration inhibition factor, leukocyte inhibitory factor, a polyclonal activator of B cells that causes production of immunoglobulins, and a fibroblast growth factor.[45, 66, 80–84] Measurable immune mediators secreted by proliferating Th cells include interleukin-2[85–88] and gamma interferon (IFN gamma), the latter being associated with activation of alveolar macrophages[83] and the growth of lung fibroblasts.[84] Pulmonary T lymphocytes from patients with active sarcoidosis, but not from normal subjects or patients with fibrosing alveolitis, secrete large quantities of a chemotactic factor for monocytes.[80, 89] In addition,

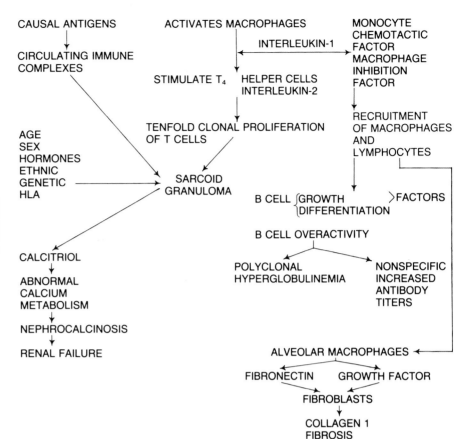

Figure 17–1. Factors Contributing to Sarcoid Granuloma Formation and to Sarcoidosis. (Reprinted from James DG: Definition and Classification of Granulomatous Disorders, Seminars in Respiratory Medicine, 8:1, 1986.)

the amount of this factor produced by T lymphocytes in BAL fluid has been estimated to be 25 times that produced by peripheral blood T lymphocytes,[89] thus establishing a gradient between lung and blood that results in a virtually continuous supply of the cells that eventually become the epithelioid cells of pulmonary granulomas (see farther on).

Activity of the effector cells in sarcoidosis is strangely parochial. Compartmentalization (anatomic localization) of the immune response as defined by the clonal proliferation of Th cells[46, 90] or by the accumulation of interleukin-2[86, 87] has been documented by several observers. Sites of involvement include not only the lungs (as reflected in BAL fluid) but also the pleura (as reflected in effusion),[91] mediastinal lymph nodes,[92] bone marrow,[82] and various other organs in which sarcoid granulomas develop.[86, 90] In such cases, the blood does not show the same Th cell proliferation and increased Th-Ts ratio as that in BAL fluid. In fact, the peripheral blood of patients with active sarcoidosis shows lymphopenia, a decrease in the number of Th cells, and a decrease in the Th-Ts ratio.[45, 49, 82, 91, 93, 94] In vitro assessment of indices of cell-mediated immunity, including interleukin-2 secretion[58] and natural killer cell activity,[95] has shown that peripheral blood T cells from patients with active sarcoidosis are lacking in response.[58, 86, 96, 97] This in vitro anergy could explain the negative

delayed hypersensitivity skin reactions to various antigens seen in sarcoidosis, although a number of studies[98–100] suggest that an inhibitor of interleukin-1 (very likely a prostaglandin) produced by bronchoalveolar inflammatory cells[101] may leak into the peripheral circulation and depress systemic immune reactivity. Despite this evidence for depression of the cell-mediated immune system, patients with sarcoidosis do not appear to be unduly susceptible to opportunistic infection, with the possible exception of those with "cyst" formation. In these patients certain infections such as invasive aspergillosis may occur as an extension of a complicating aspergilloma. On the other hand, patients with primary humoral or cell-mediated immunodeficiency can develop a generalized granulomatous process resembling sarcoidosis,[102–105] although it is probable that this association is purely coincidental.

Activated T-helper lymphocytes appear to play a role in the activation of B lymphocytes, with resultant hypergammaglobulinemia.[48, 85] In the peripheral blood, B lymphocyte overactivity is reflected in increased levels of immunoglobulins and of kappa and lambda chains, sometimes accompanied by circulating immune complexes. These manifestations of humoral immunity are usually seen in patients with more extensive organ involvement[106, 107] and are less common in those with hilar lymph node enlargement only.[106, 108] The exception appears to be patients presenting with erythema nodosum in whom an abrupt rise in immunoglobulins is associated with a rapidly developing alveolitis.[109] Immune complexes are found more often in patients with a combination of erythema nodosum, arthralgia, and uveitis;[44, 110, 111] these patients also show an increased incidence of the histocompatibility antigen, HLA-B8.[112–114]

Although immunologic abnormalities are the most consistently demonstrated and perhaps the most important in the pathogenesis of sarcoidosis, other factors also have been investigated. For example, reports of sarcoidosis occurring in more than one member of a family[115–121] and in identical twins[3, 122] have suggested the possibility of a genetic factor. In fact, the high prevalence of the disease in the Republic of Ireland has been linked to an occurrence of the disease among siblings; in one study comprising 114 index patients with biopsy-proved sarcoidosis and a total sibling pool of 534 individuals, 11 (9.6 per cent) of the index patients were found to have at least one sibling with sarcoidosis.[123] In only two instances was the temporal profile of onset of the disease considered to be suggestive of intrafamilial spread of a transmissible agent that could have offered an alternative explanation for the clustering of the disease cases. However, examples have been reported in the literature of temporal clustering of familial sarcoidosis in non-consanguineous relatives[124] and in close acquaintances,[125] thus supporting the concept of exposure to a common etiologic agent. In at least two statistical surveys,[126, 127] the incidence of sarcoidosis has been found to be significantly higher among nonsmokers than among smokers, an unexpected finding first reported by Comstock and colleagues;[128] however, in one study of American patients with sarcoidosis,[129] a "protective" effect of cigarette smoking was not confirmed. The mechanism by which such an effect might occur, if it does at all, is unknown.

The pathogenesis of the fibrosis in the lungs of patients with sarcoidosis is probably multifactorial.[81] Gamma interferon, a soluble mediator released from activated lymphocytes, is considered by some investigators to stimulate fibrogenesis;[84] a variety of substances produced by alveolar macrophages, such as gamma interferon, interleukin-1, fibronectin, an unidentified substance known as alveolar macrophage-derived growth factor (AMDGF), and platelet-derived growth factor (PDGF), also have been described as playing roles.[130–133] Prostaglandin E_2 (PGE_2) may act both as an inhibitor of fibroblast proliferation and as a modulator of the fibrotic response.[81] Alveolar macrophages from patients with sarcoidosis also produce increased amounts of the initial enzymes of both coagulation and fibrinolytic pathways, indicating that they may regulate the formation of a fibrin matrix in alveolar tissue on which subsequent fibrosis can develop.[77] There is also reason to believe that oxygen radicals, pro-

teinases, cationic proteins, and various other substances released from dying cells can contribute to the lung destruction and subsequent fibrosis as they are believed to do in fibrosing alveolitis, drug-induced pulmonary diseases, and adult respiratory distress syndrome (ARDS).[134]

PATHOLOGIC CHARACTERISTICS

The pathologic hallmark of sarcoidosis is the granuloma, which, in its early stages, is identical to that caused by many well-defined etiologic agents—a sharply circumscribed collection of epithelioid histiocytes sometimes associated with multinucleated giant cells (Fig. 17–2). The histiocytes are large cells with abundant eosinophilic cytoplasm and oval or kidney-shaped, vesicular nuclei. Lymphocytes, occasionally plasma cells, and rarely neutrophils and eosinophils can be intermingled with the epithelioid histiocytes. Monoclonal antibody studies[135] have shown that suppressor T lymphocytes tend to be located in the periphery of the granuloma whereas helper cells are distributed throughout its substance; although this implies different functional zones within the granuloma, the relationship of these to the pathogenesis is not clear.

Cytoplasmic inclusions are not infrequently present within the cells of the granuloma, especially the multinucleated giant cells; they include the asteroid body, the lamellated or conchoidal (Schaumann) body (Fig. 17–3), and small needle-shaped or ovoid, refractile particles to which a specific name is usually not applied.[136] It has been hypothesized that the refractile particles form the nucleus upon which a protein matrix, calcium salts, and iron are deposited to form the Schaumann body.[136] Although all these inclusions are more commonly identified in the granulomas of sarcoidosis, they also can be present in granulomas of other etiology[136, 137] and are of no value in differential diagnosis.

The majority of sarcoid granulomas are nonnecrotizing, but some contain small foci of necrosis, the presence of which does not exclude the diagnosis.[137, 138] The necrosis usually occupies the central one quarter of the granuloma and appears as amorphous eosinophilic material that may be associated with degenerated, hyperchromatic nuclei (Fig. 17–4); rarely, it is more extensive, occupying up to one half the diameter of the granuloma, and possesses a granular appearance more suggestive of an infectious etiology.

Although it is probable that in most patients many granulomas resolve completely over time,[138] some undergo progressive fibrosis. Fibroblasts are present in considerable numbers at the periphery of more mature granulomas,[139, 140] and it appears that the fibrosis begins at this site. In such circumstances, concentric lamellae of collagen can be seen to separate the histologically "active" central portion

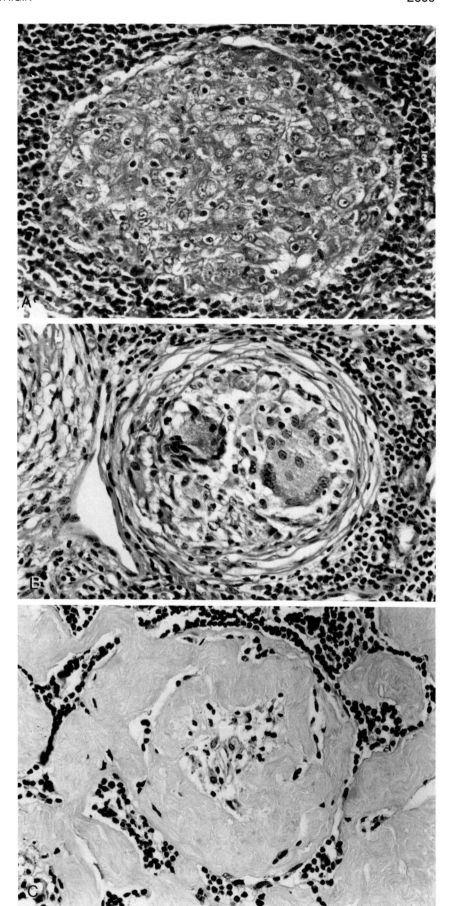

Figure 17–2. Sarcoidosis: Granulomas. Histologic sections show three well-circumscribed granulomas in different stages of activity. The most active *(A)* shows numerous epithelioid histiocytes with scattered small mononuclear cells (probably a combination of lymphocytes and monocytes); there is no fibrosis or necrosis. A later stage *(B)* shows a distinct zone of collagen possessing a clear-cut lamellated appearance at the periphery; two multinucleated giant cells are evident. An even later stage *(C)* shows almost complete replacement of the granuloma by mature fibrous tissue. *(A, B, C,* × 300.)

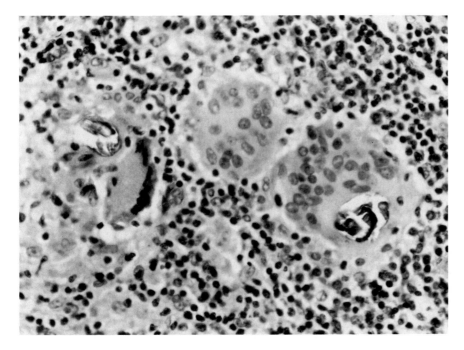

Figure 17–3. Sarcoidosis: Schaumann's Bodies. A histologic section reveals isolated multinucleated giant cells in a lymph node that elsewhere showed typical sarcoid granulomas; the giant cells contain two structures that are somewhat lamellated, irregularly shaped, and darkly stained, the characteristic appearance of Schaumann's bodies. (The presence of calcium has resulted in fracture during tissue cutting.) (×400.)

Figure 17–4. Sarcoidosis: Necrosis. A histologic section shows a well-circumscribed granuloma in the central portion of which is a cluster of necrotic cells with hyperchromatic nuclei associated with dense, eosinophilic cytoplasm *(arrow)*. (×250.)

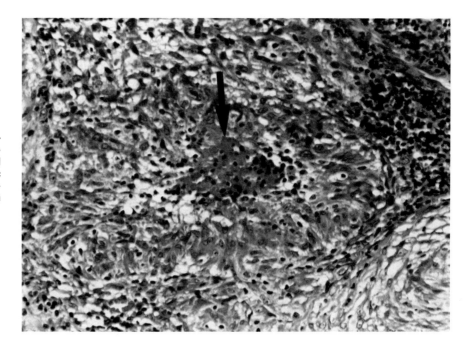

of the granuloma from the adjacent tissue (Fig. 17–2). With time, the fibrosis proceeds inwards until the entire granuloma is converted into a fibrous scar (Fig. 17–2). This pattern of peripheral lamellar fibrosis is characteristic of healing sarcoidosis and is itself strong evidence in favor of the diagnosis.

It should be emphasized that the finding of non-necrotizing granulomas does not in itself constitute absolute evidence of sarcoidosis, since such lesions are by no means specific. Local or diffuse non-necrotizing granulomas ("sarcoid lesions") can be found in various tissues or organs in association with a wide variety of conditions, including infections (particularly mycobacterial and fungal),[141] extrinsic allergic alveolitis, neoplasms (including pulmonary carcinoma,[142] leukemia, and Hodgkin's and non-Hodgkin's lymphoma), Crohn's disease,[144–146] celiac disease,[147] Whipple's disease,[148] pneumoconiosis (particularly that caused by beryllium but also by such minerals as mica[149] and talc), drugs,[150, 151] and foreign bodies. In some cases, ancillary procedures such as culture of biopsied material, special stains for mycobacteria or fungi, and polarization microscopy may clarify the nature of the granulomatous process. However, even negative results of these and other investigations do not exclude a specific etiologic agent, and it is necessary to make a careful distinction between the pathologic finding of non-necrotizing granulomatous inflammation and the clinical-roentgenographic process known as sarcoidosis.[3]

Pulmonary involvement in sarcoidosis is characteristically most prominent in the peribronchovascular, interlobular septal, and pleural interstitial tissue (Fig. 17–5). In the early stages, granulomas are typically discrete and histologically active; as the disease progresses, however, they often become confluent and associated with fibrosis, resulting in more or less diffuse interstitial thickening. The parenchymal interstitium is also affected, although typically less so than the peribronchovascular, septal, and pleural locations; in the early stage of the disease this is manifested by a nonspecific pneumonitis, comprised largely of an infiltrate of lymphocytes and histocytes in alveolar septa (Fig. 17–6).[81, 139, 152, 153] As the disease progresses, these foci appear to become granulomatous in nature[153] and can bulge into the adjacent alveolar airspaces.[154, 155] Individual foci of disease are usually microscopic in size but can conglomerate with granulomas in the peribronchovascular and septal interstitium to form relatively discrete masses 4 cm or more in diameter, an appearance sometimes referred to as "nodular sarcoidosis." Although evolution of disease from a stage of alveolitis to one of granuloma formation and eventually fibrosis is probably the rule in many cases, a number of studies indicate that such a process is by no means invariable.[156–159]

Possibly because of the prominent peribronchovascular and septal location of the granulomatous inflammation, involvement of pulmonary arteries and veins is common in sarcoidosis (Fig. 17–7);[154–155] in one study of open lung biopsy specimens from 128 patients, it was identified in 88 patients (69 per cent).[160] Although this inflammation can be associated with disruption of the elastic laminae, necrosis does not occur. Thrombosis is rare and is probably related to luminal compression rather than the inflammatory reaction itself. In addition to their location in peribronchial connective tissue, granulomas are also common in airway mucosa where they are not infrequently seen in bronchial biopsy specimens; although probably most common in small airways, they can also occur in the walls of larger bronchi.[161]

The gross appearance of pulmonary sarcoidosis depends on the stage and severity of disease. In the early, milder forms in which inflammation is most prominent in relation to peribronchovascular, interlobular, and pleural connective tissue, the appearance resembles lymphangitic carcinomatosis. As the disease progresses in both extent and time, involvement of the parenchymal interstitium becomes more evident and large portions of lung can become consolidated and eventually fibrotic. This process is usually most severe in the apical portion of the upper lobes where it can possess a honeycomb appearance characteristic of fibrosing alveolitis. More often, however, it takes the form of more or less solid areas of fibrous tissue associated with bronchiectasis (Fig. 17–8). The latter can be severe enough to result in the formation of large "cavities"; these are not infrequently the site of colonization by *Aspergillus* species,[162] a complication sometimes associated with fatal hemoptysis.[143, 162]

Lymph node involvement in sarcoidosis takes the form of more or less diffuse replacement of the node by granulomas (Fig. 17–9), often with a variable histologic appearance.[163] Initially, the granulomas are discrete and active looking; as with pulmonary disease, however, they can become confluent and undergo progressive fibrosis. In the advanced state this can result in completely fibrotic nodes in which granulomas are difficult to recognize.

ROENTGENOGRAPHIC MANIFESTATIONS

The roentgenographic changes in thoracic sarcoidosis can be usefully classified for descriptive purposes into five groups or stages:

Stage 0. No demonstrable abnormality.

Stage 1. Hilar and mediastinal lymph node enlargement unassociated with pulmonary abnormality.

Stage 2. Hilar and mediastinal lymph node enlargement associated with pulmonary abnormality.

Stage 3. Diffuse pulmonary disease unassociated with node enlargement.

Stage 4. Pulmonary fibrosis.

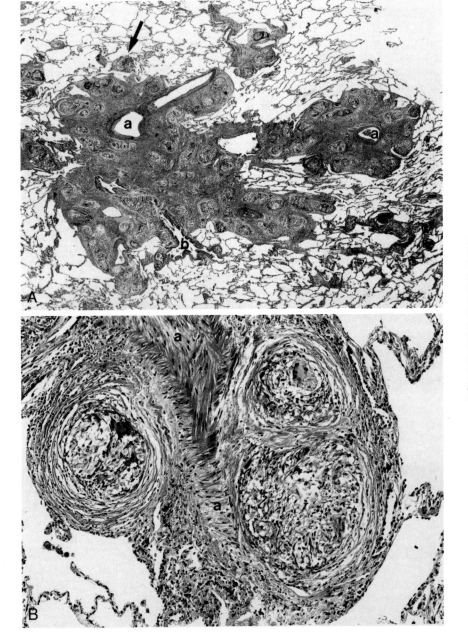

Figure 17–5. Pulmonary Sarcoidosis. A low magnification histologic section of lung parenchyma *(A)* shows numerous granulomas associated with a moderate amount of collagen; both granulomas and fibrous tissue are located predominantly in the interstitium adjacent to pulmonary arteries *(a)* and bronchioles *(b)*. Only an occasional granuloma appears to be located within parenchymal interstitium *(arrow)*. A magnified view *(B)* shows three granulomas with a peripheral rim of lamellated fibrous tissue adjacent to a tangentially sectioned pulmonary artery *(a)*. *(A, × 15; B, × 120.)*

Figure 17–6. Sarcoidosis: Interstitial Pneumonitis. A histologic section of lung parenchyma that elsewhere showed classic sarcoidosis reveals patchy interstitial thickening due to an infiltrate of mononuclear inflammatory cells. In one focus *(short arrow)*, these are predominantly lymphocytes, whereas in a second focus *(long arrow)*, the cells are larger and give the impression of early granuloma formation. (×100.)

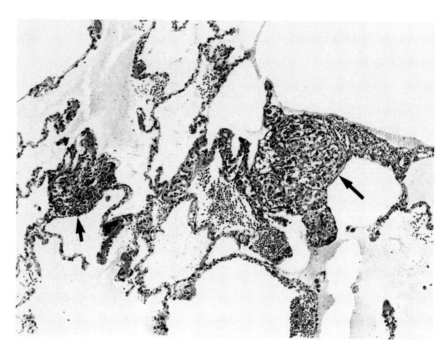

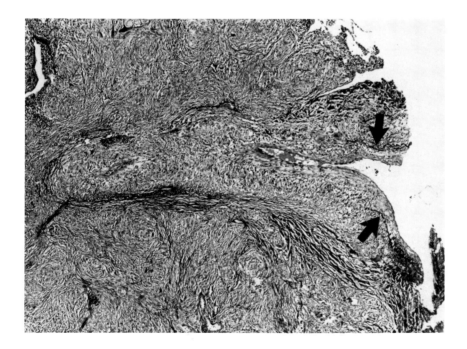

Figure 17–7. Sarcoidosis: Vasculitis. A histologic section shows replacement of lung parenchyma by numerous granulomas associated with a moderate amount of fibrous tissue. The media of a pulmonary artery is largely replaced by more or less confluent granulomas. (Residual internal elastic lamina is indicated by *arrows*.) (Verhoeff-van Gieson, ×52.)

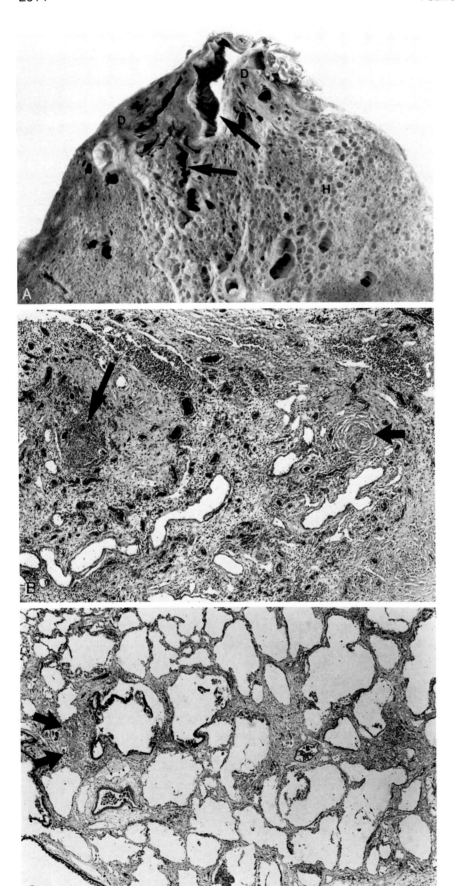

Figure 17–8. Sarcoidosis: Interstitial Fibrosis. A section of the apical portion of an upper lobe *(A)* from a patient with longstanding sarcoidosis shows foci of dense fibrosis in which the lung parenchyma is completely destroyed *(D);* extensive but less severe fibrosis with an early "honeycomb" appearance *(H)* is also present in areas where the parenchyma is still evident. Bronchi in the region of severe fibrosis are ectatic *(arrows).* A histologic section from the area of dense fibrosis *(B)* shows replacement of lung parenchyma by collagen and scattered aggregates of lymphocytes. The only evidence of sarcoidosis is two granulomas, one *(short arrow)* almost completely fibrosed and the other *(long arrow)* containing a single multinucleated giant cell. A section from the area of early "honeycombing" *(C)* shows less extensive fibrosis and numerous irregular cystic spaces representing dilated transitional airways. Two largely fibrosed granulomas are present *(arrows).* *(B, ×40; C, ×20.)*

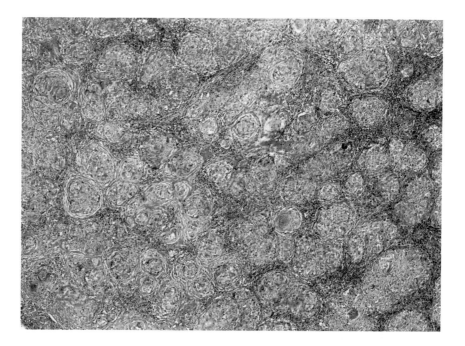

Figure 17–9. Sarcoidosis: Lymph Node Involvement. A histologic section of a mediastinal lymph node shows numerous discrete and focally confluent granulomas that virtually obliterate the normal nodal architecture. There is no necrosis. Mild fibrosis is evident at the periphery of some granulomas. (×40.)

Lymph Node Enlargement without Pulmonary Abnormality

Bilateral hilar lymph node enlargement occurs in 75 to 85 per cent of patients with sarcoidosis, in approximately equal numbers with and without diffuse parenchymal disease.[9, 164–166] Of 150 patients with proved sarcoidosis studied by Kirks and his colleagues,[167] lymph node enlargement was present as the sole abnormality in 65 patients (43.3 per cent)

and in association with pulmonary disease in 61 patients (40.7 per cent). Node enlargement usually is localized to the hilar, tracheobronchial, and paratracheal groups and is usually symmetric bilaterally (Fig. 17–10). The combination of right paratracheal and bilateral hilar lymph node enlargement (the "1–2–3" sign[168]) is considered by some to be a reliable sign of sarcoidosis; however, in our experience, paratracheal lymph node enlargement is far more often bilateral than right-sided only, an ob-

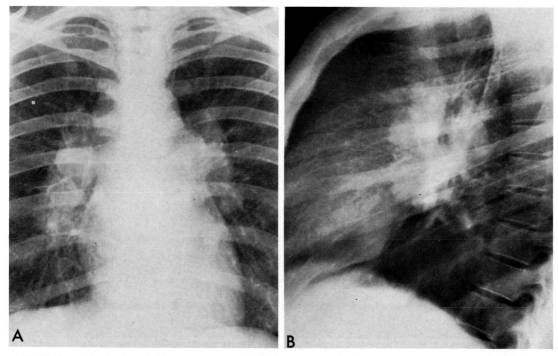

Figure 17–10. Sarcoidosis: Lymph Node Involvement Alone. Posteroanterior *(A)* and lateral *(B)* roentgenograms of a 32-year-old asymptomatic woman demonstrate marked enlargement of both hila, the lobulated contour being typical of lymph node enlargement. Nodes are also enlarged in the right paratracheal and aortopulmonary regions. The lungs are clear.

servation with which Kirks and his colleagues[167] concur. The reason for the emphasis sometimes placed on right paratracheal lymph node involvement is the fact that on posteroanterior roentgenograms this zone is seen much more clearly than the left, because the latter is obscured by the superimposed aorta and brachiocephalic vessels; tomography frequently reveals symmetric enlargement of both groups of nodes.

The contour of the outer borders of enlarged hila usually is lobulated, particularly on the right side; enlargement of right paratracheal nodes causes a loss of visibility of the right tracheal stripe and creates a smooth or slightly lobulated contour. It has been shown that computed tomography (CT) can reveal enlargement of lymph nodes in locations unsuspected on conventional roentgenograms. For example, Kuhlman and her colleagues[169] found a surprising incidence of node involvement in the anterior mediastinum, axilla, internal mammary chain, and infradiaphragmatic area. They also found that unlike node enlargement in neoplastic disorders in which coalescence is usual, the nodes of sarcoidosis tend to maintain their shape and to remain discrete as they enlarge.

Unilateral hilar lymph node enlargement is uncommon, being reported in 3 to 5 per cent of proved cases (Fig. 17–11).[170, 171] Workers at the Mayo Clinic[172] reviewed the chest roentgenograms of 800 patients with histologically proved sarcoidosis seen between 1960 and 1969 and found 38 (4.7 per cent) in which the initial unbiased roentgenographic interpretation was unilateral node enlargement. Of these 38 cases, erythema nodosum was present in 6 patients, a surprisingly high incidence. The authors suggested that mediastinal node enlargement may have its onset or may regress unilaterally or asymmetrically.[172] A single case has been reported[173] of unilateral lymph node enlargement in the left hilum, which presented as an endobronchial mass causing atelectasis of the lingula.

Occasionally, enlarged hilar and carinal nodes can compress the major bronchi (Fig. 17–12). Similarly, enlarged hilar nodes can exert extrinsic pressure upon major pulmonary arteries and result in reduction in pulmonary perfusion; two such cases have been reported.[174, 175] In each case only the truncus anterior branch of the right pulmonary artery was affected, perhaps coincidentally.

Calcification of hilar lymph nodes has been reported in roughly 5 per cent of patients in two series[171, 176] and in some cases is said to resemble the eggshell calcification of silicosis (see Fig. 4–102, page 603).[171] However, eggshell calcification must be very rare; for example, in a lateral tomographic study of 100 patients with pulmonary sarcoidosis, not a single case was discovered.[177] Nodal calcification is usually a late manifestation and is almost invariably associated with advanced disease; it has been reported also in association with corticosteroid therapy.[179] Israel and his coworkers[179] detected calcification of mediastinal lymph nodes in over 20 per cent of 111 patients with sarcoidosis followed for 10 years or more; they concluded that as a result

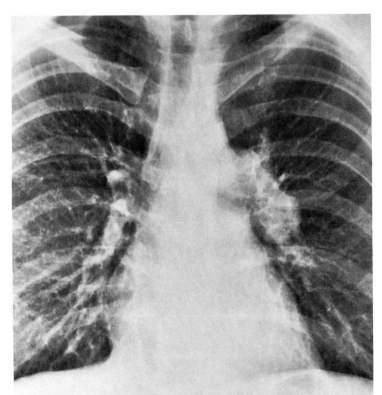

Figure 17–11. Unilateral Hilar Lymph Node Enlargement in Sarcoidosis. A posteroanterior roentgenogram of this 26-year-old asymptomatic man reveals marked enlargement of the left hilum in a configuration characteristic of enlarged lymph nodes. There is no evidence of node enlargement in the right hilum or paratracheal chain. The lungs are clear. The diagnosis was established by biopsy of a left scalene node. The patient had an uneventful recovery.

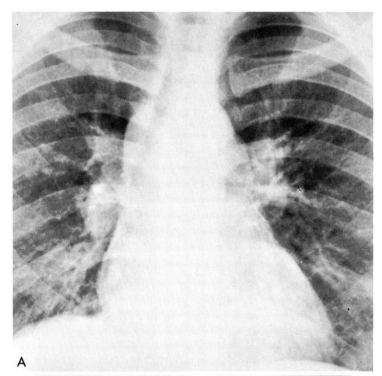

A

Figure 17-12. Lymph Node Sarcoidosis with Bronchial Compression. A posteroanterior roentgenogram *(A)* of this asymptomatic man in his 20s reveals marked enlargement of hilar and paratracheal lymph nodes bilaterally. On the original roentgenogram, there was highly suggestive evidence of blunting of the carina and narrowing of the left main bronchus. An anteroposterior tomogram *(B)* confirms the presence of upward displacement of the medial wall of the right main bronchus and marked narrowing of the lumen of the left main bronchus *(arrowheads)* due to enlarged nodes. The node enlargement and bronchial compression disappeared on corticosteroid therapy. (Courtesy of Dr. James McCort, Santa Clara Valley Medical Center, San Jose, California.)

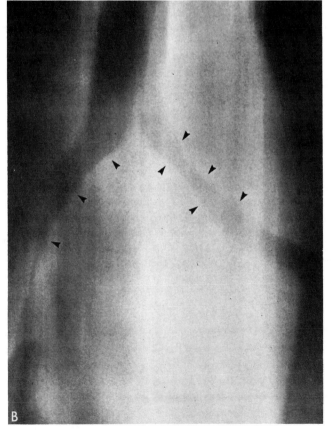

B

of the decline in the incidence of mycobacterial infection, sarcoidosis is possibly the most common cause of calcified mediastinal and hilar lymph nodes in individuals over 30 years of age.

Paratracheal node enlargement seldom, if ever, occurs without concomitant enlargement of hilar nodes.[180] This bilaterally symmetric hilar and paratracheal lymph node enlargement contrasts sharply with the node enlargement of primary tuberculosis, which tends to be unilateral and less sharply demarcated,[181] and even more with the node enlargement that characterizes the lymphomas. In Hodgkin's disease, for example, enlargement tends to occur predominantly in the anterior mediastinal and paratracheal groups; when it involves the hilar nodes, it is predominantly unilateral and asymmetric. As indicated earlier, although retrosternal node enlargement is uncommon in sarcoidosis, there are individual case reports[171, 182] of anterior mediastinal lymph node enlargement evident on conventional roentgenograms, and there is no doubt that the incidence is considerably higher on CT scans,[169] perhaps as high as 10 per cent.[183] Thus, the possibility of sarcoidosis should not be dismissed when such node enlargement is present, particularly when it is associated with enlargement of hilar nodes. An additional contrasting feature of sarcoidosis and lymphoma concerns the development of pulmonary disease: in the former, the onset of diffuse lung disease is commonly associated with a diminution in size of the lymph nodes or at least with cessation of their growth,[181] a finding not observed in lymphoma. Enlargement of posterior mediastinal nodes in sarcoidosis is very uncommon in our experience, although the incidence in reported series varies greatly (in only 1 of 62 patients in one series[184] but in 6 [20 per cent] of 30 cases in another[185]).

It is important to appreciate the fact that stages 0 and 1 refer to roentgenographic evidence alone and not to pathologic or physiologic evidence. As in other interstitial diseases, the lungs can be involved in the absence of a demonstrable abnormality on the chest roentgenogram.[186–188] One group of investigators found the incidence of pathologically proven pulmonary sarcoidosis in stage 0 to be slightly over 9 per cent, an incidence that must reflect a liberal use of biopsy.[186] Similarly, in a report of 21 consecutive patients with stage 1 disease who underwent open lung biopsy, Rosen and his colleagues[189] found typical sarcoid granulomas in all; however, the extent of granulomatous inflammation and fibrosis was significantly less than that seen in open lung biopsies of patients with roentgenographic evidence of diffuse lung involvement. These authors also cited six articles from the literature in which the results of lung biopsy of patients with stage 1 disease were reported: lung tissue containing sarcoid granulomas was obtained in 50 to 100 per cent of cases. Similar results have been obtained in studies in which CT scans have been compared with conventional roentgenograms in pa-

tients with sarcoidosis: focal pulmonary parenchymal abnormalities have been identified on CT in most patients with stage 0 or stage 1 disease. Pulmonary function impairment also can be present in the absence of roentgenographically apparent lung abnormality,[190–197] as may abnormalities in BAL fluid such as lymphocytosis and the presence of activated alveolar macrophages.[33] In fact, a case has been reported in which alveolitis was discovered on the basis of bronchoalveolar lavage of a volunteer who was to serve as a normal control; it was attributed to sarcoidosis.[198]

Seventy to 80 per cent of patients with hilar lymph node enlargement, with or without visible pulmonary involvement, will eventually show complete roentgenographic resolution without residua.[9, 181, 199] Occasionally, enlarged hilar and mediastinal nodes regress to normal size only to undergo enlargement once again at a later date.[200–202] On the other hand, hilar and paratracheal node enlargement can persist unchanged for 15 years or more.[164, 203] Israel and his colleagues[204] studied 12 patients with chronic hilar and mediastinal lymph node enlargement caused by sarcoidosis: 7 of the 12 remained asymptomatic for a mean period of 16 years despite persistent node enlargement, 2 patients had disfiguring facial sarcoid for which corticosteroid therapy was administered for 18 and 27 years, and 3 of the 12 patients developed diffuse pulmonary disease after 10 years of stable node enlargement (Fig. 17–13). Tests performed on patients with node enlargement to evaluate cellular activity after a mean interval of over 16 years included Kveim reaction (positive in 9 of 10 patients), measurement of serum angiotensin-converting enzyme (elevated in 8 of 12 patients), and gallium 67 scanning (hilar uptake in all 8 patients tested). Of considerable importance was the observation that the results of these tests were similar for patients who remained well and for those who had symptomatic or progressive disease, thus indicating that these parameters of active granulomatous inflammation do not necessarily reflect the duration of the disease, its outcome, or the need for treatment.

Diffuse Pulmonary Disease with or without Lymph Node Enlargement

A follow-up study by Smellie and Hoyle[199] of 66 patients who initially presented with roentgenologic evidence of only enlarged hilar lymph nodes showed the subsequent development of pulmonary disease in 21 patients (32 per cent). On the other hand, approximately 16[167] to 25 per cent[9, 164] of patients with pulmonary sarcoidosis present with pulmonary disease without hilar lymph node enlargement. In the majority of cases the pulmonary abnormality is diffuse and evenly distributed throughout the lungs, although sometimes there is upper zonal predominance, particularly during the

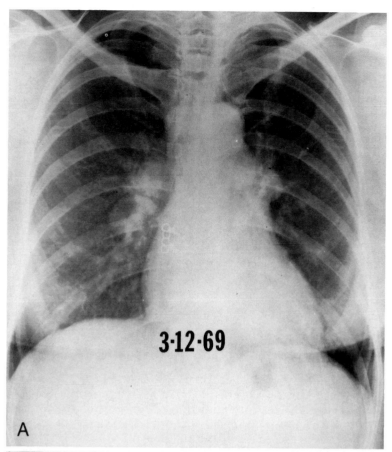

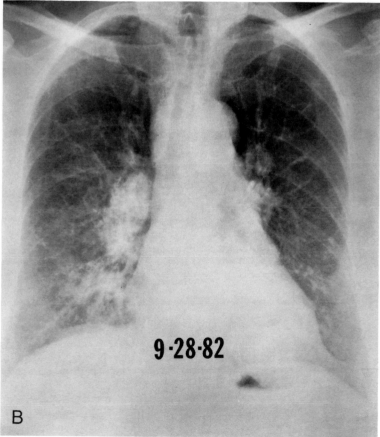

Figure 17–13. Sarcoidosis: Lymph Node Enlargement Persisting for 13 Years. A postero-anterior roentgenogram obtained in 1969 *(A)* reveals bilateral hilar and paratracheal lymph node enlargement. The lungs are clear. Thirteen years later *(B),* not only had the node enlargement persisted but there had developed diffuse interstitial pulmonary disease. The patient was a 60-year-old woman at the time of the second roentgenogram.

fibrotic stage. Occasionally the disease is asymmetric during the stage of development or during resolution[203] and, in fact, may be unilateral.[205] Although there is no question that CT can reveal parenchymal disease in the absence of abnormality on conventional roentgenograms, Müller and his colleagues[194] have shown that when roentgenograms display disease the extent and profusion of opacities are little different from that revealed by CT. Although it is probable that high-resolution CT will be capable of demonstrating the precise anatomic location of parenchymal disease with greater accuracy than conventional 10-mm collimation, the clinical and functional significance of this improvement is still open to question.

Three basic patterns of disease can be recognized on conventional roentgenograms: the reticulonodular pattern, the "acinar" pattern, and large nodules.

THE RETICULONODULAR PATTERN

This roentgenographic pattern can range from purely nodular to purely reticular but usually is a combination of both (Fig. 17–14).[9, 164, 167, 180, 206] The reticulation may be in the form of a very fine or a very coarse network and was observed in 70 (46 per cent) of the 150 patients studied by Kirks and his colleagues.[167] A so-called miliary pattern is very rare, being observed in only 2 of the 150 patients in this study. A linear pattern has been described as being

relatively common on CT scans;[169] alternatively, a reticular pattern on a conventional roentgenogram can be manifested by a nodular pattern on CT (Fig. 17–15). In fact, nodules are the most frequent CT manifestation of sarcoidosis. They were identified in all 44 patients studied by Brauner and colleagues using high-resolution CT;[207] in this series, nodules were seen occasionally in the absence of abnormality on conventional roentgenograms. Nodules tend to be related to pulmonary vessels, giving them a beaded appearance (Fig. 17–16). Müller has informed us in personal communication that this change can be seen to better advantage on 1-cm scans than on those obtained with a high-resolution algorithm (Fig. 17–17).

THE "ACINAR" PATTERN

This pattern consists chiefly of indistinctly defined opacities measuring up to 6 or 7 mm in diameter, thus possessing features of acinar shadows (Fig. 17–18). They may be discrete or coalescent and in the latter circumstance may be associated with an air bronchogram.[167] In the Kirks and colleagues study,[167] this pattern was frequently associated with a reticulonodular pattern elsewhere in the lungs and was the predominant pattern in 32 patients (twenty per cent). Sometimes confluence of acinar shadows can produce large areas of segmental consolidation (Fig. 17–19) or scattered, hazy areas of consolidation with irregular borders (Fig.

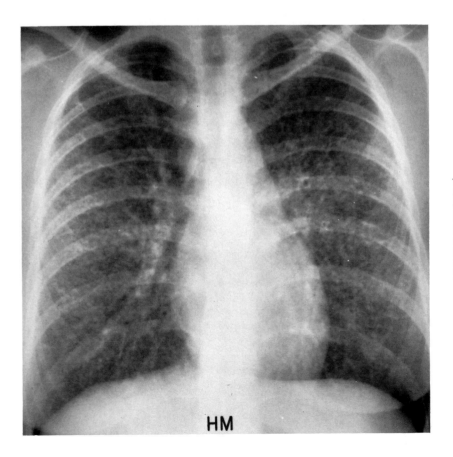

Figure 17–14. Sarcoidosis: The Diffuse Reticulonodular Pattern. A posteroanterior roentgenogram reveals a rather coarse reticulonodular pattern throughout both lungs with some mid-zonal predominance. There is no evidence of hilar or mediastinal lymph node enlargement. This 26-year-old woman complained of mild dyspnea on exertion. The diagnosis was made by open lung biopsy.

Figure 17–15. Sarcoidosis: Radiographic/CT Correlation. A view of the right lung from a conventional posteroanterior roentgenogram *(A)* reveals a coarse reticular and linear pattern with rather marked mid- and upper-zonal predominance. Hilar and tracheobronchial lymph nodes are enlarged. A CT scan just distal to the carina with 10-mm collimation *(B)* reveals a predominant nodular pattern rather than reticular. This 41-year-old man presented with an acute viral-like illness. The diagnosis was made by bronchoscopic biopsy.

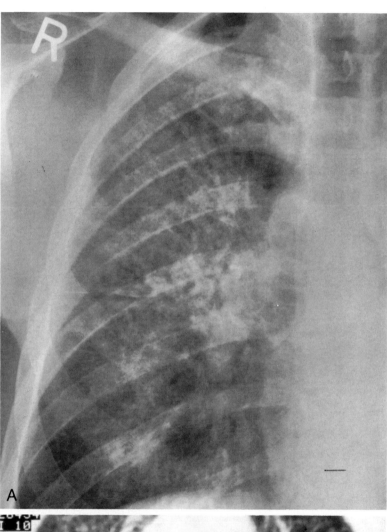

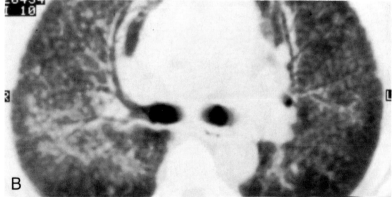

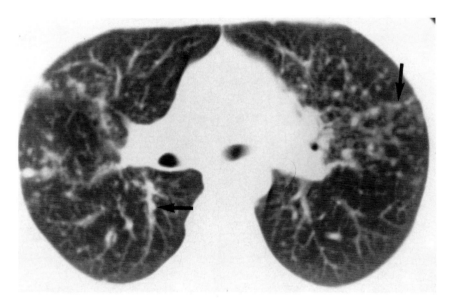

Figure 17–16. Sarcoidosis: CT Manifestations. A CT scan at the level of the mainstem bronchi with 10 mm-collimation reveals multiple ill-defined nodular areas of attenuation situated predominantly along bronchovascular bundles *(arrows)*, creating a beaded appearance. Hilar lymph node enlargement is readily apparent. (Reproduced with permission from Mathieson JR, Mayo JR, Staples CA, et al.: Chronic diffuse infiltrative lung disease: Comparison of diagnostic accuracy of CT and chest radiography. Radiology *171:*111, 1989.)

Figure 17–17. Sarcoidosis: CT Manifestations. A CT scan at a level just distal to the tracheal carina with 1.5-mm collimation shows numerous small nodules bilaterally. The majority of nodules are associated with bronchovascular bundles, giving them a beaded appearance *(arrows)*. Nodular thickening of interlobular septa is also apparent *(curved arrows)* as well as nodular thickening of the left major fissure *(arrowhead)*. (Courtesy of Dr. Nestor L. Müller, University of British Columbia, Vancouver.)

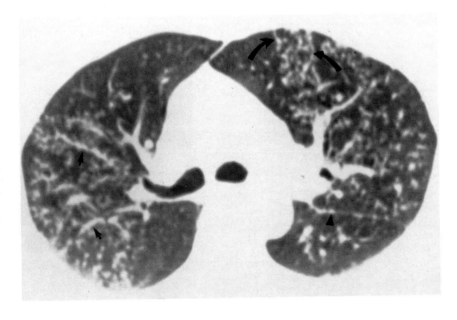

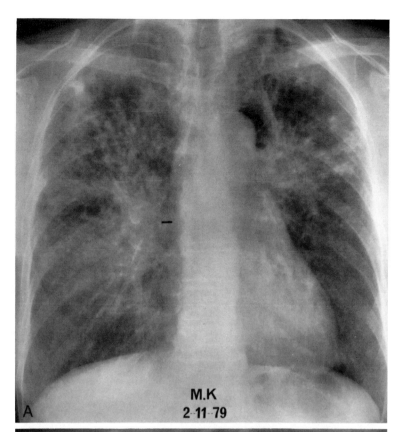

Figure 17–18. Sarcoidosis: The Acinar Pattern. A posteroanterior roentgenogram *(A)* and a detail view of the right upper lobe *(B)* reveal a combination of a coarse reticular pattern and a number of ill-defined opacities possessing characteristics of acinar shadows. Areas of homogenous consolidation are present in the parahilar zones bilaterally. (Bar = 1 cm.)

Illustration continued on following page

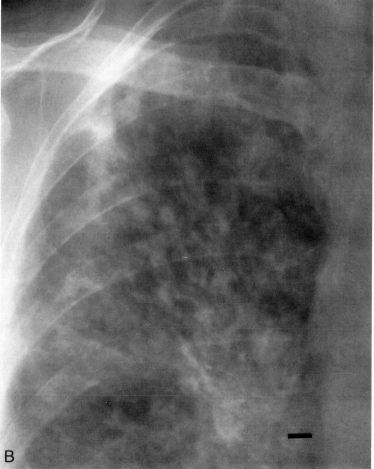

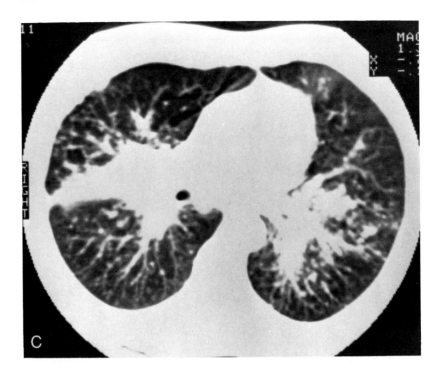

Figure 17–18 *Continued* A CT scan employing 10-mm collimation *(C)* reveals extensive consolidation of lung parenchyma in the medial and central portions of both lungs. A few nodules can be identified in the periphery, most of which relate to bronchovascular bundles.

17–20). Glazer and associates[208] have described eight cases of sarcoidosis in which the pattern consisted of peripheral nonsegmental airspace consolidation resembling chronic eosinophilic pneumonia; useful differentiating features included a lack of symptoms, an absence of blood eosinophilia, and a suggestion of a degree of nodularity in the opacities.

In patients in whom the disease is largely confined to the upper lung zones, the pattern may mimic postprimary tuberculosis. Teirstein and Siltzbach[209] identified 54 such cases (9 per cent) among 616 patients with sarcoidosis and emphasized that the combination of bullae and fibrosis in upper lung zones creates an appearance suggesting cavitary tuberculosis.

Approximately one third of the 150 patients studied by Kirks and his associates[167] eventually showed complete roentgenographic resolution of their pulmonary disease, the remainder showing either persistence of the acinar pattern for the duration of follow-up or progression to pulmonary fibrosis.

LARGE NODULES

An occasional case of sarcoidosis proved by biopsy shows large, dense, round lesions simulating metastatic neoplasm (Fig. 17–21).[210–213] This pattern, consisting of sharply marginated nodular opacities with an average diameter greater than 1 cm, was observed in only 3 of the 150 patients studied by Kirks and associates;[167] all were black. Rarely, sarcoid nodules of this type are solitary.[214–216] However, in these cases it is important to realize

that even in young patients with proven sarcoidosis a solitary nodule can be a carcinoma.[217]

When diffuse pulmonary disease and lymph node enlargement coexist, their roentgenographic appearance is no different from that of separate involvement. However, in such circumstances the two manifestations differ greatly in their temporal relationship in different patients. Diffuse pulmonary disease usually appears when hilar node enlargement is present, although the latter may be regressing. Node enlargement may disappear and be replaced by diffuse pulmonary involvement, either concurrently (Fig. 17–22) or several years later (Fig. 17–23), or it may remain and diffuse pulmonary involvement may be superimposed on it. So far as we are aware, there has been no report to indicate that hilar lymph node enlargement may develop subsequent to pulmonary parenchymal disease; however, in long-standing sarcoidosis, retraction secondary to fibrosis may produce sufficient hilar deformity to suggest lymph node enlargement.[218]

OTHER ROENTGENOGRAPHIC ABNORMALITIES

Unusual manifestations of thoracic sarcoidosis have been the subject of an excellent review by Rockoff and Rohatgi;[183] abnormalities of bone, pleura, mediastinum, lungs, and the cardiovascular system are discussed in detail. The interested reader is directed to this review for in-depth coverage of these admittedly uncommon manifestations. Only a brief description is given here. Such atypical features appear to be particularly common in older

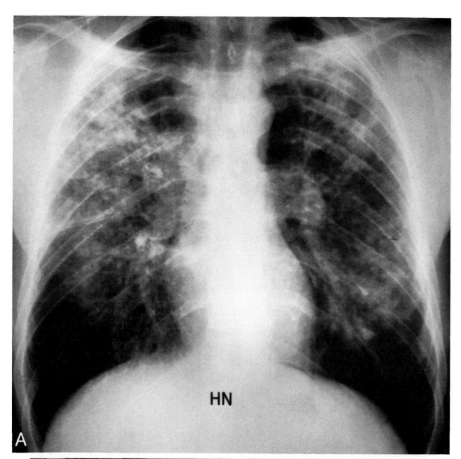

Figure 17–19. Sarcoidosis: The Acinar Pattern. A posteroanterior roentgenogram (A) reveals patchy opacities in both lungs, situated predominantly in central lung regions. This pattern simulates patchy airspace consolidation. A full-lung tomogram through the mid thorax (B) reveals fairly extensive consolidation of the right upper lobe, even to a point of a vague air bronchogram. There is evidence of enlargement of lymph nodes in the left hilum and the right paratracheal region.

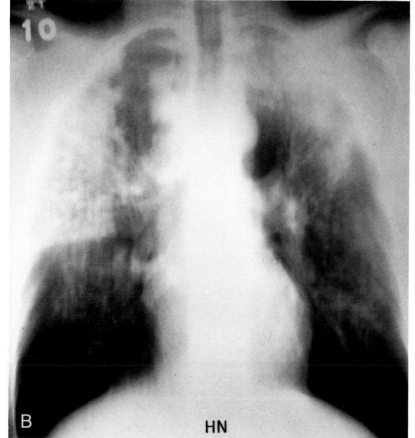

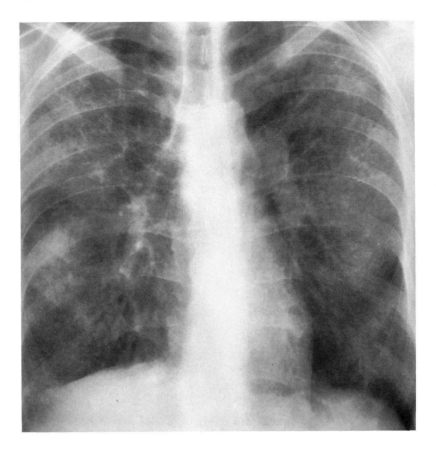

Figure 17–20. Sarcoidosis: The Acinar Pattern. A posteroanterior roentgenogram reveals extensive hazy opacities throughout both lungs with some mid- and upper-zonal predominance. The opacities are nonsegmental in distribution and are poorly defined. There is no evidence of hilar or mediastinal node enlargement. The patient is a young man who complained of mild dyspnea on exertion. The diagnosis was established by bronchoscopic biopsy.

individuals. In their study of 29 patients who presented after the age of 50 years, Conant and her colleagues[219] found 17 (59 per cent) to have atypical findings, including mediastinal node enlargement alone or in combination with unilateral hilar node enlargement in 8 patients, solitary or multiple pulmonary masses in 3, and atelectasis in 3. Extrathoracic tumors in 5 patients at presentation confused the diagnosis of sarcoidosis.

Cavitation is very uncommon (Fig. 17–24). Of 1,254 cases of sarcoidosis reviewed by Mayock and associates,[4] the thorax was involved in 94 per cent, and of these, cavitation was present in 8 cases (0.6 per cent). In their 1985 review of the literature, Rockoff and Rohatgi[183] could find only 6 well-documented cases of "true or primary" cavitation and "several" probable cases. Although cavitation was identified in 25 (12.5 per cent) of the 300 proved cases reviewed by Freundlich and associates,[220] it is probable that some of these "cavities" represented bullae, as the authors admit. In their report of 5 cases of primary cavitary pulmonary sarcoidosis in which care was taken to exclude other causes of pulmonary cavitation, Gorske and Fleming[221] usually found cavities in lung segments that were sites of diffuse infiltrative sarcoidosis *(sic)* and were in patients with the more chronic debilitating form of the disease.

Gorske and Fleming[221] emphasized the importance of eliminating all other causes of cavitation before accepting sarcoidosis as the underlying condition. Of greatest importance in this exclusion are pulmonary tuberculosis and the fungal diseases (i.e., histoplasmosis, blastomycosis, and coccidioidomycosis). Not only should infectious causes of cavitation be excluded but also the "multicystic" pattern caused by bullae or bronchiectatic segments that sometimes complicates extensive pulmonary fibrosis in sarcoidosis.[211, 212]

In 2 of Gorske and Fleming's 5 cases and in 10 of Freundlich and associates' 25 cases, mycetomas were identified. Over a period of 5 years, Israel and associates[222] recognized 10 cases of sarcoidosis associated with aspergilloma in upper lobe cystic spaces.

Atelectasis is a rare manifestation of pulmonary sarcoidosis, being observed in only 1 of 150 cases in one series,[167] in 1 of 198 cases in another,[171] and in 3 of 300 cases in a third series.[220] The atelectasis is caused by extrinsic compression by enlarged lymph nodes, by endobronchial inflammation, or perhaps most commonly by a combination of the two. Although bronchial wall involvement in sarcoidosis is common, it is seldom severe enough to result in the degree of bronchial narrowing necessary to cause atelectasis.[183] The diagnosis must be confirmed by bronchoscopy and bronchial biopsy.[223–228] Occasionally, enlarged hilar and carinal

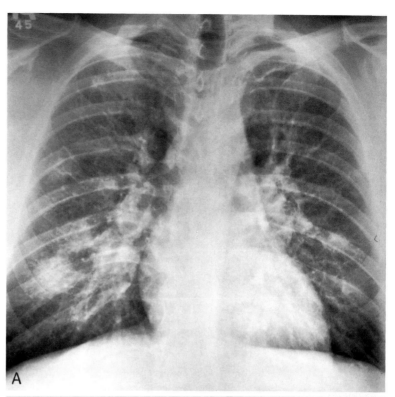

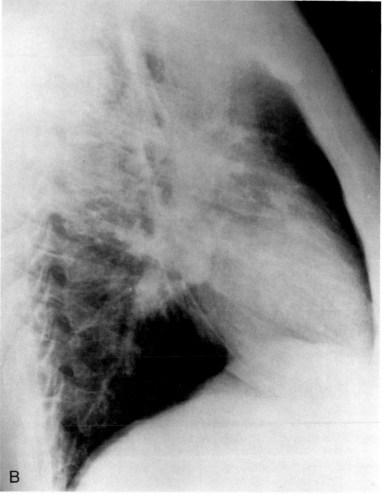

Figure 17–21. Sarcoidosis: Large Nodules.
Posteroanterior *(A)* and lateral *(B)* roentgenograms reveal several opacities in both lungs ranging in diameter from about 1 to 2 cm. The opacities have ill-defined margins but are homogeneous in density. Hilar node enlargement is present bilaterally and there is also suggestive evidence of mild enlargement of paratracheal nodes.
Illustration continued on following page

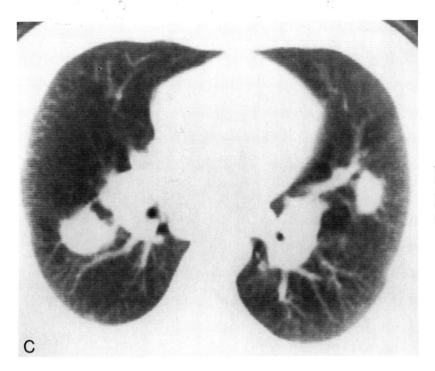

Figure 17–21 *Continued* A CT scan through the lower portion of the thorax *(C)* reveals homogeneous masses in both lungs and bilateral hilar node enlargement. The resolution of the image is insufficient to permit evaluation of lung parenchyma generally.

nodes can compress and narrow major bronchi without causing atelectasis (*see* Fig. 17–12, page 2617).[229] Both endobronchial involvement and nodal compression can cause alveolar hypoventilation and resultant hypoxic vasoconstriction and local oligemia.

Pleural effusion is uncommon but probably not to the extent that was once thought. Several reviews have reported an incidence ranging from 0.7 to 7 per cent.[167, 171, 220, 230–233] In one review of the literature,[234] only 32 reports of pleural effusion in sarcoidosis were found. One third of the cases were bilateral; most contained a preponderance of lymphocytes,[231, 232] but four were eosinophilic. In several of the patients in these reports, pleural biopsy revealed nonnecrotizing granulomas, and it has been postulated that the pathogenesis of pleural effusion is related to extensive involvement of both the visceral and parietal pleura by granulomatous disease. In a study of 227 patients with biopsy-proved sarcoidosis in which evidence of pleural involvement was specifically sought, Wilen and associates[233] found pleural effusion in 15 (7 per cent) and pleural thickening in 8 (3 per cent). All of the patients with effusion manifested moderately advanced pulmonary sarcoidosis, and nonnecrotizing granulomas were identified on pleural biopsy in 7 of the 15 cases. Pleural effusion tended to clear in 4 to 8 weeks but in some cases progressed to chronic pleural thickening. Wilen and associates[233] concluded that pleural involvement appears to be associated with progressive disease. Despite these findings, several authors have suggested that the presence of pleural effusion in association with

pulmonary sarcoidosis should raise the possibility of complicating tuberculosis,[235] coincidental pneumonia, or heart failure.[4, 164, 203, 236]

Pleural thickening and fibrothorax are undoubtedly much more common in sarcoidosis than has been emphasized in the literature, having been identified often at thoracotomy and autopsy.[183] However, the condition is seldom clinically or physiologically significant.

Spontaneous pneumothorax is a rare complication of sarcoidosis,[237–239] its estimated incidence being 1 to 2 per cent.[240, 241] Bullae tend to develop in the upper lobes in advanced fibrotic disease, and they have been said to rupture in approximately 5 per cent of cases.[240] However, it is probable that in the absence of bullae, pneumothorax represents a coincidental occurrence in patients with sarcoidosis and is of the same etiology as that which occurs spontaneously in a susceptible young male population; there have been three reports of bilateral pneumothorax in patients with sarcoidosis.[241–243]

Osseous involvement is said to occur in approximately 10 to 15 per cent of cases as judged roentgenologically.[244] However, the true incidence undoubtedly depends in large measure on the racial characteristics of the population being studied. For example, McBrine and Fisher,[245] whose experience was with a largely black population, found that abnormality of the hand phalanges was caused by sarcoidosis in 20 (40 per cent) of 48 patients; in this population group sarcoidosis was found to be the most common cause of phalangeal sclerosis. In other series also,[246–248] there is a much higher incidence of osseous involvement in blacks. Character-

Text continued on page 2633

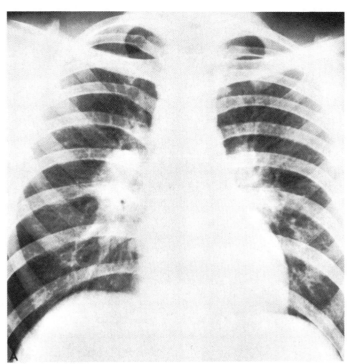

Figure 17–22. Sarcoidosis: Lymph Node Enlargement Undergoing Rapid Resolution Followed by Pulmonary Involvement. At the time of the roentgenogram illustrated in *A,* this 28-year-old man complained of recent onset of pounding occipital headaches, low-grade fever, fatigue, moderate exertional dyspnea, and pleuritic pain between the scapulae. Posteroanterior *(A)* and lateral *(B)* roentgenograms demonstrated marked enlargement of the hilar and paratracheal lymph nodes, bilaterally and symmetrically; the lungs were clear. The diagnosis of sarcoidosis was established by axillary and cervical lymph node biopsy. The patient's symptoms rapidly abated over the following 2 weeks but returned 3 months later.

Illustration continued on following page

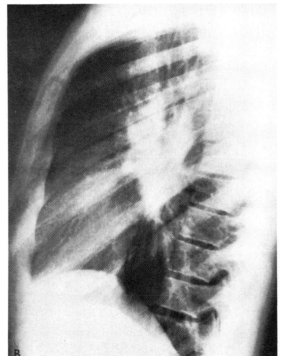

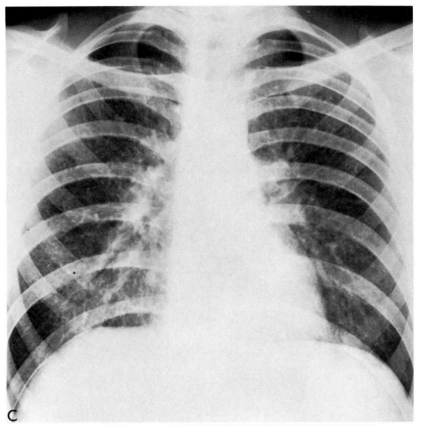

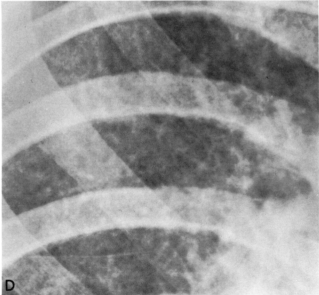

Figure 17–22 *Continued* A roentgenogram at this time *(C)* revealed complete disappearance of the mediastinal and hilar lymph node enlargement. However, in this interval there had developed a diffuse reticular pattern throughout both lungs, seen to advantage in a magnified view of the right upper lung *(D)*. Complete roentgenographic resolution occurred in 3 months without treatment.

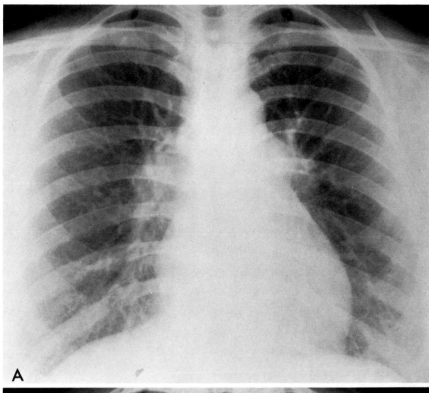
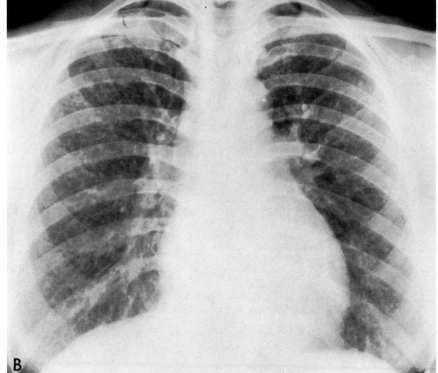

Figure 17–23. Sarcoidosis: Lymph Node Enlargement with Clearing and Subsequent Late Pulmonary Involvement. A posteroanterior roentgenogram (A) of a 31-year-old asymptomatic woman demonstrates enlargement of the tracheobronchial and hilar lymph nodes bilaterally. The diagnosis of sarcoidosis was established by scalene node biopsy. The node enlargement disappeared over the following 4 months and the chest roentgenogram returned to normal. Four years later, a posteroanterior roentgenogram (B) revealed diffuse involvement of both lungs by a coarse reticulonodular pattern compatible with a diagnosis of sarcoidosis. Although the hila are normal at this time, there is a suggestion of slight enlargement of right paratracheal nodes.

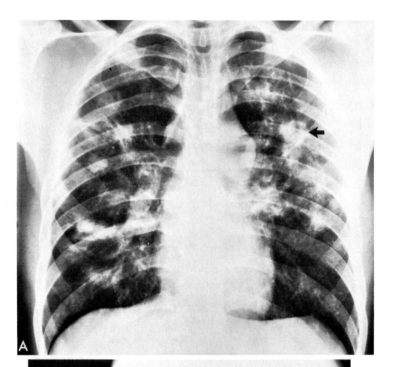

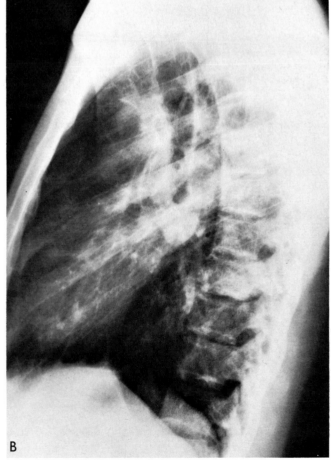

Figure 17–24. Sarcoidosis: Large Nodules with Cavitation. Posteroanterior *(A)* and lateral *(B)* roentgenograms reveal a multitude of poorly defined opacities throughout both lungs, without anatomic predilection. The opacities range up to 3 cm in diameter and most are homogeneous. A single mass *(arrow on A)* shows a central radiolucency consistent with cavitation, visualized to excellent advantage on an anteroposterior tomogram *(C)*.

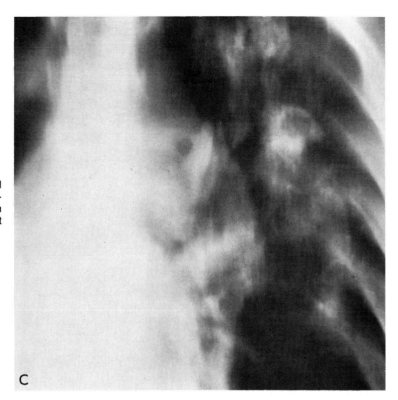

Figure 17–24 *Continued (C)* There is bilateral hilar and paratracheal lymph node enlargement. Non-necrotizing granulomas were identified histologically in tissue obtained by transbronchial biopsy. The patient is a 22-year-old asymptomatic black man.

istically, the small bones of the hands are predominantly involved, the pattern being chiefly lytic and consisting of cystic lesions and a lace-like trabecular pattern. However, a number of reports appeared in the older literature in which the predominant bony reaction was one of osteosclerosis rather than osteolysis and in which the primary involvement was of the skull, axial skeleton (occasionally accompanied by compression fractures), and proximal bones of the extremities.[249–251] Combined osteolytic and osteoblastic changes have been described in vertebral bodies,[247] as have lytic lesions in the sternum.[252] The roentgenographic, angiographic, and radionuclide manifestations of osseous sarcoidosis have been reviewed by Yaghmai[253] who illustrated five distinct types of bone lesions and called attention to the value of scintigraphy for early detection of these lesions.

Cardiovascular involvement, including abnormalities of the heart, pericardium, and pulmonary vasculature, are not uncommon pathologically but usually are of insufficient severity to cause roentgenographic manifestations. Although the incidence of cardiac involvement at autopsy ranges from 20 to 27 per cent,[254] clinically recognizable involvement of the heart occurs in only about 5 per cent of patients.[255] The only three conditions that are likely to cause enlargement of the cardiac silhouette roentgenographically are congestive cardiomyopathy, pericardial effusion, and left ventricular aneurysm.[254] Thallium has been reported to show defects in the myocardium in pathologically proven

cases,[256, 257] and in a single case report, magnetic resonance imaging (MRI) was shown to aid in diagnosis.[255] Pericardial effusion, usually small in amount, has been said to occur in 19 per cent of patients.[229] Pulmonary hypertension and cor pulmonale, caused by a combination of obliteration of the pulmonary vascular bed and hypoxic vasoconstriction, tend to occur in the late fibrobullous stage of the disease but can develop earlier.[229] Obstruction of major pulmonary arteries and veins and the superior vena cava by enlarged lymph nodes is extremely rare.[229] However, fatal hemoptysis has been reported due to erosion of a pulmonary artery in a patient with cavitary sarcoidosis[258] (we wonder whether this might have been caused by a complicating aspergilloma).

Pulmonary Fibrosis

When pulmonary changes have been present for 2 years or longer, resolution is the exception rather than the rule. Although there is disagreement as to what percentage of patients with pulmonary sarcoidosis develop irreversible pulmonary changes, an incidence of 20 per cent probably is reasonably accurate.[9, 165, 239] Scarring usually is rather coarse and in the form of irregular linear strands extending outward from the hila toward the periphery (Fig. 17–25). Commonly more uneven in its distribution than the reticulonodular pattern characteristic of the active stage, pulmonary fibrosis often shows considerable upper zonal pre-

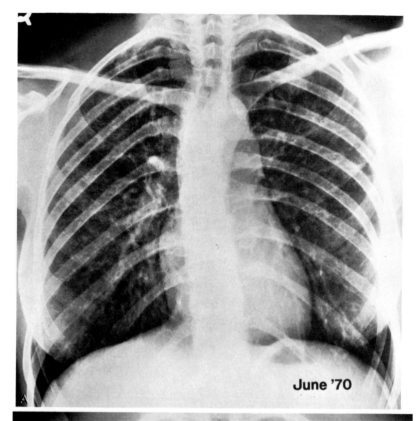

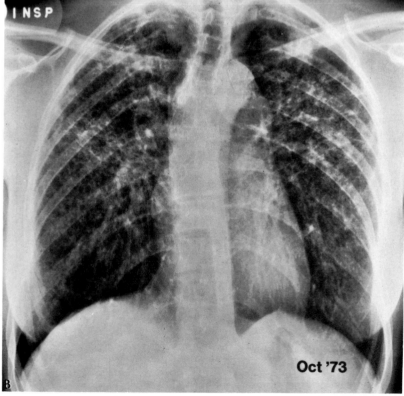

Figure 17–25. Diffuse Pulmonary Sarcoidosis with Progressive Fibrosis. The initial chest roentgenogram *(A)* of this 37-year-old woman reveals a rather coarse reticular pattern throughout both lungs with definite upper-zonal predominance. There is no evidence of hilar or mediastinal lymph node enlargement. Open lung biopsy showed nonnecrotizing granulomas consistent with a diagnosis of sarcoidosis. Three years later *(B)*, the reticulation had become more marked and there had occurred an upward displacement and flaring of lower zone vessels, indicating the fibrotic nature of the upper zone disease.

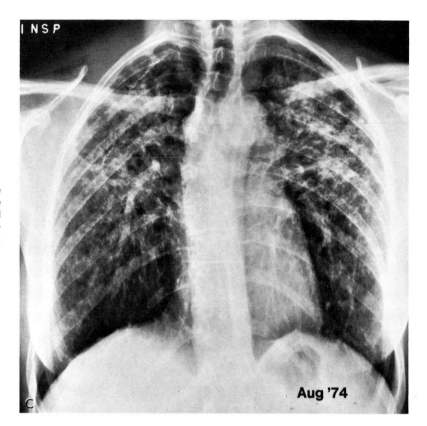

INSP

Aug '74

C

Figure 17–25 *Continued* This was still more evident 1 year later *(C)*. Note that despite the fibrotic nature of the disease, there had occurred no overall reduction in lung volume, chiefly because of overinflation of lower zone parenchyma.

dominance. It is usually associated with well-defined structural changes in the lungs, including bulla formation, bronchiectasis, and emphysema (Fig. 17–26).[239, 259] CT can be useful in evaluating the extent of disease (Fig. 17–27) and sometimes reveals evidence of fibrosis not discernible on conventional roentgenograms.[207] When fibrosis and emphysema are severe, changes in the heart and pulmonary vasculature are those of pulmonary hypertension and cor pulmonale of any cause.

CLINICAL MANIFESTATIONS

It is impossible to state precisely in what percentage of patients symptoms develop, but in our and other investigators'[2] experience they occur in approximately 50 per cent. However, others have found a considerably greater frequency of symptoms; for example, in a review of 227 patients with biopsy-proved sarcoidosis, Thrasher and Briggs[260] found only 15 per cent to be asymptomatic. We have found that patients with roentgenographic evidence of hilar and paratracheal lymph node enlargement alone are almost always asymptomatic, an observation with which some authors would disagree.[261] Since biopsy for diagnostic purposes may not be performed in these patients, they are not included in most large series in which tissue diagnosis is a prerequisite. The importance to di-

agnosis of the association of bilateral hilar lymph node enlargement and the asymptomatic state has been stressed by Winterbauer and associates.[262] In their series of 100 patients with bilateral hilar node enlargement, 30 were asymptomatic and all had proved sarcoidosis; 13 patients presented with erythema nodosum (with or without uveitis). Eleven patients with neoplastic hilar node enlargement were all symptomatic, and 9 of these had readily identifiable extrathoracic neoplasms on physical examination.

Symptoms are often associated with multisystem involvement and develop insidiously in the majority of cases. Frequently constitutional in type, symptoms include weight loss, fatigue, weakness, and malaise. Fever occurs in about 17 per cent of cases on average,[4] although a significant rise in temperature was reported in over 50 per cent of patients in one series.[263] The acute onset of symptoms, usually with erythema nodosum, is particularly common in Scandinavian women; as many as a third of these patients are said to present in this fashion.[7] A predilection for erythema nodosum has been reported also in Irish women in London and Puerto Ricans in New York City.[264]

Symptoms of *pulmonary involvement* develop in 20 to 30 per cent of patients[3, 4] and include dry cough and shortness of breath.[261] Hemoptysis is rare[265] and is usually attributable to a complicating aspergilloma in an ectatic bronchus or cystic

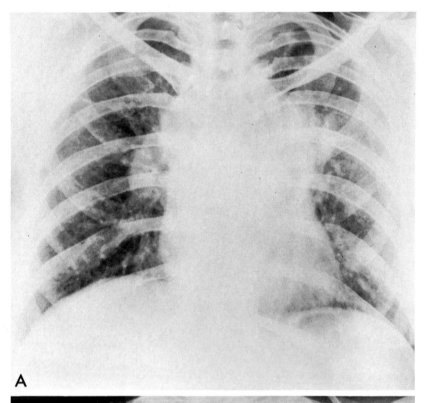

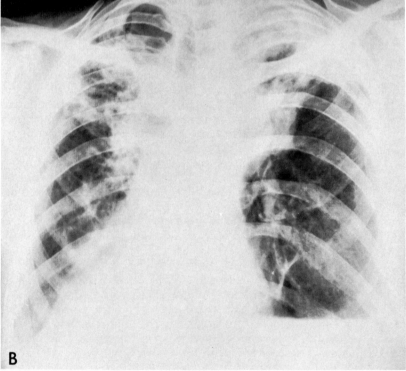

Figure 17–26. Sarcoidosis: Pulmonary and Lymph Node Involvement Followed by Severe Pulmonary Fibrosis. At the time of the roentgenogram illustrated in *(A)*, this 42-year-old woman had minor constitutional symptoms but no complaints referable to her respiratory system. This roentgenogram reveals marked enlargement of paratracheal and hilar lymph nodes. Lung involvement appears to be restricted to rather patchy shadows of increased density situated predominantly in the parahilar areas bilaterally. Six years later, the patient was readmitted to the hospital with a 2-year history of increasing exertional dyspnea, nonproductive cough, and a weight loss of 33 pounds. There was cyanosis of the nail beds. A posteroanterior roentgenogram *(B)*

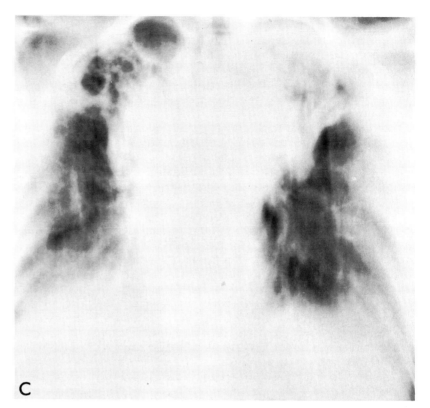

Figure 17–26 *Continued* and an antero-posterior tomogram *(C)* demonstrate marked loss of volume of both lungs, particularly of the upper lobes. Numerous cystic areas are present throughout the upper lobes, those on the right suggesting a honeycomb pattern. This picture is one of severe pulmonary fibrosis associated with compensatory overinflation of the lower lobes. Subsequent roentgenographic studies showed no change in this pattern except for the development 1 year later of spontaneous pneumothorax on the right.

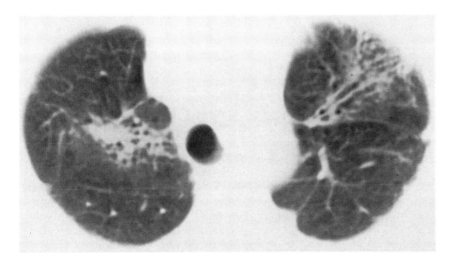

Figure 17–27. Sarcoidosis: CT Manifestations of Fibrosis. A CT scan at the level of the aortic arch with 10-mm collimation reveals irregular, poorly defined opacities in both lungs extending outwards from the mediastinum. The opacities appear to radiate along bronchovascular bundles, particularly on the left side, and are accompanied by appreciable bronchiectasis. A few subpleural nodules can be seen bilaterally. (Courtesy of Dr. Nestor L. Müller, University of British Columbia, Vancouver.)

space.[266, 267] Of 433 patients with sarcoidosis in one series,[268] 25 (6 per cent) had hemoptysis: 19, mild; 4, moderate; and 2, massive. Chest pain can be caused by excessive coughing and rarely is of pleuritic type.[269–271] Pleuropulmonary auscultatory signs usually are absent in the early stages of the disease, although a few scattered rales can be heard in some cases. Rhonchi may be audible in patients with endobronchial involvement.[272–275] With the development of pulmonary fibrosis, crepitations can become more widespread and the breath sounds can become bronchial. Rarely, involvement of mediastinal lymph nodes can result in a variety of complications such as pulmonary infarction, pulmonary arterial hypertension,[276] and pulmonary venous hypertension.[277]

The *cardiovascular system* can be affected directly or indirectly. *Indirect* involvement includes pulmonary arterial hypertension and cor pulmonale due to extensive parenchymal fibrosis, hypoxemia, or (rarely) direct compression of the pulmonary arteries[276, 278, 279] or veins[277] by enlarged hilar or mediastinal lymph nodes. Extrinsic compression by affected mediastinal lymph nodes can affect not only the pulmonary arteries and veins but also the superior vena cava[280] and left innominate vein;[281] compression of the latter vessel has been reported to cause massive left-sided pleural effusion.[281] The pulmonary hypertension that develops in the presence of diffuse parenchymal disease is generally associated with stage 3 sarcoidosis but can also occur in some patients with stage 1 or 2 disease.[282–284] *Direct* involvement of the heart is characterized by paroxysmal arrhythmias,[286–293] left ventricular failure,[294–296] and ventricular aneurysm.[295, 297] The myocardium is involved in approximately 25 per cent of cases at autopsy[3, 291, 298] but is recognized clinically in only a minority. For example, in one series of 40 patients on whom necropsy revealed cardiac lesions,[286] only 12 (32.5 per cent) had complained of symptoms referable to the heart. In another series of 84 unselected autopsied patients with systemic sarcoidosis,[298] myocardial granulomas were identified in 23 (27 per cent), in 8 of whom there were no clinical manifestations and in 15 of whom there was evidence of heart failure, arrhythmias, or conduction defects; 2 patients who died suddenly had not been recognized during life as having cardiac disease.

In a comprehensive necropsy study of 108 patients with cardiac sarcoidosis, Roberts and coworkers[295] concluded that in 89 patients cardiac dysfunction was caused by granulomatous infiltration of the heart. Sixty of the 89 had died suddenly and in 10 of these the sudden death was the initial manifestation of sarcoidosis; 20 others had died in progressive cardiac failure, 3 from recurring pericardial effusion and 6 from unknown causes. Of 163 cases of cardiac disease secondary to sarcoidosis studied in the United Kingdom,[299] the age at presentation with cardiac features ranged from 18 to 77 (mean 44.4) years, with no gender predominance. The average age of the 70 patients who died was 47 years; death was sudden in 45 patients, and in 26 of these no previous diagnosis of heart disease or sarcoidosis had been made. Most patients presented with either complete or partial heart block. The time interval from the onset of symptoms to death from myocardial involvement has been reported to range from 3 months to 15 years.[288] In the Roberts and associates series of 108 patients studied at autopsy, a ventricular aneurysm was identified in 8 patients. This complication appears to be particularly common in blacks,[300] and there is some suggestion that it is more likely to occur in those who receive corticosteroids.[295]

Electrocardiographic abnormalities occur more frequently in patients with sarcoidosis than in matched controls;[293] in one report of 80 patients with histologically confirmed sarcoidosis, but without cardiac complaints, the electrocardiogram was abnormal in 50 per cent.[291] In fact, the presence of arrhythmias in a young individual should suggest the possibility of myocardial sarcoidosis, as exemplified by the report of 2 patients with marked cardiac conduction disturbances who manifested no clinical or roentgenographic evidence of sarcoidosis. However, they both showed nonnecrotizing granulomas in scalene lymph nodes removed by biopsy.[301]

Enlargement of *peripheral lymph nodes* is said to be clinically evident in 73 per cent of cases,[4] but it is probable that such involvement occurs at some time in every case of sarcoidosis whether nodes are palpable or not; for example, lymph node biopsies from regions such as the scalene area, even when nodes are not palpable, are positive in 80 per cent of cases.[302, 303] Palpable lymph nodes are found most frequently in the cervical area but may also be felt in the axilla, epitrochlear regions, and the groin.[2]

The incidence of *ocular involvement* varies considerably from series to series, depending at least partly on the interest of the physician and ophthalmologist in sarcoidosis as a generalized disease. In reviews of the literature, Mayock[4] calculated the incidence to be 21 per cent and James[304] stated it to be 25 per cent. Scadding found uveal involvement in 39 (14 per cent) of 275 patients.[2] The characteristic lesion is uveitis, although involvement of the conjunctiva, sclera, retina, and lens may occur, resulting in cataracts and glaucoma. Patients with uveitis frequently have circulating immune complexes and show an increased incidence of HLA-B8[112–114] and HLA-B27 antigens.[305] Choroidal granulomas can be the sole manifestation of sarcoidosis and can be confused with metastatic carcinoma.[306] Bilateral exophthalmos has been reported as a presenting symptom.[307] Blindness developed in 3.5 per cent of 145 patients in one series.[4]

Once considered a prominent feature following the original description of the disease, *cutaneous involvement* is now thought to occur in no more than one third of cases; from his review of the literature,

Mayock[4] calculated the incidence to be 32 per cent. In another review of 145 patients with clinical and histologic evidence of sarcoidosis, Sharma[308] found 41 patients (28 per cent) who presented with various cutaneous manifestations of the disease, and Olive and Kataria[309] found 64 (20 per cent) of 329 patients to have skin lesions. In contrast to other forms of nonpulmonary involvement, skin lesions may be the only clinical manifestation of sarcoidosis; for example, in one series of 188 Caucasian patients with cutaneous sarcoidosis, 50 (26 per cent) lacked evidence of lesions elsewhere.[310] Skin involvement is particularly common in blacks and consists of slightly raised nodules (lupus pernio), often purplish in hue and usually occurring about the face, neck, shoulders, digits, and sometimes the mucous membrane of the nose. Large plaques resembling psoriasis may develop over the trunk or extremities. Lupus pernio and skin plaques usually are associated with a chronic persistent course. In the series reported by Sharma,[308] roentgenologic resolution of pulmonary disease occurred in only 22 per cent of the patients with skin plaques and in none of those with lupus pernio. Lupus pernio seldom, if ever, resolves completely[310, 311] and is often associated with involvement of nasal bones;[248] patients may be left with unsightly telangiectatic scars.[310] Patients with skin disease (except for erythema nodosum) are more likely to have lymph node, hepatic, and splenic involvement than patients without cutaneous lesions.[309] The infiltration of old and recent cutaneous scars by granulomatous inflammatory tissue is well recognized.[2, 312] Hancock[313] reported the development of sarcoid granulomas at the venipuncture site of six blood donors, five of whom also manifested roentgenographic evidence of bilateral hilar lymph node enlargement.

A particularly interesting form of cutaneous involvement in sarcoidosis is erythema nodosum, which consists of transitory, raised, slightly painful erythematous lesions, usually on the skin of the lower extremities. It is reported to occur in 3 to 25 per cent of patients with sarcoidosis. On the other hand, approximately 20 to 24 per cent of cases of erythema nodosum are associated with sarcoidosis,[311] at least in Europe and North America; in the Middle East, the abnormality is more often associated with streptococcal pharyngitis.[314] An acute onset of sarcoidosis characterized by fever, arthralgia, hilar lymph node enlargement, and erythema nodosum is a fairly common mode of presentation in Europe and often is referred to as Löfgren's syndrome.[315] In the original series of 212 cases reported from Scandinavia by Löfgren and Lundbäck,[315] over 50 per cent of the patients with bilateral hilar lymph node enlargement also had erythema nodosum. There was a strong female sex predominance in this association, 66 per cent of the women and only 12 per cent of the men being so affected. The maximal age in the 212 cases was 29 years, and only one patient was less than 20 years of age. This close relationship between erythema nodosum and sarcoidosis[7, 316, 317] is not so clear-cut in other countries, although one report from France[318] stated that sarcoidosis is the most common cause of the skin eruption in that country. Erythema nodosum may occur also in association with tuberculous, fungal, and bacterial infections and as a reaction to drugs.[8, 317–321] Reports from the British Isles show considerable variation in the incidence of sarcoidosis as the precipitating factor in erythema nodosum, ranging from relatively rare[319] to equal to streptococcal and tuberculosis infections[320] to the most common associated disease.[8]

The incidence of *hepatic* and *splenic* involvement depends on whether the figures are obtained from clinical or postmortem studies. Whereas necropsy reveals sarcoid granulomas at these sites in approximately 70 per cent of cases,[3, 322] the liver and spleen are palpable clinically in only about 25 per cent of patients. Although the degree of liver involvement is seldom sufficient to impair its function, it is not rare for enlargement of the spleen to be so severe as to necessitate splenectomy because of hypersplenism or because of its effects as a space-occupying mass.[3, 323] Of 32 patients with splenomegaly in one study,[324] 7 had hypersplenism and most responded to corticosteroid therapy; size decreased in all but 1 patient who required splenectomy.

The discovery of nonnecrotizing granulomas in liver tissue obtained by biopsy carried out for reasons other than to substantiate a clinical diagnosis of sarcoidosis is a rather perplexing problem. The cause can be identified in most cases[325–327] and in addition to sarcoidosis[328] may include infection, primary biliary cirrhosis (although it is possible that sarcoidosis itself can cause a syndrome that closely resembles this condition[326, 327, 329]), neoplasms (particularly Hodgkin's disease[330, 331]), and drug hypersensitivity reactions. In about 7 per cent of cases the cause is not found.[326, 327] An association with the Budd-Chiari syndrome has been reported;[332] the sarcoid granulomas narrow the hepatic veins and cause extensive thrombotic occlusions. Granulomatous hepatitis associated with prolonged fever has been described by Simon and Wolff[333] as an entity distinct from sarcoidosis, although Israel and Goldstein[325] regard such an entity with skepticism and suggest that a search for nonnecrotizing granulomas in other tissues and organs often is rewarding and results in categorizing such patients as having sarcoidosis. More difficult to classify are those patients with normal chest roentgenograms and biliary cirrhosis who show evidence in BAL fluid of subclinical alveolitis, consisting of T-lymphocytosis and activated alveolar macrophages.[334]

Symptomatic involvement of the *gastrointestinal tract* is very rare.[2, 335, 336] The esophagus can be affected by extension from contiguous mediastinal lymph nodes,[337, 338] with resulting dysphagia. A patient with a positive Kveim test has been described in whom invasion of Auerbach's plexus by nonnecrotizing granulomas resulted in achalasia.[339] A gastroscopic biopsy study of 60 patients with sarcoidosis revealed nonnecrotizing granulomas in 6 patients.[340] Cases have been reported of abdominal sarcoidosis associated with ascites[341] and perforated appendix.[342] Sarcoidosis of the bowel must be distinguished from other granulomatous diseases such as Crohn's disease and Whipple's disease. The recent discovery that most patients with Crohn's disease have BAL evidence of lymphocytic alveolitis[144-146] again raises the possibility of some interrelationship between these two diseases; this condition has been described in a child whose two siblings had sarcoidosis.[343] Two patients with Crohn's disease of the colon have been described in whom nonnecrotizing granulomas of the bronchi were demonstrated.[146] Whipple's disease also has been reported to involve the lungs occasionally (see page 872); the diagnosis can be made by finding characteristic intracytoplasmic coccobacillary rods within macrophages. Celiac disease also can be associated with sarcoidosis,[20, 147] a combination similar to that reported to occur with hypersensitivity pneumonitis (see page 1285). A study of the incidence of humoral sensitivity to dietary proteins has revealed that about 40 per cent of patients with sarcoidosis show a specific sensitization to alpha gliadin, a wheat protein; this suggests an altered gastrointestinal mucosal immune response.[344] And finally, some patients with multiorgan nonnecrotizing granulomas have overlap syndromes with various connective tissue diseases, including CREST syndrome[345] and Sjögren's syndrome.[346] Like the overlap with celiac disease and biliary cirrhosis, these can be very difficult to label with a specific diagnosis.[347] Infectious granulomas such as tuberculosis and histoplasmosis affect the gastrointestinal tract much more often than sarcoidosis and usually can be distinguished by isolation of the responsible microorganism.

Bone and joint involvement can occur with or without skin lesions.[4] Kaplan[348] has described three forms of joint involvement: (1) migratory polyarthritis associated with erythema nodosum, fever, and hilar lymph node enlargement; (2) single or recurrent episodes of polyarticular or monoarticular arthritis; and (3) persistent arthritis. The most frequent form is that which occurs acutely and is associated with fever and often with erythema nodosum. This is a polyarthralgia rather than an arthritis, and tends to involve the larger joints, particularly the ankles, wrists, elbows, and knees. Symptoms range in duration from a few days to several weeks, and the patient typically is free of disability. Arthritis is uncommon and usually is seen in patients with multiple system involvement;[349] it tends to develop during the course of chronic pulmonary sarcoidosis[350] and, although usually transient, can persist for as long as a year. When joint involvement is prominent clinically, synovial biopsy is likely to reveal non-necrotizing granulomas.[351] Bone pain is rare,[323] even in the presence of hyper-

trophic pulmonary osteoarthropathy.[352] The arthropathies that occur in adults with cystic fibrosis[353] and that are associated with fever and erythema nodosum strangely resemble those of sarcoidosis although they appear to be more incapacitating. The association between these two diseases may be more than coincidental.[354]

Involvement of *salivary glands* is not uncommon; in one study of 75 patients with sarcoidosis who underwent random biopsy of the lower lip, granulomas were found in the minor salivary gland in 44 (58 per cent).[355] The combination of parotid gland involvement, uveitis, and pyrexia is called uveoparotid fever. Although uveitis is common in the absence of parotid gland involvement and the volume of saliva and enzyme secretion from parotid and submaxillary glands often is decreased,[356] enlargement of the salivary glands is rare. Involvement of the *lacrimal glands* also is probably not uncommon, although these are rarely biopsied. In Scadding's review,[2] the glands were palpable in only 2 of 275 cases; however, such involvement may result in keratoconjunctivitis sicca and duct obstruction.[357]

Clinically evident *breast* involvement is extremely rare; we have been able to find only two reports in the literature of lumps in the breast caused by nonnecrotizing granulomas in patients with sarcoidosis.[240, 358]

Renal disease in sarcoidosis can be caused by granulomatous infiltration of the kidneys, glomerulonephritis, nephrocalcinosis, and renal artery stenosis.[359-361] Granulomas have been found in 7 to 22 per cent of necropsied patients with sarcoidosis,[362] but they rarely cause functional impairment.[363-365] The association of membranous glomerulonephritis and sarcoidosis[366-369] appears to be more than coincidental; a patient with this combination of diseases has been reported with the nephrotic syndrome.[369] Systemic hypertension can be caused by granulomatous inflammation and stenosis of the renal artery. When renal insufficiency develops, it is usually the result of hypercalcemia, nephrocalcinosis, and nephrolithiasis.

The *nervous system* is involved in 5 per cent of patients,[370, 371] with abnormalities occurring in the cranial and peripheral nerves and in the brain, spinal cord, and meninges. Although any cranial nerve can be affected, those most commonly involved are the seventh and second, presumably as a result of extension of disease from underlying basal granulomatous meningitis[372] or from nasal lesions.[373] Unilateral or bilateral facial palsy is sometimes associated with uveoparotid fever. Cerebral lesions can result in grand mal seizures and can simulate metastatic carcinoma.[374] Patients with sarcoidosis appear to be at risk for infection with the papovavirus that causes progressive multifocal leukoencephalopathy,[373, 375] a fatal disease with characteristics that can be misinterpreted as being caused by cerebral sarcoidal granulomas. Psychiatric presentations of sarcoidosis of the central nervous system include delirium, depression, personality changes, and psychosis.[371]

A characteristic intracranial localization of sarcoid granulomas involves the hypothalamus and pituitary gland;[370, 376–378] affected patients often complain of polyuria and polydipsia, symptoms usually associated with a deficiency of antidiuretic hormone (ADH) and diabetes insipidus. It has been shown, however, that many patients with hypothalamic-pituitary sarcoidosis have adequate reserves of ADH, in which case the cause of these symptoms remains obscure.[378] Direct involvement of other *endocrine glands* is relatively uncommon,[379] although there appears to be an unexplained association between sarcoidosis and either Hashimoto's thyroiditis or hyperthyroidism.[380–382]

Involvement of the *upper respiratory passages* is rare. The epiglottis is the most common site of involvement and can cause serious obstruction,[383, 384] sometimes requiring tracheostomy.[385, 386] Laryngeal lesions were identified in 1 per cent of patients in one series[4] and in 3 of 149 patients in another.[387] Symptoms include dyspnea, cough, and hoarseness. Hoarseness can also result from the extension of the inflammatory process into the recurrent laryngeal nerve from contiguous nodes.[388]

Infiltration of *skeletal muscle* can give rise to weakness. In a review of the literature, Talbot[389] found 12 patients who presented with sarcoid myopathy.

Pulmonary Function Tests

Generally, pulmonary function varies considerably among patients who manifest similar degrees of pulmonary involvement roentgenographically: those with a significant degree of disease can have normal function whereas patients with only mild disease can show substantial abnormalities on pulmonary function testing.[390] Winterbauer and Hutchinson[197] found 80 per cent of patients with pathologically proven pulmonary sarcoidosis but without roentgenographic evidence of parenchymal abnormality to have a normal vital capacity (VC) and 70 per cent to have a normal diffusing capacity; 35 per cent of those with roentgenographic evidence of parenchymal disease had a normal VC and 34 per cent a normal DL_{co}. The diffusing capacity can remain reduced when other function tests have improved and after symptoms have disappeared and the chest roentgenogram has returned to normal;[391, 392] in such cases, lung biopsy usually reveals interstitial granulomatous or fibrotic disease.[393] From studies of the fine structural morphometry of such lungs, the disturbances in blood-air gas transfer have been attributed to ventilation-perfusion $(\dot{V}/\dot{Q})$ inequality rather than to a diffusion defect,[394] a conclusion that has been substantiated by quantitative analysis of $\dot{V}/\dot{Q}$ single photon emission computed tomography (SPECT) of the lungs.[395]

Some reduction in pulmonary compliance,[396, 397] diffusing capacity, and gas transfer can be present on exercise, even in asymptomatic patients.[398–401] In patients with significant restrictive pulmonary function, exercise testing will detect a failure of the right ventricular ejection fraction to show an expected rise.[283]

Although the majority of patients with sarcoidosis show a restrictive deficiency in function, some can manifest an obstructive deficit as well; in fact, in a small percentage of cases the pattern is solely obstructive.[402] When clinical signs or routine function tests suggest the presence of airway obstruction, involvement of the bronchi by sarcoid granulomas should be suspected, with or without bronchostenosis.[275] More sophisticated tests, however, indicate that small airway function can be impaired even in asymptomatic nonsmoking patients with sarcoidosis.[403–406] Several investigators[407–409] have looked at bronchial response to methacholine in sarcoid patients, and some have found airway hyperactivity.[407, 409]

Two studies have shown clearly that despite comparable roentgenographic abnormalities and measured lung volumes, gas exchange at rest and on exercise shows a considerably greater reduction in patients with fibrosing alveolitis than in those with sarcoidosis.[410, 411]

In two recent reports, the extent and pattern of pulmonary disease on CT scans and conventional roentgenograms have been correlated with various clinical and functional parameters.[193, 194] Müller and his colleagues[194] assessed disease severity in 27 patients with pulmonary sarcoidosis, employing a visual scoring system for CT scans (0 to 100 per cent involvement of lung parenchyma) and the ILO classification for conventional roentgenograms: they found that both assessments correlated well with the severity of dyspnea and a decrease in diffusing capacity and vital capacity. Patients with predominantly irregular opacities (a reticular pattern) tended to have more severe dyspnea and lower lung volumes than those with predominantly nodular opacities. Taking a slightly different approach, Bergin and her coworkers[192] divided the CT scans of 27 patients into five categories on the basis of pattern of abnormality: (1) normal (n = 4); (2) segmental airspace disease (n = 4); (3) spherical (alveolar) mass-like opacities (n = 4); (4) multiple, discrete small nodules (n = 6); and (5) distortion of parenchymal structures (fibrotic "end-stage" disease) (n = 9). It was found that patients in CT categories 1 and 2 had normal lung function, those in category 3 had mild functional impairment, and those in categories 4 and 5 showed moderate to severe impairment. The overall CT grade correlated well with pulmonary function test results expressed as a percentage of the predicted value. Of considerable interest was the finding that CT grades did not correlate with the results of gallium scanning or BAL lymphocytosis.

Laboratory Investigation

Techniques that have been employed to support a diagnosis of sarcoidosis include differential cell counts of bronchoalveolar lavage (BAL) fluid, biochemical assay of a variety of substances that BAL fluid contains, measurement of levels of serum angiotensin-converting enzyme and lysozyme, and assessment of gallium-67 uptake by the lungs. These techniques also have been used to assess the likelihood of response to therapy, to monitor response to treatment, and to evaluate overall prognosis. Attempts have been made to correlate these indices of activity with each other and with clinical findings, roentgenographic stage, and pulmonary function tests. Innumerable reports have been published in this area, but there are so many variables to take into consideration in the interpretation of results that conclusions of the authors not only differ in many respects but in some instances are actually contradictory. The major variables include methodology employed, patient population under study, and activity of the disease.

It has been conclusively demonstrated that different techniques of BAL significantly affect the recovery of cells and proteins from the lower respiratory tract.[81] The technique we recommend involves the injection of 100 to 300 ml of normal saline (divided into 20-ml aliquots) with the scope wedged into the lingular or middle lobe bronchus. Pulmonary function tests have been performed before and after BAL:[412] it was found that small volume lavage (approximately 175 ml) did not significantly reduce function in normal subjects but did so in patients with sarcoidosis; large volume BAL (approximately 500 ml) caused decrements in function even in normal subjects. Strumpf and associates[413] performed 281 fiberoptic BALs on 119 patients and 22 controls over a period of three years and experienced no major complications; however, they recorded the presence of low-grade fever in 2.5 per cent of patients, pneumonitis in 0.4 per cent, bleeding in 0.7 per cent, and bronchospasm in 0.7 per cent (of importance was the fact that high-risk patients were excluded in this study). We agree with others[414] that BAL is a safe procedure in patients with a substantial breathing reserve. Further, we believe that it is an important investigative tool but that it plays little or no role as a diagnostic procedure or even as a routine means of determining prognosis. Chretien and his coworkers[415] came to the same conclusion on the basis of their experience with 1,188 patients with sarcoidosis.

Most investigators use albumin content as a standard to which noncellular components of BAL fluid are compared.[43] As discussed previously, quantification of cells obtained by BAL has shown that lymphocytosis, particularly of Th cells, is a characteristic feature of pulmonary sarcoidosis.[416, 417] One group of investigators[418–420] has described elevated levels of hyaluronate, a potential marker for activated pulmonary fibroblasts, in patients with sarcoidosis. This substance was not detected in the patients' serum or in the BAL fluid of normal subjects. A strong correlation was found between BAL levels of hyaluronate and recovered mast cells, which, along with activated lymphocytes and alveolar macrophages, are believed to be important in fibroblast proliferation. These same authors[419] found that mast cell and hyaluronate estimations correlated inversely with lung volume and pulmonary diffusing capacity, and that both indices increased with advancing roentgenographic stage.

Gallium-67 scanning has been used for more than 15 years[421] to detect sites of inflammation or neoplasia. Uptake in the lungs is measured 24 to 48 hours after injection, and a semiquantitative gallium-67 index can be used to minimize interpretative subjectivity.[422] Alternate methods of estimation of radioactivity include a ratio of lung-to-thigh uptake,[423] a quantitative computer index based on lung-liver activity ratios,[424] and an *in vitro* index based on radioactivity of BAL fluid and blood.[425] Many reports suggest that the correlation between the percentage of lymphocytes found in BAL fluid and gallium-67 scintiscans is good.[426, 427] The sensitivity of gallium-67 scintigraphy in detecting inflammatory lesions has been estimated to range from 80 to more than 90 per cent, but the specificity is closer to 50 per cent.[421, 428, 429] Its lack of specificity derives from its affinity for a variety of neoplastic processes and for inflammation of any cause, including that of infectious, toxin-induced, or immunologic origin. Its most useful function may be in the detection of pulmonary parenchymal disease in patients with normal chest roentgenograms who are suspected of having conditions such as *Pneumocystis carinii* pneumonia and bleomycin-induced pulmonary toxicity,[430, 431] but it may also indicate the presence of pulmonary disease in patients with stages 0 and I sarcoidosis.[429] In one study in which the values of BAL, gallium-67 scanning, angiotensin-converting enzyme (ACE) activity, and the chest roentgenogram were compared,[426] it was found that in terms of usefulness in estimating disease activity, the chest roentgenogram and ACE levels were sufficient and that gallium scanning and BAL were superfluous.

The BAL fluid concentration of *angiotensin-converting enzyme* has been found to be elevated in patients with active sarcoidosis,[270, 432] but since levels of albumin in BAL fluid are also elevated, this could simply reflect increased permeability of the alveolocapillary membrane.[433] However, in one report[432] high levels of ACE in BAL fluid were detected in all of 16 patients with active disease, some of whom had normal values for ACE in their serum.[432]

Although in drug-induced pulmonary disease and ARDS, serum ACE levels may be reduced, they are often increased in a variety of other diseases, especially sarcoidosis.[434, 435] ACE normally resides within pinocytotic vesicles in pulmonary capillary endothelial cells where it converts angiotensin I into angiotensin II as the former passes through the pulmonary circulation. Although some of the ACE in sarcoidosis probably comes from this source, there is evidence that a considerable portion derives from the granulomas themselves. Such evidence includes: (1) the demonstration by immunofluorescence of ACE in sarcoid granulomas;[436] (2) ultrastructural studies suggesting that epithelioid cells possess a synthesizing, rather than a phagocytic, function;[6] (3) the demonstration *in vitro* of enzymatic secretion of ACE from epithelioid cells;[437] (4) the observation that ACE levels are increased in granulomatous diseases other than sarcoidosis (e.g., in talc-induced pulmonary granulomas in rabbits[438]); and (5) the finding in patients with sarcoidosis of ACE activity in circulating monocytes, the precursors of epithelioid cells.[93, 439]

Both spectrophotometric and radioimmunoassay methods have been used to measure the level of serum angiotensin-converting enzyme (SACE);[439–441] in general, levels are accepted as being raised when they are two standard deviations above the control mean value. Mean values of SACE are significantly higher in healthy children and adolescents up to the age of 20 years than in adults whose SACE activity is not affected by sex or age;[442–444] blacks tend to have higher levels than whites.[445]

In various series of patients with recent onset of clinically active sarcoidosis that is not being treated with steroids, the incidence of increased SACE levels has ranged from 33 to 88 per cent.[417, 440–443, 445–450] With only two exceptions,[442, 451] normal results were found more often in stage 1 than in stage 2 disease; SACE levels were increased in only 7 (39 per cent) of 18 patients in stage 0.[34, 446, 447] There are few reports in the literature describing levels of SACE in patients who were considered on clinical grounds to have inactive sarcoidosis; 2 of 12 such patients in one series[447] and 11 per cent in another[439] had values that reflected activity.

Although measurement of SACE levels has potential value in confirming a diagnosis of sarcoidosis, it must be remembered that false positives (values for SACE that are two standard deviations above the control mean) occur in healthy individuals and in patients with a great variety of other diseases. In several published reports, 1 to 6 per cent of normal control subjects have shown values in the range considered to be indicative of active sarcoidosis.[439, 441, 442, 446, 449, 452] The following is a list of diseases in which false positive results have been observed, some being granulomatous in nature: tuberculosis,[440, 442, 452] coccidioidomycosis,[448] *M. intracellulare* infection, leprosy,[445] silicosis, asbestosis,[443, 448] berylliosis,[445] hypersensitivity pneumonitis,[452] lymphoma,[442, 445] multiple myeloma, amyloidosis,[439] osteoarthritis,[445] hepatitis and alcoholic cirrhosis,[453, 454] biliary cirrhosis,[439, 442] Gaucher's disease,[439, 445, 455] idiopathic pulmonary fibrosis,[452] lymphangioleiomyomatosis,[439] chronic granulomatous disease of

children,[456] chronic obstructive pulmonary disease (COPD), asthma,[440, 452] diabetes mellitus, and hyperthyroidism.[448] However, it should be emphasized that patients with sarcoidosis are much more likely to have higher values than those with the conditions in this rather formidable list; for example, Rømer[12] found elevated SACE levels in approximately 60 per cent of patients with sarcoidosis but in only 1 per cent of those with other conditions.

Serial measurements of SACE levels in patients with sarcoidosis show variations up and down that appear to correlate with the clinical course. Gradual falls have coincided with spontaneous improvement,[457] whereas rapid falls to normal levels have been recorded by several investigators in patients receiving corticosteroid therapy.[441, 442, 447, 449, 452, 457] Roentgenographic relapse tends to be accompanied by a return of values to pretreatment levels.[457] On the other hand, statistically significant changes in SACE levels have been observed during periods of disease stability as reflected by unchanging chest roentgenograms and pulmonary function tests.[458] Serum levels of ACE do not correlate with the number of lymphocytes found in BAL fluid or with the gallium-67 scan.[459, 460] Although SACE levels seem to reflect activity, presumably in the form of granuloma formation, they do not correlate with the usually accepted criteria for alveolitis and are often normal when these markers are present.[417]

In summary, despite the occurrence of false-positive results in many pulmonary diseases that resemble sarcoidosis, the measurement of ACE levels in blood sometimes can be useful in establishing a diagnosis. Its association with activity and the reduction in levels that occur with steroid therapy can permit monitoring of patient management.

A variety of other biochemical abnormalities have been noted in sarcoidosis. Levels of serum *alkaline phosphatase* have been found to be increased in 30 to 45 per cent of patients,[4] accompanied by elevated urinary levels of the amino acid hydroxyproline during the acute stage of the disease.[461] Serum *lysozyme* levels also have been proposed as a useful index of activity.[462, 463] From an evaluation of levels of this enzyme and of SACE in patients with sarcoidosis, Gronhagen-Riska and associates[443, 450, 464] concluded that lysozyme was more likely to be elevated in the early stages of the disease, particularly in patients with erythema nodosum.[464] They found the levels of both substances to decrease before clinical improvement could be detected.[464] Of considerable interest was their observation that serum levels of ACE and lysozyme did not correlate in normal subjects but did so when they were elevated in patients with active sarcoidosis, thus indicating separate sources for these enzymes when ACE activity is normal and a common source (i.e., macrophages) when ACE activity is increased.[443] Like ACE, lysozyme levels can be raised in pulmonary diseases that are included in the differential diagnosis of sarcoidosis.[465] In one study,[466] levels of serum *beta₂-microglobulin*, a low–molecular-weight protein associated with the histocompatibility antigens and thought to reflect activation of immunocompetent cells, particularly lymphocytes, were found to be elevated in 63 per cent of 132 patients with sarcoidosis at a time when only 32 per cent had elevated values of ACE.

Approximately 2 per cent of unselected patients with biopsy-confirmed sarcoidosis have hypercalcemia.[467] In patients with disseminated sarcoidosis who are seen as referrals,[4, 195, 379] hypercalciuria is present in approximately 30 per cent and hypercalcemia in 15 per cent, both usually in association with the chronic form of the disease. In addition, although many patients with untreated sarcoidosis have normal blood calcium levels, they can be shown by special studies to have abnormal calcium metabolism;[468] in occasional cases, the abnormal calcium metabolism may be related to the presence of granulomas within bone,[468, 469] but in most patients it probably results from an increased absorption of calcium from the gastrointestinal tract because of increased sensitivity to vitamin D. The stimulation to increased absorption can be caused by exposure to sunlight, intake of the vitamin, or overproduction of the endogenous hormonal form of vitamin D. The results of recent studies suggest that in sarcoidosis there may be an increased conversion of 25-hydroxycholecalciferol to 1,25-dihydroxycholecalciferol (1,25–dihydroxy vitamin D_3 or $1,25(OH)_2D_3$) in association with the development of hypercalcemia.[469, 470] Although this endogenous hormone was generally believed to be produced only by the kidneys, levels have been shown to be elevated in the serum of patients with sarcoidosis and hypercalcemia who are anephric[471] or who have end-stage renal disease.[472] Subsequent investigations have suggested that this stimulus of calcium metabolism may originate in secretions from granulomas.[473] The $25(OH)_2D_3$-metabolizing system has been demonstrated in pulmonary alveolar macrophages grown in culture, and synthesis could be inhibited by dexamethasone and chloroquine.[474]

Hypercalcemia in sarcoidosis is said by some investigators,[470, 475] but not by others,[467] to be more evident in the summer months, presumably as a result of increased exposure to sunlight. The hypercalcemia usually can be corrected by corticosteroid therapy, thereby serving to differentiate it from the hypercalcemia of hyperparathyroidism. In fact, some patients with proved sarcoidosis whose hypercalcemia fails to respond to corticosteroid therapy have been found subsequently to have hyperparathyroidism also.[361, 476–479] Although the majority of patients show only slight elevation of the calcium level, in a small number the levels pose a threat to life.[379] The most significant effect is on the kidneys, in which nephrocalcinosis and nephrolithiasis can develop and can impair renal function.[480] Metastatic calcification can occur in organs other than the kidney, including the eyes, lungs, stomach, blood vessels, and even the ear cartilages.[481]

Hematologic Abnormalities

Although Longcope and Freiman[3] stated that patients with sarcoidosis seldom are anemic, Mayock and associates[4] found hemoglobin values below 11 g per 100 ml in 22 per cent of their patients. In a more recent review of 75 patients with active pulmonary sarcoidosis,[482] one or more hematologic abnormalities were identified in 87 per cent. Anemia was present in 21 patients (28 per cent), in 17 of whom bone marrow examination revealed nonnecrotizing granulomas. In the majority of cases, hemoglobin levels became normal following prednisone therapy, a response that has been reported previously.[483] Some patients with anemia show evidence of increased hemolysis.[484] Leukopenia and lymphocytopenia are common; white cell counts below 5,000/cu mm are observed in approximately 30 per cent of patients. Eosinophilia greater than 5 per cent is present in about one third of cases. Thrombocytopenia is rare,[4, 483] only 24 examples having been described in the literature;[485] six of these patients died.

RELATIONSHIP OF SARCOIDOSIS TO NEOPLASM

It is well known pathologically that non-necrotizing granulomas can be found in association with a variety of neoplasms, usually well localized and often in lymph nodes draining the site of malignancy. However, Brincker[486] and Brincker and Wilbek[487] have also proposed a coexistence of sarcoidosis and malignancy that they believe cannot be attributed to pure coincidence. In reviewing the data leading to these authors' conclusions, Rømer[488] suggested that errors were made and that the number of pulmonary carcinomas and lymphomas found in the patients with sarcoidosis was not more than expected. Similarly, despite the report by Sharma and colleagues[489] of four patients with coexisting sarcoidosis and lymphoma, Snider[490] concluded on the basis of his own experience and a review of the literature that the association of these two diseases is coincidental. Our own experience and knowledge of the literature lead us to a similar conclusion with respect to all malignancies except testicular germ-cell tumors. We have seen a 33-year-old white male who developed bilateral hilar lymph node enlargement, arthralgia, and erythema nodosum 8 years after having been treated with radiotherapy for embryonal cell carcinoma of the testis. A search of the literature reveals 15 other examples of this combination of diseases.[491–500] Sarcoidosis has developed years before and years after the appearance of the testicular neoplasm; in at least two cases,[497, 499] orchiectomy was the only treatment for the testicular tumor, thus eliminating radiotherapy and chemotherapy as precipitating causes.

DIAGNOSIS AND DIFFERENTIAL DIAGNOSIS

As discussed previously, patients with sarcoidosis can present with a wide variety of symptoms and signs involving many organs and tissues.[3] In symptomatic patients, ocular disturbances, enlarged peripheral lymph nodes, skin eruptions, and respiratory symptoms are the most common reasons for a patient to consult a physician. Constitutional symptoms such as weakness and loss of weight and appetite are also frequent.[260] A small percentage of patients present with predominant involvement of the face, including such manifestations as bilateral parotid gland enlargement (with or without abnormality of other salivary glands and the lacrimal glands), iritis, uveitis, and occasionally facial nerve palsy. In our experience with the predominantly white population of Montreal, about 50 per cent of patients are asymptomatic when first seen, the disease being discovered on a screening chest roentgenogram that reveals bilateral symmetric hilar and paratracheal lymph node enlargement. Patients with metastatic malignancy, especially of renal origin, or lymphoma[501] can also present with such a pattern but usually in association with symptoms. Even when the hilar node enlargement is asymmetric, sarcoidosis is almost certainly the diagnosis if the patient is asymptomatic. The syndrome of bilateral hilar lymph node enlargement, fever, arthralgia, and erythema nodosum has been accepted as synonymous with sarcoidosis, whether or not pathologic proof is forthcoming, and with this we are in complete agreement.[502, 503]

Although the clinical picture in sarcoidosis usually is nonspecific, the diagnosis can be made with confidence in most cases when tissue biopsy reveals non-necrotizing granulomas. It should be remembered, however, that certain other granulomatous diseases, particularly tuberculosis, coccidioidomycosis, histoplasmosis, cryptococcosis, brucellosis, berylliosis, and extrinsic allergic alveolitis can present pathologic and clinical pictures similar to that of sarcoidosis.[504] This last disease, particularly, can be virtually impossible to differentiate from sarcoidosis if there is a history of exposure to antigen, with or without the presence of specific serum precipitins.[505]

Biopsy Techniques

In a minority of cases the diagnosis is established pathologically from a biopsy of a characteristic skin lesion or a palpable peripheral lymph node, most often one situated in the supraclavicular region; in the majority of patients, however, a specimen containing non-necrotizing granulomas is obtained by transbronchial biopsy. Biopsies of bronchial mucosa alone can also prove to be fruitful: in one series of 22 patients, biopsy specimens revealed granulomas in 17.[506]

The reported yield with transbronchial biopsy varies considerably depending on the stage of the disease and the number of biopsy specimens obtained. For example, in one series an average yield of 62 per cent for all stages of disease increased to 76 per cent when stage 2 was taken alone.[507] In another series, an average of 77 per cent was achieved in the three stages as follows: 69 per cent, stage 1; 80 per cent, stage 2; and 83 per cent, stage 3. These yields have been surpassed by several investigators who have taken 4 to 10 biopsies from multiple areas, with positive specimens being obtained in 88 per cent,[506, 508] 97 per cent,[509, 510] and even 100 per cent of patients.[511] In a report of 104 patients with biopsy-proved sarcoidosis on whom at least six specimens were obtained at bronchoscopy, the yield was 89 per cent in stage 1, 98 per cent in stage 2, and 88 per cent in stage 3.[260] The relative scarcity of granulomas in stage 1 disease is reflected in one study in which 7 of 10 patients showed diagnostic tissue from only one of the two lobes subjected to transbronchial biopsy.[509] Multiple biopsies of different lobes and segments are undoubtedly best performed under fluoroscopic control,[512] but even without this aid positive yields have been reported in 51 (76 per cent) of 67 patients.[513]

Bronchoscopic biopsy is usually a blind procedure that can be performed on either a proximal large bronchus or on more peripheral airways. The former site of biopsy can be potentially hazardous since significant hemorrhage can occur from relatively large bronchial or pulmonary arteries,[223, 514] and there is little doubt that biopsy of peripheral bronchi can be performed with less risk. In their series of 37 prospectively studied patients with suspected sarcoidosis on whom 10 biopsies were performed on each, Roethe and coworkers had a zero incidence of pneumothorax or serious bleeding.[509]

In patients with stage 1 disease, scalene node biopsy is generally considered to be positive in approximately 80 per cent[302, 303, 507] and may well be the diagnostic procedure of choice if for some reason pathologic confirmation is considered necessary; similarly, mediastinoscopy is positive in 95 to 100 per cent of cases.[515, 516] Transthoracic needle biopsy provides a low yield in diffuse pulmonary disease but can be of some value in cases with large nodules.[517] Open lung biopsy undoubtedly produces the most satisfactory tissue specimens but is probably associated with a higher morbidity and mortality than other biopsy procedures. Because of the high yield from peripheral transbronchial biopsies, biopsy of various other tissues of the body such as labial glands and muscle can be hardly justified in view of the low positive yield of only about 50 per cent.

Kveim Test

The Kveim test consists of the intradermal injection of 0.1 to 0.2 ml of crude saline suspension of tissue showing granulomatous inflammation, usually obtained from the spleen of patients with active sarcoidosis. The test site is marked and biopsied 4 to 6 weeks after the injection.[518] A positive reaction is indicated by the development of non-necrotizing granulomatous inflammation in the injection site. Most investigators have found the incidence of positive reactions in patients with active disease to range from 70 to 84 per cent;[519–522] however, positive reactivity has been as high as 88 per cent in patients with bilateral hilar lymph node enlargement, erythema nodosum, and arthralgia,[515] a group for whom we believe that tissue confirmation is rarely, if ever, necessary. Kveim tests performed on 74 patients with biopsy-proved pulmonary parenchymal sarcoidosis without hilar node enlargement were positive in only 53 per cent of the patients.[515] For this reason and because of the high yield afforded by transbronchial biopsy, the Kveim test has been largely abandoned as a diagnostic procedure.

CLINICAL COURSE AND PROGNOSIS

Judging from the asymptomatic condition of some patients with general lymph node enlargement and organ involvement, as well as the occasional chance finding of diffuse sarcoidosis in patients who have died from unrelated causes, it can be assumed that dissemination of sarcoidosis is much more widespread than is usually suggested by the clinical findings. Considering the number of persons in outpatient clinics in whom a presumptive diagnosis of sarcoidosis is made on the basis of bilateral hilar lymph node enlargement, it is our opinion that the majority of patients with this disease probably are asymptomatic and remain so throughout the course of the illness. However, if biopsy proof and a "characteristic" clinical picture are requisite to inclusion in any series of cases, obviously the percentage of patients with symptoms and the prognosis are different. The prognosis is also undoubtedly better in a nonreferral setting than in tertiary care institutions from which most series originate. This point was clearly made by Reich and Johnson[523] in an analysis of the course and prognosis of 86 patients with sarcoidosis seen over a 10-year period in a prepaid health maintenance organization: none died and none developed severe disability.

The assessment of prognosis in patients with sarcoidosis varies considerably in published reports, largely as a result of the selection of patients; for example, the disease is more aggressive in certain ethnic and age groups. In addition, when pathologic proof is required for entry into a specific study or when patients are chosen from a referred practice in which more difficult clinical problems are seen, it is only to be expected that the overall outcome from the disease will be somewhat worse. The length of follow-up after diagnosis is also a factor in determining prognosis: some patients may have an early remission only to relapse subsequently, and a smaller number may resolve completely even after a prolonged period of disability. The black population of the United States appears to be more susceptible to the disease, and in some,[524–526] but not all,[523, 527, 528] series they have a poorer prognosis. The elderly are more likely to be left with disability than the young.[529] It has been generally believed that sarcoidosis tends to be clinically less severe in Europe than in North America,[527] but an international retrospective comparison of 1,609 cases of sarcoidosis in London, New York, Paris, Los Angeles, and Tokyo[264] failed to demonstrate significant differences.

The incidence of severe disability appears to be increased in patients with extrathoracic involvement,[525] especially those with persistent skin lesions,[204, 311, 524, 530] bone lesions, hepatomegaly, or hypercalcemia;[529, 530] disability also tends to be more severe in patients with an intermittent course that includes frequent relapses[7] and in young children.[531, 532] Onset of the disease with erythema nodosum, arthralgia, and bilateral hilar lymph node enlargement (with or without low-grade fever) almost invariably indicates a favorable prognosis,[7, 9, 164, 264, 502, 503] although a few of these patients can pursue a chronic course.[530] In one retrospective analysis,[533] it was found that patients who presented with acute symptoms fared better than those with an asymptomatic course; we must assume that such an observation reflects a referral population of patients and that the series would not include many patients with stage 1 disease.

Most observers agree that prognosis is strongly related to the roentgenographic stage of disease on presentation; stage 1 patients fare better than stage 2 and stage 2 patients better than stage 3.[264, 529, 534] An absence of improvement in the chest roentgenogram over a 1-year period is a bad prognostic sign, whereas roentgenographic resolution that lasts for 2 years can be regarded as a cure.[529] Clearing of the chest roentgenogram is usually associated with a return to normal function,[534] although in some patients there can be a persistent diffusion defect.[535] The risk of developing abnormal pulmonary function when the initial assessment of function is normal appears small.[536] The prognosis of patients who manifest airflow obstruction on routine pulmonary function tests does not appear to differ from that of the nonobstructed group.[537]

Many attempts have been made to use the various markers of activity in sarcoidosis to indicate prognosis, to predict which patients will respond to therapy, and to monitor therapeutic management. The original impression that in untreated patients the number of lymphocytes in BAL fluid can be a useful predictor of outcome[45, 156] has not been confirmed by several subsequent studies.[81, 538–540] On the other hand, the results of at least three studies[538–541] suggest that the determination of subsets of lymphocytes in BAL fluid may be of prognostic significance, patients with greater elevation of T-helper/T-suppressor ratios (Th/Ts) being more likely to show deterioration; this effect is enhanced if the number of Ia-antigen–positive, activated T cells is also increased.[75] Turner-Warwick and her colleagues[542] were unable to obtain any indication that the degree of lymphocytosis in BAL fluid correlated with the response to corticosteroid therapy, and paradoxically Hollinger and associates[543] found that a high BAL lymphocytosis can be a predictor of therapeutic responsiveness. Although one group of investigators[544] found that the number of lymphocytes in BAL fluid is of limited value in prognosis, they correlated an increased number of mast cells with deterioration.

Gallium-67 scanning appears to be a useful indicator of activity[545, 546] but generally not a predictor of prognosis; however, the results of one long-term study[547] indicated that patients with proven pulmonary sarcoidosis on whom a gallium scan is negative are most unlikely to show a deterioration of their disease after a 2-year period. Gallium-67 can also play a useful role in documenting dissemination of the disease, particularly to mediastinal nodes, spleen, and salivary glands.[548]

Serial measurement of SACE levels appears to be a good method of monitoring activity; levels fall and rise with clinical[549] and functional[550] evidence of change, even when the initial values are within the normal range. However, evidence that measurement of SACE levels can play a role in predicting prognosis or the outcome of therapy is not good.[81] Serial chest roentgenograms, pulmonary function tests, and measurements of SACE levels are much less invasive and are cheaper than BAL and gallium-67 scanning, and are probably just as accurate in assessing activity in patients with sarcoidosis.[426]

It has been suggested that in patients with myocardial infiltration,[296] corticosteroid therapy can result in healing of granulomas with fibrosis and an increased incidence of ventricular aneurysm.

Indications for treatment include progressive pulmonary impairment, progressive loss of visual acuity, myocardial involvement associated with electrocardiographic evidence of conduction defects, central nervous system involvement, cutaneous lesions other than erythema nodosum, and persistent hypercalcemia or hypercalciuria with renal insufficiency.[551] Corticosteroid therapy appears to be beneficial for those manifestations of the disease generally considered immunologic in type, such as hypercalcemia and uveitis.[552, 553] The value of corticosteroid therapy in patients with pulmonary sarcoidosis is less obvious; although it can produce prompt roentgenographic and functional improve-

ment,[401, 554–559] long-term studies with controls have not generally confirmed benefit.[560] Once treatment is instituted, prolonged therapy is usually indicated in most patients for at least 5 years, since attempts to withdraw the drug can induce a relapse.[526] As already discussed, there are no reliable markers to identify patients who will respond to corticosteroid therapy. We consider it appropriate to observe a patient with stage 2 or 3 disease without treatment for at least a year provided that no functional deterioration is occurring;[561] then, a 3-week trial of therapy can be instituted while objectively assessing response.[562] Corticosteroid therapy suppresses such markers of activity as the gallium-67 scan, SACE levels,[563] and the immune mediators, gamma interferon[83] and interleukin-2;[564] however, it does not significantly affect BAL lymphocytosis.[563] Despite the latter observation, Hunninghake has proposed continuing corticosteroid therapy until the cytology in BAL fluid returns to accepted normal levels.[81]

The syndrome of erythema nodosum, with or without arthralgia, can usually be controlled with noncorticosteroid anti-inflammatory agents.[552]

The overall reported mortality rate ranges from 5 to 10 per cent, and in patients followed up for many years, the percentage is probably closer to 10 per cent.[264, 524, 527, 536, 565] As discussed previously, this rate very likely reflects a referred patient population with advanced disease. Most patients die in cardiac decompensation as a result of cor pulmonale secondary to pulmonary fibrosis. Pregnancy and the immediate postpartum period have been associated with an increased mortality rate.[128, 566] Sudden death can result from cardiac arrhythmias,[296, 299] central nervous system disease,[373, 375] or hemorrhage caused by complicating aspergilloma. Myocardial involvement can lead to the formation of a ventricular aneurysm and fatal cardiac failure.[296] Superimposed tuberculosis was formerly a frequent complication of sarcoidosis and often proved fatal, but this is seldom seen nowadays. Since tuberculin reactivity undergoes little change when active sarcoidosis becomes inactive, the development of tuberculin sensitivity in patients with sarcoidosis indicates the presence of superimposed tuberculosis.[567]

FIBROSING ALVEOLITIS

The subject of chronic interstitial pneumonitis and fibrosis is complex, both because of the multitude of terms that have been employed to describe the histologic appearance of the various forms (fibrosing alveolitis, chronic interstitial pneumonia, interstitial pulmonary fibrosis, usual interstitial pneumonia, desquamative interstitial pneumonia) and because of the numerous etiologies with which it has been associated. One of the most important papers to address these issues was published by

Liebow and Carrington in 1969.[568] In this paper, these authors recognized five subgroups of interstitial pneumonitis, distinguishable by histologic and, to some extent, roentgenologic and clinical criteria:

1. Classic or "usual" interstitial pneumonia (UIP), characterized by thickening of alveolar interstitium by fibrous tissue and mononuclear inflammatory cells and typically varying in severity from one focus to another.

2. Desquamative interstitial pneumonia (DIP), in which there is a striking proliferation of macrophages in the alveolar airspaces associated with a relatively mild but uniform interstitial thickening by mononuclear inflammatory cells.

3. A diffuse lesion similar to UIP but with superimposed bronchiolitis obliterans (BIP).

4. Lymphoid interstitial pneumonia (LIP), in which there is marked infiltration of parenchymal interstitium by lymphoid cells in a pattern sometimes difficult to distinguish from lymphoma.

5. Giant cell interstitial pneumonia (GIP), consisting of an interstitial infiltrate of mononuclear cells associated with large numbers of irregularly shaped multinucleated giant cells.

Each of these histologic patterns can be regarded as a tissue reaction to a variety of etiologic agents rather than as a manifestation of a specific disease process.[569–572] For example, in addition to cases in which no etiology is apparent, BIP is seen in some connective tissue disorders (particularly rheumatoid disease) and following aspiration of gastric contents; GIP is associated with viral infection (especially measles) and with exposure to heavy metals such as tungsten carbide; and LIP is seen with Sjögren's syndrome and acquired immunodeficiency syndrome (AIDS). Although there is some histologic overlap among the five forms of pneumonitis described by Liebow and Carrington,[568] the last three (BIP, LIP, and GIP) are fairly characteristic and are considered in appropriate sections elsewhere in this book. By contrast, there has been considerable debate about the distinctiveness of DIP and UIP from both clinical and pathologic perspectives. Because of this and because these forms of disease are the most common diffuse processes of unknown etiology to affect the pulmonary interstitium, the remainder of this discussion is concerned with these entities.

Liebow and Carrington[568] emphasized that their classification of interstitial pneumonitis did not necessarily imply a distinct etiology and pathogenesis of the various types; however, they suggested that the different pathologic, roentgenographic, and clinical features of DIP and UIP and the usual favorable response of DIP to corticosteroid therapy might be related to such differences and that distinction between the two was therefore justified. According to Scadding and Hinson,[573] however, these differences are not as clear as Liebow and Carrington proposed: in their study of 16 patients with diffuse interstitial pulmonary disease,

they found considerable histologic overlap among patients and suggested that the patterns of UIP and DIP simply reflected different stages of one disease process which they termed "diffuse fibrosing alveolitis." They considered this to be a broad general category of pulmonary disease characterized by an inflammatory process that possessed three essential features: (1) localization in the lung parenchyma beyond the terminal bronchiole; (2) thickening of the alveolar walls by chronic inflammatory cells, particularly lymphocytes, with a tendency to fibrosis; and (3) the presence of large mononuclear cells within the alveolar airspaces.[573] According to Scadding and Hinson, the last two essential features are present in varying proportion in virtually all cases and may represent different stages of the same disease. In support of this view are the occasional patients in whom biopsy shows the pattern of DIP but in whom subsequent biopsy or necropsy specimens show only diffuse pulmonary fibrosis.[574–576]

Although this debate about the fundamental nature of DIP and UIP has not been definitely resolved, it is probably correct to say that most authorities[571, 574, 577–585] consider these conditions to represent a spectrum of change from one in which intralveolar macrophages predominate, to one in which interstitial inflammation and fibrosis are more pronounced, to one in which there is extensive fibrosis, often with a "honeycomb" pattern. We concur with this view and consider it preferable to use the term fibrosing alveolitis to refer to each of these stages of disease. Despite this, it seems reasonable to identify those cases in which the histologic pattern of DIP is present, since there is some indication that prognosis and response to therapy are more favorable than in patients who manifest the more common UIP.

It is necessary to make one final comment regarding terminology. In 1935, Hamman and Rich[586] described an acute variety of interstitial pneumonitis and fibrosis characterized by a rapid progress of signs and symptoms leading to death in less than a year. Because the clinical features are so striking and because there is evidence that the pathologic features of this rare variety differ from those of classic fibrosing alveolitis,[587] we consider it appropriate to use the term Hamman-Rich syndrome to described this unusual entity. It should be remembered, however, that the majority of cases of fibrosing alveolitis described since the Hamman-Rich reports[586, 588] have followed a more chronic course, signs of acute disease being neither a precursor nor a feature.[589] When acute symptoms are present (e.g., with superimposed infection), they often serve simply to bring the condition to the attention of the patient and physician; in many cases a prior chest roentgenogram had shown the early stages of the diffuse pulmonary disease at a time when the patient was asymptomatic. Thus, we agree with Scadding[590] that it is a contradiction to speak of "chronic" Hamman-Rich disease and, with the exception of the occasional case in which an acute course of the disease can be accurately documented, it is recommended that the eponym be dropped in favor of the more descriptive term, fibrosing alveolitis.

Fibrosing alveolitis shows no sex predominance and has a broad age incidence. The ages of the 16 patients described by Scadding and Hinson[573] ranged from 12 to 63 years (mean 45 years); 9 were male and 7 female. In the series of 42 cases of diffuse idiopathic interstitial fibrosis reported by Stack and associates,[591] ages ranged from 12 to 77 years; almost all the younger patients were female. On average, however, the disease probably affects men slightly more often than women, and most patients are between the ages of 40 and 70 years.[577] The rare cases of fibrosing alveolitis that have been reported in neonates have been associated with a dismal prognosis.[572]

ETIOLOGY

The etiology of diffuse fibrosing alveolitis is unknown. Investigations into the etiology have focused on three areas—immunologic abnormalities, genetic abnormalities, and viral infection.

IMMUNOLOGIC ABNORMALITIES

There is much clinical, pathologic, and experimental evidence that some abnormality of immune function is involved in fibrosing alveolitis. Many patients with interstitial pneumonitis and fibrosis present with clinical and serologic evidence of autoimmunity.[591–595] In a number of these patients, the diagnosis of specific connective tissue disorders, such as rheumatoid disease, progressive systemic sclerosis, dermatomyositis/polymyositis, Sjögren's syndrome, and mixed connective tissue disease, can be made on the basis of clinical findings and the presence of a variety of autoantibodies in the blood.[596] For example, in one series of 220 patients with interstitial pneumonitis, none of whom had been exposed to external fibrogenic agents, Turner-Warwick and associates[597] found 30 per cent to have the stigmata of specific connective tissue diseases and 70 per cent to have cryptogenic (idiopathic) disease. In addition, fibrosing alveolitis is occasionally associated with tissue or organ involvement not included under the umbrella of connective tissue disorders, but in which an abnormality of immune function is implicated; these include digital vasculitis,[598] myasthenia gravis,[599] celiac disease,[600] chronic active hepatitis,[590, 601–603] renal tubular acidosis,[604] hemolytic anemia,[605, 606] IgA nephropathy,[607] and thrombocytopenic purpura.[608] Serologic abnormalities are not uncommonly documented in individuals without clinical evidence of extrapulmonary disease. For example, in one series,[609] antinuclear antibodies were identified in 21 per cent of patients

with fibrosing alveolitis unaccompanied by signs of connective tissue disease. Scadding[610] has estimated that about one third of patients with fibrosing alveolitis have antinuclear protein and one third rheumatoid factor, usually in low titers; only a few have both. Immune complexes, both circulating and bound to lung tissue, have been found in a minority of patients with "pure" fibrosing alveolitis,[611–613] but are more common in those with associated clinical findings of a specific connective tissue disease; they seem to reflect a more active cellular phase of the disease.[596, 609, 614–616]

Some pathologic and experimental animal studies also provide evidence for a possible immune pathogenesis of fibrosing alveolitis. For example, the intravenous administration of Freund's adjuvant to rabbits can result in a pattern similar to DIP,[617] and the intratracheal instillation of hapten to previously immunized hamsters causes interstitial fibrosis.[618] In humans, Schwarz and associates[609] found IgG and C3 in a granular pattern lining alveolar cells in most cases of DIP and cellular idiopathic interstitial pneumonia, although only rarely in cases judged to show "mural" fibrosis. Experimental data suggest that alveolar damage may be mediated by oxygen radicals.[619] Employing immunoperoxidase and immunofluorescent methods and monoclonal antibodies, immunohistochemical analysis supports the concept that a humoral antibody-mediated reaction is one of the pathogenetic mechanisms in the development of diffuse interstitial fibrosis.[620, 621]

GENETIC ABNORMALITIES

A genetic factor exists in a minority of patients with fibrosing alveolitis; in some of these, there is evidence for an association between inheritance and disturbed immunologic activity.[622] An example of such an association occurring in a family consists of fibrosing alveolitis, hypocalciuric hypercalcemia, and defective granulocyte function; all three disorders were inherited according to an autosomal dominant pattern.[623–625] Fibrosing alveolitis has been documented in monozygotic twins,[626] and a review of the literature in 1983[627] revealed 73 definite cases of fibrosing alveolitis in 19 families. Transmission appears to depend on a simple mendelian autosomal dominant characteristic with reduced penetrance.[626, 628–635] Designated "familial fibrocystic pulmonary dysplasia" by some authors, this condition possesses pathologic and roentgenographic characteristics identical to those of the nonfamilial form of fibrosing alveolitis (Fig. 17–28).[626, 632–634, 636]

Attempts to identify a specific gene responsible for fibrosis have not been successful; however, several studies have demonstrated abnormalities of HLA histocompatibility loci. In one study,[637] 35 antigens of HLA loci A and B were determined among 33 patients with fibrosing alveolitis and 329 healthy controls: no significant differences were observed in the phenotype frequencies. However,

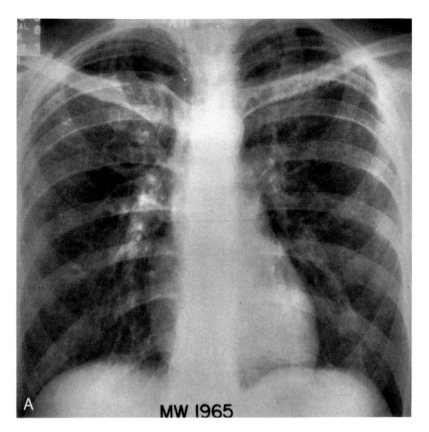

Figure 17–28. Fibrosing Alveolitis in Three Family Members: "Familial Fibrocystic Pulmonary Dysplasia". The posteroanterior roentgenogram illustrated in *(A)* is of a young female member *(MW)* of the family; it reveals a rather fine reticular pattern throughout both lungs, with a vague, hazy opacity in upper lung zones bilaterally.

other workers[638] found an increased frequency of HLA-B8 in 20 patients with cryptogenic fibrosing alveolitis, most of whom came from a subgroup of young women with the disease. Of perhaps greater interest is the finding of an increased frequency of HLA-DR2 antigen in 20 Caucasians with interstitial fibrosis compared with 200 healthy blood donors;[627] this B cell alloantigen has been associated with disorders of altered immunoreactivity such as systemic lupus erythematosus and rheumatoid disease. Kallenberg and coworkers[639] found the alveolar epithelium to react strongly with HLA-DR monoclonal antibodies in 7 of 8 patients with fibrosing alveolitis. However, in a subsequent report these investigators[640] described a similar reaction in patients with sarcoidosis and in those with microbial infections; as a consequence, the significance of their observation is unclear.

The similarity of the pulmonary pathology in fibrosing alveolitis to that of such autosomal disorders as neurofibromatosis,[641–644] oculocutaneous albinism,[645] the Hermansky-Pudlak syndrome,[646–648] and familial hypocalciuric hypercalcemia[649] also suggests a genetic role in the etiology of these diseases. Patients with the Hermansky-Pudlak syndrome (*see* page 2592) have been reported to show findings on BAL that are identical to those of patients with idiopathic fibrosing alveolitis, including increased levels of immunoglobulins and the number of IgG and IgA secreting cells.[648] In addition, results of

BAL in patients with fibrosing alveolitis have been found to be identical to those described in clinically unaffected members of three families with an autosomal dominant form of idiopathic pulmonary fibrosis,[650] including increased numbers of neutrophils and activated macrophages that released neutrophil chemoattractants and growth factors for lung fibroblasts.

Viral Infection

Although the diagnosis of fibrosing alveolitis often coincides with recognition of a viral-type syndrome[651] such as that originally described by Hamman and Rich in their cases of rapidly progressive interstitial fibrosis,[652] it is rare to document a *specific* viral infection that terminates in pathologically proven interstitial fibrosis.[653–655] Intranuclear inclusion bodies have been described,[656–658] particularly in patients labeled as having DIP, but it is believed that they represent the products of nuclear degeneration rather than bodies of viral origin.[659] Vergnon and associates[660] found specific immunoglobulins for Epstein-Barr virus (EBV) in 10 of 13 patients with fibrosing alveolitis, a finding that could either reflect a nonspecific depression of cell-mediated immunity or indicate that EBV plays a part in the production of the disease. Such reports and the results obtained with studies of pneumotoxins in mice[661] raise the possibility that cell-mediated

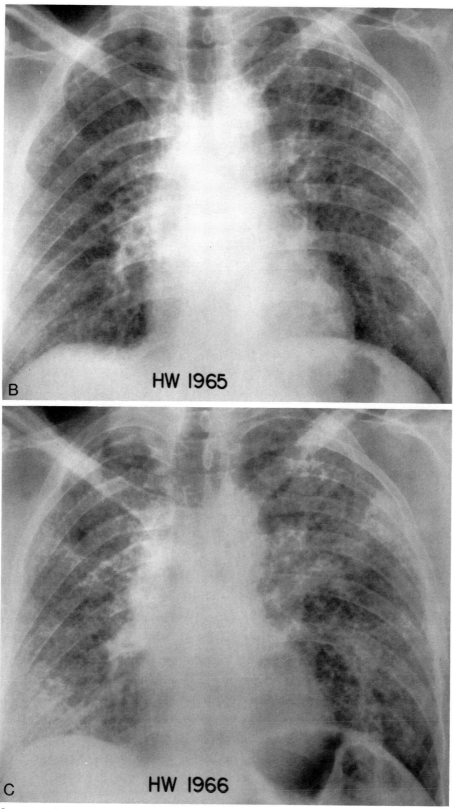

Figure 17–28 *Continued (B)* and *(C)* are from a male member *(HW)* whose 1965 roentgenogram *(B)* reveals a coarse reticular pattern without anatomic predominance; one year later *(C)*, lung volume had reduced appreciably and the reticular opacities had worsened.

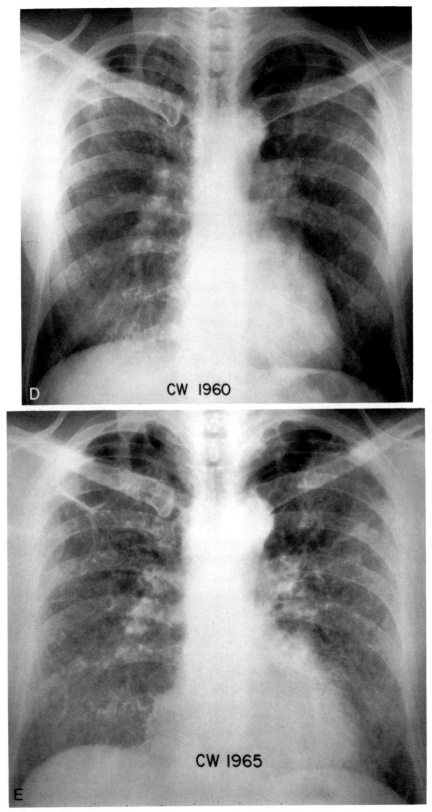

Figure 17–28 *Continued (D) and (E) are from another male member (CW) of the family whose 1960 roentgenogram (D) reveals a rather fine reticular pattern throughout both lungs similar to the changes observed in (A); five years later (E), the lungs had lost some volume and the reticular pattern had worsened considerably. Open lung biopsies of the two male members (HW and CW) of the family revealed classic changes of fibrosing alveolitis.*

immunity may play a role in the maintenance of the inflammatory response, if not in the final fibrotic process.

The histologic pattern of DIP has been seen in association with nitrofurantoin therapy,[662] (rarely) with leukemia,[663] and with a variety of inhaled particulates,[664] including aluminum[665] and tungsten carbide.[666]

PATHOGENESIS

The initial reaction to injury in fibrosing alveolitis has been hypothesized to consist of an influx of edema fluid and proteinaceous exudate in the interstitium and hyaline membrane formation in the alveoli[667] although these changes are rarely seen in tissue specimens. Activated alveolar macrophages have the potential to modulate this process, since they have been shown to synthesize the initial enzymes of both the coagulation and fibrinolytic pathways.[77] The inflammatory cell population of the lung parenchyma in fibrosing alveolitis, as revealed by both BAL and open lung biopsy, consists of alveolar macrophages, neutrophils, eosinophils, and lymphocytes.[668–670] In nonsmoking normal subjects, the neutrophil makes up less than 1 per cent of the total number of cells obtained by BAL[671, 672] whereas in fibrosing alveolitis, the percentage of neutrophils rises to 10 to 20 percent;[673] this is in contrast to other interstitial diseases, such as eosinophilic granuloma, sarcoidosis, and hypersensitivity pneumonitis, in which the neutrophil count is normal.[669] Since the neutrophil carries such a potent armamentarium of inflammatory mediators as well as oxygen radicals and proteases, it is likely that this cell is chiefly responsible for the alveolar derangement that occurs in fibrosing alveolitis.[674] The accumulation of neutrophils in the lungs has been attributed to the release of a chemotactic factor by alveolar macrophages that have been activated by immune complexes deposited in lung tissue.[675] Eosinophils and eosinophil cationic protein are also increased over values found in control groups and may play a role in pathogenesis.[676]

The role played by the T-cell lymphocyte and cell-mediated immunity in the pathogenesis of fibrosing alveolitis is less clear. Using monoclonal antibodies in conjunction with histochemical techniques on lung biopsy specimens, Campbell and associates[621] found that most of the lymphocytes in the alveolar septa were B lymphocytes, the number of T-helper and T-suppressor cells being equal. By contrast, others[677] have found T-suppressor cells to be predominant. In one study in which the population of subsets of T cells in BAL fluid was compared,[678] an association was found between fibrosing alveolitis and a predominance of T-helper cells, whereas in the connective tissue diseases with interstitial fibrosis the T-suppressor cells were more numerous; no difference was observed in blood T lymphocytes in these two groups. Cathcart and associates[679] found an excess of T-helper cells in the blood of some patients with fibrosing alveolitis and correlated this finding with the degree of neutrophilic alveolitis.

As indicated previously, on exposure to a variety of agents several animal models have been reported to develop pathologic changes similar to those of fibrosing alveolitis, an observation that may simply reflect the nonspecific and limited ability of lung parenchyma to respond to injury. Some of these studies have suggested a humoral immunologic mechanism for pulmonary damage—for example, the reaction induced by the instillation of rabbit antirat lung serum into the trachea of rats[595] or the injection of Freund's adjuvant into the lungs of pigs[680] or rabbits.[681] In others, the presence of an intra-alveolar proliferation of mononuclear cells in association with interstitial fibrosis has suggested a cell-mediated reaction. Similar pathologic changes have been observed following acute exposure to cadmium fumes in animals,[682] a single intraperitoneal injection of paraquat in rats,[683] and weekly subcutaneous administration of N-nitroso-N-methylurethane in hamsters.[684] In one study of bleomycin-induced pulmonary fibrosis in mice, in vivo blastogenesis of splenic lymphocytes and the production of migratory inhibition factor in response to the drug occurred several weeks after initial exposure;[661] the authors concluded that because of the relatively delayed onset of these cell-mediated reactions, it was probable that the autoimmune phenomenon was not associated with the fibrosis etiologically but rather with maintenance of the inflammatory response.

Although the primary mechanism of lung damage in individual cases of cryptogenic fibrosing alveolitis is unknown, the subsequent release of oxidants from both damaged epithelial lining cells and lung inflammatory cells may result in a vicious cycle of tissue destruction similar to that described in drug- and poison-induced alveolocapillary injury.[685] In addition there is considerable evidence that a variety of cellular metabolic processes can initiate fibrogenesis, chief among which are the secretions of various enzymes from alveolar macrophages and polymorphonuclear leukocytes. Activated alveolar macrophages from patients with fibrosing alveolitis have been shown to produce growth-promoting factors for lung fibroblasts;[130, 131] among those recognized are fibronectin[132] and platelet-derived growth factor.[133] Using monoclonal antibodies and cell cultures, it has been shown by phenotypic analysis of both activated alveolar macrophages[686] and fibroblasts[687] that distinct subpopulations of these cells exist, the clones of fibroblasts having intrinsic growth characteristics that could in themselves explain the fibroblast proliferation that occurs in pulmonary fibrosis. Although one study of human lung from patients with pulmonary fibrosis showed no increase in collagen compared with normal lungs,[688] more recent studies[689–691] have shown that the amount of collagen is in fact increased.

The discrepancies among the results of these studies may relate either to the selection of patients studied or to the method of expressing the results. It is difficult to know what the appropriate denominator should be for expressing collagen content. Since total lung cells and weight may be increased in the presence of disease, expressing the collagen as milligrams/milligram of DNA or as milligrams/gram of dry tissue may result in an underestimation of the amount. Ideally the results should be expressed as milligrams of collagen/anatomic lung unit (e.g., a lobe). In contrast to the regular arrangement of parallel cross-banded fibers characteristic of normal lung tissue, the collagen fibers in fibrosing alveolitis can be seen by electron microscopy to be randomly oriented, twisted, and frayed. Assays of lung collagen in patients with fibrosing alveolitis[692, 693] and in rats exposed to pneumotoxins[694] show an increase in the ratio of type 1 to type 3 fibers; in addition, type 1 fibers are less compliant than type 3 fibers. The increase in the collagen content of the lung in pulmonary fibrotic diseases could result from either increased synthesis or decreased degradation. Studies of collagen synthesis in lung biopsy specimens from patients with and without pulmonary fibrosis have found no differences.[688, 691] However, it may be that an increase in collagen synthesis occurs early in the course of the disease when tissue is not obtained, or that in vitro synthesis does not reflect in vivo synthesis. In animal models of pulmonary fibrosis,[695, 696] an increase in collagen synthesis can be detected early in the development of disease, but the rate may return to normal in the presence of established fibrosis.

An alternate explanation for increased lung collagen, as indicated previously, could be decreased degradation. Selmon and associates[691] have reported a decrease in the collagenolytic activity in samples of homogenized lung tissue from patients with idiopathic pulmonary fibrosis compared with lung tissue from a normal subject. In seeming contradiction, Gadek and associates[963] have reported the detection of collagenolytic activity in the BAL fluid of patients with pulmonary fibrosis but no activity in the fluid from normal subjects or patients with sarcoidosis. However, it is possible that results from analysis of BAL fluid do not reflect the actual concentration of enzymatic substances in the pulmonary interstitium: increased epithelial permeability could permit collagenase to reach the alveolar airspaces in patients with pulmonary fibrosis, whereas the alveolar epithelium of normal subjects might be completely impermeable to such large molecular weight substances. This newly synthesized collagen consists mostly of type 1 fibers, with differences in form and location from the normal accounting for the loss of pulmonary compliance and the restrictive defect found on physiologic assessment.[692, 693] In a study comparing fibrosing alveolitis patients with bronchial asthma patients,[697] it was found that the glycosaminoglycans, normally representing less than 1 per cent of the total parenchymal connective tissue components,[698] were increased in amount in the former patients.

In addition to the evidence for fibrinogenesis in fibrosing alveolitis, an antifibrinogenic factor has been demonstrated in mononuclear cell cultures that inhibits fibroblast growth, perhaps mediated in part by fibroblast prostaglandin production.[699]

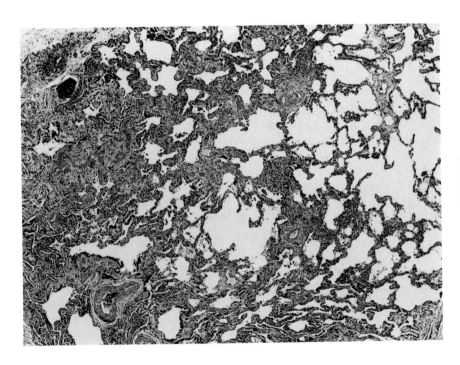

Figure 17–29. Fibrosing Alveolitis.
A low-magnification histologic section of lung parenchyma shows interstitial thickening of variable severity; some alveolar septa are almost normal whereas others show moderate or marked thickening. (×35.)

PATHOLOGIC CHARACTERISTICS

Histologically, diffuse fibrosing alveolitis is typically a condition of variable severity; areas of normal and severely diseased lung are often present in different areas of the same lobe and even in a single tissue fragment (Fig. 17–29). In the least affected areas, a mild degree of alveolar septal thickening is present, caused predominantly by an infiltrate of inflammatory cells (Fig. 17–30A); lymphocytes are usually the most numerous, although plasma cells, mast cells,[700] histiocytes, eosinophils, and, rarely, polymorphonuclear leukocytes are encountered in lesser numbers. Although the infiltrate is usually diffuse, organization of the lymphoid cells into germinal centers is seen occasionally. In more advanced disease (Fig. 17–30B), the interstitial thickening is greater and is usually associated with some degree of fibrosis. Most often this consists of mature collagen, but foci of loose fibroblastic tissue indicating active fibrogenesis are also not infrequent. Such areas of active fibrosis can be occasionally identified in alveolar airspaces and transitional airways; however, if they are present in more than an occasional focus, a diagnosis of bronchiolitis obliterans with organizing pneumonia (BOOP) should be seriously entertained.

In the most severely affected areas, interstitial thickening is so marked that alveoli are reduced to small slits (Fig. 17–30C) or are completely obliterated; fibrous tissue often is more abundant than the inflammatory cell infiltrate. It is this stage, characterized by loss of lung parenchyma and coalescence and dilatation of transitional airways (Fig. 17–31), that corresponds to the classic "honeycomb" appearance so characteristic of the gross appearance of advanced disease (*see* farther on). Often associated with the areas of severe fibrosis are smooth muscle hyperplasia (Fig. 17–32) and epithelial metaplasia (Fig. 17–33), the latter usually of squamous or columnar mucus-secreting type. Dystrophic calcification and even osseous metaplasia can also occur.[701, 702]

In contrast to normal alveoli that are lined mostly by type I epithelial cells with only scattered type II cells, the walls of alveoli affected by fibrosing alveolitis are commonly lined by cuboidal cells (Fig. 17–34); although many of these represent hyperplastic type II cells, some do not show ultrastructural features of type II cell differentiation and appear to be derived directly from bronchiolar epithelium.[703] There is some evidence that type II cells are more prominent in the least fibrotic areas and bronchiolar cells in the most fibrotic.[703, 704] Eosinophilic inclusions resembling Mallory hyaline can be seen within the cytoplasm of these hyperplastic cells (*see* Fig. 12–26, page 2323) and should not be confused with viral inclusions.[705, 706] Langerhans' cells are also present in the alveolar epithelial lining; in one study, they were identified by electron microscopic examination in 13 of 56 cases,[707] situated between or just under hyperplastic type II cells. Given the limitations of sampling with this technique, it is possible that they were also present in many of the remainder. The significance of their presence is not clear.

Although predominantly an interstitial process, fibrosing alveolitis affects the airspaces also. The most common finding is the presence of increased numbers of macrophages; in contrast to the histologic pattern of DIP (*see* farther on), they are usually variable in number from alveolus to alveolus and overall are not numerous. Occasional multinucleated giant cells also can be present,[657] both in the airspaces and in the interstitium; granulomas do not occur. The cystic spaces of "honeycomb" lung frequently contain mucus, often with fairly numerous admixed polymorphonuclear leukocytes (Fig. 17–33); the mucus is presumably related to epithelial metaplasia.

Pulmonary arteries usually show some degree of intimal fibrosis and medial muscular hyperplasia, especially in the regions of more marked interstitial fibrosis. Although such changes may be related to generalized pulmonary hypertension, they may simply reflect a reaction to locally severe disease.

Grossly, the early stages of fibrosing alveolitis consist of only a slight coarseness of the normal parenchyma, typically most severe in the subpleural region and in the lower and posterior portions of the lower lobes. As disease progresses, clear-cut areas of fibrosis alternating with small cystic spaces 1 to 2 mm in diameter appear (Fig. 17–35). Eventually, a whole lobe can be affected, resulting in innumerable 5- to 10-mm cystic spaces separated by a variable amount of firm, gray fibrous tissue (so-called honeycomb lung) (Fig. 17–36). These changes almost invariably affect the lower lobes predominantly, the central portion of the upper lobes being spared until the very last. The external surface of such a lung typically has a coarse, nodular appearance, likened by some investigators to cirrhosis,[708, 709] that is caused by bulging of the cysts and retraction of the adjacent scarred parenchyma (Fig. 17–36).

Although primarily a disease of the lung parenchyma, abnormalities of the large airways also can be seen in some cases of fibrosing alveolitis. For example, in one autopsy study of 12 patients with advanced pulmonary fibrosis, Westcott and Cole[710] identified bronchiectasis in 9 patients; its confinement to areas of advanced fibrosis suggested that its cause was traction by the fibrous tissue. The bronchiectasis was much better depicted on CT scans than on conventional roentgenograms; on the latter it was thought to contribute to the appearance of honeycombing. Another study of the proximal bronchi in 9 cases of fibrosing alveolitis showed glandular and muscle hypertrophy;[711] the authors speculated that extension of infection in fibrotic lung parenchyma might be the cause.

Unlike the characteristic variable appearance

Text continued on page 2661

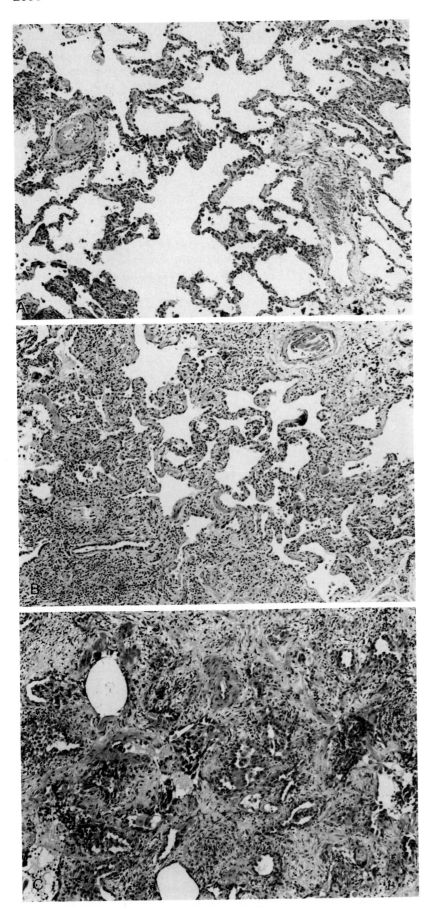

Figure 17–30. Fibrosing Alveolitis: Varying Severity. Three histologic sections demonstrate increasing degrees of severity of pathologic change in fibrosing alveolitis. An early stage (A) shows mild interstitial thickening, caused predominantly by an infiltrate of lymphocytes. More advanced disease (B) is characterized by moderate thickening of the interstitium; although there are still abundant lymphocytes, these are now associated with appreciable fibrous tissue. Still more severe disease (C) is manifested by a marked reduction in the size of alveolar airspaces and a great increase in the amount of interstitial collagen. (A, B, and C, ×80.)

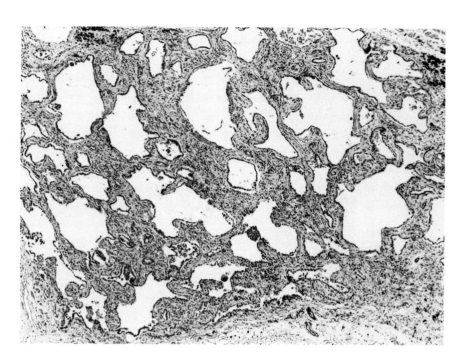

Figure 17–31. Fibrosing Alveolitis: "Honeycomb" Change. A histologic section shows that the majority of the lung parenchyma has been replaced by fibrous tissue, accompanied by a moderate infiltrate of lymphocytes. Irregularly shaped cystic spaces derived from transitional airways (representing the cells of the "honeycomb") are present at regular intervals within the fibrotic lung parenchyma. (×35.)

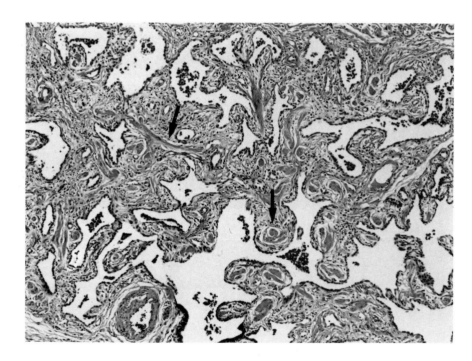

Figure 17–32. Fibrosing Alveolitis: Muscular Hyperplasia. A histologic section shows a focus of lung with advanced interstitial fibrosis, associated with haphazardly arranged bands of hyperplastic smooth muscle *(arrows)*. (×60.)

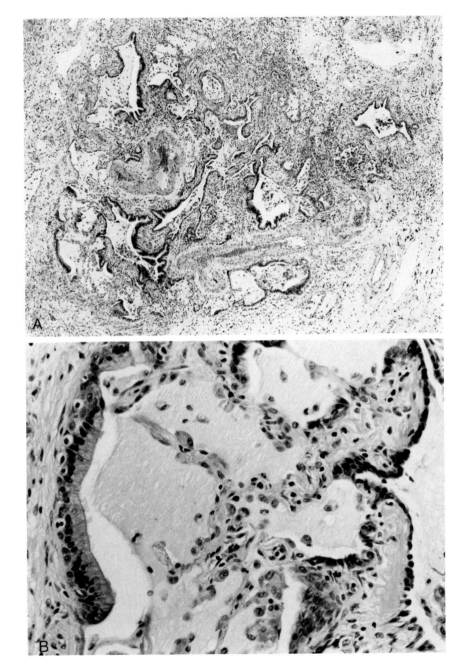

Figure 17–33. Fibrosing Alveolitis: Epithelial Metaplasia. A histologic section of another lung with advanced disease *(A)* shows several irregularly shaped cystic spaces lined by tall columnar cells. These cells are seen to better advantage at higher magnification *(B);* in this section, note the presence of mucus in the adjacent airspace, representing secretion from the metaplastic epithelium. *(A,* ×40; *B,* ×250.)

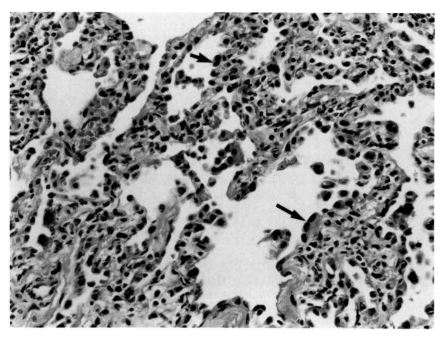

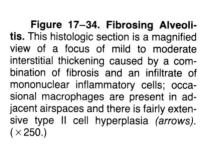

Figure 17–34. Fibrosing Alveolitis. This histologic section is a magnified view of a focus of mild to moderate interstitial thickening caused by a combination of fibrosis and an infiltrate of mononuclear inflammatory cells; occasional macrophages are present in adjacent airspaces and there is fairly extensive type II cell hyperplasia *(arrows).* (×250.)

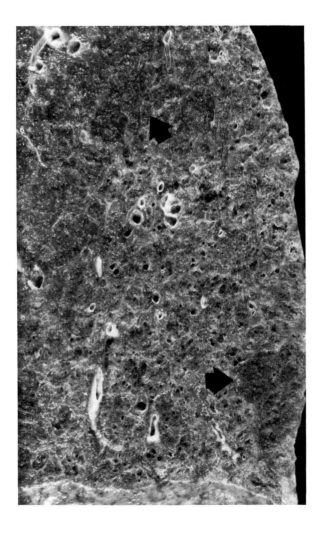

Figure 17–35. Fibrosing Alveolitis: Early Stage. A magnified view of a lower lobe of a 48-year-old man shows more or less diffuse interstitial thickening of mild to moderate degree. Relatively unaffected lung is indicated by *arrows.*

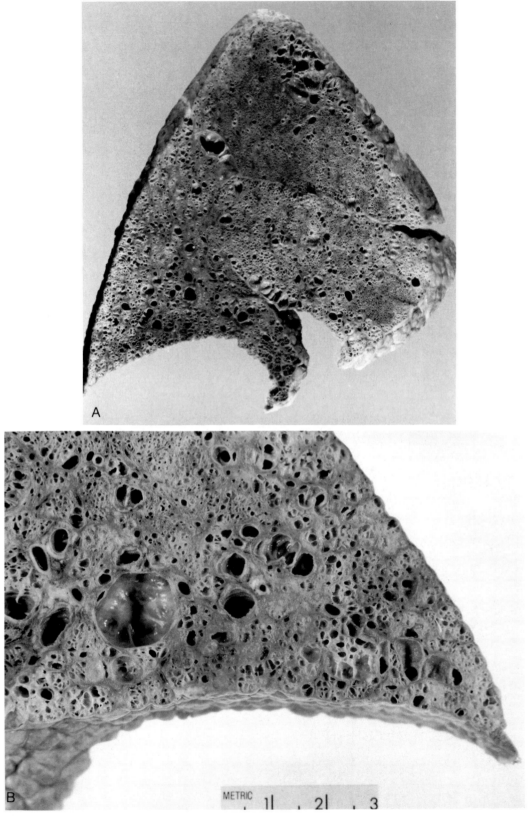

Figure 17–36. Fibrosing Alveolitis: Advanced Stage. A sagittal section of a right lung *(A)* shows advanced interstitial fibrosis with extensive "honeycomb" change. Note the relative sparing of the central portion of the upper lobe. A magnified view of the basal aspect of a lower lobe from another patient *(B)* shows severe interstitial fibrosis with virtually no remaining normal parenchyma. Note the nodular appearance of the pleural surface caused by alternating areas of fibrosis and cyst formation, sometimes referred to as pulmonary "cirrhosis."

of fibrosing alveolitis as described above, the histologic pattern of desquamative interstitial pneumonia is distinctly uniform, all portions of lung on a tissue section appearing more or less similar (Fig. 17–37). The alveolar interstitium is usually mildly to moderately thickened by an infiltrate of mononuclear inflammatory cells and a small amount of collagen, lymphoid nodules are sometimes present, and type II cell hyperplasia is extensive and again fairly uniform. Most strikingly, alveolar airspaces are filled with numerous mononuclear cells, originally believed to be desquamated type II cells but now known to be predominantly alveolar macrophages. These cells may contain small amounts of iron or other pigment and, occasionally, oval or rounded

lamellated structures resembling the Schaumann body of sarcoidosis (Fig. 17–38).[712] These structures, sometimes termed "blue bodies" because of their weak hematoxalinophilia with hematoxylin-eosin stain, are PAS-positive and contain calcium and iron; their precise nature is unclear. It is important to recognize that the histologic pattern of desquamative interstitial pneumonitis can be seen focally in association with otherwise typical cases of fibrosing alveolitis; it can also occur with other conditions such as tuberculosis, eosinophilic granuloma, and rheumatoid nodule.[713] Thus, a diagnosis of desquamative interstitial pneumonitis based on a small amount of tissue, such as that obtained by transbronchial biopsy, should be made with caution.

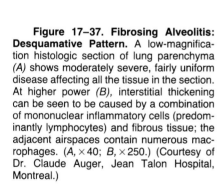

Figure 17–37. Fibrosing Alveolitis: Desquamative Pattern. A low-magnification histologic section of lung parenchyma (A) shows moderately severe, fairly uniform disease affecting all the tissue in the section. At higher power (B), interstitial thickening can be seen to be caused by a combination of mononuclear inflammatory cells (predominantly lymphocytes) and fibrous tissue; the adjacent airspaces contain numerous macrophages. (A, ×40; B, ×250.) (Courtesy of Dr. Claude Auger, Jean Talon Hospital, Montreal.)

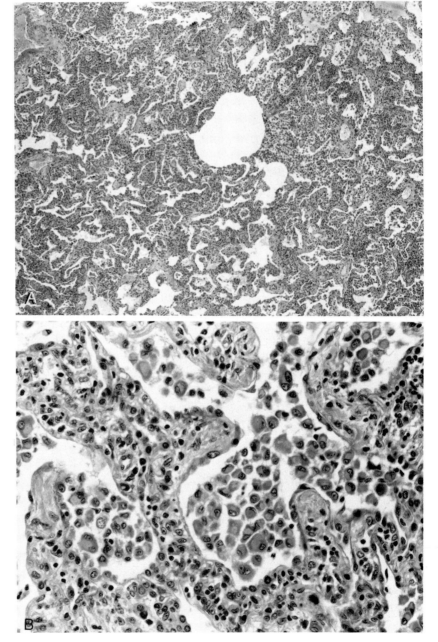

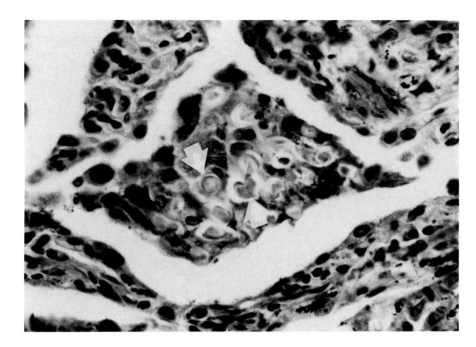

Figure 17–38. Fibrosing Alveolitis: Blue Bodies. A histologic section of an alveolar airspace at high magnification reveals a cluster of macrophages containing poorly defined, somewhat lamellated PAS-positive structures or so-called blue bodies *(arrows).* The section is from a biopsy specimen that showed the typical features of a DIP pattern. (PAS, × 600.)

Ultrastructural features of fibrosing alveolitis have been described in several reports.[703, 704, 714, 715] Basically, they document evidence of both endothelial and epithelial damage and repair associated with multilamination of alveolar septal basement membrane and an increase in collagen and elastic fibers in the interstitium; an increased number of myofibroblasts (interstitial actin-containing cells) is also seen.[715]

ROENTGENOGRAPHIC MANIFESTATIONS

As might be expected, the roentgenographic pattern varies with the stage of the disease. In desquamative interstitial pneumonitis (DIP), a pattern of symmetric "ground-glass" opacification predominant at the lung bases that was described in the early literature[656, 716] as being characteristic has not been substantiated in subsequent studies.[717, 718] For example, of 37 cases of DIP described by Feigin and Friedman,[717] this pattern was found in only 6; these investigators described the most common roentgenographic pattern as consisting of nonspecific irregular opacities most numerous in the lung bases, an appearance also observed by others (Fig. 17–39).[597]

It is probable that the earliest discernible roentgenographic changes in fibrosing alveolitis are those that can be attributed to interstitial fibrosis and that consist of a fine reticulation with lower zonal predominance. Some observers[572, 719, 720] have also described a pattern suggesting combined airspace and interstitial involvement (Fig. 17–40). At this stage, patients may be asymptomatic even though pulmonary function may be greatly impaired. On the other hand, an occasional patient with biopsy-proved disease is symptomatic and yet shows no roentgenographic abnormality,[573, 583, 642, 656, 718, 721] particularly when disease is relatively early and confined to the alveolar interstitium.

Roentgenologically, advanced disease is characterized by a coarse reticular or reticulonodular pattern throughout the lungs. Thick-walled cystic spaces 3 to 10 mm in diameter are present and create a honeycomb pattern (Fig. 17–41). The severe disorganization of lung architecture usually can be much better appreciated on CT scans than on conventional roentgenograms (Fig. 17–42). As has been emphasized previously (*see* page 562), we are strongly of the opinion that the designation honeycomb lung should not be applied to any pattern in which the cystic spaces measure less than 5 or 6 mm in diameter. If this restriction is applied, the differential diagnostic possibilities can be reduced to relatively few diseases—progressive systemic sclerosis, eosinophilic granuloma, lymphangioleiomyomatosis, fibrosing alveolitis, rheumatoid disease, and rarely, sarcoidosis and berylliosis. We submit that this is the only way to bring some order to the confusion that surrounds diffuse interstitial lung disease.

We have been repeatedly impressed by the striking loss of lung volume apparent on serial roentgenographic studies over a period of several years (Fig. 17–43) and consider that a diffuse reticulonodular pattern accompanied by progressive elevation of the diaphragm—signs that occur much less frequently in other forms of diffuse interstitial fibrosis—strongly suggests the diagnosis of either cryptogenic fibrosing alveolitis or progressive systemic sclerosis. However, except for this loss of

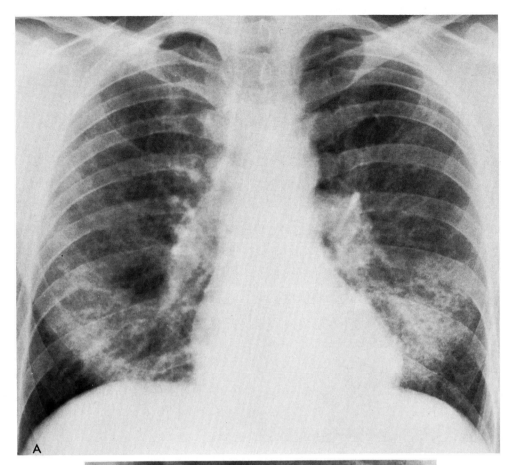

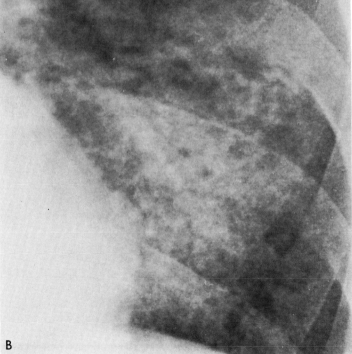

Figure 17–39. Fibrosing Alveolitis: Desquamative Phase. This 35-year-old policeman noted the onset of dyspnea 6 months previously while wrestling a suspect; the dyspnea had become progressively worse up to the time of hospital admission. A posteroanterior roentgenogram *(A)* and a magnified view of the lower portion of the left lung *(B)* reveal diffuse involvement of both lungs by a rather coarse reticular pattern, which is slightly more prominent in the bases than elsewhere. Hilar lymph nodes appear slightly enlarged.

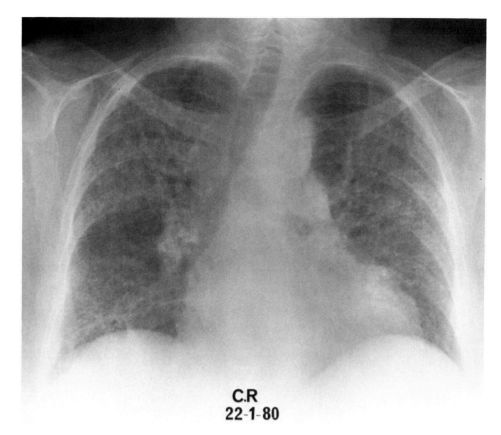

Figure 17–40. Diffuse Fibrosing Alveolitis. A posteroanterior roentgenogram reveals diffuse pulmonary disease, the pattern of which suggests a combination of interstitial and airspace abnormality, particularly in upper lung zones. The patient is a middle-aged man with recent onset of mild dyspnea.

C.R
22-1-80

volume there is nothing specific about the roentgenographic pattern of fibrosing alveolitis.[722] Hilar lymph node enlargement[657, 716, 733] and pleural effusion[656] are rare, and their presence should suggest other diagnoses or complications. Pneumothorax is uncommon;[657, 723] in one series of 82 patients, spontaneous pneumothorax was not seen in the 36 patients with interstitial pneumonitis associated with systemic disease and occurred in only 3 of the 46 patients with cryptogenic fibrosing alveolitis.[723]

In two studies carried out at the University of British Columbia in which CT findings were correlated with pathologic,[724] clinical, functional, and conventional roentgenographic[725] findings in patients with idiopathic pulmonary fibrosis, the following factors were observed: (1) disease activity on CT scans (judged by the presence or absence of opacification of airspaces) (Fig. 17–44) correlated well with the presence or absence of pathologic evidence of intra-alveolar and interstitial cellularity;[724] (2) changes were seen to better advantage on 1.5-mm than on 10-mm collimation scans, an observation that has been emphasized by others[726] (Fig. 17–44); (3) CT scans gave a better estimate of disease extent and showed more extensive honeycombing than did conventional roentgenograms (Fig. 17–45);[725] (4) a significant correlation was found between the extent of disease as assessed with

CT and the severity of dyspnea and impairment of gas exchange (diffusing capacity);[725] and (5) correlation between disease severity as assessed on conventional roentgenograms and clinical and functional variables was poor. CT also has been recommended for early diagnosis and for evaluating response to therapy.[727, 728]

Positron emission tomography has been used to measure regional lung density and fractional pulmonary blood flow in patients with fibrosing alveolitis.[729–731] Proton magnetic resonance imaging[732] is another noninvasive method that has been recommended for early diagnosis and for evaluating response to treatment; published results are encouraging, particularly with respect to sensitivity.

CLINICAL MANIFESTATIONS

Symptoms include progressive dyspnea, nonproductive cough, weight loss, and fatigue.[591, 610, 657, 658] Clubbing is common and its presence can antedate symptoms and other signs of pulmonary disease;[629] it occurs equally as often in the "desquamative" stage of the disease as in the advanced fibrotic stage. Arthralgia and myalgia have been described in patients with DIP.[658]

In the early stages, examination of the chest

Text continued on page 2670

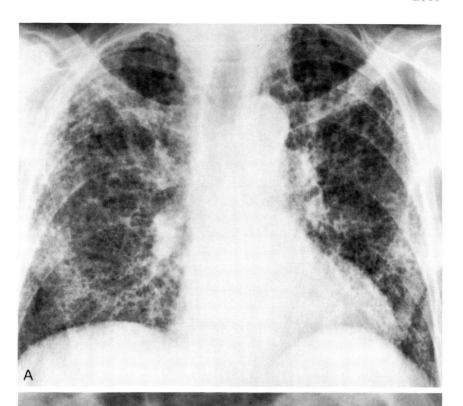

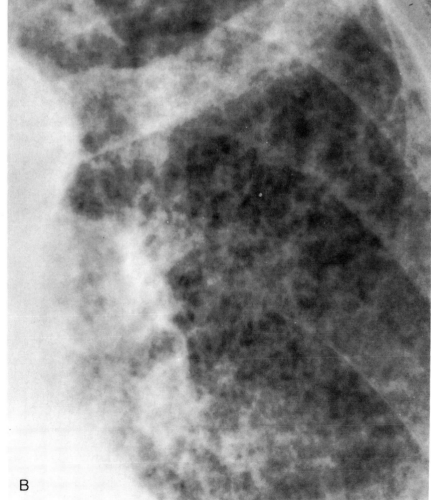

Figure 17–41. Advanced Fibrosing Alveolitis with Honeycombing. A posteroanterior roentgenogram *(A)* and a magnified view of the left mid lung *(B)* reveal a coarse reticular pattern without anatomic predominance. Honeycomb changes are present in several areas and are seen to good advantage in *B*.
Illustration continued on following page

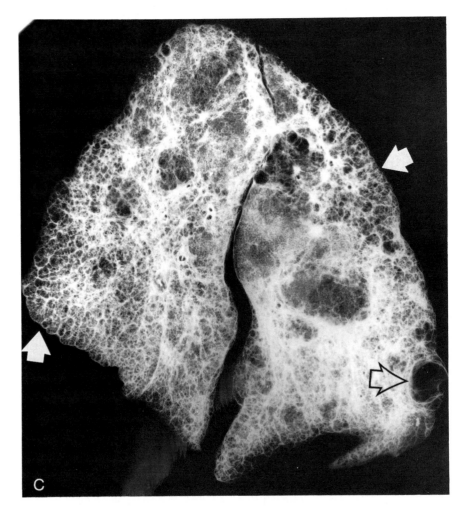

Figure 17–41 *Continued* A roentgenogram of a 1-cm thick slice of left lung removed at autopsy *(C)* shows the honeycombing well *(solid arrows)* and also reveals a large subpleural bulla in the lower lobe *(open arrow)*.

Figure 17–42. Diffuse Fibrosing Alveolitis: CT Manifestations. A CT scan at the level of the bronchus intermedius reveals extensive bilateral pulmonary disease consisting predominantly of a reticular pattern. On the left side particularly, the fibrosis involves the subpleural lung regions predominantly. (Courtesy of Dr. Nestor L. Müller, University of British Columbia, Vancouver.)

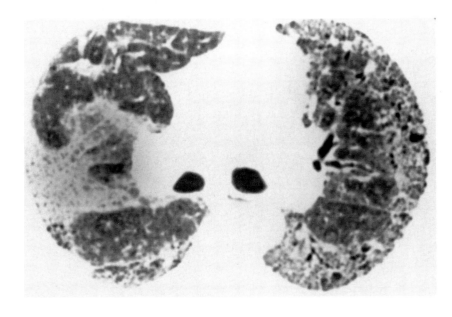

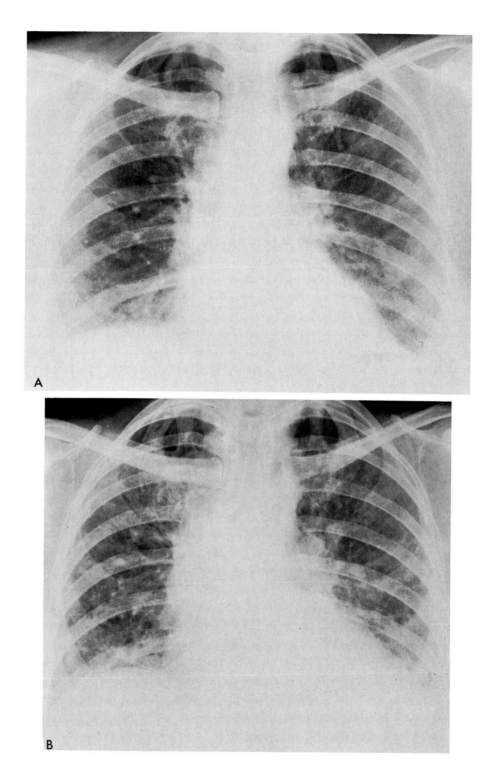

Figure 17–43. Fibrosing Alveolitis. The roentgenogram illustrated in *(A)* reveals a widespread, coarse reticular pattern superimposed upon a hazy, ground-glass opacity. (It is suggested that the latter is the result of mucus in the peripheral air spaces.) Seven years later, a roentgenogram *(B)* reveals considerable reduction in the size of the thorax, presumably as a result of diffuse cicatricial pulmonary atelectasis. The reticulonodular pattern is somewhat more prominent now. The diagnosis in this 50-year-old woman was based on open lung biopsy.

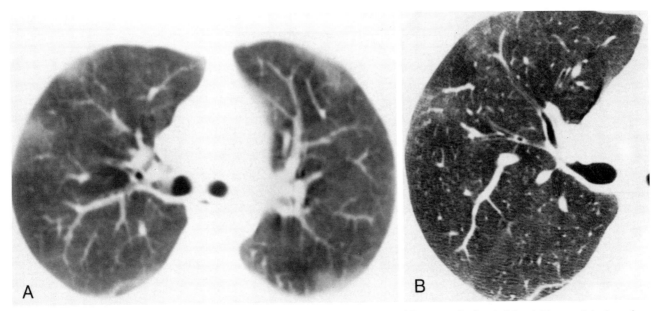

Figure 17–44. Fibrosing Alveolitis: CT Manifestations of Active Disease. A CT scan at the level of the right upper lobe bronchus with 10-mm collimation *(A)* shows patchy, ill-defined areas of airspace opacification situated predominantly in subpleural lung regions bilaterally. A high-resolution scan at the same level with 1.5-mm collimation *(B)* shows the areas of airspace opacification to be sharply demarcated from contiguous normal parenchyma. The patient is a 39-year-old man whose open lung biopsy was interpreted as "desquamative interstitial pneumonia." (Reproduced with permission from Müller NL, Staples CA, Miller RR, et al. Disease activity in idiopathic pulmonary fibrosis: CT and pathologic correlation. Radiology *165:*731, 1987.)

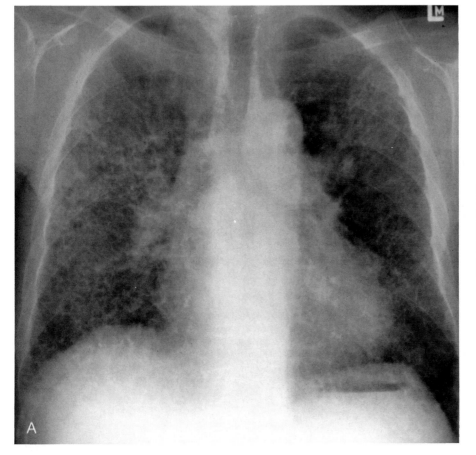

Figure 17–45. Endstage Fibrosing Alveolitis: Radiographic/CT Correlation. A conventional chest roentgenogram *(A)* reveals a rather coarse reticular pattern throughout both lungs with some basal predominance. At the right base, the changes suggest the presence of honeycombing.

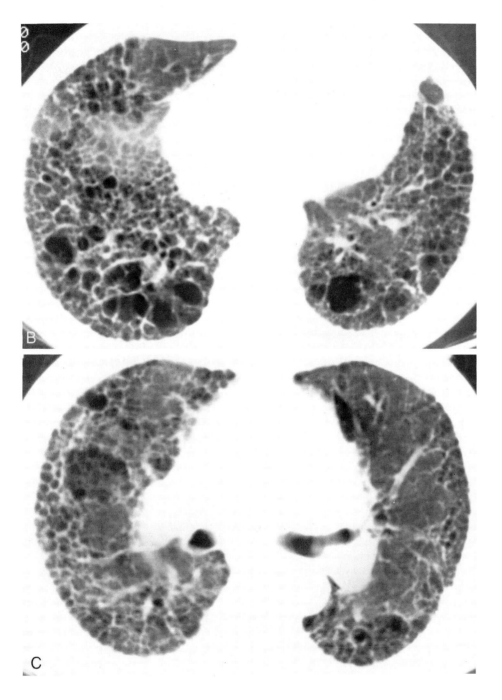

Figure 17–45 *Continued* A CT scan through the base of both lungs *(B)* reveals extensive honeycombing extending from the visceral pleura to the mediastinum on both sides. Another CT scan at the level of the bronchus intermedius *(C)* also shows severe honeycombing but at this level possessing considerable subpleural predominance. These CT changes are much more marked than would have been anticipated from the conventional roentgenogram. The patient is a 61-year-old man. (Courtesy of Dr. Nestor L. Müller, University of British Columbia, Vancouver.)

can be within normal limits, but as the disease progresses, diffuse crepitations of a very superficial quality are frequently heard, predominantly over the lung bases. DeRemee and coworkers[734] call these crepitations "Velcro" rales because of their resemblance to the sound produced by tearing apart mated strips of Velcro adhesive. When an occupational history fails to reveal asbestos exposure, the combination of these fine rales, clubbing of the fingers, and dyspnea (but no orthopnea) is virtually diagnostic of cryptogenic fibrosing alveolitis. Cyanosis and signs of pulmonary hypertension and cor pulmonale are late manifestations of the disease.

Other infrequent clinical findings include sexual impotence, presumably caused by suppression of the hypothalamo-pituitary-testicular axis by hypoxia,[735] and hyponatremia associated with the syndrome of inappropriate secretion of antidiuretic hormone.[736]

When clinical findings and the roentgenographic pattern suggest interstitial lung disease, the diagnostic possibilities are numerous. Although the combination of clubbing, slowly progressive worsening of dyspnea, serial reduction in pulmonary function, and roentgenographic evidence of progressive loss of lung volume strongly suggest the diagnosis, in most cases cryptogenic fibrosing alveolitis is a diagnosis of exclusion. Nevertheless, it is a rare occurrence for biopsy to reveal a different diagnosis when a careful history, physical examination, and laboratory investigation have reasonably excluded other diagnostic possibilities. Autoimmune conditions, such as rheumatoid disease, progressive systemic sclerosis, Sjögren's syndrome, and dermatomyositis/polymyositis, are usually readily recognized by their clinical manifestations and specific autoantibodies. Error is most likely to arise during the early stages of polymyositis when muscle weakness may be overlooked or may be ascribed to nonspecific manifestations of the pulmonary disability or to corticosteroid therapy.[737, 738]

The diagnosis of a pneumoconiosis or drug reaction usually requires little more than a searching clinical history regarding occupation and medications, a step that is often neglected in the former instance until such a possibility is suggested by the roentgenographic pattern. Similarly, a history of exposure to birds or moldy hay can raise the possibility that the interstitial lung disease is caused by extrinsic allergic alveolitis. The diagnosis of fibrosing alveolitis is virtually eliminated by the finding of hilar and paratracheal lymph node enlargement; its presence with diffuse interstitial lung disease strongly suggests the diagnosis of sarcoidosis. The clinical findings associated with other interstitial pneumonitides, such as neurofibromatosis, the Hermansky-Pudlak syndrome, tuberous sclerosis, and lymphangioleiomyomatosis, are usually sufficiently characteristic to distinguish these entities from cryptogenic fibrosing alveolitis. Eosinophilic granuloma (histiocytosis X) generally presents with normal or

increased lung volume in contrast to the classical shrunken lungs of fibrosing alveolitis and characteristically affects the upper lung zones more than the lower.

Open lung biopsy, thoracoscopic biopsy, and, in some hands, trephine biopsy[739] are the only procedures that yield sufficient tissue to support a diagnosis of fibrosing alveolitis; trephine biopsy is not without risk (see page 361). Transbronchial biopsy often does not result in a specific diagnosis,[571, 740] although the absence of granulomas virtually eliminates sarcoidosis as a diagnostic possibility.

Pulmonary Function Tests

In most series in which pulmonary function has been assessed, fibrosing alveolitis patients have been grouped with other interstitial pulmonary disease patients.[741–747] Vital capacity, diffusing capacity,[748] gas transfer, and pulmonary hemodynamics[749, 750] appear to be more severely affected in fibrosing alveolitis than in other interstitial diseases. In one study,[751] a decrease in vital capacity and transfer factor (DL_{CO}) correlated with increasing severity of the fibrotic process. In another series of 23 biopsy-proved cases,[752] lung volumes and diffusing capacity were found to be poor indicators of both the amount of fibrosis and the degree of cellularity; by contrast, parameters of lung distensibility and exercise-induced gas exchange abnormalities were judged to be useful in staging the severity of disease. It is very probable that values of PaO_2 and $P(A-a)O_2$ on exercise are the most sensitive means of assessing disability in patients with cryptogenic fibrosing alveolitis,[753–755] as they are in those exposed to asbestos.[756] Hypoxemia is caused chiefly by $\dot{V}/\dot{Q}$ inequality,[757–761] although approximately 20 per cent of the hypoxemia observed on exercise can be attributed to a diffusion defect.[651, 759] Orthodeoxia (arterial desaturation accentuated by the upright position and improved by recumbency) has been described in two patients.[762] Most patients show normal or even increased expiratory flow rates when related to absolute lung volume; however, a minority manifest a reduction in MMFR and FEV_1,[751] presumably reflecting a long history of cigarette smoking or perhaps representing a subgroup of patients with bronchiolitis obliterans.

NATURAL HISTORY AND PROGNOSIS

In the great majority of patients with fibrosing alveolitis, deterioration is gradual and inexorable with increasing shortness of breath and, in many individuals, the development of cor pulmonale. Approximately 20 per cent of patients die from a cardiac disorder[763] but most succumb to respiratory failure that is often precipitated by infection.[763, 765]

Overall mean survival is probably less than 5 years,[597, 718, 765] although individuals have been reported to live as long as 15 years after diagnosis.[766, 767] Occasional patients have an acute fulminant disease ending in early death from respiratory failure, a course similar to that described by Hamman and Rich;[651, 652, 768] this subgroup of patients has been estimated to comprise approximately 5 per cent of all cases of fibrosing alveolitis.[652]

The incidence of lung cancer is increased in patients with fibrosing alveolitis, an association between parenchymal scarring (regardless of etiology) and pulmonary neoplasia that has been discussed previously (see page 1338). It has been suggested that the neoplastic proliferation may be related to epithelial metaplasia and hyperplasia of either bronchiolar or alveolar epithelium, both processes that commonly exist in fibrosing alveolitis. Haddad and Massaro[769] studied the pathologic appearance in eight unselected cases of diffuse interstitial fibrosis and found that all of the patients had atypical epithelial proliferation in dilated terminal respiratory units; large cuboidal and columnar cells showed atypical nuclear and cytoplasmic changes. Pulmonary carcinoma developed in three of these eight cases. Meyer and Liebow[770] and Scadding[771] have also remarked on this atypical proliferation of epithelial cells. Adenocarcinoma is the most frequent histologic type, although squamous cell and anaplastic carcinoma also have been reported.[702, 772] Clubbing appears to be an almost invariable clinical finding in patients with a complicating carcinoma.[597, 773–775]

Many attempts have been made to define criteria that relate to prognosis and response to treatment of fibrosing alveolitis. There appears to be general agreement that patients fare better who have a shorter duration of symptoms before presentation[775–778] or are younger (except for infants under 1 year of age).[572] Pregnancy has been linked to rapid deterioration.[779] Patients whose lung biopsy specimens show a histologic pattern of desquamative interstitial pneumonitis usually,[572, 573, 657, 718, 721] but not always,[568, 764, 780, 781] pursue a relatively benign course. Turner-Warwick and her colleagues[597] found a number of other factors relating to longer survival: dyspnea of only mild to moderate severity, lesser grades of roentgenographic abnormality, absence of right axis deviation on the electrocardiogram, and higher levels of PaO_2. Watters and coworkers[782] have devised a clinical-roentgenographic-physiologic scoring system that they believe can be useful not only for estimating the severity of underlying pathologic derangement but also for assessing clinical impairment in a longitudinal quantitative manner. This scoring system includes an index of dyspnea, an assessment of the severity of roentgenographic abnormality, and a number of parameters of pulmonary function that could prove useful as an objective means of determining response to therapy.

There is some indication that prognosis can be improved by corticosteroid or immunosuppressive therapy or both;[673, 687, 718, 775–777, 783] however, although 50 per cent of patients are said to improve symptomatically with corticosteroid therapy,[739, 765] only half of these show roentgenographic[739] or functional[765, 775] improvement. As might be expected, pulmonary function tests performed before and after corticosteroid therapy can reveal a beneficial effect during the early stages of the disease,[721, 784, 785] but typically show a negligible response when the roentgenographic stage of honeycombing has been reached.[721, 784, 785] In view of the toxicity associated with both corticosteroid and immunosuppressive therapy, much effort has been directed toward determining the type of patient likely to respond. Estimates of the degree of cellularity in biopsy specimens do not appear to be a reliable index,[615, 775, 776, 786] although the amount of fibrosis may be an indicator of the likelihood of a lack of response.[718, 776] Using an immunohistochemical method of identifying collagen types, a group of investigators at the Brompton Hospital[786, 787] has related a good response to therapy with the presence of type 3 collagen in lung biopsy specimens. The presence of immune complexes in serum and in biopsy specimens of pulmonary parenchyma appears to correlate with less severe disease but is not associated with an increased length of survival or responsiveness to corticosteroids.[615, 616]

Determination of the type and number of cells and of the quantity of various biochemical compounds in fluid obtained by bronchoalveolar lavage has been found to be useful in the differential diagnosis of interstitial pulmonary diseases,[788] and attempts have been made to compare these elements in patients who respond to corticosteroid and immunosuppressive therapy and those who do not. Recognizing that the airways, particularly those of smokers, can contain an abundance of neutrophils[670, 671, 789] and that a proper technique for alveolar sampling is important in the interpretation of results, several investigators[668, 778, 790–792] have established that an increased percentage of neutrophils or eosinophils (or both) and a lymphocyte count of less than 11 per cent are related to a poor clinical response to therapy, whereas a lymphocyte count above 11 per cent indicates a good therapeutic response and a better prognosis. The initial good response in patients with a high BAL lymphocyte count[670] may be the result of an increased glucocorticoid receptor content that has been shown to correlate with clinical response.[793] The level of cytosolic glucocorticoid receptors also has been found to correlate with septal cellularity in open lung biopsy specimens from patients with interstitial lung diseases.[794] Phospholipid content of lavage fluid has been shown to be less than half the amount recovered from healthy volunteers.[795] In addition, patients with fibrosing alveolitis have a lower proportion of phosphatidylglycerol and a higher proportion of phosphatidylinositol in recovered phospholipids than do healthy volunteers. The severity of these alterations in phospholipid composition correlates with the degree of pulmonary fibrosis.[796]

LYMPHANGIOLEIOMYOMATOSIS

Lymphangioleiomyomatosis (*synonyms:* lymphangiomyomatosis, myomatosis, angiomyomatous hyperplasia, lymphangiomatous malformation) was first reported in 1955 by Enterline and Roberts[797] in a patient with a previously undescribed type of tumor in the retroperitoneal area that they termed "lymphangiopericytoma." Recognizing that the tumor probably originated from smooth muscle and not from pericytes, these same investigators[798] 11 years later described six additional cases under the title of lymphangiomyoma; since then, it has been recognized that involvement of small arteries and veins (particularly in the pulmonary circulation) is also a part of the myomatous proliferation, and the terms "lymphangioleiomyomatosis" and "lymphangiomyomatosis" are now in common use.

The condition is uncommon; by 1981, less than 100 cases had been documented in the literature.[799] It is virtually confined to young and middle-aged women, the average age at presentation being 43 years.[799] In patients in whom the diagnosis is made at an age generally equated with or subsequent to the menopause, it is probable that the onset of slowly progressive disease preceded clinical recognition by some years. Sinclair and associates[800] reported four patients from the literature who were over the age of 55 years at diagnosis and one woman in whom the diagnosis was made at the age of 72 years. The latter patient had had symptoms since the age of 60 years and had had a hysterectomy at the age of 55; the authors reasoned that the prolonged course in this postmenopausal woman was a consequence of oophorectomy and that the disease had begun prior to her surgery.

ETIOLOGY AND PATHOGENESIS

The precise nature of the condition is not known, but it is assumed to represent a developmental, hamartomatous abnormality. The close similarity of both pathologic and clinical features to tuberous sclerosis, a condition well characterized as a disease of disordered development, supports this hypothesis; in fact, there is persuasive evidence that pulmonary lymphangioleiomyomatosis represents simply a *form fruste* of tuberous sclerosis.[801–803] Such evidence includes the observation that roentgenologic, pathologic,[801] and functional[804, 805] abnormalities of the lungs identical to those seen in lymphangioleiomyomatosis occasionally have been documented in patients with typical features of tuberous sclerosis. In these individuals, there is a striking female preponderance,[806] and the age of onset is similar to that of lymphangioleiomyomatosis.[807] In addition, occasional patients with lymphangioleiomyomatosis show isolated abnormalities usually associated with tuberous sclerosis, such as renal angiomyolipoma.[801, 808] On the basis of these considerations, it seems reasonable to divide patients with lymphangioleiomyomatosis into three groups:[809]

1. Pulmonary parenchymal lymphangiomyoma associated with involvement of mediastinal or retroperitoneal lymph nodes (or both), usually accompanied by effusions (pleural, peritoneal, or both).

2. Localized mediastinal or retroperitoneal lymph node lymphangioma (with or without pleural or peritoneal effusions), without associated pulmonary parenchymal disease.

3. Pulmonary parenchymal and lymph node lymphangiomyomatosis associated with stigmata of tuberous sclerosis.

Since the disease is seen almost always in women during the reproductive years,[808] it is logical to suggest that there may be some association with hormone secretion or tissue response to hormones. There is both clinical and pathologic evidence to support this hypothesis: (1) exacerbations of the disease have been documented during pregnancy[810, 811] and following the administration of exogenous estrogens;[812] (2) individual case reports have shown that the disease tends not to progress following bilateral oophorectomy, with or without the administration of progesterone and tamoxifen (an antiestrogen);[810–818] and (3) receptors for estrogen and progesterone have been identified in biopsied tissue from affected patients by both cytosolic[811, 816, 819, 820] and immunohistochemical[821] techniques.

Despite this fairly persuasive evidence of an influence of estrogens in the pathogenesis of lymphangioleiomyomatosis, it is likely that other factors are involved as well; for example, in at least one patient, tamoxifen administration was associated with exacerbation of the disease.[812] In addition, therapeutic success does not always follow the elimination of estrogens, although this may be attributable in some cases to the advanced stage of the disease when this treatment is instituted.[822, 823] Perhaps related to the same effect is the observation that the few objective assessments of pulmonary function that have been made have shown little or no change following oophorectomy and antiestrogenic therapy,[811, 816, 818] regardless of subjective evidence of symptomatic improvement and a suggestion that life is prolonged.

PATHOLOGIC CHARACTERISTICS

Grossly, the lungs in advanced lymphangioleiomyomatosis show diffuse effacement of the normal architecture by cystic spaces of variable size (usually 0.2 to 2.0 cm in diameter) separated by thickened interstitial tissue (Fig. 17–46). Microscopically,[824, 825] the most striking abnormality is the presence of numerous interlacing fascicles of smooth muscle (Fig. 17–47) that form the walls of the cystic spaces observed grossly; smooth muscle also can be identified within recognizable parenchymal interstitium and in the walls of airways and pulmonary veins. It has been hypothesized that occlusion of the latter structures is related both to the formation of the parenchymal cysts and to the development of pulmonary hemorrhage (manifested pathologically by hemosiderin-laden macrophages and clinically by hemoptysis).[808]

Intrapulmonary and extrapulmonary lymphatics are often dilated and show bundles of smooth muscle in their walls. Smooth muscle proliferation is often also present in the thoracic duct, which may be totally obliterated, and in lymph nodes in the mediastinum and retroperitoneum. Involvement of all these structures causes some degree of disturbance in lymph flow and may result in the development of chylothorax, chyloperitoneum,[808, 826–829] and occasionally chylopericardium.[830]

The hyperplastic smooth muscle cells generally are elongated in shape and resemble normal adult cells; occasionally, however, they are round or polygonal and have large, somewhat pleomorphic nuclei that may contain mitotic figures.[824, 831] These latter cells have been interpreted as myoblasts and as representing evidence of ongoing proliferative activity. Support for a leiomyomatous origin was provided by one immunofluorescent study in which smooth muscle antigens were identified in the proliferating cells.[832] However, in an electron microscopic study,[833] the derivation of the proliferating cells from smooth muscle was questioned, and it was suggested that the cell of origin might be the pulmonary interstitial cell or even the pericyte as had been proposed in the initial description of the disease.[797]

ROENTGENOGRAPHIC MANIFESTATIONS

The roentgenographic pattern in the lungs in lymphangioleiomyomatosis is indistinguishable

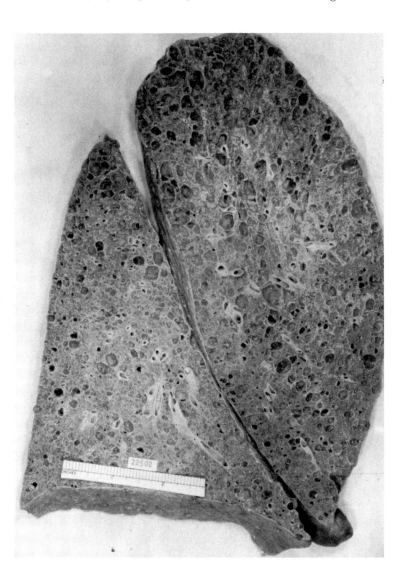

Figure 17–46. Lymphangioleiomyomatosis. A sagittal slice through the mid portion of the left lung shows numerous cystic spaces of variable size throughout both lobes.

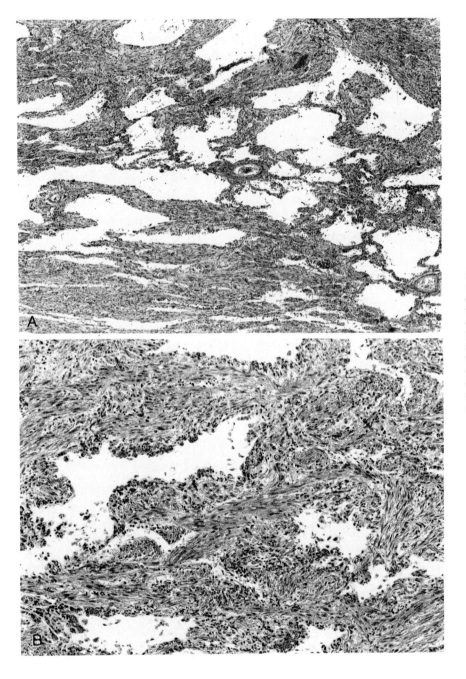

Figure 17–47. Lymphangioleio-myomatosis. A histologic section *(A)* reveals moderate to marked thickening of the parenchymal interstitium; only a few normal alveolar septa remain. Cystic changes similar to those seen in the honeycombing of fibrosing alveolitis are apparent. A section at higher magnification *(B)* shows the thickening to be caused by a proliferation of uniform spindle cells with abundant cytoplasm consistent with smooth muscle. *(A, ×30, B, ×100.)*

from that of cryptogenic fibrosing alveolitis with the exception of the effects on lung volume. Characteristically, in diffuse interstitial fibrosis there is progressive loss of lung volume, whereas in lymphangioleiomyomatosis volume tends to be increased (Fig. 17–48).[808] The basic pattern is coarse reticulonodular in type and tends to be generalized, although in two patients we studied it was more prominent in the lung bases. The late roentgenographic pattern is one of honeycombing. Although these findings on conventional roentgenograms are relatively nonspecific, two recent studies[834, 835] have shown that high-resolution CT scans can reveal abnormalities that are characteristic (Fig. 17–49): in

one study of four patients[834] and another of eight,[835] findings consisted of well-defined cystic spaces ranging in diameter from a few millimeters to 5 cm and distributed diffusely throughout both lungs; the walls of the cystic spaces were uniformly thin. The appearance was considered to be quite different from the pattern produced by fibrosing alveolitis or neurofibromatosis. Sherrier and colleagues[835] also found evidence, in four of their eight patients, of mediastinal lymph node enlargement, sometimes not apparent on conventional chest roentgenograms.

Pleural effusions may be unilateral or bilateral and typically are large and recurrent; all are chylous

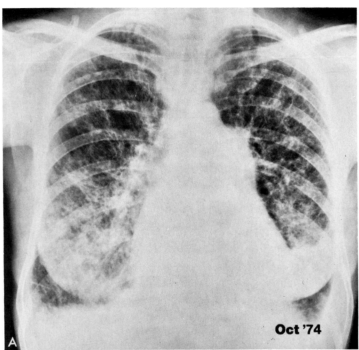

Figure 17–48. Lymphangioleiomyomatosis. The initial posteroanterior roentgenogram *(A)* of this 35-year-old white woman reveals widespread pulmonary disease showing no anatomic predominance and characterized chiefly by a very coarse, irregular reticular pattern (seen to better advantage in a detail view of the right lower zone from a primary magnification roentgenogram *[B]*). In some areas there is a suggestion of honeycombing. The central pulmonary arteries are enlarged, indicating pulmonary hypertension, and the size and configuration of the heart are consistent with the presence of cor pulmonale. Bilateral pleural effusions are present. In such a setting, these effusions could be caused by cardiac decompensation or by chylothorax secondary to leiomyomatosis (or both).

Illustration continued on following page

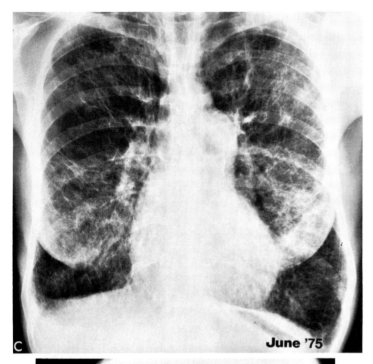

June '75

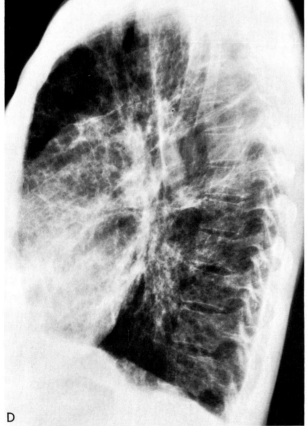

Figure 17-48 *Continued* Several months later (*C* and *D*), the pattern of disease has changed considerably in that much of the coarse reticulation has disappeared, leaving a multitude of small and large thin-walled cystic spaces or bullae. There is still evidence of pulmonary arterial hypertension and cor pulmonale, but the pleural effusions have diminished.

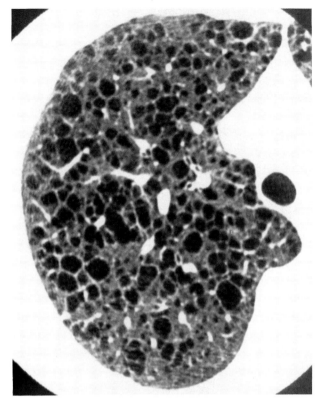

Figure 17–49. Lymphangioleiomyomatosis: CT Manifestations. A high-resolution CT scan through the right upper lobe with 1.5-mm collimation reveals a multitude of cystic spaces ranging in diameter from 5 to 20 mm. For the most part the cyst walls are very thin. Lung parenchyma between cysts is normal. (Courtesy of Dr. Nestor L. Müller, University of British Columbia, Vancouver.)

on direct examination (Fig. 17–50). Effusions may be present in the absence of lung involvement. Spontaneous pneumothorax is common. Lymphangiography can be useful in the detection of retroperitoneal disease, although it is important to use small quantities of contrast medium if the patient has advanced pulmonary disease.

CLINICAL MANIFESTATIONS

As indicated previously, all of the pulmonary lymphangioleiomyomatosis cases that have been reported have occurred in women, almost all of whom have been in childbearing age. The presenting complaint is usually shortness of breath, sometimes in association with pneumothorax or a history of repeated hemoptysis. Of the six patients reported by Carrington and his coworkers,[825] four had a total of 25 episodes of pneumothorax, three had hemoptysis, one retroperitoneal hemorrhage, and one chylothorax. The last-named is a common manifestation;[808, 836, 837] it was observed in 11 of the 28 cases studied by Corrin and associates[808] and can be unilateral or bilateral. Chyloperitoneum is less common and chylopericardium rare.[813, 814, 830, 837] Occa-

sionally, chyle is coughed up (chyloptysis) or passed in the urine (chyluria).

Lymphangiomatosis, another rare condition that usually proves fatal in childhood, is characterized by severe dilatation of lymphatic channels throughout the lungs[838, 839] and can closely resemble lymphangioleiomyomatosis clinically. Chylous effusions are caused by obstruction of lymphatic channels by a benign neoplastic proliferation of endothelial cells without smooth muscle involvement.

Pulmonary Function Tests

The pulmonary function pattern in lymphangioleiomyomatosis is one of obstruction; VC is reduced, and functional residual capacity (FRC) and residual volume (RV) are increased. Detection of the increase in total lung capacity (TLC) may require measurement of lung volumes plethysmographically.[825] FEV_1 and FEF_{25-75} are considerably decreased, and FEV_1/FVC is usually well below the predicted normal.[816, 825] DL_{CO} is reduced, and hypoxemia is common and may be severe; however, PCO_2 is almost invariably decreased.[808, 816] In the two patients we have studied personally,[826] we found pulmonary overinflation, increased rather than decreased pulmonary compliance, slightly increased resistance, and considerable loss of elastic recoil.

TUBEROUS SCLEROSIS

Tuberous sclerosis (Bourneville's disease) is an autosomal dominant familial disorder of mesodermal development that affects males and females equally; approximately 25 per cent of patients give positive family histories,[831] the remainder being sporadic in nature. The disease is characterized classically by the triad of mental retardation, epilepsy, and adenoma sebaceum, but it also includes a variety of other abnormalities, such as intracranial calcifications, retinal phacoma, angiomyolipomas of the kidneys, rhabdomyomas of the heart, sclerotic lesions of bones, and subungual fibromas. These various manifestations usually appear in infancy or early childhood, and 75 per cent of patients so affected die before their 20th year.[804]

Pulmonary involvement is very uncommon,[840, 841] occurring in only 0.1 to 1 per cent of patients;[805, 807] of 160 patients with tuberous sclerosis seen at the Mayo Clinic, only 2 had pulmonary disease.[805] In a review of the literature, Jao and associates[806] accepted 28 well-documented cases of tuberous sclerosis with diffuse lung disease, 27 being in women ranging in age from 21 to 50 years. Respiratory symptoms are usually first noted between the ages of 18 and 34 years.[807]

As discussed above, the pathologic characteristics of tuberous sclerosis and lymphangioleiomyomatosis have been generally regarded as being similar, if not identical.[805, 831, 842, 843] However, some

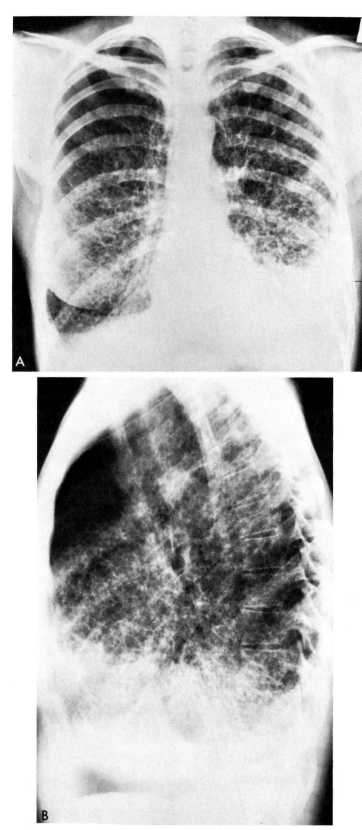

Figure 17–50. Pulmonary Lymphangioleiomyomatosis. This 24-year-old white woman presented with a 2-year history of increasing cough and dyspnea, the latter having become very severe just prior to admission. Roentgenograms in posteroanterior *(A)* and lateral *(B)* projection reveal a coarse reticulation throughout both lungs, with considerable basal and midzone predominance. In the lower lung zones particularly, there are multiple thick-walled cystic spaces ranging from 5 to 10 mm in diameter (seen to good advantage on a magnified view of the lower portion of the left lung *[C]*). This is the basic pattern of "honeycomb lung." There are bilateral pleural effusions, larger on the left. The heart is not enlarged. (Courtesy of Dr. Melvin Figley, University of Washington Hospital, Seattle.)

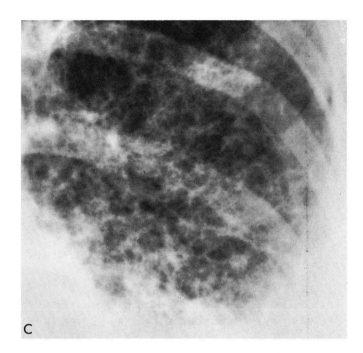

Figure 17–50 *Continued*

C

authors have found differences in the composition and distribution of the lesions:[808, 829] for example, lymphangioleiomyomatosis has been said to be characterized by intranodal and extranodal involvement of the lymphatics of the central part of the body, whereas tuberous sclerosis has been regarded as a more generalized mesodermal disorder with a special tendency to involvement of the smooth muscle of blood vessels.

Despite these possible differences, the roentgenographic manifestations of thoracic involvement in tuberous sclerosis are very similar to those of lymphangioleiomyomatosis except for the pleura (Fig. 17–51): although pneumothorax occurs,[844, 845] chylous effusions rarely have been observed in tuberous sclerosis,[806, 808, 836, 846] a scarcity that may simply reflect the paucity of patients who develop pulmonary disease. The identification of numerous sclerotic lesions (or sometimes cystic rarefactions[840]) throughout the bony skeleton, together with the other typical changes, should establish the diagnosis beyond reasonable doubt. Further confirmation may be had by the roentgenologic demonstration of renal enlargement secondary to angiomyolipomas or of intracranial calcifications. The latter were found in 35 of 68 cases (51 per cent) in one series.[840]

Clinical manifestations of pulmonary involvement in tuberous sclerosis are similar to those of isolated lymphangioleiomyomatosis. Pulmonary function tests have been described as showing severe obstruction, hyperinflation, increased airway resistance, normal static compliance, very low diffusing capacity, hypoxemia, and hypocarbia, findings that are also identical to those in lymphangioleiomyomatosis.[804, 805]

NEUROFIBROMATOSIS

Neurofibromatosis (von Recklinghausen's disease) is a relatively common familial disorder with a frequency of about 1 in 3,000; there is no sex predominance. Although it is inexorably progressive, it shows markedly variable expressivity;[847] only about 20 per cent of affected patients develop disabling disease. The most prominent manifestations are cutaneous *café au lait* spots and neurofibromas of the cutaneous and subcutaneous peripheral nerves and nerve roots; neurofibromas of viscera and blood vessels innervated by the autonomic nervous system are also seen.[847]

The condition is associated with a variety of neoplasms, including central nervous system gliomas, meningiomas, peripheral nerve sarcomas and schwannomas, pheochromocytomas, and angiosarcomas.[847–851] Thoracic neoplasms, predominantly neurogenic in type, are not uncommon. They can arise in the intercostal nerves (in which case they may be associated with rib destruction and a chest wall mass), in the mediastinum (often with characteristic CT manifestations[852]), and in the lungs themselves.[853] One unusual manifestation of these tumors is hemothorax caused by bleeding from eroded intercostal vessels.[854]

The thorax can be affected in several ways; undoubtedly the most common is the presence of cutaneous and subcutaneous neurofibromas. Roentgenographically, these can be seen in profile as nodules on the chest wall or projected over the lungs (Fig. 17–52) and are of obvious assistance in roentgenologic diagnosis. Other chest wall abnor-

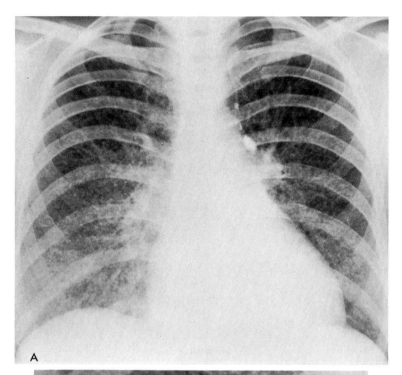

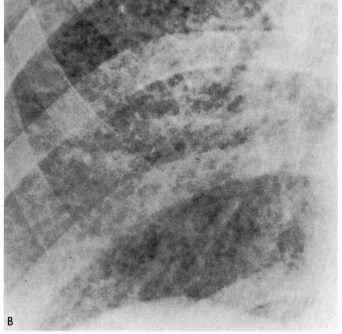

Figure 17–51. Tuberous Sclerosis. A postero-anterior roentgenogram *(A)* and a magnified view of the lower portion of the right lung *(B)* demonstrate extensive involvement of both lungs by a fine to medium reticular pattern showing no particular predominance in any lung zone. No additional findings are present. The roentgenographic appearance is not in any way diagnostic. This 37-year-old epileptic woman showed many of the stigmata of tuberous sclerosis, including intracranial calcifications, adenoma sebaceum, and multiple space-occupying lesions in the kidneys. Lung biopsy was not performed. (Courtesy of the Toronto East General and Orthopedic Hospital.)

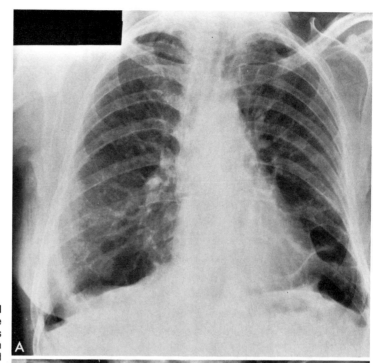

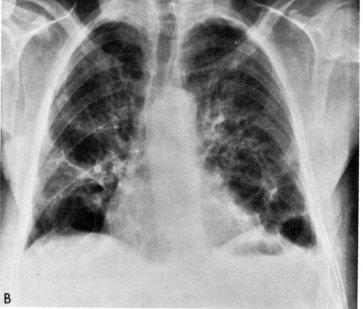

Figure 17–52. Neurofibromatosis: Pulmonary and Cutaneous Manifestations. Posteroanterior views of the chest in inspiration *(A)* and expiration *(B)* reveal numerous bullae in the lower portion of both lungs, most evident on the expiratory film because of air trapping. A background of diffuse reticulation is present, suggesting interstitial pulmonary fibrosis. Along the lateral chest wall in *(A)* and on the anterior and posterior chest walls in lateral projection *(C)* are numerous nodular opacities representing cutaneous neurofibromas.

Illustration continued on following page

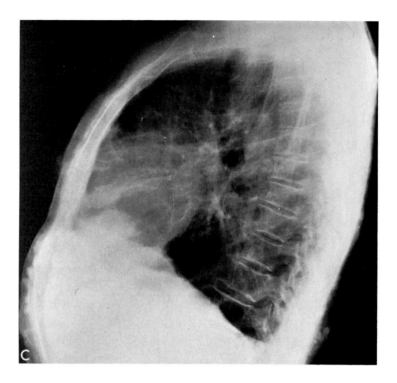

Figure 17–52 *Continued*

malities include kyphoscoliosis[847] and ribbon deformity of the ribs.

The pulmonary manifestations of neurofibromatosis consist of diffuse interstitial fibrosis and bullae, either alone or in combination (Fig. 17–52). The interstitial fibrosis characteristically involves both lungs symmetrically with some basal predominance, whereas the bullae usually are asymmetric and tend to develop in the upper lobes,[642] seldom the lower.[848] In some cases, for instance in more than one third of the 20 patients studied by Massaro and Katz,[642] bullae were unassociated with roentgenographic evidence of interstitial fibrosis, although it should be noted that fibrosis has been seen in all patients with bullae whose lungs have been examined histologically.[855, 856] Estimates of the incidence of interstitial fibrosis have ranged from less than 7[848] to 10 per cent.[642, 855]

Pathologically, the interstitial fibrosis is similar to that of many other etiologies, with variably severe parenchymal thickening usually most prominent in the immediate subpleural region. Histologically, the lungs show a spectrum of changes ranging from slight alveolar wall thickening due to a mononuclear inflammatory cell infiltrate to marked interstitial fibrosis. Increased numbers of intra-alveolar macrophages are not infrequently present and can be sufficiently numerous to suggest a diagnosis of desquamative interstitial pneumonitis.[857] Immunofluorescence studies in one case failed to show specific immunofluorescence to IgG, IgM, IgA, complement, or fibrinogen.[643] As in interstitial fibrosis associated with other conditions, the disease occa-

sionally can be complicated by the development of carcinoma.[855, 857]

Clinically, the diagnosis is readily made by the presence on the skin of multiple sessile or pedunculated neurofibromas. Despite the fact that this condition is a developmental abnormality, pulmonary disease typically does not become evident until the patient reaches adulthood. Respiratory symptoms are usually mild, the most common complaint being dyspnea on exertion.[855] The association of pulmonary hypertension and interstitial fibrosis has been reported.[858] Pulmonary function tests usually reveal evidence of obstruction, although a restrictive pattern may be dominant; diffusing capacity is often decreased.[855]

HISTIOCYTOSIS X

The grouping together by Lichenstein[859] of Letterer-Siwe disease, Hand-Schüller-Christian disease, and eosinophilic granuloma under the heading of histiocytosis X, although generally accepted, has been criticized by a number of experts.[860, 861] Despite similar morphologic characteristics, each of these three varieties of histiocytic proliferation possesses distinctive clinical features, including age of onset, organ systems involved, clinical presentation, and course of the disease process. *Letterer-Siwe disease* occurs in infants and children and is characterized by widespread dissemination and a fulminating fatal course. The structures most commonly affected are the liver, spleen, lymph nodes, lungs, and bones.[861] The histiocytic infiltrates can show prominent hemophagocytosis and a relative paucity of eosinophils. *Hand-Schüller-Christian disease* consists of a triad of osteolytic skull lesions, exophthalmos, and diabetes insipidus, and it is considered by some[861] to be a variant of multifocal eosinophilic granuloma. It becomes manifest during childhood or adolescence and progresses much more slowly than Letterer-Siwe disease, most affected persons living into adult life; occasionally it presents in adulthood.[862] *Eosinophilic granuloma* is a disease of adults; it can be widely disseminated throughout the body but is more commonly localized to the lungs or bones or both. It occurs most frequently in the white race and only rarely has been described in blacks.[863, 864] Although it was originally thought to be more common in young adult males,[865–868] recent reports have described a significant number of cases in middle-aged women.[869, 870]

It is not always possible to fit patients who have histiocytosis X into one of the four categories, Letterer-Siwe disease, Hand-Schüller-Christian disease, and focal or multifocal eosinophilic granuloma. For example, 57 of the 117 histologically proved cases of histiocytosis X reported from the Mayo Clinic could not be classified precisely.[871] The variety with which we are primarily concerned is eosinophilic granuloma.

ETIOLOGY AND PATHOGENESIS

Although the etiology and pathogenesis of the reactive histiocytoses, including eosinophilic granuloma, remain unknown, evidence recently has been obtained to suggest that some cases may reflect a primary mononuclear phagocytic immunodeficiency and others a disorder of suppressor T-lymphocyte control of autocytotoxic cells.[872–874] At one end of the spectrum are those infants with unquestioned primary immunodeficiency with secondary histiocytic changes in the thymus (familial erythrophagocytic lymphohistiocytosis),[873] a syndrome usually possessing a familial background and associated with congenital abnormalities and mental retardation.[874] This condition can be differentiated from Letterer-Siwe disease on the basis of the immunodeficiency, the pathologic evidence of prominent hemophagocytosis and minimal eosinophilic infiltration, and the absence of skeletal involvement.[861, 875] At the other end of the spectrum are the majority of patients grouped under histiocytosis X in whom evidence for impaired immunity is not at all convincing. However, there are exceptions; for example, a subset of patients has been described in whom circulating lymphocytes were spontaneously cytotoxic to cultured human fibroblasts and possessed antibody to autologous erythrocytes;[872] the patients in this series also had T cells lacking H_2 surface receptors, a finding suggestive of a suppressor-cell deficiency. The disease in 10 of the 17 patients

reported by these authors completely remitted and their immunologic abnormalities reverted to normal after intramuscular treatment with thymus extract, a response equivalent to that obtained with chemotherapy in a control group.

Additional evidence for regarding pulmonary eosinophilic granuloma as a disturbance of immunologic activity lies in the finding of circulating immune complexes in five patients with active cellular histology and in only one with fibrosis,[876] and the report of elevated levels of IgG in BAL fluid of some patients.[877] In two series,[127, 768] a highly convincing association with tobacco smoking has been described, smokers being identified in over 90 per cent of patients with eosinophilic granuloma and in less than 50 per cent of matched controls.

PATHOLOGIC CHARACTERISTICS

Grossly, the lungs in the early or active stage of eosinophilic granuloma show multiple nodules measuring up to a few millimeters in diameter. With time, these relatively discrete nodular lesions become confluent, and irregularly shaped areas of fibrosis result. In long-standing disease, the gross appearance is similar to that of advanced interstitial fibrosis of other etiology, with normal parenchymal architecture being replaced by fibrous tissue and multiple cysts of variable size. The only distinguishing feature is that eosinophilic granuloma, unlike cryptogenic fibrosing alveolitis, tends to be more severe in the upper lobes.[869, 870, 878]

Microscopically, abnormalities in the early stages are located predominantly in the interstitial connective tissue around small bronchioles and adjacent arteries and consist mainly of a cellular infiltrate (Fig. 17–53).[867, 870, 879, 880] In more advanced disease, this infiltrate extends into the adjacent alveolar interstitium; the central portion of the lesion undergoes fibrosis, resulting in more or less discrete, stellate-shaped lesions with peripheral cellularity, an appearance that is characteristic of pulmonary eosinophilic granuloma (Fig. 17–54). As the disease progresses, individual stellate foci coalesce, the fibrous tissue becomes more and more prominent, and an ever increasing amount of lung is destroyed (Fig. 17–55). In the most advanced stage, the lung consists almost entirely of fibrous tissue and cystic spaces, with only scattered "histiocytosis X" (Hx) cells (*see* farther on) and few or no eosinophils. At this stage the diagnosis of eosinophilic granuloma may be difficult, particularly in biopsy specimens.[871, 881–883]

The cellular portion of the stellate lesions contains a variety of inflammatory cells, the proportion being variable from area to area. The predominant cells are so-called Hx cells that contain large, vesicular nuclei, often with prominent nucleoli, and abundant, pale eosinophilic cytoplasm that is occasionally vacuolated (Fig. 17–54). Admixed among

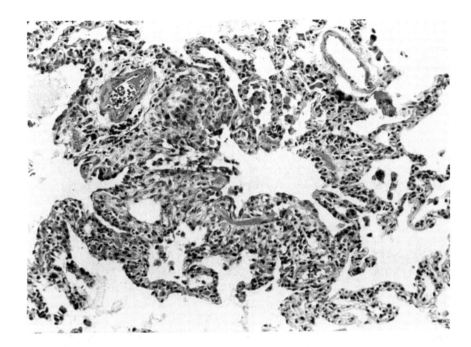

Figure 17–53. Eosinophilic Granuloma: Bronchiolar Involvement. A histologic section shows a respiratory bronchiole around which the interstitial tissue is moderately thickened by an infiltrate of histiocytes and occasional eosinophils; there is no fibrosis. (×170.)

these are fairly numerous eosinophils and lesser numbers of neutrophils, plasma cells, lymphocytes, and occasional multinucleated giant cells. Despite the designation of eosinophilic granuloma, true granuloma formation does not occur.

The diagnosis of eosinophilic granuloma is usually evident from the histologic appearance on open lung biopsy. With smaller biopsy specimens, however, the diagnosis may be difficult to make; for example, the condition has been confused with such abnormalities as desquamative interstitial pneumonitis, large cell ("histiocytic") lymphoma, and eosinophilic pneumonia.[884] In such cases, identification of Hx cells in foci of inflammation by immunohistochemical or ultrastructural means can be helpful. Several studies have reported these cells to show a positive reaction for protein S-100[885–887] in contrast to alveolar macrophages that are typically negative. Electron microscopic studies have shown the Hx cell to possess scattered surface microvilli and a moderate amount of cytoplasm that is usually rich in lysosomes and phagosomes (Fig. 17–56).[888, 889] In addition, the cytoplasm contains characteristic Birbeck or Langerhans' granules, consisting of two parallel unit membranes separated by a thin stripe of granular or striated material (Fig. 17–56); the bodies can appear to be free in the cytoplasm or attached to the plasma membrane and are sometimes expanded at one end in a form resembling a tennis racquet. Hx cells sometimes can be obtained by bronchoalveolar lavage,[878, 890, 891] a procedure that has been used for diagnosis. Although the presence of Hx cells by ultrastructural or immunohistochemical examination is suggestive of eosinophilic granuloma, these cells also can be identified in cases of pulmonary fibrosis of other etiology.[885, 887] Thus

their mere presence is not diagnostic of the condition.

ROENTGENOGRAPHIC MANIFESTATIONS

The roentgenographic pattern in the lungs varies with the stage of the disease. Involvement is characteristically diffuse and bilaterally symmetric, although unlike many other diffuse diseases of the lungs, eosinophilic granuloma tends to upper zone predominance.[863] Some observers have found maximal involvement in the mid-lung zones with sparing of the costophrenic angles.[868, 869, 892] The early and active stage of the disease is manifested by a nodular pattern with individual lesions ranging from 1 to 10 mm in diameter (Fig. 17–57); these are presumed to represent largely cellular foci with minimal fibrosis[893] and may regress or even completely resolve.[866, 879, 894, 895] In two cases, the early phase of the disease was manifested roentgenographically by fluffy alveolar consolidation in a butterfly distribution, strongly suggestive of pulmonary edema.[896] Another unusual manifestation of the active stage of the disease is the development of cavitating nodules;[897] we have seen only one example, confirmed by biopsy (Fig. 17–58).

In later stages, the pattern may become reticulonodular (Fig. 17–59). The end stage is characterized by a very coarse reticular pattern that, in the upper-lung zones particularly, often assumes a cystic appearance characteristic of the honeycomb pattern (Fig. 17–60). These cysts usually are about 1 cm in diameter but may measure up to 3 cm, especially in the periphery. We feel that this honeycomb pattern is highly suggestive of eosinophilic
Text continued on page 2691

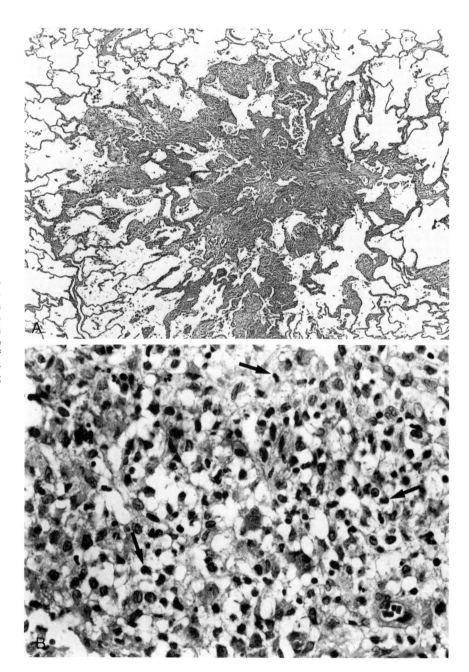

Figure 17–54. Eosinophilic Granuloma. A histologic section of lung parenchyma at low magnification *(A)* shows a vaguely stellate-shaped focus of interstitial cellular infiltration associated with mild fibrosis. A magnified view of the infiltrate *(B)* shows it to be composed of numerous histiocytes and scattered, bilobed eosinophils *(arrows).* *(A, ×32; B, ×400.)*

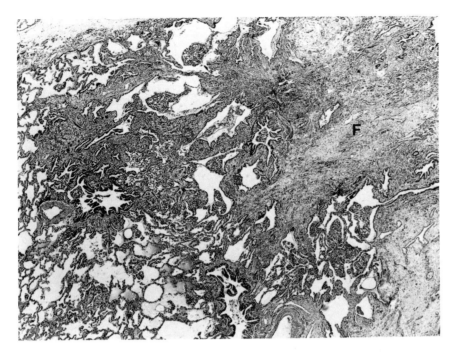

Figure 17–55. Eosinophilic Granuloma: Interstitial Fibrosis. A histologic section of lung parenchyma shows a focus of active disease on the left that blends on the right with an area of mature fibrous tissue *(F)* in which lung parenchyma is almost entirely destroyed. (×25.)

Figure 17–56. Eosinophilic Granuloma: Langerhans' Cell. An electron microscopic section *(A)* shows an intra-alveolar macrophage to resemble superficially a typical alveolar macrophage; however, several small tubular structures *(arrows)* are present in the peripheral cytoplasm. At much higher magnification *(B)*, the tubules can be seen to be composed of parallel membranous structures separated by finely granular material; one of these structures *(arrow)* shows a terminal expansion resulting in a "tennis racket" appearance. *(A,* ×7000, *B,* ×50, 650.)

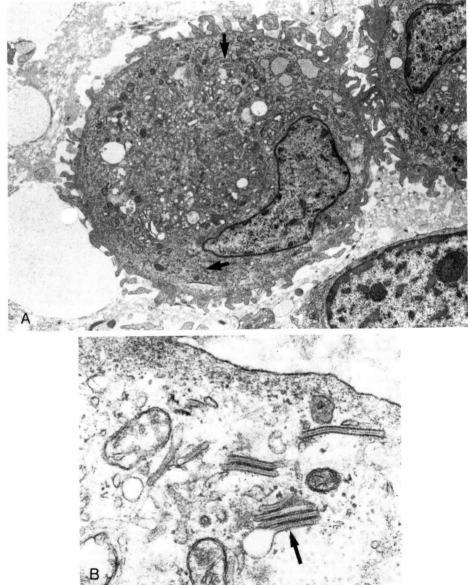

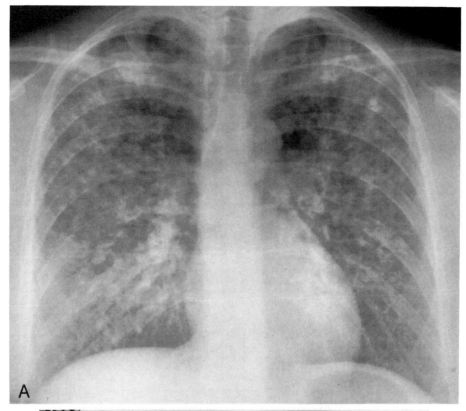

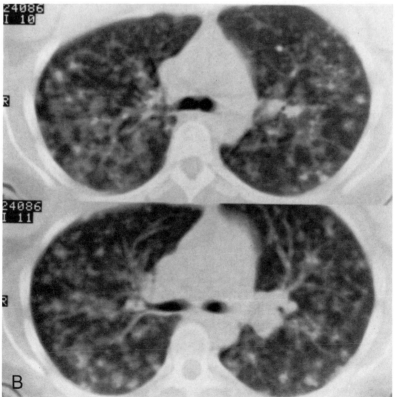

Figure 17–57. Eosinophilic Granuloma: Active Stage. A posteroanterior roentgenogram *(A)* reveals extensive bilateral pulmonary disease, the pattern of which suggests a combination of interstitial and airspace abnormality. There is some mid- and upper-zonal predominance. CT scans through the mid portion of both lungs at and just below the level of the tracheal carina *(B)* reveal a multitude of poorly defined nodular opacities ranging in diameter from about 5 to 10 mm. This 38-year-old man complained of increasing dyspnea on effort. The diagnosis was established by open lung biopsy.

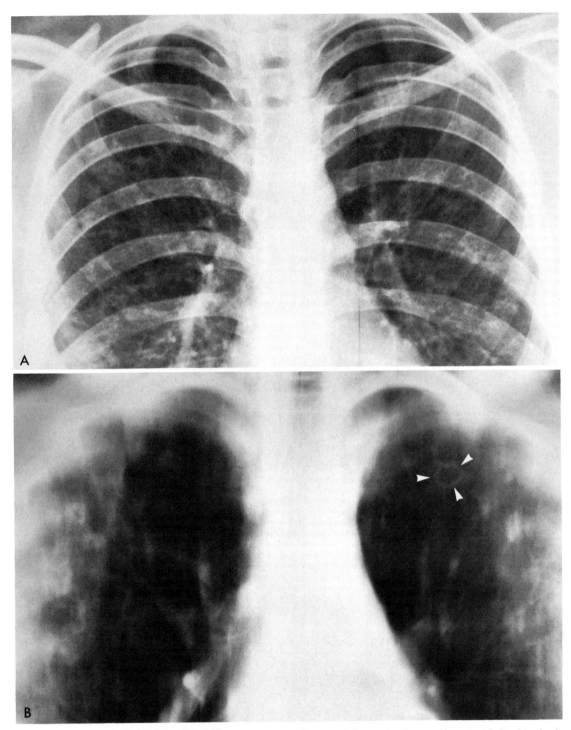

Figure 17–58. Eosinophilic Granuloma with Cavitation. This 17-year-old Caucasian housewife was admitted to the hospital for cholecystectomy. Her only complaint referable to her chest was a persistent, mild cough, attributable to fairly heavy cigarette smoking. A screening chest roentgenogram *(A)* reveals multiple, poorly defined opacities evenly distributed throughout both lungs. A tomogram in anteroposterior projection *(B)* reveals cavitation in several of the opacities (one is indicated by *arrows*). The diagnosis was established by open lung biopsy.

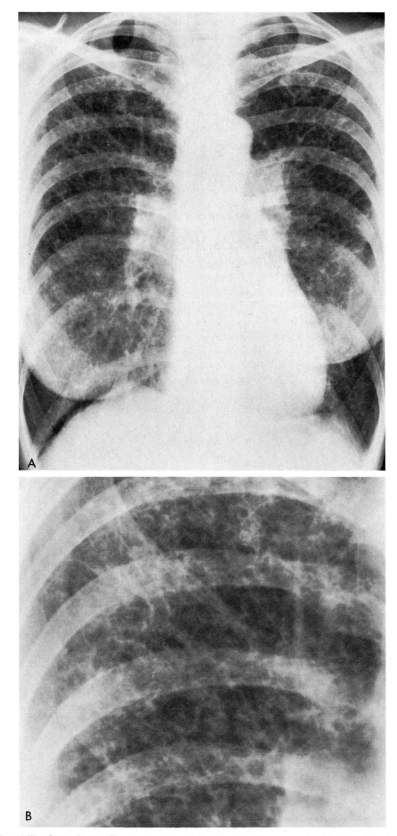

Figure 17–59. Eosinophilic Granuloma. For many years this 57-year-old woman had had a chronic cough productive of small amounts of whitish-green sputum. During the last 3 to 4 years she had experienced increasing shortness of breath on exertion, to a point that she could climb only one flight of stairs before stopping. A posteroanterior roentgenogram *(A)* and a magnified view of the upper portion of the right lung *(B)* reveal a rather coarse reticular pattern that is more prominent in the upper than in the lower lung zones. A honeycomb pattern is suggested in the upper zones. Lung volume appears slightly increased; there are no other findings of note.

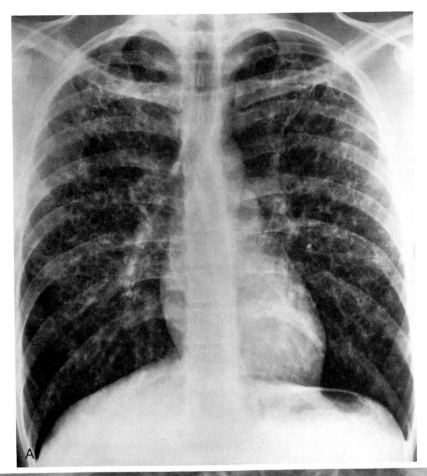

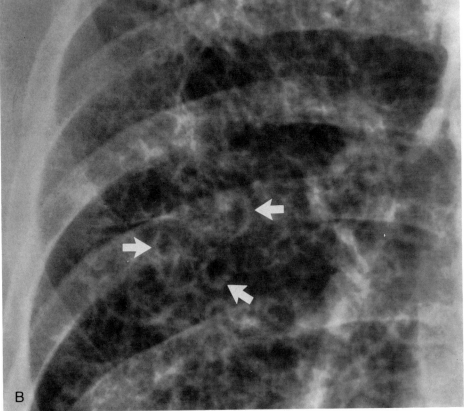

Figure 17–60. Eosinophilic Granuloma. A posteroanterior roentgenogram *(A)* and a detail view of the mid portion of the right lung *(B)* reveal a rather coarse reticulonodular pattern throughout both lungs with some upper-zonal predominance. In several areas, ring shadows are visible, measuring 7 to 10 mm in diameter and characterized by a central radiolucency surrounded by a wall of variable thickness. This honeycomb pattern is well demonstrated in the magnified view *(arrows)*.

granuloma, particularly when it is located mostly in the upper-lung zones. In fact, it is probable that the descriptive term "honeycomb lung" originally was coined to designate the severe disorganization of lung architecture seen in late eosinophilic granuloma.[898]

In three recent reports,[190, 191, 193] the CT manifestations of pulmonary eosinophilic granuloma were described in some detail, and the findings were remarkably similar. In their study of 17 patients, in 11 of whom the CT was high-resolution, Moore and colleagues[191] found that the predominant abnormality consisted of thin-walled cysts, usually less than 10 mm in diameter (n = 12). The cysts were the sole finding in half of these cases and were accompanied by multiple nodules (usually less than 5 mm in diameter) in the other half. Multiple nodules were the sole finding in 2 patients. In the 18 patients studied by high-resolution CT by Brauner and associates,[193] thin-walled cysts were again the predominant finding (Fig. 17–61), being identified in all but 1 patient. Other abnormalities in the group included nodules (n = 14), cavitated nodules (n = 3), thick-walled cysts (n = 7), reticulation (n = 4), and ground-glass opacities (n = 4). The authors of the latter study theorized that the evolution of the changes observed on CT consisted first of nodules, followed by cavitation with the formation of thick-walled cysts, then progression to thin-walled cysts, and finally to confluence of cysts.

In our experience, the progressive loss of lung volume that is so characteristic of diffuse fibrosing alveolitis is seldom seen in eosinophilic granuloma. Perhaps the tendency for the development of cysts and bullae counteracts the cicatricial effect of the diffuse fibrosis. The tendency for the lungs to maintain normal volume also has been observed by others: in one study of 50 adults with eosinophilic granuloma,[868] none was considered to have a decrease in lung volume, and some were actually regarded as being overinflated. In another review of 100 patients,[869] 60 were considered to have lung volumes within the normal range, 31 were thought to be overinflated, and only 9 were judged to have a lung volume below normal.

Hilar and mediastinal node enlargement and pleural effusion are rare in adults,[865, 868, 869, 880, 893, 899–903] although node enlargement is a recognized manifestation of the disease in children.[900, 904] Most authorities find spontaneous pneumothorax to be common:[865, 867, 868, 894, 895, 905–907] in two series comprising a total of 150 patients, 18 patients (13.5 per cent) developed this complication.[868, 869] It may be the first indicator of the disease[868] and occasionally occurs in the absence of roentgenographic abnormality in the lungs.[900] Although concomitant involvement of bones and lungs has been reported,[873, 899, 908–910] it is probably rare in adults.[868, 869]

CLINICAL MANIFESTATIONS

As might be expected of a disease in which varying manifestations become evident in many decades of life, the sex and age incidence of patients with histiocytosis differs from report to report. Selection varies from one that can be attributed to the patient population seen by a pediatrician[873] to one in which an internist sets a lower age limit on the patients included in his or her study.[869] In series limited to adults, both male[868, 878, 892] and female[869, 870] predominances have been noted.

When first seen, 20 to 25 per cent of patients are asymptomatic,[869] with the disease being discovered on a screening chest roentgenogram.[865] Somewhat less than one third of patients have nonspecific constitutional symptoms such as fatigue, weight loss, and fever.[865, 869] Respiratory symptoms are present in approximately two thirds of patients and usually consist of dry cough and dyspnea. Hemoptysis is uncommon,[865] occurring in only 6 of 100 patients in one study.[869] Chest pain can be caused by either pneumothorax or (rarely) an osteolytic rib lesion. Physical findings are of little help in diagnosis. Occasionally, rales may be heard over the lungs; there may be local tenderness over a bony lesion, and skin involvement may be apparent.[911] Finger clubbing is extremely rare.[865, 870] Hepatosplenomegaly and peripheral lymph node enlargement are seldom found in adults but are common in children.[871]

The association of diffuse lung disease with diabetes insipidus should strongly suggest the diagnosis of histiocytosis X, although this combination occasionally occurs in histoplasmosis and sarcoidosis also. Reports in the literature[865, 912] indicate that hypothalamic involvement is detected in 10 to 25 per cent of patients, an incidence much higher than we would have expected judging from our referred patient population as pulmonologists.

In contrast to the pediatric form of histiocytosis X (Letterer-Siwe disease) in which multiple organs are involved, disease in adults is generally confined to the lungs.[869, 870, 878] Although skeletal involvement is almost invariable in children,[873] it is very uncommon in adults (in only 5 of 100 patients in one series).[869]

Pulmonary function studies are said to show both restrictive and obstructive[869] patterns of insufficiency, the former being manifested by decreased vital capacity, normal residual volume, and normal flow rates.[869, 882, 913] Individual examples of severe obstructive insufficiency have been reported. In one follow-up study of 18 patients,[878] airflow limitation appeared to increase with progression of the disease. Patients tend to hyperventilate, and the combination of low diffusing capacity[878, 914] and increased physiologic dead space indicates the

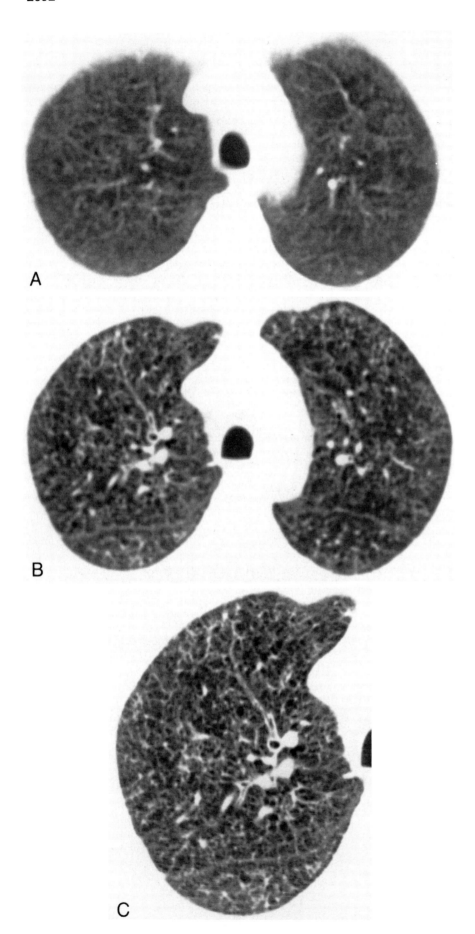

Figure 17–61. Eosinophilic Granuloma: CT Manifestations. A CT scan at the level of the aortic arch with 10-mm collimation *(A)* reveals a mixed reticular and nodular pattern, the latter predominating. A high resolution CT scan with 1.5-mm collimation *(B)* demonstrates the changes to better advantage and reveals fine parenchymal scarring associated with small cysts. Further optimization of the image by decreasing the field of view from 40 to 25 cm and using a high spatial frequency algorithm *(C)* more clearly defines the fine reticular scarring and cyst formation. The patient is a 49-year-old woman. The diagnosis was established by open lung biopsy.

presence of ventilation-perfusion inequality. Despite distinct roentgenographic abnormality, function may be within the normal predicted range in many patients, a state of affairs that seldom obtains in cryptogenic fibrosing alveolitis.[882, 913]

COURSE AND PROGNOSIS

The prognosis for infants with Letterer-Siwe disease is very bad, particularly those under 2 years of age in whom acute fulminating disease can cause death from pulmonary insufficiency.[870, 874, 895, 906, 915–917] As might be expected, the prognosis is also poor in older patients with disseminated disease and in those who show roentgenographic evidence of honeycombing, especially if associated with repeated episodes of pneumothorax; these patients tend to be more disabled and can succumb to respiratory insufficiency.[870] The outcome is considerably improved in older patients and in those with disease confined to the lungs.[874] Follow-up data in one series of adults with pulmonary eosinophilic granuloma revealed that 13 patients improved (4 returned to normal), 11 stabilized, and 13 worsened; 5 patients died.[868] In another series of 60 adult patients,[869] 16 patients were initially asymptomatic and remained so, 17 had complete remission and 11 partial remission of symptoms, 11 remained stable but symptomatic, 4 showed progression with increasing disability, and 1 patient died. An additional factor that worsens the prognosis of systemic histiocytosis X is the remote potential for the development of other systemic diseases such as monomyelocytic leukemia, histiocytic medullary reticulosis, or diffuse lymphoma.[874] There is some evidence that the prognosis is improved and progress of the disease arrested with thymosin,[872] penicillamine,[918] and chemotherapy.[919]

PULMONARY ALVEOLAR MICROLITHIASIS

This rare disease of unknown etiology and pathogenesis is characterized by the presence within the alveoli of the lungs of myriad tiny calculi ("calcispherytes"). Friedrich first described the disease in 1856.[920] The definitive work on the subject was published by Sosman and his colleagues in 1957[921] on the basis of 26 cases collected from many centers throughout the world. Two reports[922, 923] refer to approximately 160 cases published by 1983, and we are aware of another 13 in the literature since that date.

In Japan, the peak incidence occurs between the ages of 4 and 9 years,[924] but in western countries the majority of reported cases have been in patients between the ages of 30 and 50 years.[921] However, the age range is wide, the disease having been identified in premature stillborn twins[925] and in an 80-year-old woman.[926] There is no obvious sex predominance.[921]

ETIOLOGY AND PATHOGENESIS

As indicated, the etiology and pathogenesis of alveolar microlithiasis are unknown. Hypothetical mechanisms that have been invoked include an inborn error of metabolism, an unusual response to an unspecified pulmonary insult, an immune-mediated reaction to various irritants,[920] and an acquired abnormality of calcium or phosphorus metabolism.

A familial occurrence has been noted in more than half the reported cases;[921, 923, 925, 927–934] although this suggests an inborn error of metabolism, the disease has been restricted almost completely to siblings, its occurrence in a parent and child having been reported only twice.[931] Thus, environmental rather than genetic factors have been postulated to be important. Circumstantial evidence in support of this hypothesis was reported by Gómez and colleagues[927] who described a family of seven siblings in whom the disease developed in the four sisters who lived together but not in the three who had left home at an early age. Although no common history of inhalation exposure or occupation has been discovered, there has been one report of the disease in a patient who was strongly addicted to the inhalation of snuff containing over 9 per cent calcium.[935]

Theories based on an acquired metabolic disturbance have been proposed but are difficult to substantiate in view of the consistently normal serum calcium and phosphorus levels in reported series.[936, 937] Despite the lack of substantiation, several isolated case reports suggest that this occasionally may be a factor. For example, although the microliths are almost invariably confined to the lungs, one patient had multiple urinary calculi[938] and another, a 19-year-old youth, had calcific deposits in his prostate.[939] In addition, there is one report of a patient with milk-alkali syndrome in whom microliths appeared to form secondary to mineralization of desquamated epithelial cells.[940] Since calcium salts are more soluble in an acid medium and are more easily precipitated from alkaline solutions, it has been postulated that microlithiasis may result from some undefined alteration in the alveolar lining membrane or in alveolar secretions which promotes alkalinity at the alveolar interface and thus predisposes to the deposition or precipitation of calcium phosphate within the alveoli.[921, 937]

Alveolar microlithiasis is not confined to humans; a case report has appeared of the disease in an exotic animal, an adult male binturong,[941] and the condition is said to occur in orangutans.[920]

PATHOLOGIC CHARACTERISTICS

Microliths range from 0.01 to 3.0 mm in diameter[922] and are located almost invariably within alveolar airspaces. Despite this, there is evidence suggesting that they are formed in the alveolar walls, possibly in relation to type II cells,[925] and are extruded into the adjacent airspaces.[942, 943] Occasionally, microliths are present outside the alveolar lumen; for example, in one patient reported by Sears and associates,[926] pathologic examination revealed them in bronchial walls and fibrotic interstitium. Rarely, they can be found in extrapulmonary sites.[920]

Individual microliths are round, oval, or irregular in shape and have a concentric laminated appearance.[944-946] In a scanning electron microscopic study, Kawakami and colleagues[945] found them to be globular or irregular in shape and their outer surface to be granular or rough. Chemical analysis and energy-dispersive x-ray microanalysis have shown them to be composed of calcium phosphate.[920, 922] Two descriptions of patients with the disease[924, 926] suggest that there may be a noncalcified stage before the development of the typical dense calcification.

In the early stages of the disease, the alveolar walls appear perfectly normal;[921] later on, interstitial fibrosis results in alveolar wall thickening, sometimes associated with giant cell formation. It has been postulated that this may be due to irritation caused by the physical presence of the microliths.[920] Blebs and bullae often form, particularly in the lung apices;[921, 927, 938] how these relate to the presence of microliths is unclear.

ROENTGENOGRAPHIC MANIFESTATIONS

There is no other pulmonary disease with a roentgenographic pattern as characteristic and diagnostic as that of alveolar microlithiasis. Although there is considerable variation from patient to patient depending on the severity of affliction, the fundamental pattern is one of a very fine sand-like micronodulation diffusely involving both lungs (Fig. 17–62). Regardless of the effect of superimposition or summation of shadows, individual deposits are usually identifiable, particularly with magnification roentgenography. Very sharply defined, they measure less than 1 mm in diameter and are so discrete as to give the impression that one could "pick out" individual microliths with a pair of fine tweezers. The overall density is greater over the lower than upper zones, probably because of increased thickness of lung rather than selectively greater involvement. The opacities may be so numerous as to appear confluent, in which circumstance a normally exposed chest roentgenogram shows the lungs as almost uniformly white, often with total obliteration of the mediastinal and diaphragmatic contours;

however, employment of an overexposed roentgenographic technique with stationary or moving grid usually reveals the underlying pattern to better advantage. At least six cases have been described in which previous chest roentgenograms revealed no abnormality, but they appear to be the exceptions rather than the rule. In most reported cases, earlier normal chest roentgenograms were not discovered.[922, 924, 947–949]

Pleural thickening has been described both roentgenologically[927, 948] and pathologically,[950] but it is probable that this roentgenographic appearance is caused not by actual thickening of the pleural membrane but by a visual effect produced by an exceptionally heavy concentration of microliths in the subpleural parenchyma, thus creating a dense white line adjacent to the pleural surface.[921, 951] In fact, the contrast between the extreme density of the lung parenchyma on one side of the pleura and the ribs on the other may create the illusion of a "black" pleural line. Spontaneous pneumothorax may result from rupture of apical bullae or blebs;[933] in one 18-year-old girl with biopsy-confirmed disease, five episodes of pneumothorax were experienced.[934] Calcification in the pericardium was described in a 13-year-old child with this disease.[952]

In their classic paper, Sosman and his colleagues[921] suggested that in many patients the microliths continue to form and perhaps increase in size as the disease progresses rather than appear as a single massive deposit at one time. In their follow-up of three sisters with the disease, Oka and associates[921, 953] observed a definite increase in the micronodularity of the lungs in two sisters and no obvious change in the other. However, there is no doubt that the disease may become "arrested" and the deposition of microliths cease. We have had the opportunity of studying two brothers in whom the extensive changes apparent roentgenographically were stationary for 30 years.

Scintigraphy with Tc 99m diphosphonate has shown uptake of the tracer by microliths.[922, 954, 954] This indicates the presence of an active metabolic exchange across the alveolocapillary membrane.

CLINICAL MANIFESTATIONS

The majority of patients are asymptomatic when alveolar microlithiasis is first discovered, as was the case in 70 per cent of the 26 patients reported by Sosman and his colleagues.[921] The diagnosis is usually made on the basis of the typical pattern on a screening chest roentgenogram or in the investigation of persons whose siblings are known to have the disease. Symptoms may be absent even when the chest roentgenogram reveals the lungs to be almost solid and white, with little visible air-containing parenchyma. In no other condition is the lack of association between roentgenologic

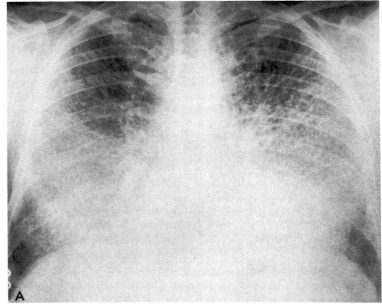

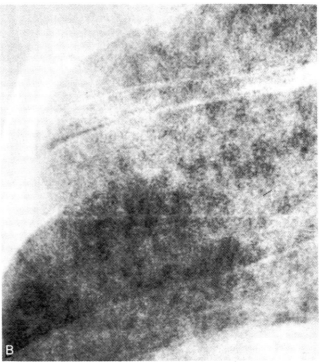

Figure 17–62. Alveolar Microlithiasis. A posteroanterior roentgenogram *(A)* of this 40-year-old asymptomatic man reveals a remarkably uniform opacification of both lungs. On close scrutiny *(B)*, this can be seen to be produced by a multitude of tiny, discrete opacities of calcific density *(B* is a detail view of the right lower zone from a two to one primary magnification image). Multiple function tests were normal except for a reduction in RV of 800 ml, representing the displacement of pulmonary volume by the calcispherytes.

and clinical findings so striking as in pulmonary alveolar microlithiasis.

Follow-up of three of Sosman and colleagues' patients (cases 4, 5, and 6)[921] who were asymptomatic in 1954 revealed the subsequent development of dyspnea, hemoptysis, finger clubbing, and cyanosis.[937] Our follow-up study of two brothers (cases 2 and 12)[921] showed one as remaining asymptomatic over a period of 28 years and the other as having remained well except for an increased susceptibility to chest infection.

The first symptom to develop in advanced cases is dyspnea on exertion; cough and expectoration are uncommon.[921, 927, 931] As the disease progresses, respiratory insufficiency may develop, with cyanosis, clubbing of the fingers, and clinical signs of right ventricular hypertrophy and failure. The physical signs usually are unrevealing, except in the late stages when breath sounds may be decreased, particularly at the bases.

The diagnosis usually can be made with confidence from the classic roentgenographic pattern and the striking roentgenologic-clinical dissociation; some patients cough up a microlith.[954] Microliths have been identified in BAL fluid[950, 956] and in transbronchial biopsy specimens.[923, 957] In fact, BAL has been tried as a therapeutic procedure, but unfortunately it has not been successful.[950, 956] Open lung biopsy to confirm the diagnosis is seldom, if ever, indicated.[930, 935]

Chemical analysis of blood is invariably within the normal range.[921] In the late stages right ventricular strain may become apparent electrocardiographically, and secondary polycythemia may develop.

Pulmonary function studies vary considerably from case to case, depending upon both the extent of replacement of alveolar air by concretions and the presence or absence of interstitial fibrosis. During the several years in which we have followed our two cases, the only significant finding has been a reduction in residual volume caused by the physical presence of calculi in the pulmonary airspaces.

Similar findings were noted in the five patients reported by Fuleihan and associates,[958] four of whom were asymptomatic; residual volume ranged from 0.35 to 1 liter. Although all five patients had an increased alveolar-arterial gradient for oxygen, the arterial oxygen saturation at rest was lowered in only one and the diffusing capacity was decreased in one. Other investigators[953] have observed a decrease in maximal breathing capacity, an increase in residual volume, and a decrease in diffusing capacity. O'Neill and colleagues[937] found decreased vital capacity, diffusing capacity, and arterial PO_2 in all three of their patients, with low dynamic compliance and high maximal inspiratory pressures in two. In all three patients, mixing was impaired as judged by the single-breath nitrogen test. In a series of eight patients studied at the Mayo Clinic,[922] most values for lung volumes were on the low side of predicted normal. In another patient,[959] mild to moderate pulmonary hypertension was detected with supine leg exercise.

DESERT LUNG

This term has been applied to a diffuse interstitial pulmonary disease that occurs in Bedöuin females in the Negev desert of Israel and that is believed to be caused by the presence of silica in the lungs, unassociated with a fibrotic reaction. A similar, if not identical, disease was originally reported in the inhabitants of the Saharan regions.[960] More recently, a new syndrome has been described by Hawass[961] that is characterized by an unusual association of cataracts and a roentgenographic pattern of diffuse micronodular opacities (the reproduced chest roentgenograms resemble alveolar microlithiasis). The author proposed that these cases of diffuse micronodular disease occurring in the various deserts might be similar in pathogenesis; in his own patients the etiology was unclear, although "tandoor" baking was suggested as a likely cause.

REFERENCES

1. James DG, Turiaf J, Hosoda Y, et al: Description of sarcoidosis: Report of the subcommittee on classification and definition. Ann NY Acad Sci 278:742, 1976.
2. Scadding JG: Sarcoidosis. London, Eyre and Spottiswoode, 1967.
3. Longcope WT, Freiman DG: A study of sarcoidosis. Based on a combined investigation of 160 cases including 30 autopsies from The Johns Hopkins Hospital and Massachusetts General Hospital. Medicine, 31:1, 1952.
4. Mayock RL, Bertrand P, Morrison CE, et al: Manifestations of sarcoidosis. Analysis of 145 patients, with a review of nine series selected from the literature. Am J Med 35:67, 1963.
5. Terris M, Chaves AD: An epidemiologic study of sarcoidosis. Am Rev Respir Dis 94:50, 1966.
6. Israel HL, Sones M: Sarcoidosis: Clinical observations on one hundred and sixty cases. AMA Arch Intern Med 102:766, 1958.
7. Rudberg-Roos I: The course and prognosis of sarcoidosis as observed in 296 cases. Acta Tuberc Scand 52(Suppl):1, 1962.
8. James DG: Erythema nodosum. Br Med J 1:853, 1961.
9. Scadding JG: Prognosis of intrathoracic sarcoidosis in England. A review of 136 cases after five years' observation. Br Med J 2:1165, 1961.
10. Akisada M, Tasaka A, Mikami R: Lymphography in sarcoidosis: Comparison with roentgen findings in the chest. Am J Roentgenol 93:1273, 1969.
11. Da Costa JL: Geographic epidemiology of sarcoidosis in Southeast Asia. Am Rev Respir Dis 108:1269, 1973.
12. Rømer FK: Clinical and biochemical aspects of sarcoidosis. With special reference to angiotensin-converting enzyme (ACE). Acta Med Scand (Suppl)3:690, 1984.
13. Hsing CT, Han FC, Liu HC, et al: Sarcoidosis among Chinese. Am Rev Respir Dis 89:917, 1964.
14. Panna LN, Man CA, Guan BO: Sarcoidosis among Chinese. Chest 80:74, 1981.
15. Lee SK, Narendran K, Chiang GS: Pulmonary sarcoidosis in Singapore. Ann Acad Med Singapore 14:446, 1985.
16. Present DH, Siltzbach LE: Sarcoidosis among the Chinese and a review of the worldwide epidemiology of sarcoidosis. Am Rev Respir Dis 95:285, 1967.
17. Purriel P, Navarrete E: Epidemiology of sarcoidosis in Uruguay and other countries of Latin America. Am Rev Respir Dis 84:155, 1961.
18. Zaki MH, Addrizzo JR, Patton JM, et al: Further exploratory studies in sarcoidosis. An epidemiologic investigation to compare the prevalence of tuberculous infection and/or disease among contacts of matched sarcoidosis and asthmatic patients. Am Rev Respir Dis 103:539, 1971.
19. Keller AZ: Anatomic sites, age attributes, and rates of sarcoidosis in U.S. veterans. Am Rev Respir Dis 107:615, 1973.
20. Honeybourne D: Ethnic differences in the clinical features of sarcoidosis in south-east London. Br J Dis Chest 74:63, 1980.
21. Cummings MM, Dunner E, Williams JH Jr: Epidemiologic and clinical observations in sarcoidosis. Ann Intern Med 50:879, 1959.
22. Seiler E: Über die epidemiologie der Sarcoidose (Morbus Boeck) in der Schweiz. Statistische untersuchungen über die geographische und berufliche Verteilung von 108 Militärpatienten mit Sarcoidose. (Epidemiology of sarcoidosis in Switzerland.) Schweiz Z Tuberk 17:205, 1960.
23. Michael M Jr, Cole RM, Beeson PB, et al: Sarcoidosis: Preliminary report on a study of 350 cases with special reference to epidemiology. Am Rev Tuberc 62:403, 1950.
24. Cummings MM, Dunner E, Schmidt RH Jr, et al: Concepts of epidemiology of sarcoidosis. Preliminary report of 1,194 cases reviewed with special reference to geographic ecology. Postgrad Med 19:437, 1956.
25. Brown IG, Hamblin TJ, Mikhail JR: Oldest case of sarcoidosis in the world. Br Med J 283:190, 1981.
26. Kendig EL Jr, Niitu Y: Sarcoidosis in Japanese and American children. Chest 77:514, 1980.
27. Kendig EL, Brummer DL: The prognosis of sarcoidosis in children. Chest 70:351, 1976.
28. Kendig EL Jr: Sarcoidosis. Am J Dis Child 136:11, 1982.
29. Merten DF, Kirks DR, Grossman H: Pulmonary sarcoidosis in childhood. Am J Roentgenol 135:673, 1980.
30. Hetherington S: Sarcoidosis in young children. Am J Dis Child 136:13, 1982.
31. Longcope WT, Freiman DG: A study of sarcoidosis. Based on a combined investigation of 160 cases including 30 autopsies from The Johns Hopkins Hospital and Massachusetts General Hospital. Medicine 31:1, 1952.
32. Mayock RL, Bertrand P, Morrison CE, et al: Manifestations of sarcoidosis. Analysis of 145 patients, with a review of nine series selected from the literature. Am J Med 35:67, 1963.
33. Wallaert B, Ramon P, Fournier EC, et al: Activated alveolar macrophage and lymphocyte alveolitis in extrathoracic sarcoidosis without radiological mediastinopulmonary involvement. Ann NY Acad Sci 465:201, 1986.
34. Wallaert B, Ramon P, Fournier EC, et al: Bronchoalveolar lavage, serum angiotensin-converting enzyme and gallium-67 scanning in extrathoracic sarcoidosis. Chest 82:553, 1982.
35. Scadding JG: Sarcoidosis. London, Eyre and Spottiswoode, 1967.
36. Mankiewicz E: The relationship of sarcoidosis to anonymous bacteria. [Proceedings of Third International Conference on Sarcoidosis. Acta Med Scand 425(Suppl):68, 1964.
37. Mitchell DN, Rees RJW, Goswami KKA: Transmissible agents from human sarcoid and Crohn's disease tissues. Lancet 2:761, 1976.
38. Mitchell DN, Rees RJW: The nature and physical characteristics of a transmissible agent from human sarcoid tissue. Ann NY Acad Sci 278:233, 1976.
39. Mitchell DN, Rees RJW: Further observations on the nature and physical characteristics of transmissible agents from human sarcoid and Crohn's disease tissues. In Williams WJ, Davies BH (eds): Eighth International Conference on Sarcoidosis and Other Granulomatous Disease. Cardiff, UK, Alpha Omega Publishing Ltd, 1978, p 121.
40. Wang N–S, Schraufnagel DE, Sampson MG: The tadpole-shaped structure in human non-necrotizing granulomas. Am Rev Respir Dis 123:560, 1981.
41. Agner E, Larsen JH: Yersinia enterocolitica infection and sarcoidosis. A report of seven cases. Scand J Respir Dis 60:230, 1979.
42. Williams WJ: Aetiology of sarcoidosis. Pathol Res Pract 175:1, 1982.
43. Keogh BA, Crystal RG: Alveolitis: The key to the interstitial lung disorders. Thorax 37:1, 1982.
44. James DG, Williams WJ: Immunology of sarcoidosis. Am J Med 72:5, 1982.
45. Hunninghake GW, Crystal RG: Pulmonary sarcoidosis: A disorder mediated by excess helper T-lymphocyte activity at sites of disease activity. N Engl J Med 305:429, 1981.
46. Rossi GA, Sacco O, Cosulich E, et al: Pulmonary sarcoidosis: Excess of helper T lymphocytes and T-cell subset imbalance at sites of disease activity. Thorax 39:143, 1984.
47. Ceuppens JL, Lacquet LM, Mariën G, et al: Alveolar T-cell subsets in pulmonary sarcoidosis. Correlation with disease activity and effect of steroid treatment. Am Rev Respir Dis 129:563, 1984.
48. Rossi GA, Sacco O, Cosulich E, et al: Helper T lymphocytes in pulmonary sarcoidosis. Functional analysis of a lung T-cell subpopulation in patients with active disease. Am Rev Respir Dis 133:1086, 1986.
49. Ginns LC, Goldenheim PD, Burton RC, et al: T-lymphocyte subsets in peripheral blood and lung lavage in idiopathic pulmonary fibrosis and sarcoidosis: Analysis by monoclonal antibodies and flow cytometry. Clin Immunol Immunopathol 25:11, 1982.
50. White DA, Rankin JA, Stover DE, et al: Methotrexate pneumonitis. Bronchoalveolar lavage findings suggest an immunologic disorder. Am Rev Respir Dis 139:18, 1989.
51. Akoun GM, Milleron BJ, Mayaud CM, et al: Provocation test coupled with bronchoalveolar lavage in diagnosis of propanolol-induced hypersensitivity pneumonitis. Am Rev Respir Dis 139:247, 1989.
52. Morgan JE, McCaul DS, Rodriguez FH, et al: Pulmonary immunologic features of alveolar septal amyloidosis associated with multiple myeloma. Chest 92:704, 1987.
53. Robinson BW, Rose AH, Thompson PJ, et al: Comparison of bronchoalveolar lavage helper/suppressor T-cell ratios in sarcoidosis versus other interstitial lung diseases. Aust NZ J Med 17:9, 1987.
54. Hunninghake GW: Release of interleukin-1 by alveolar macrophages of patients with active pulmonary sarcoidosis. Am Rev Respir Dis 129:569, 1984.
55. Lecossier D, Valeyre D, Loiseau A, et al: T-lymphocytes recovered by bronchoalveolar lavage from normal subjects and patients with sarcoidosis are refractory to proliferative signals. Am Rev Respir Dis 137:592, 1988.
56. Saltini C, Spurzem JR, Kirby MR, et al: Sarcoidosis is not associated with a generalized defect in T cell suppressor function. J Immunol 140:1854, 1988.

17

57. Spurzem JR, Saltini C, Crystal RG: Functional significance of anti-T-lymphocyte antibodies in sarcoidosis. Am Rev Respir Dis 137:600, 1988.

58. Hudspith BN, Flint KC, Geraint-James D, et al: Lack of immune deficiency in sarcoidosis: Compartmentalisation of the immune response. Thorax 42:250, 1987.

59. Gallagher RB, Guckian M, van Breda A, et al: Altered immunological reactivity in alveolar macrophages from patients with sarcoidosis. Eur Respir J 1:153, 1988.

60. Sandron D, Reynolds HY, Venet A, et al: Human alveolar macrophage subpopulations isolated on discontinuous albumin gradients: Functional data in normals and sarcoid patients. Eur J Respir Dis 69:226, 1986.

61. Venet A, Hance AJ, Saltini C, et al: Enhanced alveolar macrophage-mediated antigen-induced T-lymphocyte proliferation in sarcoidosis. J Clin Invest 75:293, 1985.

62. Campbell DA, Poulter LW, du Bois RM: Immunocompetent cells in bronchoalveolar lavage reflect the cell populations in transbronchial biopsies in pulmonary sarcoidosis. Am Rev Respir Dis 132:1300, 1985.

63. Hance AJ, Douches S, Winchester RJ, et al: Characterization of mononuclear phagocyte subpopulations in the human lung by using monoclonal antibodies: Changes in alveolar macrophage phenotype associated with pulmonary sarcoidosis. J Immunol 134:284, 1985.

64. Razma AG, Lynch JP III, Wilson BS, et al: Expression of Ia-like (DR) antigen on human alveolar macrophages isolated by bronchoalveolar lavage. Am Rev Respir Dis 129:419, 1984.

65. Lem VM, Lipscomb MF, Weissler JC, et al: Bronchoalveolar cells from sarcoid patients demonstrate enhanced antigen presentation. J Immunol 135:1766, 1985.

66. Toews GB, Lem VM, Weissler JC, et al: Antigen presentation by alveolar macrophages in patients with sarcoidosis. Ann NY Acad Sci 465:74, 1986.

67. Campbell DA, du Bois RM, Butcher RG, et al: The density of HLA-DR antigen expression on alveolar macrophages is increased in pulmonary sarcoidosis. Clin Exp Immunol 65:165, 1986.

68. Abe S, Yamaguchi E, Makimura S, et al: Association of HLA-DR with sarcoidosis. Correlation with clinical course. Chest 92:488, 1987.

69. Costabel U, Bross KJ, Andreesen R, et al: HLA-DR antigens on human macrophages from bronchoalveolar lavage fluid. Thorax 41:261, 1986.

70. Hunninghake GW, Kawanami O, Ferrans VJ, et al: Characterization of the inflammatory and immune effector cells in the lung parenchyma of patients with interstitial lung disease. Am Rev Respir Dis 123:407, 1981.

71. Wallace JM, Oishi JS, Barbers RG, et al: Bronchoalveolar lavage cell and lymphocytic phenotype profiles in healthy asbestos-exposed shipyard workers. Am Rev Respir Dis 139:33, 1989.

72. Roth C, Huchon GJ, Arnoux A, et al: Bronchoalveolar cells in advanced pulmonary sarcoidosis. Am Rev Respir Dis 124:9, 1981.

73. Mornex JF, Cordier G, Pages J, et al: Pulmonary sarcoidosis: Flow cytometry measurement of lung T cell activation. J Lab Clin Med 105:70, 1985.

74. Costabel U, Bross KJ, Ruhle KH, et al: Ia-like antigens on T-cells and their subpopulations in pulmonary sarcoidosis and in hypersensitivity pneumonitis. Analysis of bronchoalveolar and blood lymphocytes. Am Rev Respir Dis 131:337, 1985.

75. Costabel U, Bross KJ, Guzman J, et al: Predictive value of bronchoalveolar T cell subsets for the course of pulmonary sarcoidosis. Ann NY Acad Sci 465:418, 1986.

76. Flint KC, Leung KB, Hudspith BN, et al: Bronchoalveolar mast cells in sarcoidosis: Increased numbers and accentuation of mediator release. Thorax 41:94, 1986.

77. Chapman HA, Allen CL, Stone OL: Abnormalities in pathways of alveolar fibrin turnover among patients with interstitial lung disease. Am Rev Respir Dis 133:437, 1986.

78. Danel C, Dewar A, Corrin B, et al: Ultrastructural changes in bronchoalveolar lavage cells in sarcoidosis and comparison with the tissue granuloma. Am J Pathol 112:7, 1983.

79. Davis GS, Brody AR, Craighead JE: Analysis of airspace and interstitial mononuclear cell populations in human diffuse interstitial lung disease. Am Rev Respir Dis 118:7, 1978.

80. Gadek JE: Maintenance of the alveolitis of sarcoidosis. In Crystal RG, moderator: Pulmonary sarcoidosis: A disease characterized and perpetuated by activated lung T-lymphocytes. Ann Intern Med 94:73, 1981.

81. Thomas PD, Hunninghake GW: Current concepts of the pathogenesis of sarcoidosis. Am Rev Respir Dis 135:747, 1987.

82. Hunninghake GW, Fulmer JD, Young RC Jr, et al: Localization of the immune response in sarcoidosis. Am Rev Respir Dis 120:49, 1979.

83. Robinson BW, McLemome TE, Crystal RG: Gamma interferon is spontaneously released by alveolar macrophages and lung lymphocytes in patients with pulmonary sarcoidosis. J Clin Invest 75:1488, 1985.

84. Moseley PL, Hemken C, Monick M, et al: Interferon and growth factor activity for human lung fibroblasts. Release from bronchoalveolar cells from patients with active sarcoidosis. Chest 89:657, 1986.

85. Hunninghake GW, Bedell GN, Zavala DC, et al: Role of interleukin-2 release by lung T-cells in active pulmonary sarcoidosis. Am Rev Respir Dis 128:634, 1983.

86. Semenzato G, Agostini C, Trentin L, et al: Evidence of cells bearing interleukin-2 receptor at sites of disease activity in sarcoid patients. Clin Exp Immunol 57:331, 1984.

87. Muller-Quernheim J, Saltini C, Sondermeyer P, et al: Compartmentalized activation of the interleukin-2 gene by lung T lymphocytes in active pulmonary sarcoidosis. J Immunol 137:3475, 1986.

88. Konishi K, Moller DR, Saltini C, et al: Spontaneous expression of the interleukin-2 receptor gene and presence of functional interleukin-2 receptors on T lymphocytes in the blood of individuals with active pulmonary sarcoidosis. J Clin Invest 82:775, 1988.

89. Hunninghake GW, Gadek JE, Young RC Jr, et al: Maintenance of granuloma formation in pulmonary sarcoidosis by T-lymphocytes within the lung. N Engl J Med 302:594, 1980.

90. Semenzato G, Agostini C, Zambello R, et al: Activated T cells with immunoregulatory functions at different sites of involvement in sarcoidosis. Phenotypic and functional evaluations. Ann NY Acad Sci 465:56, 1986.

91. Groman GS, Castele RJ, Altose MD, et al: Lymphocyte subpopulations in sarcoid pleural effusion. Ann Intern Med 100:75, 1984.

92. Semenzato G, Pezzutto A, Chilosi M, et al: Redistribution of T lymphocytes in the lymph nodes of patients with sarcoidosis. N Engl J Med 306:48, 1982.

93. Rómer FK, Christiansen SE, Kragballe K, et al: Studies of peripheral blood monocytes in pulmonary sarcoidosis. Clin Exp Immunol 58:357, 1984.

94. Powell S, Eisenberg H, Siegal J, et al: Characterization of peripheral blood lymphocyte subsets in pulmonary sarcoidosis. Sarcoidosis 4:28, 1987.

95. Tartof D, Curran JJ, Yang SL, et al: NK cell activity and skin test antigen stimulation of NK-like CMC in vitro are decreased to different degrees in pregnancy and sarcoidosis. Clin Exp Immunol 57:502, 1984.

96. Arnoux A, Stanislas-Leguern G, Marsac J, et al: Immunocompetent cells and delayed hypersensitivity reaction in sarcoidosis. Lung 159:137, 1981.

97. Walters CS, Young RC Jr, Hutchinson J: Relationship between peripheral blood lymphocytes and their functional capacity in sarcoidosis. Clin Immunol Immunopathol 16:103, 1980.

98. Hudspith BN, Brostoff J, McNicol MW, et al: Anergy in sarcoidosis: The role of interleukin-1 and prostaglandins in the depressed in vitro lymphocyte response. Clin Exp Immunol 57:324, 1984.

99. Kleinhenz ME, Fujiwara H, Rich EA: Interleukin-1 production by blood monocytes and bronchoalveolar cells in sarcoidosis. Ann NY Acad Sci 465:91, 1986.

100. Baughman RP, Gallon LS, Barcelli U: Prostaglandins in the bronchoalveolar lavage fluid. Possible block of immunoregulation in sarcoidosis. Ann NY Acad Sci 465:41, 1986.

101. Baughman RP, Gallon LS, Barcelli U: Prostaglandins and thrombaxanes in the bronchoalveolar lavage fluid: Possible immunoregulation in sarcoidosis. Am Rev Respir Dis 130:933, 1984.

102. Perks WH, Petheram IS: Familial combined cellular and humoral immune defect with multisystem granulomata. Thorax 33:101, 1978.

103. Rubinstein I, Baum GL: Selective IgA deficiency associated with recurrent sinopulmonary infections in sarcoidosis. Eur J Respir Dis 65:550, 1984.

104. Burmester GR, Gramatzki M, von Gernler J, et al: Pulmonary sarcoidosis associated with acquired humoral and cellular immunodeficiency. Clin Immunol Immunopathol 37:406, 1985.

105. Leen CL, Bath JC, Brettle RP, et al: Sarcoidosis and primary hypogammaglobulinaemia: A report of two cases and a review of the literature. Sarcoidosis 2:91, 1985.

106. Saint-Remy J-MR, Mitchell DN, Cole PJ: Variation in immunoglobulin levels and circulating immune complexes in sarcoidosis. Correlation with extent of disease and duration of symptoms. Am Rev Respir Dis 127:23, 1983.

107. Rómer FK, Solling K: Repeated measurements of serum immunoglobulin-free light chains in early sarcoidosis. Eur J Respir Dis 65:292, 1984.

108. Glikmann G, Nielsen H, Pallisgaard G, et al: Circulating immune complexes, free antigen and alpha-1 antitrypsin levels in sarcoidosis patients. Scand J Respir Dis 60:317, 1979.

109. Valeyre D, Saumon G, Georges R, et al: The relationship between disease duration and noninvasive pulmonary explorations in sarcoidosis with erythema nodosum. Am Rev Respir Dis 129:938, 1984.

110. Johnson NM, McNicol MW, Burton-Kee JE, et al: Circulating immune complexes in sarcoidosis. Thorax 35:286, 1980.

111. Williams JD, Smith MD, Davies BH: Interaction of immune complexes and T suppressor cells in sarcoidosis. Thorax 37:602, 1982.

112. Smith MJ, Turton CWG, Mitchell DN, et al: Association of HLA-B8 with spontaneous resolution in sarcoidosis. Thorax 36:296, 1981.
113. Neville E: HLA antigens and disease. Mt Sinai J Med 44:772, 1977.
114. Olenchock SA, Heise ER, Marx JJ Jr, et al: HLA-B8 in sarcoidosis. Ann Allergy 47:151, 1981.
115. Buck AA: Epidemiologic investigations of sarcoidosis. I. Introduction; material and methods. Am J Hyg 74:137, 1961.
116. Buck AA, Sartwell PE: Epidemiologic investigations of sarcoidosis. II. Skin sensitivity and environmental factors. Am J Hyg 74:152, 1961.
117. Buck AA, McKusick VA: Epidemiologic investigations of sarcoidosis. III. Serum proteins; syphilis; association with tuberculosis; familial aggregation. Am J Hyg 74:174, 1961.
118. Buck AA: Epidemiologic investigations of sarcoidosis. IV. Discussion and summary. Am J Hyg 74:189, 1961.
119. Baer RB: Familial sarcoidosis. Epidemiological aspects with notes of a possible relationship to the chewing of pine pitch. AMA Arch Intern Med 105:60, 1960.
120. Sharma OP, Johnson CS, Balchum OJ: Familial sarcoidosis, report of four siblings with acute sarcoidosis. Am Rev Respir Dis 104:255, 1971.
121. Priestley S, Delaney JC: Familial sarcoidosis presenting with stridor. Thorax 36:636, 1981.
122. Plummer NS, Symmers WS, Winner HI: Sarcoidosis in identical twins: With torulosis as a complication in one case. Br Med J 2:599, 1957.
123. Brennan NJ, Crean P, Long JP, et al: High prevalence of familial sarcoidosis in an Irish population. Thorax 39:14, 1984.
124. Edmondstone WM, Wilson AG: Temporal clustering of familial sarcoidosis in nonconsanguineous relatives. Br J Dis Chest 78:184, 1984.
125. Stewart IC, Davidson NM: Clustering of sarcoidosis. Thorax 37:398, 1982.
126. Douglas JG, Middleton WG, Gaddie J, et al: Sarcoidosis: A disorder commoner in non-smokers? Thorax 41:787, 1986.
127. Hance AJ, Basset P, Saumon G, et al: Smoking and interstitial lung disease. The effect of cigarette smoking on the incidence of pulmonary histiocytosis X and sarcoidosis. Ann NY Acad Sci 465:643, 1986.
128. Comstock GW, Keltz H, Sencer DJ: Clay eating and sarcoidosis: A controlled study in the state of Georgia. Am Rev Respir Dis 84(Suppl):130, 1961.
129. Bresnitz EA, Stolley PD, Israel HL, et al: Possible risk factors for sarcoidosis: A case-control study. Ann NY Acad Sci 465:632, 1986.
130. Bitterman PB, Adelberg S, Crystal RG: Mechanisms of pulmonary fibrosis: Spontaneous release of the alveolar macrophage-derived growth factor in the interstitial lung disorders. J Clin Invest 72:1801, 1983.
131. Cantin AM, Boileau R, Begin R: Increased procollagen III amino-terminal peptide-related antigens and fibroblast growth signals in the lungs of patients with idiopathic pulmonary fibrosis. Am Rev Respir Dis 137:572, 1988.
132. Yamauchi K, Martinet Y, Crystal RG: Modulation of fibronectin gene expression in human mononuclear phagocytes. J Clin Invest 80:1720, 1987.
133. Martinet Y, Rom WN, Grotendorst GR, et al: Exaggerated spontaneous release of platelet-derived growth factor by alveolar macrophages from patients with idiopathic pulmonary fibrosis. N Engl J Med 317:202, 1987.
134. Calhoun WJ, Salisbury SM, Chosy LW, et al: Increased alveolar macrophage chemiluminescence and airspace cell superoxide production in active pulmonary sarcoidosis. J Lab Clin Med 112:147, 1988.
135. Sharma OP: Sarcoidosis: Clinical, laboratory, and immunologic aspects. Semin Roentgenol 20:340, 1985.
136. Reid JD, Andersen ME: Calcium oxalate in sarcoid granulomas. With particular reference to the small ovoid body and a note on the finding of dolomite. Am J Clin Pathol 90:545, 1988.
137. Rosen Y, Vuletin JC, Pertschuk LP, et al: Sarcoidosis: From the pathologist's vantage point. Pathol Ann (I):405, 1979.
138. Mitchell DN, Scadding JG, Heard BE, et al: Sarcoidosis: Histopathological definition and clinical diagnosis. J Clin Pathol 30:395, 1977.
139. Rosen Y, Athanassiades TJ, Moon S, et al: Nongranulomatous interstitial pneumonitis in sarcoidosis. Relationship to development of epithelioid granulomas. Chest 74:122, 1978.
140. Arnoux AG, Jaubert F, Stanislas-Leguern G, et al: In vitro granuloma-like formations in bronchoalveolar cell cultures from patients with sarcoidosis. Ann NY Acad Sci 465:183, 1986.
141. James DG: Definition and classification of granulomatous disorders. Semin Respir Med 8:1, 1986.
142. Laurberg P: Sarcoid reactions in pulmonary neoplasms. Scand J Respir Dis 56:20, 1975.
143. Edelman RR, Johnson TS, Jhaveri HS, et al: Fatal hemoptysis resulting from erosion of a pulmonary artery in cavitary sarcoidosis. Am J Roentgenol 145:37, 1985.
144. Smiéjan JM, Cosnes J, Chollet-Martin S, et al: Sarcoid-like lymphocytosis of the lower respiratory tract in patients with active Crohn's disease. Ann Intern Med 104:17, 1986.
145. Bonniere P, Wallaert B, Cortot A, et al: Latent pulmonary involvement in Crohn's disease: Biological, functional, bronchoalveolar lavage and scintigraphic studies. Gut 27:919, 1986.
146. Lemann M, Messing B, D'Agay P, et al: Crohn's disease with respiratory tract involvement. Gut 28:1669, 1987.
147. Douglas JG, Gillon J, Logan RF, et al: Sarcoidosis and coeliac disease: An association? Lancet 2:13, 1984.
148. Cho C, Linscheer WG, Hirschkorn MA, et al: Sarcoidlike granulomas as an early manifestation of Whipple's disease. Gastroenterology 87:941, 1984.
149. Pimental CJ, Menezes PA: Pulmonary and hepatic granulomatous disorders due to the inhalation of cement and mica dusts. Thorax 33:219, 1978.
150. Wood GM, Bolton RP, Muers MF, et al: Pleurisy and pulmonary granulomas after treatment with acebutolol. Br Med J 285:936, 1982.
151. Rubenstein I, Baum GL, Hiss Y, et al: Does prolonged use of diphenylhydantoin predispose to pulmonary sarcoidosis? Eur Neurol 25:281, 1986.
152. Crystal RG, Roberts WC, Hunninghake GW, et al: Pulmonary sarcoidosis: A disease characterized and perpetuated by activated lung T-lymphocytes. Ann Intern Med 94:73, 1981.
153. Rosen Y, Athanassiades TJ, Moon S, et al: Nongranulomatous interstitial pneumonitis in sarcoidosis. Chest 74:122, 1978.
154. Shigematsu N, Emori K, Matsuba K, et al: Clinicopathologic characteristics of pulmonary acinar sarcoidosis. Chest 73:186, 1978.
155. Battesti JP, Saumon G, Valeyre D, et al: Pulmonary sarcoidosis with an alveolar radiographic pattern. Thorax 37:448, 1982.
156. Keogh BA, Hunninghake GW, Line BR, et al: The alveolitis of pulmonary sarcoidosis. Evaluation of natural history and alveolitis-dependent changes in lung function. Am Rev Respir Dis 128:256, 1983.
157. Cantin A, Begin R, Rola-Pleszozynski M, et al: Heterogeneity of bronchoalveolar lavage cellularity in stage III pulmonary sarcoidosis. Chest 83:485, 1983.
158. Staton GW Jr, Check IJ, Fajman WA, et al: Analysis of homogeneity of alveolitis in pulmonary sarcoidosis by bilateral bronchoalveolar lavage, gallium-67 lung uptake, and chest radiograph. Sarcoidosis 4:8, 1987.
159. Sanguinetti CM, Montroni M, Balbi B, et al: Does activity of pulmonary sarcoidosis depend on disease duration: A correlation between bronchoalveolar lavage, scintigraphic, radiologic, and physiologic parameters and time of onset of the disease. Sarcoidosis 4:18, 1987.
160. Rosen Y, Moon S, Huang C-T, et al: Granulomatous pulmonary angiitis in sarcoidosis. Arch Pathol Lab Med 101:170, 1977.
161. Rossman MD, Daniele RP, Dauber JH: Nodular endobronchial sarcoidosis: A study comparing blood and lung lymphocytes. Chest 79:427, 1981.
162. Wollschlager C, Khan F: Aspergillomas complicating sarcoidosis. A prospective study in 100 patients. Chest 86:585, 1984.
163. Maarsseveen ACM Th v, Veldhuizen RW, Stam J, et al: A quantitative histomorphologic analysis of lymph node granulomas in sarcoidosis in relation to radiological stage I and II. J Pathol 134:441, 1983.
164. Ellis K, Renthal G: Pulmonary sarcoidosis: Roentgenographic observations on course of disease. Am J Roentgenol 88:1070, 1962.
165. Smellie H, Hoyle C: The natural history of pulmonary sarcoidosis. Q J Med 29:539, 1960.
166. Finestone AW: Sarcoidosis. An analysis of twenty-one proved cases. Am J Roentgenol 74:455, 1955.
167. Kirks DR, McCormick VD, Greenspan RH: Pulmonary sarcoidosis. Roentgenologic analysis of 150 patients. Am J Roentgenol 117:777, 1973.
168. Theros EG: RPC of the month from the AFIP. Radiology 92:1557, 1969.
169. Kuhlman JE, Fishman EK, Hamper UM, et al: The computed tomographic spectrum of thoracic sarcoidosis. RadioGraphics 9:449, 1989.
170. Kent DC: Recurrent unilateral hilar adenopathy in sarcoidosis. Am Rev Respir Dis 91:272, 1965.
171. Rabinowitz JG, Ulreich S, Soriano C: The usual unusual manifestations of sarcoidosis and the "hilar-haze"—A new diagnostic aid. Am J Roentgenol 120:821, 1974.
172. Spann RW, Rosenow EC III, DeRemee RA, et al: Unilateral hilar or paratracheal adenopathy in sarcoidosis: A study of 38 cases. Thorax 26:296, 1971.
173. Hsu JT, Cottrell TS: Pulmonary sarcoidosis: Unilateral hilar adenopathy presenting as an endobronchial tumor. Case report. Radiology 98:385, 1971.
174. Westcott JL, Graff AC Jr: Sarcoidosis, hilar adenopathy, and pulmonary artery narrowing. Radiology 108:585, 1973.

17

175. Faunce HF, Ramsay GC, Sy W: Protracted yet variable major pulmonary artery compression in sarcoidosis. Radiology 119:313, 1976.
176. Scadding JG: The late stages of pulmonary sarcoidosis. Postgrad Med J 46:530, 1970.
177. Tsou E, Romano MC, Kerwin DM, et al: Sarcoidosis of anterior mediastinal nodes, pancreas, and uterine cervix: Three unusual sites in the same patient. Am Rev Respir Dis 122:333, 1980.
178. McLoud TC, Putman CE, Pascual R: Eggshell calcification with systemic sarcoidosis. Chest 66:515, 1974.
179. Israel HL, Lenchner G, Steiner RM: Late development of mediastinal calcification in sarcoidosis. Am Rev Respir Dis 124:302, 1981.
180. Wurm K, Reindell H: On the differential roentgenological diagnosis of sarcoidosis (Boeck's disease) and lymphogranulomatosis. Radiologe 2:134, 1962.
181. Wurm K: The stages of pulmonary sarcoidosis. Ger Med Monthly 5:386, 1960.
182. Berkmen YM, Javors BR: Anterior mediastinal lymphadenopathy in sarcoidosis. Am J Roentgenol 127:983, 1976.
183. Rockoff SD, Rohatgi PK: Unusual manifestations of thoracic sarcoidosis. Am J Roentgenol 144:513, 1985.
184. Bein ME, Putman CE, McCloud TC, et al: A re-evaluation of intrathoracic lymphadenopathy in sarcoidosis. Am J Roentgenol 131:409, 1978.
185. Schabel SI, Foote GA, McKee KA: Posterior lymphadenopathy in sarcoidosis. Radiology 129:591, 1978.
186. Epler GR, McLoud TC, Gaensler EA, et al: Normal chest roentgenograms in chronic diffuse infiltrative lung disease. N Engl J Med 298:934, 1978.
187. Schlossberg O, Sfedu E: Disseminated sarcoidosis. Sarcoidosis 4:149, 1987.
188. Israel RH: Diagnosing sarcoidosis (letter). JAMA 241:1791, 1979.
189. Rosen Y, Amorosa JK, Moon S, et al: Occurrence of lung granulomas in patients with stage I sarcoidosis. Am J Roentgenol 129:1083, 1977.
190. Austin JHM: Pulmonary sarcoidosis: What are we learning from CT? Radiology 171:603, 1989.
191. Moore ADA, Godwin JD, Müller NL, et al: Pulmonary histiocytosis X: Comparison of radiographic and CT findings. Radiology 172:249, 1989.
192. Bergin CJ, Bell DY, Coblentz CL, et al: Sarcoidosis: Correlation of pulmonary parenchymal pattern at CT with results of pulmonary function tests. Radiology 171:619, 1989.
193. Brauner MW, Grenier P, Mouelhi MM, et al: Pulmonary histiocytosis X: Evaluation with high-resolution CT. Radiology 172:255, 1989.
194. Müller NL, Mawson JB, Mathieson JR, et al: Sarcoidosis: Correlation of extent of disease at CT with clinical, functional, and radiographic findings. Radiology 171:613, 1989.
195. Conference at Royal Northern Hospital on Sarcoidosis, held January 28, 1966: Contribution by Davies PDB. Lancet 1:423, 1966.
196. Young RL, Krumholz RA, with the technical assistance of Harkleroad LE: A physiologic roentgenographic disparity in sarcoidosis. Dis Chest 50:81, 1966.
197. Winterbauer RH, Hutchinson JF: Use of pulmonary function tests in the management of sarcoidosis. Chest 78:640, 1980.
198. Eklund A, Blaschke E, Persson U, et al: Sarcoidosis in an apparently healthy volunteer. Chest 89:615, 1986.
199. Smellie H, Hoyle C: The hilar lymph nodes in sarcoidosis: With special reference to prognosis. Lancet 2:66, 1957.
200. Symmons DPM, Woods KL: Recurrent sarcoidosis. Thorax 35:879, 1980.
201. Baughman RP: Sarcoidosis. Usual and unusual manifestations (clinical conference). Chest 94:165, 1988.
202. Steiger V, Fanburg BL: Recurrence of thoracic lymphadenopathy in sarcoidosis (letter). N Engl J Med 314:1512, 1986.
203. Stone DJ, Schwartz A: A long-term study of sarcoid and its modification by steroid therapy. Lung function and other factors in prognosis. Am J Med 41:528, 1966.
204. Israel HL, Sperber M, Steiner RM: Course of chronic hilar sarcoidosis in relation to markers of granulomatous activity. Invest Radiol 18:1, 1983.
205. Mesbahi SJ, Davies P: Unilateral pulmonary changes in the chest x-ray in sarcoidosis. Clin Radiol 32:283, 1981.
206. Hartweg H: Chest x-rays in the diagnosis of sarcoidosis. J Coll Radiol Aust 10:344, 1966.
207. Brauner MW, Grenier P, Mompoint D, et al: Pulmonary sarcoidosis: Evaluation with high-resolution CT. Radiology 172:467, 1989.
208. Glazer HS, Levitt RG, Shackelford GD: Peripheral pulmonary infiltrates in sarcoidosis. Chest 86:741, 1984.
209. Teirstein AS, Siltzbach LE: Sarcoidosis of the upper lung fields simulating pulmonary tuberculosis. Chest 64:303, 1973.
210. Turiaf J: Les inscriptions radiographiques inattendues de la sarcoidose pulmonaire. (Unexpected roentgenographic appearance of pulmonary sarcoidosis.) Rev Tuberc (Paris) 28:971, 1964.
211. Felson B: Uncommon roentgen patterns of pulmonary sarcoidosis. Dis Chest 34:357, 1958.
212. Felson B: Less familiar roentgen patterns of pulmonary granulomas. Sarcoidosis, histoplasmosis and noninfectious necrotizing granulomatosis (Wegener's syndrome). Am J Roentgenol 81:211, 1959.
213. Rubinstein I, Solomon A, Baum GL, et al: Pulmonary sarcoidosis presenting with unusual roentgenographic manifestations. Eur J Respir Dis 67:335, 1985.
214. Pinsker KL: Solitary pulmonary nodule in sarcoidosis. JAMA 240:1379, 1978.
215. Pinsker KL: Solitary pulmonary nodule in sarcoidosis. JAMA 240:1379, 1978.
216. Rose RM, Lee RG, Costello P: Solitary nodular sarcoidosis. Clin Radiol 36:589, 1985.
217. Hasan FM, Mark EJ: A young man with a diagnosis of sarcoidosis and a pulmonary mass. N Engl J Med 306:412, 1982.
218. Rakower J: Sarcoidal bilateral hilar lymphoma (Löfgren's syndrome): A review of 31 cases. Am Rev Respir Dis 87:518, 1963.
219. Conant EF, Glickstein MF, Mahar P, et al: Pulmonary sarcoidosis in the older patient: Conventional radiographic features. Radiology 169:315, 1988.
220. Freundlich IM, Libshitz HI, Glassman LM, et al: Sarcoidosis. Typical and atypical thoracic manifestations and complications. Clin Radiol 21:376, 1970.
221. Gorske KJ, Fleming RJ: Mycetoma formation in cavitary pulmonary sarcoidosis. Radiology 95:279, 1970.
222. Israel HL, Ostrow A: Sarcoidosis and aspergilloma. Am J Med 47:243, 1969.
223. Kalbian VV: Bronchial involvement in pulmonary sarcoidosis. Thorax 12:18, 1957.
224. Marland P, Rose Y: Étude anatomique et clinique des lésions bronchiques de la sarcoidose de BBS. (Anatomic and clinical study of bronchial lesions in sarcoidosis of BBS.) J Fr Med Chir Thorac 9:530, 1955.
225. Honey M, Jepson E: Multiple bronchostenoses due to sarcoidosis. Report of two cases. Br Med J 2:1330, 1957.
226. Goldenberg GJ, Greenspan RH: Middle-lobe atelectasis due to endobronchial sarcoidosis with hypercalcemia and renal impairment. N Engl J Med 262:1112, 1960.
227. Schermuly W, Behrend H: Atelektasen bei Sarkoidose. (Atelectasis in sarcoidosis.) Fortschr Roentgenstr 105:208, 1966.
228. Citron KM, Scadding JG: Stenosing non-caseating tuberculosis (sarcoidosis) of the bronchi. Thorax 12:10, 1957.
229. Henry DA, Kiser PE, Scheer CE, et al: Multiple imaging evaluation of sarcoidosis. RadioGraphics 6:75, 1986.
230. Sharma OP, Gordonson J: Pleural effusion in sarcoidosis: A report of six cases. Thorax 30:95, 1975.
231. Chusid EL, Siltzbach LE: Sarcoidosis of the pleura. Ann Intern Med 81:190, 1974.
232. Beekman JF, Zimmet SM, Chun BK, et al: Spectrum of pleural involvement in sarcoidosis. Arch Intern Med 136:323, 1976.
233. Wilen SB, Rabinowitz JG, Ulreich S, et al: Pleural involvement in sarcoidosis. Am J Med 57:200, 1974.
234. Durand DV, Dellinger A, Guerin C, et al: Pleural sarcoidosis: One case presenting with an eosinophilic effusion. Thorax 39:468, 1984.
235. Knox AJ, Wardman AG, Page RL: Tuberculous pleural effusion occurring during corticosteroid treatment of sarcoidosis. Thorax 41:651, 1986.
236. Berte SJ, Pfotenhauer MA: Massive pleural effusion in sarcoidosis. Am Rev Respir Dis 86:261, 1962.
237. Clements JA: Surface tension of lung extracts. Proc Soc Exp Biol Med 95:170, 1957.
238. Aho A, Heinivaara O, Mähönen H: Boeck's sarcoid as a cause of spontaneous pneumothorax. Ann Med Int Fenn 47:163, 1958.
239. McCort JJ, Paré JAP: Pulmonary fibrosis and cor pulmonale in sarcoidosis. Radiology 62:496, 1954.
240. Whitcomb ME, Hawley PC, Domby WR, et al: The role of fiberoptic bronchoscopy in the diagnosis of sarcoidosis. Clinical conference in pulmonary disease from Ohio State University, Columbus. Chest 74:205, 1978.
241. Gomm SA: An unusual presentation of sarcoidosis: Spontaneous haemopneumothorax. Postgrad Med J 60:621, 1984.
242. Ross RJ, Empey DW: Bilateral spontaneous pneumothorax in sarcoidosis. Postgrad Med J 59:106, 1983.
243. Sharma SK, Pande JN, Mukhopadhay AK, et al: Bilateral recurrent spontaneous pneumothoraces in sarcoidosis. Jpn J Med 26:69, 1987.
244. Murray RO, Jacobson HG: The Radiology of Skeletal Disorders. Baltimore, Williams & Wilkins, 1971.
245. McBrine CS, Fisher MS: Acrosclerosis in sarcoidosis. Radiology 115:279, 1975.
246. Young DA, Laman ML: Radiodense skeletal lesions in Boeck's sarcoid. Am J Roentgenol 114:553, 1972.
247. Stump D, Spock A, Grossman H: Vertebral sarcoidosis in adolescents. Radiology 121:153, 1976.

248. Spiteri MA, Matthey F, Gordon T, et al: Lupus pernio: A clinico-radiological study of thirty-five cases. Br J Dermatol *112*:315, 1985.
249. Lin S-R, Levy W, Go EB, et al: Unusual osteosclerotic changes in sarcoidosis, simulating osteoblastic metastases. Radiology *106*:311, 1973.
250. Weston M, Duffy P: Osteosclerosis in sarcoidosis. Australas Radiol *19*:191, 1975.
251. Bonakdarpour A, Levy W, Aegerter EE: Osteosclerotic changes in sarcoidosis. Am J Roentgenol *113*:646, 1971.
252. Oven TJ, Sones M, Morrissey WL: Lytic lesion of the sternum. Rare manifestation of sarcoidosis. Am J Med *80*:285, 1986.
253. Yaghmai I: Radiographic, angiographic and radionuclide manifestations of osseous sarcoidosis. RadioGraphics *3*:375, 1983.
254. Chiles C, Adams GW, Ravin CE: Radiographic manifestations of cardiac carcoid. Am J Roentgenol *145*:711, 1985.
255. Riedy K, Fisher MR, Belic N, et al: MR imaging of myocardial sarcoidosis. Am J Roentgenol *151*:915, 1988.
256. Bulkley BH, Rouleau JR, Whitaker JQ, et al: The use of 201 Thallium for myocardial perfusion imaging in sarcoid heart disease. Chest *72*:27, 1977.
257. Kinney EL, Jackson GL, Reeves WC, et al: Thallium-scan myocardial defects and echocardiographic abnormalities in patients with sarcoidosis without clinical cardiac dysfunction: An analysis of 44 patients. Am J Med *68*:497, 1980.
258. Edelman RR, Johnson TS, Jhaveri HS, et al: Fatal hemoptysis resulting from erosion of a pulmonary artery in cavitary sarcoidosis. Am J Roentgenol *145*:37, 1985.
259. Miller A: The vanishing lung syndrome associated with pulmonary sarcoidosis. Br J Dis Chest *75*:209, 1981.
260. Thrasher DR, Briggs DD Jr: Pulmonary sarcoidosis. Clin Chest Med *3*:537, 1982.
261. Kataria YP, Shaw RA, Campbell PB: Sarcoidosis: An overview II. Clin Notes Respir Dis *20*:3, 1982.
262. Winterbauer RH, Belic N, Moores KD: A clinical interpretation of bilateral hilar adenopathy. Ann Intern Med *78*:65, 1973.
263. Nolan JP, Klatskin G: The fever of sarcoidosis. Ann Intern Med *61*:455, 1964.
264. Siltzbach LE, James DG, Neville E, et al: Course and prognosis of sarcoidosis around the world. Am J Med *57*:847, 1974.
265. Rubinstein I, Baum GL, Hiss Y, et al: Hemoptysis in sarcoidosis. Eur J Respir Dis *66*:302, 1985.
266. Israel HL, Lenchner GS, Atkinson GW: Sarcoidosis and aspergilloma: The role of surgery. Chest *82*:430, 1982.
267. Johns CJ: Management of hemoptysis with pulmonary fungus ball in sarcoidosis. Chest *82*:400, 1982.
268. Chang JC, Driver AG, Townsend CA, et al: Hemoptysis in sarcoidosis. Sarcoidosis *4*:49, 1987.
269. Gardiner IT, Uff JS: Acute pleurisy in sarcoidosis. Thorax *33*:124, 1978.
270. Kanada DJ, Scott D, Sharma OP: Unusual presentations of pleural sarcoidosis. Br J Dis Chest *74*:203, 1980.
271. Liss HP: Pleuropericarditis in sarcoidosis. South Med J *79*:258, 1986.
272. Benatar SR, Clark TJH: Pulmonary function in a case of endobronchial sarcoidosis. Am Rev Respir Dis *110*:490, 1974.
273. Olsson T, Bjornstad-Pettersen H, Stjernberg NL: Bronchostenosis due to sarcoidosis: A cause of atelectasis and airway obstruction simulating pulmonary neoplasm and chronic obstructive pulmonary disease. Chest *75*:663, 1979.
274. Hadfield JW, Page RL, Flower CDR, et al: Localised airway narrowing in sarcoidosis. Thorax *37*:443, 1982.
275. Stjernberg N, Thunell M: Pulmonary function in patients with endobronchial sarcoidosis. Acta Med Scand *215*:121, 1984.
276. Damuth TE, Bower JS, Cho K, et al: Major pulmonary artery stenosis causing pulmonary hypertension in sarcoidosis. Chest *78*:888, 1980.
277. Hoffstein V, Ranganathan N, Mullen JB: Sarcoidosis simulating pulmonary veno-occlusive disease. Am Rev Respir Dis *134*:809, 1986.
278. Martin JM, Dowling GP: Sudden death associated with compression of pulmonary arteries in sarcoidosis. Can Med Assoc J *133*:423, 1985.
279. Khan MM, Gill DS, McConkey B: Myopathy and external pulmonary compression caused by sarcoidosis. Thorax *36*:703, 1981.
280. Morgans WE, Al-Jilahawi AN, Mbatha PB: Superior vena caval obstruction caused by sarcoidosis. Thorax *35*:397, 1980.
281. Javaheri S, Hales CA: Sarcoidosis: A cause of innominate vein obstruction and massive pleural effusion. Lung *157*:81, 1980.
282. Thunell M, Bjerle P, Olofsson BO, et al: Cardiopulmonary function in sarcoidosis. Acta Med Scand *215*:215, 1984.
283. Baughman RP, Gerson M, Bosken CH: Right and left ventricular function at rest and with exercise in patients with sarcoidosis. Chest *85*:301, 1984.
284. Guskowski J, Hawrykiewicz I, Zych D, et al: Pulmonary haemodynamics at rest and during exercise in patients with sarcoidosis. Respiration *46*:26, 1984.

285. Dewar A, Corrin B, Turner-Warwick M: Tadpole shaped structures in a further patient with granulomatous lung disease. Thorax *39*:466, 1984.
286. Kircheiner B: Sarcoidosis cordis. Acta Med Scand *168*:223, 1960.
287. Iwai K, Oka H: Sarcoidosis: Report of ten autopsy cases in Japan. Am Rev Respir Dis *90*:612, 1964.
288. Botti RE, Young FE: Myocardial sarcoid, complete heart block and aortic stenosis. Ann Intern Med *51*:811, 1959.
289. Porter GH: Sarcoid heart disease. N Engl J Med *263*:1350, 1960.
290. Bashour FA, McConnell T, Skinner W, et al: Myocardial sarcoidosis. Dis Chest *53*:413, 1968.
291. Editorial. Myocardial sarcoidosis. Lancet *2*:1351, 1972.
292. Schuster EH, Conrad G, Morris F, et al: Systemic sarcoidosis and electrocardiographic conduction abnormalities: Electrophysiologic evaluation of 2 patients. Chest *78*:601, 1980.
293. Thunell M, Bjerle P, Stjernberg N: ECG abnormalities in patients with sarcoidosis. Acta Med Scand *213*:115, 1983.
294. Miller A, Jackler I, Chuang M: Onset of sarcoidosis with left ventricular failure and multisystem involvement. Chest *70*:302, 1976.
295. Roberts WC, McAllister HA Jr, Ferrans VJ: Sarcoidosis of the heart: A clinicopathologic study of 35 necropsy patients (group I) and review of 78 previously described necropsy patients (Group II). Am J Med *63*:86, 1977.
296. Virmani R, Bures JC, Roberts WC: Cardiac sarcoidosis: Major cause of sudden death in young individuals. Chest *77*:423, 1980.
297. Ahmed SS, Rozefort R, Taclob LT, et al: Development of ventricular aneurysm in cardiac sarcoidosis. Angiology *28*:323, 1977.
298. Silverman KJ, Hutchins GM, Buckley BH: Cardiac sarcoid: A clinicopathologic study of 84 unselected patients with systemic sarcoidosis. Circulation *58*:1204, 1978.
299. Fleming HA: Sarcoid heart disease: A review and an appeal. Thorax *35*:641, 1980.
300. Chun SK, Andy JJ, Jilly P, et al: Ventricular aneurysm in sarcoidosis. Chest *68*:392, 1975.
301. Strauss GS, Lawton BR, Wenzel FJ, et al: Detection of covert myocardial sarcoidosis by scalene node biopsy. Chest *69*:790, 1976.
302. Lillington GA, Jamplis RW: Scalene node biopsy. Ann Intern Med *59*:101, 1963.
303. Editorial. "Diagnosis" of sarcoidosis. N Engl J Med *267*:103, 1962.
304. James DG: Ocular sarcoidosis. Am J Med *26*:331, 1959.
305. Wakefield D, Schrieber L, Penny R: Immunological factors in uveitis. Med J Aust *1*:229, 1982.
306. Campo RV, Aaberg TM: Choroidal granuloma in sarcoidosis. Am J Ophthalmol *97*:419, 1984.
307. Melmon KJ, Goldberg JS: Sarcoidosis with bilateral exophthalmos as the initial symptom. Am J Med *33*:158, 1962.
308. Sharma OP: Cutaneous sarcoidosis: Clinical features and management. Chest *61*:320, 1972.
309. Olive KE, Kataria YP: Cutaneous manifestations of sarcoidosis. Relationships to other organ system involvement, abnormal laboratory measurements, and disease course. Arch Intern Med *145*:1811, 1985.
310. Veien NK, Stahl D, Brodthagen H: Cutaneous sarcoidosis in Caucasians. J Am Acad Dermatol *16*(3 Pt 1):534, 1987.
311. Hanno R, Callen JP: Sarcoidosis: A disorder with prominent cutaneous features and their interrelationship with systemic disease. Med Clin North Am *64*:847, 1980.
312. James DG: Dermatological aspects of sarcoidosis. Q J Med *28*:109, 1959.
313. Hancock BW: Cutaneous sarcoidosis in blood donation venipuncture sites. Br Med J *4*:706, 1972.
314. Erez A, Horowitz J, Sukenik S: Erythema nodosum in the Negev area: A survey of 50 patients. Isr J Med Sci *23*:1228, 1987.
315. Löfgren S, Lundbäck H: The bilateral hilar lymphoma syndrome. I. A study of the relation to age and sex in 212 cases. II. A study of the relation to tuberculosis and sarcoidosis in 212 cases. Acta Med Scand *142*:259, 1952.
316. Hedvall E: The prognosis of sarcoidosis. Acta Tuberc Scand *39*:249, 1960.
317. Similä S, Pietilä J: The changing etiology of erythema nodosum in children. Acta Tuberc Pneumol Scand *46*:159, 1965.
318. Lebacq E, Verhaegen H, Baert L: Erythema nodosum. A study of seventy cases and a review of the literature. Semin Hôp Paris *40*:2103, 1964.
319. MacPherson P: Erythema nodosum in Argyll. Tubercle *42*:341, 1961.
320. Wynn-Williams N: On erythema nodosum, bilateral hilar lymphadenopathy and sarcoidosis. Tubercle *42*:57, 1961.
321. Ford FDC: Puerperal erythema nodosum after liver extract injections. Treatment with prednisone. Br Med J *1*:400, 1960.
322. Freiman DG: Sarcoidosis. N Engl J Med *239*:664, 709, 743, 1948.
323. Joseph RR, Cohen RV: Sarcoidosis: An exercise in differential diagnosis. Dis Chest *52*:458, 1967.
324. Kataria YP, Whitcomb ME: Splenomegaly in sarcoidosis. Arch Intern Med *140*:35, 1980.

17

325. Israel HL, Goldstein RA: Hepatic granulomatosis and sarcoidosis. Ann Intern Med 79:669, 1973.

326. Cunningham D, Mills PR, Quigley EMM, et al: Hepatic granulomas: Experience over a 10-year period in the west of Scotland. Q J Med 51:162, 1982.

327. Scheuer PJ: Hepatic granulomas. Br Med J 285:833, 1982.

328. Maddrey WC, Johns CJ, Boitnott JK, et al: Sarcoidosis and chronic hepatic disease: A clinical and pathologic study of 20 patients. Medicine 49:375, 1970.

329. Rudzki C, Ishak KG, Zimmerman HJ: Chronic intrahepatic cholestasis of sarcoidosis. Am J Med 59:373, 1975.

330. Kadin ME, Donaldson SS, Dorfman RF: Isolated granulomas in Hodgkin's disease. N Engl J Med 283:859, 1970.

331. Bagley CM, Roth JA, Thomas LB, et al: Liver biopsy in Hodgkin's disease. Ann Intern Med 76:219, 1972.

332. Russi EW, Bansky G, Pfaltz M, et al: Budd-Chiari syndrome in sarcoidosis. Am J Gastroenterol 81:71, 1986.

333. Simon HB, Wolff SM: Granulomatous hepatitis and prolonged fever of unknown origin: A study of 13 patients. Medicine 52:1, 1973.

334. Wallaert B, Bonniere P, Prin L, et al: Primary biliary cirrhosis. Subclinical inflammatory alveolitis in patients with normal chest roentgenograms. Chest 90:842, 1986.

335. McLaughlin JS, Van Eck W, Thayer W, et al: Gastric sarcoidosis. Ann Surg 153:283, 1961.

336. Sprague R, Harper P, McClain S, et al: Disseminated gastrointestinal sarcoidosis. Case report and review of the literature. Gastroenterology 87:421, 1984.

337. Cook DM, Dines DE, Dycus DS: Sarcoidosis: Report of a case presenting as dysphagia. Chest 57:84, 1970.

338. Davies RJ: Dysphagia, abdominal pain, and sarcoid granulomata. Br Med J 3:564, 1972.

339. Dufresne CR, Jeyasingham K, Baker RR: Achalasia of the cardia associated with pulmonary sarcoidosis. Surgery 94:32, 1983.

340. Palmer ED: Note on silent sarcoidosis of the gastric mucosa. J Lab Clin Med 52:231, 1958.

341. Papowitz AJ, Li JKH: Abdominal sarcoidosis with ascites. Chest 59:692, 1971.

342. Munt PW: Sarcoidosis of the appendix presenting as appendiceal perforation and abscess. Chest 66:295, 1974.

343. Willoughby JMT, Mitchell DN, Wilson JD: Sarcoidosis and Crohn's disease in siblings. Am Rev Respir Dis 104:249, 1971.

344. McCormick PA, Feighery C, Dolan C, et al: Altered gastrointestinal immune response in sarcoidosis. Gut 29:1628, 1988.

345. Sharma OP, Ahamad I: The CREST syndrome and sarcoidosis. Another example of an overlap syndrome. Sarcoidosis 5:71, 1988.

346. Deheinzelin D, de Carvalho CR, Tomazini ME, et al: Association of Sjögren's syndrome and sarcoidosis. Report of a case. Sarcoidosis 5:68, 1988.

347. Fagan EA, Moore-Gillon JC, Turner-Warwick M: Multiorgan granulomas and mitochondrial antibodies. N Engl J Med 308:572, 1983.

348. Kaplan H: Sarcoid arthritis: A review. Arch Intern Med 112:924, 1963.

349. Grigor RR, Hughes GRV: Chronic sarcoid arthritis. Br Med J 2:1044, 1976.

350. Perruquet JL, Harrington TM, Davis DE, et al: Sarcoid arthritis in a North American Caucasian population. J Rheumatol 11:521, 1984.

351. Sokoloff L, Bunim JJ: Clinical and pathological studies of joint involvement in sarcoidosis. N Engl J Med 260:841, 1959.

352. Halevy J, Segal I, Pitlik S, et al: Unusual clinical presentation of acute sarcoidosis. Respiration 40:237, 1981.

353. Dixey J, Redington AN, Butler RC, et al: The arthropathy of cystic fibrosis. Ann Rheum Dis 47:218, 1988.

354. Cooper TJ, Day AJ, Weller PH, et al: Sarcoidosis in two patients with cystic fibrosis: A fortuitous association? Thorax 42:818, 1987.

355. Nessan VJ, Jacoway JR: Biopsy of minor salivary glands in the diagnosis of sarcoidosis. N Engl J Med 301:922, 1979.

356. Bhoola KD, McNicol MW, Oliver S, et al: Changes in salivary enzymes in patients with sarcoidosis. N Engl J Med 281:877, 1969.

357. Fisher OE, Burton GG, Bryan WF: Sarcoidosis involving the lacrimal sac. Am Rev Respir Dis 103:708, 1971.

358. Rigden B: Sarcoid lesion in breast after probable sarcoidosis in lung. Br Med J 2:1533, 1978.

359. Muther RS, McCarron DA, Bennett WM: Renal manifestations of sarcoidosis. Arch Intern Med 141:643, 1981.

360. Godin M, Fillastre J-P, Ducastelle T, et al: Sarcoidosis: Retroperitoneal fibrosis, renal arterial involvement and unilateral focal glomerulosclerosis. Arch Intern Med 140:1240, 1980.

361. Rømer FK: Renal manifestations and abnormal calcium metabolism in sarcoidosis. Q J Med 49:233, 1980.

362. King BP, Esparza AR, Kahn SI, et al: Sarcoid granulomatous nephritis occurring as isolated renal failure. Arch Intern Med 136:241, 1976.

363. King BP, Esparza AR, Kahn SI, et al: Sarcoid granulomatous nephritis occurring as isolated renal failure. Arch Intern Med 136:241, 1976.

364. Bear RA, Handelsman S, Lang A, et al: Clinical and pathological features of six cases of sarcoidosis presenting with renal failure. Can Med Assoc J 121:1367, 1979.

365. van Dorp WT, Jie K, Lobatto S, et al: Renal failure due to granulomatous interstitial nephritis after pulmonary sarcoidosis. Nephrol Dial Transplant 2:573, 1987.

366. Taylor RG, Fisher C, Hoffbrand BI: Sarcoidosis and membranous glomerulonephritis: A significant association. Br Med J 284:1297, 1982.

367. Taylor TK, Senekjian HO, Knight TF, et al: Membranous nephropathy with epithelial crescents in a patient with pulmonary sarcoidosis. Arch Intern Med 139:1183, 1979.

368. Molle D, Baumelou A, Beaufils H, et al: Membranoproliferative glomerulonephritis associated with pulmonary sarcoidosis. Am J Nephrol 6:386, 1986.

369. Vidal F, Oliver JA, Campanya E, et al: Sarcoidosis presenting as multiple pulmonary nodules and nephrotic syndrome. Postgrad Med J 62:1147, 1986.

370. Delaney P: Neurologic manifestations in sarcoidosis. Review of the literature, with a report of 23 cases. Ann Intern Med 87:336, 1977.

371. Stoudemire A, Linfors E, Houpt JL: Central nervous system sarcoidosis. Gen Hosp Psychiatry 5:129, 1983.

372. Grizzanti JN, Knapp AB, Schecter AJ, et al: Treatment of sarcoid meningitis with radiotherapy. Am J Med 73:605, 1982.

373. Delaney P: Neurologic manifestations in sarcoidosis. Review of the literature, with a report of 23 cases. Ann Intern Med 87:336, 1977.

374. Karnik AS: Nodular cerebral sarcoidosis simulating metastatic carcinoma. Arch Intern Med 142:385, 1982.

375. Rosenbloom MA, Uphoff DF: The association of progressive multifocal leukoencephalopathy and sarcoidosis. Chest 83:572, 1983.

376. Cariski AT: Isolated CNS sarcoidosis. JAMA 245:62, 1981.

377. Ismail F, Miller JL, Kahn SE, et al: Hypothalamic-pituitary sarcoidosis: A case report. S Afr Med J 67:139, 1985.

378. Stuart CA, Neelon FA, Lebovitz HE: Disordered control of thirst in hypothalamic-pituitary sarcoidosis. N Engl J Med 303:1078, 1980.

379. Winnacker JL, Becker KL, Katz S: Endocrine aspects of sarcoidosis. N Engl J Med 278:427, 483, 1968.

380. Karlish AJ, MacGregor GA: Sarcoidosis, thyroiditis, and Addison's disease. Lancet 2:330, 1970.

381. Lender M, Dollberg L: Coincidence of sarcoidosis and Hashimoto's thyroiditis. Am Rev Respir Dis 112:113, 1975.

382. Rubinstein I, Baum GL, Hiss Y, et al: Sarcoidosis and Hashimoto's thyroiditis: A chance occurrence? Respiration 48:136, 1985.

383. Bower JS, Belen JE, Weg JG, et al: Manifestations and treatment of laryngeal sarcoidosis. Am Rev Respir Dis 122:325, 1980.

384. Fogel TD, Weissberg JB, Dobular K, et al: Radiotherapy in sarcoidosis of the larynx: Case report and review of the literature. Laryngoscope 94:1223, 1984.

385. Di Benedetto R, Lefrak S: Systematic sarcoidosis with severe involvement of the upper respiratory tract. Am Rev Respir Dis 102:801, 1970.

386. Carasso B: Sarcoidosis of the larynx causing airway obstruction. Chest 65:693, 1974.

387. Firooznia H, Young R, Lee T: Sarcoidosis of the larynx. Radiology 95:425, 1970.

388. Chijimatsu Y, Tajima J, Washizaki M, et al: Hoarseness as an initial manifestation of sarcoidosis. Chest 78:779, 1980.

389. Talbot PS: Sarcoid myopathy. Br Med J 4:465, 1967.

390. Keogh BA, Crystal RG: Pulmonary function testing in interstitial pulmonary disease: What does it tell us? Chest 78:856, 1980.

391. Boushy SF, Kurtzman RS, Martin ND, et al: The course of pulmonary function in sarcoidosis. Ann Intern Med 62:939, 1965.

392. Leading article. Pulmonary function in sarcoidosis. Br Med J 1:710, 1967.

393. Young RC Jr, Carr C, Shelton TG, et al: Sarcoidosis: Relationship between changes in lung structure and function. Am Rev Respir Dis 95:224, 1967.

394. Divertie MB, Cassan SM, O'Brien PC, et al: Fine structural morphometry of diffuse lung diseases with abnormal blood-air gas transfer. Mayo Clin Proc 51:42, 1976.

395. Zwijnenburg A, Alberts C, Jansen HM, et al: Distribution of ventilation-perfusion ratios in pulmonary sarcoidosis. Sarcoidosis 4:122, 1987.

396. Snider GL, Doctor L: The mechanics of ventilation in sarcoidosis. Am Rev Respir Dis 89:897, 1964.

397. Sellers RD, Siebens AA: The effects of sarcoidosis on pulmonary function with particular reference to changes in pulmonary compliance. Am Rev Respir Dis 91:660, 1965.

398. Ingram CG, Reid PC, Johnston RN: Exercise testing in pulmonary sarcoidosis. Thorax 37:129, 1982.

399. Matthews JI, Hooper RG: Exercise testing in pulmonary sarcoidosis. Chest 83:75, 1983.

400. Athos L, Mohler JG, Sharma Om. P: Exercise testing in the physiologic assessment of sarcoidosis. Ann NY Acad Sci 465:491, 1986.

401. Demeter SL: Gas exchange across abnormal interstitial tissue in pulmonary sarcoidosis: Results of therapy. Angiology 38:256, 1987.
402. Dines DE, Stubbs SE, McDougall JC: Obstructive disease of the airways associated with stage I sarcoidosis. Mayo Clin Proc 53:788, 1978.
403. Renzi GD, Renzi PM, Lopez-Majano V, et al: Airway function in sarcoidosis: Effect of short-term steroid therapy. Respiration 42:98, 1981.
404. Radwan L, Grebska E, Koziorowski A: Small airways function in pulmonary sarcoidosis. Scand J Respir Dis 59:37, 1978.
405. Angyropoulou PK, Patakas DA, Louridas GE: Airway function in stage I and stage II pulmonary sarcoidosis. Respiration 46:17, 1984.
406. Scano G, Monechi GC, Stendardi L, et al: Functional evaluation in stage I pulmonary sarcoidosis. Respiration 49:195, 1986.
407. Bechtel JT, Starr T III, Dantzker DR, et al: Airway hyperreactivity in patients with sarcoidosis. Am Rev Respir Dis 1241:759, 1981.
408. Olafsson M, Simonsson BG, Hansson SB: Bronchial reactivity in patients with recent pulmonary sarcoidosis. Thorax 40:51, 1985.
409. Manresa Presas F, Romero Colomer P, Rodriguez Sanchon B: Bronchial hyperreactivity in fresh stage I sarcoidosis. Ann NY Acad Sci 465:523, 1986.
410. Spiro SG, Dowdeswell IRG, Clark TJH: An analysis of submaximal exercise responses in patients with sarcoidosis and fibrosing alveolitis. Br J Dis Chest 75:169, 1981.
411. Dunn TL, Watters LC, Hendrix C, et al: Gas exchange at a given degree of volume restriction is different in sarcoidosis and idiopathic pulmonary fibrosis. Am J Med 85:221, 1988.
412. Tilles DS, Goldenheim PD, Ginns LC, et al: Pulmonary function in normal subjects and patients with sarcoidosis after bronchoalveolar lavage. Chest 89:244, 1986.
413. Strumpf IJ, Feld MK, Cornelius MJ, et al: Safety of fiberoptic bronchoalveolar lavage in evaluation of interstitial lung disease. Chest 80:268, 1981.
414. Smith LJ: Bronchoalveolar lavage today. Chest 80:251, 1981.
415. Chretien J, Venet A, Danel C, et al: Bronchoalveolar lavage in sarcoidosis. Respiration 48:222, 1985.
416. Abe S, Munakata M, Nishimura M, et al: Gallium-67 scintigraphy, bronchoalveolar lavage, and pathologic changes in patients with pulmonary sarcoidosis. Chest 85:650, 1984.
417. Rossman MD, Dauber JH, Cardillo ME, et al: Pulmonary sarcoidosis: Correlation of serum angiotensin-converting enzyme with blood and bronchoalveolar lymphocytes. Am Rev Respir Dis 125:366, 1982.
418. Hallgren R, Eklund A, Engstrom-Laurent A, et al: Hyaluronate in bronchoalveolar lavage fluid: A new marker in sarcoidosis reflecting pulmonary disease. Br Med J 290:1778, 1985.
419. Bjermer L, Engstrom-Laurent A, Thunell M, et al: Hyaluronic acid in bronchoalveolar lavage fluid in patients with sarcoidosis: Relationship to lavage mast cells. Thorax 42:933, 1987.
420. Eklund A, Hallgren R, Blaschke E, et al: Hyaluronate in bronchoalveolar lavage fluid in sarcoidosis and its relationship to alveolar cell populations. Eur J Respir Dis 71:30, 1987.
421. Ebright JR, Soin JS, Manoli RS: The gallium scan: Problems and misuse in examination of patients with suspected infection. Arch Intern Med 142:246, 1982.
422. Line BR, Fulmer JD, Reynolds HY, et al: Gallium-67 citrate scanning in the staging of idiopathic pulmonary fibrosis: Correlation with physiologic and morphologic features and bronchoalveolar lavage. Am Rev Respir Dis 118:355, 1978.
423. Duffy GJ, Thirumurthi K, Casey M, et al: Semi-quantitative gallium lung scanning as a measure of the intensity of alveolitis in pulmonary sarcoidosis. Eur J Nucl Med 12:187, 1986.
424. Johnson DG, Johnson SM, Harris CC, et al: Ga-67 uptake in the lung in sarcoidosis. Radiology 150:551, 1984.
425. Braude AC, Cohen R, Rahmani R, et al: An in vitro gallium-67 lung index for the evaluation of sarcoidosis. Am Rev Respir Dis 130:783, 1984.
426. Okada M, Takahashi H, Nukiwa T, et al: Correlative analysis of longitudinal changes in bronchoalveolar lavage, 67 gallium scanning, serum angiotensin-converting enzyme activity, chest x-ray, and pulmonary function tests in pulmonary sarcoidosis. Jpn J Med 26:360, 1987.
427. Line BR, Hunninghake GW, Keogh BA, et al: Gallium-67 scanning to stage the alveolitis of sarcoidosis: Correlation with clinical studies, pulmonary function studies and bronchoalveolar lavage. Am Rev Respir Dis 123:440, 1981.
428. Forgacs P: The gallium scan and inflammatory lesions. Arch Intern Med 142:231, 1982.
429. Klech H, Kohn H, Kummer F, et al: Assessment of activity in sarcoidosis. Sensitivity and specificity of 67 gallium scintigraphy, serum ACE levels, chest roentgenography, and blood lymphocyte populations. Chest 82:732, 1982.
430. Staab EV, McCartney WH: Role of gallium 67 in inflammatory disease. Semin Nucl Med 8:219, 1978.
431. MacMahon H, Bekerman C: The diagnostic significance of gallium lung uptake in patients with normal chest radiographs. Radiology 127:189, 1978.
432. Perrin-Fayolle M, Pacheco Y, Harf R, et al: Angiotensin-converting enzyme in bronchoalveolar lavage fluid in pulmonary sarcoidosis. Thorax 36:790, 1981.
433. Mordelet-Dambrine MS, Stanislas-Leguern GM, Huchon GJ, et al: Elevation of the bronchoalveolar concentration of angiotensin-I converting enzyme in sarcoidosis. Am Rev Respir Dis 126:472, 1982.
434. Lieberman J: Elevation of serum angiotensin-converting-enzyme (ACE) level in sarcoidosis. Am J Med 59:365, 1975.
435. Fanburg BL, Schoenberger MD, Bachus B, et al: Elevated serum angiotensin-I converting enzyme in sarcoidosis. Am Rev Respir Dis 114:525, 1976.
436. Pertschuk LP, Silverstein E, Friedland J: Immunohistologic diagnosis of sarcoidosis. Am J Clin Pathol 75:350, 1981.
437. Okabe T, Suzuki A, Ishikawa H, et al: Cells originating from sarcoid granulomas in vitro. Am Rev Respir Dis 124:608, 1981.
438. Horowitz J, Kueppers F, Rosen S: Angiotensin-converting enzyme concentrations in rabbits with talc-induced pulmonary granulomas. Am Rev Respir Dis 124:306, 1981.
439. Rohrbach MS, DeRemee RA: Pulmonary sarcoidosis and serum angiotensin-converting enzyme. Mayo Clin Proc 57:64, 1982.
440. Sandron D, LeCossier D, Moreau F, et al: Angiotensin-converting enzyme in sarcoidosis and other pulmonary diseases: A comparison of two methods of determination. Lung 157:31, 1979.
441. Rohatgi PK, Ryan JW: Simple radioassay for measuring serum activity of angiotensin-converting enzyme in sarcoidosis. Chest 78:69, 1980.
442. Studdy P, Bird R, James DG: Serum angiotensin-converting enzyme (SACE) in sarcoidosis and other granulomatous disorders. Lancet 2:1331, 1978.
443. Gronhagen-Riska C: Angiotensin-converting enzyme. I. Activity and correlations with serum lysozyme in sarcoidosis, other chest or lymph node diseases and healthy persons. Scand J Respir Dis 60:83, 1979.
444. Glatt A: Angiotensin-converting enzyme in sarcoidosis (letter). Mayo Clin Proc 58:140, 1983.
445. Lieberman J, Nosal A, Schlessner LA, et al: Serum angiotensin-converting enzyme for diagnosis and therapeutic evaluation of sarcoidosis. Am Rev Respir Dis 120:329, 1979.
446. Bhigjee AI, Pillay NL, Omar MAK, et al: Serum angiotensin-converting in sarcoidosis. S Afr Med J 58:615, 1980.
447. Allen R, Mendelsohn FAO, Csicsmann J, et al: A clinical evaluation of serum angiotensin-converting enzyme in sarcoidosis. Aust NZ J Med 10:496, 1980.
448. Rohatgi PK: Serum angiotensin-converting enzyme in pulmonary disease (review). Lung 160:287, 1982.
449. Rohatgi PK, Ryan JW, Lindeman P: Value of serial measurement of serum angiotensin-converting enzyme in the management of sarcoidosis. Am J Med 70:44, 1981.
450. Gronhagen-Riska C, Selroos O, Wagar G, et al: Angiotensin-converting enzyme. II. Serum activity in early and newly diagnosed sarcoidosis. Scand J Respir Dis 60:94, 1979.
451. Bunting PS, Szalai JP, Katic M: Diagnostic aspects of angiotensin-converting enzyme in pulmonary sarcoidosis. Clin Biochem 20:213, 1987.
452. Baur X, Fruhmann G, Dahlheim H: Follow-up of angiotensin-converting enzyme in serum of patients with sarcoidosis. Respiration 41:133, 1981.
453. Matsuki K, Sakata T: Angiotensin-converting enzyme in diseases of the liver. Am J Med 73:549, 1982.
454. Borowsky SA, Lieberman J, Strome S, et al: Elevation of serum angiotensin-converting enzyme level: Occurrence in alcoholic liver disease. Arch Intern Med 142:893, 1982.
455. Silverstein E, Pertschuk LP, Friedland J: Immunofluorescent detection of angiotensin-converting enzyme (ACE) in Gaucher cells. Am J Med 69:408, 1980.
456. Römer FK, Faber V, Koch C, et al: Serum-angiotensin-enzyme in chronic granulomatous disease (letter). Lancet 1:1237, 1979.
457. Yotsumoto H: Longitudinal observations of serum angiotensin-converting enzyme activity in sarcoidosis with and without treatment. Chest 82:556, 1982.
458. Selroos O, Gronhagen-Riska C: Angiotensin-converting enzyme. III. Changes in serum level as an indicator of disease activity in untreated sarcoidosis. Scand J Respir Dis 60:328, 1979.
459. Schoenberger CI, Line BR, Keogh BA, et al: Lung inflammation in sarcoidosis: Comparison of serum angiotensin-converting enzyme with bronchoalveolar lavage and gallium-67 scanning assessment of the T-lymphocyte alveolitis. Thorax 37:19, 1982.
460. Radermecker M, Gustin M, Saint-Remy P: Lack of correlation between serum angiotensin-converting enzyme. Eur J Respir Dis 65:189, 1984.
461. Massaro D, Handler AE, Katz S, et al: Excretion of hydroxyproline in patients with sarcoidosis. Am Rev Respir Dis 93:929, 1966.
462. Pascual RS, Gee JBL, Finch SC: Usefulness of serum lysozyme

17

measurement in diagnosis and evaluation of sarcoidosis. N Engl J Med 289:1074, 1973.

463. Zorn SK, Stevens CA, Schachter EN, et al: The angiotensin-converting enzyme in pulmonary sarcoidosis and the relative diagnostic value of serum lysozyme. Lung 157:87, 1980.

464. Gronhagen-Riska C, Selroos O: Angiotensin-converting enzyme. IV. Changes in serum activity and in lysozyme concentrations as indicators of the course of untreated sarcoidosis. Scand J Respir Dis 60:337, 1979.

465. Turton CWG, Grundy E, Firth G, et al: Value of measuring serum angiotensin-I converting enzyme and serum lysozyme in the management of sarcoidosis. Thorax 34:57, 1979.

466. Parrish RW, Williams JD, Davies BH: Serum beta-2-microglobulin and angiotensin-converting enzyme activity in sarcoidosis. Thorax 37:936, 1982.

467. Goldstein RA, Israel HL, Becker KL, et al: The infrequency of hypercalcemia in sarcoidosis. Am J Med 51:21, 1971.

468. Reiner M, Sigurdsson G, Nunziata V, et al: Abnormal calcium metabolism in normocalcaemic sarcoidosis. Br Med J 2:1473, 1976.

469. Meyrier A, Valeyre D, Bouillon R, et al: Different mechanisms of hypercalciuria in sarcoidosis. Correlations with disease extension and activity. Ann NY Acad Sci 465:575, 1986.

470. Papapoulos SE, Clemens TL, Fraher LJ, et al: 1,25-dihydroxycholecalciferol in the pathogenesis of the hypercalcaemia of sarcoidosis. Lancet 1:627, 1979.

471. Barbour GL, Coburn JW, Slatopolsky E, et al: Hypercalcemia in an anephric patient with sarcoidosis: Evidence for extrarenal generation of 1,25-dihydroxyvitamin D. N Engl J Med 305:440, 1981.

472. Maesaka JK, Batuman V, Pablo NC, et al: Elevated 1,25-dihydroxyvitamin D levels: Occurrence with sarcoidosis with end-stage renal disease. Arch Int Med 142:1206, 1982.

473. Mason RS, Frankel T, Chan Y-L, et al: Vitamin D conversion by sarcoid lymph node homogenate. Ann Intern Med 100:59, 1984.

474. Reichel H, Koeffler HP, Barbers R, et al: Regulation of 1,25-dihydroxyvitamin D_3 production by cultured alveolar macrophages from normal human donors and from patients with pulmonary sarcoidosis. J Clin Endocrinol Metab 65:1201, 1987.

475. Taylor RL, Lynch HJ Jr, Wysor WG Jr: Seasonal influence of sunlight on the hypercalcemia of sarcoidosis. Am J Med 34:221, 1963.

476. Lief PD, Bogartz LJ, Koerner SK, et al: Sarcoidosis and primary hyperparathyroidism. An unusual association. Am J Med 47:825, 1969.

477. Burr JM, Farrell JJ, Hills AG: Sarcoidosis and hyperparathyroidism with hypercalcemia. Special usefulness of the cortisone test. N Engl J Med 261:1271, 1959.

478. Dent CE, Watson L: Hyperparathyroidism and sarcoidosis. Br Med J 1:646, 1966.

479. Robinson RG, Kerwin DM, Tsou E: Parathyroid adenoma with coexistent sarcoid granulomas: A hypercalcemic patient. Arch Intern Byrd 140:1547, 1980.

480. Löfgren S, Snellman B, Lindgren AGH: Renal complications in sarcoidosis. Functional and biopsy studies. Acta Med Scand 159:295, 1957.

481. Batson JM: Calcification of the ear cartilage associated with the hypercalcemia of sarcoidosis. Report of a case. N Engl J Med 265:876, 1961.

482. Lower EE, Smith JT, Martelo OJ, et al: The anemia of sarcoidosis. Sarcoidosis 5:51, 1988.

483. Semple P d'A: Thrombocytopenia, hemolytic anaemia, and sarcoidosis. Br Med J 4:440, 1975.

484. West WO: Acquired hemolytic anemia secondary to Boeck's sarcoid. Report of a case and review of the literature. N Engl J Med 261:688, 1959.

485. Knodel AR, Beekman JF: Severe thrombocytopenia and sarcoidosis. JAMA 243:258, 1980.

486. Brincker H: Sarcoid reactions and sarcoidosis in Hodgkin's disease and other malignant lymphomata. Br J Cancer 26:120, 1972.

487. Brincker H, Wilbek E: The incidence of malignant tumours in patients with respiratory sarcoidosis. Br J Cancer 29:247, 1974.

488. Rómer FK: Case 7–1982: Sarcoidosis and cancer (letter). N Engl J Med 306:1490, 1982.

489. Sharma OP, Meyer PR, Akil B, et al: Sarcoidosis and lymphoma: An unusual association. Sarcoidosis 4:58, 1987.

490. Case records of the Massachusetts General Hospital. Weekly clinicopathological exercises. Case 11–1984. Long-standing sarcoidosis with the recent onset of the superior-vena-cava syndrome. N Engl J Med 310:708, 1984.

491. Gefter WB, Glick JH, Epstein DM, et al: Sarcoidosis: A cause of intrathoracic lymphadenopathy after treatment of testicular carcinoma. Am J Roentgenol 139:820, 1982.

492. Geller RA, Kuremsky DA, Copeland JS, et al: Sarcoidosis and testicular neoplasm: An unusual association. J Urol 118:487, 1977.

493. Trump DL, Ettinger DS, Feldman MJ, et al: Sarcoidosis and sarcoid-like lesions: Their occurrence after cytotoxic and radiation therapy of testis cancer. Arch Intern Med 141:37, 1981.

494. Gefter WB, Glick JH, Epstein DM, et al: Sarcoidosis: A cause of intrathoracic lymphadenopathy after treatment of testicular carcinoma. Am J Roentgenol 139:820, 1982.

495. O'Connell M, Powell S, Horwich A: Sarcoid-like lymphadenopathy in malignant teratoma. Postgrad Med J 59:108, 1983.

496. Colebunders R, Bultinck J, Servais J, et al: A patient with testis seminoma, sarcoidosis, and neutropenic enterocolitis. Hum Pathol 15:394, 1984.

497. Blacher EJ, Maynard JF: Seminoma and sarcoidosis: An unusual association. Urology 26:288, 1985.

498. Fossa SD, Abeler V, Marton PF, et al: Sarcoid reaction of hilar and paratracheal lymph nodes in patients treated for testicular cancer. Cancer 56:2212, 1985.

499. Urbanski SJ, Alison RE, Jewett MAS, et al: Association of germ cell tumours of the testis and intrathoracic sarcoid-like lesions. Can Med Assoc J 137:416, 1987.

500. Heffner JE, Milam MG: Sarcoid-like hilar and mediastinal lymphadenopathy in a patient with metastatic testicular cancer. Cancer 60:1545, 1987.

501. Bogaerts Y, Van Der Straeten M, Tasson J, et al: Sarcoidosis or malignancy: A diagnostic dilemma. Eur J Respir Dis 64:541, 1983.

502. Meyer A, Raugel M, Jullien JL, et al: Nontuberculous mediastinal adenopathies with erythema nodosum (Löfgren's syndrome). Four new case reports. Rev Tuberc (Paris) 23:357, 1959.

503. Rajasuriya K, Nagaratnam N, Somasunderam M: Syndrome of erythema nodosum, bilateral hilar enlargement and polyarthritis. Br J Dis Chest 53:314, 1959.

504. Bacharach T, Zalis EG: Sarcoid syndrome associated with coccidioidomycosis. Am Rev Respir Dis 88:248, 1963.

505. Cohen SH, Fink JN, Garancis JC, et al: Sarcoidosis in hypersensitivity pneumonitis. Chest 72:588, 1977.

506. Mitchell DM, Mitchell DN, Collins JV, et al: Transbronchial lung biopsy through fibreoptic bronchoscope in diagnosis of sarcoidosis. Br Med J 280:679, 1980.

507. Stjernberg N, Thunell M, Lundgren R: Comparison of flexible fibreoptic bronchoscopy and scalene lymph node biopsy in the diagnosis of sarcoidosis. Endoscopy 15:300, 1983.

508. Mitchell DM, Mitchell DN, Collins JV, et al: Transbronchial lung biopsy through fibreoptic bronchoscope in diagnosis of sarcoidosis. Br J Dis Chest 74:320, 1980.

509. Roethe RA, Fuller PB, Byrd RB, et al: Transbronchoscopic lung biopsy in sarcoidosis: Optimal number and sites for diagnosis. Chest 77:400, 1980.

510. Pinsker KL, Kamholz SL: Diagnosis of sarcoidosis by transbronchial lung biopsy. Chest 79:123, 1981.

511. Gilman MJ, Wang KP: Transbronchial lung biopsy in sarcoidosis: An approach to determine the optimal number of biopsies. Am Rev Respir Dis 122:721, 1980.

512. Byrd RB, Roethe RA, Hafermann DR, et al: Diagnosis of sarcoidosis by transbronchial lung biopsy. Chest 79:125, 1981.

513. Puar HS, Young RC Jr, Armstrong EM: Bronchial and transbronchial lung biopsy without fluoroscopy in sarcoidosis. Chest 87:303, 1985.

514. Friedman OH, Blaugrund SM, Siltzbach LE: Biopsy of the bronchial wall as an aid in diagnosis of sarcoidosis. JAMA 183:646, 1963.

515. Mikhail JR, Mitchell DN, Drury RAB, et al: A comparison of the value of mediastinal lymph node biopsy and the Kveim test in sarcoidosis. Am Rev Respir Dis 104:544, 1971.

516. Koontz CH, Joyner LR, Nelson RA: Transbronchial lung biopsy via the fiberoptic bronchoscope in sarcoidosis. Ann Intern Med 85:64, 1976.

517. Vernon SE: Nodular pulmonary sarcoidosis. Diagnosis with fine needle aspiration biopsy. Acta Cytologica 29:473, 1985.

518. James DG, Sharma OP, Bradstreet P: The Kveim-Siltzbach test. Report of a new British antigen. Lancet 2:1274, 1967.

519. Anderson R, James DG, Peters PM, et al: The Kveim test in sarcoidosis. Lancet 2:650, 1963.

520. Hirsch JG, Cohn ZA, Morse SI, et al: Evaluation of the Kveim reaction as a diagnostic test for sarcoidosis. N Engl J Med 265:827, 1961.

521. American Thoracic Society: Brummer DI, chairman; Chaves AD, Cugell DW, et al: The Kveim test. A statement by the committee on therapy. Am Rev Respir Dis 103:435, 1971.

522. Siltzbach LE: The Kveim test in sarcoidosis. A study of 750 patients. JAMA 178:476, 1961.

523. Reich JM, Johnson RE: Course and prognosis of sarcoidosis in a nonreferral setting. Analysis of 86 patients observed for 10 years. Am J Med 78:61, 1985.

524. Sones M, Israel HL: Course and prognosis of sarcoidosis. Am J Med 29:84, 1960.

525. Israel HL, Karlin P, Menduke H, et al: Factors affecting outcome of sarcoidosis. Influence of race, extrathoracic involvement, and initial radiologic lung lesions. Ann NY Acad Sci 465:609, 1986.

526. Johns CJ, Schonfeld SA, Scott PP, et al: Longitudinal study of chronic sarcoidosis with low-dose maintenance corticosteroid therapy. Outcome and complications. Ann NY Acad Sci 465:702, 1986.

527. Israel HL: Prognosis of sarcoidosis. Ann Intern Med 73:1038, 1970.

528. Young RC Jr, Titus-Dillon PY, Schneider ML, et al: Sarcoidosis in Washington, D.C. Clinical observations in 105 black patients. Arch Intern Med 125:102, 1970.

529. Editorial. Management of pulmonary sarcoidosis. Lancet 1:890, 1982.

530. Neville E, Walker AN, James DG: Prognostic factors predicting the outcome of sarcoidosis: An analysis of 818 patients. Q J Med 52:525, 1983.

531. Siltzbach LE, Greenberg GM: Childhood sarcoidosis—a study of 18 patients. N Engl J Med 279:1239, 1968.

532. Kendig EL, Brummer DL: The prognosis of sarcoidosis in children. Chest 70:351, 1976.

533. Zych D, Krychniak W, Pawlicka L, et al: Sarcoidosis of the lung. Natural history and effects of treatment. Sarcoidosis 4:64, 1987.

534. Huhti E, Poukkula A, Lilja M: Prognosis for sarcoidosis in a defined geographical area. Br J Dis Chest 81:381, 1987.

535. Johnston RN: Pulmonary sarcoidosis after ten to twenty years. Scott Med J 31:72, 1986.

536. McLoud TC, Epler GR, Gaensler EA, et al: A radiographic classification for sarcoidosis: Physiologic correlation. Invest Radiol 17:129, 1982.

537. Meier-Sydow J, Rust MG, Kappos A, et al: The long-term course of airflow obstruction in obstructive variants of the fibrotic stage of sarcoidosis and of idiopathic pulmonary fibrosis. Ann NY Acad Sci 465:515, 1986.

538. Israel-Biet D, Venet A, Chretien J: Persistent high alveolar lymphocytosis as a predictive criterion of chronic pulmonary sarcoidosis. Ann NY Acad Sci 465:395, 1986.

539. Buchalter S, App W, Jackson L, et al: Bronchoalveolar lavage cell analysis in sarcoidosis. A comparison of lymphocyte counts and clinical course. Ann NY Acad Sci 465:678, 1986.

540. Baughman RP, Fernandez M, Bosken CH, et al: Comparison of gallium-67 scanning, bronchoalveolar lavage, and serum angiotensin-converting enzyme levels in pulmonary sarcoidosis. Predicting response to therapy. Am Rev Respir Dis 129:676, 1984.

541. Rust M, Bergmann L, Kuhn T, et al: Prognostic value of chest radiograph, serum angiotensin-converting enzyme and T helper cell count in blood and in bronchoalveolar lavage of patients with pulmonary sarcoidosis. Respiration 48:231, 1985.

542. Turner-Warwick M, McAllister W, Lawrence R, et al: Corticosteroid treatment in pulmonary sarcoidosis: Do serial lavage lymphocyte counts, serum angiotensin-converting enzyme measurements, and gallium-67 scans help management? Thorax 41:903, 1986.

543. Hollinger WM, Staton GW Jr, Fajman WA, et al: Prediction of therapeutic response in steroid-treated pulmonary sarcoidosis. Evaluation of clinical parameters, bronchoalveolar lavage, gallium-67 lung scanning, and serum angiotensin-converting enzyme levels. Am Rev Respir Dis 132:65, 1985.

544. Bjermer L, Rosenhall L, Angstrom T, et al: Predictive value of bronchoalveolar lavage cell analysis in sarcoidosis. Thorax 43:284, 1988.

545. Rohatgi PK, Bates HR, Noss RW: Computer-assisted sequential quantitative analysis of gallium scans in pulmonary sarcoidosis. Eur J Respir Dis 66:248, 1985.

546. Niden AH, Mishkin FS, Salem F, et al: Prognostic significance of gallium lung scans in sarcoidosis. Ann NY Acad Sci 465:435, 1986.

547. Baughman RP, Shipley R, Eisentrout CE: Predictive value of gallium scan, angiotensin-converting enzyme level, and bronchoalveolar lavage in two-year follow-up of pulmonary sarcoidosis. Lung 165:371, 1987.

548. Beaumont D, Herry JY, Sapene M, et al: Gallium-67 in the evaluation of sarcoidosis: Correlations with serum angiotensin-converting enzyme and bronchoalveolar lavage. Thorax 37:11, 1982.

549. Ueda E, Kawabe T, Tachibana T, et al: Serum angiotensin-converting enzyme activity as an indicator of prognosis in sarcoidosis. Am Rev Respir Dis 121:667, 1980.

550. Weaver LJ, Solliday NH, Celic L, et al: Serial observations of angiotensin-converting enzyme and pulmonary function in sarcoidosis. Arch Intern Med 141:931, 1981.

551. American Thoracic Society: Brummer DL, chairman; Chaves AD; Cugell DW; et al: Treatment of sarcoidosis. A statement by the committee on therapy. Am Rev Respir Dis 103:433, 1971.

552. Mitchell DN, Scadding JG: Sarcoidosis. Am Rev Respir Dis 110:774, 1974.

553. Leading article. Steroids and sarcoid. Br Med J 4:757, 1969.

554. Israel HL, Fouts DW, Beggs RA: A controlled trial of prednisone treatment of sarcoidosis. Am Rev Respir Dis 107:609, 1973.

555. Young RI, Harkleroad LE, Lordon RE, et al: Pulmonary sarcoidosis: A prospective evaluation of glucocorticoid therapy. Ann Intern Med 73:207, 1970.

556. Sharma OP, Colp C, Williams MH Jr: Course of pulmonary sarcoidosis with and without corticosteroid therapy as determined by pulmonary function studies. Am J Med 41:541, 1966.

557. Selroos O, Sellergren TL, Vuorio M, et al: Sarcoidosis in identical twins. Observations on the course of treated and untreated identical diseases. Am Rev Respir Dis 108:1401, 1973.

558. Spratling L, Tenholder MF, Underwood GH, et al: Daily vs alternate day prednisone therapy for stage II sarcoidosis. Chest 88:687, 1985.

559. Odlum CM, FitzGerald MX: Evidence that steroids alter the natural history of previously untreated progressive pulmonary sarcoidosis. Sarcoidosis 3:40, 1986.

560. Harkleroad LE, Young RL, Savage PJ, et al: Pulmonary sarcoidosis: Long-term follow-up of the effects of steroid therapy. Chest 82:84, 1982.

561. Eule H, Weinecke A, Roth I, et al: The possible influence of corticosteroid therapy on the natural course of pulmonary sarcoidosis. Late results of a continuing clinical study. Ann NY Acad Sci 465:695, 1986.

562. Goldstein DS, Williams MH: Rate of improvement of pulmonary function in sarcoidosis during treatment with corticosteroids. Thorax 41:473, 1986.

563. Lawrence EC, Teague RB, Gottlieb MS, et al: Serial changes in markers of disease activity with corticosteroid treatment in sarcoidosis. Am J Med 74:747, 1983.

564. Pinkston P, Saltini C, Muller-Quernheim J, et al: Corticosteroid therapy suppresses spontaneous interleukin-2 release and spontaneous proliferation of lung T lymphocytes of patients with active pulmonary sarcoidosis. J Immunol 139:755, 1987.

565. O'Brien LE, Forsman PJ, Wiltse HE: Early onset sarcoidosis with pulmonary function abnormalities. Chest 65:472, 1974.

566. Haynes de Regt R: Sarcoidosis and pregnancy. Obstet Gynecol 70(3 Pt 1):369, 1987.

567. Chusid EL, Shah R, Siltzbach LE: Tuberculin tests during the course of sarcoidosis in 350 patients. Am Rev Respir Dis 104:13, 1971.

568. Liebow AA, Carrington CB: The interstitial pneumonias. In Simon M, Potchen EJ, LeMay M (eds): Frontiers of Pulmonary Radiology. New York, Grune & Stratton, 1969, p 102.

569. Bhagwat AG, Wentworth P, Conen PE: Observations on the relationship of desquamative interstitial pneumonia and pulmonary alveolar proteinosis in childhood: A pathologic and experimental study. Chest 58:326, 1970.

570. Bedrossian CW, Kuhn C 3d, Luna MA, et al: Desquamative interstitial pneumonia-like reaction accompanying pulmonary lesions. Chest 72:166, 1977.

571. Henderson DW: The morphogenesis and classification of diffuse interstitial lung diseases: A clinicopathological approach, based on tissue reaction patterns. Aust NZ J Med 14(Suppl):735, 1984.

572. Stilwell PC, Norris DG, O'Connell EJ, et al: Desquamative interstitial pneumonitis in children. Chest 77:165, 1980.

573. Scadding JG, Hinson KFW: Diffuse fibrosing alveolitis (diffuse interstitial fibrosis of the lungs). Thorax 22:291, 1967.

574. Patchefsky AS, Israel HL, Hoch WS, et al: Desquamative interstitial pneumonia: Relationship to interstitial fibrosis. Thorax 28:680, 1973.

575. McCann BG, Brewer DB: A case of desquamative interstitial pneumonia progressing to "honeycomb lung." J Pathol 112:199, 1974.

576. Patchefsky AS, Israel HL, Hoch WS, et al: Desquamative interstitial pneumonia: Relationship to interstitial fibrosis. Thorax 28:680, 1973.

577. Crystal RG, Fulmer JD, Roberts WC, et al: Idiopathic pulmonary fibrosis. Ann Intern Med 85:769, 1976.

578. Bone RC, Wolfe J, Sobonya RE, et al: Desquamative interstitial pneumonia following long-term nitrofurantoin therapy. Am J Med 60:697, 1976.

579. Farr GH, Harley RA, Hennigar GR: Desquamative interstitial pneumonia: An electron microscopic study. Am J Pathol 60:347, 1970.

580. Brewer DB, Heath D, Asquith P: Electron microscopy of desquamative interstitial pneumonia. J Pathol 97:317, 1969.

581. Valdivia E, Hensley G, Wu J, et al: Morphology and pathogenesis of desquamative interstitial pneumonitis. Thorax 32:7, 1977.

582. Stachura I, Singh G, Whiteside TL: Mechanisms of tissue injury in desquamative interstitial pneumonitis. Am J Med 68:733, 1980.

583. Scadding JG, Hinson KFW: Diffuse fibrosing alveolitis (diffuse interstitial fibrosis of the lungs). Thorax 22:291, 1967.

584. Crystal RG, Fulmer JD, Roberts WC, et al: Idiopathic pulmonary fibrosis. Ann Intern Med 85:769, 1976.

585. Fromm GB, Dunn LJ, Harris JO: Desquamative interstitial pneumonitis: Characterization of free intra-alveolar cells. Chest 77:552, 1980.

586. Hamman L, Rich AR: Fulminating diffuse interstitial fibrosis of the lungs. Trans Am Clin Climatol Assoc 51:154, 1935.

587. Katzenstein A-LA, Myers JL, Mazur MT: Acute interstitial pneumonia. A clinicopathologic, ultrastructural, and cell kinetic study. Am J Surg Pathol 10(4):256, 1986.

588. Hamman L, Rich AR: Acute diffuse interstitial fibrosis of the lungs. Bull Hopkins Hosp 74:177, 1944.

17

589. Gross P: The concept of the Hamman-Rich syndrome: A critique. Am Rev Respir Dis 85:828, 1962.
590. Scadding JG: Chronic diffuse interstitial fibrosis of the lungs. Br Med J 1:443, 1960.
591. Stack BHR, Grant IWB, Irvine WJ, et al: Idiopathic diffuse interstitial lung disease: A review of 42 cases. Am Rev Respir Dis 92:939, 1965.
592. Bonanni PP, Frymoyer JW, Jacox RJ: A family study of idiopathic pulmonary fibrosis. A possible dysproteinemic and genetically determined disease. Am J Med 39:411, 1965.
593. Moore FH, Hamlin JW, Lindsay S: Progressive diffuse interstitial fibrosis of the lungs (Hamman-Rich syndrome). Report of a case of seven years' duration. AMA Arch Intern Med 100:651, 1957.
594. MacKay IR, Ritchie B: Diffuse fibrosing alveolitis (diffuse interstitial fibrosis of the lungs): Two cases with autoimmune features. Thorax 20:200, 1965.
595. Read J: The pathogenesis of the Hamman-Rich syndrome. A review from the standpoint of possible allergic etiology. Am Rev Tuberc 78:353, 1958.
596. Chapman JR, Charles PJ, Venables PJW, et al: Definition and clinical relevance of antibodies to nuclear ribonucleoprotein and other nuclear antigens in patients with cryptogenic fibrosing alveolitis. Am Rev Respir Dis 130:439, 1984.
597. Turner-Warwick M, Burrows B, Johnson A: Cryptogenic fibrosing alveolitis: Clinical features and their influence on survival. Thorax 35:171, 1980.
598. Hodson ME, Haslam PL, Spiro SG, et al: Digital vasculitis in patients with cryptogenic fibrosing alveolitis. Br J Dis Chest 78:140, 1984.
599. McFadden RG, Craig ID, Paterson NAM: Interstitial pneumonitis in myasthenia gravis. Br J Dis Chest 78:187, 1984.
600. Smith MJL, Benson MK, Strickland ID: Coeliac disease and diffuse interstitial lung disease. Lancet 1:473, 1971.
601. Turner-Warwick M: Fibrosing alveolitis and chronic liver disease. QJ Med 37:133, 1968.
602. Golding PL, Smith M, Williams R: Multisystem involvement in chronic liver disease. Studies on the incidence and pathogenesis. Am J Med 55:772, 1973.
603. Capron JP, Marti R, Rey JL, et al: Fibrosing alveolitis and hepatitis B surface antigen-associated chronic active hepatitis in a patient with immunoglobulin A deficiency. Am J Med 66:874, 1979.
604. Mason AMS, McIllmurray MB, Golding PL, et al: Fibrosing alveolitis associated with renal tubular acidosis. Br Med J 4:596, 1970.
605. Williams AJ, Marsh J, Stableforth DE: Cryptogenic fibrosing alveolitis, chronic active hepatitis, and autoimmune haemolytic anaemia in the same patient. Br J Dis Chest 79:200, 1985.
606. Scadding JW: Fibrosing alveolitis with autoimmune haemolytic anaemia: Two case reports. Thorax 32:134, 1977.
607. Endo Y, Hara M: Glomerular IgA deposition in pulmonary diseases. Kidney Int 29:557, 1986.
608. May JJ, Schwarz MI, Dreisin RB: Idiopathic thrombocytopenic purpura occurring with interstitial pneumonitis. Ann Intern Med 90:199, 1979.
609. Schwarz MI, Dreisin RB, Pratt DS, et al: Immunofluorescent patterns in the idiopathic interstitial pneumonias. J Lab Clin Med 91:929, 1978.
610. Scadding JG: Diffuse pulmonary alveolar fibrosis. Thorax 29:271, 1974.
611. Nagaya H, Buckley EC III, Sieker HO: Positive antinuclear factor in patients with unexplained pulmonary fibrosis. Ann Intern Med 70:1135, 1969.
612. Nagaya H, Sieker HO: Pathogenic mechanisms of interstitial pulmonary fibrosis in patients with serum antinuclear factor. A histologic and clinical correlation. Am J Med 52:51, 1972.
613. Nagaya H, Elmore M, Ford CD: Idiopathic interstitial pulmonary fibrosis. An immune complex disease. Am Rev Respir Dis 107:826, 1973.
614. Holgate ST, Haslam P, Turner-Warwick M: The significance of antinuclear and DNA antibodies in cryptogenic fibrosing alveolitis. Thorax 38:67, 1983.
615. Gelb AF, Dreisen RB, Epstein JD, et al: Immune complexes, gallium lung scans, and bronchoalveolar lavage in idiopathic interstitial pneumonitis-fibrosis. Chest 84:148, 1983.
616. Martinet Y, Haslam PL, Turner-Warwick M: Clinical significance of circulating immune complexes in "lone" cryptogenic fibrosing alveolitis and those with associated connective tissue disorders. Clin Allergy 14:491, 1984.
617. Deodhar SD, Bhagwat AG: Desquamative interstitial pneumonia-like syndrome in rabbits. Arch Pathol 84:54, 1967.
618. Stein-Streilein J, Lipscomb MF, Fisch H, et al: Pulmonary interstitial fibrosis induced in hapten-immune hamsters. Am Rev Respir Dis 136:119, 1987.
619. McCormick JR, Harkin MM, Johnson KJ, et al: Suppression by superoxide dismutase of immune-complex–induced pulmonary alveolitis and dermal inflammation. Am J Pathol 102:55, 1981.

620. Fan K, D'Orsogna DE: Diffuse pulmonary interstitial fibrosis. Evidence of humoral antibody mediated pathogenesis. Chest 85:150, 1984.
621. Campbell DA, Poulter LW, Janossy G, et al: Immunohistological analysis of lung tissue from patients with cryptogenic fibrosing alveolitis suggesting local expression of immune hypersensitivity. Thorax 40:405, 1985.
622. Barzo P: Familial idiopathic fibrosing alveolitis. Eur J Respir Dis 66:350, 1985.
623. Auwerx J, Demedts M, Bouillon R, et al: Coexistence of hypocalciuric hypercalcaemia and interstitial lung disease in a family: A cross-sectional study. Eur J Clin Invest 15:6, 1985.
624. Demedts M, Auwerx J, Goddeeris P, et al: The inherited association of interstitial lung disease, hypocalciuric hypercalcemia, and defective granulocyte function. Am Rev Respir Dis 131:470, 1985.
625. Auwerx J, Boogaerts M, Ceuppens JL, et al: Defective host defense mechanisms in a family with hypocalciuric hypercalcaemia and coexisting interstitial lung disease. Clin Exp Immunol 62:57, 1985.
626. Solliday NH, Williams JA, Gaensler EA, et al: Familial chronic interstitial pneumonia. Am Rev Respir Dis 108:193, 1973.
627. Libby DM, Gibofsky A, Fotino M, et al: Immunogenetic and clinical findings in idiopathic pulmonary fibrosis: Association with the B-cell alloantigen HLA-DR2. Am Rev Respir Dis 127:618, 1983.
628. Koch B: Familial fibrocystic pulmonary dysplasia: Observations in one family. Can Med Assoc J 92:801, 1965.
629. McKusick VA, Fisher AM: Congenital cystic disease of the lung with progressive pulmonary fibrosis and carcinomatosis. Ann Intern Med 48:774, 1958.
630. Hughes EW: Familial interstitial pulmonary fibrosis. Thorax 19:515, 1964.
631. Young WA: Familial fibrocystic pulmonary dysplasia: A new case in a known affected family. Can Med Assoc J 94:1059, 1966.
632. Laski B, Donohue WL, Uchida I, et al: Familial pulmonary fibrosis and its relationship with the Hamman-Rich syndrome. AMA J Dis Child 98:503, 1959.
633. Donohue WL, Laski B, Uchida I, et al: Familial fibrocystic pulmonary dysplasia and its relation to the Hamman-Rich syndrome. Pediatrics 24:786, 1959.
634. Swaye P, Van Ordstrand HS, McCormack LJ, et al: Familial Hamman-Rich syndrome. Dis Chest 55:7, 1969.
635. Musk AW, Zilko PJ, Manners P, et al: Genetic studies in familial fibrosing alveolitis. Possible linkage with immunoglobulin allotypes (Gm). Chest 89:206, 1986.
636. Wagley PF: A new look at the Hamman-Rich syndrome. Johns Hopkins Med J 131:412, 1972.
637. Fulmer JD, Sposovska MS, von Gal ER: Distribution of HLA antigens in idiopathic pulmonary fibrosis. Am Rev Respir Dis 118:141, 1978.
638. Turton CWG, Morris LM, Lawler SD, et al: HLA in cryptogenic fibrosing alveolitis (letter). Lancet 1:507, 1978.
639. Kallenberg CG, Schilizzi BM, Beaumont F, et al: Expression of class II MHC antigens on alveolar epithelium in fibrosing alveolitis. Clin Exp Immunol 67:182, 1987.
640. Kallenberg CG, Schilizzi BM, Beaumont F, et al: Expression of class II major histocompatibility complex antigens on alveolar epithelium in interstitial lung disease: Relevance to pathogenesis of idiopathic pulmonary fibrosis. J Clin Pathol 40:725, 1987.
641. Israël-Asselain R, Chebat J, Sors CH, et al: Diffuse interstitial pulmonary fibrosis in a mother and son with von Recklinghausen's disease. Thorax 20:153, 1965.
642. Massaro D, Katz S: Fibrosing alveolitis: Its occurrence, roentgenographic and pathologic features in von Recklinghausen's neurofibromatosis. Am Rev Respir Dis 93:934, 1966.
643. Patchefsky AS, Atkinson WG, Hoch WS, et al: Interstitial pulmonary fibrosis and von Recklinghausen's disease: An ultrastructural and immunofluorescent study. Chest 64:459, 1973.
644. Davis SA, Kaplan RL: Neurofibromatosis and interstitial lung disease. Arch Dermatol 114:1368, 1978.
645. Hoste P, Willems J, Devriendt J, et al: Familial diffuse interstitial pulmonary fibrosis associated with oculocutaneous albinism: Report of two cases with a family study. Scand J Respir Dis 60:128, 1979.
646. Davies BH, Tuddenham EGD: Familial pulmonary fibrosis associated with oculocutaneous albinism and platelet function defect: A new syndrome. Q J Med 45:219, 1976.
647. Garay SM, Gardella JE, Fazzini EP, et al: Hermansky-Pudlak syndrome: Pulmonary manifestations of a ceroid storage disorder. Am J Med 66:737, 1979.
648. White DA, Smith GJW, Cooper JAD Jr, et al: Hermansky-Pudlak syndrome and interstitial lung disease: Report of a case with lavage findings. Am Rev Respir Dis 130:138, 1984.
649. Auwerx J, Demedts M, Bouillon R, et al: Coexistence of hypocalciuric hypercalcaemia and interstitial lung disease in a family: A cross-sectional study. Eur J Clin Invest 15:6, 1985.
650. Bitterman PB, Rennard SI, Keogh BA, et al: Familial idiopathic pulmonary fibrosis. Evidence of lung inflammation in unaffected family members. N Engl J Med 314:1343, 1986.

651. Campbell EJ, Harris B, Avioli LV: Idiopathic pulmonary fibrosis. Arch Intern Med 141:771, 1981.
652. Hamman L, Rich AR: Acute diffuse interstitial fibrosis of the lungs. Bull Hopkins Hosp 74:177, 1944.
653. Pinsker KL, Schneyer B, Becker N, et al: Usual interstitial pneumonia following Texas A2 influenza infection. Chest 80:123, 1981.
654. Kawai T, Fujiwara T, Aoyama Y, et al: Diffuse interstitial fibrosing pneumonitis and adenovirus infection. Chest 69:692, 1976.
655. Pinsker KL, Schneyer B, Becker N, et al: Usual interstitial pneumonia following Texas A2 influenza infection. Chest 80:123, 1981.
656. Liebow AA, Steer A, Billingsley J: Desquamative interstitial pneumonia. Am J Med 39:369, 1965.
657. Gaensler EA, Goff AM, Prowse CM: Desquamative interstitial pneumonia. N Engl J Med 274:113, 1966.
658. Patchefsky AS, Banner M, Freundlich IM: Desquamative interstitial pneumonia. Significance of intranuclear viral-like inclusion bodies. Ann Intern Med 74:322, 1971.
659. McNary WF Jr, Gaensler EA: Intranuclear inclusion bodies in desquamative interstitial pneumonia. Ann Intern Med 74:404, 1971.
660. Vergnon JM, Vincent M, de The G, et al: Cryptogenic fibrosing alveolitis and Epstein-Barr virus: An association? Lancet 2:768, 1984.
661. Carvajal RE, Gonzalez R, Vargas AF, et al: Cell-mediated immunity against connective tissue in experimental pulmonary fibrosis. Lung 160:131, 1982.
662. Bone RC, Wolfe J, Sobonya RE, et al: Desquamative interstitial pneumonia following long-term nitrofurantoin therapy. Am J Med 60:697, 1976.
663. Goldstein JD, Godleski JJ, Herman PG: Desquamative interstitial pneumonitis associated with monomyelocytic leukemia. Chest 81:321, 1982.
664. Abraham JL, Hertzberg MA: Inorganic particulates associated with desquamative interstitial pneumonia. Chest 80:67S, 1981.
665. Herbert A, Sterling G, Abraham J, et al: Desquamative interstitial pneumonia in an aluminum welder. Hum Pathol 13:694, 1982.
666. Coates EO, Watson JHL: Diffuse interstitial lung disease in tungsten carbide workers. Ann Intern Med 75:709, 1971.
667. Porte A, Stoeckel ME, Mantz JM, et al: Acute interstitial pulmonary fibrosis: Comparative light and electron microscopic study of 19 cases: Pathogenic and therapeutic implications. Intensive Care Med 4:181, 1978.
668. Haslam PL, Turton CWG, Lukoszek A, et al: Bronchoalveolar lavage fluid cell counts in cryptogenic fibrosing alveolitis and their relation to therapy. Thorax 35:328, 1980.
669. Weinberger SE, Kelman JA, Elson NA, et al: Bronchoalveolar lavage in interstitial lung disease. Ann Intern Med 89:459, 1978.
670. Haslam PL, Turton CWG, Heard B, et al: Bronchoalveolar lavage in pulmonary fibrosis: Comparison of cells obtained with lung biopsy and clinical features. Thorax 35:9, 1980.
671. Yasuoka S, Nakayama T, Kawano T, et al: Comparison of cell profiles of bronchial and bronchoalveolar lavage fluids between normal subjects and patients with idiopathic pulmonary fibrosis. Tohoku J Exp Med 146:33, 1985.
672. Hunninghake GW, Gadek JE, Kawanami O, et al: Inflammatory and immune processes in the human lung in health and disease: Evaluation of bronchoalveolar lavage. Am J Pathol 97:149, 1979.
673. O'Donnell K, Keogh B, Cantin A, et al: Pharmacologic suppression of the neutrophil component of the alveolitis in idiopathic pulmonary fibrosis. Am Rev Respir Dis 136:288, 1987.
674. Keogh BA, Bernardo J, Hunninghake GW, et al: Effect of intermittent high dose parenteral corticosteroids on the alveolitis of idiopathic pulmonary fibrosis. Am Rev Respir Dis 127:18, 1983.
675. Hunninghake GW, Gadek JE, Lawley TJ: Mechanisms of neutrophil accumulation in the lungs of patients with idiopathic pulmonary fibrosis. J Clin Invest 68:259, 1981.
676. Hällgren R, Bjermer L, Lundgren R, et al: The eosinophil component of the alveolitis in idiopathic pulmonary fibrosis. Signs of eosinophil activation in the lung are related to impaired pulmonary function. Am Rev Respir Dis 139:373, 1989.
677. Kradin RL, Divertie MB, Colvin RB, et al: Usual interstitial pneumonitis is a T-cell alveolitis. Clin Immunol Immunopathol 40:224, 1986.
678. Nagai S, Fujimura N, Hirata T, et al: Differentiation between idiopathic pulmonary fibrosis and interstitial pneumonia associated with collagen vascular diseases by comparison of the ratio of OKT4 + cells and OKT8 + cells in BALF T lymphocytes. Eur J Respir Dis 67:1, 1985.
679. Cathcart MK, Emdur LI, Ahtiala-Stewart K, et al: Excessive helper T-cell function in patients with idiopathic pulmonary fibrosis: Correlation with disease activity. Clin Immunol Immunopathol 43:382, 1987.
680. Phillipson EA: Pathophysiology of experimental canine interstitial lung disease. Chest 69:280, 1976.
681. Deodhar SD, Bhagwat AG: Desquamative interstitial pneumonia-like syndrome in rabbits. Arch Pathol 84:54, 1967.
682. Palmer KC, Snider GL, Hayes JA: An association between alveolar cell proliferation and interstitial fibrosis following acute lung injury. Chest 69:307, 1976.
683. Wasan SM, McElligott TF: An electron microscopic study of experimentally induced interstitial pulmonary fibrosis. Am Rev Respir Dis 105:276, 1972.
684. Ryan SF: Experimental fibrosing alveolitis. Am Rev Respir Dis 105:776, 1972.
685. Cantin AM, North SL, Fells GA, et al: Oxidant-mediated epithelial cell injury in idiopathic pulmonary fibrosis. J Clin Invest 79:1665, 1987.
686. Campbell DA, Poulter LW, Du Bois RM: Phenotypic analysis of alveolar macrophages in normal subjects and in patients with interstitial lung diseases. Thorax 41:429, 1986.
687. Jordana M, Schulman J, McSharry C, et al: Heterogeneous proliferative characteristics of human adult lung fibroblast lines and clonally derived fibroblasts from control and fibrotic lung. Am Rev Respir Dis 137:579, 1988.
688. Fulmer JD, Bienkowski RS, Cowan MJ, et al: Collagen concentration and rates of synthesis in idiopathic pulmonary fibrosis. Am Rev Respir Dis 122:289, 1980.
689. Selman M, Chapela R, Montaño M, et al: Changes of collagen content in fibrotic lung disease. Arch Invest Med (Méx) 13:93, 1982.
690. Kirk JME, Da Costa PE, Turner-Warwick M, et al: Biochemical evidence for an increased and progressive deposition of collagen in lungs of patients with pulmonary fibrosis. Clin Sci 70:39, 1986.
691. Selman M, Montaño M, Ramos C, et al: Concentration, biosynthesis and degradation of collagen in idiopathic pulmonary fibrosis. Thorax 41:355, 1986.
692. Fulmer JD, Bienkowski RS, Cowan MJ, et al: Collagen concentration and rates of synthesis in idiopathic pulmonary fibrosis. Am Rev Respir Dis 122:289, 1980.
693. Editorial. Collagen in idiopathic pulmonary fibrosis. Lancet 2:1277, 1979.
694. Reiser KM, Last JA: Pulmonary fibrosis in experimental acute respiratory disease. Am Rev Respir Dis 123:58, 1981.
695. Phan SH, Thrall RS, Ward PA: Bleomycin-induced pulmonary fibrosis in rats: Biochemical demonstration of increased rate of collagen synthesis. Am Rev Respir Dis 121:501, 1980.
696. Lee YCC, Kehrer JP: Increased pulmonary collagen synthesis in mice treated with cyclophosphamide. Drug Chem Toxicol 8:503, 1985.
697. Masuda H, Ozeki T, Takazono I, et al: Tissue content of glycosaminoglycans in the diffuse idiopathic interstitial fibrosis patient. Am J Med Sci 295:507, 1988.
698. Hance AJ, Horwitz AL, Cowan MJ, et al: Biochemical approaches to investigation of fibrotic lung disease. Chest 69:257, 1976.
699. Elias JA, Rossman MD, Daniele RP: Inhibition of human lung fibroblast growth by mononuclear cells. Am Rev Respir Dis 125:701, 1982.
700. Kawanami O, Ferrans VJ, Fulmer JD, et al: Ultrastructure of pulmonary mast cells in patients with fibrotic lung disorders. Lab Invest 40:717, 1979.
701. Mendeloff J: Disseminated nodular pulmonary ossification in the Hamman-Rich lung. Am Rev Respir Dis 103:269, 1971.
702. Genereux GP: The end-stage lung. Radiology 116:279, 1975.
703. Kawanami O, Ferrans VJ, Crystal RG: Structure of alveolar epithelial cells in patients with fibrotic lung disorders. Lab Invest 46:39, 1982.
704. Sutinen S, Rainio P, Sutinen S, et al: Ultrastructure of terminal respiratory epithelium and prognosis in chronic interstitial pneumonia. Eur J Respir Dis 61:325, 1980.
705. Shimizu S, Kobayashi H, Watanabe H, et al: Mallory body-like structures in the lung. Acta Pathol Jpn 36(1):105, 1986.
706. Nonomura A, Kono N, Ohta G: Pulmonary cytoplasmic hyalin resembling Mallory's alcoholic hyalin in the liver. Acta Pathol Jpn 36(6):869, 1986.
707. Kawanami O, Basset F, Ferrans VJ, et al: Pulmonary Langerhans' cells in patients with fibrotic lung disorders. Lab Invest 44:227, 1981.
708. Kuisk H, Sanchez JS: Diffuse bronchiolectasis with muscular hyperplasia ("muscular cirrhosis of the lung"): Relationship to chronic form of Hamman-Rich syndrome. Am J Roentgenol 96:979, 1966.
709. Fisher JH: Bronchiolar emphysema (diffuse bronchiolectasis)—So-called muscular cirrhosis of the lungs. Can Med Assoc J 93:681, 1965.
710. Westcott JL, Cole SR: Traction bronchiectasis in end-stage pulmonary fibrosis. Radiology 161:665, 1986.
711. Edwards CW, Carlile A: The larger bronchi in cryptogenic fibrosing alveolitis: A morphometric study. Thorax 37:828, 1982.
712. Gardiner IT, Uff JS: "Blue bodies" in a case of cryptogenic fibrosing alveolitis (desquamative type): An ultra-structural study. Thorax 33:806, 1978.
713. Bedrossian CWM, Kuhn C III, Luna MA, et al: Desquamative interstitial pneumonia-like reaction accompanying pulmonary lesions. Chest 72:166, 1977.

17

714. Coalson JJ: The ultrastructure of human fibrosing alveolitis. Virchows Arch (Pathol Anat) 395:181, 1982.

715. Adler KB, Craighead JE, Vallyathan NV, et al: Actin-containing cells in human pulmonary fibrosis. Am J Pathol 102:427, 1981.

716. Schneider RM, Nevius DB, Brown HZ: Desquamative interstitial pneumonia in a four-year-old child. N Engl J Med 277:1056, 1967.

717. Feigin DS, Friedman PJ: Chest radiography in desquamative interstitial pneumonitis: A review of 37 patients. Am J Roentgenol 134:91, 1980.

718. Carrington CB, Gaensler EA, Coutu RE, et al: Natural history and treated course of usual and desquamative interstitial pneumonia. N Engl J Med 298:801, 1978.

719. Woodruff CE, Barrett RJ, Champan PT, et al: Carcinoma of the chest with bone destruction. Am Rev Respir Dis 93:442, 1966.

720. Lemire P, Bettez P, Gelinas M, et al: Patterns of desquamative interstitial pneumonia (DIP) and diffuse interstitial pulmonary fibrosis (DIPF). Am J Roentgenol 115:479, 1972.

721. Davis GS, Brody AR, Landis JN, et al: Quantitation of inflammatory activity in interstitial pneumonitis by bronchofiberscopic pulmonary lavage. Chest 69:265, 1976.

722. Feigin DS: New perspectives on interstitial lung disease. Radiol Clin North Am 21:683, 1983.

723. Picado C, Gomez de Almeida R, Xaubet A, et al: Spontaneous pneumothorax in cryptogenic fibrosing alveolitis. Respiration 48:77, 1985.

724. Müller NL, Staples CA, Miller RR, et al: Disease activity in idiopathic pulmonary fibrosis: CT and pathologic correlation. Radiology 165:731, 1987.

725. Staples CA, Müller NL, Vedal S, et al: Unusual interstitial pneumonia: Correlation of CT with clinical, functional, and radiologic findings. Radiology 162:377, 1987.

726. Klein J, Gamsu G: High resolution computed tomography of diffuse lung disease. Invest Radiol 24:805, 1989.

727. Müller NL, Staples CA, Miller RR, et al: Disease activity in idiopathic pulmonary fibrosis: CT and pathologic correlation. Radiology 165:731, 1987.

728. Vedal S, Welsh EV, Miller RR, et al: Desquamative interstitial pneumonia. Computed tomographic findings before and after treatment with corticosteroids. Chest 93:215, 1988.

729. Wollmer P, Rhodes CG, Hughes JM: Regional extravascular density and fractional blood volume of the lung in interstitial disease. Thorax 39:286, 1984.

730. Peacock A, Alchanat M, Valind S, et al: A non-invasive method for estimation of lung tissue volume in patients with fibrosing lung disease: Comparison with lung density measurement by positron transmission tomography. Lancet 2:785, 1984.

731. Pantin CF, Valind SO, Sweatman M, et al: Measures of the inflammatory response in cryptogenic fibrosing alveolitis. Am Rev Respir Dis 138:1234, 1988.

732. McFadden RG, Carr TJ, Wood TE: Proton magnetic resonance imaging to stage activity of interstitial lung disease. Chest 92:31, 1987.

733. Cruz E, Rodriguez J, Lisboa C, et al: Desquamative alveolar disease (desquamative interstitial pneumonia): Case report. Thorax 24:186, 1969.

734. DeRemee RA, Harrison EG Jr, Andersen HA: The concept of classic interstitial pneumonitis-fibrosis (CIP-F) as a clinicopathologic syndrome. Chest 61:213, 1972.

735. Semple P d'a, Beastall GH, Brown TM, et al: Sex hormone suppression and sexual impotence in hypoxic pulmonary fibrosis. Thorax 39:46, 1984.

736. Snell NJC, Coysh HL: Persistent hyponatremia complicating fibrosing alveolitis. Thorax 33:820, 1978.

737. Webb DR, Currie GD: Pulmonary fibrosis masking polymyositis. JAMA 222:1146, 1972.

738. Thompson PL, Mackay IR: Fibrosing alveolitis and polymyositis. Thorax 25:504, 1970.

739. Wright PH, Heard BE, Steel SJ, et al: Cryptogenic fibrosing alveolitis: Assessment by graded trephine lung biopsy. Histology compared with clinical, radiographic, and physiological features. Br J Dis Chest 745:61, 1981.

740. Chuang MT, Raskin J, Krellenstein DJ, et al: Bronchoscopy in diffuse lung disease: Evaluation by open lung biopsy in nondiagnostic transbronchial lung biopsy. Ann Otol Rhinol Laryngol 96:654, 1987.

741. Bye PTP, Anderson SD, Woolcock AJ, et al: Bicycle endurance performance of patients with interstitial lung disease breathing air and oxygen. Am Rev Respir Dis 126:1005, 1982.

742. Burdon JG, Killian KJ, Jones NL: Pattern of breathing during exercise in patients with interstitial lung disease. Thorax 38:778, 1983.

743. Bye PTP, Issa F, Berthon-Jones M, et al: Studies of oxygenation during sleep in patients with interstitial lung disease. Am Rev Respir Dis 129:27, 1984.

744. Finucane KE, Prichard MG: Lung function in diffuse interstitial lung disease of unknown cause. Aust NZ J Med 14(Suppl):749, 1984.

745. Finucane KE, Prichard MG: Mechanical properties of the lung in diffuse interstitial lung disease. Aust NZ J Med 14(Suppl):755, 1984.

746. Anderson SD, Bye PTP: Exercise testing in the evaluation of diffuse interstitial lung disease. Aust NZ J Med 14(Suppl):762, 1984.

747. DiMarco AF, Kelsen SG, Cherniack NS, et al: Occlusion pressure and breathing pattern in patients with interstitial lung disease. Am Rev Respir Dis 127:425, 1983.

748. Epler GR, Saber FA, Gaensler EA: Determination of severe impairment (disability) in interstitial lung disease. Am Rev Respir Dis 121:647, 1980.

749. Weitzenblum E, Ehrart M, Rasaholinjanahary J, et al: Pulmonary hemodynamics in idiopathic pulmonary fibrosis and other interstitial pulmonary diseases. Respiration 44:118, 1983.

750. Zapletal A, Houstek J, Samanek M, et al: Lung function in children and adolescents with idiopathic pulmonary fibrosis. Pediatr Pulmonol 1:154, 1985.

751. Pande JN: Interrelationship between lung volume, expiratory flow, and lung transfer factor in fibrosing alveolitis. Thorax 36:858, 1981.

752. Fulmer JD, Roberts WC, von Gal ER, et al: Morphologic-physiologic correlates of the severity of fibrosis and degree of cellularity in idiopathic pulmonary fibrosis. J Clin Invest 63:665, 1979.

753. Fulmer JD, Roberts WC, Crystal RG: Diffuse fibrotic lung disease: A correlative study. Chest 69:263, 1976.

754. Green GM, Graham WGB, Hanson JS, et al: Correlated studies of interstitial pulmonary disease. Chest 69:263, 1976.

755. Risk C, Epler GR, Gaensler EA: Exercise alveolar-arterial oxygen pressure difference in interstitial lung disease. Chest 85:69, 1984.

756. Sue DY, Oren A, Hansen JE, et al: Diffusing capacity for carbon monoxide as a predictor of gas exchange during exercise. N Engl J Med 316:1301, 1987.

757. Lemle A, Teirstein AS, Bader RA, et al: The distribution of inspired air in interstitial lung disease. Dis Chest 49:502, 1966.

758. Hamer J: Cause of low arterial oxygen saturation in pulmonary fibrosis. Thorax 19:507, 1964.

759. Cassan SM, Divertie MB, Brown AL Jr: Fine structural morphometry on biopsy specimens of human lung. 2. Diffuse idiopathic pulmonary fibrosis. Chest 65:275, 1974.

760. McCarthy D, Cherniack RM: Regional ventilation-perfusion and hypoxia in cryptogenic fibrosing alveolitis. Am Rev Respir Dis 107:200, 1973.

761. Wagner PD, Dantzker DR, Dueck R, et al: Distribution of ventilation-perfusion ratios in patients with interstitial lung disease. Chest 69:256, 1976.

762. Tenholder MF, Russell MD, Knight E, et al: Orthodeoxia: A new finding in interstitial fibrosis. Am Rev Respir Dis 136:170, 1987.

763. Stack BHR, Choo-Kang YFJ, Heard BE: The prognosis of cryptogenic fibrosing alveolitis. Thorax 27:535, 1972.

764. Patchefsky AS, Israel HL, Hoch WS, et al: Desquamative interstitial pneumonia: Relationship to interstitial fibrosis. Thorax 28:680, 1973.

765. Louw SJ, Bateman ED, Benatar SR: Cryptogenic fibrosing alveolitis: Clinical spectrum and treatment. S Afr Med J 65:195, 1984.

766. Carabasi RJ: Diffuse interstitial pulmonary fibrosis (Hamman-Rich syndrome). Report of three cases. Am Rev Tuberc 78:610, 1958.

767. Muschenheim C: Some observations on the Hamman-Rich disease. Am J Med Sci 241:279, 1961.

768. Katzenstein AL, Myers JL, Mazur MT: Acute interstitial pneumonia. A clinicopathologic, ultrastructural, and cell kinetic study. Am J Surg Pathol 10:256, 1986.

769. Haddad R, Massaro D: Idiopathic diffuse interstitial pulmonary fibrosis (fibrosing alveolitis), atypical epithelial proliferation and lung cancer. Am J Med 45:211, 1968.

770. Meyer EC, Liebow AA: Relationship of interstitial pneumonia, honeycombing and atypical epithelial proliferation to cancer of the lung. Cancer 18:322, 1965.

771. Scadding JG: Chronic diffuse interstitial fibrosis of the lungs. Br Med J 1:443, 1960.

772. Lutwyche VU: Another presentation of fibrosing alveolitis and alveolar cell carcinoma. Chest 70:292, 1976.

773. Beaumont F, Jansen HM, Elema JD, et al: Simultaneous occurrence of pulmonary interstitial fibrosis and alveolar cell carcinoma in one family. Thorax 36:252, 1981.

774. Turner-Warwick M, Lebowitz M, Burrows B, et al: Cryptogenic fibrosing alveolitis and lung cancer. Thorax 35:496, 1980.

775. Tukiainen P, Taskinen E, Holsti P, et al: Prognosis of cryptogenic fibrosing alveolitis. Thorax 38:349, 1983.

776. Winterbauer RH, Hammar SP, Hallman KO, et al: Diffuse interstitial pneumonitis: Clinicopathologic correlations in 20 patients treated with prednisone/azathioprine. Am J Med 65:661, 1978.

777. Turner-Warwick M, Burrows B, Johnson A: Cryptogenic fibrosing alveolitis: Response to corticosteroid treatment and its effect on survival. Thorax 35:593, 1980.

778. Rudd RM, Haslam PL, Turner-Warwick M: Cryptogenic fibrosing

alveolitis: Relationships of pulmonary physiology and bronchoalveolar lavage to response to treatment and prognosis. Am Rev Respir Dis 124:1, 1981.
779. Prichard MG, Musk AW: Adverse effect of pregnancy on familial fibrosing alveolitis. Thorax 39:319, 1984.
780. Genereux GP, Merriman JE: Desquamative interstitial pneumonia: Progression to the end-stage lung and the unusual complication of alveolar cell carcinoma. Case report. J Can Assoc Radiol 24:144, 1973.
781. Gaensler EA, Carrington CB, Coutu RE: Chronic interstitial pneumonias. Clin Notes Respir Dis 10:3, 1972.
782. Watters LC, King TE, Schwarz MI, et al: A clinical, radiographic, and physiologic scoring system for the longitudinal assessment of patients with idiopathic pulmonary fibrosis. Am Rev Respir Dis 133:97, 1986.
783. Editorial. Interstitial pneumonia (fibrosing alveolitis). Lancet 2:191, 1978.
784. Rhodes ML: Desquamative interstitial pneumonia. New ultrastructural findings. Am Rev Respir Dis 108:950, 1973.
785. Chester EH, Fleming GM, Montenegro H: Effect of steroid therapy on gas exchange abnormalities in patients with diffuse interstitial lung disease. Chest 69:269, 1976.
786. Bateman ED, Turner-Warwick M, Haslam PL, et al: Cryptogenic fibrosing alveolitis: Prediction of fibrogenic activity from immunohistochemical studies of collagen types in lung biopsy specimens. Thorax 38:93, 1983.
787. Bateman ED, Turner-Warwick M, Adelmann-Grill BC: Immunohistochemical study of collagen types in human foetal lung and fibrotic lung disease. Thorax 36:645, 1981.
788. Studdy PR, Rudd RM, Gellert AR, et al: Bronchoalveolar lavage in the diagnosis of diffuse pulmonary shadowing. Br J Dis Chest 78:46, 1984.
789. Watters LC, King TE, Cherniack RM, et al: Bronchoalveolar lavage fluid neutrophils increase after corticosteroid therapy in smokers with idiopathic pulmonary fibrosis. Am Rev Respir Dis 133:104, 1986.
790. Strumpf IJ, Feld MK, Cornelius MJ, et al: Safety of fiberoptic bronchoalveolar lavage in evaluation of interstitial lung disease. Chest 80:268, 1981.
791. Shindoh Y, Shimura S, Tomioka M, et al: Cellular analysis in bronchoalveolar lavage fluids in infiltrative and fibrotic stages of idiopathic pulmonary fibrosis. Tohoku J Exp Med 149:47, 1986.
792. Peterson MW, Monick M, Hunninghake GW: Prognostic role of eosinophils in pulmonary fibrosis. Chest 92:51, 1987.
793. Ozaki T, Nakayama T, Ishimi H, et al: Glucocorticoid receptors in bronchoalveolar cells from patients with idiopathic pulmonary fibrosis. Am Rev Respir Dis 126:968, 1982.
794. Saldiva PH, Brentani MM, de Carvalho CR, et al: Changes in the pulmonary glucocorticoid receptor content in the course of interstitial disease. Chest 88:417, 1985.
795. Robinson PC, Watters LC, King TE, et al: Idiopathic pulmonary fibrosis, abnormalities in bronchoalveolar lavage fluid phospholipids. Am Rev Respir Dis 137:585, 1988.
796. Robinson PC, Watters LC, King TE, et al: Idiopathic pulmonary fibrosis. Abnormalities in bronchoalveolar lavage fluid phospholipids. Am Rev Respir Dis 137:585, 1988.
797. Enterline HT, Roberts B: Lymphangiopericytoma: Case report of a previously undescribed tumor type. Cancer 8:582, 1955.
798. Cornog JL Jr, Enterline HT: Lymphangiomyoma, a benign lesion of chyliferous lymphatics synonymous with lymphangiopericytoma. Cancer 19:1909, 1966.
799. Berger JL, Shaff MI: Pulmonary lymphangioleiomyomatosis. J Comput Assist Tomog 5(4):565, 1981.
800. Sinclair W, Wright JL, Churg A: Lymphangioleiomyomatosis presenting in a postmenopausal woman. Thorax 40:475, 1985.
801. Capron F, Ameille J, Leclerc P, et al: Pulmonary lymphangioleiomyomatosis and Bourneville's tuberous sclerosis with pulmonary involvement: The same disease? Cancer 52:851, 1983.
802. Valensi QJ: Pulmonary lymphangiomyoma, a probable Forme Frust of tuberous sclerosis. A case report and survey of the literature. Am Rev Respir Dis 108:1411, 1973.
803. Monteforte WJ, Kohnen PW: Angiomyolipomas in a case of lymphangiomyomatosis syndrome: Relationships to tuberous sclerosis. Cancer 34:317, 1974.
804. Harris JO, Waltuck BL, Swenson EW: The pathophysiology of the lungs in tuberous sclerosis. A case report and literature review. Am Rev Respir Dis 100:379, 1969.
805. Lie JT, Miller RD, Williams DE: Cystic disease of the lungs in tuberous sclerosis: Clinicopathologic correlation, including body plethysmographic lung function tests. Mayo Clin Proc 55:547, 1980.
806. Jao J, Gilbert S, Messer R: Lymphangiomyoma and tuberous sclerosis. Cancer 29:1188, 1972.
807. Dwyer JM, Hickie JB, Garvan J: Pulmonary tuberous sclerosis. Report of three patients and a review of the literature. Q J Med 40:115, 1971.
808. Corrin B, Liebow AA, Friedman PJ: Pulmonary lymphangiomyomatosis. Am J Pathol 79:347, 1975.
809. Silverstein EF, Ellis K, Wolff M, et al: Pulmonary lymphangiomyomatosis. Am J Roentgenol 120:832, 1974.
810. Kitzsteiner KA, Mallen RG: Pulmonary lymphangiomyomatosis: Treatment with castration. Cancer 46:2248, 1980.
811. Hughes E, Hodder RV: Pulmonary lymphangiomyomatosis complicating pregnancy. A case report. J Reprod Med 32:553, 1987.
812. Shen A, Iseman MD, Waldron JA, et al: Exacerbation of pulmonary lymphangioleiomyomatosis by exogenous estrogens. Chest 91:782, 1987.
813. Kanbe A, Hajiro K, Adachi Y, et al: Lymphangiomyomatosis associated with chylous ascites and high serum CA-125 levels: A case report. Jpn J Med 26:237, 1987.
814. Sheth RA, Greenberg SD, Jenkins DE, et al: Lymphangiomyomatosis with chylous effusions. South Med J 77:1032, 1984.
815. Svendsen TL, Viskum K, Hansborg N, et al: Pulmonary lymphangioleiomyomatosis: A case of progesterone receptor positive lymphangioleiomyomatosis treated with medroxyprogesterone, oophorectomy and tamoxifen. Br J Dis Chest 78:264, 1984.
816. McCarty KS Jr, Mossler JA, McLelland R, et al: Pulmonary lymphangiomyomatosis responsive to progesterone. N Engl J Med 303:1461, 1980.
817. Dishner W, Cordasco EM, Blackburn J, et al: Pulmonary lymphangiomyomatosis. Chest 85:796, 1984.
818. Sawicka EH, Morris AJ: A report of two long-surviving cases of pulmonary lymphangioleiomyomatosis and the response to progesterone therapy. Br J Dis Chest 79:400, 1985.
819. Graham ML II, Spelsberg TC, Dines DE, et al: Pulmonary lymphangiomyomatosis: With particular reference to steroid-receptor assay studies and pathologic correlation. Mayo Clin Proc 59:3, 1984.
820. Brentani MM, Carvalho CR, Saldiva PH, et al: Steroid receptors in pulmonary lymphangiomyomatosis. Chest 85:96, 1984.
821. Colley MH, Geppert E, Franklin WA: Immunohistochemical detection of steroid receptors in a case of pulmonary lymphangioleiomyomatosis. Am J Surg Pathol 13:803, 1989.
822. El Allaf D, Borlee G, Hadjoudj H, et al: Pulmonary lymphangiomyomatosis. Eur J Respir Dis 65:147, 1984.
823. Oxorn DC, Landrigan P: Anaesthetic management for oophorectomy in pulmonary lymphangiomyomatosis. Can J Anaesth 34:512, 1987.
824. Corrin B, Liebow AA, Friedman PJ: Pulmonary lymphangiomyomatosis. Am J Pathol 79:348, 1975.
825. Carrington CB, Cugell DW, Gaensler EA, et al: Lymphangioleiomyomatosis. Physiologic-pathologic-radiologic correlations. Am Rev Respir Dis 116:977, 1977.
826. Vadas G, Paré JAP, Thurlbeck WM: Pulmonary and lymph node myomatosis: Review of the literature and report of a case. Can Med Assoc J 96:420, 1967.
827. Laipply TC, Sherrick JC: Intrathoracic angiomyomatous hyperplasia associated with chronic chylothorax. Lab Invest 7:387, 1958.
828. Burrell LST, Ross JM: A case of chylous effusion due to leiomyosarcoma. Br J Tuberc 31:38, 1937.
829. Roujeau J, Delarue J, Depierre R: Lymphangiectasie pulmonaire diffuse, pneumonie chyleuse et chylothorax, après thrombose puerpérale de la veine sousclaviére gauche. (Diffuse pulmonary lymphangiectasia, chylous pneumonia and chylothorax, after postpartum thrombosis of the left subclavian vein.) J Fr Med Chir Thorac 4:488, 1950.
830. Jenner RE, Oo HLA: Isolated chylopericardium due to mediastinal lymphangiomatous hamartoma. Thorax 30:113, 1975.
831. Valensi QJ: Pulmonary lymphangiomyoma, a probable forme fruste of tuberous sclerosis. A case report and survey of the literature. Am Rev Respir Dis 108:1411, 1973.
832. Steffelaar JW, Nijkamp DA, Hilvering C: Pulmonary lymphangiomyomatosis. Demonstration of smooth muscle antigens by immunofluorescence technique. Scand J Respir Dis 58:103, 1977.
833. Kane PB, Lane BP, Cordice JWV, et al: Ultrastructure of the proliferating cells in pulmonary lymphangiomyomatosis. Arch Pathol Lab Med 102:618, 1978.
834. Rappaport DC, Weisbrod GL, Herman SJ, et al: Pulmonary lymphangioleiomyomatosis: High-resolution CT findings in four cases. Am J Roentgenol 152:961, 1989.
835. Sherrier RH, Chiles C, Roggli V: Pulmonary lymphangioleiomyomatosis: CT findings. Am J Roentgenol 153:937, 1989.
836. Stovin PGI, Lum LC, Flower CDR, et al: The lungs in lymphangiomyomatosis and in tuberous sclerosis. Thorax 30:497, 1975.
837. Chew QT, Nouri MS: Pulmonary and retroperitoneal lymphangiomyomatosis. Clinical and radiographic features. NY State J Med 79:250, 1979.
838. Bhatti MA, Ferrante JW, Gielchinsky I, et al: Pleuropulmonary and skeletal lymphangiomatosis with chylothorax and chylopericardium. Ann Thorac Surg 40:398, 1985.
839. Carlson KC, Parnassus WH, Klatt EC: Thoracic lymphangiomatosis. Arch Pathol Lab Med 111:475, 1987.

17

840. Lagos JC, Gomez MR: Tuberous sclerosis: Reappraisal of a clinical entity. Mayo Clin Proc *42*:26, 1967.
841. Dawson J: Pulmonary tuberous sclerosis and its relationship to other forms of the disease. Q J Med *23*:113, 1954.
842. Capron F, Ameille J, Leclerc P, et al: Pulmonary lymphangioleiomyomatosis and Bourneville's tuberous sclerosis with pulmonary involvement: The same disease? Cancer *52*:851, 1983.
843. Liberman BA, Chamberlain DW, Goldstein RS: Tuberous sclerosis with pulmonary involvement. Can Med Assoc J *130*:287, 1984.
844. Babcock TL, Snyder BA: Spontaneous pneumothorax associated with tuberous sclerosis. J Thorac Cardiovasc Surg *83*:100, 1982.
845. Mestres CA, Catalan M, Letang E, et al: Tuberous sclerosis and associated pleuropulmonary lesions. Thorac Cardiovasc Surg *31*:243, 1983.
846. Broughton RBK: Pulmonary tuberous sclerosis presenting with pleural effusion. Br Med J *1*:477, 1970.
847. Riccardi VM: von Recklinghausen neurofibromatosis. N Engl J Med *305*:1617, 1981.
848. Burkhalter JL, Morano JU, McCay MB: Diffuse interstitial lung disease in neurofibromatosis. South Med J *79*:944, 1986.
849. Larrieu AJ, Hashimoto SA, Allen P: Spontaneous massive haemothorax in von Recklinghausen's disease. Thorax *37*:151, 1982.
850. Riccardi VM, Wheeler TM, Pickard LR, et al: The pathophysiology of neurofibromatosis. II. Angiosarcoma as a complication. Cancer Genet Cytogenet *12*:275, 1984.
851. Arpornchayanon O, Hirota T, Itabashi M, et al: Malignant peripheral nerve tumors: A clinicopathological and electron microscopic study. Jpn J Clin Oncol *14*:57, 1984.
852. Bourgouin PM, Shepard JA, Moore EH, et al: Plexiform neurofibromatosis of the mediastinum: CT appearance. Am J Roentgenol *151*:461, 1988.
853. Unger PD, Geller SA, Anderson PJ: Pulmonary lesions in a patient with neurofibromatosis. Arch Pathol Lab Med *108*:654, 1984.
854. Larrieu AJ, Hashimoto SA, Allen P: Spontaneous massive haemothorax in von Recklinghausen's disease. Thorax *37*:151, 1982.
855. Webb WR, Goodman PC: Fibrosing alveolitis in patients with neurofibromatosis. Radiology *122*:289, 1977.
856. Klatte EC, Franken EA, Smith JA: The radiographic spectrum in neurofibromatosis. Semin Roentgenol *11*:17, 1976.
857. De Scheerder I, Elinck W, Van Renterghem D, et al: Desquamative interstitial pneumonia and scar cancer of the lung complicating generalized neurofibromatosis. Eur J Respir Dis *65*:623, 1984.
858. Porterfield JK, Pyeritz RE, Traill TA: Pulmonary hypertension and interstitial fibrosis in von Recklinghausen neurofibromatosis. Am J Med Genet *25*:531, 1986.
859. Lichtenstein L: Histiocytosis X: Integration of eosinophilic granuloma of bone. "Letterer-Siwe disease" and "Schüller-Christian disease" as related manifestations of a single nosologic entity. Arch Pathol *56*:84, 1953.
860. Lieberman PH, Jones CR, Dargeon HW, et al: A reappraisal of eosinophilic granuloma of bone, Hand-Schüller-Christian syndrome and Letterer-Siwe syndrome. Medicine *48*:375, 1969.
861. Groopman JE, Golde DW: The histiocytic disorders: A pathophysiologic analysis. Ann Intern Med *94*:95, 1981.
862. Kaufman A, Bukberg PR, Werlin S, et al: Multifocal eosinophilic granuloma ("Hand-Schüller-Christian disease"). Report illustrating H-S-C chronicity and diagnostic challenge. Am J Med *60*:541, 1976.
863. Dunmore LA Jr, El-Khoury SA: Eosinophilic granuloma of the lung. A report of three cases in Negro patients. Am Rev Respir Dis *90*:789, 1964.
864. Avery ME, McAfee JG, Guild HG: The course and prognosis of reticuloendotheliosis (eosinophilic granuloma) (Schüller-Christian disease and Letterer-Siwe disease). Am J Med *22*:636, 1957.
865. Lewis JG: Eosinophilic granuloma and its variants with special reference to lung involvement. A report of 12 patients. Q J Med *33*:337, 1964.
866. Williams AW, Dunnington WG, Berte SJ: Pulmonary eosinophilic granuloma: A clinical and pathologic discussion. Ann Intern Med *54*:30, 1961.
867. Nadeau PJ, Ellis FH Jr, Harrison EG Jr, et al: Primary pulmonary histiocytosis X. Dis Chest *37*:325, 1960.
868. Lacronique J, Roth C, Battesti J-P, et al: Chest radiological features of pulmonary histiocytosis X: A report based on 50 adult cases. Thorax *37*:104, 1982.
869. Friedman PJ, Liebow AA, Sokoloff J: Eosinophilic granuloma of lung: Clinical aspects of primary pulmonary histiocytosis in the adult. Medicine *60*:385, 1981.
870. Colby TV, Lombard C: Histiocytosis X in the lung. Human Pathol *14*:847, 1983.
871. Enriquez P, Dahlin DC, Hayles AB, et al: Histiocytosis X: A clinical study. Mayo Clin Proc *42*:88, 1967.
872. Osband ME, Lipton JM, Lavin P, et al: Histiocytosis X: Demonstration of abnormal immunity, T-cell histamine H$_2$-receptor deficiency, and successful treatment with thymic extract. N Engl J Med *304*:146, 1981.
873. Favara BE, McCarthy RC, Mierau GW: Histiocytosis X. Human Pathol *14*:663, 1983.
874. Greenberger JS, Crocker AC, Vawter G, et al: Results of treatment of 127 patients with systemic histiocytosis (Letterer-Siwe's syndrome, Schuller-Christian syndrome and multifocal eosinophilic granuloma). Medicine *60*:311, 1981.
875. Shapiro DN, Hutchinson RJ: Familial histiocytosis in offspring of two pregnancies after artificial insemination. N Engl J Med *304*:757, 1981.
876. King TE Jr, Schwarz MI, Dreisin RE, et al: Circulating immune complexes in pulmonary eosinophilic granuloma. Ann Intern Med *91*:397, 1979.
877. Weinberger SE, Kelman JA, Elson NA, et al: Bronchoalveolar lavage in interstitial lung disease. Ann Intern Med *89*:459, 1978.
878. Basset F, Corrin B, Spencer H, et al: Pulmonary histiocytosis X. Am Rev Respir Dis *118*:811, 1978.
879. Bickers JN, Buechner HA, Ekman PJ: Pulmonary eosinophilic granuloma. Its natural history and prognosis. Am Rev Respir Dis *85*:211, 1962.
880. Knudson RJ, Badger TL, Gaensler EA: Eosinophilic granuloma of the lung. Med Thorac *23*:248, 1966.
881. Spencer H: Pathology of the Lung: Excluding Pulmonary Tuberculosis. London–New York, Pergamon Press, 1962.
882. Hoffman L, Cohn JE, Gaensler EA: Respiratory abnormalities in eosinophilic granuloma of the lung. Long-term study of five cases. N Engl J Med *267*:577, 1962.
883. Powers MA, Askin FB, Cresson DH: Pulmonary eosinophilic granuloma. 25-year follow-up. Am Rev Respir Dis *129*:503, 1984.
884. Pomeranz SJ, Proto AV: Histiocytosis X. Unusual-confusing features of eosinophilic granuloma. Chest *89*:88, 1986.
885. Flint A, Lloyd RV, Colby TV, et al: Pulmonary histiocytosis X. Immunoperoxidase staining for HLA-DR antigen and S100 protein. Arch Pathol Lab Med *110*:930, 1986.
886. Soler P, Chollet S, Jacque C, et al: Immunocytochemical characterization of pulmonary histiocytosis X cells in lung biopsies. Am J Pathol *118*:439, 1985.
887. Webber D, Tron V, Askin F, et al: S-100 staining in the diagnosis of eosinophilic granuloma of lung. Am J Clin Pathol *84*:447, 1985.
888. Akhtar M, Ali MA, Sabbah R: Ultrastructure of histiocytosis X. A study of 9 cases with review of the literature. King Faisal Specialist Hospital Medical Journal *4*:137, 1984.
889. Ide F, Iwase T, Saito I, et al: Immunohistochemical and ultrastructural analysis of the proliferating cells in histiocytosis X. Cancer *53*:917, 1984.
890. Verea-Hernando H, Fontan-Bueso J, Martin-Egana MT, et al: Langerhans' cells in bronchoalveolar lavage in the late stages of pulmonary histiocytosis X. Chest *81*:130, 1982.
891. Basset F, Soler P, Jaurand MC, et al: Ultrastructural examination of broncho-alveolar lavage for diagnosis of pulmonary histiocytosis X: preliminary report on 4 cases. Thorax *32*:303, 1977.
892. Tellis CJ, Hunt KK Jr: Eosinophilic granuloma with pulmonary involvement: A review. Military Med *143*:256, 1978.
893. Arnett NL, Schulz DM: Primary pulmonary eosinophilic granuloma. Radiology *69*:224, 1957.
894. Thompson J, Buechner RHA, Fishman R: Eosinophilic granuloma of the lung. Ann Intern Med *48*:1134, 1958.
895. Kittredge RD, Geller A, Finby N: The reticuloendothelioses in the lung. Am J Roentgenol *100*:588, 1967.
896. Weber WN, Margolin FR, Nielsen SL: Pulmonary histiocytosis X. A review of 18 patients with reports of 6 cases. Am J Roentgenol *107*:280, 1969.
897. Clark RL, Margulies SI, Mulholland JH: Histiocytosis X. A fatal case with unusual pulmonary manifestations. Radiology *95*:631, 1970.
898. McLetchie NGB, Reynolds DP: Histiocytic reticulosis and honeycomb lungs. Can Med Assoc J *71*:44, 1954.
899. Takahashi M, Martel W, Oberman HA: The variable roentgenographic appearance of idiopathic histiocytosis. Clin Radiol *17*:48, 1966.
900. Carlson RA, Hattery RR, O'Connell EJ, et al: Pulmonary involvement by histiocytosis X in the pediatric age group. Mayo Clin Proc *51*:542, 1976.
901. Tittel PW, Winkler CF: Chronic recurrent pleural effusion in adult histiocytosis X. Br J Radiol *54*:68, 1981.
902. Tittel PW, Winkler CF: Chronic recurrent pleural effusion in adult histiocytosis X. Br J Radiol *54*:68, 1981.
903. Guardia J, Pedreira J-D, Esteban R, et al: Early pleural effusion in histiocytosis X. Arch Intern Med *139*:934, 1979.
904. Matlin AH, Young LW, Klemperer MR: Pleural effusion in two children with histiocytosis X. Chest *61*:33, 1972.
905. Roland AS, Merdinger WF, Froeb HF: Recurrent spontaneous pneumothorax. A clue to the diagnosis of histiocytosis X. N Engl J Med *270*:73, 1964.
906. Laios NC, Lovelock FJ: Eosinophilic granuloma of the lung. Am Rev Respir Dis *83*:394, 1961.

907. Gelfand ET, Sheiner NM: Pneumothorax in pulmonary eosinophilic granuloma. Can Med Assoc J 110:937, 1974.
908. Konno K, Hayashi I, Oka S: Eosinophilic granuloma (histiocytosis X) involving anterior chest wall and lung. Am Rev Respir Dis 100:391, 1969.
909. Meier B, Rhyner K, Medici TC, et al: Eosinophilic granuloma of the skeleton with involvement of the lung: A report of three cases. Eur J Respir Dis 64:551, 1983.
910. Langer A, Fettes I: Multifocal eosinophilic granuloma with a pituitary stalk lesion. West J Med 142:829, 1985.
911. Bank A, Christensen C: Unusual manifestation of Langerhans' cell histiocytosis. Acta Med Scand 223:479, 1988.
912. Pongor F, Viragh Z: Pulmonary histiocytosis X with diabetes insipidus. Am Rev Tuberc 79:652, 1959.
913. Bates DV, Macklem PT, Christie RV: Respiratory Function in Disease; an Introduction to the Integrated Study of the Lung, 2nd ed. Philadelphia, WB Saunders, 1971.
914. Divertie MB, Cassan SM, Brown AL Jr: Application of ultrastructural morphometry to lung biopsy specimens in pulmonary histiocytosis X. Thorax 30:326, 1975.
915. Melhem RE, Hajjar JJ, Balassanian N: Histiocytosis X. A report of 15 cases in the paediatric age group. Br J Radiol 37:898, 1964.
916. Recant L, Hartroft WS (eds, case report): Rapidly progressive pulmonary infiltration, fever and coma. Am J Med 24:437, 1958.
917. Pruzanski W, Altman R: Histiocytosis X in adult with predominant pulmonary manifestation. Arch Intern Med 113:261, 1964.
918. Petheram IS, Holmes P, Turner-Warwick M: Penicillamine in eosinophilic granuloma. Br J Dis Chest 75:410, 1981.
919. Komp DM, Herson J, Starling KA, et al: A staging system for histiocytosis X: A Southwest Oncology Group study. Cancer 47:798, 1981.
920. Barnard NJ, Crocker PR, Blainey AD, et al: Pulmonary alveolar microlithiasis. A new analytical approach. Histopathology 11:639, 1987.
921. Sosman MC, Dodd GD, Jones WD, et al: The familial occurrence of pulmonary alveolar microlithiasis. Am J Roentgenol 77:947, 1957.
922. Prakash UBS, Barham SS, Rosenow EC III, et al: Pulmonary alveolar microlithiasis. A review including ultrastructural and pulmonary function studies. Mayo Clin Proc 58:290, 1983.
923. Miro JM, Moreno A, Coca A, et al: Pulmonary alveolar microlithiasis with an unusual radiological pattern. Br J Dis Chest 76:91, 1982.
924. Kino T, Kohara Y, Tsuji S: Pulmonary alveolar microlithiasis. A report of two young sisters. Am Rev Respir Dis 105:105, 1972.
925. Caffrey PR, Altman RS: Pulmonary alveolar microlithiasis occurring in premature twins. J Pediatr 66:758, 1965.
926. Sears MR, Chang AR, Taylor AJ: Pulmonary alveolar microlithiasis. Thorax 26:704, 1971.
927. Gómez GE, Lichtemberger E, Santamaria A, et al: Familial pulmonary alveolar microlithiasis: Four cases from Colombia, S.A. Is microlithiasis also an environmental disease? Radiology 72:550, 1959.
928. Oka S, Shiraishi K, Ogata K, et al: Clinical course, roentgenographic findings and pulmonary function in pulmonary alveolar microlithiasis. Jap J Chest Dis 24:263, 1965.
929. Häberlin F: Beitrag zur Ikonographie miliarer Lungenerkrankungen. (Contribution to the iconography of miliary lung disease.) Schweiz Z Tuberk 15:226, 1958.
930. Doehnett HR, Gomez L: Pulmonary microlithiasis. Rev Tisiol Neumonol 5:63, 1963.
931. Drinković I, Strohal K, Sabljica B: Mikrolithiasis alveolaris pulmonum. (Pulmonary alveolar microlithiasis.) Fortschr Roentgenstr 97:180, 1962.
932. Viswanathan R: Pulmonary alveolar microlithiasis. Thorax 17:251, 1962.
933. Waters MH: Microlithiasis alveolaris pulmonum. Tubercle 41:276, 1960.
934. Winzelberg GG, Boller M, Sachs M, et al: CT evaluation of pulmonary alveolar microlithiasis. J Comput Assist Tomogr 8:1029, 1984.
935. Chinachoti N, Tangchai P: Pulmonary alveolar microlithiasis associated with the inhalation of snuff in Thailand. Dis Chest 32:687, 1957.
936. Greenberg MJ: Miliary shadows in the lungs due to microlithiasis alveolaris pulmonum. Thorax 12:171, 1957.
937. O'Neill RP, Cohn JE, Pellegrino ED: Pulmonary alveolar microlithiasis—A family study. Ann Intern Med 67:957, 1967.
938. Badger TL, Gottlieb L, Gaensler EA: Pulmonary alveolar microlithiasis, or calcinosis of the lungs. N Engl J Med 253:709, 1955.
939. Bünger P, Fassbender CW, Schültze G: Zur Mikrolithiasis alveolaris pulmonum. (Pulmonary alveolar microlithiasis.) Fortschr Roentgenstr 97:775, 1962.
940. Portnoy LM, Amadeo B, Hennigar GR: Pulmonary alveolar microlithiasis. An unusual case (associated with milk-alkali syndrome). Am J Clin Pathol 41:194, 1964.
941. Bush M, James AE Jr, Montali RJ, et al: Pulmonary alveolar microlithiasis in a binturong (Arctictis binturong): A case report. J Am Vet Radiol Soc 17:157, 1976.
942. Greenspan R: Personal communication, 1968.
943. Bab I, Rosenmann E, Ne'eman Z, et al: The occurrence of extracellular matrix vesicles in pulmonary alveolar microlithiasis. Virchows Arch (Pathol Anat) 391:357, 1981.
944. Tao L-C: Microliths in sputum specimens and their relationship to pulmonary alveolar microlithiasis. Am J Clin Pathol 69:482, 1978.
945. Kawakami M, Sato S, Takishima T: Electron microscopic studies on pulmonary alveolar microlithiasis. Tohoku J Exp Med 126:343, 1978.
946. Hawass ND, Noah MS: Pulmonary alveolar microlithiasis. Eur J Respir Dis 69:199, 1986.
947. Krokowski E, Michel H: Das Röntgenbild im Verlauf der Mikrolithiasis alveolaris pulmonum. (The roentgenogram in the course of microlithiasis alveolaris pulmonum.) Fortschr Roentgenstr 105:201, 1966.
948. Rotem Y, Solomon M, Hertz-Frankenhuis M: Pulmonary alveolar microlithiasis. Ann Paediat 201(Suppl):4, 1963.
949. Thind GS, Bhatia JL: Pulmonary alveolar microlithiasis. Br J Dis Chest 72:151, 1978.
950. Chalmers AG, Wyatt J, Robinson PJ: Computed tomographic and pathological findings in pulmonary alveolar microlithiasis. Br J Radiol 59:408, 1986.
951. Cole WR: Pulmonary alveolar microlithiasis. J Fac Radiol 10:54, 1959.
952. Varma BN: Pulmonary alveolar microlithiasis in a child of thirteen years. Br J Dis Chest 57:213, 1963.
953. Oka S, Shiraishi K, Ogata K, et al: Pulmonary alveolar microlithiasis. Report of three cases. Am Rev Respir Dis 93:612, 1966.
954. Brown ML, Swee RG, Olson RJ, et al: Pulmonary uptake of 99mTc diphosphonate in alveolar microlithiasis. Am J Roentgenol 131:703, 1978.
955. Garty I, Giladi N, Flatau E: Bone scintigraphy in two siblings with pulmonary alveolar microlithiasis. Br J Radiol 58:763, 1985.
956. Palombini BC, Porto NS, Wallau CV, et al: Bronchopulmonary lavage in alveolar microlithiasis (letter). Anaesth Intensive Care 6:265, 1978.
957. Cale WF, Petsonk EL, Boyd CB: Transbronchial biopsy of pulmonary alveolar microlithiasis. Arch Intern Med 143:358, 1983.
958. Fuleihan FJD, Abboud RT, Balikian JP, et al: Pulmonary alveolar microlithiasis: Lung function in five cases. Thorax 24:84, 1969.
959. Brown J, Leon W, Felton C: Hemodynamic and pulmonary studies in pulmonary alveolar microlithiasis. Am J Med 77:176, 1984.
960. Policard A, Collet A: Deposition of siliceous dust in the lungs of the inhabitants of the Saharan regions. Arch Ind Hyg Occup Med 5:527, 1952.
961. Hawass ND: An association "between desert lung" and cataract—A new syndrome. Br J Ophthalmol 71:694, 1987.
962. Wirostko E, Johnson L, Wirostko B: Sarcoidosis-associated uveitis. Parasitization of vitreous leucocytes by mollicute-like organisms. Acta Ophthalmol 67:415, 1989.
963. Gadek JE, Kelman JA, Fells G, et al: Collagenase in the lower respiratory tract of patients with idiopathic pulmonary fibrosis. N Engl J Med 301:737, 1979.

18

The Pleura

The precise incidence of pleural abnormality in association with chest disease is unknown, but it is seen in a sufficient proportion of roentgenograms of hospital patients that its importance cannot be overestimated. Pleural effusion—the most important, if not the most frequent, abnormality observed—may occur alone without other changes in the thorax or may accompany abnormalities of the lungs, mediastinum, or chest wall. In the former circumstance, diagnosis may prove exceedingly difficult, even with bacteriologic, biochemical, and pathologic investigative techniques. When effusion occurs as part of a complex of roentgenographic changes, however, it may provide an important diagnostic clue. Often its cause is immediately apparent—for example, when it accompanies enlargement of the heart and is the result of cardiac decompensation, or when it occurs as a hemothorax in association with multiple rib fractures following trauma to the chest wall. Just as often, however, an effusion constitutes one facet of a complex of roentgen signs that tries the diagnostic skills of the physician.

This chapter is concerned with the diagnosis and differential diagnosis of diseases of the pleura. The physiologic mechanisms underlying the formation and absorption of pleural fluid (see page 175), the roentgenologic signs of pleural disease (see page 663), the use of ultrasound in the detection of loculated effusion[1-4] (see pages 349 and 677), and the diagnostic methods used in analyzing pleural fluid (see pages 354 and 422) should be studied in conjunction with this chapter. The value of various procedures as aids to the diagnosis of specific causes of pleural disease is discussed in appropriate sections.

PLEURAL EFFUSION

As discussed in Chapter 1, fluid movement at both the parietal and the visceral layers of pleura is determined not only by the Starling (fluid transport) equation but by lymphatic drainage and the surface area of the parietal and visceral pleural membranes.[5] In disease states, alteration in one or more of these factors results in the accumulation of excess fluid within the pleural space. Inflammation results in an increase in both filtration coefficient and local blood flow, the latter causing a rise in capillary hydrostatic pressure. Protein loss into the pleural space increases both intrapleural colloid osmotic pressure and intrapleural hydrostatic pressure. When protein concentration in the pleural fluid increases to 4 g per 100 ml or more, absorption pressure in the visceral pleural capillaries reaches zero, so that any subsequent absorption of pleural fluid must be by way of the lymphatics until protein concentration is lowered. Transudation into the pleural space occurs when hydrostatic pressure rises in both the visceral and parietal pleural capillaries or when there is a severe fall in colloid osmotic pressure of the plasma. The efficiency of lymphatic drainage may be diminished by fibrosis or neoplastic involvement of mediastinal lymph nodes, by thickening of pleural membranes, by hypoplasia of draining lymphatics, by obstruction in the thoracic duct, or by systemic venous hypertension.

The character of fluid in the pleural space—transudate, exudate, pus, blood, chyle, or any combination of these—is seldom, if ever, discernible roentgenologically; therefore "increase in pleural fluid," and not "pleural effusion," should be the correct term for reporting these roentgenographic appearances. Because it is in common usage, however, the term "pleural effusion" is used here. Where appropriate, the precise terms *hydrothorax* (for serous effusions, either transudate or exudate), *pyothorax, hemothorax,* and *chylothorax* are employed.

Since the etiologic diagnosis of pleural effusion depends largely on whether or not there is other disease in the lungs, mediastinum, diaphragm, or chest wall, the approach to differential diagnosis must be along different lines when effusion is the sole abnormality and when one or more of these structures is affected. Justification for this approach can be found in a report by Rabin and Blackman[6] of 78 cases of bilateral pleural effusion of widely varying etiology. Only 29 showed additional roentgenographic shadows that directed attention to a specific etiology. In the remaining 49 cases, almost two thirds of the series, no other abnormalities were apparent that might aid in diagnosis of the disease causing the effusion. Detailed reference to this excellent analysis is made later in this chapter. It is important to note that underlying pulmonary or mediastinal disease is not always detectable on the first available roentgenograms. Large effusions may mask parenchymal shadows or mediastinal masses, and these may become evident only when fluid has been removed or when special roentgenography in the supine or lateral decubitus position renders the underlying lung or mediastinal contour visible.

"Associated findings" include *any* abnormality on the chest roentgenogram other than the pleural fluid. For example, an elevated hemidiaphragm (not to be confused with infrapulmonary effusion) constitutes a significant additional finding in that it may point to acute subphrenic disease as the etiologic basis for a small effusion. Similarly, an enlarged spleen, despite its extrathoracic position, may be visible on a chest roentgenogram and is of potential significance in differential diagnosis. Finally, an absent breast shadow bears clear testimony to the possibility of metastatic carcinoma as the provocative agent.

As in preceding chapters in this book, the contents of this chapter are presented in two ways, each designed to complement the other. In the text, conditions with which effusion is commonly associated are discussed on the basis of etiologic classification, such as infections, neoplasms, immunologic disease, thromboembolism, trauma, congestion, and incidental causes. The tables in the Appendix give a classification on the basis of roentgenographic patterns. Table A–14 presents the causes of pleural effusion occurring as the sole abnormality on the chest roentgenogram, and Table A–15 indicates the causes when effusion is associated with specific abnormalities in the lungs, mediastinum, or chest wall. Reference to the tables is recommended as the first step in narrowing down possibilities of differential diagnosis to a few diseases on the strength of a specific roentgenographic pattern. Further discussion of each entity is given in the text.

CLINICAL MANIFESTATIONS

Pleural pain is a frequent manifestation of "dry" pleurisy (see page 280) but often diminishes when effusion develops. In some cases the pain is not accentuated by breathing and is felt as a dull ache. The parietal pleura is innervated by branches of the intercostal nerves; thus, pleural pain usually is well localized, although it may be referred to the abdomen. When the phrenic nerve endings are irritated by inflammation of the diaphragmatic pleura, the pain may be felt in the shoulder. A dry cough may become productive if there is an associated pneumonia. Dyspnea is common; if it is severe and associated with decreased respiratory reserve, immediate thoracentesis may be required for relief. The severe mediastinal displacement that occurs in tension hydrothorax can cause respiratory distress, dysphagia, engorged neck veins, a tender liver, and edema of the lower extremities;[7] thoracentesis is characteristically followed by immediate relief of symptoms and signs.

Physical examination reveals dullness or flatness on percussion and a decrease or absence of breath sounds. When dullness on percussion is shifting, this sign by itself is diagnostic. Breath sounds may persist even when the effusion is large, and may sound distant and be bronchial in type. The explanation for this discrepancy is not always apparent. In 13 of 21 patients with protracted unilateral pleural effusion, examination showed edema of the ipsilateral chest wall; these patients proved to have either empyema or a malignant effusion.[8] Another rare cause of ipsilateral chest wall "edema" is illustrated in Figure 18–1.

PULMONARY FUNCTION STUDIES

The results of pulmonary function studies in cases of pleural effusion depend on the presence and nature of underlying pulmonary disease and are so variable that little information of value has been published. In the absence of underlying pulmonary disease, the effects of pleural effusion on pulmonary function reflect the combination of a space-occupying process and a reduction in lung volume as a consequence of relaxation atelectasis. The space-occupying process reduces all subdivisions of lung volume, including total lung capacity (TLC), functional residual capacity (FRC), and vital capacity (VC), although ventilatory ability may be little impaired when the other lung is normal and there is no pleural pain inhibiting chest movement.[9] Depending on the amount of fluid and, therefore, on the degree of ipsilateral pulmonary collapse, diffusing capacity may be moderately diminished but often remains within the predicted normal range. Blood gas concentrations may be normal; arterial oxygen saturation usually is unaffected, even with a major degree of relaxation atelectasis, since perfusion adjusts downward in response to the reduction in ventilation. Arterial PCO_2 may decrease if unilateral pulmonary collapse results in hyperventilation, but otherwise it remains unaffected.

Arterial oxygen saturation can fall significantly in the lateral decubitus position when the hemithorax with the pleural effusion is dependent, a phenomenon that can also occur in the presence of parenchymal consolidation.[10, 11] The slight but significant increase in PaO_2 and lung volumes and the decrease in $P(A-a)O_2$ that occur in some patients following thoracentesis are insufficient to explain the relief of dyspnea that is commonly experienced. Estenne and coworkers[12] have suggested that this results from a reduction in the size of the thoracic cage that allows the inspiratory muscles to operate on a more advantageous portion of their length-tension curve. In some patients, thoracentesis results in hypoxemia, presumably as a result of the development of pulmonary edema: Brandstetter and Cohen[13] reported this phenomenon in 15 patients in whom a significant drop in PaO_2 was recorded 20 minutes and 2 hours after thoracentesis; pre-aspiration levels had returned within 24 hours.

Using radioactive xenon, Anthonisen and Martin[14] studied the regional lung function of six patients with a small unilateral pleural effusion and found a reduction in count rate at the base of the lung that they considered to be the result of displacement rather than compression of lung. This conclusion was based on the observation that the distribution of boluses that were inhaled slowly from residual volume was no different on the side with the effusion than on the contralateral normal side.

LABORATORY PROCEDURES

The biochemical and other characteristics of pleural effusions were discussed in Chapter 3 (see

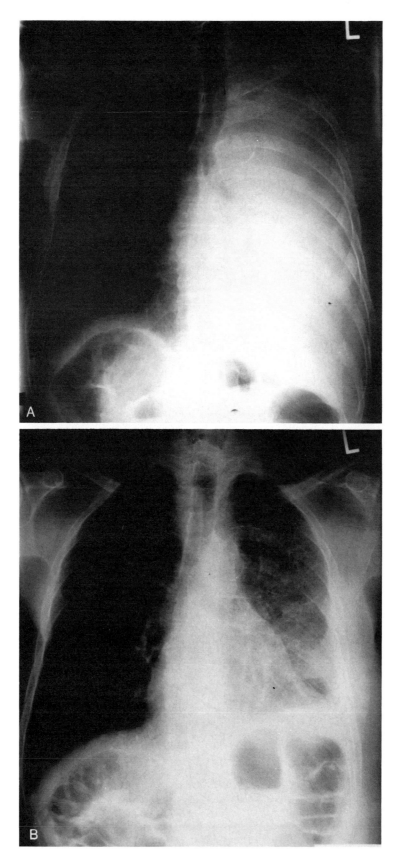

Figure 18–1. Ipsilateral Chest Wall Swelling Following Thoracentesis. A posteroanterior roentgenogram *(A)* reveals a massive left pleural effusion; note the markedly depressed left hemidiaphragm. Thoracentesis was attempted, but only 50 ml of straw-colored fluid could be removed. Despite this, a roentgenogram obtained following thoracentesis *(B)* shows virtually no fluid remaining in the pleural space; however, note that a marked increase in the thickness of the left chest wall has occurred.

Illustration continued on following page

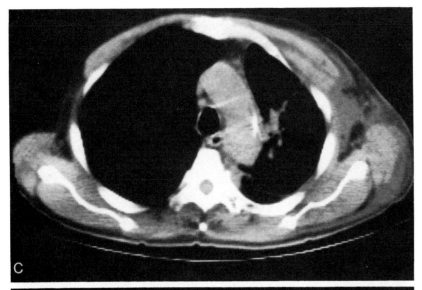

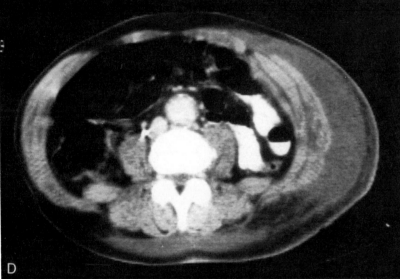

Figure 18–1 *Continued* CT scans at the level of the aortic arch *(C)* and upper abdomen *(D)* show a marked increase in the volume of soft tissue in the left chest wall and abdomen that was caused by drainage of pleural fluid through the needle tract created for thoracentesis. The cause of the pleural effusion in this 62-year-old man was metastatic adenocarcinoma from a primary in the bowel.

page 422) and were summarized in Table 3–5 (*see* pages 424 and 425). Although in most cases the combination of clinical presentation and appropriate laboratory tests will lead to a positive diagnosis, sometimes the etiology of pleural effusion remains undetermined even after complete diagnostic evaluation. In patients in whom associated clinical and roentgenographic findings fail to indicate the etiology, the usual sequence of diagnostic procedures includes thoracentesis (with hematologic, cytologic, and biochemical analysis of fluid), closed pleural biopsy, and finally thoracoscopic (pleuroscopic) or open pleural biopsy. However, since 25 to 30 per cent of pleural effusions do not recur and follow-up indicates benign causes,[15–18] patients would obviously benefit if certain clinical characteristics could be found that would reflect benignity and thus serve to prevent the morbidity and mortality associated with invasive procedures. In one study of 119 patients in whom closed pleural biopsy and subsequent follow-up established the pleural effusion as being

malignant (n = 41), granulomatous (n = 25), or nonspecific (n = 53) in nature,[19] certain findings appeared to distinguish the patients with tuberculosis and malignancy from those with nonspecific pleuritis. These findings included weight loss, fever greater than 38° C, a positive PPD, pleural lymphocytosis greater than 95 per cent, and an effusion that occupied more than half a hemithorax. Based on the results of this study, the authors recommended a conservative approach for patients in whom closed pleural biopsy reveals only nonspecific pleuritis and in whom the clinical criteria are all negative. An aggressive diagnostic workup is indicated for patients with two or more positive findings. In a retrospective assessment of 27 patients with pleural effusion in whom the etiology was not obvious, Gunnels[16] concluded that when neoplastic or granulomatous disease is not suspected before surgery, pleuroscopic or open biopsy (or both) is usually nondiagnostic and that such patients are best managed conservatively. However, in a review of 28 cases of pleural effusion of unknown etiology out of a consecutive series of 110 patients subjected to needle biopsy, Black[20] obtained a definitive diagnosis following thoracotomy in 16 cases (57 per cent), the rest showing nonspecific inflammation.

The etiology of effusion is multifactorial in some cases. For example, the transformation of a transudate to an exudate following treatment of heart failure may indicate the presence of underlying thromboembolic disease or malignancy.[21] Rarely, bilateral pleural effusions have a different etiology; this combination is known as "Contarini's condition," a reference to the 95th doge of Venice who died in 1625 with orthopnea, foul-smelling sputum, cardiac arrhythmia, and clear pleural fluid on one side and pus on the other.[22] Examples of this unusual combination have been reported in the more recent literature.[22, 23]

PLEURAL EFFUSION CAUSED BY INFECTION

Pleural infections usually produce an exudative effusion (i.e., with a protein content greater than 3 g per 100 ml). The inflammatory reaction results in increased capillary permeability, causing protein loss from capillaries. According to Black,[5] reabsorption of fluid and protein by the lymphatics may be impaired when fibrin deposition and inflammatory thickening of the pleural membrane occur. By far the most common etiologic agents of infectious pleural effusion are the bacteria; the fungi, viruses, and parasites are much less frequent causes.

PLEURAL EFFUSION CAUSED BY BACTERIA

Mycobacterium tuberculosis

In many areas of the world, tuberculosis remains the most common cause of pleural effusion in the absence of demonstrable pulmonary disease.[24] However, in other areas such as parts of the United States, tuberculous pleural effusion is becoming a rarity. For example, of 108 patients with pleural effusion studied at the Mayo Clinic,[15] only 1 had effusion of tuberculous etiology. Even in inner city areas in the United States where tuberculosis is not uncommon, tuberculous pleural effusion is surprisingly unusual. Light and his colleagues[25] found only 13 per cent of 103 exudative pleural effusions in Baltimore to be of this etiology.

Tuberculous pleural effusion occurs most commonly in young adults, a fact that was emphasized by Stead.[26] Although it may complicate established pulmonary tuberculosis—when its presence invariably indicates activity of the pulmonary disease—it also presents as uncomplicated "pleurisy with effusion." Pleural effusion as a manifestation of primary tuberculosis occurs more commonly in adults than

in children. Both Weber and coworkers[27] and Durham[28] observed effusion in only 10 per cent of their child patients, whereas Stead and his associates[29] reported it in 38 per cent of their adult cases. In eight of Weber and associates' nine cases, the effusion was mild to moderate in degree and was associated with roentgenographic evidence of pulmonary disease; in the ninth case it was the sole manifestation of disease. In some cases of well-established postprimary infection of the lungs, the development of pleural effusion has been well documented, even after the initiation of chemotherapy.[30]

Tuberculous pleural effusion is believed to result from rupture of subpleural foci of caseous necrosis into the adjacent pleural space, initiating a delayed hypersensitivity reaction.[31, 32] Several investigators[33–35] have demonstrated T lymphocytes in tuberculous pleural fluid that are specifically sensitized to PPD. This delayed hypersensitivity reaction can occur in the pleura of some patients who fail to react to cutaneous PPD, a fact that is explained by the presence in the circulation of suppressor cells that inhibit response in the skin; these suppressor cells are apparently lacking in the pleural fluid.[33] The small caseous foci that spill their contents into the pleural space usually cannot be seen on conventional chest roentgenograms but have been documented pathologically[31] and more recently on CT scans:[36] in a CT study of patients with proved "acute" tuberculous pleurisy, Hulnick and his colleagues[36] found areas of pulmonary cavitation not apparent on conventional chest roentgenograms and were able to detect or confirm the presence of hilar and mediastinal lymph node enlargement. In 10 patients with "chronic" tuberculous pleural disease, these authors were able to distinguish active from inactive infection by the presence of a collection of fluid within the pleural rind.

The onset of tuberculous pleurisy with effusion is usually acute, with chest pain, fever, and prostration, and suggests acute pneumonia;[37] Sibley reported an acute onset of this type in 147 of 200 consecutive cases.[38] Occasionally the onset is insidious and heralded only by mild pleuritic pain, sometimes with low-grade fever, nonproductive cough, weight loss, and easy fatigability.

The effusion is almost invariably unilateral and seldom massive. Thoracentesis typically yields clear, straw-colored fluid containing more than 3 g protein per 100 ml. If the aspirate is bloody, serosanguineous, or even pink, a tuberculous etiology is unlikely. Lymphocytes predominate, amounting to more than 70 per cent of the total white blood cell count; on preparations examined cytologically, they can appear to be the only cell type, a finding that may result in a mistaken diagnosis of lymphoma.[39] Although polymorphonuclear leukocytes may be fairly numerous during the early stages, it is reasonable to assume that effusions containing more than

50 per cent of these cells are of nontuberculous etiology. Eosinophils rarely are present in significant numbers unless there is an associated pneumothorax, a complication that may have been caused by an earlier thoracentesis. In tuberculous pleural fluid, the percentage and absolute numbers of T lymphocytes are higher and of B lymphocytes significantly lower than in blood.[34, 35, 40] Analysis of T cell subpopulations reveals that this is caused by a selective increase of T-helper cells, the percentage of suppressor cells being similar in pleural fluid and peripheral blood.[41] Natural killer (NK) cell activity is much more evident in tuberculous than in carcinomatous pleural effusions,[42] but like T-cell lymphocyte predominance it is unlikely to prove useful in differential diagnosis.

Light[32] considers a paucity of mesothelial cells to be of some value in indicating a tuberculous etiology of primary effusion. Other investigators have stated that a tuberculous etiology is unlikely if the percentage of mesothelial cells is higher than 5 per cent;[43, 44] however, it should be emphasized that any inflammatory process involving the pleural membrane can limit the number of mesothelial cells in pleural fluid. Guzman and associates[44] have proposed that a determination of macrophage size can be helpful in diagnosis; in their experience, macrophages are considerably smaller in tuberculous effusion than in effusion associated with malignancy or heart failure.

Pleural fluid glucose content can be low in tuberculous effusion, but this finding does not help to differentiate this etiology from that of bacterial pneumonia, rheumatoid disease, or pulmonary carcinoma in which pleural fluid glucose levels are often lower than those in blood. In fact, the majority of patients with effusions of tuberculous etiology have pleural fluid glucose levels above 60 mg per 100 ml.[32] It has been reported that intravenous infusion of glucose will increase glucose levels in tuberculous effusions but not in those of rheumatoid origin.[45] The original impression that a pH value below 7.30 was more characteristic of a tuberculous than a neoplastic effusion[46] has not been supported by further experience.[32] Brook[47] found lactic acid content of pleural effusion to be significantly higher in tuberculous, bacterial, and neoplastic effusions than in congestive heart failure, cirrhosis, nephrosis, trauma, and systemic lupus erythematosus.[47] Other workers have reported a raised pleural fluid lactate concentration measured by an enzymatic method[48] or by gas chromatography[49] to be suggestive, but not diagnostic, of nontuberculous empyema. In a small series of patients, the level of lysozyme in pleural fluid has been shown to be useful in distinguishing tuberculous from nontuberculous effusions,[50] the concentration being significantly higher in the former presumably because of secretion from epithelioid cells.[50] The activity of adenosine deaminase has been reported to be increased in tuberculous pleural effusions,[51, 52]

but there is some overlap in activity with effusions of other origin, particularly those of rheumatoid disease;[53] simultaneous determination of adenosine deaminase and of pleural fluid lysozyme/serum lysozyme ratio has been recommended as a more sensitive and specific biochemical approach to diagnosis.[54]

A *presumptive* diagnosis of tuberculous pleural effusion may be made with a combination of a positive tuberculin test and a predominantly lymphocytic response in the pleural fluid.[55] However, a negative PPD reaction does not exclude the diagnosis, and the skin test should be repeated in any patient suspected of having tuberculosis whose initial reaction is negative. In roughly 60 to 80 per cent of patients with proved tuberculosis, pleural biopsy specimens reveal granulomas.[56] Although this finding is virtually diagnostic, *definitive* diagnosis requires the identification of acid-fast organisms in the tissue specimen or a positive culture of pleural fluid or tissue. The incidence of positive culture from pleural fluid is surprisingly low, being found in only 20 to 25 per cent of proved cases,[57] whereas cultures of biopsy specimens are positive in 55 to 80 per cent of patients.[50, 58] Image-guided pleural biopsies can be useful in patients with small pleural effusions.[59]

The long-term prognosis in patients with tuberculous pleurisy with effusion is influenced to a considerable degree by the method of treatment. Simple bed rest often results in complete absorption of the pleural fluid and apparently complete restoration of the patient's health to normal, but the incidence of the subsequent development of active pulmonary tuberculosis is high. In a prechemotherapy follow-up study of 141 military personnel with pleural effusion and a positive PPD reported by Roper and Waring,[60] 92 patients (65 per cent) subsequently developed some form of active tuberculosis. By contrast, the incidence of the subsequent development of pulmonary tuberculosis is much less with the use of chemotherapy, although short-term results are similar to those of bed rest alone and occur no more rapidly. In one series, tuberculosis developed subsequently in 9 of 32 patients (28 per cent) with tuberculous pleural effusion treated by bed rest alone, in contrast to only 2 of 24 patients (8 per cent) who received chemotherapy.[61]

Nontuberculous mycobacteria rarely cause pleural effusion, either in the form of primary disease or as a complication of pulmonary involvement.[62]

Bacteria Other than Mycobacterium tuberculosis

The incidence of bacterial pneumonia in the United States is estimated to be over 1.2 million cases annually that result in 70,000 deaths. Parapneumonic pleural effusion occurred in 40 per cent of cases, and tube thoracostomy was required for drainage in about 10 per cent of these.[63] Pleural effusion accompanying acute pneumonia is undoubtedly even more common than these figures suggest, since its presence is frequently unrecognized because of the small amount. As discussed previously, it is likely that the recorded incidence of parapneumonic effusion would increase sharply if roentgenograms were obtained in the lateral decubitus position in all cases (Fig. 18–2). This supposition was borne out by a prospective evaluation of 203 patients with acute bacterial pneumonia on whom bilateral decubitus roentgenograms were obtained within 72 hours of the onset of the pneumonia:[64] 90 patients (44 per cent) were found to have roentgenographically demonstrable pleural effusion. Parapneumonic effusions usually are "benign" serous exudates (sympathetic) that resolve spontaneously.[64]

When the underlying pneumonia is of bacterial (nontuberculous) origin, a predominance of poly-

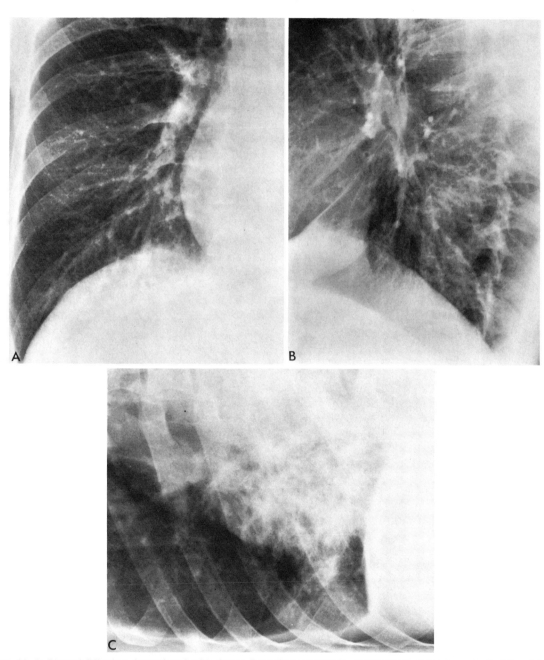

Figure 18–2. Pleural Effusion Associated with Acute Bronchopneumonia. Detail views of the lower half of the right lung from posteroanterior *(A)* and lateral *(B)* roentgenograms reveal inhomogeneous consolidation of all basal segments of the right lower lobe. Note that the parenchymal abnormality extends from the hilum to the diaphragmatic pleural surface in strict segmental distribution. Although no pleural effusion is evident on these roentgenograms exposed in the erect position, a lateral decubitus view *(C)* shows a small free pleural effusion extending along the lateral chest wall. Such a combination provides suggestive, but by no means conclusive, evidence for a staphylococcal etiology of the acute bronchopneumonia.

morphonuclear leukocytes will be present and in a few patients the fluid will become grossly cloudy and then frankly purulent (empyema). The major pathogenesis of empyema is as a complication of pneumonia,[65–69] but it can also represent a nidus of infection secondary to bacteremia, a subphrenic abscess, thoracotomy, or a traumatic episode (see farther on). A few cases have been reported of pleural effusion or empyema in patients with documented bacteremia, in the absence of evidence of pulmonary disease. Two young adults with group A beta-hemolytic streptococcal pharyngitis and a normal chest roentgenogram developed persistent high fever and severe pleuritic pain secondary to empyema caused by this organism.[70] Pneumococcal empyema, presumed to have been hematogenously seeded from an unexplained pneumococcemia, has been reported in a patient without evidence of pulmonary infection.[71] Clostridium perfringens was cultured from an empyema unassociated with pneumonia or subphrenic infection in a patient with cirrhosis.[72]

Drainage is required when empyema develops or when a serous effusion becomes loculated.[73] According to Light,[63, 74] there are four main indications for tube drainage: (1) the presence of gross pus, (2) the demonstration of organisms on Gram staining, (3) a glucose level in the pleural fluid of less than 40 mg per 100 ml, or (4) a pleural fluid pH level of less than 7.00. Potts and associates[73] measured the pH of pleural fluid of 24 consecutive patients with pneumonia and found that when it was greater than 7.30 (in 10 patients), the effusion resolved spontaneously; in contrast, when the pH was less than 7.30 (10 patients with empyema and 4 patients with loculated effusion), drainage was required. As pointed out by Light,[74] this criterion for closed drainage applies only when parapneumonic effusions are collected anaerobically and only when the pH of the pleural fluid is at least 0.15 units lower than a simultaneous arterial blood pH. Serial measurements of pH can prove useful in making management decisions when the level of the initial specimen is between 7.00 and 7.20: according to Light and colleagues,[63, 64] if the pH is above 7.20, complicated effusions usually do not develop and drainage is seldom required.

The management of parapneumonic effusions also can be based on the amount of fluid present: all 53 of Light's patients on whom the thickness of pleural fluid on a decubitus roentgenogram was less than 10 mm had spontaneous resolution of their effusions;[63] if the fluid measures more than 10 mm in depth, thoracentesis is probably indicated and the decision to insert a tube is based on the criteria previously enunciated. In about one third of patients with empyema, tube drainage proves inadequate and open drainage with rib resection is required.[75]

Although most patients with empyema are febrile and have blood neutrophilia, the compromised host[76] and patients receiving corticosteroid therapy[77, 78] can be afebrile and can have a normal white count. Penetration of the chest wall and "pointing" under the skin (empyema necessitatis) now are rare complications of empyema.[79]

As in the bacterial pneumonias, the types of organisms responsible for empyema vary with the host's state of health. In the western world, as a result of the control of tuberculosis and the availability of antibiotics effective against bacteria such as Streptococcus pneumoniae, most empyemas are now caused by Staphylococcus aureus and enteric gram-negative bacilli.[76, 80–84] Cultures frequently reveal multiple organisms, sometimes consisting of a combination of aerobic and anaerobic bacteria.[65, 68, 75, 85] Acid-fast bacteria are rarely isolated; although still found in a significant proportion of cases,[67, 80, 83, 84, 86] S. pneumoniae and Streptococcus pyogenes are much less common causes than in the past. Welch and associates[87] identified pleural effusion in 19 of 20 patients with acute beta-hemolytic streptococcal pneumonia in a military population. In another study,[88] 14 of 123 patients (11 per cent) with pneumococcal pneumonia, diagnosed on the basis of sputum smears and roentgenologic appearance, were found to have effusion or empyema. In infants and young children, empyema develops in almost every case of staphylococcal pneumonia, being observed in approximately 90 per cent of cases in several series.[89–93] In young patients, roentgenologic appearances characteristically progress rapidly—from minimal to extensive involvement within a few hours. The confluent bronchopneumonia can be partly or completely obscured by the massive effusion.

In patients who acquire infection in the community, the most frequent organisms are cocci, particularly staphylococci but also the gram-negative coccobacillus, Haemophilus influenzae; the latter organism is a common cause of empyema in children[83, 84] and is accompanied by pleural effusion in approximately 50 per cent of adults with H. influenzae pneumonia (see page 853).[94, 95–97] Pleural effusion or empyema occurs in roughly 50 per cent of adult patients with staphylococcal pneumonia. In hospitalized patients, gram-negative organisms predominate as the responsible etiologic agents of empyema.[66] Rarely, these microorganisms are the cause of community-acquired pneumonia: in an acutely debilitated population of New York City hospitalized for pneumonia, the incidence of nontuberculous bacterial empyema was 6.8 per cent; the majority of these cases were caused by gram-negative organisms.[76] Most cases of Klebsiella-Enterobacter-Serratia infection occur in elderly hospitalized patients whose immune status has been compromised by major medical or surgical illnesses. Pneumonia caused by Klebsiella types I, III, IV, and V develops in alcoholic or otherwise debilitated patients and is rarely hospital-acquired;[98] empyema frequently complicates acute pneumonia caused by these organisms. Other hospital-acquired gram-negative pneumonias that are associated with a high incidence of empyema include those caused by *Escherichia coli*[32, 99–101] and *Pseudomonas aeruginosa;*[32] small effusions can be identified in many cases of *P. aeruginosa* pneumonia[102] and are an almost invariable finding at necropsy.

Not uncommonly, pus aspirated from the pleural cavity in patients with empyema is sterile on culture, a finding that may reflect the administration of antimicrobial drugs before admission. In such circumstances, the etiologic agent may be determined by counter-immunoelectrophoresis, since soluble bacterial antigens can persist in body fluids after organisms no longer can be isolated.[103] Perhaps more often, negative results are caused by a failure to culture pleural fluid anaerobically: of 83 cases of empyema studied in three different hospitals with a special interest in anaerobic infection, pleural fluid culture isolated anaerobic bacteria exclusively in 29 cases (35 per cent), anaerobes mixed with aerobes in 34 cases (41 per cent), and aerobic or facultative bacteria exclusively in the remaining 20 cases (24 per cent).[80] In this series the most commonly encountered anaerobic bacteria were *Fusobacterium nucleatum; Bacteroides melaninogenicus; Bacteroides fragilis;* anaerobic and microaerophilic gram-positive cocci; *Clostridia;* and catalase-negative, non–spore-forming, gram-positive bacteria. It is possible that this study reflected some selection, since other series cite an incidence of anaerobic etiology in the range of 6 to 38 per cent.[65, 75, 86, 104, 105]

Some rather uncommon causes of pneumonia have a relatively high incidence of empyema. For example, pneumonia caused by the gram-negative bacillus, *Francisella tularensis,* is associated with pleural effusion in 25 to 50 per cent of patients (*see* page 870);[106–109] the diagnosis can be suspected from a history of contact with animals and can be confirmed by a rise in specific serum agglutinins or a positive culture from sputum or pleural fluid. *Proteus* pneumonia (*see* page 850) has been reported to cause empyema in which an elevated pH is believed to be due to ammonia production by the organism.[110] Group B streptococcal empyema (*see* page 836) occurs in neonates, in women after parturition, and in elderly diabetics.[111] Although it was once thought that pleural effusion is not a prominent manifestation of Legionnaires' pneumonia,[112] in two series[113, 114] the incidence was approximately 50 per cent. Other bacterial infections prone to the development of empyema include those caused by *Bacillus anthracis* (*see* page 842), *Pseudomonas mallei* (*see* page 861), *Salmonella* (*see* page 850),[115, 116] and *Brucella* species (*see* page 869).[117] Uncommon causes are *Yersinia pestis* and *enterocolitica* (*see* page 850),[118] *Neisseria meningitidis* (*see* page 868), and the gram-negative organism associated with Whipple's disease (*see* page 873).[119]

In the vast majority of cases of empyema, no roentgenologic criteria exist to permit diagnosis of a specific etiology; in most instances diagnosis is made by isolation of the organism from the pleural fluid. However, infections caused by two organisms, *Clostridium perfringens* and *Bacteroides fragilis,* have roentgenographic manifestations that can permit a presumptive diagnosis. These gas-forming bacteria not only cause pneumonia and pleural effusion but can also produce gas in the soft tissues of the chest wall or in the pleural space (pyopneumothorax).

PROGNOSIS IN PARAPNEUMONIC PLEURAL EFFUSION AND EMPYEMA

Uncomplicated pleural effusions—those that clear spontaneously—do not alter the prognosis of pneumonia. By contrast, pleural effusions that require drainage or thoracotomy are associated with an increased morbidity and mortality.[83, 84, 120, 121] Prognosis also varies with the age of the patient, the presence or absence of underlying disease, and the cause of the empyema. Parapneumonic empyema in children usually responds to simple closed drainage,[83, 122] whereas hospital-acquired empyema in the elderly is associated with considerable morbidity and a high mortality.[69, 123] Loculation of pleural fluid always indicates an exudate but not necessarily an empyema.[124] Occasionally a loculated empyema is situated adjacent to a pocket of sterile parapneumonic effusion; such pockets were shown by one group[125] to contain complement breakdown products, alerting them to the presence of a contiguous empyema. Ultrasonography and computed tomography[126–130] are not only useful in detecting an empyema but can be essential for positioning of a catheter for adequate drainage. Following diagnostic thoracentesis, it is appropriate to attempt therapeutic aspiration in selected patients with empyema, especially in children.[69, 122] If this fails to resolve the empyema, dependent thoracostomy closed underwater seal drainage is used; if the fluid is loculated, more than one tube may be needed.[63, 68] If this measure does not obliterate the empyema cavity, open drainage, with or without an Eloesser flap, is indicated; in the majority of patients this will effect a cure.[69] When all other measures fail, thoracotomy with pleural decortication is indicated; the literature suggests that in many cases procrastination in arriving at this decision results in increased morbidity and mortality.[63, 69, 121, 123, 131–133]

Actinomyces israelii and Nocardia Species

Pleural disease caused by these organisms can be considered together, since their roentgenologic characteristics are identical. Pulmonary involvement is an invariable accompaniment, usually in the form of acute airspace pneumonia, homogeneous in density and nonsegmental in distribution. Abscess formation is common. The infection extends into the pleura, producing empyema, and subsequently may transgress the parietal pleura to involve the chest wall, with rib destruction and subcutaneous abscess formation (empyema necessitatis).[134]

In one series of 15 cases,[135] pleural effusion in the form of either empyema or pleural "thickening" was observed in 12 patients and chest wall involvement in 9. Although extension across the pleural fissures or into the chest wall is common, it is not unique to these diseases—it may also occur in blastomycosis, cryptococcosis, and, of course, tuberculosis. The extension of *Actinomyces israelii* and *Nocardia* species without respect for usual anatomic boundaries may be related to the organisms' proteolytic activity. The manifestations of chest wall involvement include a soft tissue mass and osteomyelitis or periostitis of the ribs; the former was seen in almost half the patients with this type of involvement in one series,[135] sometimes without pulmonary spread.[136-138] Periosteal proliferation along the ribs may have a peculiar wavy configuration.[135] Although acute airspace pneumonia is the usual pulmonary manifestation of nocardiosis and is usually associated with empyema, chest wall involvement and widespread dissemination now are rare.[139] Isolation of either *Actinomyces israelii* or *Nocardia* species from pleural fluid or a chest wall abscess is necessary for positive diagnosis. Patients with empyema due to *Actinomyces israelii* frequently have poor oral hygiene.[141]

Fungi

Pleural effusion caused by fungi is very uncommon. *Histoplasma capsulatum* rarely shows pleural effusion at the time of primary infection, the associated pneumonia being localized predominantly to the lower lobes and being frequently associated with lymph node enlargement. Only 2 of 100 cases of pulmonary histoplasmosis reported by Curry and Wier[140] had pleural effusion. When it occurs, pleural disease can be caused by direct infection by *Histoplasma* organisms or by a reaction to antigen that diffuses into the pleural space from a histoplasmoma; the nodule may require resection to prevent impairment of ventilation from pleural fibrosis.[142]

Pleural effusion occurs in 7 per cent of symptomatic patients with primary *Coccidioides immitis* infection; the effusion may be associated with erythema nodosum and peripheral blood eosinophilia (rarely pleural fluid eosinophilia).[143] In addition, hydropneumothorax can develop when a coccidioidal cavity ruptures into the pleural space, said to occur in 1 to 5 per cent of patients with chronic cavitary coccidiodomycosis.[32]

Effusions caused by *Blastomyces dermatitidis* and *Cryptococcus neoformans* are very uncommon and are usually associated with acute airspace pneumonia.[144, 145] Isolation of the fungus or, in the case of *Cryptococcus,* detection of antigen in the pleural fluid[145] is essential for definitive diagnosis.

Pleural invasion by *Aspergillus* species occurs most commonly in two clinical situations: (1) as a late complication of thoracoplasty for tuberculosis, often in association with a bronchopleural fistula;[32, 146] or (2) as a complication of resectional surgery.[147, 148] In the latter situation, it can be caused either by direct infection of the pleural space or by extension of organisms from an aspergilloma that forms in a bronchial stump.[149, 150] As an opportunistic invader, the infection can develop rapidly in the pleural cavity after an operative procedure; a characteristic finding is the lack of any tendency to form pus.

Viruses, Mycoplasma, and Rickettsiae

Although roentgenographic demonstration of pleural effusion in viral and *Mycoplasma* pneumonia was formerly considered rare,[151-153] Fine and his coworkers[154] achieved this in 12 (20 per cent) of 59 patients with serologically proved *Mycoplasma,* viral, or cold agglutinin-positive pneumonia. In 4 cases, however, this required roentgenography of patients in the lateral decubitus position, which probably accounts for the low reported incidence of effusion in pneumonias of viral etiology and possibly in those of other etiologies, including bacterial. The overall incidence of effusion in their series (20 per cent) was roughly the same in *Mycoplasma* pneumonia (6 of 29), influenzal pneumonia (1 of 4), and pneumonia associated with elevated cold agglutinin titers (4 of 19) but occurred in only 1 of 7 cases of adenoviral pneumonia. In two other series of patients with acute *Mycoplasma* pneumonia, small effusions were noted in 4 of 20 cases[155] and in 9 of 48 cases.[156] In children with underlying disease, the pneumonia is often more severe and is usually accompanied by effusion.[157, 158]

Pleural effusion, large in some cases, is said to be a common accompaniment of the acute pneumonia of "atypical measles"[159] (*see* page 1051). This "altered measles syndrome" occurs in children in whom measles develops or who receive live measles virus vaccine[160, 161] after being immunized with killed measles vaccine. Roentgenographically there is extensive parenchymal consolidation, usually bilateral and consistently nonsegmental.[159, 162] Pleural effusion and pericarditis have been reported in *influenza A* infection.[163] Lander and Palayew[164] reviewed the chest roentgenograms of 59 patients with *infectious mononucleosis* and found 3 (5 per cent) to have pleural effusion. Pleural effusion is described as occurring in 3 per cent of patients with *Lassa fever,*[165] and in 0.16 per cent of those with *viral hepatitis.*[32] It also occurs in some cases of acute *Q fever pneumonia,*[166, 167] the effusion sometimes being eosinophilic.[168]

Parasites

ENTAMEBA HISTOLYTICA

Pleuropulmonary involvement in amebiasis is almost invariably secondary to liver abscess, with transmission of the infection into the thorax by direct extension through the diaphragm into the pleural space and eventually into the lung;[169] occasionally this occurs via the portal vein or diaphragmatic lymphatics. Pleuropulmonary disease is said to occur in 15 to 20 per cent of patients with liver involvement.[170, 171] Of 153 cases of pleuropulmonary amebiasis described by Ochsner and DeBakey in 1936,[172] 27 (17.6 per cent) presented as empyema that extended from liver abscesses. In a review from Mexico City of 88 patients with extension of hepatic amebiasis into the pleural cavity,[173] all had symptoms and signs that could be attributed to liver abscesses; the clinical course ran from 3 days to 8 months (average 71 days) before the onset of pleural complications. Chest roentgenograms revealed total or near-total opacification of the right hemithorax with shift of the mediastinum to the left. On thoracentesis, the color of the fluid was not constant but ranged from clear to dark brown, green, or yellow. The clinical picture of rupture into the pleural cavity consisted of the abrupt onset of sharp, tearing lower thoracic pain or worsening of the already present right upper quadrant pain, frequently radiating to the ipsilateral shoulder; rapidly progressing dyspnea was common.

The pleural effusion usually is serofibrinous. When the infestation extends into lung parenchyma, the pulmonary lesion may cavitate, providing communication between the bronchial tree and the liver abscess—a bronchohepatic fistula. In this case, fluid of typical "chocolate sauce" appearance may be seen on thoracentesis or in the sputum. This fluid contains blood and fragments of liver parenchyma. Identification of these substances in pleural fluid or sputum is diagnostic. The pleural space may become secondarily infected, with the development of frankly purulent empyema. Roentgenography commonly reveals elevation and fixation of the right hemidiaphragm, right-sided pleural effusion, and consolidation of the right lower lobe with or without abscess formation. This combination of findings should suggest the possibility of this etiology, particularly when the liver is enlarged (the differential diagnosis usually is from subphrenic abscess of other etiology). The necessity for a high index of suspicion was emphasized by Daniels and Childress[171] in their report of 10 patients, 4 of whom died before a diagnosis was made. The rapid response to specific antiamebic therapy makes early diagnosis vital.[174]

PARAGONIMUS WESTERMANI

The route of entry of this organism into the thorax is identical to that of *Entameba histolytica*—through the diaphragm. Despite this, roentgenographically detectable pleural effusion is rare; in a comprehensive study of the roentgenographic changes in 100 cases of pulmonary disease caused by *Paragonimus,* Ogakwu and Nwokolo[175] found only

1 case of free pleural effusion, and that was in the form of empyema from which *Paragonimus* ova were recovered. Pleural thickening was apparent in 4 other cases.

ECHINOCOCCUS GRANULOSUS (HYDATID DISEASE)

Pleural effusion is uncommon in hydatid disease, being observed in only 3 of 100 cases studied by Rakower and Milwidsky.[176] It occurs when a pulmonary hydatid cyst ruptures into the pleural space rather than into its usual site, the bronchial tree. In most cases, since air also is present, the roentgenographic appearance is of a hydropneumothorax. Scoleces and daughter cysts floating on the surface of the fluid produce irregularities of the fluid surface, creating the "water lily" sign or "sign of the camalote" (Fig. 18–3). A partly or wholly collapsed hydatid cyst may be visible in the pulmonary parenchyma, possibly associated with solid cysts. Diagnosis may be confirmed by a positive Casoni skin test or complement fixation test. It is relatively easy to recover hooklets from the pleural fluid or sputum in cases in which a cyst has ruptured.

MISCELLANEOUS PARASITES

Empyema due to *Trichomonas* has been reported following esophageal surgery,[177] and pleural effusion has been described in association with infestation by *Dracunculus medinensis*.[178] Roentgenographic evidence of pleural effusion in *Pneumocystis carinii* infestation is rare[179–181] but does occur.[182]

PLEURAL EFFUSION CAUSED BY IMMUNOLOGIC DISEASE

Only two of the connective tissue diseases are important causes of pleural effusion, systemic lupus erythematosus (SLE) and rheumatoid disease. In patients with progressive systemic sclerosis, dermatomyositis, and Sjögren's syndrome, effusion probably results from other causes (e.g., heart failure) rather than from the primary disease. Pleural effusion is said to occur fairly frequently in Wegener's granulomatosis[183] (in 6 of 11 cases in one series[184]) but its presence in other pulmonary vasculitides most likely results from other causes. Effusion occurring as a result of nitrofurantoin sensitivity[185, 186] and hypocomplementemic urticardial vasculitis[187] perhaps belongs in this category but is very uncommon.

Systemic Lupus Erythematosus

The reported incidence of pleural effusion in this disease varies widely, from 33 per cent of cases studied by Bulgrin and his associates[188] to 74 per

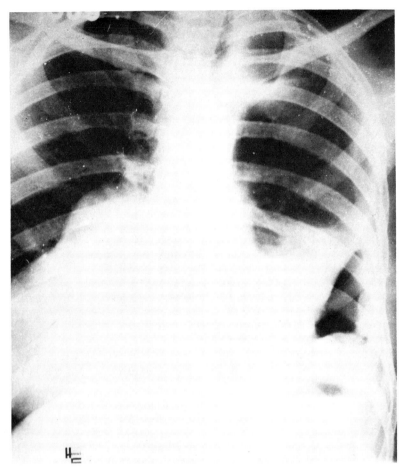

Figure 18–3. Perforation of Pulmonary Hydatid Cyst into the Pleural Space. A posteroanterior roentgenogram reveals a left hydropneumothorax, the surface of the fluid being irregular as a result of the presence of collapsed membranes (the sign of the camalote). A large hydatid cyst is present in the right lung. (Courtesy of Dr. Manuel Gonzalez Maseda, Uruguay, and Dr. Luis Suarez Halty, Rio Grande, Brazil.)

cent of cases investigated by Gould and Daves.[189] In the former series, the effusion occurred as an isolated abnormality in 12.6 per cent of patients and in combination with cardiac enlargement and pulmonary abnormalities in 20 per cent. Effusions are bilateral in about half the cases and when unilateral are predominantly left-sided.[191] They are usually small but may be massive.[188–190, 766] Winslow and his colleagues[191] stress the importance of pleuritis as an early manifestation of SLE. Of 57 cases reported by these authors, pleural effusion occurred in 42; in 3 of these cases, pleuritis appeared as an isolated first sign, and in 16 others it was associated with only minor antecedent symptoms. In 23 of the 42 cases the effusion was bilateral, either simultaneously or alternately, and in 13 of the 19 cases of unilateral effusion it was on the left side.

Levin[192] has emphasized the importance of distinguishing pleural effusion due to direct involvement of the pleura by SLE from that associated with lupus-induced renal disease. The former characteristically is accompanied by pain and splinting, whereas the serous effusions of nephrosis are painless.

The protein concentration of pleural effusion in SLE is variable. When the effusion is attributable to direct pleural involvement, it is probable that inflammation, possibly mediated by immune complexes,[193, 194] causes increased capillary permeability, resulting in pleural effusion with a relatively high protein concentration.[195] By contrast, when the effusion results from the nephrotic syndrome secondary to SLE, it will be a transudate.

The fluid usually possesses no diagnostic biochemical findings. Carr and associates[196] have shown that the glucose concentration of pleural fluid in SLE is approximately equal to blood glucose concentration, in contrast to the low levels characteristic of rheumatoid disease. Also in contrast to rheumatoid pleural effusion, the pH is greater than 7.35 and levels of rheumatoid factor are not significantly elevated.[197] Lupus erythematosus cells can be present.[198, 199]

The most common associated roentgenologic finding is enlargement of the cardiovascular silhouette, which is said to occur in 35 to 50 per cent of all cases.[188, 189] This is usually nonspecific in character and minimal to moderate in degree. It has been ascribed to pericardial effusion, endocarditis or myocarditis, or secondary effects of hypertension, renal disease, or anemia. Variation in heart size usually takes place over a period of weeks but may occur with startling abruptness. When it is sudden, pericardial effusion is the most likely cause.

Although there is nothing specific about the roentgenographic pattern of SLE, the combination of bilateral pleural effusion with nonspecific cardiac enlargement should at least suggest the diagnosis, particularly in young women. Confirmation depends upon the demonstration of antinuclear or anti-DNA antibodies.

Rheumatoid Disease

Pleural abnormality probably is the most frequent manifestation of rheumatoid disease in the thorax.[200, 201] Of 516 patients with rheumatoid arthritis in one series,[202] 108 (21 per cent) gave a history of pleurisy and 17 (3.3 per cent) had pleural effusions for which no other cause could be found. These figures are in contrast to those observed in 301 controls with degenerative joint disease, of whom only 36 (12 per cent) gave a history of pleurisy and only 1 had pleural effusion.

The most noteworthy clinical aspect of pleural effusion in rheumatoid disease is its predominance in men. For example, 24 of 25 patients studied by Carr and Mayne[203] were males, a sex incidence similar to that of all reported series and especially remarkable since the incidence of rheumatoid arthritis in females is about twice that in males. Middle-aged patients are most often affected, the average age of 52 years in one large series being identical to that usually reported for rheumatoid arthritis as a whole.[203] Although effusions usually appear some time after the clinical onset of rheumatoid arthritis, they may antedate both signs and symptoms of joint disease. They are usually unilateral, slightly more often on the right side. The only unique characteristic of the pleural effusion roentgenographically is its tendency to remain relatively unchanged for many months or even years.[203-205]

The fluid is typically an exudate, usually turbid and greenish yellow,[203] with a predominance of lymphocytes and a paucity of mesothelial cells;[206] in some cases polymorphonuclear leukocytes are found in abundance.[207] Cytologic examination of filter specimens may reveal the presence of elongated cells with vesicular nuclei, irregularly shaped multinucleated giant cells, and clumps of amorphous granular material (Fig. 18–4); this appearance is caused by rupture of a subpleural necrobiotic (rheumatoid) nodule into the pleural space and is diagnostic of the rheumatoid etiology of the effusion.[208, 209] So-called rheumatoid arthritis cells (mostly polymorphonuclear leukocytes with cytoplasm containing minute black granules believed to be lipids) also can be found in some pleural effusions in rheumatoid disease. Although it has been suggested that their presence is evidence in favor of a diagnosis of rheumatoid disease,[210-212] it is now clear that they also can be seen in effusions of other etiology, such as tuberculosis[213] and malignancy.[214]

Characteristically, the glucose content of rheumatoid pleural effusion is very low; in fact, it has been estimated that glucose levels below 30 mg per 100 ml are found in 70 to 80 per cent of patients with rheumatoid disease.[215] Typically a low pleural fluid glucose level is associated with a normal blood level and does not rise following intravenous infusion of glucose.[45, 203, 207, 216-218] This latter fact is important in the differential diagnosis from tuberculous effusion: whereas the sugar content of tuberculous fluid also is characteristically low, its level rises following intravenous loading with glucose. The mechanism of the low pleural fluid glucose is unknown; it has been suggested that some factor associated with rheumatoid pleural inflammation interferes with glucose transfer across the pleural space.[45] In support of this hypothesis is the observation that low glucose values also have been recorded in joint fluid of patients with rheumatoid arthritis.[203] Regardless of the mechanism, a low pleural fluid glucose level should suggest the diagnosis, especially when the pleural fluid is nonpurulent, contains no bacteria on smear and culture, and shows no malignant cells on cytologic examination; if the possibility of tuberculosis has been excluded by pleural biopsy, the diagnosis is almost certain.

Rheumatoid factor is frequently present in the pleural fluid of rheumatoid disease, typically when there is a concomitant increase in the serum.[219] Its presence, however, is not diagnostic of a rheumatoid etiology, since elevated levels also have been described in parapneumonic, carcinomatous, and tuberculous effusions.[197, 219-221] The pH of the pleural fluid is also reduced in rheumatoid disease, usually below 7.20; when accompanied by low glucose and complement levels and high rheumatoid factor levels, this finding is virtually diagnostic of rheumatoid pleural effusion.[197, 221, 222] It has been shown that the detection of immune complex levels in pleural fluid by various techniques can be useful also in confirming whether or not the etiology of an effusion is of connective tissue type; it may even help in distinguishing SLE from rheumatoid disease as the initiating cause.[223] Less valuable diagnostic laboratory tests include the measurement of hydroxyproline[222] and lactate dehydrogenase (LDH)[207, 217, 224] levels, said to be higher in the pleural fluid than in the blood of patients with rheumatoid disease, and a paucity of mesothelial cells, also a feature of tuberculous effusions.[206]

Empyema is surprisingly common in rheumatoid pleuropulmonary disease.[77] The most plausible causes for its development include a deficiency of host defense, the discharge into the pleural cavity of necrotic material from rheumatoid nodules situated in the subpleural parenchyma, and perhaps most commonly a complication of corticosteroid therapy.[77]

The incidence of coexistent pulmonary disease and pleural effusion in rheumatoid disease is not known, but it seems that they tend to occur independently. For example, there was no evidence of pulmonary disease in 19 of Carr and Mayne's 25 patients with rheumatoid effusion[203] and in only one other patient, who had had known silicosis for

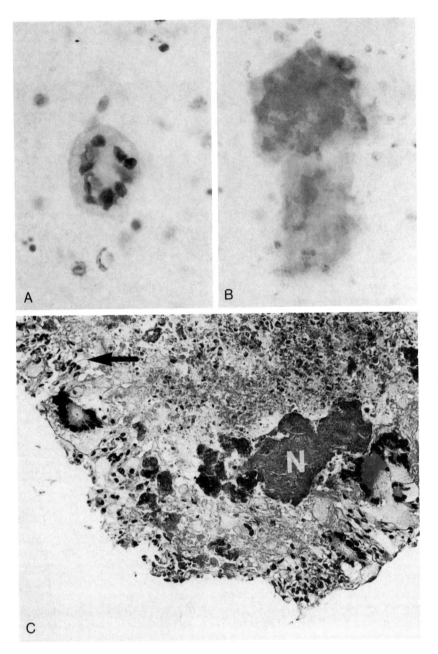

Figure 18–4. Rheumatoid Pleural Effusion: Cytologic Appearance. Highly magnified views of a filter preparation of pleural fluid show a multinucleated giant cell and scattered mononuclear cells *(A)* and an irregular fragment of more or less amorphous, acellular material *(B)*. Taken together, these findings are highly suggestive of a rheumatoid etiology. A histologic section of a closed pleural biopsy specimen from the same patient *(C)* shows that the likely origin of the material seen on the filter preparation is a fairly typical necrobiotic nodule composed of necrotic material *(N)*, epithelioid histocytes *(arrow)*, and multinucleated giant cells. (*A* and *B*, Papanicolaou × 450; *C*, hematoxylin-eosin × 130.)

18 years, could a definite relationship be established between the pulmonary abnormality and rheumatoid disease. Martel and his colleagues,[225] who studied 35 cases of rheumatoid disease with pulmonary and pleural involvement, recorded the following incidence and sex ratios of the three forms of pleuropulmonary disease: pleural effusion, 2 (male to female, 2:0); pulmonary nodules, 12 (8:4); and "chronic pneumonitis with interstitial fibrosis," 21 (10:11). However, one of the patients with pleural effusion had coexistent diffuse pulmonary fibrosis, and pulmonary nodules developed later in the other.

Symptoms relating to the effusion vary and often are absent. Of 25 patients described by Carr and Mayne,[203] 13 were asymptomatic, 6 had typical pleural pain, and 2 experienced a dull ache in the thorax. Shortness of breath was the presenting complaint in 6 patients, and in only 2 patients did chills and fever, suggestive of acute infection, herald the onset.

It is clear that rheumatoid disease merits a prominent place in the differential diagnosis of pleural effusion, especially in middle-aged men and in association with recent or developing joint symptoms. Since there are no distinctive roentgenologic characteristics of the pleural effusion, the diagnosis can be suggested only when there are clinical or roentgenologic manifestations of rheumatoid arthritis or when the serum contains a high titer of rheumatoid factor. The value of laboratory procedures in the diagnosis of rheumatoid pleural effusion is exemplified by the not uncommon occurrence of nonrheumatoid effusion in patients with rheumatoid arthritis.[226]

PLEURAL EFFUSION ASSOCIATED WITH ASBESTOS EXPOSURE

Four types of roentgenographic changes occur in the pleura as a result of asbestos exposure: plaque formation, diffuse pleural thickening, calcification, and pleural effusion; each may occur alone or in combination with the others.[227–229] The first three of these are discussed later in this chapter. Pleural effusion is probably more common than is generally recognized, and is often not appreciated.[230–233] The most comprehensive report of the prevalence and incidence of pleural effusion in an asbestos-exposed population was by Epler and his colleagues,[231] who studied 1,134 exposed workers and 717 control subjects. Benign asbestos effusion was defined by (1) exposure to asbestos, (2) confirmation by roentgenograms or thoracentesis, (3) no other disease related to pleural effusion, and (4) no malignant tumor within 3 years. These authors found 34 benign effusions among the exposed workers (3 per cent), compared with no unexplained effusions among the control subjects. In another study by Martensson and associates,[234] the incidence of asbestos exposure was compared between 64 consecutive men with idiopathic pleural effusions and 129 randomly sampled age-matched controls without effusions; asbestos exposure was significantly more frequent in men with idiopathic effusions than in controls.

The presence of benign asbestos effusion appears to be dose-related.[231] In the study by Epler and colleagues,[231] the latency period was shorter than for other asbestos-related disorders, and benign effusion was the most common abnormality during the first 20 years after exposure. Most effusions were small, 28 per cent recurred, and 66 per cent did not cause symptoms. Chest pain was the most common symptom; some patients had fever suggesting a viral infection.

In most, if not all, cases the fluid is a sterile serous or blood-tinged exudate. The differential diagnosis must include tuberculosis and mesothelioma. Large effusions are more likely to be caused by mesothelioma than to have a benign origin;[235] by contrast, painful and bloody effusions are just as likely to have a benign as a malignant cause. Of the 12 patients described by Gaensler and Kaplan,[236] the presence of mesothelioma was recognized in 1 patient 9 years after the first documented effusion. Of four cases in another series,[237] 2 eventually developed mesothelioma.

DRUG-INDUCED PLEURAL EFFUSION

Some drugs, such as bromocriptine, methysergide, and dantrolene sodium, appear to affect the pleura almost selectively.[238] Since the original description by Rinne in 1981 of the pleuropulmonary manifestations of long-term *bromocriptine* treatment for Parkinson's disease,[239] over 20 such cases have been described in the literature. Complications consisting mainly of pleural effusion have their onset from 9 months to 4 years after initiation of therapy;[240, 241] in most cases the effusion is lymphocyte-predominant and resolves following withdrawal of the drug. This medication has a chemical structure similar to *methysergide,* an ergot drug used in the treatment of migraine and well known as a cause of pleural effusion and fibrosis.[242] *Dantrolene sodium* is a long-acting skeletal muscle relaxant used in the treatment of spastic neurological disorders. Sterile exudative pleural and pericardial effusions have been described in four patients after long-term therapy with this drug. The effusions were associated with eosinophilia in both pleural fluid and peripheral blood[243] but resolved on cessation of medication. Dantrolene sodium is structurally similar to *nitrofurantoin,* which also causes an eosinophilia and pleural effusion but usually after a shorter period of treatment. Additional information about drug-induced pleural disease is found in Chapters 7 (*see* page 1191) and 14.

PLEURAL EFFUSION CAUSED BY NEOPLASMS

The most common cause of exudative pleural effusion is malignancy.[15, 32] In the Mayo Clinic series of 83 patients with pleural exudates,[15] the cause was cancer in 64 patients (77 per cent) (this percentage may indicate some selection in that the majority of patients were referred). In another series of 96 patients with neoplastic involvement of the pleura,[244] the presence of pleural effusion was the abnormality that led to the diagnosis of carcinoma in 44 patients (46 per cent). Several series[32, 244–246] clearly indicate that the major causes of malignant pleural effusion are pulmonary, breast, ovarian, and gastric carcinoma and lymphoma; primary lung and metastatic breast malignancies head the list. Of 96 cases of malignant pleural effusion seen at the Colorado General Hospital from 1960 to 1975,[244] 32 cases (33 per cent) originated in the lung, 20 (20.9 per cent) in the breast, 9 (9.3 per cent) in the ovaries, and 7 (7.3 per cent) in the stomach. These sites of origin represented 32 of 459 (7 per cent) carcinomas of the lung, 20 of 645 (3.1 per cent) neoplasms of the breast, 9 of 303 (2.9 per cent) carcinomas of the ovary, and 7 of 195 (3.6 per cent) carcinomas of the stomach seen over this period of time. Ninety-two percent of the lung, breast, and ovarian malignant effusions were on the same side as the primary lesions.[244] (However, in a review of 105 cases of metastatic breast carcinoma, Fentiman and associates[309] found the incidence of ipsilateral and contralateral pleural effusion to be almost equal, 50 and 40 per cent respectively; *see* farther on.) An additional important, although relatively infrequent, cause of malignant pleural effusion is mesothelioma; effusion is invariably associated with this neoplasm. Mesothelioma is considered in greater detail farther on (*see* page 2763).

The importance of cancer as a cause of pleural effusion is also reflected in the etiology of bilateral effusions associated with normal heart size; Rabin and Blackman[6] described 78 such cases: 35 cases (44.9 per cent) were due to cancer, 19 being metastatic, 13 lymphoma, and 3 primary carcinoma of the lung. Of these 35 patients, 13 (37 per cent) showed no roentgenographic abnormality of the thorax other than the bilateral pleural effusions.

There has been considerable speculation as to the pathogenesis of pleural effusion in malignancy, and it is likely that in most cases it is multifactorial.[32, 247] Possible mechanisms include the following: (1) tumor invasion of the pleura stimulates an inflammatory reaction associated with capillary leakage; (2) tumor invasion of the pulmonary or pleural lymphatics and bronchopulmonary, hilar, or mediastinal lymph nodes hinders the return of lymphatic fluid to the systemic circulation; (3) bronchial obstruction creates an increased negative intrapleural pressure, thus increasing transudation; (4) the hypoproteinemia present in many patients debilitated by cancer leads to increased transudation; (5) the development of infection in association with obstructive pneumonitis results in a parapneumonic effusion; and (6) deposition of immune complexes related to circulating tumor antigens causes increased pleural capillary permeability.[193]

In a detailed autopsy report of 52 patients with pleural metastases (29 from the lung, 9 from the breast, 4 from the pancreas, 5 from the stomach, and 5 miscellaneous), Meyer[248] found effusions in only 31 patients (60 per cent). He concluded that the effusions bore no relation to the extent of pleural involvement by metastases and that fluid accumulated principally as a result of neoplastic infiltration of mediastinal lymph nodes. If Meyer's conclusion is valid, it would lend some support to Stewart's hypothesis (*see* page 176)[249] that a pleural exudate of high protein content is removed from the pleural space by the lymphatics through bulk flow. Provided that the lymphatic channels are not obstructed and that the rate of fluid formation is not too great, it might be logically assumed that in this way the pleural space could be kept dry (or ideally moist) and that if lymphatic drainage were obstructed pleural fluid would accumulate. Meyer[248] provided further support for a close link between lymphatic obstruction and pleural effusion when he observed that effusions do not develop with metastatic sarcomas, tumors that seldom spread via the lymphatics. It should be emphasized that mediastinal nodes may be affected by metastatic neoplasm and thereby create lymphatic obstruction and resultant pleural effusion without convincing evidence of their enlargement on conventional chest roentgenograms. In such cases computed tomography may reveal enlarged nodes compatible with the possibility of lymphatic obstruction. Meyer[248] stressed that, regardless of primary site, bilateral pleural involvement in metastatic carcinoma is frequently associated with hepatic metastases with spread to the pleura from the liver deposits.

The diagnosis of carcinoma as the etiology of pleural effusion may be strongly suspected from the chest roentgenogram, the manifestation being one of either primary pulmonary cancer or diffuse nodular opacities characteristic of metastatic carcinoma. If, in addition, the patient complains of hemoptysis, a definitive diagnosis usually can be made with the aid of fiberoptic bronchoscopy.[250] Bronchoscopy can occasionally yield the diagnosis even in patients whose chest roentgenograms reveal nothing more than pleural effusion; however, in such cases thoracentesis and pleural biopsy are more likely to prove fruitful.[250]

The incidence of positive cytologic examination of malignant pleural effusion ranges from 33 to 87 per cent in various series (*see* page 355). Light[32] is of the opinion that an experienced cytologist will make a positive diagnosis in 80 per cent of cases if three separate specimens are submitted. As a diagnostic procedure, cytologic examination of pleural fluid gives a higher yield than needle pleural biopsy, although these procedures are complementary.[245, 251, 252]

Pleural effusions associated with malignancy are almost invariably exudates; those that meet exudative criteria by the LDH level but not by the protein level are usually malignant.[32] Although lymphocytes predominate, polymorphonuclear leukocytes are frequent. A minority are grossly bloody, as in 9 of the 31 cases in Meyer's series.[248] The great majority have normal glucose levels and pH above 7.30.[32, 244] Those with glucose levels below 60 mg per 100 ml and a pH below 7.30 are more likely to be large, to have a positive cytology, and to carry a poor prognosis.[32, 253, 254]

There have been numerous reports of attempts to differentiate between benign and malignant effusions by using a variety of tumor markers.[255–266] In the great majority of cases, considerable overlap has been found in the levels of these markers in pleural fluid to the extent that, as at the time of this writing, it can be said that they serve little, if any, useful purpose. The sensitivity and specificity can be improved by using various combinations of markers. For example, setting a high cutoff level for carcinoembryonic antigen (CEA) raises the specificity to almost 100 per cent, although even this marker has not been found particularly sensitive.

When pleural fluid persists and cytology is negative for malignant cells, open pleural biopsy or thoracoscopy with biopsy may be required for diagnosis. Some investigators feel that thoracoscopy for the identification of suitable areas for direct pleural biopsy is underused.[267–271] Chromosome analysis of pleural fluid cells[272–274] may also prove useful when malignancy is suspected and cytology and pleural biopsy fail to provide a diagnosis. In some cases, electron microscopy can permit identification of the primary site of a metastatic neoplasm.[275]

Pulmonary Carcinoma

Pleural involvement in primary pulmonary carcinoma is not uncommon by the time patients first seek medical attention; effusion has been observed in 7 per cent,[244] 8 per cent,[276] and 15 per cent[277] of patients in three series. During the course of the disease, at least 50 per cent of patients with disseminated lung cancer develop a pleural effusion.[32] As a cause of pleural effusion, these neoplasms are nearly always associated with roentgenographically demonstrable pulmonary abnormality. Rarely, the abnormality presents as a hilar mass, and the roentgenographic evidence may be very subtle; perhaps more frequently, a diminutive peripheral carcinoma manifests itself by disproportionate metastatic enlargement of mediastinal and hilar lymph nodes. The primary lesion may be so small as to be almost invisible roentgenologically except with such special techniques as CT. A high index of suspicion may allow a *presumptive* diagnosis, although differentiation from lymphoma, especially Hodgkin's disease, may be impossible without pleural or mediastinal lymph node biopsy. *Positive* diagnosis requires recovery of malignant cells from the sputum or pleural fluid or from pleural, bronchoscopic, or mediastinal lymph node biopsy.

The recovery of malignant cells from pleural fluid of patients with proved pulmonary carcinoma is generally regarded as evidence of inoperability.[278] If cells are not found—a common event judging from the series reported by Rosenblatt and Lisa[279] in which 22 per cent of patients with pleural effusion and pulmonary carcinoma had no evidence of metastatic pleural involvement—the significance of the effusion is controversial. If a reasonable explanation exists for fluid formation without direct neoplastic involvement and if no other findings contraindicate surgery, a thoracotomy is probably justified. However, in patients with negative pleural fluid cytology and otherwise operable pulmonary carcinoma, pleural effusion is an ominous finding; for example, Brinkman[280] described 21 such patients, 17 of whom were found to have extrapulmonary spread of the disease at thoracotomy. Pleural effusion with proved carcinomatous involvement has a very poor prognosis; in Chernow and Sahn's series of 96 patients,[244] 54 per cent were dead within 1 month and 84 per cent within 6 months.

The cytologic features of pleural fluid in small cell carcinoma[281, 282] and pulmonary neuroendocrine carcinoma[283] have been described.

Lymphoreticular Neoplasms and Leukemia

The term lymphoreticular here includes Hodgkin's disease, non-Hodgkin's lymphoma, Waldenström's macroglobulinemia, and multiple myeloma.

HODGKIN'S AND NON-HODGKIN'S LYMPHOMA

Although there are some differences in the incidence of pleural effusion and of pulmonary and mediastinal abnormalities between these lymphomas, the general pattern is similar. Opinion differs concerning the precise mechanisms by which pleural fluid accumulates in cases of lymphoma, the main point of controversy being the obstructive influence of mediastinal lymph nodes. In a study of 50 patients with Hodgkin's disease, Stolberg and coworkers[284] found a 26 per cent incidence of pleural effusion, and in almost all of these patients the mediastinal lymph nodes were enlarged. These authors concluded that the effusions were the result of lymphatic obstruction, either centrally or peripherally. However, in another study of 154 patients with histologically proved Hodgkin's disease reported by Fisher and coworkers,[285] pleural effusion was observed in 44 (28 per cent), but these authors found no convincing evidence that even massive enlargement of lymph nodes severely obstructed lymph flow; their observation that peripheral septal edema was seldom present lent some support to their conclusion. Martin[286] observed pleural effusion in only 3 of 61 patients with mediastinal node enlargement in Hodgkin's disease. (It is interesting to note that in two cases the effusion disappeared after irradiation of the mediastinal nodes.) Vieta and Craver[287] found mediastinal lymph node enlargement in 48 per cent and pleural fluid in only 16 per cent of 335 cases of Hodgkin's disease. The same authors found enlarged lymph nodes in 27 per cent and pleural fluid in 16 per cent of 239 cases of non-Hodgkin's lymphoma and in 36 per cent and 12 per cent, respectively, of 150 cases of leukemia. Of interest is the report of Molander and Pack,[288] who found enlarged mediastinal lymph nodes in 30 per cent and pleural effusion in 20 per cent of cases of non-Hodgkin's lymphoma but reported no correlative incidence of the two findings. In the Vieta and Craver series,[287] although 29 per cent of patients with Hodgkin's disease had pleural involvement at necropsy, only 16 per cent of these had had pleural effusions during the course of the disease. Pleural effusion has been reported as the initial presentation of lymphoma related to acquired immunodeficiency syndrome (AIDS) in 3 patients.[289]

Pleural fluid may be serous or serosanguineous with the characteristics of a transudate or exudate; specific gravity is between 1.015 and 1.018.[290] Wong and associates[291] found pleural fluid protein concentration to range from 0.8 to 6.2 g per 100 ml in patients with Hodgkin's disease. Thus, it must be concluded that the cause of pleural effusion in Hodgkin's disease is highly variable, possibly being lymphatic obstruction, venous obstruction, secondary pulmonary infection, direct involvement of the pleura by neoplasm, or a combination of these.

The cytologic diagnosis of lymphoma in pleural fluid specimens can be difficult, particularly in the small lymphocytic (well-differentiated) form; as indicated previously, cytologically atypical lymphocytes can be virtually the only cell in tuberculous effusions, resulting in an appearance that can be mistaken for lymphoma.[39] Despite this, some investigators report a high degree of accuracy in diagnosis and, to some extent, even in classification of types of lymphoma by this means.[292] Immunohistochemical analysis can be most helpful in difficult cases in determining the true nature of an effusion.[294]

Chylothorax in association with lymphoma results largely from obstruction of the thoracic duct. Such effusions contain high concentrations of neutral fat and fatty acid (see farther on for discussion of chylous effusions).

LEUKEMIA

Pleural effusion is usually unilateral in leukemia. As a roentgenographic abnormality it is second in frequency only to mediastinal lymph node enlargement and is identified in up to 25 per cent of patients.[295] It is probably caused by leukemic infiltration of the pleura in no more than 5 per cent,[296] the majority of cases being due to obstructed lymphatics, cardiac failure, or infection.[295, 296] Despite this, general or local pleural thickening simulating plaques may be caused by leukemic infiltration,[297] particularly in children. Cytochemical and immunocytochemical studies of cells obtained from the fluid may be helpful in diagnosis.[293, 298, 299]

MULTIPLE MYELOMA

Pleural effusion in multiple myeloma is uncommon[300–303] but can be associated with other roentgenographic changes that are sufficiently distinctive to permit a strongly *presumptive* diagnosis. Destructive lesions in one or more ribs are frequently accompanied by soft tissue masses that typically protrude into the thorax and indent the pleura and lung. The ribs may be expanded, a finding that is almost pathognomonic of myeloma. Destructive lesions may be apparent also in the shoulder girdles or thoracic spine. Despite the characteristic appearance of these chest wall abnormalities, a similar roentgenographic appearance can occur with a variety of primary and metastatic neoplasms, and a *positive* diagnosis of myeloma rests on the finding of abnormal plasma cells in bone marrow or pleural fluid. A high level of the specific immunoglobulin produced by the myeloma cells can be identified in blood and sometimes in pleural fluid.[301, 304] In contrast to most cases of lymphoma, the pleural exudate is probably caused in many cases by direct infiltration by myeloma cells.[300]

WALDENSTRÖM'S MACROGLOBULINEMIA

Pleural effusion is not an uncommon finding in Waldenström's macroglobulinemia and can occur in the absence of parenchymal disease.[305–307] A gamma peak will be found in the serum protein, as well as lymphocytes and a high level of immunoglobulin M in the pleural fluid.[306, 307] Pleural effusion also has been reported in two patients with alpha chain disease,[308] a lymphomatous disorder characterized by the synthesis and secretion of an abnormal IgA immunoglobulin devoid of light chains; this condition more commonly involves the gastrointestinal tract.

Nonpulmonary Metastatic Carcinoma

As previously stated, the major sites of origin of malignant pleural effusion from extrathoracic neoplasms are breast, ovary, and stomach,[244] but the breast is the most common site. In breast carcinoma, the effusion is usually unilateral; as noted previously, in a review of 105 cases, Fentiman and associates[309] found 90 per cent to be unilateral, 50 per cent ipsilateral, and 40 per cent contralateral. However, this rough equality of ipsilateral and contralateral effusion has not been the experience of all investigators: of 122 cases of pleural effusion caused by metastatic breast carcinoma reviewed by Raju and Kardinal,[310] 101 (83 per cent) were ipsilateral. If this incidence of ipsilaterality is accepted, it obviously indicates that spread is via the lymphatics rather than the bloodstream, a conclusion that was supported in an autopsy study.[311] Contiguous spread through the chest wall to the parietal pleura is extremely rare, having been identified in only one patient in another autopsy series reported by Meyer.[248] Direct spread is also rare in patients with primary carcinoma of the liver[312] and pancreas.[313]

Although bilateral pleural effusion was found in only 10 per cent of the 105 patients with breast carcinoma reported by Fentiman and colleagues,[309] it must be considered among the major causes of this relatively uncommon form of presentation. Of the 78 cases of bilateral pleural effusion associated with normal heart size reported by Rabin and Blackman, 35 (45 per cent) were caused by cancer and the major site of origin of metastatic cancer was breast.[6] It is believed that this manifestation of pleural malignancy represents secondary metastases from the liver.[248]

In Fentiman and colleagues' series, the mean lag time between the diagnosis of the primary tumor and the identification of effusion was 41.5 months.[309] In Raju and Kardinal's series of 122 cases,[310] it was 22 months, ranging from 1 month to as long as 23 years after diagnosis of the primary tumor. Whenever it occurs, the development of pleural effusion carries a dismal prognosis, especially if the pleural fluid cytology is positive[310] or if there is evidence for metastases elsewhere;[314] death usually occurs within a period of 6 to 14 months.[310]

The incidence of pleural effusion is higher in cases of metastatic carcinoma of the breast when pulmonary lymphatic involvement is present. Goldsmith and his associates, in their retrospective study[315] of 365 consecutive necropsies of patients who died from breast carcinoma, recorded pleural effusion in 52 (60 per cent) of the 87 patients who had lymphangitic spread and in 117 (42 per cent) of those who did not, a variation in incidence that supports Meyer's thesis[248] of the influence of lymphatic obstruction in the pathogenesis of effusion in metastatic cancer. The cytologic features of breast carcinoma cells in pleural fluid have been described in several reports.[316, 317]

PLEURAL EFFUSION CAUSED BY THROMBOEMBOLIC DISEASE

As a roentgenographic manifestation of thromboembolic disease, pleural effusion is as common as parenchymal consolidation.[318–321] In a prospective study of 62 patients with pulmonary embolism and effusion, Bynum and Wilson[322] found roentgenographic evidence of infarction in only half of the patients. In another series of 10 patients with bilateral pleural effusion caused by thromboembolism, the effusion was the only manifestation of disease in seven.[6] However, in our experience pleural effusion nearly always indicates infarction. The parenchymal shadow may be diminutive or hidden by the fluid;[323, 324] this can confuse the diagnostic possibilities to such an extent that an embolic episode will be suggested only if there is a high index of suspicion. The amount of pleural fluid is frequently small, but may be abundant, and is most often unilateral.[32, 322, 325, 326] When predominantly infrapulmonary, it may be mistaken for hemidiaphragmatic elevation.[325] Pleural fluid usually develops and absorbs synchronously with the infarction but sometimes appears later and clears sooner.[327]

Light[32] has stated categorically that analysis of the pleural fluid in pulmonary embolism is not helpful in diagnosis, since it can have the features of either a transudate or an exudate and in only a minority of cases is it grossly bloody. We concur that transudates can occur but suspect that in most, if not all, such cases they are caused by clinically unrecognized heart failure. We also feel that in a patient suspected on clinical grounds of having pulmonary embolism, a bloody pleural effusion is strong confirmatory evidence for associated infarction. Thoracentesis was performed early in the course of the disease in 26 of the 62 patients described by Bynum and Wilson:[322] the effusion was bloody in 15 of 18 patients (83 per cent) with

evidence of infarction but in only 3 of the 8 patients (38 per cent) without parenchymal abnormality.

The pulmonary changes of thromboembolism and infarction (described in detail in Chapter 9) are varied. The combination of diaphragmatic elevation, basal pulmonary opacity of almost any type (but usually homogeneous), and a small pleural effusion constitutes a triad of roentgenologic signs highly suggestive of the diagnosis.

PLEURAL EFFUSION CAUSED BY CARDIAC DECOMPENSATION

Probably one of the most common forms of pleural effusion is that associated with increase in hydrostatic pressure in the venous circulation, either pulmonary or systemic (or both). It occurs most commonly with cardiac decompensation but may be seen also with constrictive pericarditis[328, 329] or obstruction of the superior vena cava or azygos vein. It has been reported to occur in 60 per cent of patients with constrictive pericarditis and may be the presenting clinical finding.[329, 330] The mechanisms whereby the effusions develop are complex and are related not only to increased hydrostatic pressure but also to influences such as altered capillary permeability (secondary to hypoxia) and reduced lymphatic drainage.

Considerable confusion and difference of opinion have existed as to whether the development of hydrothorax in human cardiac decompensation is attributable predominantly to failure of the right side of the heart (systemic venous hypertension), the left side of the heart (pulmonary venous hypertension), or a combination of the two. Although Logue and coworkers[331] reported 66 instances of pleural effusion in 114 patients with "left-sided heart failure," we have felt for some time that right-sided or left-sided cardiac failure in relatively "pure" form seldom leads to hydrothorax and that decompensation of both sides of the heart is required.

In 1970, Mellins and his colleagues reported a study on dogs that cast considerable light on this controversy.[332] In all of the animals, elevation of pulmonary and systemic venous pressures was achieved by inflation of balloon catheters appropriately placed in the left atrium or in the superior vena cava (SVC) and inferior vena cava (IVC), respectively. Simultaneously, plasma colloid osmotic pressure was reduced by intravenous saline infusion. Three experimental arrangements were used in order to bring about pulmonary venous hypertension (left atrial balloon inflated), systemic venous hypertension (SVC and IVC balloons inflated), and combined venous hypertension (all balloons inflated). Pulmonary venous hypertension (mean left atrial pressure 24.5 mm Hg) resulted in an average accumulation of pleural fluid of 25.5 ml, only slightly more than the nonhypertensive control group. With systemic venous hypertension (mean pressure in the venae cavae 26.5 mm Hg), the average volume of pleural fluid was 67.5 ml. When pulmonary and systemic venous hypertension co-existed (mean pressure in the left atrium and venae cavae 23.6 mm Hg), the average pleural fluid volume was 87.5 ml. Thus, a significantly larger amount of pleural fluid accumulated after systemic venous hypertension than after pulmonary venous hypertension, and the largest amount of fluid accumulated with combined systemic and venous hypertension. Although one cannot categorically apply these results to humans, they at least lend considerable support to the contention that the clinical situation most favorable for the development of pleural effusion is decompensation of both sides of the heart.

For some unknown reason unilateral hydrothorax in congestive heart failure is more prone to be right-sided than left-sided, although it is frequently bilateral; in fact, Race and colleagues[333] found 88 per cent of patients to have bilateral effusions at autopsy. Light[32] has suggested that unilateral effusion in congestive heart failure should alert the physician to look for some other cause. We concur with this position but only if the unilateral effusion is confined to the left hemithorax.[331] Associated clinical and roentgenologic evidence of cardiac enlargement, with or without pulmonary venous hypertension, usually makes the diagnosis obvious in most cases. The fluid, usually clear and light yellow, is a transudate with low protein and LDH content and a specific gravity of 1.015 or less. At least two groups of investigators[334, 335] have shown that when pleural fluid is subjected to serial assays while a patient is undergoing treatment, it can develop the characteristics of an exudate.

A roentgenologic finding peculiar to hydrothorax associated with congestive heart failure is the so-called "phantom tumor," in which fluid tends to localize (not loculate) in an interlobar pleural fissure (Fig. 18–5). These "disappearing tumors" occur most frequently in the right horizontal fissure. The mechanism of this localization is not clear. In a case studied by Sanghvi and Misra,[336] pneumothorax was induced after the phantom tumor had disappeared, and this clearly showed the absence of any pleural adhesions. Cases also have been described in which localized interlobar effusion associated with cardiac decompensation has been followed by the development of free bilateral pleural effusions without localization, an observation lending further support to the contention that the mechanism has nothing to do with pleural adhesions, at least in some cases.[337]

PLEURAL EFFUSION CAUSED BY TRAUMA

Hemothorax is a common manifestation of penetrating and nonpenetrating trauma and may develop from a variety of causes. Blood may originate in vessels within the chest wall, diaphragm, lung, or mediastinum. Reynolds and Davis[340] have emphasized the importance of the site of hemorrhage in relation to the size of a hemothorax: when bleeding occurs from a systemic vessel in the chest wall, diaphragm, or mediastinum, the hemothorax tends to increase despite the quantity of blood present; by contrast, when the blood comes from the pulmonary vasculature the expanding hemothorax compresses the lung, with resultant pulmonary tamponade that may produce hemostasis. Although hemorrhage may result from laceration of the parietal or visceral pleura by fractured ribs, it can also occur (with or without associated pneumothorax) in closed chest trauma without evidence of fracture. Hemothorax complicating traumatic rupture of the aorta is common and is almost invariably left-sided.[339] It must not be attributed erroneously to left-sided rib fracture.

When blood enters the pleural space it coagulates rapidly, but, presumably as a result of physical agitation produced by movement of the heart and lungs, the clot may be defibrinated and leave fluid indistinguishable roentgenologically from effusion of any other cause.[339, 340] Tube drainage is indicated in most patients with hemothorax and is usually effective.[341] If residual clots remain, further management is controversial. Some surgical authorities[342] recommend early evacuation by thoracotomy, and others[341] find that such remaining blood clears with time and can be treated conservatively. Intrapleural streptokinase has been recommended to dissolve clots[343] but has been reported also to induce severe intrapleural hemorrhage.[344] Loculation tends to occur early, further increasing the difficulty of needle drainage.

Empyema complicating hemothorax is usually caused by *Staphylococcus aureus*. By contrast, empyema that complicates serous effusions or pneumothorax in traumatized patients is usually caused by hospital-acquired gram-negative organisms, and there is reason to believe that chest tube thoracostomy may be responsible for the infection, at least in some cases.[85] Once post-traumatic empyema becomes well established and refractory to tube drainage, decortication with evacuation of the empyema cavity should be performed as soon as possible.[345]

Pleural effusion or hydropneumothorax, almost always left-sided, frequently develops following esophageal perforation. Rupture of the esophagus from closed chest trauma is rare and results in changes localized to the mediastinum and pleura.[339] Of considerably greater frequency is the rupture that occurs as a complication of esophagoscopy or gastroscopy,[346] overzealous dilatation of a stricture or achalasia, disruption of the suture line following esophageal resection and anastomosis, or, as in two reported cases,[347] passage of an esophageal obturator airway used by paramedical personnel during cardiopulmonary resuscitation. In any of

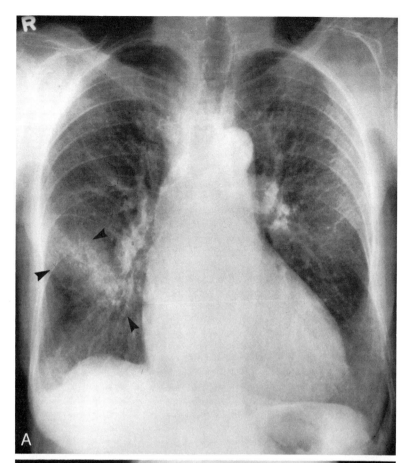

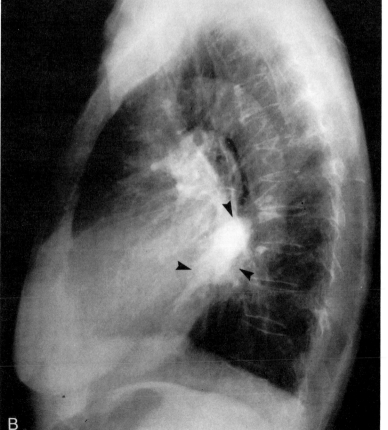

Figure 18–5. Focal Interlobar Pleural Effusion (Pseudotumor) in Cardiac Decompensation. Posteroanterior *(A)* and lateral *(B)* roentgenograms reveal a moderately enlarged left ventricle and diffuse interstitial edema. An elliptical, obliquely oriented opacity *(arrowheads)* present on the right is suggestive of fluid in the interlobar fissure; minimal blunting of the ipsilateral costophrenic sulcus signifies only a small effusion.

Illustration continued on following page

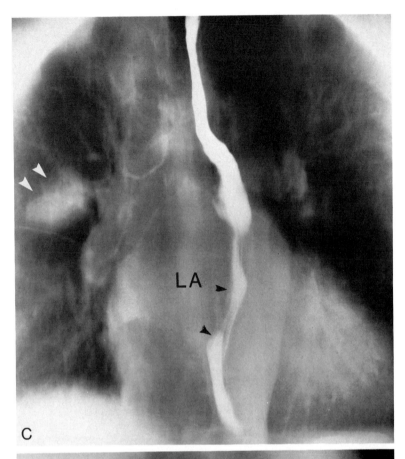

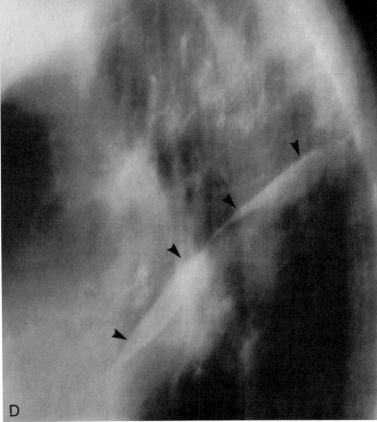

Figure 18–5 *Continued* Conventional linear tomograms in anteroposterior projection through the hila *(C)* and in lateral projection through the midpoint of the right lung *(D)* reveal an elliptical interlobar pleural effusion *(white arrowheads)* that is more extensive than might be suspected from the conventional roentgenograms. Enlargement of the left atrium *(LA)* displaces the barium-filled esophagus *(arrowheads)*.

these circumstances, identification of ingested material (such as milk) in pleural fluid is diagnostic. Pleural fluid amylase levels are raised in most,[348] but not all,[349, 350] patients; the amylase originates in the salivary glands. The pH of the effusion is reduced.[32] In the majority of cases the site of rupture must be identified precisely (and sometimes with considerable difficulty) by roentgenographic evidence of extravasation of ingested contrast material.

Rupture of the thoracic duct, resulting in chylothorax, may develop from surgical trauma, a nonpenetrating injury, or a penetrating wound from a bullet or knife.[339, 340] Chylothorax is considered in greater detail in the next section of this chapter. Small exudative effusions sometimes develop following endoscopic sclerotherapy of esophageal varices, presumably as a result of inflammation of the mediastinal parietal pleura; Bacon and associates[351] identified this complication following 31 of 65 sclerotherapy sessions in 30 patients. These episodes were associated with more pain and a greater volume of sclerosant than obtained in the patients who did not develop effusion.

The most common pleural effusion of "traumatic" etiology is that caused by thoracotomy. Chest roentgenograms 2 or 3 days after thoracotomy usually show no fluid, since the pleural space is effectively drained. Following removal of the drainage tube, however, often a small amount of fluid appears, only to disappear quite quickly during convalescence. Minimal residual pleural thickening may remain. The accumulation of fluid in larger than expected amounts may be attributable to a variety of causes, including poor positioning of the drainage tube, hemorrhage from an intercostal vessel, or infection (empyema). Hemorrhage from an intercostal vessel has been reported to be a significant complication in patients undergoing heart-lung transplantation.[352] Empyema can develop shortly after lung resection or can be delayed for several months and often results from a complicating bronchopleural fistula. In one series of 75 patients with empyema of varied etiology,[353] 15.5 per cent developed empyema after pneumonectomy and 3.7 per cent after lobectomy. In four of nine cases of late onset empyema that presented at least three months following surgery,[354] the roentgenographic demonstration of gas in a previously opaque hemithorax led to the diagnosis of fistulae, one being bronchial, two esophageal, and the fourth both bronchial and esophageal; in the remaining five, the presence of empyema was established only following the development of empyema necessitatis. The belief that empyema complicating resectional surgery for pulmonary carcinoma improves the prognosis of this disease[355–360] has not been confirmed by more recent studies.[361–364]

Malpositioning of percutaneous central venous and Swan-Ganz catheters[365] can cause perforation of a vessel, either at the time of insertion or some time later as a result of gradual erosion of a relatively thin-walled intrathoracic vessel by the catheter tip. Depending on the vein involved and on the reason for catheter insertion (monitoring of pressure or hyperalimentation), the result may be mediastinal hemorrhage, hemothorax,[366] pneumothorax, massive hydrothorax,[367, 371] or extrapleural hematoma.[368–370] In patients receiving hyperalimentation, the infusion of toxic or potentially toxic solutions obviously increases the hazard.

An uncommon cause of pleural effusion is subarachnoid-pleural fistula, usually secondary to accidental trauma;[372–374] rarely such a fistula follows surgery[375] or a neurogenic tumor related to the vertebral column.[376] One case has been described in which a combination of subarachnoid-pleural fistula and chylothorax followed trauma.[377]

An unusual cause of hemothorax following severe trauma has been reported[378] in which a lacerated spleen herniated into the thorax through a traumatic rupture of the diaphragm. Splenic arteriography revealed the ruptured spleen within the left hemithorax and showed extravasation of contrast medium into the pleural space. An association also has been reported between recurrent left-sided pleural effusion and silent splenic hematomas following trauma.[379]

Roentgenographically demonstrable pleural effusion following radiation therapy to the thorax is very uncommon.[380–382] However, fairly extensive thickening of the pleura may be seen both roentgenologically and pathologically.[380, 383]

Although trauma (including thoracotomy) is by far the most common cause of hemothorax, spontaneous intrapleural bleeding can occur from a variety of causes. If Light's definition of hemothorax as fluid with a hematocrit of over 50 per cent is accepted, some malignancies involving the pleura can result in hemothorax rather than a simple serosanguineous effusion.[32] In addition, hemothorax occurs occasionally as a result of anticoagulation,[384] endometriosis,[385–387] hemophilia,[388] and neurofibromatosis in pregnancy.[389]

PLEURAL EFFUSION SECONDARY TO DISEASE BELOW THE DIAPHRAGM

A variety of intra-abdominal or pelvic disorders are associated with pleural effusion, the pathogenesis of which is complex; it can be caused by secondary effects on cardiac function, changes in plasma oncotic pressure, or the production of ascites or secretions that are transferred through diaphragmatic lymphatics or deficiencies into the pleural space.

In 1929 Lemon and Higgins[390] described lymphatic channels that carry particulate matter from the peritoneum to the thorax and found that those of the right hemidiaphragm are larger and carry more fluid than those of the left. Experimental work confirmed these observations. For example, it was shown that, in the presence of ascites, carbon particles or radioiodinated serum albumin instilled into the peritoneal space passes into the pleural space[391] and that flow is always from the peritoneum to the pleura, never in the reverse direction.[391, 392] Although it seems probable that most fluid transfer occurs by way of diaphragmatic lymphatic channels, it is possible that defects within the diaphragm may permit fluid passage in some patients.[393, 394] In a study of 18 patients with hydrothorax associated with cirrhosis, Lieberman and associates[395] injected air into the peritoneal space of 5 patients and subsequently were able to confirm the presence of hydropneumothorax in all 5 patients; a defect in the diaphragm was identified on thoracoscopic examination of 1 patient and at necropsy in 2 others. The conclusion must be drawn that in some patients fluid transfer from the peritoneal to the pleural space occurs by way of diaphragmatic lymphatics and in others by way of diaphragmatic defects. The question inevitably arises as to why all cases of ascites are not associated with pleural effusion, and, to the best of our knowledge, the answer has not been found.

Pancreatitis

Acute or chronic pancreatitis is sometimes associated with pleural effusion, often without roentgenographic evidence of other intrathoracic abnormality. Effusions are predominantly left-sided: of 31 cases reviewed by Hammarsten and his colleagues[396] the effusion was on the left in 21, on the right in 3, and bilateral in 7. In another series of 80 cases of pleural effusion secondary to pancreatic disease, Kaye[397] found that 48 effusions (60 per cent) were left-sided, 24 (30 per cent) right-sided, and 8 (10 per cent) bilateral. In the majority of patients with acute pancreatitis, symptoms will suggest an acute upper abdominal disorder, but in some the clinical presentation can be confused with a primary or parapneumonic pleural effusion.[398, 399] A minority of patients with acute pancreatitis develop an abscess[32, 398] that only becomes apparent 2 to 3 weeks after the acute episode; the abscess itself can be responsible for the pleural effusion.

Chronic pancreatitis is associated with pleural effusion even more often than the acute disease.[400–412] The effusion is often recurrent, and symptoms frequently direct attention to the thorax rather than the abdomen. In many cases the patient has a history of heavy alcohol consumption that has been responsible for the pancreatitis. Duct disruption can lead to the creation of a pancreaticopleural fistula, with or without pseudocyst formation. The fistulous tract can also communicate with the peritoneal cavity (causing ascites),[400, 405] the mediastinum (resulting in bilateral pleural effusions and sometimes pericarditis),[409] and even occasionally a bronchus.[411, 413]

The pleural fluid in both acute and chronic pancreatitis has the characteristics of an exudate and is sometimes serosanguineous and occasionally bloody.[399, 404, 407] In acute pancreatitis, the effusion is more likely to be slight or moderate in amount and bloody,[32, 399] whereas in chronic pancreatitis it tends to be serous, massive, and recurrent.[402, 404, 407, 414] The amylase content of the pleural fluid is characteristically very high and is almost invariably higher than that of the serum.[400–402, 404, 406, 407, 410, 411] Elevated levels of pleural fluid amylase can be found also in esophageal perforation[348] and in neoplasm-related pleural effusion,[415] including carcinoma of the pancreas.[416]

With proper positioning, the pancreatico-pleural fistula in either acute or chronic pancreatitis can be demonstrated with contrast medium by endoscopic retrograde cholangiopancreatography (ERCP) or computed tomography (CT);[399, 401–403, 406, 408–412, 417] the latter technique appears to be more profitable. McCarthy and her colleagues[417] demonstrated such fistulae in four patients by CT that were not demonstrable by ERCP. However, ERCP is not only important in diagnosis but also permits a precise evaluation of the ductal morphology that is indispensable for proper surgical management.

Three cases have been reported in which pleural calcification occurred in association with pancreatitis, the calcification being bilateral and basal in situation and curvilinear in configuration;[418] there was no known history of asbestos exposure.

Following Abdominal Surgery

The development of small pleural effusions is common after abdominal surgery. Light and George[419] carried out a study of 200 patients 48 to 72 hours following surgery in whom roentgenograms were obtained in the right and left lateral decubitus positions. Pleural effusion was identified in 97 patients (49 per cent), being less than 4 mm in thickness in 50 patients, 4 to 10 mm in 26, and greater than 10 mm in 21. The incidence was higher following surgery on the upper abdomen, in patients with postoperative atelectasis on the side on which the surgery was performed, and in patients with free abdominal fluid. Thoracentesis was carried out on 20 of the 97 patients and 16 of these revealed an exudate. All but one of these effusions resolved spontaneously, the exception being associated with staphylococcal infection.

Subphrenic Abscess

Small pleural effusions are often found in cases of acute subphrenic infection; they were observed in 37 of 47 cases (79 per cent) reported by Miller and Talman.[420] Associated findings include elevation and restriction of movement of the ipsilateral hemidiaphragm (95 per cent in the above series) and basal plate atelectasis or pneumonitis (79 per cent). This combination of findings should strongly suggest the diagnosis, especially in the postoperative period after laparotomy or following rupture of a hollow abdominal viscus.

Subphrenic abscess secondary to infection of abdominal viscera, with or without perforation, is often misdiagnosed.[32, 421] The diagnosis should be suspected in any patient with pleural effusion who has recently undergone abdominal surgery or whose effusion is exudative with a high neutrophilic leukocyte count. Most patients have fever, leukocytosis, and abdominal pain; upper abdominal tenderness is generally present but is not invariable. The effusions are usually negative on culture and probably result from diaphragmatic inflammation; however, this is not necessarily the case, as illustrated by a report of 10 patients with empyema secondary to intra-abdominal sepsis.[422] CT scans, ultrasonography, and gallium scans may prove useful in establishing the diagnosis.[423]

Two patients have been reported[423] who had recently undergone major abdominal surgery and who were suspected of having pulmonary embolism; in each case a pulmonary angiogram showed a hemidiaphragm clearly outlined by contrast medium, a phenomenon that was interpreted as being caused by hyperperfusion as a consequence of subdiaphragmatic inflammation.

Meigs-Salmon Syndrome

In 1934 Salmon[424] described the association of pleural effusion with benign pelvic tumors in a report that antedated by 3 years the results of the study by Meigs and Cass[425] of seven cases of ovarian fibromas associated with ascites and hydrothorax. The syndrome is now known to be associated with a wide variety of primary ovarian neoplasms, including fibroma, thecoma, granulosa cell tumor, Brenner tumor, cystadenoma,[426, 427] and even adenocarcinoma;[428] occasionally, extraovarian pelvic tumors such as uterine leiomyomas have been implicated.[429, 430] According to Meigs,[392] the first four of these neoplasms are those with which the syndrome is most commonly associated. It is believed that the tumor size, rather than the specific histologic type of tumor, is the most important factor leading to the formation of sufficient fluid to cause ascites and accompanying pleural effusion.[32] Supporting this hypothesis is a 1945 review by Dockerty,[431] in which almost 40 per cent of ovarian neoplasms measuring more than 6 cm in diameter were associated with ascites; however, hydrothorax occurred in only 2 to 3 per cent of these cases.

The effusions vary widely in amount and may be massive; they occur more frequently on the right but may be left-sided or bilateral. Although usually a transudate, the fluid occasionally contains blood.[430] Removal of the pelvic tumor is usually followed by disappearance of the ascites and hydrothorax. In a woman with a pelvic mass and hydrothorax, the absence of malignant cells in the pleural fluid may be considered presumptive evidence of Meigs-Salmon syndrome, although absolute proof rests upon disappearance of the fluid following resection of the neoplasm. Perhaps the most important feature of Meigs-Salmon syndrome is the fact that neither pleural effusion nor ascites is necessarily an ominous sign in patients with a pelvic neoplasm, even when the tumor is malignant.[428]

Intra-Abdominal Malignancy (Other than Pelvic)

Both primary carcinoma of the pancreas[432] and retroperitoneal lymphoma[433] may be associated with pleural effusion without direct invasion of the thorax. The implications in regard to therapy are of obvious importance.

Dialysis

Since ascites may be associated with pleural effusion, it might be reasonably anticipated that peritoneal dialysis would sometimes lead to hydrothorax, and several such cases have been reported.[434, 435] Patients receiving chronic hemodialysis may also develop pleural effusion,[436, 437] the fluid often being serosanguineous as a consequence of the use of heparin during hemodialysis. Because such patients are uremic, it may not be possible to distinguish effusion occurring as a complication of hemodialysis from that associated with uremia itself (*see* farther on).

Hydronephrosis and Urinothorax

Corriere and his colleagues[438] described two patients who presented with right-sided pleural effusion and were found subsequently to have hydronephrosis of the right kidney. Relief of the obstruction to urinary flow resulted in disappearance of the effusion in both cases. This association of urinary tract obstruction and the development of unilateral or bilateral pleural effusion has been subsequently described by several other investigators.[439–448] The majority of published reports attribute the source of the urine collection in the thorax to retroperitoneal collections of urine (urinomas). Urinomas form as a result of extravasation of urine from the urinary tract secondary to obstruction in the renal pelvis, ureters, bladder, or urethra. The diagnosis of urinothorax is made by the demonstration of a level of creatinine in pleural fluid that is higher than in the blood.[440, 442, 443, 448] Surgical drainage of the urinomas results in rapid clearing of effusions. Despite the foregoing, it is probable that in some cases the pleural fluid represents a reaction to inflammation of the diaphragmatic pleura from an adjacent hydronephrosis or urinoma;[32, 445, 448] in such cases the effusion will be a transudate.

Nephrotic Syndrome

Pleural effusion is common in the nephrotic syndrome, having been observed in 21 per cent of 52 patients studied by Cavina and Vichi.[450] The main influence leading to pleural transudation is diminution in the plasma osmotic pressure, thereby upsetting the fine balance that normally keeps the pleural space "dry." The fluid is a transudate. The nephrotic syndrome is one of the few disorders associated with a high incidence of atypical location of pleural effusion, commonly in the infrapulmonary space.[449] Of 19 cases of pleural effusion associated with the nephrotic syndrome and acute glomerulonephritis studied by Cavina and Vichi,[450] the effusion was infrapulmonary in 10 patients. The reasons underlying this high incidence are obscure. Clearly, the fact that the effusion is a transudate is not significant in this regard, since a wide variety of fluids (including blood) sometimes behave similarly. Recurrent pleural effusion may require obliteration of the pleural spaces for adequate control.[451] In patients with the nephrotic syndrome and pleural effusion, it is important to exclude thromboembolic disease as a cause of the effusion.[452] Two cases of empyema and mesangiocapillary glomerulonephritis with nephrotic syndrome have been described;[453] in one the nephrotic syndrome resolved with treatment of the empyema.

Cirrhosis

Of 200 consecutive cases of cirrhosis associated with ascites, Johnston and Loo[391] found 12 patients (6 per cent) to have hydrothorax. The effusion was right-sided in 8, bilateral in 2, and left-sided in 2 patients. In most reports of cirrhosis with pleural effusion, the effusion is right-sided.[454-456] According to Black,[5] there are at least three possible mechanisms for the development of pleural effusion in patients with cirrhosis—hypoproteinemia, azygos hypertension, and transfer of peritoneal fluid to the pleural cavity. For a variety of reasons, azygos hypertension is unlikely to be a major factor. It is probable that the chief mechanism is the transfer of ascitic fluid through the diaphragm by way of either the lymphatics or diaphragmatic defects, although hypoproteinemia may be a contributing factor; for example, some cases of effusion have been reported in the absence of ascites.[456] The rapidity with which radioisotope injected into the peritoneal space appears in the pleural fluid may provide evidence as to which of these two routes is effective, being more rapid in the presence of diaphragmatic defects.[454]

Acute Glomerulonephritis

The incidence of pleural effusion in association with acute glomerulonephritis in children is fairly high; it was observed in 42 of 76 children studied by Kirkpatrick and Fleisher.[457] The effusion may be associated with a variety of pulmonary changes, including segmental or lobar atelectasis, pneumonia, and pulmonary edema.[458] It is postulated that these effusions relate to alterations in extracellular fluid volume, but the evidence that they are not infectious in origin has not been clearly documented.

Uremic Pleuritis

Both the pericardium and pleura may become inflamed in patients with uremia. Hopps and Wissler[459] found fibrinous pleuritis in 20 per cent of uremic patients at necropsy. The pleuritis is not necessarily fibrinous, however; in some patients, the fluid is an exudate containing high levels of protein and LDH, suggesting that there must be some disruption of the pleural membrane.[460, 461] Affected patients sometimes complain of pain, and friction rubs frequently are heard on auscultation.[461] If the patient is receiving chronic hemodialysis the effusion usually clears slowly. The fluid frequently contains blood, possibly as a result of the anticoagulation associated with hemodialysis.[436, 437] A patient on hemodialysis who had fibrosing uremic pleuritis and developed empyema has been described.[462]

MISCELLANEOUS CAUSES OF PLEURAL EFFUSION

Myxedema

Abnormal accumulations of pleural fluid are known to occur in patients with myxedema even in the absence of cardiovascular, renal, or other causes of fluid retention. Most often the effusion occurs in the pericardium, but it may also develop in the pleural space.[463] It has no distinctive roentgenographic characteristics.

Lymphatic Hypoplasia

Pleural effusion may develop as a result of hypoplasia of the lymphatic system. In some instances the clinical presentation is that of Milroy's disease;[464] in others the effusion is associated with lymphedema of an extremity, yellow nails, and sometimes bronchiectasis (see page 2206).[465] The pleural fluid characteristically has a high protein content and accumulates as a result of an underlying congenital or inherited lymphatic dysplasia. Two siblings with this syndrome have been described in whom pleural effusion was associated with immunologic deficiency manifested by hypogammaglobulinemia and episodes of lymphopenia. One of the siblings suffered from repeated infections and eventually died of cor pulmonale; the other subsequently developed Hodgkin's disease.[466] Recurrent pleural effusion also has been reported in a patient with protein-losing enteropathy, malabsorption, mosaic warts, and generalized lymphatic hypoplasia.[467] Lymphography revealed the lymphatic hypoplasia to be asymmetric. Intestinal lymphangiectasis was demonstrated on jejunal biopsy.

Dressler's Syndrome

The postpericardiectomy and postmyocardial infarction syndromes, known eponymously as Dressler's syndrome, are characterized by chest pain, fever, and pericardial and pleural effusion. Dressler[468] estimated the incidence to be 3 to 4 per cent of patients following myocardial infarction, and it is probable that the incidence is even higher following surgical procedures involving the pericardium.[32] The pathogenesis is unknown but is suspected to represent a manifestation of an immunologic reaction.

Symptoms appear 2 to 3 weeks after the infarct or pericardial surgery; in patients with myocardial infarction, the syndrome is particularly apt to occur in the presence of transmural myocardial damage with epicardial extension.[469] In a comprehensive retrospective study of 35 patients with Dressler's syndrome (21 patients following cardiac surgery and 14 after myocardial infarction), Stelzner and associates[470] found the onset of symptoms to occur, on average, 20 days after the injury. The major clinical findings were pleurisy (91 per cent), fever (66 per cent), pericardial rub (63 per cent), dyspnea (57 per cent), rales (51 per cent), pleural rub (46 per cent), and leukocytosis (49 per cent). The chest roentgenogram was abnormal in 94 per cent of the patients: pleural effusion was present in 83 per cent, parenchymal opacities in 74 per cent, and an enlarged cardiopericardial silhouette in 49 per cent. Analysis of pleural fluid was performed on 16 samples from 12 patients and revealed a bloody exudate with a pH greater than 7.40. The syndrome can recur several years after the initial episode.[471]

Familial Paroxysmal Polyserositis

This disease, known also as familial Mediterranean fever[472, 473] and recurrent hereditary polyserositis,[474] is a rare cause of paroxysmal attacks of pleurisy. It occurs predominantly in Sephardic Jews, Arabs, Turks, and Armenians. Although there appears to be a genetic factor in etiology, the incidence of the disease in North America in the same racial population at risk apparently is considerably less than in the Mediterranean area. The actual cause of the precipitation of attacks is unknown. One group of investigators[475] found that leukocyte chemotaxis was increased during attacks and that it decreased by about 50 per cent with colchicine therapy. Abnormalities in catecholamine metabolism[474] and a defect in serum complement[478] also have been proposed as factors in the pathogenesis.

In one large study of 175 Arabs with the disease,[474] the most common manifestation was peritonitis (93.7 per cent), followed by arthritis (33.7 per cent) and pleurisy (32 per cent). An erysipelas-like rash and pericarditis are less frequent manifestations.[476] Pulmonary atelectasis was reported in one patient,[477] with response to colchicine and recurrence on cessation of medication. Seventy five to 80 per cent of the attacks of pleurisy are associated with arthritis and arthralgia, usually involving the large joints; joint pain typically lasts for 12 to 24 hours and occasionally for as long as 3 days. Fever, sometimes as high as 104° F, persists for 12 to 48 hours. Remissions may last for months to years. One ophthalmologic study[479] reported tiny white colloid bodies in the retina of 50 per cent of patients. Despite the recurrent disability, the prognosis is apparently excellent in most cases.[480, 481] An exception to this rule is the rare patient who develops renal amyloidosis.

Incidental Causes of Pleural Effusion

Perforation of an abdominal viscus can lead to pleural effusion, usually as a consequence of a subphrenic abscess; occasionally a gastric or duodenal ulcer communicates directly with the pleural cavity through the diaphragm, resulting in an effusion that can be bilious or at least can contain a high bilirubin level.[475, 482] Roentgenographic evidence of a left pleural effusion in a patient with a history suggesting the possibility of a *traumatic diaphragmatic hernia* should alert the physician to the likelihood of this etiology; the presence of intestinal loops within the hemithorax virtually confirms the diagnosis. Since fluid seldom accumulates in the pleural space in the absence of bowel strangulation (it leaks through the diaphragmatic rent), a pleural effusion should alert the physician to the presence of vascular compromise, and immediate therapeutic intervention is indicated.[483] Rarely pleural effusion occurs in *inflammatory bowel disease* such as Crohn's disease or chronic ulcerative colitis, presumably as a manifestation of a multisystem immunologic disorder.[484, 485] Right-sided or bilateral pleural effusions also have been reported following *liver transplantation;*[486, 487] postoperative mechanical ventilation appears to prevent this complication.[487]

In addition to the effusion that can accompany malignant neoplasms of ribs and vertebrae, *eosinophilic granuloma* can be complicated rarely by effusion.[488] *Suppurative spondylitis* caused by *S. aureus* and other organisms can initiate a pleural effusion that is high in neutrophil content.[489] *Gorham's disease,* a rare nonmalignant proliferation of vascular or lymphatic tissue, has been reported to cause a serious complicating hemorrhagic pleural effusion secondary to involvement of the thoracic skeleton.[490]

Pleural effusion is a common manifestation of *hydrops fetalis.* The prognosis in such cases is generally poor because of pulmonary hypoplasia. Ultrasonography can detect the presence of pleural fluid that can be removed either *in utero* or immediately on delivery, with benefit to those newborns whose lungs are functioning.[491-493]

CHYLOTHORAX

Chylothorax designates an increase in pleural fluid that is high in lipid content. The fluid is characteristically "milky" in appearance, although not all milky effusions are truly chylous in nature[290, 494] and not all chylous effusions are milky.[495] Several terms have been employed to describe these fluids. *Chylous effusion* is caused by the escape of chyle into the pleural space from obstruction or laceration of the thoracic duct. *Chyliform effusion* results from degeneration of malignant and other cells in pleural fluid. *Pseudochylous effusion* results from the presence of cholesterol crystals and occurs most commonly in tuberculosis and the nephrotic syndrome. We agree with Light[32] that the separation of pseudochylous and chyliform effusions on the basis of the presence or absence of cholesterol crystals serves little useful purpose, and we propose to designate all high-lipid nonchylous effusions as chyliform.

Chylous effusion is high in neutral fat and fatty acid but low in cholesterol, whereas chyliform effusions are low in neutral fat and high in cholesterol and lecithin.[494] The simultaneous analysis of fasting samples of serum and pleural fluid by lipoprotein electrophoresis readily distinguishes the two forms.[496] Williams and Burford[497] have described another simple test—the ingestion of a coal-tar dye (labeled "drug and cosmetic green #6") with a high-fat meal that colors the chyle a distinctive green. In an analysis of 141 patients with chylous effusions based on the presence of chylomicrons, Staats and coworkers[495] found that the gross appearance indicated chylothorax in only 50 per cent. However, triglyceride levels in the fluid readily differentiated almost all chylous from serous effusions, and the authors recommended that a triglyceride level should be obtained in all pleural effusions of undetermined pathogenesis.

Pseudochylothorax with its associated chyliform pleural fluid is uncommon: in one review of 53 nontraumatic effusions of high lipid content, only 6 (11 per cent) were chyliform. They have a milky appearance similar to that of chylothorax,[498-500] and may contain some triglycerides; cholesterol crystals probably derive from breakdown products of blood cells and can be readily identified on smear. Although the clinical situation will usually indicate whether an effusion is chylous or chyliform, the detection of chylomicrons by lipoprotein analysis may be necessary in some cases to identify a true chylous effusion. Patients with chyliform effusions are often asymptomatic, but a patient may give a history of a disease that was the cause of the effusion; rheumatoid disease and tuberculosis are the most commonly associated diseases.[32, 500] Chyliform pleural effusions secondary to paragonimiasis have been reported in three Hmong immigrants to the United States.[501]

Schulman and associates have described the lymphographic abnormalities that occur in association with chylothorax in detail[502] and reached a number of conclusions that deserve repetition here. They pointed out that the lymphatic drainage of the small intestine (chyle) is carried entirely by the thoracic duct; thus, chylothorax can occur only with obstruction or laceration of this duct. Lesions that obstruct the right lymphatic duct or pulmonary lymphatics can cause pleural effusion but never chylothorax.

In a review of 143 cases of chylothorax from five separate series, Light[32] found the most common causes to be neoplasm and trauma, the former being responsible twice as often as the latter. Lymphoma is the most common neoplasm,[503] and was the cause in 75 per cent of the patients with malignancy in Light's series.[32] However, pulmonary carcinoma and metastatic cancer from virtually every organ in the body have been reported to obstruct the thoracic duct and cause chylothorax; the effusion is often bilateral and is usually accompanied by chylous ascites.[503-507] Sometimes, chylothorax occurs spontaneously:[508, 509] of 92 cases of chylothorax reviewed by Schmidt,[508] fully one third were idiopathic.

When the thoracic duct is blocked by neoplasm, chylous effusion tends to be very uncommon, almost certainly as a result of the presence of collaterals between the thoracic duct and the right posterior intercostal lymphatics and of the opening up of pre-existing lymphovenous channels.[502] In such circumstances, therefore, in order for chylothorax to occur there must be a developmental or acquired deficiency of one or both of these channels of communication. Chyle may reflux from an obstructed thoracic duct by two routes—the left posterior intercostal lymphatics to the parietal pleural lymphatics, and the left bronchomediastinal trunk to lymphatics of the pulmonary parenchyma and visceral pleura. From either the visceral or parietal lymphatics, chyle then extravasates into the pleural cavity.

Trauma is the second most common cause of chylothorax, most episodes being related to surgery but some to penetrating or nonpenetrating thoracic injury.[510] Since the thoracic duct crosses to the left of the spine between the fifth and seventh thoracic vertebrae, disruption tends to cause right-sided chylothorax when the lower portion is affected and left-sided chylothorax when the upper half is involved. Once the thoracic duct has been disrupted, chyle can leak into the mediastinum and thence into the pleural cavity, either because of damage to the parietal pleura by the initial trauma or because the pleura breaks down under the pressure of the mediastinal fluid collection. Because of its anatomic course, the thoracic duct is particularly vulnerable to traumatic injury during surgery on the vertebral column[511, 512] or on the left hemithorax near the hilum. Postoperative chylothorax is particularly common in children undergoing surgery for congenital heart disease[509, 513–516] but has been reported also in adults following aortocoronary bypass.[517] Sometimes surgical intervention below the diaphragm[518–521] or in the neck[522–524] can also cause leakage of chyle with resultant unilateral or bilateral fluid accumulation; very occasionally, pancreatitis can produce chylothorax.[433, 525] A most unusual cause of traumatic bilateral chylothorax occurred in a patient following an episode of yawning and stretching; the chylothorax presumably resulted from sudden hyperextension of the spine.[526]

Chylothorax in neonates and infants is usually secondary to congenital defects[527–530] but is sometimes idiopathic or traumatic in origin. Even adults have been described with chylothorax and chylopericardium secondary to congenital defects, one in association with congenital lymphedema[531] and another in a patient with localized lymphangiectasia.[532] Generalized lymphatic dysplasia is a serious condition that is usually fatal.[530] Bilateral chylothorax has been diagnosed and successfully drained in utero.[529] The association of chylothorax with Noonan's syndrome[533] is likely attributable to some kind of outlet obstruction to the thoracic duct as well as to other lymphatic or lymphaticovenous abnormalities.

Miscellaneous causes of chylothorax include tuberculosis of the vertebral column,[534] pleura, or lymph nodes;[535] sclerosing mediastinitis;[536] and Gorham's syndrome.[490, 537, 538] The high incidence of chylothorax in patients with lymphangioleiomyomatosis is also well recognized and was described in detail in Chapter 17 (see page 2672).

Lymphangiography is said to play an important role in the investigation of patients with chylothorax.[539–541] It has been pointed out, however, that roentgenographic visualization of intrapulmonary and pleural lymphatics following lymphangiography, while usually associated with chylothorax,[540] can occasionally occur without it.[542] Persistent or recurrent chylous effusions lead to a depletion of lymphocytes and the appearance of immature forms in the peripheral circulation. These findings should not be confused with those of lymphoma.[543]

The prognosis of chylothorax is generally good with the exception of those patients in whom it is caused by neoplasm; in these circumstances it is usually a late manifestation of disease.[509] Considerable difference of opinion exists as to when surgical intervention is indicated. Many authorities report success with conservative management, including aspiration or drainage, restriction of oral fat intake, and intravenous replacement. This approach will probably prove successful in most cases of iatrogenic and traumatic etiology,[519] but in other situations procrastination is not recommended and early surgery with supradiaphragmatic ligature of the thoracic duct or pleurodesis may be lifesaving.[516, 544–547]

PNEUMOTHORAX

The presence of air within the pleural space, or pneumothorax, is one of the more common forms of thoracic disease. It is caused most often by trauma, either accidental or iatrogenic. In the absence of a history of a trauma, pneumothorax is traditionally referred to as *spontaneous:* in this situation, it can be either *primary* (unassociated with clinical or roentgenographic evidence of significant pulmonary disease) or *secondary* (in which such disease is present). This section is concerned predominantly with the incidence, etiology, pathogenesis, and clinical manifestations of the spontaneous form; roentgenographic signs of pneumothorax were discussed in detail in Chapter 4 (*see* page 683).

Incidence

Primary spontaneous pneumothorax occurs most commonly in men in the third and fourth decades of life.[548–550] In a 1967 study of 176 episodes in 153 patients,[551] there was a male-to-female predominance of eight to one. There was no unilateral predominance and only 5 episodes were bilateral. In a 1985 report from Singapore,[552] the male-to-female predominance was as high as 15 to 1. This extraordinary male prevalence has not been the experience in the western world where the male-to-female predominance range is between about 6 to 1[553] and 2 to 1.[554] A study of the overall incidence of spontaneous pneumothorax in Olmsted County, Minnesota, by Melton and his colleagues[553] identified 318 patients on whom a diagnosis of an initial episode of pneumothorax or pneumomediastinum was made during a 25-year period from 1950 to 1974. Of these episodes, 75 were attributed to trauma and 102 to iatrogenic causes; in the remaining 141 patients, the pneumothorax was spontaneous. As a further distinction, the 141 cases were broken down into 77 with primary spontaneous pneumothorax (no roentgenographic evidence of pulmonary disease) and 64 with secondary spontaneous pneumothorax (demonstrable pulmonary disease). The age-adjusted incidence of primary spontaneous pneumothorax was 7.4/100,000 per year for males and 1.2/100,000 per year for females (male-to-female predominance, 6.2 to 1); the incidence of secondary spontaneous pneumothorax was 6.3/100,000 per year and 2.0/100,000 per year, respectively (male-to-female predominance, 3.2 to 1). In an epidemiologic study of 15,204 persons domiciled in the county of Stockholm, Sweden, the annual incidence of first spontaneous pneumothorax was somewhat higher, 18/100,000 for men and 6/100,000 for women.[555]

In several reports a familial incidence of spontaneous pneumothorax has been described:[556–561] in one family of 23 members, 6 had repeated episodes of pneumothorax, an incidence that appeared to relate to the presence of HLA haplotype A2, B40 and the alpha 1-antitrypsin phenotype M1M2.[558] In one series, the incidence of a familial tendency to spontaneous pneumothorax was significantly higher in women than in men.[562]

Etiology and Pathogenesis

The details of the pathogenesis of spontaneous pneumothorax are not clear. The primary form appears to be caused by rupture of an air-containing space within or immediately deep to the visceral pleura. Pathologic studies of resected lung from patients with spontaneous pneumothorax frequently show one or both of two types of air-containing space, a bleb and a bulla. The bulla is lined partly by a thickened fibrotic pleura, partly by fibrous tissue within the lung itself, and partly by emphysematous lung (Fig. 18–6),[563] whereas the bleb is situated entirely within the pleura (Fig. 18–6). The mechanisms behind the formation of each of these are not well understood. In the case of

blebs, the pathogenesis usually is attributed to the dissection of air from a ruptured alveolus through interstitial tissue into the thin fibrous layer of visceral pleura where it accumulates in the form of a "cyst."[564, 565] This is analogous to the mechanism for the development of mediastinal emphysema proposed by Macklin and Macklin in 1944[566] and elaborated upon by Cooley and Gillespie in 1966.[567] The latter authors suggested that pulmonary alveoli are of two types—*marginal*, relating to the perivascular sheaths and having no intercommunicating pores or "safety valves," and *partitional*, representing all other alveoli and possessing intercommunicating pores. These authors further proposed that with overdistention of the marginal alveoli, intra-alveolar pressure becomes greater than that within contiguous tissue, thus establishing a pressure gradient that results in rupture of the alveoli and escape of air into perivascular sheaths.

Alveolar rupture may also relate to check-valve obstruction of a small airway, leading to distention

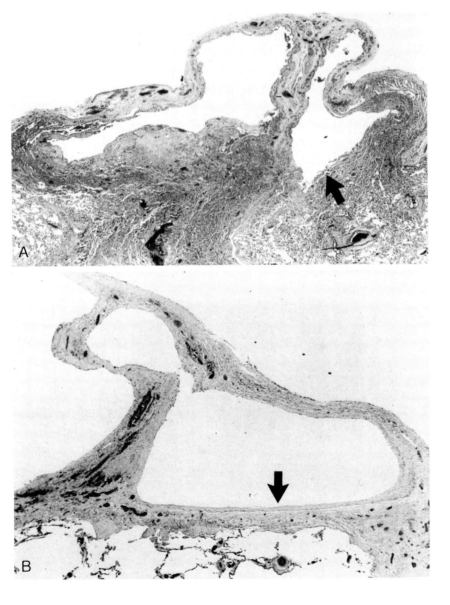

Figure 18–6. Blebs and Bullae: Pathologic Distinction. Lung tissue resected from an individual with spontaneous pneumothorax *(A)* shows two cystic spaces lined by fibrous tissue. Although these spaces appear to be largely within the pleura, one *(arrow)* is in direct contact with lung parenchyma, indicating that it represents a bulla. A section of lung from another patient *(B)* shows similar cystic spaces but in this instance completely surrounded by pleura *(arrow)*, indicating that they are true blebs. (*A*, × 12; *B*, × 18.)

of distal airspaces. Theoretically, airway obstruction could have several causes, including recent or remote infection and a local accumulation of mucus within bronchioles; in addition, full-term infants are capable of generating pleural pressures ranging from -40 to -100 cm H_2O, and it has been postulated that alveolar rupture may occur following airway obstruction by aspirated meconium.[568, 569] Support for this obstructive hypothesis is provided by the high incidence of cigarette smoking in patients with spontaneous pneumothorax; tobacco smoke is clearly associated with increased mucus production.[554, 555, 570] In addition, in one study of 11 nonsmokers with healed spontaneous pneumothorax, assessment of lung function by ventilation-perfusion scintigraphy produced results compatible with the presence of airway obstruction.[571]

The mechanisms behind the formation of bullae are even less clear than those of blebs. Most speculation has centered about the possibility of regional damage to the apical portion of the lung, related either to ischemia or to the greater distensive forces on apical alveoli caused by more negative pleural pressure.[572] In support of both of these mechanisms is the pathologic and roentgenologic identification of apical bullae in many individuals with spontaneous pneumothorax, and the well-documented clinical observation that *primary* spontaneous pneumothorax occurs predominantly in tall, thin men.[553, 573–575] For example, in the series of Melton and associates,[553] an increased incidence of primary spontaneous pneumothorax was found with increased height and reached more than 200 per 100,000 person-years for individuals 76 inches (193 cm) tall or more; the authors considered that this finding could explain the greater incidence of pneumothorax in men. In another series,[575] the average height of affected patients was 2 inches more than that of the general population. Other investigators[576] have measured chest dimensions in young adults with spontaneous pneumothorax and concluded that, on average, the men had longer chests and greater height-to-width ratios than matched controls, whereas the women had a diminished anteroposterior diameter only.

An intrinsic abnormality of connective tissue resulting in an increased tendency to bulla or bleb formation is probably also important in occasional individuals. For example, spontaneous pneumothorax is a known complication of Marfan's syndrome[577–579] and also shows a strong association with mitral valve prolapse, especially in subjects with an abnormal body build.[580]

Even in the presence of pneumothorax, blebs or bullae are sometimes not identifiable on conventional chest roentgenograms,[551, 589] although their visualization may be facilitated by roentgenography in expiration or at the time of maximal pulmonary collapse. Tomography, both conventional and computed, may reveal small blebs or bullae that are invisible on plain roentgenograms. Gobbel and associates[590] found subpleural blebs or bullae at thoracotomy in all 31 patients operated on for primary spontaneous pneumothorax, a clear indication that even if these air-containing spaces are not detected roentgenographically they are nevertheless frequently, if not invariably, present.

The immediate cause of rupture of a bleb or bulla is often unknown. It is clearly not related to exertional effort, because the majority of patients are at rest when the pneumothorax occurs.[581] Blebs and bullae distend with decrease in atmospheric pressure (for example, with increasing altitude during flight[582] and with rapid surfacing after diving[583, 584]) and this mechanism may be important in some cases. In fact, in one comprehensive study a change in atmospheric pressure was chronologically correlated with the development of pneumothorax.[585] West[586] and his colleagues[587] have postulated that the mechanical stress to which the apex of the lung is subjected with increasing lung height causes rupture of apical blebs in addition to acting as a mechanism in their formation. An ultrastructural examination of bullae in spontaneous pneumothorax has even led to the suggestion that air can leak through the walls of Reid type I bullae because of the paucity of lining mesothelial cells.[588]

As noted above, spontaneous pneumothorax occurs most frequently in otherwise healthy young adults as a result of rupture of visceral pleural blebs or subpleural bullae, but it also can be associated with innumerable pulmonary diseases and hence the designation *secondary* spontaneous pneumothorax. The pathogenesis of the pneumothorax in these diseases is probably multifactorial. Many are associated with the formation of subpleural cystic spaces related to diffuse interstitial fibrosis or emphysema; rupture of one of these is likely the immediate cause of pneumothorax in many cases. As might be expected from a knowledge of the pathogenesis of emphysema and interstitial fibrosis, patient height is not nearly as important a factor in the secondary as in the primary form. Although there was a suggestion of an increased incidence with increased height among the patients with secondary spontaneous pneumothorax in the study by Melton and associates,[553] this was not nearly as clear as it was for the primary condition, and height alone was not a strong predictor of risk. The most common concurrent condition in patients with secondary spontaneous pneumothorax in this study was chronic obstructive pulmonary disease. Presumably reflecting this association, the incidence of pneumothorax increased with age, whereas that of primary spontaneous pneumothorax peaked among young adults aged 25 to 34 years and then rapidly declined.

The pathogenesis of cyst or bulla rupture in secondary spontaneous pneumothorax is probably also multifactorial. Since by definition patients with secondary pneumothorax have underlying pulmonary disease, local airway obstruction caused by pneumonia, mucous plugs, or physiologic abnormalities may be important. In addition, many episodes occur during artificial ventilation used as therapy for the underlying disease, and this is undoubtedly a factor (*see* farther on).

In adults, the following list gives some idea of the broad spectrum of diseases associated with spontaneous pneumothorax but is by no means complete (no attempt is made to indicate incidence): asthma,[591, 592] staphylococcal septicemia,[593] pulmonary infarction,[594–597] sarcoidosis (Fig. 18–7),[598] idiopathic pulmonary hemorrhage,[599] pulmonary alveolar proteinosis,[600] familial fibrocystic pulmonary dysplasia,[601] tuberous sclerosis,[602] cryptogenic fibrosing alveolitis,[603] eosinophilic granuloma,[604] coccidioidomycosis,[605, 606] echinococcal disease,[607] chronic obstructive pulmonary disease (COPD) and emphysema (Fig. 18–8),[608] Shaver's disease (bauxite pneumoconiosis),[609, 610] lymphangioleiomyomatosis,[611] von Recklinghausen's disease,[612] gastropleural and colopleural fistulas through the diaphragm into the left pleural cavity,[613–617] radiation therapy to the thorax,[618] Wegener's granulomatosis,[619] cystic fibrosis (in which pneumothorax is a common and ominous development),[620, 621] acute bacterial pneumonia (Fig. 18–9), *Pneumocystis carinii* pneumonia in patients with AIDS,[622, 623] pulmonary carcinoma,[624–626] a complication of the chemotherapy used in the treatment of malignancy,[627–629] and pulmonary metastases (particularly from osteogenic and other types of sarcoma[630–636] but also from carcinoma of the pancreas, adrenal carcinoma,[637] Wilms' tumor,[630] and germ cell malignancies[638]). Pneumothorax can occur following blunt abdominal trauma and is sometimes evidenced on CT scans but not on conventional roentgenograms or on clinical examination.[639]

CATAMENIAL PNEUMOTHORAX

Recurrent pneumothorax in association with menstrual periods has been recognized since 1958;[648] by 1982, 59 cases had been reported in the English literature.[649] The mechanism by which air enters the pleural space in catamenial pneumo-

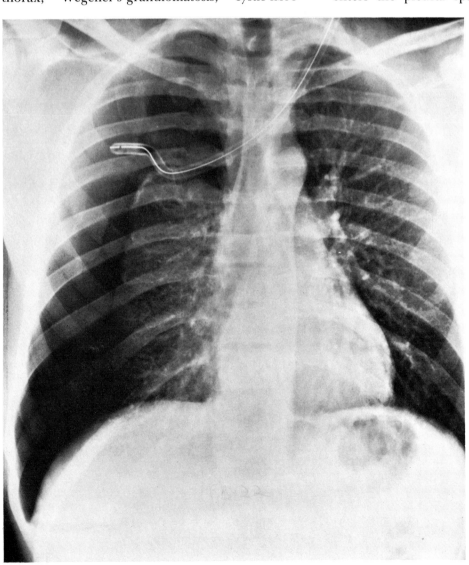

Figure 18–7. Spontaneous Pneumothorax Associated with Pulmonary Sarcoidosis. A posteroanterior roentgenogram reveals a large right pneumothorax. A chest tube has been introduced, but the lung is still collapsed to less than 50 per cent of its normal volume. Although the left lung looks normal on this roentgenogram, within the following few weeks widespread interstitial disease developed that proved pathologically to be sarcoidosis. The patient is a 24-year-old man who had no symptoms referable to his chest other than those occasioned by the spontaneous pneumothorax.

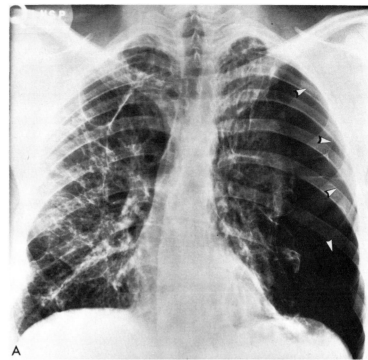

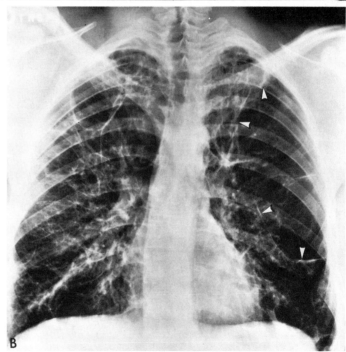

Figure 18–8. Spontaneous Pneumothorax Associated with Diffuse Bullous Emphysema. A posteroanterior roentgenogram *(A)* reveals a left pneumothorax amounting to approximately 50 per cent. Both lungs contain a multitude of small and large thin-walled bullae, several of which have failed to collapse because of air trapping *(arrowheads)*. A chest tube was promptly inserted and the pneumothorax evacuated. Following removal of the chest tube 4 days later *(B)*, the pneumothorax is no longer evident. The large bullae that failed to collapse at the time of the pneumothorax are again indicated by *arrowheads*.

thorax is controversial. Several mechanisms have been proposed:

1. Air migrates through the vagina, uterus, and fallopian tubes into the peritoneal cavity and thence through diaphragmatic defects into the pleural space.[648] As discussed previously *(see* page 1621), these defects have been found in about one third of patients with pneumothorax associated with pleural endometriosis and have been considered to represent both developmental anomalies and acquired lesions secondary to endometriosis itself. In support of this mechanism is the occasional case in which diagnostic pneumoperitoneum has been associated with pneumothorax, the observation that air can be found within the peritoneum in postpartum women carrying out exercises in the knee-chest position,[650] and the observation that tubal ligation cures the condition in some patients.[651] It is clear, however, that intraperitoneal migration of air cannot be the sole mechanism of catamenial pneumothorax since diaphragmatic defects are not present in all individuals with the condition. For example, in one study of 18 patients subjected to thoracotomy, Lillington and associates[652] identified defects

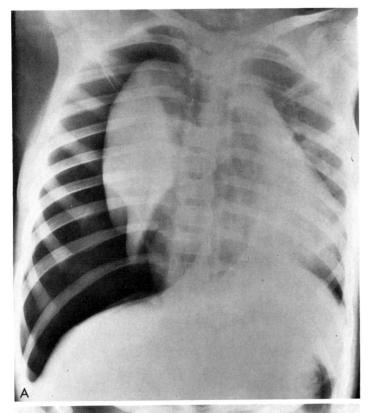

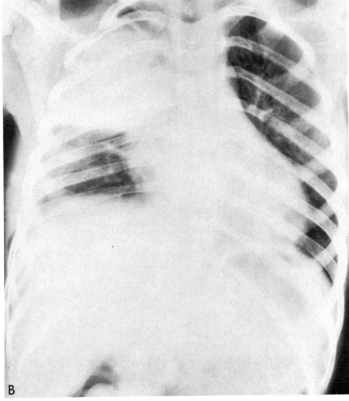

Figure 18–9. Spontaneous Pneumothorax Associated with Massive Pneumonia. This 6-year-old girl was admitted to the hospital following a 2-day history of acute respiratory illness and the abrupt onset 2 hours before of severe right-sided chest pain and shortness of breath. An anteroposterior roentgenogram on admission *(A)* reveals a massive right pneumothorax associated with marked shift of the mediastinum to the left, an appearance consistent with the presence of "tension." Despite this, the volume of the airless right lung is obviously greater than could be accounted for by relaxation atelectasis alone. Note that an air bronchogram is not visualized. A chest tube was promptly inserted and the pneumothorax drained. A roentgenogram obtained 24 hours later *(B)* reveals homogeneous consolidation of the right upper lobe caused by acute pneumonia of probable staphylococcal etiology. (Courtesy of St. Joseph's General Hospital, Blind River, Ontario.)

in only 3 patients. Even more convincing in this regard is the report by Soderberg and Dahlquist[650] of recurrent catamenial pneumothorax in 8 patients who had undergone hysterectomy.

2. Most patients with catamenial pneumothorax have endometriosis, frequently involving the diaphragm or parietal pleura and occasionally the visceral pleura.[648, 653–655] It has been hypothesized

that necrosis of endometrial tissue at the latter site during menses might result in the formation of an air leak between lung and pleura, thus causing pneumothorax. Although initially this was an attractive hypothesis, it is nevertheless unusual to find such foci at thoracotomy, either grossly or microscopically. Rossi and Goplerud[656] have proposed instead that prostaglandin $F_{2\alpha}$-mediated vasospasm and bronchoconstriction may be involved: according to these authors, this substance is present in menstrual debris of some women and has been shown to have these effects on the lungs. The authors speculated that rupture of parenchyma damaged by local vasoconstriction might be the source of the air leak.

3. The failure to detect pleural endometriosis or diaphragmatic defects in some cases, even at thoracotomy, has suggested that other factors might be important. In some patients with catamenial pneumothorax, the only pathologic finding is apical pulmonary fibrosis or blebs (or both); it has been speculated that some unidentified factor associated with menses may make these more liable to rupture.[657]

Catamenial pneumothorax usually occurs between the ages of 30 and 36 years, an age distribution that is similar to that of patients with pelvic endometriosis.[658]

The condition has been reported in two sisters[659] and in a 39-year-old woman in whom the episode occurred during or shortly after sexual intercourse in proximity to the beginning of the menstrual cycle;[651] this patient was successfully treated by tubal ligation. A patient has been described in whom pleural endometriosis was demonstrated by CT and ultrasonography;[660] the abnormal tissue was shown to extend into the pleural space via defects in the diaphragm.

THE VALSALVA MANEUVER AND PNEUMOTHORAX

The Valsalva maneuver has resulted in pneumomediastinum and pneumothorax during emesis, coughing,[661] and perhaps most commonly, during pregnancy and labor.[662–665] The increasing incidence of marijuana and cocaine smoking in recent years, and the use of a prolonged Valsalva maneuver to augment the "high," have been associated with these complications in drug users.[661, 666–668] However, a more frequent mechanism for the production of pneumothorax in addicts is needle puncture while mainlining into neck veins (see farther on).

TRAUMATIC PNEUMOTHORAX

As indicated previously, trauma is probably the most common etiology of pneumothorax: of the 318 cases of pneumothorax described by Melton and associates,[573] trauma was the responsible mechanism in 177 (56 per cent), iatrogenic in 102 cases and noniatrogenic in 75. In these circumstances,

pneumothorax can be caused by direct communication of the pleural space with the atmosphere via chest wall puncture or by disruption of the proximal tracheobronchial tree or the visceral pleura.

With the increasing use of invasive diagnostic procedures, we can expect *iatrogenic pneumothorax* to be even more common in the future, although the majority of these episodes are of minor degree and of little clinical significance. A variety of procedures can be complicated by pneumothorax, the most common being transbronchial biopsy, transthoracic needle aspiration, central venous catheterization,[669–673] and faulty feeding tube insertion.[674–677] Less common iatrogenic causes include tracheal intubation,[678, 679] the use of a tracheoesophageal voice prosthesis,[680] diagnostic colonoscopy,[681] electromyographic electrode insertion,[682] acupuncture,[562, 683] fine needle aspiration of the breast,[684] and percutaneous nephrolithotomy.[685, 686]

Patients being assisted by artificial ventilation are at special risk for the development of pneumothorax, particularly when volume-cycled machines and positive end-expiratory pressure (PEEP) are used or when marginal alveoli are damaged as a result of infection, infarction, or aspiration of gastric contents.[687] The incidence of pneumothorax in these situations has been estimated to be between 0.5 and 15 per cent, depending on the duration of ventilation, the nature of the underlying disease, and the use of PEEP.[688] Alveolar rupture is more likely to occur when very high peak inspiratory pressures are employed to ventilate patients with severely obstructed airways or noncompliant lungs; in such circumstances, pneumothorax (sometimes associated with pneumomediastinum or pneumoperitoneum) may be a terminal event. In one autopsy study, pneumothorax was frequently attributed to mechanical ventilation or attempts at cardiorespiratory resuscitation.[596]

Noniatrogenic traumatic pneumothorax can result from either penetrating or nonpenetrating chest injury. There need not be roentgenographic evidence of rib fracture, in which circumstances the likely pathogenesis is an abrupt increase in intrathoracic pressure that results in interstitial emphysema and tracking of air to the visceral pleura. This explanation also provides adequate reason for the occurrence of pneumomediastinum and subcutaneous emphysema, conditions that frequently accompany pneumothorax in these circumstances. When rib fractures are present, the likely mechanism is laceration of the visceral pleura by rib fragments; in such circumstances hemothorax can be expected as a concomitant finding.

One unusual mechanism of traumatic pneumothorax has recently been recognized in drug addicts: individuals whose peripheral veins are thrombosed tend to use the internal jugular vein to inject drugs directly (the so-called pocket shot). In some areas, such as Detroit,[689–691] this procedure has been responsible for a significant increase in the incidence of pneumothorax. In 1986, Douglass and Levison[689] found reports of 19 such cases in the literature. The authors reviewed their own experience at the Detroit Receiving Hospital; of 525 episodes of pneumothorax seen over a 2-year period, they found that 113 (21.5 per cent) had occurred as a result of drug abuse. Not infrequently this complication is bilateral, presumably as a result of sequential insertion of needles.[689, 690, 692–694] Such a clinical presentation in a young person should lead to a suspicion of this mechanism of development.

Pathologic Characteristics

Pathologic characteristics of the pleura and subpleural lung parenchyma clearly depend to some extent on the presence and type of underlying disease. As indicated previously, it is our experience that the most common abnormality of lung excised from individuals with *primary* spontaneous pneumothorax is a bulla, usually 0.5 to 1.5 cm in diameter and located adjacent to fibrotic pleura (*see* Fig. 18–6, page 2742); true blebs (i.e., entirely intrapleural cystic spaces) are relatively uncommon. Like bullae, the latter are usually isolated abnormalities measuring 0.5 to 1.5 cm in diameter; in neonates who have undergone vigorous ventilatory support, they may be associated with the presence of air cysts in the peribronchovascular and interlobular interstitial tissue (Fig. 18–10).[640] Histologic examination of these interstitial cysts may reveal the presence of multinucleated giant cells,[640, 641] representing a tissue manifestation of the reaction to air.

Pathologic findings in *secondary* spontaneous pneumothorax depend on the nature of the underlying disease; emphysematous bullae and cystic spaces associated with interstitial fibrosis are the most common. Tomashefski and his colleagues[641] have also described subpleural cystic spaces in patients with cystic fibrosis that appeared to be caused by localized exaggerated bronchiectasis ("bronchiectatic cysts"); although there was often a zone of compressed, fibrotic lung between the cyst wall and the pleura, the authors suggested that their rupture might sometimes be the mechanism of pneumothorax in these individuals.

Histologic examination of pleura excised at thoracotomy in the therapy of pneumothorax often reveals characteristic changes believed to represent a reaction to the presence of air.[642–645] These consist of a fibrinous exudate within and adjacent to which are large numbers of mononuclear cells (probably mostly macrophages), eosinophils, and occasional multinucleated giant cells (Fig. 18–11). This so-called reactive eosinophilic pleuritis resembles the inflammatory infiltrate of eosinophilic granuloma, a condition known to have an increased incidence of spontaneous pneumothorax and with which it should not be confused; the presence or absence of the characteristic parenchymal histologic changes of eosinophilic granuloma should suffice to make the pathologic distinction. It must be remembered, however, that reactive eosinophilic pleuritis and eosinophilic granuloma can coexist.[646]

Pneumothorax can also occur secondary to pneumomediastinum, air tracking from that location into the pleural space via the mediastinal pleura. In this situation, there is evidence that the most likely sites of rupture are small areas just above the root of the left lung and at the junction with the pericardium.[647] Conditions associated with pneumothorax that merit additional comments are those that occur coincidentally with menses (catamenial pneumothorax), that follow a Valsalva maneuver, and that occur with trauma.

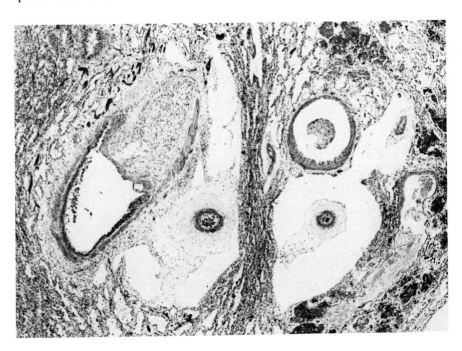

Figure 18–10. Interstitial Emphysema. A histologic section shows that the interstitial tissue surrounding two bronchioles and their accompanying pulmonary arteries is expanded by irregularly shaped spaces that *in vivo* contained air. The section is from a neonate who had had positive pressure ventilatory support for several days before death. (× 35.)

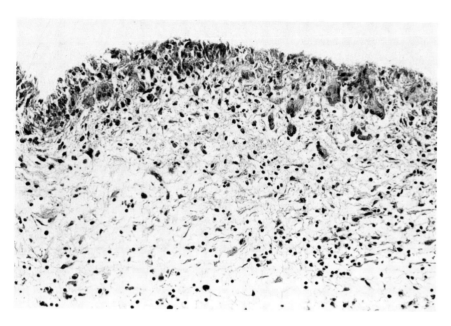

Figure 18–11. Pleuritis Associated with Pneumothorax. A histologic section of parietal pleura removed at thoracotomy for spontaneous pneumothorax shows it to be thickened by loose fibroblastic tissue and a cellular infiltrate composed of histiocytes, multinucleated giant cells, and numerous smaller inflammatory cells, many of which are eosinophils. (× 200.)

Clinical Manifestations

Chest pain and dyspnea, either alone or in combination, are the classic symptoms of spontaneous pneumothorax; pain was the sole complaint of 69 per cent of 72 patients studied by Lindskog and Halasz.[550] Dyspnea, which can be severe, may disappear within 24 hours regardless of whether the collapsed lung undergoes partial re-expansion. The major physical sign suggesting pneumothorax is a marked decrease or absence of breath sounds despite normal or increased resonance on percussion. Even with a small pneumothorax (approximately 20 per cent) in patients with otherwise normal lungs, the relative difference in breath sounds between the two hemithoraces should suggest the diagnosis. However, in patients with emphysema whose breath sounds are already greatly reduced and in whom percussion is normal or increased, the presence of pneumothorax may be very difficult to recognize by physical signs.

Hamman's sign, originally considered to be caused by pneumomediastinum, is now thought to be associated much more frequently with left pneumothorax. The sign results from the presence of gas in close contact with the heart and has been described as a variety of "clicks" and "whoops" occurring throughout the entire cardiac cycle but influenced by the respiratory phase and the position of the patient.[695, 696] In some cases the sounds disappear completely when the patient is moved from the left to the right lateral decubitus position.

Unusual manifestations of pneumothorax include ptosis (extension from subcutaneous emphysema),[697] pneumocephalus (secondary to tension pneumothorax associated with a comminuted fracture of the thoracic spine),[698] and recurrent pneumopericardium; this last manifestation occurred in a patient with recurrent pneumothorax in whom a pleuropericardial defect was identified.[699] Bilateral

pneumothorax is uncommon[700, 701] and, as indicated above, should suggest the possibility of intravenous drug injection into neck veins. The frequency of recurrence of spontaneous pneumothorax on the same side is surprisingly high, amounting to roughly 30 per cent in most reported series.[548, 573, 589, 702] In approximately 10 per cent of cases, spontaneous pneumothorax will develop subsequently on the contralateral side.[548, 702]

Occasionally inspired air becomes trapped in a pleural space, presumably on the basis of a bronchopleural check-valve mechanism, leading to a tension pneumothorax. Immediate recognition of this complication is essential, since these patients rapidly become severely hypoxic and acidotic, not uncommonly with fatal outcomes.[703, 704] In one series of 3,500 autopsies,[596] unsuspected tension pneumothorax was found in 12 patients; 10 of these had been supported by mechanical ventilators, and 9 had undergone cardiopulmonary resuscitation.

Pleural effusion coincident with pneumothorax appears to occur less frequently than might be anticipated. For example, Lindskog and Halasz[550] found fluid in only 19 (26 per cent) of their 72 patients before diagnostic or therapeutic manipulation; of the 15 effusions aspirated, 11 were serous and four were bloody. Spontaneous hemopneumothorax is especially rare:[705] of 228 cases of spontaneous pneumothorax seen over a 10-year period, Abyholm and Storen[705] observed hemopneumothorax in only 5 patients (2.2 per cent). According to these authors, bleeding results from the rupture or tearing of vascularized adhesions between the parietal and visceral layers of pleura as the lung collapses. They emphasize that if the lung does not fully expand and the hemorrhage does not cease within a few days, thoracotomy is probably indicated.

Pneumothorax is considered to be the major cause of an eosinophilic effusion,[32, 645, 706] an association that was substantiated by Adelman and colleagues[706] in a review of 343 cases of eosinophilic pleural effusion in the literature.

PULMONARY FUNCTION TESTS

The effect of pneumothorax on pulmonary function depends largely on its size, although reduction in lung volumes and flow rates also can be influenced at least partly by pleural pain. In a study of 12 patients with spontaneous pneumothorax, Norris and associates[707] found 9 to have a Po_2 below 80 mm Hg. The physiologic dead space was normal, but there was an increased A-a gradient for oxygen. The authors concluded that there was an increased anatomic shunt. Anthonisen[708] measured regional lung function in three young men with pneumothorax ranging in size from 25 to 40 per cent. He found that the lung with the pneumothorax showed uniform airway closure at low lung volumes, an abnormality that appeared to be the chief cause of ventilation maldistribution.

At long-term follow-up, patients who are subjected to unilateral pleurodesis for pneumothorax have normal pulmonary function[709] or, at most, mild restriction.[710] However, they show a change in regional lung ventilation manifested by distribution of boluses of xenon more to the apex and less to the base on the operated than on the unoperated side.[709] In addition, a recent assessment of diaphragmatic motion using ultrasonography has shown a measurable reduction in excursion of the chemically sclerosed hemithorax.[711]

The complication of re-expansion pulmonary edema[712, 713] that may occur after removal of air in patients with pneumothorax is reviewed in Chapter 10 (see page 1952).

PLEURAL FIBROSIS

After effusion, fibrosis is undoubtedly the most common pleural abnormality. As with the former condition, fibrosis has numerous etiologies and is the outcome of many primary diseases of the pleura, as well as a potential complication of virtually every inflammatory condition to affect the lungs. In the majority of cases, the fibrosis is patchy or is localized to a single relatively small area; in these circumstances clinical and functional abnormalities are absent and the condition is recognized on a screening roentgenogram, during the investigation of other intrathoracic disease, or at necropsy. Less commonly, the fibrosis is more or less diffuse in one or both pleural cavities, in which case functional abnormalities may be apparent. Because of this important difference, the two forms are discussed separately.

LOCAL PLEURAL FIBROSIS

HEALED PLEURITIS

The most common cause of localized pleural fibrosis is organized fibrinous or fibrinopurulent pleuritis secondary to pneumonia. Since pleural effusions of infectious etiology are almost invariably basal, it is not surprising that this is the anatomic location of most cases of residual pleural thickening of this type. The usual roentgenographic abnormality is partial obliteration or blunting of the posterior and lateral costophrenic sulci, in some cases associated with line shadows. Thickening of the pleural line may extend for a variable distance up the lateral and posterior thoracic walls, diminishing gradually toward the apex and seldom amounting to more than 1 to 2 mm in width. Obliteration of the costophrenic sulci sometimes has a roentgenographic appearance difficult to differentiate from that of a small pleural effusion. Roentgenography in the lateral decubitus position is required for clarification.

THE "APICAL CAP"

Somewhat similar roentgenographically to fibrosis due to healed pleuritis but in a different location are curved shadows of unit density situated at the apex of one or both hemithoraces in the concavity formed by the first and second ribs. The morphologic counterpart of these shadows, often called "apical caps," is not uncommon; in one review of 183 lungs derived from a consecutive series of 183 necropsies, they were identified in 48 (26 per cent).[714] They occur with equal frequency in men and women[714] and are more common and larger in older individuals.[714, 715]

Pathologically, apical caps consist of a combination of pleural and pulmonary parenchymal fibrosis, the latter usually predominating (Fig. 18–12).[714] Histologically, the pleura shows dense, sometimes hyalinized collagen, accompanied by small foci of chronic inflammatory cells. The architecture of the underlying lung parenchyma is preserved, but the airspaces are obliterated by fibrous tissue (Fig. 18–12); elastic tissue of the alveolar walls is typically increased in amount and quite prominent, even with hematoxylin-eosin (H&E) stained sections. Although focal areas of calcification or ossification can be seen, evidence of prior granulomatous inflammation and necrosis, such as that occurring in tuberculosis, is invariably absent.[714, 715]

The pathogenesis of the abnormality is not certain. Although it has been ascribed to tuberculosis,[716] as indicated above pathologic evidence is clearly against this in the great majority of, if not all, cases.[714, 715, 717] In their autopsy study, Butler and Kleinerman[714] found an association with histologic evidence of chronic bronchitis and pulmonary artery narrowing and suggested that intermittent or

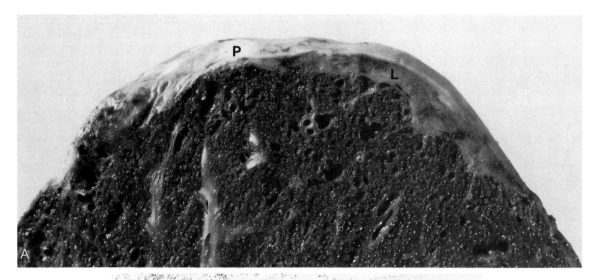

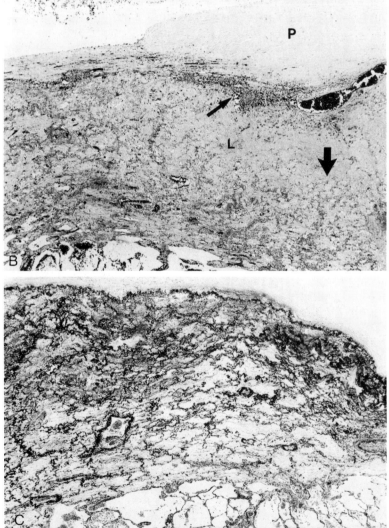

Figure 18–12. Apical Pleural Cap. A magnified view of the apex of the right upper lobe *(A)* shows a mild degree of fibrosis affecting both the pleura *(P)* and underlying lung parenchyma *(L)*. A histologic section *(B)* reveals fibrosis within the pleura *(P)* and lung *(L)* associated with focal chronic inflammation *(thin arrow)*. Despite the parenchymal fibrosis, the underlying lung architecture is clearly preserved as demonstrated in sections stained with hematoxylin-eosin *(large arrow* in *B)* and with elastic tissue stain *(C)*. *(B,* × 25; *C,* Verhoeff–van Gieson × 25.)

continuing low-grade infection combined with relative apical ischemia might be responsible for the fibrosis.

Care should be taken not to confuse the apical cap with the companion shadows of the first and second ribs or to fail to recognize apparent apical pleural thickening as an early manifestation of much more serious disease—apical pulmonary cancer or Pancoast's tumor. Early apical carcinoma of the Pancoast type can closely mimic pleural thickening, and only a high index of suspicion will permit early diagnosis. Suspicion should be enhanced when the apical abnormality is predominantly unilateral.

PLEURAL PLAQUES

Four types of roentgenographic change occur in the pleura of patients exposed to asbestos or talc—plaque formation, calcification, diffuse pleural thickening, and pleural effusion. Plaque formation is by far the most common. Pleural plaques are usually, but not invariably, bilateral: in a review of the roentgenographic changes in 200 patients with known or suspected asbestos exposure, pleural plaques or thickening (with or without calcification) occurred solely or predominantly on the left side in 90 patients, on the right side in 32, and equally on the two sides in 44.[718] This unexplained left-sided predominance for pleural plaques also has been described by Withers and associates;[719] in their study, there was a left-to-right predominance of approximately 3 to 1. Plaques are more prominent in the lower half of the thorax and tend to follow the rib contours.

Pleural plaques are found in the parietal pleura where they appear as well-circumscribed foci of fibrosis that are typically ivory white in color (see Fig. 12–23, page 2320). They may be smooth or nodular in contour and can measure up to 1 cm in thickness, although they usually are much thinner. They occur most commonly on the aponeurotic portion of the diaphragm, on the posterolateral chest wall between the seventh and tenth ribs, and on the lateral chest wall between the sixth and ninth ribs.[720–724] Origin from the parietal pleura is in contrast to the visceral pleural involvement that characterizes previous hemothorax or empyema. Adhesions between visceral and parietal pleural membranes develop infrequently.[725]

Roentgenographically, the earliest appearance of a pleural plaque occurs as a thin line of unit density visible under a rib in the axillary region, usually the seventh or eighth rib, on one or both sides. The plaques may be very difficult to visualize, particularly when viewed *en face,* and tangential roentgenograms may be necessary. In fact, the frequency with which plaques occur along the posterolateral or anterolateral portion of the thorax suggested to Fletcher and Edge[723] that oblique projections of the thorax should be standard in the roentgenographic investigation of patients suspected of having asbestos-related disease. The value of 45° oblique projections has been stressed also by MacKenzie,[726] who regards as an important diagnostic area the space between the inner border of the ribs and the lung margin, where a localized expansion occurs in the presence of plaques. Despite the foregoing, other investigators[727] have concluded that oblique views add little to the detection of asbestos-induced disease in exposed workers: in a series of 489 male pipefitters examined in a screening program, the oblique views represented the sole evidence of an asbestos-related roentgenographic abnormality in only 8 (1.6 per cent). A comparison of roentgenographic findings during life with observations at autopsy indicates that a significant number of pleural plaques are missed on premortem roentgenograms.[728] Although pleural thickening posteriorly may be difficult to recognize roentgenographically, its presence may be detected by ultrasonic examination.[729] Differentiation of plaques from diffuse pleural thickening can be difficult at times when using the present guidelines of the ILO 1980 classification,[730] and caution should be exercised in attributing diffuse pleural thickening to asbestos exposure.

The greatest problem in the diagnosis of early plaque formation lies in distinguishing plaques from normal companion shadows of the chest wall—not those that are associated with the first three ribs (since this area is rarely involved in asbestos-related disease) but those muscle and fat shadows that may be identified in as many as 75 per cent of normal posteroanterior roentgenograms along the convexity of the thorax inferiorly. In fact, sometimes it is impossible to differentiate pleural plaques from companion shadows with conviction.

The identification of pleural plaques can be regarded as highly suggestive (if not conclusive) evidence of asbestos-related disease. In several series in which they have been discovered on randomized or consecutive autopsies, a history of asbestos exposure has been obtained in approximately 80 per cent of cases. Even without such a history, evidence of an asbestos etiology sometimes can be obtained by lung digestion studies. For example, in one retrospective study in which the number of asbestos bodies in the lung at necropsy was correlated with roentgenologic appearances premortem,[731] positive roentgenographic features of asbestos-related disease (most often calcified and noncalcified pleural plaques) were found in eight of nine cases in which asbestos bodies exceeded 40 in number; in only one of these cases had such exposure been recognized during life. However, such findings need not reflect direct occupational exposure as evidenced by asbestos-induced disease acquired in the environment in the Metsovo area of Northwest Greece,[732, 733] in isolated villages in Turkey,[734–736] in Corsica,[737] and in Quebec.[738] Tremolite-contaminated soil was considered to be responsible for the plaques in Greece, Turkey, and Quebec.

Although in most patients pleural plaques do not interfere with pulmonary function, some authors have suggested that they are sometimes responsible for mild restrictive insufficiency.[739, 740] In a review of this subject, Jones and collaborators[741] concluded: (1) pleural plaques are not associated with a clinically significant reduction in pulmonary function; (2) diffuse pleural thickening, when extensive, can severely impair ventilation; and (3) when pleural lesions are responsible for reduced pulmonary function, the expected pattern is restriction with preserved diffusing capacity.

Although noncalcified pleural plaques are probably the most common roentgenographic manifestation of asbestos-related disease, the most striking abnormality is calcification of pleural plaques (Fig. 18–13). The frequency of such calcification is variable. Anton[742] found calcified and noncalcified plaques in roughly equal numbers in his 40 patients, whereas Freundlich and Greening[743] observed calcification in only 21 per cent of their 56 patients. In an American survey of 261 workers exposed to asbestos in industry, none had calcified pleura,[744] whereas in Finland calcification is common,[722] a difference in incidence probably relating to the variety of asbestos concerned. Calcified plaques vary from small linear or circular shadows usually situated over the diaphragmatic domes[745] to large shadows that completely encircle the lower portion of the lungs.[746] When calcification is minimal, a roentgenogram overexposed at maximal inspiration facilitates visibility.[747]

There appears to be a dose-response relationship in the development of pleural plaques and calcification. A period of at least 20 years is generally required after the first exposure to asbestos for pleural calcification to develop,[723, 745] although the occupational exposure can be relatively short. Two patients have been described in whom isolated calcific diaphragmatic pleural plaques developed approximately 20 years after occupational exposure of only 8 and 11 months.

GENERAL PLEURAL FIBROSIS (FIBROTHORAX)

Healing of a massive hemothorax or empyema may be associated with deposition of a thick layer of dense fibrous tissue. The thickness of the pleural "peel" may be 2 cm or more around a whole lung, resulting in marked decrease in volume of the hemithorax and creating a severe impediment to ventilation. Calcification occurs frequently on the *inner* aspect of the peel and provides an indicator by which the thickness of the peel may be accurately measured (Fig. 18–14).

The degree to which unilateral fibrothorax impairs ventilation of the underlying lung can be gauged, at least roughly, by assessing pulmonary vascularity. If the pulmonary vessels of the affected lung are smaller than those of the opposite side, it can be assumed that the reduction in perfusion has occurred in response to reduced ventilation, presumably as a result of hypoxic vasoconstriction (Fig. 18–15). If the vascularity of the two lungs is roughly symmetric, it is reasonable to assume that reflex vasoconstriction has not occurred and that ventilation is therefore preserved. We have frequently been impressed by the fact that the degree of pleural thickening does not bear a close relationship to reduced ventilation and perfusion. In other words, a thick pleural peel does not necessarily imply reduced ventilation and perfusion any more than a thin peel.

Assessment of the underlying lungs may indicate the original etiology of the fibrothorax. If the lung appears relatively normal, the antecedent insult probably was traumatic hemothorax. If there is local scarring and loss of volume, the pleural change probably was the result of a remote empyema secondary to *M. tuberculosis* or some pyogenic organism. Severe fibrosing pleuritis may occur as a late complication of uremia, resulting in extreme incarceration of both lungs and disabling restriction of pulmonary function.[460] Buchanan and associates have described four patients with disabling bilateral pleural effusions that progressed to diffuse pleural thickening; all four were HLA-B44 positive and none gave a history of asbestos exposure. Both layers of pleura were severely thickened, requiring decortication. The authors refer to this disorder as cryptogenic bilateral fibrosing pleuritis.[748]

In addition to pleural plaques, asbestos exposure can cause diffuse pleural fibrosis indistinguishable from that caused by other etiologies.[749, 750] Rarely, this type of pleural fibrosis can cause some degree of restrictive pulmonary insufficiency in the absence of roentgenographic evidence of pulmonary disease.[741, 751, 752] Such restrictive impairment of pulmonary function caused by fibrothorax, whether or not related to asbestos exposure, usually can be alleviated in varying degree by pleural decortication.[753–755]

The majority of cases of round or helical atelectasis occur in patients who have a history of asbestos exposure, some of whom have had a previous clinically recognized episode of pleural effusion.[756–758] Hillerdal[757] described 74 patients with this entity, 64 of whom had a history of asbestos exposure. Mintzer and Cugell[758] identified 18 cases over a period of 20 months, 15 of which involved historical information confirming contact with asbestos. Recent pathologic[759, 760] and roentgenographic studies, including high-resolution CT[756, 760–763] have clearly revealed this distortion of pleuropulmonary architecture to be caused by invagination of the pleura into the lung with production of localized atelectasis. The characteristic "comet tail" is caused by vessels and bronchi sweeping into the margins of the mass (Fig. 18–16). This subject was considered in more detail in Chapters 4 (*see* page 487) and 12 (*see* page 2328).

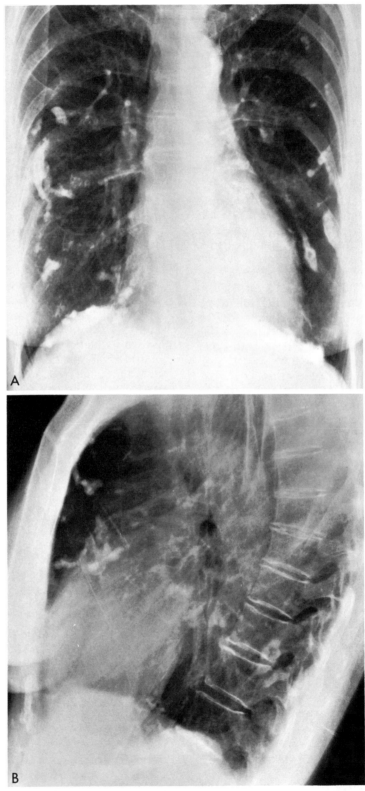

Figure 18–13. Multiple Calcified Pleural Plaques. Posteroanterior *(A)* and lateral *(B)* roentgenograms of this asymptomatic 70-year-old woman reveal a multitude of irregular opacities of calcific density scattered randomly over the peripheral portions of both lungs. Fluoroscopic examination showed all opacities to be related to the pleura. There was no history of asbestos exposure. The etiology of the calcific plaque formation was not established.

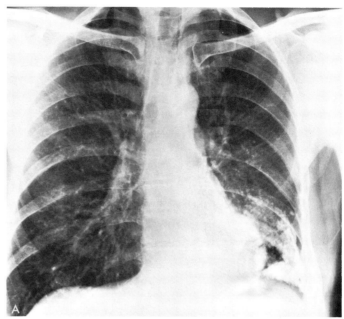

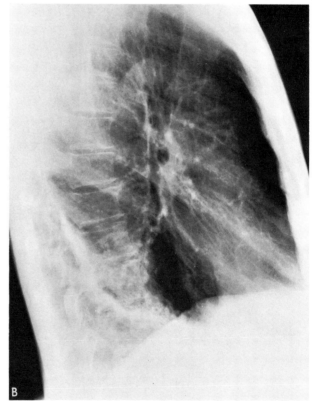

Figure 18–14. Pleural Calcification Caused by Remote Hemothorax. Posteroanterior *(A)* and lateral *(B)* roentgenograms reveal a thick, irregular calcific plaque overlying the posterolateral portion of the left lower lobe. The pleura is markedly thickened. Note the loss of volume of the lower half of the left lung as a result of cicatrization. Several years previously, the patient had developed a moderate-sized left hemothorax following blunt nonpenetrating trauma to the chest.

PRIMARY NEOPLASMS
OF THE PLEURA

LOCALIZED FIBROUS TUMOR

Localized (solitary) fibrous tumor is an uncommon neoplasm of the pleura known by a variety of terms, including local, fibrous, or benign mesothelioma; subpleural or pleural fibroma or fibromyxoma; and fibrosarcoma. We prefer the relatively nonspecific term "localized fibrous tumor" for several reasons: (1) although in the vast majority of cases the neoplasm is histologically and biologically benign, malignant forms clearly exist,[764] and in some tumors the histologic distinction between benign and malignant forms can be exceedingly difficult, if not impossible; (2) the neoplasm typically shows evidence of fibroblastic differentiation; (3) the tumor must be distinguished from the rare case of localized pleural neoplasm of pure epithelial type;[765] and (4) anatomic and experimental evidence suggests that the tumor originates in submesothelial

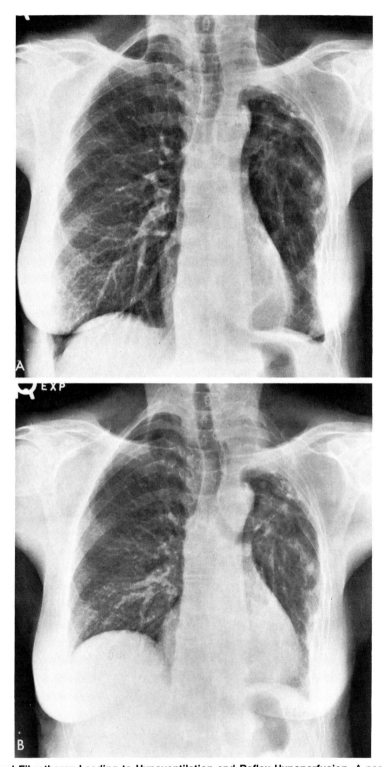

Figure 18–15. Unilateral Fibrothorax Leading to Hypoventilation and Reflex Hypoperfusion. A posteroanterior roentgenogram *(A)* of this 73-year-old asymptomatic woman reveals moderate thickening of the pleura over the whole of the left lung. The pleura is calcified over the lower axillary lung zone. The volume of the left lung is moderately reduced and its vessel markings diminutive. A posteroanterior roentgenogram exposed at full expiration *(B)* shows excellent movement of the right hemidiaphragm, whereas elevation of the left hemidiaphragm has been minimal. Thus, the volume of the left lung has shown little change from inspiration to expiration, indicating hypoventilation.

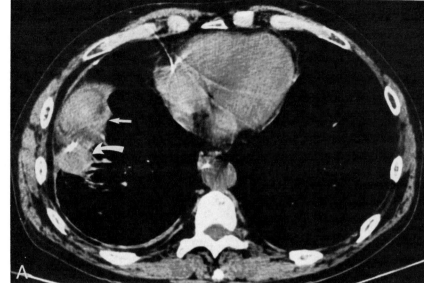

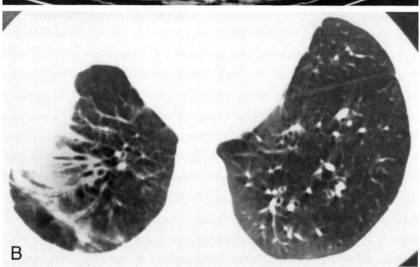

Figure 18–16. Round Atelectasis in Asbestos-Related Pleural Disease. A CT scan *(A)* at the level of the dome of the right hemidiaphragm *(arrow)* shows a 3-cm diameter soft tissue opacity *(curved arrow)* with a peripheral area of calcification. The lesion is pleural based. A CT scan with lung windows at the same level *(B)* shows a characteristic comet tail sign with vessels and bronchi converging toward the soft tissue mass. The patient is a 66-year-old man. (Courtesy of Dr. Nestor Müller, University of British Columbia, Vancouver.)

connective tissue of the pleura rather than the mesothelium itself *(see* farther on). For these reasons, use of the term mesothelioma and of specific modifiers implying a benign or malignant behavior are inappropriate.

The tumor is probably less common than diffuse malignant mesothelioma, although over 350 cases had been documented in the literature by 1980[767] and an additional 223 cases were reported from the files of the Armed Forces Institute of Pathology (AFIP) in 1989.[764] It occurs slightly more often in women than in men and the mean age at presentation is about 50 years.[767] The etiology is unknown; in one patient, the occurrence of the tumor 23 years after external radiation therapy for a chest wall keloid suggested that this could be a factor in some cases.[768] There is no association with asbestos exposure.[764, 767]

The histogenesis of the neoplasm has been debated. On the basis of ultrastructural[769, 770] and tissue culture[771] studies, it has been suggested by some investigators that the tumor is derived from mesothelial cells (hence the designation benign or solitary "mesothelioma"). However, the results of additional ultrastructural and immunohistochemical investigations[772–775] have not supported this hypothesis, and most authors now believe that the tumor originates in a submesothelial mesenchymal cell that possesses the capacity for fibroblastic differentiation.[764, 773–776]

PATHOLOGIC CHARACTERISTICS

Pathologically, 66 to 80 per cent of localized fibrous tumors arise in relation to the visceral pleura.[764, 767, 777, 778] Most project into the pleural space and compress the adjacent lung to a variable degree (Fig. 18–17). Occasionally, tumors arising in the medial pleura extend into the mediastinum[777, 779] and those in a fissure into the pulmonary parenchyma;[764, 767] rarely, they can be located entirely within the lung[780] or mediastinum[779] without evident pleural derivation. The majority are spherical or oblong in shape and well circumscribed or

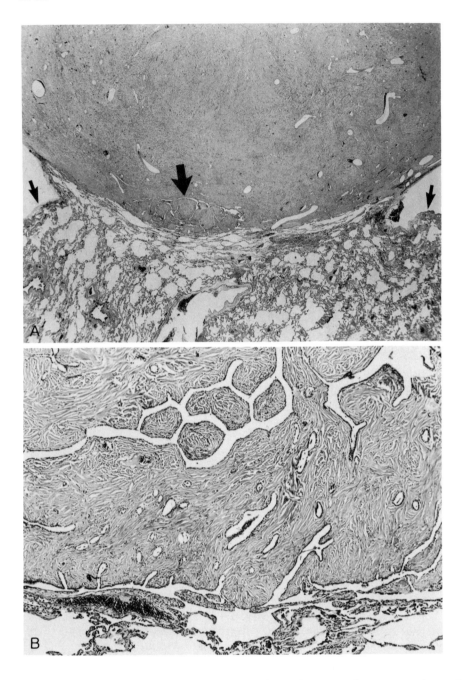

Figure 18–17. Localized Fibrous Tumor of the Pleura. A low-power histologic section of a small fibrous tumor discovered incidentally at autopsy *(A)* shows a well-circumscribed mass compressing, but not invading, the adjacent lung parenchyma. The tumor is clearly related to the normal pleura as indicated by the *small arrows* on either side of the mass. Occasional slit-like spaces lined by a thin layer of attenuated cells are present focally at the junction of the tumor and lung parenchyma *(large arrow)*. At greater magnification *(B)*, these appear to represent mesothelial inclusions entrapped within the expanding tumor. *(A, × 10; B, × 50.)*

encapsulated; many are attached to the pleura by a short vascular pedicle. They can grow to a huge size, examples up to 36 cm in diameter having been reported.[767] Cut sections show a firm, tan or grey mass, often possessing a lobulated or whorled appearance reminiscent of a leiomyoma (Fig. 18–18). Cysts, hemorrhage, necrosis, and calcification can be present, especially in the larger tumors.

Histologically, the tumors are usually well delimited from contiguous compressed lung parenchyma or soft tissues of the chest wall or mediastinum, and may appear to arise directly from the pleura (*see* Fig. 18–17). They consist of haphazardly arranged or interlacing fascicles of spindle cells, occasionally with a storiform pattern (Fig. 18–19). Between the cells is a variable amount of collagen,

in some regions virtually undetectable and in others so abundant that the spindle cells themselves are almost inapparent (Fig. 18–19); myxoid change or hyalinization is often present. In most clinically benign tumors, nuclear atypia is minimal and mitotic figures are sparse; however, in many tumors that behave in an aggressive fashion, mitotic figures (often abnormal) are more abundant and there is an appreciable degree of nuclear atypia.[764] Admixed neoplastic epithelial cells are not a feature of pleural fibrous tumor; if such cells are present, the tumor probably should be interpreted as a localized malignant mesothelioma of mixed type.[778] In this regard, it is important to distinguish true neoplastic epithelial elements from alveolar epithelium or mesothelium entrapped within the tumor.[764, 780, 781] Such

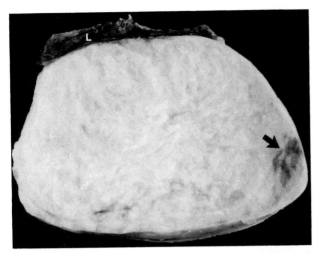

Figure 18-18. Localized Fibrous Tumor of the Pleura. A cut section of the pleural tumor illustrated in Figure 18-20 shows a well circumscribed, lobulated mass compressing a small amount of attached lung parenchyma *(L)*. There is focal hemorrhage *(arrow)* but no necrosis.

inclusions are not uncommon at the junction between the expanding edge of the neoplasm and adjacent lung parenchyma *(see* Fig. 18–17).

Ultrastructural examination of pleural fibrous tumor typically reveals primitive intercellular junctions, a small amount of cytoplasmic filaments, and an absence of features usually present in tumors with mesothelial differentiation.[764] Immunohistochemical studies have generally shown a negative reaction for keratin[772, 773, 775, 776] in contrast to the sarcomatous form of diffuse malignant mesothelioma in which the reaction is often positive.[782, 783] Vimentin positivity is often present.[764, 776] One flow-cytometric study of DNA from 16 tumors showed that all were diploid, including 2 that were recurrences.[776]

ROENTGENOGRAPHIC MANIFESTATIONS

Roentgenologically, localized fibrous tumors are sharply defined, somewhat lobulated masses of homogeneous density ranging in diameter from 2 to 14 cm (Fig. 18–20). In one series of 17 cases,[784] there was no predilection for either side but only two lesions were in the upper half of the chest; five lesions were located within a fissure, three along the mediastinal pleural reflection, two contiguous with the diaphragm, two anteriorly, and one posteriorly. All but one of these lesions formed an obtuse angle with the chest wall or mediastinum, a finding important to the establishment of the extrapulmonary origin of a thoracic mass (Fig. 18–21). When a tumor is very large, however, its site of origin is frequently difficult or impossible to establish on conventional roentgenograms or even on CT. In such circumstances, Hahn and his colleagues[785] recommend arteriography to determine the blood supply of the mass; should it opacify following injection of the inferior phrenic, intercos-

tal, or internal mammary arteries, its extrapulmonary origin may be considered to be reasonably (although perhaps not conclusively) established. Calcification was evident in 4 (7 per cent) of 58 cases reviewed in the AFIP series,[764] and pleural effusion was demonstrated in 10 cases (17 per cent). The CT characteristics have been described in six patients,[786] in none of whom were the findings considered pathognomonic.

Of considerable diagnostic value is the tendency for these lesions to change position with respiration or needling,[787] regardless of their site of origin. If they originate from the visceral pleura, movement is detected by relating the position of the tumor to contiguous ribs or mediastinal structures; if origin is from the parietal pleura, movement may occur because of the frequency of pedunculation (in 30 to 50 per cent of cases according to Berne and Heitzman[788]). In occasional cases, the pedicle becomes twisted, resulting in detachment of the tumor from the pleura and the formation of a free intrapleural body.[789, 790]

CLINICAL MANIFESTATIONS

Clinically, most patients with localized fibrous tumors are asymptomatic;[764, 767, 781, 791] cough, chest pain, and dyspnea occur occasionally.[767] Dyspnea occurs especially with larger tumors.[792] One particularly common finding is hypertrophic osteoarthropathy, which Briselli and colleagues noted in an astounding 35 per cent of the 360 patients they reviewed in the literature.[767] The association of this abnormality with pleural fibrous tumor is much stronger than with pulmonary carcinoma; in fact, its presence in a patient with a large intrathoracic mass should suggest the diagnosis. Surgical removal of the tumor relieves the symptoms of arthropathy in most cases.[794] Another interesting association with pleural fibrous tumor is symptomatic hypoglycemia that occurs in 4 per cent of patients;[792, 793] in the AFIP series,[764] it was somewhat more common in malignant than in benign tumors (11 versus 3 per cent) and three times more frequent in women than in men.[764]

The majority of localized fibrous tumors behave in a benign fashion, intrathoracic growth resulting in compression of contiguous structures but no true invasion. Most tumors grow slowly *(see* Fig. 18–21); in one case, a 12-cm tumor was excised 20 years after it was first identified roentgenographically.[777] Surgical excision usually results in complete cure, particularly when the tumor possesses a well-defined pedicle; however, local recurrence can occur if initial surgery is inadequate. Death caused by extensive intrathoracic disease was documented in 13 per cent of the patients reviewed by Briselli and colleagues.[767] Patients with unresectable primary or recurrent disease usually die within 2 years.[767] Extrathoracic metastases are rare.

Prediction of the aggressive or benign behavior

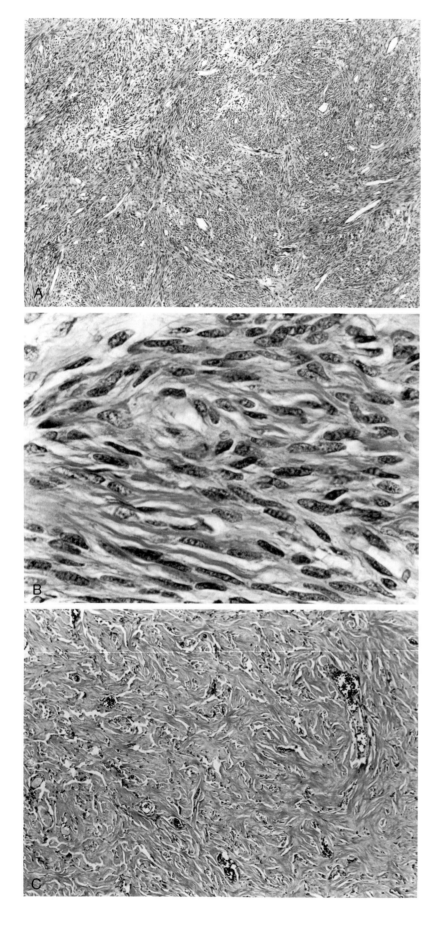

Figure 18–19. Localized Fibrous Tumor of the Pleura. A histologic section (A) shows interlacing fascicles of spindle cells with little intercellular collagen. A magnified view (B) demonstrates minimal pleomorphism of cell nuclei. A section from another tumor (C) shows a less cellular neoplasm with abundant intercellular collagen. (A, × 60; B, × 600; C, × 60.)

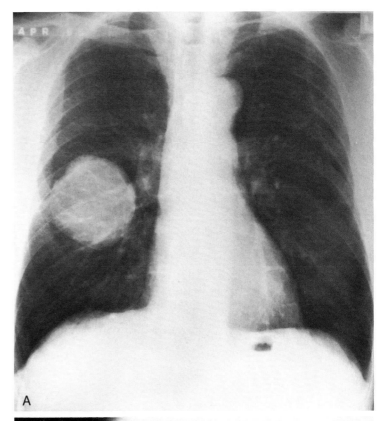

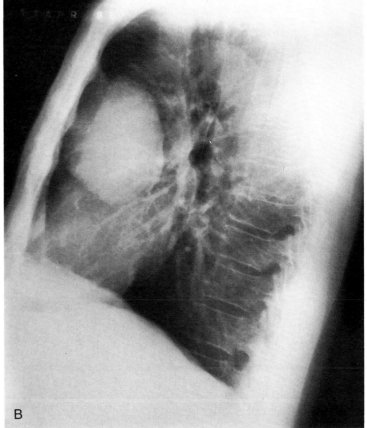

Figure 18–20. Localized Fibrous Tumor of the Pleura. Posteroanterior (A) and lateral (B) roentgenograms reveal a homogeneous, somewhat lobulated mass in the right upper lobe. The relationship of the mass to the visceral pleura cannot be established from these two projections and would have required fluoroscopic examination, oblique roentgenograms, or CT. The patient is an asymptomatic 50-year-old man. The resected specimen is shown in Figure 18–18.

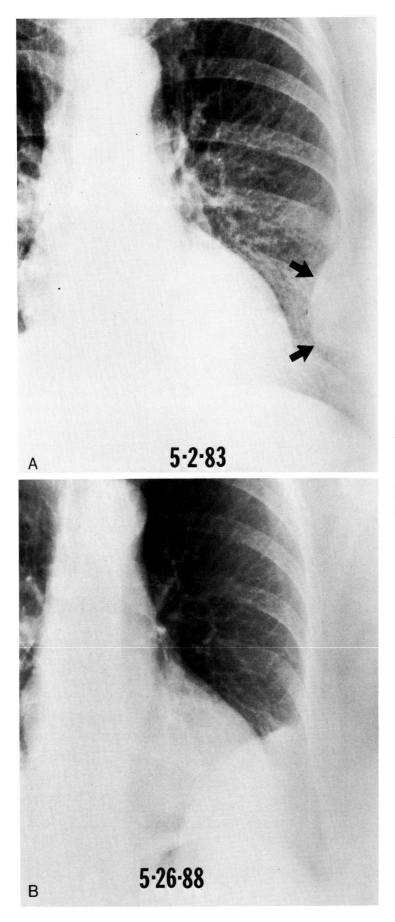

A 5·2·83

B 5·26·88

Figure 18–21. Localized Fibrous Tumor Showing Growth. A view of the left lung from a posteroanterior roentgenogram *(A)* reveals a sharply defined opacity in the axillary region inferiorly *(arrows)*. The mass is homogeneous and possesses a broad pleural base. Note the obtuse angle the mass makes with the pleural surface, indicating its extrapulmonary location. Five years later *(B)*, the tumor had undergone remarkable growth.

of these neoplasms can be difficult. In the AFIP series,[764] a considerably greater proportion of malignant tumors was associated with pleural effusion and arose in the parietal pleura; chest wall invasion was present in almost half the cases. In their review, Briselli and colleagues[767] stated that the presence of cellular pleomorphism and a high mitotic rate do not necessarily imply a bad prognosis. This was confirmed in the AFIP review by England and colleagues[764] in which 32 (45 per cent) of the patients judged to have a malignant neoplasm by light microscopic criteria were considered to be cured. Compounding the difficulty in histologic prediction is the observation that occasional tumors with a bland histologic appearance ultimately recur. On the whole, it would seem prudent to regard localized fibrous tumors of the pleura that possess atypical cytologic features and a significant mitotic rate as malignant. Although some of these tumors are associated with a good prognosis, especially those in which apparent complete excision has been accomplished, it is perhaps advisable to adopt a cautious approach in predicting cure.

DIFFUSE MALIGNANT MESOTHELIOMA

Diffuse mesothelioma is an uncommon, but increasingly recognized, malignant neoplasm of the pleura.[795, 796] Before 1960, it was a rarity and its very existence was questioned by some prominent pathologists.[797] In the 1970s, the incidence in England and the United States was estimated to be 2.2 cases per million per year,[798] but more recently this estimate has been increased to 7 to 13 individuals per million per year.[799] It has been predicted that in Australia the peak in mortality will not occur until the mid-1990s[800] and in Great Britain until around the turn of the century.[801] This neoplasm is important not only because of its almost invariable lethality, usually within a short time from diagnosis, but also because of the potential economic impact of litigation and the almost inevitable workers' compensation cases that will result.

Etiology and Pathogenesis

There is good evidence that in the majority of cases the etiologic agent of diffuse mesothelioma is asbestos; in a small number of cases, other minerals such as erionite have been implicated. In addition, factors such as radiation, pleural scarring, and hereditary susceptibility may be occasionally important.

ASBESTOS

The close association between asbestos and mesothelioma was first reported by Wagner and colleagues in 1960.[802] Since that time, abundant evidence has been published confirming their ob-

servation, and it is now clear that exposure to asbestos is by far the most important risk factor for the development of this neoplasm. This evidence can be summarized under three categories.

Epidemiologic Studies and Clinical Experience Showing a Strong Relationship Between Asbestos Exposure and Mesothelioma. A history of exposure to asbestos is obtained in over 50 per cent of individuals in most series of patients with mesothelioma;[803–811] in some studies[812, 813] the frequency is as high as 85 per cent. In those reports in which the frequency of asbestos exposure is relatively small, the lack of a strong association may be due to an inadequate search for an appropriate occupational or environmental history;[814] it is well known that the neoplasm can develop with minimal asbestos exposure[804, 815, 816] and many years after the initial contact.[817–819] Epidemiologic studies show a high incidence of the tumor in individuals involved both in the mining and production of asbestos and in the numerous secondary occupations associated with its use (see Table 12–1, page 2318); however, the risk appears to be greater in manufacturing and secondary uses than in mining and milling.[820–823] Some occupations are especially at risk. For example, a number of studies have shown a dramatic clustering of cases in the vicinity of shipyards throughout the world, including the United States,[795] Ireland,[824] Scotland,[825] England,[812, 826] Japan,[827] and Canada.[828]

There is also good evidence that contact with asbestos in the environment can be hazardous. Such contact can be secondarily related to occupation; for example, mesothelioma has been reported in wives of individuals who work in asbestos plants, probably contracted through their laundering of the workers' clothes,[829] and in individuals who reside near factories that process asbestos,[830] presumably contracted from contaminants in the atmosphere. Nonoccupational environmental contact also can be related to the presence of asbestos in the soil. For example, some cases of mesothelioma in Greece,[831, 832] Corsica,[833] and Cyprus[834] have been found to be associated with significant quantities of tremolite in the soil, and it is probable that contact occurred incidentally from this source.

Studies of Asbestos Fiber Burden in the Lungs of Patients with Mesothelioma. Several reports document an association between a large number of asbestos fibers in lung tissue and the presence of mesothelioma.[810] For example, of 100 patients with mesothelioma described by Davies,[812] 88 gave a history of asbestos exposure, and in all but 1 of these patients light microscopy showed over 20,000 coated and uncoated asbestos fibers per gram of dried lung. By contrast, of the 7 patients in the group who could confidently deny exposure to asbestos, 6 had fiber counts below 20,000. Despite the finding of an increased number of asbestos fibers in the lungs of many patients with malignant mesothelioma, several workers[805, 835, 836] have found this number to be intermediate between those found in the general population and in patients with asbestosis; those patients in whom the counts overlapped with those of the general population lacked identifiable occupational exposure.[819] In one study of patients with asbestosis,[837] an increased incidence of pulmonary carcinoma was found in those with moderate to severe asbestosis and of mesothelioma in those with minimal or slight disease. It has been speculated that this finding may reflect a dose relationship between asbestos burden and the development of asbestosis and lung cancer that does not exist for mesothelioma;[838, 839] this in turn suggests that there may be no threshold of asbestos burden below which there is no risk for the development of mesothelioma. Although this hypothesis has not been proven conclusively, some experimental evidence supports it.[840]

Experimental Studies in Animals Showing the Development of Mesothelioma after Asbestos Exposure. Diffuse mesothelioma morphologically similar to that seen in humans has been shown to develop following instillation of asbestos fibers into the pleural space[799, 841] or trachea[842] of various animals.

Although there is now no question regarding the association of mesothelioma with asbestos, the risk varies considerably with the type of asbestos, the majority of evidence indicating the greatest risk with the amphiboles crocidolite and amosite, substantially less with chrysotile, and virtually none with anthophyllite.[837, 843–849] The relative importance of chrysotile has been the subject of some debate:[799] because the use of amphiboles has decreased dramatically since their toxicity was recognized, the vast majority of asbestos used in primary and secondary occupations today is chrysotile; thus, mesotheliomas that develop 30 years from now almost certainly will be related to exposure to this substance. Although the bulk of evidence suggests that such exposure does lead to an increased risk of mesothelioma, there is evidence that the risk may be related to the presence of contaminating amphiboles,[799] particularly tremolite.[850, 851]

The variable pathogenicity of the different types of asbestos may be related to their different physicochemical characteristics. Long straight fibers, such as those of the amphiboles, tend to be transported in the center of the airway lumen to the periphery of the lung; by contrast, the irregular curly shape of the chrysotile fiber predisposes to its deposition in the more central airways.[799] Thus, amosite and crocidolite tend to accumulate in relatively large numbers in the peripheral portions of the lung close to the pleura. There is also evidence that chrysotile fibers fragment with time and are transported out of the lung via the mucociliary escalator or lymphatics.[799, 852] Amphiboles, on the other hand, are relatively stable and remain either constant in number in an individual who is no longer exposed or continue to accumulate over the lifetime of an individual who is continually exposed. For example, in one study in a Norwegian cement plant,[853] analysis of fiber types showed 91.7 per cent of the fibers to be chrysotile, 3.1 per cent amosite, 4.1 per cent crocidolite, and 1.1 per cent anthophyllite. However, electron microscopic and x-ray microanalysis of lung tissue samples from workers who had died of mesothelioma or pulmonary carcinoma showed a completely inverse proportion, the percentage of chrysotile asbestos fibers ranging from 0 to 9 per cent and of amphiboles from 76 to 99 per cent. There is also experimental evidence that chrysotile and crocidolite fibers interact differently with chromosomes of mesothelial cells,[854] possibly reflecting a different carcinogenic potential.

The pathogenesis of asbestos-related mesothelioma is far from clear. Several possible mechanisms have been discussed by Craighead.[799] Experimental studies have shown that the size and shape of the fibers are important determinants of carcinogenicity.[841, 847, 855] For example, it is possible to prepare samples of chrysotile that are long and straight (in contrast to their natural state) and that are at least as carcinogenic as amosite both in inhalation experiments and after introduction of the fiber into the pleural space.[841] In addition to amphiboles, other fibers such as fiberglass, anthophyllite, and certain metals[799] can also induce cancer when introduced directly into the pleural space of animals; however, inhalation of these substances by humans does not appear to be associated with an increased risk of mesothelioma. This suggests that factors associated with deposition or clearance of these particles may be at least as important as their physical properties. Whether the asbestos fibers are responsible for malignant transformation by means of an inflammatory reaction, as some experiments suggest,[799] or by a mechanism similar to that of foreign body carcinogenesis is not clear.

OTHER ETIOLOGIC AGENTS

Despite the presence of a large asbestos burden in the lungs of many individuals with mesothelioma, there are some patients in whom the burden is relatively slight[836] and, in fact, overlaps that of the general population.[819] In addition, the tumor was recognized at the turn of the century when little asbestos was being used,[812] and sporadic cases occur in children too young to have had significant asbestos exposure within the usually accepted latent period.[856, 857] Although, as discussed above, these observations may reflect the existence of a very low (or even nonexistent) threshold of asbestos burden, there is evidence that other explanations may be valid. Because the pathogenesis of asbestos-related mesothelioma appears to be intimately associated with the size and shape of the fiber, attention has been directed to the possibility that other minerals with the same physical characteristics as asbestos also may be pathogenic. The most clearly implicated of these is *erionite*, a nonasbestos mineral of the zeolite group found in the soil of central Turkey and the western United States (*see* page 2357). Strong epidemiologic[858–860] and experimental[861] evidence has accumulated that implicates this substance in the production of pleural plaques and mesothelioma. Although other natural and man-made fibers[799] can also cause mesothelioma when placed in the pleural cavity of experimental animals, as mentioned previously there is no evidence that inhalation of such fibers by humans leads to an increased risk of developing this neoplasm.

On the basis of several reports,[862, 863] it is probable that *radiation* is also responsible for occasional cases of mesothelioma; in fact, experimental evidence suggests that the risk is significantly increased when radiation is combined with asbestos exposure.[864] Malignant neoplasms occasionally arise in relation to a *chronically scarred pleura*, such as can occur following chronic empyema or therapeutic pneumothorax for tuberculosis.[975] Although most of these neoplasms are squamous cell carcinomas, occasional tumors morphologically similar to mesothelioma have been described.[975]

A familial occurrence of mesothelioma has been documented in several studies;[866–870] although this may be largely explained by asbestos dust brought to the home or by a common source of exposure, it is also possible that there is a degree of *genetic susceptibility*. The risk of developing mesothelioma appears to be independent of *cigarette smoking*.[871, 872]

Pathologic Characteristics

The pathologic characteristics of malignant mesothelioma have been described in detail in several reports[873, 874] and monographs.[875] Although it can occur as a solitary, more or less spherical intrapleural mass,[876, 877] in the vast majority of cases it appears as a diffuse, plaque-like thickening that usually encases the entire lung, at least in autopsy specimens (Fig. 18–22). Discrete cyst-like spaces containing gelatinous or hemorrhagic fluid can be occasionally identified within the tumor and probably represent portions of the original pleural space. Extension of the neoplasm along fissures and into adjacent tissues, such as the chest wall, diaphragm, and pericardium, is not uncommon. Despite this, the border between the tumor and underlying lung parenchyma is usually well defined, although nodular expansions occasionally project from the thickened pleura into the lung itself (Fig. 18–23). The tumor can be soft and fleshy or, in the case of desmoplastic forms, quite firm and gritty, resembling mature fibrous tissue.

Histologically, mesothelioma is usually classified in three forms—*epithelial, mesenchymal* (sarcomatous, fibrous, or spindle-cell), and *biphasic* (mixed). Although the first form is the most common in the majority of series, careful search will reveal many tumors to be mixed. The epithelial form has a

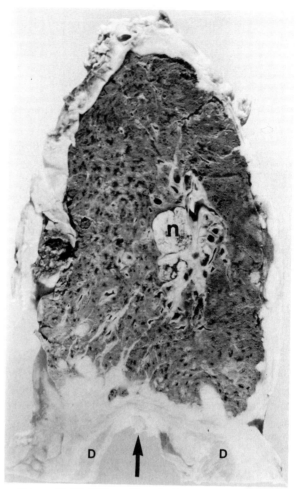

Figure 18–22. Diffuse Mesothelioma. A sagittal section of left lung shows mild to moderate thickening of the pleura over almost its entire surface; lung parenchyma is unremarkable. The tumor has extended into the adjacent hemidiaphragm *(D)* to involve the peritoneum *(arrow)*. Metastases are evident in peribronchial lymph nodes *(N)*.

variable appearance, cells being organized in papillary projections, tubular or acinar clusters, and solid sheets (Fig. 18–24); an elongated, slit-like space lined on either side by a single layer of neoplastic cells is characteristic. The tumor cells are usually cuboidal in shape and possess a moderate amount of eosinophilic cytoplasm (Fig. 18–25); occasionally they have a foamy or clear (signet ring) appearance due to the presence of lipid.[873, 878] Squamous differentiation is seen rarely.[879] Nuclei are often rather uniform in size and shape, although pleomorphism is common in the less differentiated forms.

The mesenchymal form typically consists of spindle cells that can be arranged either haphazardly or in a fascicular or storiform pattern (Fig. 18–26). Interstitial collagen may be apparent, suggesting fibroblastic differentiation; occasionally this tissue is abundant, leading to the designation "desmoplastic" mesothelioma.[880] In this case differentiation from benign fibrous proliferation can be difficult, particularly with small biopsy specimens. Other

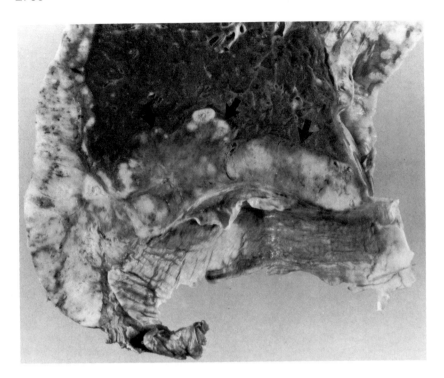

Figure 18–23. Diffuse Mesothelioma: Parenchymal Extension. A cut section of the basal aspect of a lower lobe shows marked pleural thickening by a tumor that possesses a somewhat variegated appearance. It has extended from the diaphragmatic portion of the pleura into adjacent lung parenchyma along a broad front *(arrows)*.

forms of mesenchymal differentiation, especially cartilage and bone, occur occasionally.[881–883] A rare variant of the sarcomatous form, termed "lymphohistiocytoid" mesothelioma by Henderson and colleagues,[884] shows an intense lymphocytic infiltrate admixed with neoplastic mesothelial cells, a pattern that can be confused with lymphoma.

There are two major practical problems in the pathologic diagnosis of mesothelioma: (1) distinguishing mesothelial hyperplasia from neoplasia, and (2) distinguishing mesothelioma from metastatic carcinoma, especially adenocarcinoma (Fig. 18–27). Both of these problems are particularly troublesome with the small tissue fragments commonly obtained by closed chest pleural biopsy.

MESOTHELIAL HYPERPLASIA VERSUS NEOPLASIA

Although there is evidence that significant mesothelial hyperplasia is infrequent in association with common pleural abnormalities,[885] it is clear that mesothelial cells can react to pleural injury by proliferating, sometimes to a marked degree. This proliferation can result in a variety of morphologic appearances, including simple or complex papillary projections and aggregates of cells of variable thickness covering the pleural surface (Fig. 18–28).[886, 887] Occasionally, there are features suggesting neoplasia, such as mitotic figures, cytologic atypia,[888] and entrapment of mesothelial cell clusters in underlying fibrous tissue, simulating invasion (Fig. 18–28).[887] Each of these features also can be present in mesothelioma; consequently, the distinction between a reactive and a neoplastic process can be extremely difficult, particularly if only a small

amount of mesothelial tissue is present in a biopsy specimen. Although histologic criteria have been proposed to aid in such differentiation,[873, 887, 889, 890] in some cases it may be impossible to be definitive. Indeed, it is possible that some represent examples of dysplastic mesothelium analogous to the preinvasive neoplastic process that commonly occurs in epithelia throughout the body.

In addition to simple light microscopic examination of H&E stained sections, several ancillary procedures have been investigated in an attempt to distinguish reactive from neoplastic mesothelium. For example, morphometric analysis of the nuclear and cytoplasmic area of cells both in tissue sections[891] and in filter preparations of pleural fluid[892, 893] has shown that reactive cells possess a significantly smaller mean area than neoplastic ones. There is overlap between the two, however, and the practical advantage of performing measurements in a particular case is not clear. Herbert and Gallagher[894] reported evidence that the immunohistochemical demonstration of alpha$_1$-antichymotrypsin may be a feature of reactive, as opposed to neoplastic, mesothelial cells, but their results have not been replicated by others.[887] It has also been proposed that analysis of DNA content by flow cytometry can be helpful;[895, 896] however, reactive mesothelial cells themselves can be polyploid, suggesting that interpretation of specimens based on this feature alone can be hazardous.[897] Other techniques that have been proposed, but have yet to be conclusively shown to be of value, are the use of specific antimesothelial cell antibodies[898] and the staining of proteins associated with the nucleolar organizer region.[899]

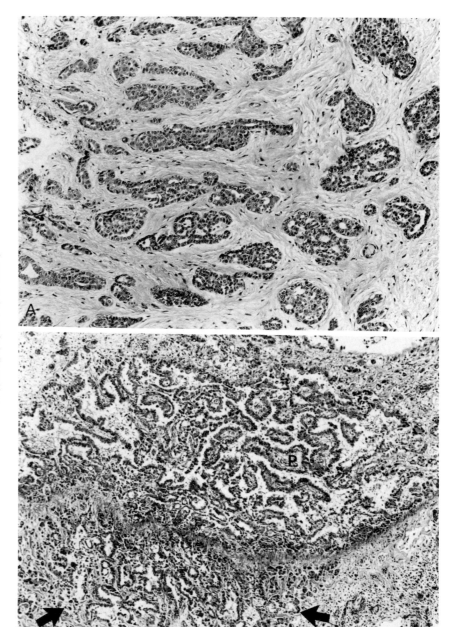

Figure 18–24. Diffuse Mesothelioma: Epithelial Type. A histologic section *(A)* reveals small nests of cells separated by a fibroblastic stroma, associated with round or elongated slit-like spaces. The neoplastic cells have abundant eosinophilic cytoplasm and fairly uniform round to oval nuclei. A section from another tumor *(B)* demonstrates multiple papillary projections *(P)* lined by a single layer of malignant mesothelial cells and protruding into a small cystic space. The adjacent pleura is focally invaded *(arrows)*. (*A, ×* 100; *B, ×* 60.)

MESOTHELIOMA VERSUS METASTATIC CARCINOMA

The second major problem in the pathologic diagnosis of mesothelioma lies in distinguishing it from metastatic carcinoma. As with hyperplasia and neoplasia, a variety of ancillary studies have been employed to aid in the solution of this problem, including histochemistry, immunohistochemistry, ultrastructural analysis, biochemistry, and lectin binding.

Histochemistry. Many malignant mesothelial cells contain glycogen and thus show a positive reaction to para-amino salicylic acid (PAS),[900] a feature that is characteristic, but not diagnostic, of the neoplasm. Of greater differential diagnostic value is the reaction to PAS with diastase,[900, 901, 902] which is positive in many adenocarcinomas and almost never in mesothelioma. For example, the reaction was positive in 15 of 25 cases of adenocarcinoma in one series[903] and in 8 of 39 cases in another[904] but was negative in all 57 cases of mesothelioma in the two series. As might be expected, the mucicarmine stain is also typically negative in mesothelioma.[904] The demonstration of acid-mucopolysaccharides, specifically hyaluronic acid, within tumor cells is quite suggestive of mesothelioma.[878, 902, 904–906] This substance can be detected by a positive reaction to stains such as colloidal iron or alcian blue and its presence confirmed by a negative reaction after treatment of the tissue with hyaluronidase.

Immunohistochemistry. Numerous studies were performed in the 1980s documenting the

THE PLEURA

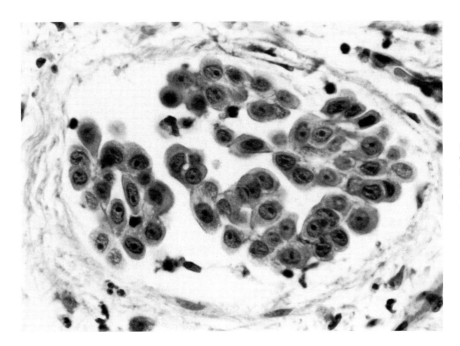

Figure 18–25. Mesothelioma: Cytologic Appearance. A magnified view of a well-differentiated epithelial mesothelioma shows several clusters of cells with moderately abundant cytoplasm, fairly uniform round or oval nuclei, and prominent nucleoli. (× 600.)

immunohistochemical features of mesothelioma and adenocarcinoma in an attempt to find consistent differences between the two; these were performed on both paraffin-embedded tissue sections[903–905, 907–918] and on exfoliated cells present in pleural fluid.[919–923] Although there is no doubt that some of these investigations (such as those involving CEA) proved to be extremely useful, the results of tests on many of the antibodies were conflicting and left the somewhat perplexed diagnostic pathologist little better off than he or she would have been without them. The reasons for this variability of results are several: (1) individual differences in the interpretation of a positive or negative reaction;[911] (2) the use of different tissue fixatives;[912, 919] (3) the use by investigators of different antibodies supposedly directed to the same antigen, but probably reacting with different proteins (for example, polyclonal versus monoclonal anti-CEA[911] and high versus low molecular weight antikeratin antibodies[911, 920]); (4) the use of different techniques in carrying out the immunohistochemical reactions;[924] and (5) the possibility that not all cases reported as mesothelioma truly represent this neoplasm (the criteria for diagnosis in some studies were not well documented).

The most extensively studied antibodies have been those directed against CEA and cytoplasmic keratins. Many investigators have reported a positive reaction of adenocarcinoma for CEA (in 60 to 100 per cent of cases),[903, 904, 907–911, 914–916, 918, 923, 925] whereas the reaction in mesothelioma is almost always negative; when the latter is positive, it is usually described as weak.[914–916] It can be reasonably concluded, therefore, that a clearly positive reaction for CEA is very much against a diagnosis of mesothelioma; however, since as many as 40 per cent of adenocarcinomas in some series are negative for this substance, the lack of a reaction does not establish the diagnosis of mesothelioma.

The presence of a positive reaction to antikeratin antibodies is characteristic of mesothelioma and is detected in virtually all tumors in many series.[904, 905, 907, 911, 914–916, 923] However, a positive reaction is also seen in many adenocarcinomas so that its presence is not of differential diagnostic value. It has been suggested, however, that certain features of the reaction for keratins might have some specificity, particularly the presence of high molecular weight keratins in mesothelioma[911, 920] and a peripheral as opposed to a central or diffuse cytoplasmic keratin reaction in adenocarcinoma.[904, 914] These distinctions, however, have not been replicated by all investigators,[910] and their value has yet to be definitively proven. Of some interest is the observation that the spindle cells of the biphasic and mesenchymal forms of mesothelioma also react strongly with antikeratin antibodies.[782, 783]

Several additional antibodies are also of potential value in distinguishing mesothelioma from adenocarcinoma, although they have not been as extensively studied as those against CEA and the keratins. The reaction to Leu-M1, a sugar linked to membranes in intercellular proteins and lipids,[910] has been found to be almost always negative in mesothelioma and often positive in adenocarcinoma.[901, 910, 911, 922, 925] For example, in a study by Ordonez,[910] the reaction was negative in all 19 mesotheliomas and positive in 14 of 23 (61 per cent) adenocarcinomas. We are aware of only one study in which an antisurfactant lipoprotein antibody has been utilized;[918] in all 9 cases of mesothelioma the reaction was negative, whereas in 13 of 21 (62 per cent) peripheral pulmonary adenocarcinomas it was positive. Other antibodies used in attempts to differentiate mesothelioma and adenocarcinoma but that have given results of unproved or equivocal value include vimentin,[908, 910, 912, 913, 923] epithelial membrane antigen (EMA),[904, 905, 908, 910, 921, 922] protein S-100,[908, 910, 926] pregnancy-specific antigen,[908–910] hu-

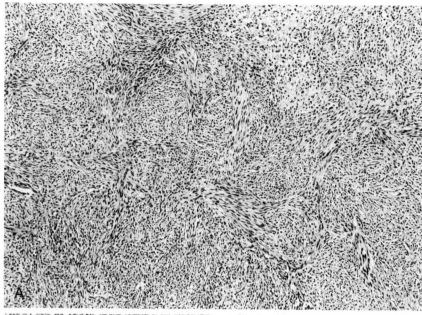

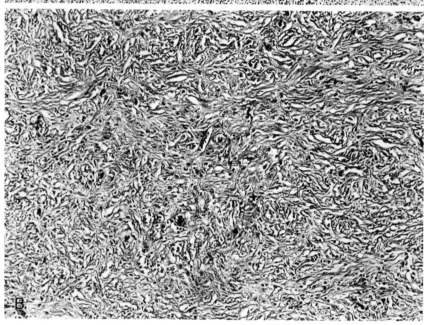

Figure 18–26. Diffuse Mesothelioma: Mesenchymal Type. A histologic section *(A)* reveals fascicles of spindle-shaped cells arranged in an interdigitating pattern; a storiform appearance is present focally. A section of another tumor *(B)* shows moderately abundant, intercellular collagen. *(A, × 80; B, × 120.)*

man milk fat globulin,[904, 905, 907, 910, 911, 915, 925, 927] human placental lactogen,[909, 910] secretory component,[907, 910] and Lewis[a] blood groups (or related antigen CA 19–9).[910, 918, 928] It is possible that further investigations using monoclonal[929–931] or polyclonal[932] antibodies that are more specifically related to mesothelioma may prove to be of greater diagnostic value.

Ultrastructure. The ultrastructural features of mesothelioma, especially the better differentiated epithelial forms, are so characteristic as to be almost diagnostic.[902, 933] As summarized in a recent review by Coleman and colleagues,[933] they include (1) the absence of microvillous core rootlets, glycocalyceal bodies, and secretory granules (three structures that are characteristic of adenocarcinoma); and (2) the presence of intercellular desmosomes and junc-

tional complexes, intracytoplasmic lumina (sometimes containing flocculent material thought to be hyaluronic acid), glycogen, intermediate filaments (often aggregated in a perinuclear location), and microvilli (Fig. 18–29). Of all these features, the appearance of the microvilli is the most important diagnostically: in mesothelioma they are numerous and are characteristically long and thin, whereas in adenocarcinoma they are typically much less frequent and are usually short and stubby.[902, 933, 934] Several attempts have been made to quantify this subjective impression by measuring the length and width of microvilli; in general, the mean length-to-width ratio has been found to be 10:1 in mesotheliomas and about 5:1 in adenocarcinomas.[933] Microvilli are usually most prominent on the apical cell surface where they project into empty lumina, but

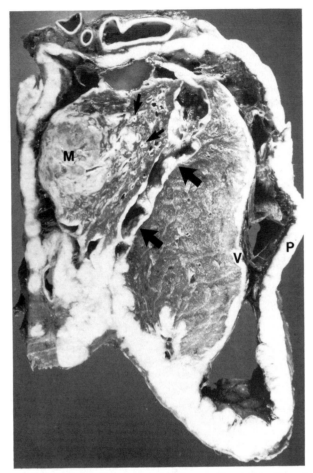

Figure 18–27. Pulmonary Carcinoma Simulating Pleural Mesothelioma. A sagittal section of a left lung and attached pleura shows marked thickening of both visceral *(V)* and parietal *(P)* pleura by a solid white tumor. The neoplasm extends into the major fissure *(large arrows)*. This appearance is highly suggestive of diffuse mesothelioma; however, a nodular mass is present in the upper lobe *(M)* and is associated with fairly extensive lymphangitic spread *(small arrows)*, both features being very unusual for mesothelioma. Histologic sections showed the tumor to be a mucin-secreting adenocarcinoma, considered to originate in the upper lobe.

Biochemistry. As with the histochemical detection of hyaluronic acid in mesothelioma cells, the demonstration of this substance in tissue fragments by digestion and electrophoresis is evidence in favor of the diagnosis of mesothelioma.[906, 936, 937] A second glycosaminoglycan, chondroitin sulfate, is also elaborated by some mesotheliomas[937, 938] and is sometimes the principal substance present;[939] it is also suggestive of mesothelioma.

Lectin Binding. Kawai and colleagues[940] studied the reaction of various lectins (a form of non-immune glycoprotein that binds specifically to carbohydrate groups) in mesotheliomas and pulmonary adenocarcinomas. They found that the pattern of positive reactions to a variety of lectins differed in the two forms of tumor; this suggests that these substances may be useful in differential diagnosis.

Roentgenographic Manifestations

Although malignant mesothelioma can be manifested by a solitary mass simulating peripheral pulmonary carcinoma (Fig. 18–30), the most common roentgenographic presentation is of irregular, nodular opacities around the periphery of the lung, either over the convexity or along the mediastinum or diaphragm. Such opacities may or may not be associated with pleural effusion. When effusion is present, it frequently obscures the underlying neoplasm (Fig. 18–31). In contrast to other forms of pleural effusion, that associated with mesothelioma is frequently not accompanied by significant shift of the mediastinum to the contralateral side, a peculiarity that has two possible explanations: (1) the formation of a large pleural "peel" acts in a restrictive capacity and prevents inflation of the lung on full inspiration, thus reducing volume; and (2) local invasion of the medial aspect of the lung by the neoplasm can occlude bronchi and result in atelectasis. This pattern of massive pleural effusion unassociated with mediastinal shift can also occur with primary pulmonary carcinoma accompanied by obstructive atelectasis and pleural metastases, and it is obviously important to differentiate these two causes.

Computed tomography is generally superior to conventional roentgenograms in determining the extent of the neoplasm. For example, in one study of five patients with proven pleural mesothelioma,[941] it was shown that in each case conventional chest roentgenography underestimated the extent of disease. However, in each case, CT revealed an extensive, pleural-based mass surrounding the lung (Fig. 18–32), spreading into the fissures and extending into the mediastinum and sometimes the contralateral chest, abdomen, and chest wall. In a similar comparative study in which CT and conventional radiography were performed on 27 patients with mesothelioma and 13 patients with advanced asbestosis, Rabinowitz and his colleagues[942] found that,

they can be seen also between adjacent cells and directly interdigitating with collagen fibers of the adjacent stroma.[902, 933] As expected, ultrastructural features of mesothelial differentiation are not as well seen in poorly differentiated as in well-differentiated tumors, but other criteria suggestive of mesothelioma have been described for the former neoplasms.[935]

The spindle cells of the mesenchymal form of mesothelioma show few intercellular junctions, focal basal lamina, absent or occasional microvilli (usually much shorter than those in the epithelial form), abundant rough endoplasmic reticulum, and numerous randomly oriented intermediate filaments.[933] As expected, most cells of biphasic mesotheliomas show ultrastructural features that are either epithelial or mesenchymal; in addition, a variable number of cells possess intermediate (or transitional) features.[933]

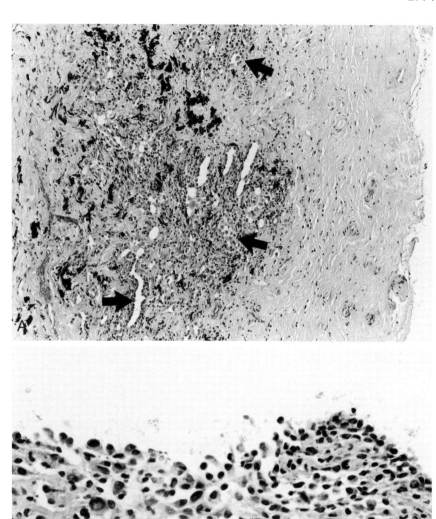

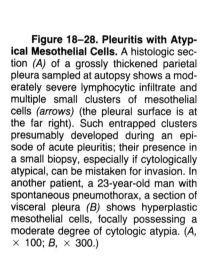

Figure 18–28. Pleuritis with Atypical Mesothelial Cells. A histologic section *(A)* of a grossly thickened parietal pleura sampled at autopsy shows a moderately severe lymphocytic infiltrate and multiple small clusters of mesothelial cells *(arrows)* (the pleural surface is at the far right). Such entrapped clusters presumably developed during an episode of acute pleuritis; their presence in a small biopsy, especially if cytologically atypical, can be mistaken for invasion. In another patient, a 23-year-old man with spontaneous pneumothorax, a section of visceral pleura *(B)* shows hyperplastic mesothelial cells, focally possessing a moderate degree of cytologic atypia. (*A*, × 100; *B*, × 300.)

although the major pathologic features of both diseases were well demonstrated by both modalities, CT demonstrated the findings more frequently and in greater detail. They noted that nodular involvement of the pleural fissures, pleural effusion, and ipsilateral volume loss were features that predominated in mesothelioma, findings that supported the observations of Alexander and her associates.[941] However, Solomon[943] has taken exception to the statement that involvement of the pleural fissures tends to be a sign that favors a diagnosis of mesothelioma. This author referred to a South African study of 1,692 men employed in the crocidolite and amosite asbestos mines in whom the prevalence of thickened interlobar fissures showed a strong relationship to the duration of asbestos exposure; in

this group, thickened fissures were seen in 25 per cent of persons with more than 15 years' exposure to asbestos and were not indicative of the presence of mesothelioma.

Calcification occasionally can be identified in both primary tumors and metastases on conventional roentgenograms and CT.[881, 882, 944, 945] In primary tumors, it probably reflects incorporation of calcified pleural plaques into the neoplasm, whereas in metastases it is perhaps more likely caused by osseous differentiation.

The diagnosis of mesothelioma may be suggested by the finding of parenchymal fibrosis or pleural plaques (Fig. 18–33) (or both), but these clues are often absent. Gallium-67 scanning has been reported to be helpful in determining the

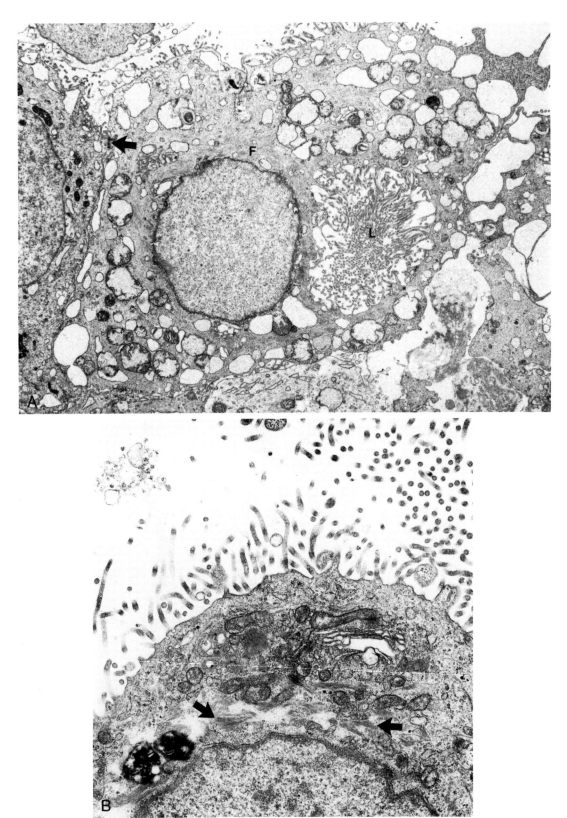

Figure 18–29. Diffuse Mesothelioma: Ultrastructure. An electron micrograph of a well-differentiated epithelial mesothelioma *(A)* shows a large cell with a more or less round nucleus and finely granular nuclear material. The cell cytoplasm contains a moderate number of intermediate filaments *(F)*, focally in clusters adjacent to the nucleus. A poorly developed intercellular junction is evident *(arrow)*. Long thin microvilli are present on the cell surface and are especially numerous within an intracellular lumen *(L)*. A magnified view of another cell from the same patient *(B)* reveals perinuclear clusters of intermediate filaments *(arrows)* and long thin surface microvilli. *(A,* × 7200; *B,* × 21,700.)

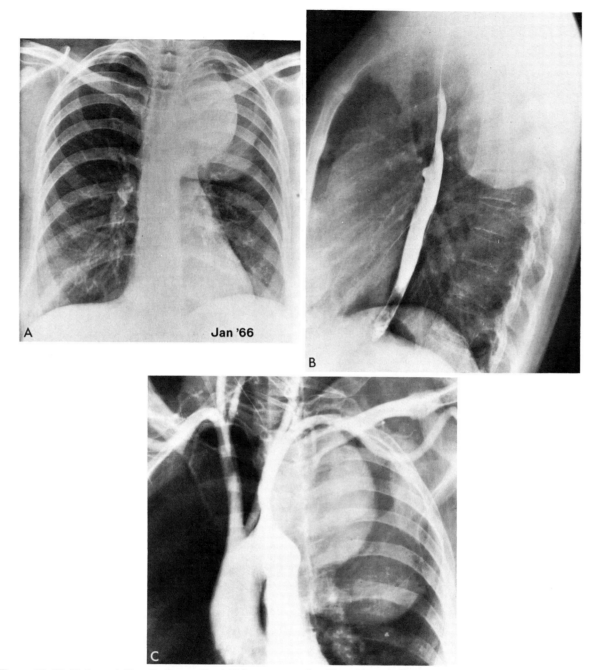

Figure 18–30. Malignant Mesothelioma. The initial posteroanterior *(A)* and lateral *(B)* roentgenograms of this 45-year-old woman reveal a large homogeneous mass arising from the mediastinal aspect of the left upper hemithorax. The obtuse angle at which the mass relates to the mediastinum suggests an origin from either the pleura or the mediastinum. Since one of the differential diagnostic possibilities was aortic aneurysm, an aortogram *(C)* was performed but was normal except for displacement of the aorta and its major branches by the mass. A large malignant mesothelioma was resected at thoracotomy.

Illustration continued on following page

extent of disease.[946] Basal linear opacities may be seen in some cases and when combined with a pleural effusion can lead to a misdiagnosis of pulmonary embolism.[947]

Clinical Manifestations

Patients with diffuse pleural mesothelioma can present with either vague chest or shoulder ache or true pleuritic pain.[948, 949] As the disease progresses, shortness of breath, weight loss, and dry hacking cough can develop.[825] Physical examination often reveals clubbing, retraction of the thorax, and dullness on percussion. Cardiac abnormalities are common:[950] in one series of 64 patients, ECG abnormalities were present in 55 patients (89 per cent) and consisted of arrhythmia (60 per cent) and a conduction abnormality (37 per cent). Echocardi-

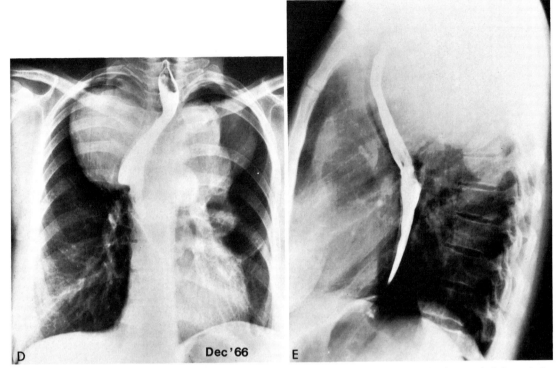

Dec '66

Figure 18–30 *Continued* Almost 1 year later (*D* and *E*) the left-sided mass had recurred and had extended through the posterior mediastinum into the right hemithorax. Note the marked anterior displacement of the esophagus and trachea. We regard this case as a most unusual manifestation of malignant mesothelioma.

ography revealed pericardial effusion in 13 patients. In the 19 patients who were autopsied, cardiac invasion was found in 14 cases (74 per cent), the pericardium being involved in more than half and the myocardium in over a fourth. Extension of tumor through the myocardium to form an intraluminal obstructing mass has been reported.[951]

Occasionally the neoplasm invades the chest wall along the needle tract used for prior thoracentesis or biopsy; in this circumstance a localized tumor may be palpated in relation to the puncture site, a finding highly suggestive of the diagnosis. Although metastases outside the thorax are not uncommonly identified at autopsy,[809, 862, 952, 953] they are infrequently detected clinically;[862, 954, 955] they usually occur in tumors with a sarcomatous morphology.[800, 956, 957] Rare presentations or complications include the superior vena cava syndrome[958] and the syndrome of inappropriate secretion of antidiuretic hormone.[959, 960]

An occupational history of asbestos exposure may suggest the diagnosis. However, as discussed previously, some patients give a history of minimal exposure,[804, 815, 816] and careful questioning may be necessary to elicit evidence of the asbestos association. Compounding this difficulty is the latent period between exposure and the development of clinical signs that usually exceeds 20 years[812, 961] and sometimes may be 40 years or longer.[817–819]

Laboratory Investigation

Pleural effusion is present in the majority of patients with mesothelioma and is often considerable in amount;[800] it may be either straw-colored or serosanguineous, in roughly equal numbers.[804] Examination of the fluid by either biochemistry or cytology can be helpful in making the diagnosis. Low or nonexistent levels of CEA (less than 12 mg/ml) in aspirated fluid were found in two studies[962, 963] to be characteristic of mesothelioma (as in all 35 patients in the two studies), whereas values greater than 15 mg/ml were indicative of metastatic carcinoma. Measurement of other substances, such as alpha$_1$–acid-glycoprotein and phosphohexose isomerase, also has been advocated.[964]

Cytologic features of malignant mesothelioma cells in pleural fluid have been described in several reports;[873, 965–967] as with histologic diagnosis, problems are encountered in distinguishing reactive from neoplastic mesothelial cells and mesothelioma from metastatic adenocarcinoma. Although a variety of ancillary procedures have been investigated in an attempt to overcome these problems[968] and some observers report a high degree of accuracy in the cytologic diagnosis of mesothelioma,[873] we and others[968] find that a diagnosis based on cytology alone can be quite difficult and that examination of pleural tissue specimens obtained at thoracoscopy or thoracotomy or by transthoracic needle aspira-

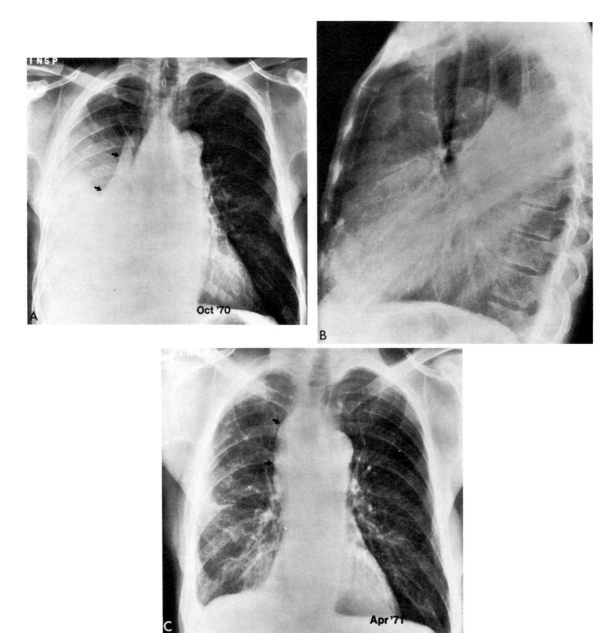

Figure 18–31. Malignant Mesothelioma Presenting with a Massive Pleural Effusion. The initial roentgenograms of this 56-year-old man (*A* and *B*) reveal a massive right pleural effusion whose upper configuration in lateral projection is somewhat atypical, suggesting the presence of pulmonary disease underlying the effusion. In addition, in the posteroanterior view there is an unusual opacity in the medial portion of the right hemithorax contiguous to the mediastinum *(arrows)*. Thoracotomy was performed and a large mediastinal mesothelioma removed. This was followed by a course of antineoplastic drug therapy. Six months later, a roentgenogram *(C)* reveals a smooth, sharply circumscribed mass in the right paramediastinal zone *(arrows)*; there is still a small pleural effusion.

Illustration continued on following page

tion is usually necessary to establish a confident diagnosis.[969, 970]

Prognosis

The prognosis of diffuse pleural mesothelioma is extremely poor; many patients die within the first year of the onset of symptoms.[804, 971] "Long-term" survival is almost unheard of; in two series of 167[971] and 114[862] patients, only 7 (2.5 per cent) lived more than 5 years. It has been suggested that prognosis tends to be somewhat better in a patient whose neoplasm possesses an epithelial, rather than a mesenchymal, morphology,[800, 862, 880, 900] although at least one study found no evidence for this association.[971]

Extrapleural pneumonectomy, consisting of *en bloc* excision of parietal pleura, lung, pericardium, diaphragm, and attached tumor, has been said to offer some benefit in selected patients. Of 33 patients subjected to this procedure,[972] 8 patients (24 per cent) survived for 2 years, 5 for 3 years, and 3 for 5 years or longer. As might be expected, however, the operation is not without risk; in the same

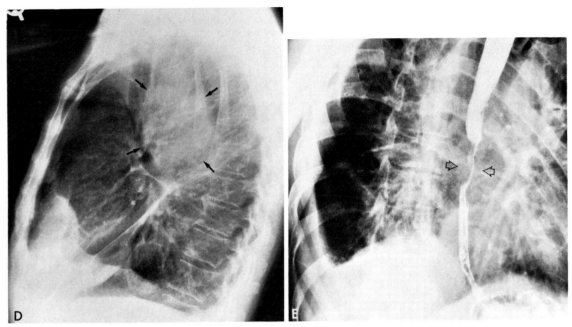

Figure 18–31 *Continued* In lateral projection *(D)*, the mass is rather indistinctly defined *(arrows)* but is obviously displacing the lower trachea and main bronchi anteriorly. Proof of invasion of the mediastinum was provided by a barium swallow *(E)*, which revealed concentric narrowing of the esophagus *(arrows)*.

series, there were three operative deaths and eight serious postoperative complications.

MISCELLANEOUS MALIGNANT NEOPLASMS

Very rarely, squamous cell carcinoma can arise in the pleura[973] and is usually associated with either persistent empyema that has been drained by a pleurocutaneous fistula[974] or long-standing extra-pleural pneumothorax without fistula.[975] Primary pleural melanoma also has been reported,[976] although such cases must be exceedingly rare.

In addition to localized fibrous tumors, a variety of soft tissue neoplasms have been reported to develop in the pleura. Although it is conceivable that some of these are derived from the submeso-thelial mesenchymal cells of the pleura itself and thus indeed arise in this location, it is probable that some originate in the chest wall and simply expand into the pleural space. The most common of these is lipoma, a tumor that is usually small but can become sufficiently large to erode contiguous ribs.[977] Gramiak and Koerner[978] drew attention to the fact that the shape of these lesions may change during respiration, presumably as a result of the relatively fluid nature of their content. Sarcomas that have been reported to arise in the pleura include leio-

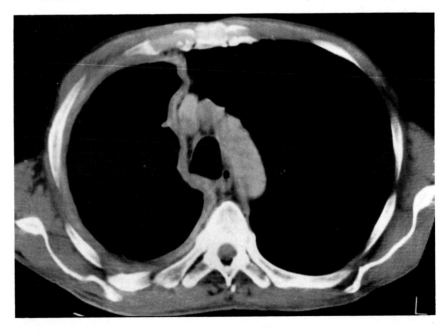

Figure 18–32. Malignant Mesothelioma: CT Manifestations. A CT scan at the level of the aortic arch shows circumferential pleural thickening (pleural rind). Mild nodularity is noted posteromedial to the trachea. Also noted is moderate loss of volume of the right hemithorax. The patient is a 75-year-old man. (Courtesy of Drs. Ann Leung, RR Miller, and Nestor Müller, University of British Columbia, Vancouver.)

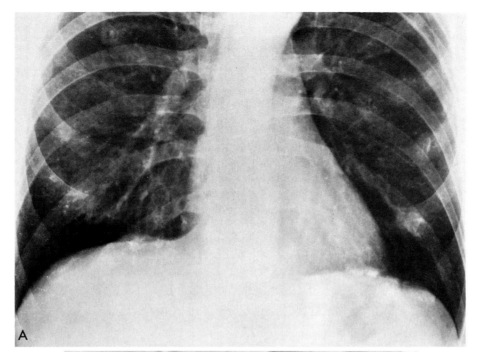

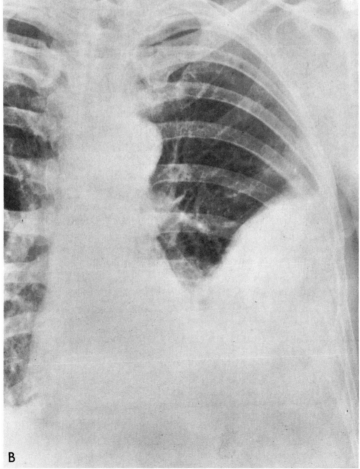

Figure 18–33. Malignant Mesothelioma Associated with Asbestos Exposure. This 60-year-old man had worked in the asbestos mines of Quebec for many years and showed roentgenographic evidence of calcification of the diaphragmatic pleura bilaterally *(A)*. There was no convincing evidence of pulmonary disease roentgenologically. Approximately 6 months after the roentgenogram illustrated in *(A)*, the patient presented with pain in the left side of his chest. Posteroanterior *(B)* and lateral *(C)* roentgenograms revealed a large left-sided pleural effusion associated with an irregular, poorly defined mass in the lateral portion of the left hemithorax *(arrows in C)*.

Illustration continued on following page

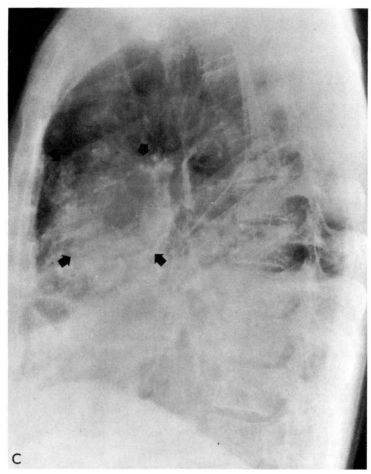

Figure 18–33 *Continued*

myosarcoma,[979] rhabdomyosarcoma,[980] malignant fibrous histiocytoma,[981] and liposarcoma.[982]

MISCELLANEOUS NON-NEOPLASTIC TUMORS

Pleural amyloidosis is a very rare condition[983] that can present as more or less diffuse involvement, sometimes associated with effusion, or as a localized tumor-like nodule or mass.[984] There are no specific roentgenographic features to suggest the diagnosis.

Although *oleothorax* as a method of therapy for pulmonary tuberculosis was largely abandoned in the 1950s, patients are still seen occasionally in whom the instilled paraffin is visible as a mass within the pleural space. In four examples reported by Hutton,[985] the mass increased considerably in size over time, thus creating some confusion in differential diagnosis.

Intrathoracic splenosis is a rare condition in which tissue from a traumatized spleen crosses an injured diaphragm and proliferates within the left pleural space,[942, 986, 987] thus creating nodules of possibly more ominous consequence. As pointed out by Scales and Lee,[942] once the diagnosis is suspected it can be easily confirmed by radionuclide imaging but also has been made by transthoracic needle aspiration.[988]

Fibrin bodies are tumor-like concentrations of fibrin that sometimes develop in a serofibrinous pleural effusion. These bodies are round, oval, or of irregular shape and are seldom more than 3 to 4 cm in diameter. They usually become evident following absorption of a pleural effusion. They may disappear spontaneously and fairly rapidly[989] or may remain unchanged in size, position, or shape for many years.[990] They tend to be situated near the lung base and when viewed *en face* can simulate a solitary pulmonary nodule. Their anatomic relationship to the pleura may be established by fluoroscopy, tangential roentgenography, or CT.

REFERENCES

1. Adams FV, Galati V: M-mode ultrasonic localization of pleural effusion. Use in patients with nondiagnostic physical and roentgenographic examinations. JAMA 239:1761, 1978.
2. Lipscomb DJ, Flower CDR: Ultrasound in the diagnosis and management of pleural disease. Br J Dis Chest 74:353, 1980.
3. Pugatch RD, Spirn PW: Radiology of the pleura. Clin Chest Med 6:17, 1985.
4. Dorne HL: Differentiation of pulmonary parenchymal consolidation from pleural disease using the sonographic fluid bronchogram. Radiology 158:41, 1986.
5. Black LF: The pleural space and pleural fluid. Mayo Clin Proc 47:493, 1972.
6. Rabin CB, Blackman NS: Bilateral pleural effusion. Its significance in association with a heart of normal size. J Mt. Sinai Hosp 24:45, 1957.
7. DeSouza R, Lipsett N, Spagnolo SV: Mediastinal compression due to tension hydrothorax. Chest 72:782, 1977.
8. Naschitz JE, Yeshurun D: Unilateral chest wall edema in carcinomatous pleurisy. Respiration 47:73, 1985.
9. Gilmartin JJ, Wright AJ, Gibson GJ: Effects of pneumothorax or pleural effusion on pulmonary function. Thorax 40:60, 1985.
10. Sonnenblick M, Melzer E, Rosin AJ: Body positional effect on gas exchange in unilateral pleural effusion. Chest 83:784, 1983.
11. Neagley SR, Zwillich CW: The effect of positional changes on oxygenation in patients with pleural effusions. Chest 88:714, 1985.
12. Estenne M, Yernault JC, De Troyer A: Mechanism of relief of dyspnea after thoracocentesis in patients with large pleural effusions. Am J Med 74:813, 1983.
13. Brandstetter RD, Cohen RP: Hypoxemia after thoracentesis. A predictable and treatable condition. JAMA 242:1060, 1979.
14. Anthonisen NR, Martin RR: Regional lung function in pleural effusion. Am Rev Respir Dis 116:201, 1977.
15. Storey DD, Dines DE, Coles, DT: Pleural effusion. A diagnostic dilemma. JAMA 236:2183, 1976.
16. Gunnels JJ: Perplexing pleural effusion. Chest 74:390, 1978.
17. Hirsch A, Ruffie P, Nebut M, et al: Pleural effusion: Laboratory tests in 300 cases. Thorax 34:106, 1979.
18. Ryan CJ, Rodgers RF, Unni KK, et al: The outcome of patients with pleural effusion of indeterminate cause at thoracotomy. Mayo Clin Proc 56:145, 1981.
19. Leslie WK, Kinasewitz GT: Clinical characteristics of the patient with nonspecific pleuritis. Chest 94:603, 1988.
20. Black LF: Pleural effusions. Mayo Clin Proc 56:201, 1981.
21. Leading article. Pleural effusion. Br Med J 3:192, 1975.
22. Kutty CP, Varkey B: "Contarini's condition": Bilateral pleural effusions with markedly different characteristics. Chest 74:679, 1978.
23. Lawton F, Blackledge G, Johnson R: Co-existent chylous and serous pleural effusions associated with ovarian cancer: A case report of Contarini's syndrome. Eur J Surg Oncol 11:177, 1985.
24. Sinzobahamvya N, Bhakta HP: Pleural exudate in a tropical hospital. Eur Respir J 2:145, 1989.
25. Light RW, MacGregor MI, Luchsinger PC, et al: Pleural effusions: The diagnostic separation of transudates and exudates. Ann Intern Med 77:507, 1972.
26. Stead WW: Pleural effusion (letter). JAMA 237:2469, 1977.
27. Weber AL, Bird KT, Janower ML: Primary tuberculosis in childhood with particular emphasis on changes affecting the tracheobronchial tree. Am J Roentgenol 103:123, 1968.
28. Durham RJ: Postprimary intrathoracic tuberculosis in childhood with special reference to its sequelae. Texas J Med 52:583, 1956.
29. Stead WW, Kerby GR, Schlueter DP, et al: The clinical spectrum of primary tuberculosis in adults: Confusion with reinfection in the pathogenesis of chronic tuberculosis. Ann Intern Med 68:731, 1968.
30. Matthay RA, Neff TA, Iseman MD: Tuberculous pleural effusions developing during chemotherapy for pulmonary tuberculosis. Am Rev Respir Dis 109:469, 1974.
31. Stead WW, Eichenholz A, Stauss HK: Operative and pathologic findings in twenty-four patients with syndrome of idiopathic pleurisy with effusion, presumably tuberculous. Am Rev Respir Dis 71:473, 1955.
32. Light RW: Pleural Diseases. Philadelphia, Lea and Febiger, 1983.
33. Ellner JJ: Pleural fluid and peripheral blood lymphocyte function in tuberculosis. Ann Intern Med 89:932, 1978.
34. Shimokata K, Kawachi H, Kishimoto H, et al: Local cellular immunity in tuberculous pleurisy. Am Rev Respir Dis 126:822, 1982.

35. Fujiwara H, Tsuyuguchi I: Frequency of tuberculin-reactive T-lymphocytes in pleural fluid and blood from patients with tuberculous pleurisy. Chest 89:530, 1986.
36. Hulnick DH, Naidich DP, McCauley DI: Pleural tuberculosis evaluated by computed tomography. Radiology 149:759, 1983.
37. Levine H, Szanto PB, Cugell DW: Tuberculous pleurisy—An acute illness. Arch Intern Med 122:329, 1968.
38. Sibley JC: A study of 200 cases of tuberculous pleurisy with effusion. Am Rev Tuberc 62:314, 1950.
39. Spieler P: The cytologic diagnosis of tuberculosis in pleural effusions. Acta Cytol 23:374, 1979.
40. Pettersson T, Klockars M, Hellström PE, et al: T and B lymphocytes in pleural effusions. Chest 73:49, 1978.
41. Lucivero G, Pierucci G, Bonomo L: Lymphocyte subsets in peripheral blood and pleural fluid. Eur Respir J 1:337, 1988.
42. Okubo Y, Nakata M, Kuroiwa Y, et al: NK cells in carcinomatous and tuberculous pleurisy. Phenotypic and functional analyses of NK cells in peripheral blood and pleural effusion. Chest 92:500, 1987.
43. Hurwitz S, Leiman G, Shapiro C: Mesothelial cells in pleural fluid: TB or not TB? S Afr Med J 57:937, 1980.
44. Guzman J, Costabel U, Bross KJ, et al: Macrophage size determinations in the diagnosis of tuberculous effusions. Anal Quant Cytol Histol 10:371, 1988.
45. Dodson WH, Hollingsworth JW: Pleural effusion in rheumatoid arthritis. Impaired transport of glucose. N Engl J Med 275:1337, 1966.
46. Light RW, MacGregor MI, Ball WC Jr, et al: Diagnostic significance of pleural fluid pH and P_{CO_2}. Chest 64:591, 1973.
47. Brook I: Measurement of lactic acid in pleural fluid. Respiration 40:344, 1980.
48. Pettersson T, Ojala K, Weber TH: Diagnostic significance of pleural fluid lactate concentrations. Infection 13:257, 1985.
49. Jokipii AM, Kiviranta K, Jokipii L: Gas chromatographically quantitated lactate in empyema and other pleural effusions. Eur J Clin Microbiol 6:731, 1987.
50. Klockars M, Pettersson T, Riska H, et al: Pleural fluid lysozyme in tuberculous and non-tuberculous pleurisy. Br Med J 1:1381, 1976.
51. Piras MA, Gakis C, Budroni M, et al: Adenosine deaminase activity in pleural effusions: An aid to differential diagnosis. Br Med J 2:1751, 1978.
52. Pettersson T, Ojala K, Weber TH: Adenosine deaminase in the diagnosis of pleural effusions. Acta Med Scand 215:299, 1984.
53. Ocāna I, Ribera E, Martinez-Vázquez JM, et al: Adenosine deaminase activity in rheumatoid pleural effusion. Ann Rheum Dis 47:394, 1988.
54. Fontan Bueso J, Verea Hernando H, Garcia-Buela JP, et al: Diagnostic value of simultaneous determination of pleural adenosine deaminase and pleural lysozyme/serum lysozyme ratio in pleural effusions. Chest 93:303, 1988.
55. Mestitz P, Pollard AC: The diagnosis of tuberculosis pleural effusion. Br J Dis Chest 53:86, 1959.
56. Scerbo J, Keltz H, Stone DJ: A prospective study of closed pleural biopsies. JAMA 218:377, 1971.
57. Schub HM, Spivey CG Jr, Baird GD: Pleural involvement in histoplasmosis. Am Rev Respir Dis 94:225, 1966.
58. Levine H, Metzger W, Lacera D, et al: Diagnosis of tuberculous pleurisy by culture of pleural biopsy specimen. Arch Intern Med 126:269, 1970.
59. Mueller PR, Saini S, Simeone JF, et al: Image-guided pleural biopsies: Indications, technique, and results in 23 patients. Radiology 169:1, 1988.
60. Roper WH, Waring JJ: Primary serofibrinous pleural effusion in military personnel. Am Rev Respir Dis 71:616, 1955.
61. Pines A: The results of chemotherapy in the treatment of tuberculous pleural effusions. Br Med J 2:863, 1957.
62. Pfeutze K: Pulmonary disease caused by photochromogenic mycobacteria. General Practitioner 35:85, 1967.
63. Light RW: Management of parapneumonic effusions. Arch Intern Med 141:1339, 1981.
64. Light RW, Girard WM, Jenkinson SG, et al: Parapneumonic effusions. Am J Med 69:507, 1980.
65. Delikaris PG, Conlan AA, Abramor E, et al: Empyema thoracis: A prospective study on 73 patients. S Afr Med J 65:47, 1984.
66. Benfield GFA: Recent trends in empyema thoracis. Br J Dis Chest 75:358, 1981.

18

67. Davis WC, Johnson LF: Adult thoracic empyema revisited. Am Surg 44:362, 1978.
68. Mavroudis C, Symmonds JB, Minagi H, et al: Improved survival in management of empyema thoracis. J Thorac Cardiovasc Surg 82:49, 1981.
69. Wehr CJ, Adkins RB Jr: Empyema thoracis: A ten-year experience. South Med J 79:171, 1986.
70. Braman SS, Donat WE: Explosive pleuritis. Manifestations of group A beta-hemolytic streptococcal infection. Am J Med 81:723, 1986.
71. Bennett MR, Fiehler PC, Weinbaum DL: Occult pneumococcal bacteremia and empyema without preceding pulmonary parenchymal involvement. South Med J 80:774, 1987.
72. Streifler J, Pitlik S, Dux S, et al: Spontaneous bacterial pleuritis in a patient with cirrhosis. Respiration 46:382, 1984.
73. Potts DE, Levin DC, Sahn SA: Pleural fluid pH in parapneumonic effusions. Chest 70:328, 1976.
74. Light RW: Management of parapneumonic effusions. Chest 70:325, 1976.
75. Varkey B, Rose HD, Kutty CPK, et al: Empyema thoracis during a 10-year period: Analysis of 72 cases and comparison to a previous study (1952 to 1967). Arch Intern Med 141:1771, 1981.
76. Vianna NJ: Nontuberculous bacterial empyema in patients with and without underlying diseases. JAMA 215:69, 1971.
77. Jones FL Jr, Blodgett RC Jr: Empyema in rheumatic pleuropulmonary disease. Ann Intern Med 74:665, 1971.
78. Sahn SA, Lakshminarayan S, Char DC: "Silent" empyema in patients receiving corticosteroids. Am Rev Respir Dis 107:873, 1973.
79. Marks MI, Eickhoff TC: Empyema necessitatis. Am Rev Respir Dis 101:759, 1970.
80. Bartlett JG, Gorbach SL, Thadepalli H, et al: Bacteriology of empyema. Lancet 1:338, 1974.
81. Béchamps GF, Lynn HB, Wenzl JE: Empyema in children: Review of Mayo Clinic experience. Mayo Clin Proc 45:43, 1970.
82. Weese WC, Shindler ER, Smith IM, et al: Empyema of the thorax then and now. A study of 122 cases over four decades. Arch Intern Med 131:516, 1973.
83. McLaughlin FJ, Goldmann DA, Rosenbaum DM, et al: Empyema in children: Clinical course and long-term follow-up. Pediatrics 73:587, 1984.
84. Fajardo JE, Chang MJ: Pleural empyema in children: A nationwide retrospective study. South Med J 80:593, 1987.
85. Caplan ES, Hoyt NJ, Rodriguez A, et al: Empyema occurring in the multiple traumatized patient. J Trauma 24:785, 1984.
86. Chonmaitree T, Powell KR: Parapneumonic pleural effusion and empyema in children. Review of a 19-year experience, 1962–1980. Clin Pediatr 22:414, 1983.
87. Welch CC, Tombridge TL, Baker WJ, et al: Beta-hemolytic streptococcal pneumonia: Report of an outbreak in a military population. Am J Med Sci 242:157, 1961.
88. Brewin A, Arango L, Hadley WK, et al: High-dose penicillin therapy and pneumococcal pneumonia. JAMA 230:409, 1974.
89. Hendren WH III, Haggerty RJ: Staphylococcic pneumonia in infancy and childhood: Analysis of seventy-five cases. JAMA 168:6, 1958.
90. Dines DE: Diagnostic significance of pneumatocele of the lung. JAMA 204:1169, 1968.
91. Meyers HI, Jacobsen G: Staphylococcal pneumonia in children and adults. Radiology 72:665, 1959.
92. Schultze G: Unusual roentgen manifestations of primary staphylococcal pneumonia in infants and young children. Am J Roentgenol 81:290, 1959.
93. Huxtable KA, Tucker AS, Wedgwood RJ: Staphylococcal pneumonia in childhood. Long-term follow-up. Am J Dis Child 108:262, 1964.
94. Vinik M, Altman DH, Parks RE: Experience with Haemophilus influenzae pneumonia. Radiology 86:701, 1966.
95. Wallace RJ Jr, Musher DM, Martin RR: Haemophilus influenzae pneumonia in adults. Am J Med 64:87, 1978.
96. Berk SL, Holtsclaw SA, Wiener SL, et al: Nontypeable Haemophilus influenzae in the elderly. Arch Intern Med 134:537, 1982.
97. Stratton CW, Hawley HB, Horsman TA, et al: Haemophilus influenzae pneumonia in adults: Report of five cases caused by ampicillin-resistant strains. Am Rev Respir Dis 121:595, 1980.
98. Steinhauer BW, Eickhoff TC, Kislak JW, et al: The Klebsiella-Enterobacter-Serratia division: Clinical and epidemiologic characteristics. Ann Intern Med 65:1180, 1966.
99. Tillotson JR, Lerner AM: Pneumonias caused by gram-negative bacilli. Medicine 45:65, 1966.
100. Unger JD, Rose HD, Unger GF: Gram-negative pneumonia. Radiology 107:283, 1973.
101. Tillotson JR, Lerner AM: Characteristics of pneumonias caused by Escherichia coli. N Engl J Med 277:115, 1967.
102. Iannini PB, Claffey T, Quintiliani R: Bacteremic Pseudomonas pneumonia. JAMA 230:558, 1974.
103. Coonrod JD, Wilson HD: Etiologic diagnosis of intrapleural empyema by counterimmunoelectrophoresis. Am Rev Respir Dis 113:637, 1976.
104. Sullivan KM, O'Toole RD, Fisher RH, et al: Anaerobic empyema thoracis. Arch Intern Med 131:521, 1973.
105. Abramor EJ, Baptista L, McHendry JA, et al: The microflora of chronic pleural empyema. An analysis of 89 patients. S Afr Med J 68:80, 1985.
106. Miller RP, Bates JH: Pleuropulmonary tularemia. A review of 29 patients. Am Rev Respir Dis 99:31, 1969.
107. Overholt EL, Tigertt WD: Roentgenographic manifestations of pulmonary tularemia. Radiology 74:758, 1960.
108. Dennis JM, Boudreau RP: Pleuropulmonary tularemia: Its roentgen manifestations. Radiology 68:25, 1957.
109. Ivie JM: Roentgenological observations on pleuropulmonary tularemia. Am J Roentgenol 74:466, 1955.
110. Pine JR, Hollman JL: Elevated pleural fluid pH in Proteus mirabilis empyema. Chest 84:109, 1983.
111. George AL Jr, Savage AM: Fatal group B streptococcal empyema in an adult. South Med J 80:1436, 1987.
112. Swartz MN: Clinical aspects of Legionnaires' disease. Ann Intern Med 90:492, 1979.
113. Kirby BD, Snyder KM, Meyer RD, et al: Legionnaires' disease: Report of sixty-five nosocomially acquired cases and review of the literature. Medicine 59:188, 1980.
114. Kroboth FJ, Yu VL, Reddy SC, et al: Clinicoradiographic correlation with the extent of Legionnaires' disease. Am J Roentgenol 141:263, 1983.
115. Weiss W, Eisenberg GM, Flippin HF: Salmonella pleuropulmonary disease. Am J Med Sci 233:487, 1957.
116. Hahne OH: Lung abscess due to Salmonella typhi. Am Rev Respir Dis 89:566, 1964.
117. Garcia-Rodriguez JA, Garcia-Sanchez JE, Munoz Bellido JL, et al: Review of pulmonary brucellosis: A case report on brucellar pulmonary empyema. Diagn Microbiol Infect Dis 11:53, 1988.
118. Clarridge J, Roberts C, Peters J, et al: Sepsis and empyema caused by Yersinia enterocolitica. J Clin Microbiol 17:936, 1983.
119. Pollock JJ: Pleuropulmonary Whipple's disease. South Med J 78:216, 1985.
120. Jess P, Brynitz S, Friis Møller A: Mortality in thoracic empyema. Scand J Thorac Cardiovasc Surg 18:85, 1984.
121. Muskett A, Burton NA, Karwande SV, et al: Management of refractory empyema with early decortication. Am J Surg 156:529, 1988.
122. LeBlanc KA, Tucker WY: Empyema of the thorax. Surg Gynecol Obstet 158:66, 1984.
123. Mayo P: Early thoracotomy and decortication for nontuberculous empyema in adults with and without underlying disease. A twenty-five year review. Am Surg 51:230, 1985.
124. Himelman RB, Callen PW: The prognostic value of loculations in parapneumonic pleural effusions. Chest 90:852, 1986.
125. Lew PD, Perrin LH, Waldvogel FA, et al: Loculated pleural empyema: Identification of complement breakdown products in contiguous sterile pleural fluid. Scand J Infect Dis 14:225, 1982.
126. Shin MS, Ho KJ: Computed tomographic characteristics of pleural empyema. CT 7:179, 1983.
127. van Sonnenberg E, Nakamoto SK, Mueller PR, et al: CT- and ultrasound-guided catheter drainage of empyemas after chest-tube failure. Radiology 151:349, 1984.
128. Mace AH, Elyaderani MK: Ultrasonography in the diagnosis and management of empyema of the thorax. South Med J 77:294, 1984.
129. Hunnam GR, Flower CD: Radiologically guided percutaneous catheter drainage of empyemas. Clin Radiol 39:121, 1988.
130. Glasier CM, Leithiser RE Jr, Williamson SL, et al: Extracardiac chest ultrasonography in infants and children: Radiographic and clinical implications. J Pediatr 114:540, 1989.
131. Morin JE, Munro DD, MacLean LD: Early thoracotomy for empyema. J Thorac Cardiovasc Surg 44:530, 1972.
132. Hoover EL, Hsu HK, Ross MJ, et al: Reappraisal of empyema thoracis. Surgical intervention when the duration of illness is unknown. Chest 90:511, 1986.
133. Iioka S, Sawamura K, Mori T, et al: Surgical treatment of chronic empyema. A new one-stage operation. J Thorac Cardiovasc Surg 90:179, 1985.
134. Murray JF, Finegold SM, Froman S, et al: The changing spectrum of nocardiosis. A review and presentation of nine cases. Am Rev Respir Dis 83:315, 1961.
135. Flynn MW, Felson B: The roentgen manifestations of thoracic actinomycosis. Am J Roentgenol 110:707, 1970.
136. Greer AE: Disseminating Fungus Diseases of the Lung. Springfield, Ill, Charles C Thomas, 1962.
137. Conant NF, Martin DS, Smith DT, et al: Manual of Clinical Mycology. (Prepared under the auspices of the Division of Medical Sciences of the National Research Council.) 3rd ed. Philadelphia, WB Saunders, 1971.

138. Harvey JC, Cantrell JR, Fisher AM: Actinomycosis: Its recognition and treatment. Ann Intern Med 46:868, 1957.

139. Neu HC, Silva M, Hazen E, et al: Necrotizing nocardial pneumonitis. Ann Intern Med 66:274, 1967.

140. Curry FJ, Wier JA: Histoplasmosis: A review of one hundred consecutively hospitalized patients. Am Rev Tuberc 77:749, 1958.

141. Matthay MA, Addison TE, Ellinger G, et al: Chest mass with pleurisy. Chest 76:453, 1979.

142. Swinburne AJ, Fedullo AJ, Wahl GW, et al: Histoplasmoma, pleural fibrosis, and slowly enlarging pleural effusion in an asymptomatic patient. Am Rev Respir Dis 135:502, 1987.

143. Lonky SA, Catanzaro A, Moser KM, et al: Acute coccidioidal pleural effusion. Am Rev Respir Dis 114:681, 1976.

144. Arora NS, Oblinger MJ, Feldman PS: Chronic pleural blastomycosis with hyperprolactinemia, galactorrhea, and amenorrhea. Am Rev Respir Dis 120:451, 1979.

145. Young EJ, Hirsh DD, Fainstein V, et al: Pleural effusions due to Cryptococcus neoformans: A review of the literature and report of two cases with cryptococcal antigen determinations. Am Rev Respir Dis 121:743, 1980.

146. Case records of the Massachusetts General Hospital. Weekly clinicopathological exercises. Case 38–1983. Empyema 40 years after a thoracoplasty. N Engl J Med 309:715, 1983.

147. Monod O, Dieudonné P, Tardieu P: Les aspergilloses pulmonaires post-opératoires. (Postoperative pulmonary aspergillosis.) J Fr Med Chir Thorac 18:579, 1964.

148. Meredith HC, Corgan BM, McLaulin B: Pleural aspergillosis. Am J Roentgenol 130:164, 1978.

149. Sawasaki H, Horie K, Yamada M, et al: Bronchial stump aspergillosis. Experimental and clinical study. J Thorac Cardiovasc Surg 58:198, 1969.

150. Parry MF, Coughlin FR, Zambetti FX: Aspergillus empyema. Chest 81:768, 1982.

151. George RB, Ziskind M, Rasch JR, et al: Mycoplasma and adenovirus pneumonias. Comparison with other atypical pneumonias in a military population. Ann Intern Med 65:931, 1966.

152. Rytel MW: Primary atypical pneumonia: Current concepts. Am J Med Sci 247:84, 1964.

153. Rosmus HH, Paré JAP, Masson AM, et al: Roentgenographic patterns of acute Mycoplasma and viral pneumonitis. J Can Assoc Radiol 19:74, 1968.

154. Fine NL, Smith LR, Sheedy PF: Frequency of pleural effusions in Mycoplasma and viral pneumonias. N Engl J Med 283:790, 1970.

155. Lambert HP: Mycoplasma pneumoniae infections. J Clin Pathol 21(Suppl 2):52, 1968.

156. Putnam CE, Curtis AM, Simeone JF, et al: Mycoplasma pneumonia. Clinical and roentgenographic patterns. Am J Roentgenol 124:417, 1975.

157. Shulman ST, Bartlett J, Clyde WA Jr, et al: The unusual severity of mycoplasmal pneumonia in children with sickle-cell disease. N Engl J Med 287:164, 1972.

158. Grix A, Giammona ST: Pneumonitis with pleural effusion in children due to Mycoplasma pneumoniae. Am Rev Respir Dis 109:665, 1974.

159. Gokeirt JG, Beamish WE: Altered reactivity to measles virus in previously vaccinated children. Can Med Assoc J 103:724, 1970.

160. Editorial. Pneumonia in atypical measles. Br Med J 2:235, 1971.

161. McLean DM, Kettyls GDM, Hingston J, et al: Atypical measles following immunization with killed measles vaccine. Can Med Assoc J 103:743, 1970.

162. Young LW, Smith DI, Glasgow LA: Pneumonia of atypical measles: Residual nodular lesions. Am J Roentgenol 110:439, 1970.

163. Proby CM, Hackett D, Gupta S, et al: Acute myopericarditis in influenza A infection. Q J Med 60:887, 1986.

164. Lander P, Palayew MJ: Infectious mononucleosis—a review of chest roentgenographic manifestations. J Can Assoc Radiol 25:303, 1974.

165. McCormick JB, King IJ, Webb PA, et al: A case-control study of the clinical diagnosis and course of Lassa fever. J Infect Dis 155:445, 1987.

166. Johnson JE III, Perry JE, Fekety FR, et al: Laboratory-acquired Q fever: A report of 50 cases. Am J Med 41:391, 1966.

167. Ramos HS, Hodges RE, Meroney WH: Q fever: Report of a case simulating lymphoma. Ann Intern Med 47:1030, 1957.

168. Murphy PP, Richardson SG: Q fever pneumonia presenting as an eosinophilic pleural effusion. Thorax 44:228, 1989.

169. Delahaye RP, Pannier R, Laaban J, et al: Les aspects radiologiques des localisations thoraciques de l'amibase: 17 observations metropolitaines. (Radiologic aspects of thoracic amebiasis: 17 metropolitan observations.) J Radiol Electrol Med Nucl 48:173, 1967.

170. Webster BH: Pleuropulmonary amebiasis. A review with an analysis of ten cases. Am Rev Respir Dis 81:683, 1960.

171. Daniels AC, Childress ME: Pleuropulmonary amebiasis. Calif Med 85:369, 1956.

172. Ochsner A, DeBakey M: Pleuropulmonary complications of ame-

173. Ibarra-Perez C, Selman-Lama M: Diagnosis and treatment of amebic "empyema." Report of eighty-eight cases. Am J Surg 134:283, 1977.

174. Herrera-Llerandi R: Thoracic repercussions of amebiasis. J Thorac Cardiovasc Surg 52:361, 1966.

175. Ogakwu M, Nwokolo C: Radiological findings in pulmonary paragonimiasis as seen in Nigeria. A review based on one hundred cases. Br J Radiol 46:699, 1973.

176. Rakower J, Miwidsky H: Hyatid pleural disease. Am Rev Respir Dis 90:623, 1964.

177. Miller MJ, Leith DE, Brooks JR, et al: Trichomonas empyema. Thorax 37:384, 1982.

178. Pancholia AK, Jain SM: Pleural effusion due to dracunculosis. Indian J Chest Dis Allied Sci 27:122, 1985.

179. Capitanio MA, Kirkpatrick JA Jr: Pneumocystis carinii pneumonia. Am J Roentgenol 97:174, 1966.

180. Schultz JC, Ross SW, Abernathy RS: Diagnosis of Pneumocystis carinii pneumonia in an adult with survival. Am Rev Respir Dis 93:943, 1966.

181. Feinberg SB, Lester RG, Burke B: The roentgen findings in Pneumocystis carinii pneumonia. Radiology 76:954, 1961.

182. Forrest JV: Radiographic findings in Pneumocystis carinii pneumonia. Radiology 103:539, 1972.

183. Maguire R, Fauci AS, Doppman JL, et al: Unusual radiographic features of Wegener's granulomatosis. Am J Roentgenol 130:233, 1978.

184. Gonzalez L, Van Ordstrand HS: Wegener's granulomatosis: Review of 11 cases. Radiology 107:295, 1973.

185. Bahk YW: Pulmonary paragonimiasis as a cause of Löffler's syndrome. Radiology 78:598, 1962.

186. Robinson BR: Pleuropulmonary reaction to nitrofurantoin. JAMA 189:239, 1964.

187. Knobler H, Admon D, Leibovici V, et al: Urticarial vasculitis and recurrent pleural effusion: A systemic manifestation of urticarial vasculitis. Dermatologica 172:120, 1986.

188. Bulgrin JG, Dubois EL, Jacobson G: Chest roentgenographic changes in systemic lupus erythematosus. Radiology 74:42, 1960.

189. Gould DM, Daves ML: A review of roentgen findings in systemic lupus erythematosus. (SLE). Am J Med Sci 235:596, 1958.

190. Taylor TL, Ostrum H: The roentgen evaluation of systemic lupus erythematosus. Am J Roentgenol 82:95, 1959.

191. Winslow WA, Ploss LN, Loitman B: Pleuritis in systemic lupus erythematosus: Its importance as an early manifestation in diagnosis. Ann Intern Med 49:70, 1958.

192. Levin DC: Proper interpretation of pulmonary roentgen changes in systemic lupus erythematosus. Am J Roentgenol 111:510, 1971.

193. Andrews BS, Arora NS, Shadforth MF, et al: The role of immune complexes in the pathogenesis of pleural effusions. Am Rev Respir Dis 124:115, 1981.

194. Albini B, Ossi E, Andres G: The pathogenesis of pericardial, pleural, and peritoneal effusions in rabbits with serum sickness. Lab Invest 37:64, 1977.

195. Black LF: The pleural space and pleural fluid. Mayo Clin Proc 47:493, 1972.

196. Carr DT, Lillington GA, Mayne JG: Pleural fluid glucose in systemic lupus erythematosus. Mayo Clin Proc 45:409, 1970.

197. Halla JT, Schronhenloher RE, Volanakis JE: Immune complexes and other laboratory features of pleural effusions. Ann Intern Med 92:748, 1980.

198. Good JT Jr, King TE, Antony VB, et al: Lupus pleuritis: Clinical features and pleural fluid antinuclear antibodies. Chest 84:714, 1983.

199. Osamura RY, Shioya S, Handa K, et al: Lupus erythematosus cells in pleural fluid: Cytologic diagnosis in two patients. Acta Cytol 21:216, 1977.

200. Rubin EH: Pulmonary lesions in "rheumatoid disease" with remarks on diffuse interstitial pulmonary fibrosis. Am J Med 19:569, 1955.

201. Sievers K, Aho K, Hurri L, et al: Studies of rheumatoid pulmonary disease. A comparison of roentgenological findings among patients with high rheumatoid factor titers and with completely negative reactions. Acta Tuberc Scand 45:21, 1964.

202. Walker WC, Wright V: Rheumatoid pleuritis. Ann Rheum Dis 26:467, 1967.

203. Carr DT, Mayne JG: Pleurisy with effusion in rheumatoid arthritis, with reference to the low concentration of glucose in pleural fluid. Am Rev Respir Dis 85:345, 1962.

204. Locke CB: Rheumatoid lung. Clin Radiol 14:43, 1963.

205. Lee PR, Sox HC, North FS, et al: Pleurisy with effusion in rheumatoid arthritis. Arch Intern Med 104:634, 1959.

206. Engel U, Aru A, Francis D: Rheumatoid pleurisy. Specificity of cytological findings. Acta Pathol Microbiol Immunol Scand (A)94:53, 1986.

207. Campbell GD, Ferrington E: Rheumatoid pleuritis with effusion. Dis Chest 53:521, 1968.

18

208. Nosanchuk JS, Naylor B: A unique cytologic picture in pleural fluid from patients with rheumatoid arthritis. Am J Clin Pathol 50:330, 1968.
209. Engel U, Aru A, Francis D: Rheumatoid pleurisy. Acta Pathol Microbiol Immunol Scand 94:53, 1986.
210. Shinto R, Prete P: Characteristic cytology in rheumatoid pleural effusion. Am J Med 85:587, 1988.
211. Berger HW, Seckler SG: Pleural and pericardial effusions in rheumatoid disease. Ann Intern Med 64:1291, 1966.
212. Mays EE: Rheumatoid pleuritis: Observations in eight cases and suggestions for making the diagnosis in patients without the "typical findings." Dis Chest 53:202, 1968.
213. Faurschou P, Faarup P: Granulocytes containing cytoplasmic inclusions in human tuberculous pleuritis. Scand J Respir Dis 54:341, 1973.
214. Faarup P, Faurschou P: Rheumatoid arthritis cells in experimental pleuritis in mice. Acta Pathol Microbiol Immunol Scand 93:209, 1985.
215. Lillington GA, Carr DT, Mayne JG: Rheumatoid pleurisy with effusion. Arch Intern Med 128:764, 1971.
216. Grossman LA, Kaplan HJ, Ownby FD, et al: Acute pericarditis: With subsequent clinical rheumatoid arthritis. Arch Intern Med 109:665, 1962.
217. Stengel BF, Watson RA, Darling RJ: Pulmonary rheumatoid nodule with cavitation and chronic lipid effusion. JAMA 198:1263, 1966.
218. Berger HW, Seckler SG: Pleural and pericardial effusions in rheumatoid disease. Ann Intern Med 64:1291, 1966.
219. Leading article. Pleurisy and rheumatoid arthritis. Br Med J 2:1, 1968.
220. Levine H, Szanto M, Grieble HG, et al: Rheumatoid factor in nonrheumatoid pleural effusion. Ann Intern Med 69:487, 1968.
221. Leading article. Laboratory features of pleural effusions. Br Med J 281:763, 1980.
222. Pettersson T, Klockars M, Hellström P-E: Chemical and immunological features of pleural effusion: Comparison between rheumatoid arthritis and other diseases. Thorax 37:354, 1982.
223. Halla JT, Schrohenloher RE, Volanakis JE: Immune complexers and other laboratory features of pleural effusions: A comparison of rheumatoid arthritis, systemic lupus erythematosus, and other diseases. Ann Intern Med 92:748, 1980.
224. Mays EE: Rheumatoid pleuritis: Observations in eight cases and suggestions for making the diagnosis in patients without the "typical findings." Dis Chest 53:202, 1968.
225. Martel W, Abell MR, Mikkelsen WM, et al: Pulmonary and pleural lesions in rheumatoid disease. Radiology 90:641, 1968.
226. Sheridan AQ, Berger HW: Nonrheumatoid pleural effusions in patients with rheumatoid arthritis. Mt Sinai J Med 45:271, 1978.
227. Hillerdal G: Nonmalignant pleural disease related to asbestos exposure. Clin Chest Med 6:141, 1985.
228. Luther R, Wetzer K, Kuhne W, et al: Asbestos-induced pleural disease—Thoracoscopic aspects. Endoscopy 20:104, 1988.
229. Smith WHR, Davies D: Nonmalignant pleural disease and asbestos. Br J Dis Chest 74:180, 1980.
230. Robinson BWS, Musk AW: Benign asbestos pleural effusion: Diagnosis and course. Thorax 36:896, 1981.
231. Epler GR, McCloud TC, Gaensler EA: Prevalence and incidence of benign asbestos pleural effusion in a working population. JAMA 247:617, 1982.
232. Gaensler EA, Kaplan AI: Asbestos pleural effusion. Ann Intern Med 74:178, 1971.
233. Sluis-Cremer GK, Webster I: Acute pleurisy in asbestosis exposed persons. Environ Res 5:380, 1972.
234. Martensson G, Hagberg S, Pettersson K, et al: Asbestos pleural effusion: A clinical entity. Thorax 42:646, 1987.
235. Editorial. Mysterious pleural effusion. Lancet 1:1226, 1982.
236. Gaensler EA, Kaplan AI: Asbestos pleural effusion. Ann Intern Med 74:178, 1971.
237. Eisenstadt HB: Benign asbestos pleurisy. JAMA 192:419, 1965.
238. Jurivich DA: Iatrogenic pleural effusions. South Med J 81:1417, 1988.
239. Rinne UK: Pleuropulmonary changes during long-term bromocriptine treatment for Parkinson's disease. Lancet 1:44, 1981.
240. McElvaney NG, Wilcox PG, Churg A, et al: Pleuropulmonary disease during bromocriptine treatment of Parkinson's disease. Arch Intern Med 148:2231, 1988.
241. Kinnunen E, Viljanen A: Pleuropulmonary involvement during bromocriptine treatment. Chest 94:1034, 1988.
242. Gefter WB, Epstein DM, Bonavita JA, et al: Pleural thickening caused by Sansert and Ergotrate in the treatment of migraine. Am J Roentgenol 135:375, 1980.
243. Petusevsky ML, Faling LJ, Rocklin RE, et al: Pleuropericardial reaction to treatment with dantrolene. JAMA 242:2772, 1979.
244. Chernow B, Sahn SA: Carcinomatous involvement of the pleura: An analysis of 96 patients. Am J Med 63:695, 1977.
245. Hsu C: Cytologic detection of malignancy in pleural effusion: A review of 5,255 samples from 3,811 patients. Diagn Cytopathol 3:8, 1987.
246. Johnston WW: The malignant pleural effusion. A review of cytopathologic diagnoses of 584 specimens from 472 consecutive patients. Cancer 56:905, 1985.
247. Editorial. Treatment of malignant effusions. Lancet 1:198, 1981.
248. Meyer PC: Metastatic carcinoma of the pleura. Thorax 21:437, 1966.
249. Stewart PB: The rate of formation and lymphatic removal of fluid in pleural effusions. J Clin Invest 42:258, 1963.
250. Chang SC, Perng RP: The role of fiberoptic bronchoscopy in evaluating the causes of pleural effusions. Arch Intern Med 149:855, 1989.
251. Salyer WR, Eggleston JC, Erozan YS: Efficacy of pleural needle biopsy and pleural fluid cytopathology in the diagnosis of malignant neoplasm involving the pleura. Chest 67:536, 1975.
252. Irani DR, Underwood RD, Johnson EH, et al: Malignant pleural effusions. A clinical cytopathologic study. Arch Intern Med 147:1133, 1987.
253. Berger HW, Maher G: Decreased glucose concentration in malignant pleural effusions. Am Rev Respir Dis 103:427, 1971.
254. Sahn SA, Good JT Jr: Pleural fluid pH in malignant effusions. Diagnostic, prognostic, and therapeutic implications. Ann Intern Med 108:345, 1988.
255. McKenna JM, Chandrasekhar AJ, Henkin RE: Diagnostic value of carcinoembryonic antigen in exudative pleural effusions. Chest 78:587, 1980.
256. Vladutiu AO, Brason FW, Adler RH: Differential diagnosis of pleural effusions: Clinical usefulness of cell marker quantitation. Chest 79:297, 1981.
257. Wardman AG, Bowen M, Struthers LP, et al: The diagnosis of pleural effusions—Are cancer markers clinically helpful? Med Pediatr Oncol 12:68, 1984.
258. Siri A, Carnemolla B, Raffanti S, et al: Fibronectin concentrations in pleural effusions of patients with malignant and nonmalignant diseases. Cancer Lett 22:1, 1984.
259. Niwa Y, Kishimoto H, Shimokata K: Carcinomatous and tuberculous pleural effusions. Comparison of tumor markers. Chest 87:351, 1985.
260. Faravelli B, Nosenzo M, Razzetti A, et al: The role of concurrent determinations of pleural fluid and tissue carcinoembryonic antigen in the distinction of malignant mesothelioma from metastatic pleural malignancies. Eur J Cancer Clin Oncol 21:1083, 1985.
261. Tamura S, Nishigaki T, Moriwaki Y, et al: Tumor markers in pleural effusion diagnosis. Cancer 61:298, 1988.
262. Shimokata K, Totani Y, Nakanishi K, et al: Diagnostic value of cancer antigen 15–3 (CA15–3) detected by monoclonal antibodies (115D8 and DF3) in exudative pleural effusions. Eur Respir J 1:341, 1988.
263. Pettersson T, Klockars M, Fröseth B: Neuron-specific enolase in the diagnosis of small-cell lung cancer with pleural effusion: A negative report. Eur Respir J 1:698, 1988.
264. Yinnon A, Konijn AM, Link G, et al: Diagnostic value of ferritin in malignant pleural and peritoneal effusions. Cancer 62:2564, 1988.
265. Delpuech P, Desch G, Fructus F: Fibronectin is unsuitable as a tumor marker in pleural effusions. Clin Chem 35:166, 1989.
266. Iguchi H, Hara N, Miyazaki K, et al: Elevation of sialyl stage-specific mouse embryonic antigen levels in pleural effusion in patients with adenocarcinoma of the lung. Cancer 63:1327, 1989.
267. Boutin C, Viallat JR, Cargnino P, et al: Thoracoscopy in malignant pleural effusions. Am Rev Respir Dis 124:588, 1981.
268. Williams T, Thomas P: The diagnosis of pleural effusions by fiberoptic bronchoscopy and pleuroscopy. Chest 80:566, 1981.
269. Loddenkemper R: Thoracoscopy: Results in noncancerous and idiopathic pleural effusions. Poumon-Coeur 37:261, 1981.
270. Rusch VM, Mountain C: Thoracoscopy under regional anesthesia for the diagnosis and management of pleural disease. Am J Surg 154:274, 1987.
271. Kaiser LR: Diagnostic and therapeutic uses of pleuroscopy (thoracoscopy) in lung cancer. Surg Clin North Am 67:1081, 1987.
272. Falor WH, Ward RM, Brezler MR: Diagnosis of pleural effusions by chromosome analysis. Chest 81:193, 1982.
273. Falor WH, Ward RM, Brezler MR: Diagnosis of pleural effusions by chromosome analysis. Chest 81:193, 1982.
274. Høstmark J, Vigander T, Skaarland: Characterization of pleural effusions by flow-cytometric DNA analysis. Eur J Respir Dis 66:315, 1985.
275. Legrand M, Pariente R: Electron microscopy in the cytological examination of metastatic pleural effusions. Thorax 31:443, 1976.
276. Emerson GL, Emerson MS, Sherwood CE: The natural history of carcinoma of the lung. J Thorac Cardiovasc Surg 37:291, 1959.
277. Cohen S, Hossain MS-A: Primary carcinoma of the lung. A review of 417 histologically proved cases. Dis Chest 49:67, 1966.
278. Maier HC: Surgical treatment (of pulmonary carcinoma). In Mayer

E, Maier HC (eds): Pulmonary Carcinoma. Pathogenesis, Diagnosis, and Treatment. New York, New York University Press, 1956, p. 298.

279. Rosenblatt MB, Lisa JR: Cancer of the Lung. Pathology, Diagnosis and Treatment. New York, Oxford University Press, 1956.

280. Brinkman GL: The significance of pleural effusion complicating otherwise operable bronchogenic carcinoma. Dis Chest 36:152, 1959.

281. Spriggs AI, Boddington MM: Oat cell bronchial carcinoma. Identification of cells in pleural fluid. Acta Cytol 20:525, 1976.

282. Salhadin A, Nasiell M, Nasiell K, et al: The unique cytologic picture of oat cell carcinoma in effusions. Acta Cytol 20:298, 1976.

283. Banner BF, Warren WH, Gould VE: Cytomorphology and marker expression of malignant neuroendocrine cells in pleural effusions. Acta Cytol 30:99, 1986.

284. Stolberg HO, Patt NL, MacEwen KF, et al: Hodgkin's disease of the lung: Roentgenologic-pathologic correlation. Am J Roentgenol 92:96, 1964.

285. Fisher AMH, Kendall B, Van Leuven BD: Hodgkin's disease. A radiological survey. Clin Radiol 13:115, 1962.

286. Martin JJ: The Nisbet Symposium: Hodgkin's disease. Radiological aspects of the disease. Australas Radiol 11:206, 1967.

287. Vieta JD, Craver LF: Intrathoracic manifestations of the lymphomatoid diseases. Radiology 37:138, 1941.

288. Molander DW, Pack GT: Treatment of lymphosarcoma. In Pack GT, Ariel IM (eds): Treatment of Cancer and Allied Diseases, 2nd ed. Vol 9. Lymphomas and Related Diseases. New York, Harper & Row, 1964, pp. 131–167.

289. Sider L, Horton ES: Pleural effusion as a presentation of AIDS-related lymphoma. Invest Radiol 24:150, 1989.

290. Bruneau R, Rubin P: The management of pleural effusions and chylothorax in lymphoma. Radiology 85:1085, 1965.

291. Wong F, Grace WJ, Rottino A: Pleural effusions, ascites, pericardial effusions and edema in Hodgkin's disease. Am J Med Sci 246:678, 1963.

292. Spriggs AI, Vanhegan RI: Cytological diagnosis of lymphoma in serous effusions. J Clin Pathol 34:1311, 1981.

293. Yam LT: Granulocytic sarcoma with pleural involvement. Identification of neoplastic cells with cytochemistry. Acta Cytol 29:63, 1985.

294. Spieler P, Kradolfer D, Schmid U: Immunocytochemical characterization of lymphocytes in benign and malignant lymphocyte-rich serous effusions. Virchows Arch (Pathol Anat) 409:211, 1986.

295. Hartweg H: Das röntgenbild des thorax bei den chronischen leukosen. (The roentgenogram of the thorax in chronic leukoses.) Fortschr Roentgenstr 92:477, 1960.

296. Green RA, Nichols NJ: Pulmonary involvement in leukemia. Am Rev Respir Dis 80:833, 1959.

297. Siegel MJ, Shackelford GD, McAlister WH: Pleural thickening: An unusual feature of childhood leukemia. Radiology 138:367, 1981.

298. Janckila AJ, Yam LT, Li C-Y: Immunocytochemical diagnosis of acute leukemia with pleural involvement. Acta Cytol 29:67, 1985.

299. Krause JR, Dekker A: Hairy cell leukemia (leukemic reticuloendotheliosis) in serous effusions. Acta Cytol 22:80, 1978.

300. Kapadia SB: Cytological diagnosis of malignant pleural effusion in myeloma. Arch Pathol Lab Med 101:534, 1977.

301. Shoenfeld Y, Pick AI, Weinberger A, et al: Pleural effusion—Presenting sign in multiple myeloma. Respiration 36:160, 1978.

302. Hughes JC, Votaw ML: Pleural effusion in multiple myeloma. Cancer 44:1150, 1979.

303. Kamal MK, Williams E, Poskitt TR: IgD myeloma with malignant pleural effusion. South Med J 80:657, 1987.

304. Favis E, Kerman H, Shildecker W: Multiple myeloma manifested as a problem in the diagnosis of pulmonary disease. Am J Med 28:323, 1960.

305. Winterbauer RH, Riggins RCK, Griesman FA, et al: Pleuropulmonary manifestations of Waldenström's macroglobulinemia. Chest 66:368, 1974.

306. Teo SK, Lee SK: Recurrent pleural effusion in Waldenström's macroglobulinemia. Br Med J 2:607, 1978.

307. Simos A, Asseo P, Hadjidimitriou G, et al: Waldenström's macroglobulinemia presented as pleurisy of unknown origin. A case report. Acta Haematol 59:246, 1978.

308. Kumar PV, Esfahani FN, Tabei SZ, et al: Cytopathology of alpha chain disease involving the central nervous system and pleura. Acta Cytol 32:902, 1988.

309. Fentiman IS, Millis R, Sexton S, et al: Pleural effusion in breast cancer: A review of 105 cases. Cancer 47:2087, 1981.

310. Raju RN, Kardinal CG: Pleural effusion in breast carcinoma: Analysis of 122 cases. Cancer 48:2524, 1981.

311. Thomas JM, Redding WH, Sloane JP: The spread of breast cancer: Importance of the intrathoracic lymphatic route and its relevance to treatment. Br J Cancer 40:540, 1979.

312. DeVita VT, Trujillo NP, Blackman AH, et al: Pulmonary manifestations of primary hepatic carcinoma. Am J Med Sci 250:428, 1965.

313. Ward P: Pulmonary and oesophageal presentations of pancreatic carcinoma. Br J Radiol 37:27, 1964.

314. Poe RH, Qazi R, Israel RH, et al: Survival of patient with pleural involvement by breast carcinoma. Am J Clin Oncol 6:523, 1983.

315. Goldsmith HS, Bailey HD, Callahan EL, et al: Pulmonary lymphangitic metastases from breast carcinoma. Arch Surg 94:483, 1967.

316. Danner DE, Gmelich JT: A comparative study of tumor cells from metastatic carcinoma of the breast in effusions. Acta Cytol 19:509, 1975.

317. Ashton PR, Hollingsworth AS Jr, Johnston WW: The cytopathology of metastatic breast cancer. Acta Cytol 19:1, 1975.

318. Williams JR, Wilcox WC: Pulmonary embolism: Roentgenographic and angiographic considerations. Am J Roentgenol 89:333, 1963.

319. Wiener SN, Edelstein J, Charms BL: Observations on pulmonary embolism and the pulmonary angiogram. Am J Roentgenol 98:859, 1966.

320. Stein GN, Chen JT, Goldstein F, et al: The importance of chest roentgenography in the diagnosis of pulmonary embolism. Am J Roentgenol 81:255, 1959.

321. Kaye J, Cohen G, Sandler A, et al: Massive pulmonary embolism without infarction. Br J Radiol 31:326, 1958.

322. Bynum LJ, Wilson JE III: Radiographic features of pleural effusions in pulmonary embolism. Am Rev Respir Dis 117:829, 1978.

323. Fleischner FG: Pulmonary embolism. Can Med Assoc J 78:653, 1958.

324. Torrance DJ Jr: Roentgenographic signs of pulmonary artery occlusion. Am J Med Sci 237:651, 1959.

325. Fleischner FG: Roentgenology of the pulmonary infarct. Semin Roentgenol 2:61, 1967.

326. Fleischner FG: Pulmonary embolism. Clin Radiol 13:169, 1962.

327. Figley MM, Gerdes AJ, Ricketts HJ: Radiographic aspects of pulmonary embolism. Semin Roentgenol 2:389, 1967.

328. Cornell SH, Rossi NP: Roentgenographic findings in constrictive pericarditis. Analysis of 21 cases. Am J Roentgenol 102:301, 1968.

329. Plum GE, Bruwer AJ, Clagett OT: Chronic constrictive pericarditis: Roentgenologic findings in 35 surgically proved cases. Mayo Clin Proc 32:555, 1957.

330. Tomaselli G, Gamsu G, Stulbarg MS: Constrictive pericarditis presenting as pleural effusion of unknown origin. Arch Intern Med 149:201, 1989.

331. Logue RB, Rogers JV Jr, Gay BB Jr: Subtle roentgenographic signs of left heart failure. Am Heart J 65:464, 1963.

332. Mellins RB, Levine OR, Fishman AP: Effect of systemic and pulmonary venous hypertension on pleural and pericardial fluid accumulation. J Appl Physiol 29:142, 1970.

333. Race GA, Scheifley CH, Edwards JE: Hydrothorax in congestive heart failure. Am J Med 22:83, 1957.

334. Pillay VKG: Total proteins in serous fluids in cardiac failure. S Afr Med J 39:142, 1965.

335. Chakko SC, Caldwell SH, Sforza PP: Treatment of congestive heart failure. Its effect on pleural fluid chemistry. Chest 95:798, 1989.

336. Sanghvi LM, Misra SN: Loculated pleural effusion in congestive heart failure due to severe anemia: Report of a case. Am Heart J 55:421, 1958.

337. Millard CE: Vanishing or phantom tumor of the lung: Localized interlobar effusion in congestive heart failure. Chest 59:675, 1971.

338. Mearns M, Longbottom J, Batten J: Precipitating antibodies to Aspergillus fumigatus in cystic fibrosis. Lancet 1:538, 1967.

339. Williams JR, Bonte FJ: The Roentgenologic Aspect of Nonpenetrating Chest Injuries. Springfield, Ill, Charles C Thomas, 1961.

340. Reynolds J, Davis JT: Injuries of the chest wall, pleura, pericardium, lungs, bronchi and esophagus. Radiol Clin North Am 4:383, 1966.

341. Wilson JM, Boren CH Jr, Peterson SR, et al: Traumatic hemothorax: Is decortication necessary? J Thorac Cardiovasc Surg 77:489, 1979.

342. Coselli JS, Mattox KL, Beall AC Jr: Reevaluation of early evacuation of clotted hemothorax. Am J Surg 148:786, 1984.

343. Weil PH, Margolis IB: Systematic approach to traumatic hemothorax. Am J Surg 142:692, 1981.

344. Godley PJ, Bell RC: Major hemorrhage following administration of intrapleural streptokinase. Chest 86:486, 1984.

345. Villalba M, Lucas CE, Ledgerwood AM, et al: The etiology of post-traumatic empyema and the role of decortication. J Trauma 19:414, 1979.

346. Leading article. Traumatic perforation of oesophagus. Br Med J 1:524, 1972.

347. Scholl DG, Tsai SH: Esophageal perforation following the use of the esophageal obturator airway. Radiology 122:315, 1977.

348. Abbott OA, Mansour KA, Logan WD Jr, et al: Atraumatic so-called "spontaneous" rupture of the esophagus. A review of 47 personal cases with comments on a new method of surgical therapy. J Thorac Cardiovasc Surg 59:67, 1970.

349. Faling LJ, Pugatch RD, Robbins AH: Case report: The diagnosis of unsuspected esophageal perforation by computed tomography. Am J Med Sci 281:31, 1981.

18

350. Rudin JS, Ellrodt AG, Phillips EH: Low pleural fluid amylase associated with spontaneous rupture of the esophagus. Arch Intern Med 143:1034, 1983.

351. Bacon BR, Bailey-Newton RS, Connors AF Jr: Pleural effusions after endoscopic variceal sclerotherapy. Gastroenterology 88:1910, 1985.

352. Tazelaar HD, Yousem SA: The pathology of combined heart-lung transplantation: An autopsy study. Hum Pathol 19:1403, 1988.

353. de la Rocha AG: Empyema thoracis. Surg Gynecol Obstet 155:839, 1982.

354. Kerr WF: Late-onset post-pneumonectomy empyema. Thorax 32:149, 1977.

355. Ruckdeschel JC, Codish JD, Stranahan A, et al: Postoperative empyema improves survival in lung cancer. Documentation and analysis of a natural experiment. N Engl J Med 287:1013, 1972.

356. Sensenig DM, Rossi NP, Ehrenhaft JL: Results of the surgical treatment of bronchogenic carcinoma. Surg Gynecol Obstet 116:279, 1963.

357. Takita H: Effect of postoperative empyema on survival of patients with bronchogenic carcinoma. J Thorac Cardiovasc Surg 59:642, 1970.

358. Le Roux BT: Empyema thoracis. Br J Surg 52:89, 1965.

359. Editorial. Empyema in lung cancer. JAMA 224:1644, 1973.

360. Leading article. Postoperative empyema and survival in lung cancer. Br Med J 1:504, 1973.

361. Goldstraw P: Postpneumonectomy empyema: The cloud with a silver lining? J Thorac Cardiovasc Surg 79:851, 1980.

362. Minasian H, Lewis CT, Evans SJW: Influence of postoperative empyema on survival after pulmonary resection for bronchogenic carcinoma. Br Med J 2:1329, 1978.

363. Peterson A, Kirsh M, Sloan H: Bronchogenic carcinoma and postoperative empyema: Is survival really enhanced? Ann Thorac Surg 31:240, 1981.

364. Pastorino U, Valente M, Piva L, et al: Empyema following lung cancer resection: Risk factors and prognostic value on survival. Ann Thorac Surg 33:320, 1982.

365. Hart U, Ward DR, Gillilian R, et al: Fatal pulmonary hemorrhage complicating Swan-Ganz catheterization. Surgery 91:24, 1982.

366. Carbone K, Gimenez LF, Rogers WH, et al: Hemothorax due to vena caval erosion by a subclavian dual-lumen dialysis catheter. South Med J 80:795, 1987.

367. Rudge CJ, Bewick M, McColl I: Hydrothorax after central venous catheterization. Br Med J 3:23, 1973.

368. Paskin DL, Hoffman WS, Tuddenham WJ: A new complication of subclavian vein catheterization. Ann Surg 179:266, 1974.

369. Knight L, Tobin J Jr, L'Heureux P: Hydrothorax: A complication of hyperalimentation with radiologic manifestations. Radiology 111:693, 1974.

370. Holt S, Kirkham N, Myrescough E: Haemothorax after subclavian vein cannulation. Thorax 32:101, 1977.

371. Usselman JA, Seat SG: Superior caval catheter displacement causing bilateral pleural effusions. Am J Roentgenol 133:738, 1979.

372. Higgins CB, Mulder DG: Traumatic subarachnoid-pleural fistula. Chest 61:189, 1972.

373. Lovaas ME, Castillo RG, Deutschman CS: Traumatic subarachnoid-pleural fistula. Neurosurgery 17:650, 1985.

374. Beutel EW, Roberts JD, Langston HT, et al: Subarachnoid-pleural fistula. J Thorac Cardiovasc Surg 80:21, 1980.

375. Qureshi MM, Roble DC, Gindin RA, et al: Subarachnoid-pleural fistula. Case report and review of the literature. J Thorac Cardiovasc Surg 91:238, 1986.

376. Qureshi MM, Roble DC, Gindin A, et al: Subarachnoid-pleural fistula. J Thorac Cardiovasc Surg 91:238, 1986.

377. Azambuja PC, Fragomeni LS: Traumatic chylothorax associated with subarachnoid-pleural fistula. Thorax 36:699, 1981.

378. Tempero SJ, Bookstein JJ: Angiographic demonstration of a ruptured spleen causing hemothorax. Case report. J Can Assoc Radiol 24:78, 1973.

379. Koehler PR, Jones R: Association of left-sided pleural effusions and splenic hematomas. Am J Roentgenol 135:851, 1980.

380. Lougheed MN, Maguire GH: Irradiation pneumonitis in the treatment of carcinoma of the breast. J Can Assoc Radiol 11:1, 1960.

381. Bachman AL, Macken K: Pleural effusions following supervoltage radiation for breast carcinoma. Radiology 72:699, 1959.

382. Whitcomb ME, Schwarz MI: Pleural effusion complicating intensive mediastinal radiation therapy. Am Rev Respir Dis 103:100, 1971.

383. Deeley TJ: The effects of radiation on the lungs in the treatment of carcinoma of the bronchus. Clin Radiol 11:33, 1960.

384. Rostand RA, Feldman RL, Block ER: Massive hemothorax complicating heparin anticoagulation for pulmonary embolus. South Med J 70:1128, 1977.

385. Heneghan MA, Teixidor HS: Pleuroperitoneal endometriosis. Case reports. Am J Roentgenol 133:727, 1979.

386. Wilkins SB, Bell-Thomson J, Tyras DH: Hemothorax associated with endometriosis. J Thorac Cardiovasc Surg 89:636, 1985.

387. Jung-Gi I, Heung Sik Kang, Byung Ihn Choi, et al: Pleural endometriosis: CT and sonographic findings. Am J Roentgenol 148:523, 1987.

388. Wilimas JA, Presbury G, Orenstein D, et al: Hemothorax and hemomediastinum in patients with hemophilia. Acta Haematol 73:176, 1985.

389. Brady DB, Bolan JC: Neurofibromatosis and spontaneous hemothorax in pregnancy: Two case reports. Obstet Gynecol 63(3 Suppl):35S, 1984.

390. Lemon WS, Higgins GM: Lymphatic absorption of particulate matter through the normal and paralyzed diaphragm: An experimental study. Am J Med Sci 178:536, 1929.

391. Johnston RF, Loo RV: Hepatic hydrothorax. Studies to determine the source of the fluid and report of thirteen cases. Ann Intern Med 61:385, 1964.

392. Meigs JV: Pelvic tumors other than fibromas of the ovary with ascites and hydrothorax. Obstet Gynecol 3:471, 1954.

393. Stanley NN, Williams AJ, Dewar CA, et al: Hypoxia and hydrothoraces in a case of liver cirrhosis: Correlation of physiological, radiographic, scintigraphic, and pathological findings. Thorax 32:457, 1977.

394. Lieberman FL, Peters RL: Cirrhotic hydrothorax—Further evidence that an acquired diaphragmatic defect is at fault. Arch Intern Med 125:114, 1970.

395. Lieberman FL, Hidemura R, Peters RL, et al: Pathogenesis and treatment of hydrothorax complicating cirrhosis with ascites. Ann Intern Med 64:341, 1966.

396. Hammarsten JF, Honska WL Jr, Limes BJ: Pleural fluid amylase in pancreatitis and other diseases. Am Rev Respir Dis 79:606, 1959.

397. Kaye MD: Pleuropulmonary complications of pancreatitis. Thorax 23:297, 1968.

398. Falk A, Gustafsson L, Gamklou R: Silent pancreatitis. Report of 4 cases of acute pancreatitis with atypical symptomatology. Acta Chir Scand 150:341, 1984.

399. Belfar HL, Radecki PD, Friedman AC, et al: Pancreatitis presenting as pleural effusions: Computed tomography demonstration of pleural space extension of pancreatitis exudate. J Comput Tomogr 11:184, 1987.

400. Cameron JL: Chronic pancreatic ascites and pancreatic pleural effusions. Gastroenterology 74:134, 1978.

401. Strimlan CV, Turbiner EH: Pleuropericardial effusions associated with chest and abdominal pain. Chest 81:493, 1982.

402. Liedberg G, Lindmark G, Struwe I: Pleural effusion with dyspnea as the presenting symptom in chronic pancreatitis. A case report. Acta Chir Scand 149:209, 1983.

403. Faling LJ, Gerzof SG, Daly BD, et al: Treatment of chronic pancreatitic pleural effusion by percutaneous catheter drainage of abdominal pseudocyst. Am J Med 76:329, 1984.

404. Dewan NA, Kinney WW, O'Donohue WJ Jr: Chronic massive pancreatic pleural effusion. Chest 85:497, 1984.

405. Gertsch P, Marquis C, Diserens H, et al: Chronic pancreatic pleural effusions and ascites. Int Surg 69:145, 1984.

406. Rotman N, Fagniez PL: Chronic pancreaticopleural fistulas. Arch Surg 119:1204, 1984.

407. Bedingfield JA, Anderson MC: Pancreatopleural fistula. Pancreas 1:283, 1986.

408. Bronner MH, Marsh WH, Stanley JH: Pancreaticopleural fistula: Demonstration by computed tomography and endoscopic retrograde cholangiopancreatography. J Comput Tomogr 10:167, 1986.

409. Louie S, McGahan JP, Frey C, et al: Pancreatic pleuropericardial effusions. Fistulous tracts demonstrated by computed tomography. Arch Intern Med 145:1231, 1985.

410. Becx MC, van den Berg W, Bruggink ED, et al: Relapsing pleural exudate complicating chronic pancreatitis. Neth J Med 34:88, 1989.

411. Izbicki JR, Wilker DK, Waldner H, et al: Thoracic manifestations of internal pancreatic fistulas: Report of five cases. Am J Gastroenterol 84:265, 1989.

412. Ihse I, Lindström E, Evander A, et al: The value of preoperative imaging techniques in patients with chronic pancreatic pleural effusions. Int J Pancreatol 2:269, 1987.

413. Cooper CB, Bardsley PA, Rao SS, et al: Pleural effusions and pancreaticopleural fistulae associated with asymptomatic pancreatic disease. Br J Dis Chest 82:315, 1988.

414. Anderson WJ, Skinner DB, Zuidema GD, et al: Chronic pancreatic pleural effusions. Surg Gynecol Obstet 137:827, 1973.

415. Kramer MR, Saldana MJ, Cepero RJ, et al: High amylase levels in neoplasm-related pleural effusion. Ann Intern Med 110:567, 1989.

416. Sankarankutty M, Baird JL, Dowse JA, et al: Adenocarcinoma of the pancreas with massive pleural effusion. Br J Clin Pract 32:294, 1978.

417. McCarthy S, Pellegrini CA, Moss AA, et al: Pleuropancreatic fistula: Endoscopic retrograde cholangiopancreatography and computed tomography. Am J Roentgenol 142:1151, 1984.

418. Bydder GM, Kreel L: Pleural calcification in pancreatitis demon-

strated by computed tomography. J Comput Assist Tomogr 5:161, 1981.

419. Light RW, George RB: Incidence and significance of pleural effusion after abdominal surgery. Chest 69:621, 1976.

420. Miller WT, Talman EA: Subphrenic abscess. Am J Roentgenol 101:961, 1967.

421. Buscaglia AJ: Empyema due to splenic abscess with Salmonella newport. JAMA 240:1990, 1978.

422. Ballantyne KC, Sethia B, Reece IJ, et al: Empyema following intra-abdominal sepsis. Br J Surg 71:723, 1984.

423. Banham SW, Howie AD, Stevenson RD, et al: The pulmonary angiographic appearance of pleurisy associated with subdiaphragmatic inflammation. Thorax 34:241, 1979.

424. Salmon VJ: Benign pelvic tumors associated with ascites and pleural effusion. J Mt Sinai Hosp 1:169, 1934.

425. Meigs JV, Cass JW: Fibroma of the ovary with ascites and hydrothorax. With a report of seven cases. Am J Obstet Gynecol 33:249, 1937.

426. Millett J, Shell J: Meigs' syndrome in a case of multilocular pseudomucinous cystadenoma of the ovary. Am J Med Sci 209:327, 1945.

427. Carson SA, Mazur MT: Atypical endometrioid cystadenofibroma with Meigs' syndrome: Ultrastructure and S-phase fraction. Cancer 49:472, 1982.

428. Mokrohisky JF: So-called "Meigs' syndrome" associated with benign and malignant ovarian tumors. Radiology 70:578, 1958.

429. Solomon S, Farber SJ, Caruso LJ: Fibromyomata of the uterus with hemothorax—Meigs' syndrome? Arch Intern Med 127:307, 1971.

430. Handler CE, Fray RE, Snashall PD: Atypical Meigs' syndrome. Thorax 37:396, 1982.

431. Dockerty MB: Ovarian neoplasms. A collective review of the recent literature. Int Abstr Surg 81:179, 1945.

432. Rothstein E: Benign pleural effusion and ascites associated with adenocarcinoma of the body of the pancreas. Dis Chest 15:603, 1949.

433. Swensson NL, Kurohara SS, George FW III: Complete regression, following abdominal irradiation alone, of chylothorax complicating lymphosarcoma with ascites. Radiology 87:635, 1966.

434. Edwards SR, Unger AM: Acute hydrothorax—a new complication of peritoneal dialysis. JAMA 199:853, 1967.

435. Rudnick MR, Coyle JF, Beck LH, et al: Acute massive hydrothorax complicating peritoneal dialysis, report of 2 cases and a review of the literature. Clin Nephrol 12:38, 1979.

436. Galen MA, Steinberg SM, Lowrie EG, et al: Hemorrhagic pleural effusion in patients undergoing chronic hemodialysis. Ann Intern Med 82:359, 1975.

437. Berger HW, Rammohan G, Neff MS, et al: Uremic pleural effusion—A study in 14 patients on chronic dialysis. Ann Intern Med 82:362, 1975.

438. Corriere JN Jr, Miller WT, Murphy JJ: Hydronephrosis as a cause of pleural effusion. Radiology 90:79, 1968.

439. Barek LB, Cigtay OS: Urinothorax—An unusual pleural effusion. Br J Radiol 48:685, 1975.

440. Baron RL, Stark DD, McClennan BL, et al: Intrathoracic extension of retroperitoneal urine collections. Am J Roentgenol 137:37, 1981.

441. Leung FW, Williams AJ, Oill PA: Pleural effusion associated with urinary tract obstruction: Support for a hypothesis. Thorax 36:632, 1981.

442. Shanes JG, Senior RM, Stark DD, et al: Pleural effusion associated with urinary tract obstruction. Thorax 37:160, 1982.

443. Stark DD, Shanes JG, Baron RL, et al: Biochemical features of urinothorax. Arch Intern Med 142:1509, 1982.

444. Ralston MD, Wilkinson RH Jr: Bilateral urinothorax identified by technetium-99m DPTA renal imaging. J Nucl Med 27:56, 1986.

445. Nusser RA, Culhane RH: Recurrent transudative effusion with an abdominal mass. Urinothorax. Chest 90:263, 1986.

446. Weiss Z, Shalev E, Zuckerman H, et al: Obstructive renal failure and pleural effusion caused by the gravid uterus. Acta Obstet Gynecol Scand 65:187, 1986.

447. Salcedo JR: Urinothorax: Report of 4 cases and review of the literature. J Urol 135:805, 1986.

448. Miller KS, Wooten S, Sahn SA: Urinothorax: A cause of low pH transudative pleural effusions. Am J Med 85:448, 1988.

449. Dunbar JS, Favreau M: Infrapulmonary pleural effusion with particular reference to its occurrence in nephrosis. J Can Assoc Radiol 10:24, 1959.

450. Cavina C, Vichi G: Radiological aspects of pleural effusions in medical neuropathy in children. Ann Radiol Diag 31:163, 1958.

451. Jenkins PG, Shelp WD: Recurrent pleural transudate in the nephrotic syndrome. A new approach to treatment. JAMA 230:587, 1974.

452. Llach F, Arieff AL, Massry SG: Renal vein thrombosis and nephrotic syndrome: A prospective study of 36 adult patients. Ann Intern Med 83:8, 1975.

453. Frew AJ, Higgins RM: Empyema and mesangiocapillary glomerulonephritis with nephrotic syndrome. Br J Dis Chest 82:93, 1988.

454. Verreault J, Lepage S, Bisson G, et al: Ascites and right pleural effusion: Demonstration of a peritoneopleural communication. J Nucl Med 27:1706, 1986.

455. Noseda A, Adler M, Ketelbant P, et al: Massive vitamin A intoxication with ascites and pleural effusion. J Clin Gastroenterol 7:344, 1985.

456. Frazer IH, Lichtenstein M, Andrews JT: Pleuroperitoneal effusion without ascites. Med J Aust 2:520, 1983.

457. Kirkpatrick JA Jr, Fleisher DS: The roentgenographic appearance of the chest in acute glomerulonephritis in children. J Pediatr 64:492, 1964.

458. Holzel A, Fawcitt J: Pulmonary changes in acute glomerulonephritis in childhood. J Pediatr 57:695, 1960.

459. Hopps HC, Wissler RW: Uremic pneumonitis. Am J Pathol 31:261, 1955.

460. Gilbert L, Ribot S, Frankel H, et al: Fibrinous uremic pleuritis—Surgical entity. Chest 67:53, 1975.

461. Nidus BD, Matalon R, Cantacuzino D, et al: Uremic pleuritis—A clinicopathological entity. N Engl J Med 281:255, 1969.

462. McCabe TA, Radowski TA, Argy WP, et al: Fibrosing uremic pleuritis complicated by thoracic empyema. Arch Intern Med 142:1369, 1982.

463. Schneierson SJ, Katz M: Solitary pleural effusion due to myxedema. JAMA 168:1003, 1958.

464. Hurwitz PA, Pinals DJ: Pleural effusion in chronic hereditary lymphedema (Nonne, Milroy, Meige's disease). Report of two cases. Radiology 82:246, 1964.

465. Emerson PA: Yellow nails, lymphoedema, and pleural effusions. Thorax 21:247, 1966.

466. Siegelman SS, Heckman BH, Hasson J: Lymphedema, pleural effusions and yellow nails: Associated immunologic deficiency. Dis Chest 56:114, 1969.

467. Ross JD, Reid KDG, Ambujakshan VP, et al: Recurrent pleural effusion, protein-losing enteropathy, malabsorption, and mosaic warts associated with generalized lymphatic hypoplasia. Thorax 26:119, 1971.

468. Dressler W: The post-myocardial infarction syndrome. Arch Intern Med 103:28, 1959.

469. Wen JY, Baughman KL: The Dressler syndrome. Johns Hopkins Med J 148:179, 1981.

470. Stelzner TJ, King TE Jr, Antony VB, et al: The pleuropulmonary manifestations of the postcardiac injury syndrome. Chest 84:383, 1983.

471. Domby WR, Whitcomb ME: Pleural effusion as a manifestation of Dressler's syndrome in the distant post-infarction period. Am Heart J 96:243, 1978.

472. Heller H, Sohar E, Sherf L: Familial Mediterranean fever. Arch Intern Med 102:50, 1958.

473. Sohar E, Gafni J, Pras M, et al: Familial Mediterranean fever. Am J Med 43:227, 1967.

474. Barakat MH, Karnik AM, Majeed HW, et al: Familial Mediterranean fever (recurrent hereditary polyserositis) in Arabs—A study of 175 patients and review of the literature. Q J Med 60:837, 1986.

475. Brandstetter RD, Klass SC, Gutherz P, et al: Pleural effusion due to communicating gastric ulcer. NY State J Med 85:706, 1985.

476. Dabestani A, Noble LM, Child JS, et al: Pericardial disease in familial Mediterranean fever: An echocardiographic study. Chest 81:592, 1982.

477. Brauman A, Gilboa Y: Recurrent pulmonary atelectasis as a manifestation of familial Mediterranean fever. Arch Intern Med 147:378, 1987.

478. Reimann HA, Coppola ED, Villegas GR: Serum complement defects in periodic diseases. Ann Intern Med 73:737, 1970.

479. Michaelson I, Eliakam M, Ehrenfeld EN, et al: Fundal changes resembling colloid bodies in recurrent polyserositis (periodic disease). AMA Arch Ophthalmol 62:1, 1959.

480. Mancini JL: Familial paroxysmal polyserositis, phenotype I (familial Mediterranean fever). A rare cause of pleurisy. A case report and review of the literature. Am Rev Respir Dis 107:461, 1973.

481. Siegal S: Familial paroxysmal polyserositis. Am J Med 36:893, 1964.

482. Daee SA, Wagner R, Boneval H: Bilious pleural effusion. An unusual consequence of gastrointestinal perforation. Md State Med J 31:54, 1982.

483. Aronchick JM, Epstein DM, Gefter WB, et al: Chronic traumatic diaphragmatic hernia: The significance of pleural effusion. Radiology 168:675, 1988.

484. Patwardhan RV, Heilpern RJ, Brewster AC, et al: Pleuropericarditis: An extraintestinal complication of inflammatory disease. Report of three cases and review of literature. Arch Intern Med 143:94, 1983.

485. Rosenbaum AJ, Murphy PJ, Engel JJ: Pleurisy during the course of ulcerative colitis. J Clin Gastroenterol 5:517, 1983.

486. Olutola PS, Hutton L, Wall WJ: Pleural effusion following liver transplantation. Radiology 157:594, 1985.

487. Matsumata T, Kanematsu T, Okudaira Y, et al: Postoperative

18

mechanical ventilation preventing the occurrence of pleural effusion after hepatectomy. Surgery 102:493, 1987.

488. Pappas CA, Rheinlander HF, Stadecker MJ: Pleural effusion as a complication of solitary eosinophilic granuloma of the rib. Hum Pathol 11:675, 1980.

489. Horn BR, Byrd RB: Simulation of pleural disease by disk space infection. Chest 74:575, 1978.

490. Feigl D, Seidel L, Marmor A: Gorham's disease of the clavicle with bilateral pleural effusions. Chest 79:242, 1981.

491. Castillo RA, Devoe LD, Hadi HA, et al: Nonimmune hydrops fetalis: Clinical experience and factors related to a poor outcome. Am J Obstet Gynecol 155:812, 1986.

492. Castillo RA, Devoe LD, Falls G, et al: Pleural effusions and pulmonary hypoplasia. Am J Obstet Gynecol 157:1252, 1987.

493. Adams H, Jones A, Hayward C: The sonographic features and implications of fetal pleural effusions. Clin Radiol 39:398, 1988.

494. Latner AL: Cantarow and Trumper Clinical Biochemistry, 7th ed. Philadelphia, WB Saunders, 1975.

495. Staats BA, Ellefson RD, Budahn LL, et al: The lipoprotein profile of chylous and nonchylous pleural effusions. Mayo Clin Proc 55:700, 1980.

496. Seriff NS, Cohen ML, Samuel P, et al: Chylothorax: Diagnosis by lipoprotein electrophoresis of serum and pleural fluid. Thorax 32:98, 1977.

497. Williams KR, Burford TH: The management of chylothorax. Ann Surg 160:131, 1964.

498. Hughes RL, Mintzer RA, Hidvegi DF, et al: The management of chylothorax. Clinical conference in pulmonary disease from Northwestern University Medical School, Chicago. Chest 76:212, 1979.

499. Sassoon CS, Light RW: Chylothorax and pseudochylothorax. Clin Chest Med 6:163, 1985.

500. Hillerdal G: Chyliform (cholesterol) pleural effusion. Chest 88:426, 1985.

501. Johnson JR, Falk A, Iber C, et al: Paragonimiasis in the United States: A report of 9 cases in Hmong immigrants. Chest 82:168, 1982.

502. Schulman A, Fataar S, Dalrymple R, et al: The lymphographic anatomy of chylothorax. Br J Radiol 51:420, 1978.

503. Strausser JL, Flye MW: Management of nontraumatic chylothorax. Ann Thorac Surg 31:520, 1981.

504. Segal R, Waron M, Reif R, et al: Chylous ascites and chylothorax as presenting manifestations of stomach carcinoma. Isr J Med Sci 22:897, 1986.

505. Pandya K, Lal C, Tuchschmidt J, et al: Bilateral chylothorax with pulmonary Kaposi's sarcoma (letter). Chest 94:1316, 1988.

506. Quinonez A, Halabe J, Avelar F, et al: Chylothorax due to metastatic prostatic carcinoma. Br J Urol 63:325, 1989.

507. Tani K, Ogushi F, Sone S, et al: Chylothorax and chylous ascites in a patient with uterine cancer. Jpn J Clin Oncol 18:175, 1988.

508. Schmidt A: Chylothorax. Review of 5 years' cases in the literature and report of a case. Acta Chir Scand 118:5, 1959.

509. Macfarlane JR, Holman CW: Chylothorax. Am Rev Respir Dis 105:287, 1972.

510. Dulchavsky SA, Ledgerwood AM, Lucas CE: Management of chylothorax after blunt chest trauma. J Trauma 28:1400, 1988.

511. Fine PG, Bubela C: Chylothorax following celiac plexus block. Anesthesiology 63:454, 1985.

512. Nakai S, Zielke K: Chylothorax—A rare complication after anterior and posterior spinal correction. Report of six cases. Spine 11:830, 1986.

513. Higgins CB, Reinke RT: Postoperative chylothorax in children with congenital heart disease. Clinical and roentgenographic features. Radiology 119:409, 1976.

514. Kaul TK, Bain WH, Turner MA, et al: Chylothorax: Report of a case complicating ductus ligation through a median sternotomy, and review. Thorax 31:610, 1976.

515. Verunelli F, Giorgini V, Luisi VS, et al: Chylothorax following cardiac surgery in children. J Cardiovasc Surg 24:227, 1983.

516. Fairfax AJ, McNabb WR, Spiro SG: Chylothorax: A review of 18 cases. Thorax 41:880, 1986.

517. Zakhour BJ, Drucker MH, Franco AA: Chylothorax as a complication of aortocoronary bypass. Two case reports and a review of the literature. Scand J Thorac Cardiovasc Surg 22:93, 1988.

518. Czerniak A, Dreznik Z, Neuman Y, et al: Chylothorax complicating repair of a left diaphragmatic hernia in a neonate. Thorax 36:701, 1981.

519. Kostiainen S, Meurala H, Mattila S, et al: Chylothorax. Clinical experience in nine cases. Scand J Thorac Cardiovasc Surg 17:79, 1983.

520. Dharman K, Temes SP, Wetherell FE, et al: Chyloperitoneum and chylothorax: A combined rare occurrence after retroperitoneal lymphadenectomy and radiotherapy for testis tumor. J Urol 131:346, 1984.

521. van der Vliet JA, van der Linden CJ, Greep JM: Chylothorax after gastric resection. Neth J Surg 37:16, 1985.

522. Har-El G, Segal K, Sidi J: Bilateral chylothorax complicating radical neck dissection: Report of a case with no concurrent external chylous leakage. Head Neck Surg 7:225, 1985.

523. Ng RS, Kerbavaz RJ, Hilsinger RL Jr: Bilateral chylothorax from radical neck dissection. Otolaryngol Head Neck Surg 93:814, 1985.

524. Sinclair D, Woods E, Saibil EA, et al: "Chyloma": A persistent post-traumatic collection in the left supraclavicular region. J Trauma 27:567, 1987.

525. Goldfarb JP: Chylous effusions secondary to pancreatitis: Case report and review of the literature. Am J Gastroenterol 79:133, 1984.

526. Reilly KM, Tsou E: Bilateral chylothorax. JAMA 233:536, 1975.

527. Wojciech J: Chylothorax in infancy. Thorax 23:214, 1968.

528. Koffler H, Papile L-A, Burstein RL: Congenital chylothorax: Two cases associated with maternal polyhydramnios. Am J Dis Child 132:638, 1978.

529. Petres RE, Redwine FO, Cruikshank DP: Congenital bilateral chylothorax: Antepartum diagnosis and successful intrauterine surgical management. JAMA 248:1360, 1982.

530. Smeltzer DM, Stickler GB, Fleming RE: Primary lymphatic dysplasia in children: Chylothorax, chylous ascites, and generalized lymphatic dysplasia. Eur J Pediatr 145:286, 1986.

531. Pauwels R, Oomen C, Huybrechts W, et al: Chylothorax in adult age in association with congenital lymphedema. Eur J Respir Dis 69:285, 1986.

532. Wilmshurst PT, Burnie JP, Turner PR, et al: Chylopericardium, chylothorax, and hypobetalipoproteinaemia. Br Med J 293:483, 1986.

533. Noonan JA, Walters LR, Reeves JT: Congenital pulmonary lymphangiectasia. Am J Dis Child 120:314, 1970.

534. Menzies R, Hidvegi R: Chylothorax associated with tuberculous spondylitis. J Can Assoc Radiol 39:238, 1988.

535. Vennera MC, Moreno R, Cot J, et al: Chylothorax and tuberculosis. Thorax 38:694, 1983.

536. Bristo LD, Mandal AK, Oparah SS, et al: Bilateral chylothorax associated with sclerosing mediastinitis. Int Surg 68:273, 1983.

537. Takamoto RM, Armstrong RG, Stanford W, et al: Chylothorax with multiple lymphangiomata of the bone. Chest 59:687, 1971.

538. Pedicelli G, Mattia P, Zorzoli AA, et al: Gorham syndrome. JAMA 252:1449, 1984.

539. Freundlich, IM: The role of lymphangiography in chylothorax. A report of six nontraumatic cases. Am J Roentgenol 125:617, 1975.

540. Weidner WA, Steiner RM: Roentgenographic demonstration of intrapulmonary and pleural lymphatics during lymphangiography. Radiology 100:533, 1971.

541. Ngan H, Fok M, Wong J: The role of lymphography in chylothorax following thoracic surgery. Br J Radiol 61:1032, 1988.

542. Grant T, Levin B: Lymphangiographic visualization of pleural and pulmonary lymphatics in a patient without chylothorax. Radiology 113:49, 1974.

543. Camiel MR, Benninghoff DL, Alexander LL: Chylous effusions, extravasation of lymphographic contrast material, hypoplasia of lymph nodes and lymphocytopenia. Chest 59:107, 1971.

544. Adler RH, Levinsky L: Persistent chylothorax. Treatment by talc pleurodesis. J Thorac Cardiovasc Surg 76:859, 1978.

545. Patterson GA, Todd TRJ, Delarue NC, et al: Supradiaphragmatic ligation of the thoracic duct in intractable chylous fistula. Ann Thorac Surg 32:44, 1981.

546. Robinson CL: The management of chylothorax. Ann Thorac Surg 39:90, 1985.

547. Milsom JW, Kron IL, Rheuban KS, et al: Chylothorax: An assessment of current surgical management. J Thorac Cardiovasc Surg 89:221, 1985.

548. Smith WG, Rothwell PPG: Treatment of spontaneous pneumothorax. Thorax 17:342, 1962.

549. Hyde L: Benign spontaneous pneumothorax. Ann Intern Med 56:746, 1962.

550. Lindskog GE, Halasz NA: Spontaneous pneumothorax. A consideration of pathogenesis and management with review of seventy-two hospitalized cases. Arch Surg 75:693, 1957.

551. Inouye WY, Berggren RB, Johnson J: Spontaneous pneumothorax—treatment and mortality. Dis Chest 51:67, 1967.

552. Chan TB, Tan WC, Tech PC: Spontaneous pneumothorax in medical practise in a general hospital. Ann Acad Med Singapore 14:457, 1985.

553. Melton LJ III, Hepper NGG, Offord KP: Influence of height on the risk of spontaneous pneumothorax. Mayo Clin Proc 56:678, 1981.

554. Primrose WR: Spontaneous pneumothorax: A retrospective review of aetiology, pathogenesis and management. Scott Med J 29:15, 1984.

555. Bense L, Eklund G, Wiman LG: Smoking and the increased risk of contracting spontaneous pneumothorax. Chest 92:1009, 1987.

556. Wilson WG, Aylsworth AS: Familial spontaneous pneumothorax. Pediatrics 64:172, 1979.

557. Pierce JA, Suarez B, Reich T: More on familial spontaneous pneumothorax. Chest 78:263, 1980.
558. Sharpe IK, Ahmad M, Braun W: Familial spontaneous pneumothorax and HLA antigens. Chest 78:264, 1980.
559. Sugiyama Y, Maeda H, Yotsumoto H, et al: Familial spontaneous pneumothorax. Thorax 41:969, 1986.
560. Rashid A, Sendi A, Al-Kadhimi A, et al: Concurrent spontaneous pneumothorax in identical twins. Thorax 41:971, 1986.
561. Gibson GJ: Familial pneumothoraces and bullae. Thorax 32:88, 1977.
562. Nakamura H, Konishiike J, Sugamura A, et al: Epidemiology of spontaneous pneumothorax in women. Chest 89:378, 1986.
563. Lichter I, Gwynne JF: Spontaneous pneumothorax in young subjects. Thorax 26:409, 1971.
564. Grimes OF, Farber SM: Air cysts of the lung. Surg Gynecol Obstet 113:720, 1961.
565. Feraru F, Morrow CS: Surgery of subpleural blebs: Indications and contraindications. Am Rev Respir Dis 79:577, 1959.
566. Macklin MT, Macklin CC: Malignant interstitial emphysema of the lungs and mediastinum as an important occult complication in many respiratory diseases and other conditions: An interpretation of the clinical literature in the light of laboratory experiment. Medicine 23:281, 1944.
567. Cooley JC, Gillespie JB: Mediastinal emphysema: Pathogenesis and management. Report of a case. Dis Chest 49:104, 1966.
568. Editorial. Neonatal pneumothorax. Lancet 2:1304, 1973.
569. Price HV: Neonatal pneumothorax: Survey and prevention. Br Med J 2:456, 1976.
570. Jansveld CAF, Dijkman JH: Primary spontaneous pneumothorax and smoking. Br Med J 4:559, 1975.
571. Bense L, Hedenstierna G, Lewander R, et al: Regional lung function of nonsmokers with healed spontaneous pneumothorax. A physiologic and emission radiologic study. Chest 90:352, 1986.
572. Leading Article. Spontaneous pneumothorax and apical lung disease. Br Med J 4:573, 1971.
573. Melton LJ III, Hepper NGG, Offord KP: Incidence of spontaneous pneumothorax in Olmsted County, Minnesota: 1950 to 1974. Am Rev Respir Dis 120:1379, 1979.
574. Kawakami Y, Irie T, Kamishima K: Stature, lung height, and spontaneous pneumothorax. Respiration 43:35, 1982.
575. West JB: Distribution of mechanical stress in the lung, a possible factor in localisation of pulmonary disease. Lancet 1:839, 1971.
576. Peters RM, Peters BA, Benirschke SK, et al: Chest dimensions in young adults with spontaneous pneumothorax. Ann Thorac Surg 25:193, 1978.
577. Hall JR, Pyeritz RE, Dudgeon DL, et al: Pneumothorax in the Marfan syndrome: prevalence and therapy. Ann Thorac Surg 37:500, 1984.
578. Dwyer EM Jr, Troncale F: Spontaneous pneumothorax and pulmonary disease in the Marfan syndrome. Report of two cases and review of the literature. Ann Intern Med 62:1285, 1965.
579. Lipton RA, Greenwald RA, Seriff NS: Pneumothorax and bilateral honeycombed lung in Marfan syndrome. Report of a case and review of the pulmonary abnormalities in this disorder. Am Rev Respir Dis 104:924, 1971.
580. Margaliot SZ, Barzilay J, Bar-David M, et al: Spontaneous pneumothorax and mitral valve prolapse. Chest 89:93, 1986.
581. Bense L, Wiman LG, Hedenstierna G: Onset of symptoms in spontaneous pneumothorax: Correlations to physical activity. Eur J Respir Dis 71:181, 1987.
582. Dermksian G, Lamb LE: Spontaneous pneumothorax in apparently healthy flying personnel. Ann Intern Med 51:39, 1959.
583. Rose DM, Jarczyk PA: Spontaneous pneumoperitoneum after scuba diving. JAMA 239:223, 1978.
584. Saywell WR: Submarine escape training, lung cysts and tension pneumothorax. Br J Radiol 62:276, 1989.
585. Scott GC, Berger R, McKean HE: The role of atmospheric pressure variation in the development of spontaneous pneumothoraces. Am Rev Respir Dis 139:659, 1989.
586. West J: Distribution of mechanical stress in the lung, a possible factor in localisation of pulmonary disease. Lancet 1:839, 1971.
587. Vawter DL, Matthews FL, West JB: Effect of shape and size of lung and chest wall on stresses in the lung. J Appl Physiol 39:9, 1975.
588. Ohata M, Suzuki H: Pathogenesis of spontaneous pneumothorax: With special reference to the ultrastructure of emphysematous bullae. Chest 77:771, 1980.
589. Ruckley CV, McCormack RJM: The management of spontaneous pneumothorax. Thorax 21:139, 1966.
590. Gobbel WG Jr, Rhea WG Jr, Nelson IA, et al: Spontaneous pneumothorax. J Thorac Cardiovasc Surg 46:331, 1963.
591. Bierman CW: Pneumomediastinum and pneumothorax complicating asthma in children. Am J Dis Child 114:42, 1967.
592. Sugita K, Koya E: Bronchial asthma and spontaneous pneumothorax. Jpn J Dis Chest 6:1188, 1962.
593. Schweich A, Fierstein J: Staphylococcal septicemia with recurrent spontaneous pneumothorax. Ann Intern Med 50:819, 1959.
594. Blundell JE: Pneumothorax complicating pulmonary infarction. Br J Radiol 40:226, 1967.
595. Hall FM, Salzman EW, Ellis BI, et al: Pneumothorax complicating aseptic cavitating pulmonary infarction. Chest 72:232, 1977.
596. Ludwig J, Kienzle GD: Pneumothorax in a large autopsy population. A study of 77 cases. Am J Clin Pathol 70:24, 1978.
597. Hall FM, Salzman EW, Ellis BI, et al: Pneumothorax complicating aseptic cavitating pulmonary infarction. Chest 72:232, 1977.
598. Aho A, Heinivaara O, Mähönen H: Boeck's sarcoid as a cause of spontaneous pneumothorax. Ann Med Int Fenn 47:163, 1958.
599. Nickol KH: Idiopathic pulmonary haemosiderosis presenting with spontaneous pneumothorax. Tubercle 41:216, 1960.
600. Anton HC, Gray B: Pulmonary alveolar proteinosis presenting with pneumothorax. Clin Radiol 18:428, 1967.
601. Young WA: Familial fibrocystic pulmonary dysplasia: A new case in a known affected family. Can Med Assoc J 94:1059, 1966.
602. Babcock TL, Snyder BA: Spontaneous pneumothorax associated with tuberous sclerosis. J Thorac Cardiovasc Surg 83:100, 1982.
603. Beyer A, Richter K, Eribo O: Zwei verlaufsbeobachtungen eines Hamman-Rich-syndromes mit rezidivierendem spontanpneumothorax. (Two observations of the Hamman-Rich syndrome with recurrent spontaneous pneumothorax.) Fortschr Roentgenstr 94:568, 1961.
604. Kittredge RD, Geller A, Finby N: The reticuloendothelioses in the lung. Am J Roentgenol 100:588, 1967.
605. Haber K, Freundlich IM: Spontaneous pneumothorax with unusual manifestations. Chest 65:675, 1974.
606. Edelstein G, Levitt RG: Cavitary coccidioidomycosis presenting as spontaneous pneumothorax. Am J Roentgenol 141:533, 1983.
607. Bakir F, Al-Omeri MM: Echinococcal tension pneumothorax. Thorax 24:547, 1969.
608. Dines DE, Clagett OT, Payne WS: Spontaneous pneumothorax in emphysema. Mayo Clin Proc 45:481, 1970.
609. Shaver CG, Riddell AR: Lung changes associated with the manifestation of alumina abrasives. J Industr Hyg Toxicol 29:145, 1947.
610. Bohlig H: Röntgenologische lungenbefunde bei korundschmelzern. (Roentgenologic findings in the lungs of corundum melters.) Fortschr Roentgenstr 83:678, 1955.
611. Graham ML II, Spelsberg TC, Dines DE, et al: Pulmonary lymphangiomyomatosis: With particular reference to steroid-receptor assay studies and pathologic correlation. Mayo Clin Proc 59:3, 1984.
612. Torrington KG, Ashbaugh DG, Stackle EG: Recklinghausen's disease. Occurrence with intrathoracic vagal neurofibroma and contralateral spontaneous pneumothorax. Arch Intern Med 143:568, 1983.
613. Price BA, Elliott MJ, Featherstone G, et al: Perforation of intrathoracic colon causing acute pneumothorax. Thorax 38:959, 1983.
614. McDonald CF, Walbaum PR, Sircus W, et al: Intrapleural perforation of peptic ulcer in association with diaphragmatic hernia. Br J Dis Chest 79:196, 1985.
615. Rotstein OD, Pruett TL, Simmons RL: Gastropleural fistula. Report of three cases and review of the literature. Am J Surg 150:392, 1985.
616. Reddy SA, Vemuru R, Padmanabhan K, et al: Colopleural fistula presenting as tension pneumothorax in strangulated diaphragmatic hernia. Report of a case. Dis Colon Rectum 32:165, 1989.
617. Phipps RF, Jackson BT: Faeco-pneumothorax as the presenting feature of a traumatic diaphragmatic hernia. JR Soc Med 81:549, 1988.
618. Twiford TW Jr, Zornoza J, Libshitz HI: Recurrent spontaneous pneumothorax after radiation therapy to the thorax. Chest 73:387, 1978.
619. Epstein DM, Gefter WB, Miller WT, et al: Spontaneous pneumothorax: An uncommon manifestation of Wegener granulomatosis. Radiology 135:327, 1980.
620. Luck SR, Raffensperger JG, Sullivan HJ, et al: Management of pneumothorax in children with chronic pulmonary disease. J Thorac Cardiovasc Surg 74:834, 1977.
621. Spector ML, Stern RC: Pneumothorax in cystic fibrosis: A 26-year experience. Ann Thorac Surg 47:204, 1989.
622. Goodman PC, Daley C, Minagi H: Spontaneous pneumothorax in AIDS patients with Pneumocystis carinii pneumonia. Am J Roentgenol 147:29, 1986.
623. Sherman M, Levin D, Breidbart D: Pneumocystis carinii pneumonia with spontaneous pneumothorax. A report of three cases. Chest 90:609, 1986.
624. Heimlich HJ, Rubin M: Spontaneous pneumothorax as a presenting feature of primary carcinoma of the lung. Dis Chest 27:457, 1955.
625. Citron KM: Spontaneous pneumothorax complicating bronchial carcinoma. Tubercle 40:384, 1959.
626. Khan F, Seriff NS: Pneumothorax. A rare presenting manifestation of lung cancer. Am Rev Respir Dis 108:1397, 1973.
627. Schulman P, Cheng E, Cvitkovic E, et al: Spontaneous pneumo-

18

thorax as a result of intensive cytotoxic chemotherapy. Chest 75:194, 1979.

628. Lote K, Dahl O, Vigander T: Pneumothorax during combination chemotherapy. Cancer 47:1743, 1981.

629. Lesser JE, Carr D: Fatal pneumothorax following bleomycin and other cytotoxic drugs. Cancer Treat Rep 69:344, 1985.

630. D'Angio GJ, Iannaccone G: Spontaneous pneumothorax as a complication of pulmonary metastases in malignant tumors of childhood. Am J Roentgenol 86:1092, 1961.

631. Dines DE, Cortese DA, Brennan MD, et al: Malignant pulmonary neoplasms predisposing to spontaneous pneumothorax. Mayo Clin Proc 48:541, 1973.

632. D'Ettorre A, Babini L: Pneumothorax from pulmonary metastases. Ann Radiol Diag (Bologna) 38:595, 1965.

633. Janetos GP, Ochsner SF: Bilateral pneumothorax in metastatic osteogenic sarcoma. Am Rev Respir Dis 88:73, 1963.

634. Smevik B, Klepp O: The risk of spontaneous pneumothorax in patients with osteogenic sarcoma and testicular cancer. Cancer 49:1734, 1982.

635. Kader HA, Bolger JJ, Goepel JR: Bilateral pneumothorax secondary to metastatic angiosarcoma of the breast. Clin Radiol 38:201, 1987.

636. Lobo AJ, Butland RJ, Stewart S, et al: Primary cardiac angiosarcoma causing rupture of the heart and spontaneous bilateral pneumothorax. Thorax 44:78, 1989.

637. Michelassi PL, Sbragia S: Clinicoradiological considerations on 2 cases of spontaneous pneumothorax, apparently idiopathic, secondary to pulmonary metastases. Ann Radiol Diag 33:39, 1960.

638. Slasky BS, Deutsch M: Germ cell tumors complicated by pneumothorax. Urology 22:39, 1983.

639. Wall SD, Federle MP, Jeffrey RB, et al: CT diagnosis of unsuspected pneumothorax after blunt abdominal trauma. Am J Roentgenol 141:919, 1983.

640. Brewer LL, Moskowitz PS, Carrington CB, et al: Pneumatosis pulmonalis. A complication of the idiopathic respiratory distress syndrome. Am J Pathol 95:171, 1979.

641. Tomashefski JF, Bruce M, Stern RC, et al: Pulmonary air cysts in cystic fibrosis: Relation of pathologic features to radiologic findings and history of pneumothorax. Hum Pathol 16:253, 1985.

642. Tomashefski JF, Dahms B, Bruce M: Pleura in pneumothorax. Comparison of patients with cystic fibrosis and "idiopathic" spontaneous pneumothorax. Arch Pathol Lab Med 109:910, 1985.

643. Askin FB, McCann BG, Kuhn C: Reactive eosinophilic pleuritis. A lesion to be distinguished from pulmonary eosinophilic granuloma. Arch Pathol Lab Med 101:187, 1977.

644. Askin FB, McCann BG, Kuhn C: Reactive eosinophilic pleuritis. A lesion to be distinguished from pulmonary eosinophilic granuloma. Arch Pathol Lab Med 101:187, 1977.

645. McDonnell TJ, Crouch EC, Gonzalez JG: Reactive eosinophilic pleuritis. A sequela of pneumothorax in pulmonary eosinophilic granuloma. Am J Clin Pathol 91:107, 1989.

646. McDonnell TJ, Crouch EC, Gonzalez JG: Reactive eosinophilic pleuritis. A sequela of pneumothorax in pulmonary eosinophilic granuloma. Am J Clin Pathol 91:107, 1989.

647. Riemann R, Jakse R: Pneumothorax nach mediastinalemphysem. über den ort und den mechanismus der pleuraruptur. Acta Anat 128:115, 1986.

648. Maurer ER, Schaal JA, Mendez FL: Chronic recurrent spontaneous pneumothorax due to endometriosis of the diaphragm. JAMA 168:2013, 1958.

649. Slasky BS, Siewers RD, Lecky JW, et al: Catamenial pneumothorax: The roles of diaphragmatic defects and endometriosis. Am J Roentgenol 138:639, 1982.

650. Soderberg CH Jr, Dahlquist EH Jr: Catamenial pneumothorax. Surgery 79:236, 1976.

651. Müller NL, Nelems B: Postcoital catamenial pneumothorax. Report of a case not associated with endometriosis and successfully treated with tubal ligation. Am Rev Respir Dis 134:803, 1986.

652. Lillington GA, Mitchell SP, Wood GA: Catamenial pneumothorax. JAMA 219:1328, 1972.

653. Balasingham S, Arulkumaran S, Nadarajah K, et al: Catamenial pneumothorax. Aust NZ J Obstet Gynaecol 26:88, 1986.

654. Stern H, Toole AL, Merino M: Catamenial pneumothorax. Chest 78:480, 1980.

655. Furman WR, Wang KP, Summer WR, et al: Catamenial pneumothorax: Evaluation by fiberoptic pleuroscopy. Am Rev Respir Dis 121:137, 1980.

656. Rossi NP, Goplerud CP: Recurrent catamenial pneumothorax. Arch Surg 109:173, 1974.

657. Editorial. Spontaneous pneumothorax and menstruation. Br Med J 1:269, 1969.

658. Davies R: Recurring spontaneous pneumothorax concomitant with menstruation. Thorax 23:370, 1968.

659. Hinson JM, Brigham KL, Daniell J: Catamenial pneumothorax in sisters. Chest 80:634, 1981.

660. Im J-G, Kang HS, Choi BI, et al: Pleural endometriosis: CT and sonographic findings. Am J Roentgenol 148:523, 1987.

661. Birrer RB, Calderon J: Pneumothorax, pneumomediastinum, and pneumopericardium following Valsalva's maneuver during marijuana smoking. NY State J Med 84:619, 1984.

662. Najafi JA, Guzman LG: Spontaneous pneumothorax in labor. Am J Obstet Gynecol 129:463, 1977.

663. Najafi JA, Guzman LG: Spontaneous pneumothorax in labor: Case report. Milit Med 143:341, 1978.

664. Bending JJ: Spontaneous pneumothorax in pregnancy and labour. Postgrad Med J 58:711, 1982.

665. Farrell SJ: Spontaneous pneumothorax in pregnancy: A case report and review of the literature. Obstet Gynecol 62(3 Suppl):43s, 1983.

666. Miller WE, Spiekerman RE, Hepper NG: Pneumomediastinum resulting from performing Valsalva maneuvers during marihuana smoking. Chest 62:233, 1972.

667. Bush MN, Rubenstein R, Hoffman I, et al: Spontaneous pneumomediastinum as a consequence of cocaine use. NY State J Med 84:618, 1984.

668. Luque MA III, Cavallaro DL, Torres M, et al: Pneumomediastinum, pneumothorax, and subcutaneous emphysema after alternate cocaine inhalation and marijuana smoking. Pediatr Emerg Care 3:107, 1987.

669. Arnold S, Feathers RS, Gibbs E: Bilateral pneumothoraces and subcutaneous emphysema: A complication of internal jugular venipuncture. Br Med J 1:211, 1973.

670. Maggs PR, Schwaber JR: Fatal bilateral pneumothoraces complicating subclavian vein catheterization. Chest 71:552, 1977.

671. Matz R: Complications of determining the central venous pressure. N Engl J Med 273:703, 1965.

672. Schapira M, Stern WZ: Hazards of subclavian vein cannulation for central venous pressure monitoring. JAMA 201:327, 1967.

673. Slezak FA, Williams GB: Delayed pneumothorax: A complication of subclavian vein catheterization. J Parenter Enteral Nutr 8:571, 1984.

674. Saltzberg DM, Goldstein M, Levine GM: Feeding tube-induced pneumothorax. J Parenter Enteral Nutr 8:714, 1984.

675. Sheffner SE, Gross BH, Birnberg FA, et al: Iatrogenic bronchopleural fistula caused by feeding tube insertion. J Can Assoc Radiol 36:52, 1985.

676. Konarzewski WH, Richards GD, Thomson SJ: Pneumothorax following insertion of a nasogastric tube (letter). Anaesthesia 41:678, 1986.

677. Scholten DJ, Wood TL, Thompson DR: Pneumothorax from nasoenteric feeding tube insertion. A report of five cases. Am Surg 52:381, 1986.

678. Padovan IF, Dawson CA, Henschel EO, et al: Pathogenesis of mediastinal emphysema and pneumothorax following tracheotomy (experimental approaches). Chest 66:553, 1974.

679. Biswas C, Jana N, Maitra S: Bilateral pneumothorax following tracheal intubation. Br J Anaesth 62:338, 1989.

680. Odland R, Adams G: Pneumothorax as a complication of tracheoesophageal voice prosthesis use. Ann Otol Rhinol Laryngol 97:537, 1988.

681. Schmidt G, Börsch G, Wegener M: Subcutaneous emphysema and pneumothorax complicating diagnostic colonoscopy. Dis Colon Rectum 29:136, 1986.

682. Honet JE, Honet JC, Cascade P: Pneumothorax after electromyographic electrode insertion in the paracervical muscles: Case report and radiographic analysis. Arch Phys Med Rehabil 67:601, 1986.

683. Ritter HG, Tarala R: Pneumothorax after acupuncture. Br Med J 2:602, 1978.

684. Catania S, Boccato P, Bono A, et al: Pneumothorax: A rare complication of fine needle aspiration of the breast. Acta Cytol 33:140, 1989.

685. Munshi CA, Bardeen-Henschel A: Hydropneumothorax after percutaneous nephrolithotomy. Anesth Analg 64:840, 1985.

686. O'Donnell A, Schoenberger C, Weiner J, et al: Pulmonary complications of percutaneous nephrostomy and kidney stone extraction. South Med J 81:1002, 1988.

687. de Latorre FJ, Tomasa A, Klamburg J, et al: Incidence of pneumothorax and pneumomediastinum in patients with aspiration pneumonia requiring ventilatory support. Chest 72:141, 1977.

688. Albelda SM, Gefter WB, Kelley MA, et al: Ventilator-induced subpleural air cysts: Clinical, radiographic, and pathologic significance. Am Rev Respir Dis 127:360, 1983.

689. Douglass RE, Levison MA: Pneumothorax in drug abusers. An urban epidemic? Am Surg 52:377, 1986.

690. Wisdom K, Nowak RM, Richardson HH, et al: Alternate therapy for traumatic pneumothorax in "pocket shooters." Ann Emerg Med 15:428, 1986.

691. Lewis JW Jr, Groux N, Elliot JP Jr, et al: Complications of attempted central venous injections performed by drug abusers. Chest 78:613, 1980.

692. Cohen HL, Cohen SW: Spontaneous bilateral pneumothorax in drug addicts. Chest 86:645, 1984.

693. Savitt D, Oblinger P, Levy RC: Bilateral pneumothorax in an intravenous drug abuser. J Emerg Med 2:405, 1985.
694. Zorc TG, O'Donnell AE, Holt RW, et al: Bilateral pneumothorax secondary to intravenous drug abuse. Chest 93:645, 1988.
695. Roelandt J, Willems J, van der Hauwaert LG, et al: Clicks and sounds (whoops) in left-sided pneumothorax: A clinical and phonocardiographic study. Dis Chest 56:31, 1969.
696. Desser KB, Benchimol A: Clicks secondary to pneumothorax confounding diagnosis of mitral valve prolapse. Chest 71:523, 1977.
697. Widder D: Ptosis associated with iatrogenic pneumothorax: A false lateralizing sign. Arch Intern Med 142:145, 1982.
698. McCall CS, Nguyen TQ, Vines FS, et al: Pneumocephalus secondary to tension pneumothorax associated with comminuted fracture of the thoracic spine. Neurosurgery 19:120, 1986.
699. Bogaert MG, van der Straeten M: Relapsing spontaneous pneumopericardium and pneumothorax with proven pleuropericardial defect. A case report. Scand J Respir Dis 60:17, 1979.
700. Pettersson GB, Gatzinsky P, Selin K: A case of total bilateral spontaneous pneumothorax. Scand J Thorac Cardiovasc Surg 17:175, 1983.
701. Donovan PJ: Bilateral spontaneous pneumothorax: A rare entity. Ann Emerg Med 16:1277, 1987.
702. Hickok DF, Ballenger FP: The management of spontaneous pneumothorax due to emphysematous blebs. Surg Gynecol Obstet 120:499, 1965.
703. Peatfield RC, Edwards PR, Johnson NM: Two unexpected deaths from pneumothorax. Lancet 1:356, 1979.
704. Woodruff WW III, Gamba JL, Putman CE, et al: Chronic tension pneumothorax presumably due to a "ball valve" bronchopleural fistula. South Med J 79:510, 1986.
705. Abyholm FE, Storen G: Spontaneous haemopneumothorax. Thorax 28:376, 1973.
706. Adelman M, Albelda SM, Gottlieb J, et al: Diagnostic utility of pleural fluid eosinophilia. Am J Med 77:915, 1984.
707. Norris RM, Jones JG, Bishop JM: Respiratory gas exchange in patients with spontaneous pneumothorax. Thorax 23:427, 1968.
708. Anthonisen NR: Regional lung function in spontaneous pneumothorax. Am Rev Respir Dis 115:873, 1977.
709. Fleetham JA, Forkert L, Clarke H, et al: Regional lung function in the presence of pleural symphysis. Am Rev Respir Dis 122:33, 1980.
710. Lange P, Mortensen J, Groth S: Lung function 22–35 years after treatment of idiopathic spontaneous pneumothorax with talc poudrage or simple drainage. Thorax 43:559, 1988.
711. Loring SH, Kurachek SC, Wohl ME: Diaphragmatic excursion after pleural sclerosis. Chest 95:374, 1989.
712. Yamazaki S, Ogawa J, Shohzu A, et al: Pulmonary blood flow to rapidly re-expanded lung in spontaneous pneumothorax. Chest 81:118, 1982.
713. Pavlin DJ, Raghu G, Rogers TR, et al: Reexpansion hypotension. A complication of rapid evacuation of prolonged pneumothorax. Chest 89:70, 1986.
714. Butler C II, Kleinerman J: The pulmonary apical cap. Am J Pathol 60:205, 1970.
715. Renner RR, Markarian B, Pernice NJ, et al: The apical cap. Radiology 110:569, 1974.
716. Fraser RG, Paré JAPP: Diagnosis of Diseases of the Chest: An Integrated Study Based on the Abnormal Roentgenogram. Philadelphia, WB Saunders, 1970.
717. Jamison HW: An anatomic-roentgenographic study of the pleural domes and pulmonary apices: With special reference to apical subpleural scars. Radiology 36:302, 1941.
718. Fisher MS: Asymmetrical changes in asbestos-related disease. J Can Assoc Radiol 36:110, 1985.
719. Withers BF, Ducatman AM, Yang WN: Roentgenographic evidence for predominant left-sided location of unilateral pleural plaques. Chest 95:1262, 1989.
720. Lawson JP: Pleural calcification as a sign of asbestosis: A report of three cases. Clin Radiol 14:414, 1963.
721. Schneider L, Wimpfheimer F: Multiple progressive calcific pleural plaque formation; a sign of silicosis. JAMA 189:328, 1964.
722. Kiviluoto R: Pleural calcification as a roentgenologic sign of nonoccupational endemic anthophyllite-asbestosis. Acta Radiol (Suppl)194, 1960.
723. Fletcher DE, Edge JR: The early radiological changes in pulmonary and pleural asbestosis. Clin Radiol 21:355, 1970.
724. Oosthuizen SF, Theron CP, Sluis-Cremer GK: Calcified pleural plaques in asbestosis. An investigation into their significance. Med Proc (Johannesburg) 10:496, 1964.
725. Roberts WC, Ferrans VJ: Pure collagen plaques on the diaphragm and pleura—gross, histologic and electron microscopic observations. Chest 61:357, 1972.
726. MacKenzie FAF: The radiological investigation of the early manifestations of exposure to asbestos dust. Proc R Soc Med 64:834, 1971.
727. Sherman CB, Barnhart S, Rosenstock L: Use of oblique chest roentgenograms in detecting pleural disease in asbestos-exposed workers. J Occup Med 30:681, 1988.
728. Svenes KB, Borgersen A, Haaversen O, et al: Parietal pleural plaques: A comparison between autopsy and X-ray findings. Eur J Respir Dis 69:10, 1986.
729. Vückeri M, Jääskeläinen J, Tähti E: Ultrasonic examination of pleural thickenings and calcifications in occupational asbestosis. Dis Chest 54:17, 1968.
730. Bourbeau J, Ernst P: Between- and within-reader variability in the assessment of pleural abnormality using the ILO 1980 international classification of pneumoconiosis. Am J Ind Med 14:537, 1988.
731. MacPherson P, Davidson JK: Correlation between lung asbestos count at necropsy and radiological appearances. Br Med J 1:355, 1969.
732. Constantopoulos SH, Goudevenos JA, Saratzis NA, et al: Metsovo lung: Pleural calcification and restrictive lung function in northwestern Greece. Environmental exposure to mineral fiber as etiology. Environ Res 38:319, 1985.
733. Constantopoulos SH, Saratzis NA, Kontogiannis D, et al: Tremolite whitewashing and pleural calcification. Chest 92:709, 1987.
734. Yazicioglu S, Ilcayto R, Balci K, et al: Pleural calcification, pleural mesotheliomas, and bronchial cancers caused by tremolite dust. Thorax 35:564, 1980.
735. Baris YI, Sahin AA, Erkan ML: Clinical and radiological study in sepiolite workers. Arch Environ Health 35:343, 1980.
736. De Vuyst P, Mairesse M, Gaudichet A, et al: Mineralogical analysis of bronchoalveolar lavage fluid as an aid to diagnosis of "imported" pleural asbestosis. Thorax 38:628, 1983.
737. Boutin C, Viallat JR, Steinbauer J, et al: Bilateral pleural plaques in Corsica: A nonoccupational asbestos exposure marker. Eur J Respir Dis 69:4, 1986.
738. Churg A, DePaoli L: Environmental pleural plaques in residents of a Quebec chrysotile mining town. Chest 94:58, 1988.
739. Fridriksson HV, Hedenstrom H, Hillerdal G, et al: Increased lung stiffness in persons with pleural plaques. Eur J Respir Dis 62:412, 1981.
740. Hjortsberg U, Orbaek P, Aborelius M Jr, et al: Railroad workers with pleural plaques: I. Spirometric and nitrogen washout investigation on smoking and nonsmoking asbestos-exposed workers. Am J Ind Med 14:635, 1988.
741. Jones RN, McLoud T, Rockoff SD: The radiographic pleural abnormalities in asbestos exposure: Relationship to physiologic abnormalities. J Thorac Imaging 3:57, 1988.
742. Anton HC: Multiple pleural plaques, part II. Br J Radiol 41:341, 1968.
743. Freundlich IM, Greening RR: Asbestosis and associated medical problems. Radiology 89:224, 1967.
744. Smith AR: Pleural calcification resulting from exposure to certain dusts. Am J Roentgenol 67:375, 1952.
745. Solomon A: Radiology of asbestosis. Environ Res 3:320, 1970.
746. Kleinfeld M: Pleural calcification as a sign of silicosis. Am J Med Sci 251:215, 1966.
747. Krige L: Asbestosis—With special reference to the radiological diagnosis. S Afr J Radiol 4:13, 1966.
748. Buchanan DR, Johnston ID, Kerr IH, et al: Cryptogenic bilateral fibrosing pleuritis. Br J Dis Chest 82:186, 1988.
749. McLoud TC, Woods BO, Carrington CB, et al: Diffuse pleural thickening in an asbestos-exposed population: Prevalence and causes. Am J Roentgenol 144:9, 1985.
750. Bohlig H, Calavrezos A: Development, radiological zone patterns, and importance of diffuse pleural thickening in relation to occupational exposure to asbestos. Br J Ind Med 44:673, 1987.
751. Corris PA, Best JJ, Gibson GJ: Effects of diffuse pleural thickening on respiratory mechanics. Eur Respir J 1:248, 1988.
752. Picado C, Laporta D, Grassino A, et al: Mechanisms affecting exercise performance in subjects with asbestos-related pleural fibrosis. Lung 165:45, 1987.
753. Bates DV, Macklem PT, Christie RV: Respiratory Function in Disease; an Introduction to the Integrated Study of the Lung, 2nd ed. Philadelphia, WB Saunders, 1971.
754. Nieminen MM, Antila P, Markkula H, et al: Effect of decortication in fibrothorax on pulmonary function. Respiration 48:94, 1985.
755. Toomes H, Vogt—Moykopf I, Ahrendt J: Decortication of the lung. Thorac Cardiovasc Surg 31:338, 1983.
756. Lynch DA, Gamsu G, Ray CS, et al: Asbestos-related focal lung masses: Manifestations on conventional and high-resolution CT scans. Radiology 169:603, 1988.
757. Hillerdal G: Rounded atelectasis. Clinical experience with 74 patients. Chest 95:836, 1989.
758. Mintzer RA, Cugell DW: The association of asbestos-induced pleural disease and rounded atelectasis. Chest 81:457, 1982.
759. Menzies R, Fraser R: Round atelectasis. Pathologic and pathogenetic features. Am J Surg Pathol 11:674, 1987.

18

760. Ren H, Hruban RH, Kuhlman JE, et al: Computed tomography of rounded atelectasis. J Comput Assist Tomogr 12:1031, 1988.

761. Schneider HJ, Felson B, Gonzalez LL: Rounded atelectasis. Am J Roentgenol 134:225, 1980.

762. Cho S-R, Henry DA, Beachley MC, et al: Round (helical) atelectasis. Br J Radiol 54:643, 1981.

763. Doyle TC, Lawler GA: CT features of rounded atelectasis of the lung. Am J Roentgenol 143:225, 1984.

764. England DM, Hochholzer L, McCarthy MJ: Localized benign and malignant fibrous tumors of the pleura. A clinicopathologic review of 223 cases. Am J Surg Pathol 13(8):640, 1989.

765. Yesner R, Hurwitz A: Localized pleural mesothelioma of epithelial type. J Thorac Surg 26:325, 1953.

766. Elborn JS, Conn P, Roberts SD: Refractory massive pleural effusion in systemic lupus erythematosus treated by pleurectomy. Ann Rheum Dis 46:77, 1987.

767. Briselli M, Mark EJ, Dickerson GR: Solitary fibrous tumors of the pleura: Eight new cases and review of 360 cases in the literature. Cancer 47:2678, 1981.

768. Bilbey JH, Müller NL, Miller RR, et al: Localized fibrous mesothelioma of pleura following external ionizing radiation therapy. Chest 94:1291, 1988.

769. Kawai T, Mikata A, Torikata C, et al: Solitary (localized) pleural mesothelioma. A light- and electron-microscopic study. Am J Surg Pathol 2:365, 1978.

770. Doucet J, Dardick I, Srigley JR, et al: Localized fibrous tumour of serosal surfaces. Immunohistochemical and ultrastructural evidence for a type of mesothelioma. Virchows Arch (Pathol Anat) 409:349, 1986.

771. Stout AP, Murray MR: Localized pleural mesothelioma. Arch Pathol 34:951, 1942.

772. Carter D, Otis CN: Three types of spindle cell tumors of the pleura. Fibroma, sarcoma, and sarcomatoid mesothelioma. Am J Surg Pathol 12:747, 1988.

773. Dervan PA, Tobin B, O'Connor M: Solitary (localized) fibrous mesothelioma: Evidence against mesothelial cell origin. Histopathol 10:867, 1986.

774. Hernandez FJ, Fernandez BB: Localized fibrous tumors of pleura: A light and electron microscopic study. Cancer 34:1667, 1974.

775. Said JW, Nash G, Banks-Schlegel S, et al: Localized fibrous mesothelioma: An immunohistochemical and electron microscopic study. Hum Pathol 15:440, 1984.

776. El-Naggar AK, Ro JY, Ayala AG, et al: Localized fibrous tumor of the serosal cavities. Immunohistochemical, electron-microscopic, and flow-cytometric DNA study. Am J Clin Pathol 92:561, 1989.

777. Scharifker D, Kaneko M: Localized fibrous "mesothelioma" of pleura (submesothelial fibroma). A clinicopathologic study of 18 cases. Cancer 43:627, 1979.

778. Okike N, Bernatz PE, Woolner LB: Localized mesothelioma of the pleura. Benign and malignant variants. J Thorac Cardiovasc Surg 75(3):363, 1978.

779. Witkin GB, Rosai J: Solitary fibrous tumor of the mediastinum. A report of 14 cases. Am J Surg Pathol 13(7):547, 1989.

780. Yousem SA, Flynn SD: Intrapulmonary localized fibrous tumor. Intraparenchymal so-called localized fibrous mesothelioma. Am J Clin Pathol 89:365, 1988.

781. Janssen JP, Wagenaar SS, van den Bosch JM, et al: Benign localized mesothelioma of the pleura. Histopathology 9:309, 1985.

782. Blobel GA, Moll R, Franke WW, et al: The intermediate filament cytoskeleton of malignant mesotheliomas and its diagnostic significance. Am J Pathol 121:235, 1985.

783. Epstein JI, Budin RE: Keratin and epithelial membrane antigen immunoreactivity in non-neoplastic pleural lesions: Implications for the diagnosis of desmoplastic mesothelioma. Hum Pathol 17:514, 1986.

784. Hutchinson WB, Friedenberg MJ: Intrathoracic mesothelioma. Radiology 80:937, 1963.

785. Hahn PF, Novelline RA, Mark EJ: Arteriography in the localization of massive pleural tumors. Am J Roentgenol 139:814, 1982.

786. Dedrick CG, McLoud TC, Shepard JO, et al: Computed tomography of localized pleural mesothelioma. Am J Roentgenol 144:275, 1985.

787. Hayward RH: Migrating lung tumor. Chest 66:77, 1974.

788. Berne AS, Heitzman ER: The roentgenologic signs of pedunculated pleural tumors. Am J Roentgenol 87:892, 1962.

789. Zamperlin A, Drigo R, Famulare CI, et al: A vagabond pleural pebble. Respiration 51:155, 1987.

790. Mengeot PM, Gailly CH: Spontaneous detachment of benign mesothelioma into the pleural space and removal during pleuroscopy. Eur J Respir Dis 68:141, 1986.

791. Nathan H, Seiden D: Localized fibrous mesothelioma of the pleura. Int Surg 63:161, 1978.

792. Kniznik DO, Roncoroni AJ, Rosenberg M, et al: Giant fibrous pleural mesothelioma associated with myocardial restriction and hypoglycemia. Respiration 37:346, 1979.

793. Mandal AK, Rozer MA, Salem FA, et al: Localized benign mesothelioma of the pleura associated with a hypoglycemic episode. Arch Intern Med 143:1608, 1983.

794. Okike N, Bernatz PE, Woolner LB: Localized mesothelioma of the pleura: Benign and malignant variants. J Thorac Cardiovasc Surg 75:363, 1978.

795. Connelly RR, Spirtas R, Myers MH, et al: Demographic patterns for mesothelioma in the United States. JNCI 78:1053, 1987.

796. Spirtas R, Beebe GW, Connelly RR, et al: Recent trends in mesothelioma incidence in the United States. Am J Ind Med 9:397, 1986.

797. Willis RA: Pathology of Tumours, 3rd Ed. London, Butterworths, 1960.

798. Legha SS, Muggia FM: Pleural mesothelioma: Clinical features and therapeutic implications. Ann Intern Med 87:613, 1977.

799. Craighead JE: Current pathogenetic concepts of diffuse malignant mesothelioma. Hum Pathol 18:544, 1987.

800. Law MR, Hodson ME, Heard BE: Malignant mesothelioma of the pleura: Relation between histological type and clinical behaviour. Thorax 37:810, 1982.

801. Jones RD, Smith DM, Thomas PG: Mesothelioma in Great Britain in 1968–1983. Scand J Work Environ Health 14:145, 1988.

802. Wagner JC, Sleggs CA, Marchand P: Diffuse pleural mesothelioma and asbestos exposure in the northwestern Cape Province. Br J Ind Med 7:260, 1960.

803. Wright GW: Asbestos and health in 1969. Am Rev Respir Dis 100:467, 1969.

804. Borow M, Couston A, Livornese L, et al: Mesothelioma following exposure to asbestos. A review of 72 cases. Chest 64:641, 1973.

805. Whitwell F, Rawcliffe RM: Diffuse malignant pleural mesothelioma and asbestos exposure. Thorax 26:6, 1971.

806. Armstrong BK, Musk AW, Baker JE, et al: Epidemiology of malignant mesothelioma in Western Australia. Med J Aust 141:86, 1984.

807. Teta MJ, Lewinsohn HC, Meigs JW, et al: Mesothelioma in Connecticut, 1955–1977. Occupational and geographic associations. J Occup Med 25:749, 1983.

808. Solomons K: Malignant mesothelioma—Clinical and epidemiological features. A report of 80 cases. S Afr Med J 66:407, 1984.

809. Edge JR, Choudhury SL: Malignant mesothelioma of the pleura in Barrow-in-Furness. Thorax 33:26, 1978.

810. Hasan FM, Nash G, Kazemi H: The significance of asbestos exposure in the diagnosis of mesothelioma: A 28-year experience from a major urban hospital. Am Rev Respir Dis 115:761, 1977.

811. Wolf KM, Piotrowski ZH, Engel JD, et al: Malignant mesothelioma with occupational and environmental asbestos exposure in an Illinois community hospital. Arch Intern Med 147:2145, 1987.

812. Davies D: Are all mesotheliomas due to asbestos? (Editorial.) Br Med J 289:1164, 1984.

813. Churg A: Malignant mesothelioma in British Columbia in 1982. Cancer 55:672, 1985.

814. Hasan FM, Nash G, Kazemi H: The significance of asbestos exposure in the diagnosis of mesothelioma: A 28-year experience from a major urban hospital. Am Rev Respir Dis 115:761, 1977.

815. Gracey DR, Cugell DW, Bazley ES, et al: Pulmonary complications of asbestos exposure. Chest 59:77, 1971.

816. Chen W-J, Mottet NK: Malignant mesothelioma with minimal asbestos exposure. Hum Pathol 9:253, 1978.

817. Jefferys DB, Vale JA: Malignant mesothelioma and gas-mask assemblers. Br Med J 2:607, 1978.

818. Ferguson DA, Berry G, Jelihovsky T, et al: The Australian Mesothelioma Surveillance Program 1979–1985. Med J Aust 147:166, 1987.

819. Mowé G, Gylseth B, Hartveit F, et al: Occupational asbestos exposure, lung-fiber concentration and latency time in malignant mesothelioma. Scand J Work Environ Health 10:293, 1984.

820. Elmes PC, Wade OL: Relationship between exposure to asbestos and pleural malignancy in Belfast. Ann NY Acad Sci 132:549, 1965.

821. McDonald AD, Harper A, El-Attar OA, et al: Epidemiology of primary malignant mesothelial tumors in Canada. Cancer 26:914, 1970.

822. Acheson ED, Bennett C, Gardner MJ, et al: Mesothelioma in a factory using amosite and chrysotile asbestos. Lancet 2:1403, 1981.

823. Churg A, Wiggs B: Fiber size and number in amphibole asbestos-induced mesothelioma. Am J Pathol 115:437, 1984.

824. Elmes P: Asbestosis and mesothelioma (proceedings). Br J Dis Chest 73:50, 1979.

825. Dorward AJ, Stack BHR: Diffuse malignant pleural mesothelioma in Glasgow. Br J Dis Chest 75:397, 1981.

826. Sheers G, Coles RM: Mesothelioma risks in a naval dockyard. Arch Environ Health 35:276, 1980.

827. Kishimoto T, Okada K, Sato T, et al: Evaluation of the pleural malignant mesothelioma patients with the relation of asbestos exposure. Environ Res 48:42, 1989.

828. Morrison HI, Band PR, Gallagher R, et al: Recent trends in incidence rates of pleural mesothelioma in British Columbia. Can Med Assoc J 131:1069, 1984.

829. Epler GR, FitzGerald MX, Gaensler EA, et al: Asbestos-related disease from household exposure. Respiration 39:229, 1980.
830. Fischbein A, Rohl AN: Pleural mesothelioma and neighborhood asbestos exposure. Findings from micro-chemical analysis of lung tissue. JAMA 252:86, 1984.
831. Constantopoulos SH, Malamou-Mitsi VD, Goudevenos JA, et al: High incidence of malignant pleural mesothelioma in neighbouring villages of Northwestern Greece. Respiration 51:266, 1987.
832. Langer AM, Nolan RP, Constantopoulos SH, et al: Association of Metsovo lung and pleural mesothelioma with exposure to tremolite-containing whitewash. Lancet 1:965, 1987.
833. Magee F, Wright JL, Chan N, et al: Malignant mesothelioma caused by childhood exposure to long-fiber low aspect ratio tremolite. Am J Ind Med 9:529, 1986.
834. McConnochie K, Simonato L, Mavrides P, et al: Mesothelioma in Cyprus: The role of tremolite. Thorax 42:342, 1987.
835. Whitwell F, Scott J, Grimshaw M: Relationship between occupation and asbestos-fibre content of the lungs in patients with pleural mesothelioma, lung cancer, and other diseases. Thorax 32:377, 1977.
836. Roggli VL, McGavran MH, Subach J, et al: Pulmonary asbestos body counts and electron probe analysis of asbestos body cores in patients with mesothelioma: A study of 25 cases. Cancer 50:2423, 1982.
837. Wagner JC, Moncrieff CB, Coles R, et al: Correlation between fibre content of the lungs and disease in naval dockyard workers. Br J Ind Med 43:391, 1986.
838. Antman KH, Corson JM: Benign and malignant pleural mesothelioma. Clin Chest Med 6:127, 1985.
839. Mowé G, Gylseth B, Hartveit F, et al: Fiber concentration in lung tissue of patients with malignant mesothelioma. A case-control study. Cancer 56:1089, 1985.
840. Churg A, Wiggs B: Fiber size and number in amphibole asbestos-induced mesothelioma. Am J Pathol 115:437, 1984.
841. Editorial. Amosite asbestos and mesothelioma. Lancet 2:1397, 1981.
842. Humphrey EW, Ewing SL, Wrigley JV, et al: The production of malignant tumors of the lung and pleura in dogs from intratracheal asbestos instillation and cigarette smoking. Cancer 47:1994, 1981.
843. Meurman LO, Kiviluoto R, Hakama M: Mortality and morbidity among the working population of anthophyllite asbestos miners in Finland. Br J Ind Med 31:105, 1974.
844. Becklake MR: Asbestos-related diseases of the lung and other organs: Their epidemiology and implications for clinical practice. Am Rev Respir Dis 114:187, 1976.
845. Webster I: Asbestosis. S Afr Med J 38:870, 1964.
846. Editorial. Asbestosis and malignant disease. N Engl J Med 72:590, 1965.
847. Elmes PC: Mesotheliomas, minerals, and man-made mineral fibres. Thorax 35:561, 1980.
848. McDonald AD, Fry JS, Woolley AJ, et al: Dust exposure and mortality in an American chrysotile textile plant. Br J Ind Med 40:361, 1983.
849. Hughes JM, Weill H, Hammad YY: Mortality of workers employed in two asbestos cement manufacturing plants. Br J Ind Med 44:161, 1987.
850. Churg A, Wiggs B, Depaoli L, et al: Lung asbestos content in chrysotile workers with mesothelioma. Am Rev Respir Dis 130:1042, 1984.
851. McDonald JC, Armstrong B, Case B, et al: Mesothelioma and asbestos fiber type. Evidence from lung tissue analysis. Cancer 63:1544, 1989.
852. Churg A: Asbestos fiber content of the lungs in patients with and without asbestos airways disease. Am Rev Respir Dis 127:470, 1983.
853. Gylseth B, Mowé G, Wannag A: Fibre type and concentration in the lungs of workers in an asbestos cement factory. Br J Ind Med 40:375, 1983.
854. Wang NS, Jaurand MC, Magne L, et al: The interactions between asbestos fibers and metaphase chromosomes of rat pleural mesothelial cells in culture. A scanning and transmission electron microscopic study. Am J Pathol 126:343, 1987.
855. Wagner JC: Mesothelioma and mineral fibers. Cancer 57:1905, 1986.
856. Marcinski A, Cieslak H, Swiatkowska I: Mesothelioma of the pleura in children. Ann Radiol 17:327, 1974.
857. Lin-Chu M, Lee Y-J, Ho MY: Malignant mesothelioma in infancy. Arch Pathol Lab Med 113:409, 1989.
858. Baris YI, Sahin AA, Ozesmi M, et al: An outbreak of pleural mesothelioma and chronic fibrosing pleurisy in the village of Karain/ Urgüp in Anatolia. Thorax 33:181, 1978.
859. Baris YI, Sarracci R, Simonato L, et al: Malignant mesothelioma and radiological chest abnormalities in two villages in central Turkey. Lancet 1:984, 1981.
860. Hillerdal G, Baris YI: Radiological study of pleural changes in relation to mesothelioma in Turkey. Thorax 38:443, 1983.
861. Wagner JC, Skidmore JW, Hill RJ, et al: Erionite exposure and mesotheliomas in rats. Br J Cancer 51:727, 1985.
862. Brenner J, Sordillo PP, Magill GB, et al: Malignant mesothelioma of the pleura: Review of 123 patients. Cancer 49:2431, 1982.
863. Austin MB, Fechner RE, Roggli VL: Pleural malignant mesothelioma following Wilms' tumor. Am J Clin Pathol 86:227, 1986.
864. Warren S, Brown CE, Chute RN, et al: Mesothelioma relative to asbestos, radiation, and methylcholanthrene. Arch Pathol Lab Med 105:305, 1981.
865. Nauta RJ, Osteen RT, Antman KH, et al: Clinical staging and the tendency of malignant pleural mesotheliomas to remain localized. Ann Thorac Surg 34:66, 1982.
866. Li FP, Lokich J, Lapey J, et al: Familial mesothelioma after intense asbestos exposure at home. JAMA 240:467, 1978.
867. Hammar SP, Bockus D, Remington F, et al: Familial mesothelioma: A report of two families. Hum Pathol 20:107, 1989.
868. Risberg B, Nickels J, Wagermark J: Familial clustering of malignant mesothelioma. Cancer 45:2422, 1980.
869. Martensson G, Larsson S, Zettergren L: Malignant mesothelioma in two pairs of siblings: Is there a hereditary predisposing factor? Eur J Respir Dis 65:179, 1984.
870. Krousel T, Garcas N, Rothschild H: Familial clustering of mesothelioma: A report on three affected persons in one family. Am J Prev Med 2:186, 1986.
871. Hillerdal G: Malignant mesothelioma 1982: Review of 4,710 published cases. Br J Dis Chest 77:321, 1983.
872. Berry G, Newhouse ML, Antonis P: Combined effect of asbestos and smoking on mortality from lung cancer and mesothelioma in factory workers. Br J Ind Med 42:12, 1985.
873. Whitaker D, Shilkin KB: Diagnosis of pleural malignant melothelioma in life—A practical approach. J Pathol 143:147, 1984.
874. Suzuki Y: Pathology of human malignant mesothelioma. Sem Oncol 8:268, 1980.
875. McCaughey WTE, Kannerstein M, Churg J: Tumors and pseudo-tumors of the serous membranes. Atlas of Tumor Pathology, Chapter 18. Washington DC, Armed Forces Institute of Pathology, 1985.
876. Gotfried MH, Quan SF, Sobonya RE: Diffuse epithelial pleural mesothelioma presenting as a solitary lung mass. Chest 84:99, 1983.
877. Okike N, Bernatz PE, Woolner LB: Localized mesothelioma of the pleura. Benign and malignant variants. J Thorac Cardiovasc Surg 75:363, 1978.
878. Martensson G, Hagmar B, Zettergren L: Diagnosis and prognosis in malignant pleural mesothelioma: A prospective study. Eur J Respir Dis 65:169, 1984.
879. Kwee WS, Veldhuizen RW, Golding RP, et al: Primary "adenosquamous" mesothelioma of the pleura. Virchows Arch (Pathol Anat) 393:353, 1981.
880. Cantin R, Al-Jabi M, McCaughey WTE: Desmoplastic diffuse mesothelioma. Am J Surg Pathol 6:215, 1982.
881. Donna A, Betta PG: Differentiation towards cartilage and bone in a primary tumour of pleura. Further evidence in support of the concept of mesodermoma. Histopathology 10:101, 1986.
882. Yousem SA, Hochholzer L: Malignant mesotheliomas with osseous and cartilaginous differentiation. Arch Pathol Lab Med 111:62, 1987.
883. Andrion A, Mazzucco G, Bernardi P, et al: Sarcomatous tumor of the chest wall with osteochondroid differentiation. Evidence of mesothelial origin. Am J Surg Pathol 13(8):707, 1989.
884. Henderson DW, Attwood HD, Constance TJ, et al: Lymphohistiocytoid mesothelioma: A rare lymphomatoid variant of predominantly sarcomatoid mesothelioma. Ultrastruct Pathol 12:367, 1988.
885. Sheldon CD, Herbert A, Gallagher PJ: Reactive mesothelial proliferation: A necropsy study. Thorax 36:901, 1981.
886. Hansen RM, Caya JG, Clowry LJ Jr, et al: Benign mesothelial proliferation with effusion. Clinicopathologic entity that may mimic malignancy. Am J Med 77:887, 1984.
887. McCaughey WTE, Al-Jabi M: Differentiation of serosal hyperplasia and neoplasia in biopsies. Path Annual 1:271, 1986.
888. Rosai J, Dehner LP: Nodular mesothelial hyperplasia in hernia sacs. A benign reactive condition simulating a neoplastic process. Cancer 35:165, 1975.
889. Herbert A, Gallagher PJ: Pleural biopsy in the diagnosis of malignant mesothelioma. Thorax 37:816, 1982.
890. Tuder RM: Malignant disease of the pleura: A histopathological study with special emphasis on diagnostic criteria and differentiation from reactive mesothelium. Histopathology 10:851, 1986.
891. Kwee WS, Veldhuizen RW, Golding RP, et al: Histologic distinction between malignant mesothelioma, benign pleural lesion and carcinoma metastasis. Virchows Arch (Pathol Anat) 397:287, 1982.
892. Kwee WS, Veldhuizen RW, Alons CA, et al: Quantitative and qualitative differences between benign and malignant mesothelial cells in pleural fluid. Acta Cytol 26:401, 1982.
893. Gavin FM, Gray C, Sutton J, et al: Morphometric differences between cytologically benign and malignant serous effusions. Acta Cytol 32:175, 1988.
894. Herbert A, Gallagher PJ: Interpretation of pleural biopsy specimens and aspirates with the immunoperoxidase technique. Thorax 37:822, 1982.
895. Krivinkova H, Pontén J, Blöndai T: The diagnosis of cancer from

18

body fluids. A comparison of cytology, DNA measurement, tissue culture, scanning and transmission microscopy. Acta Pathol Microbiol Scand A 84:455, 1976.

896. Frierson HF, Mills SE, Legier JF: Flow cytometric analysis of ploidy in immunohistochemically confirmed examples of malignant epithelial mesothelioma. Am J Clin Pathol 90:240, 1988.

897. Isoda K, Hamamoto Y: Polyploid mesothelial cells in pleural fluid. Acta Pathol Jpn 33(4):733, 1983.

898. Donna A, Betta PG, Robutti P: Use of antimesothelial cell antibody and computer assisted quantitative analysis for distinguishing between reactive and neoplastic serosal tissues. J Clin Pathol 40:1428, 1987.

899. Ayres JG, Crocker JG, Skilbeck NQ: Differentiation of malignant from normal and reactive mesothelial cells by the argyrophil technique for nucleolar organiser region associated proteins. Thorax 43:366, 1988.

900. Griffiths MH, Riddell RJ, Xipell JM: Malignant mesothelioma: A review of 35 cases with diagnosis and prognosis. Pathology 12:591, 1980.

901. Warnock ML, Stoloff A, Thor A: Differentiation of adenocarcinoma of the lung from mesothelioma. Periodic acid-Schiff, monoclonal antibodies B72.3, and Leu-M1. Am J Pathol 133:30, 1988.

902. Dewar A, Valente M, Ring NP, et al: Pleural mesothelioma of epithelial type and pulmonary adenocarcinoma: An ultrastructural and cytochemical comparison. J Pathol 152:309, 1987.

903. Kwee WS, Veldhuizen RW, Golding RP, et al: Histologic distinction between malignant mesothelioma, benign pleural lesion and carcinoma metastasis. Virchows Arch (Pathol Anat) 397:287, 1982.

904. Cibas ES, Corson JM, Pinkus GS: The distinction of adenocarcinoma from malignant mesothelioma in cell blocks of effusions: The role of routine mucin histochemistry and immunohistochemical assessment of carcinoembryonic antigen, keratin proteins, epithelial membrane antigen, and milk fat globule-derived antigen. Hum Pathol 18:67, 1987.

905. Strickler JG, Herndier BG, Rouse RV: Immunohistochemical staining in malignant mesotheliomas. Am J Clin Pathol 88:610, 1987.

906. Arai H, Kang K-Y, Sato H, et al: Significance of the quantification and demonstration of hyaluronic acid in tissue specimens for the diagnosis of pleural mesothelioma. Am Rev Respir Dis 120:529, 1979.

907. Loosli H, Hurlimann J: Immunohistological study of malignant diffuse mesotheliomas of the pleura. Histopathology 8:793, 1984.

908. Pfaltz M, Odermatt B, Christen B, et al: Immunohistochemistry in the diagnosis of malignant mesothelioma. Virchows Arch A 411:387, 1987.

909. Gibbs AR, Harach R, Wagner JC, et al: Comparison of tumour markers in malignant mesothelioma and pulmonary adenocarcinoma. Thorax 40:91, 1985.

910. Ordóéz NG: The immunohistochemical diagnosis of mesothelioma. Differentiation of mesothelioma and lung adenocarcinoma. Am J Surg Pathol 13(4):276, 1989.

911. Otis CN, Carter D, Cole S, et al: Immunohistochemical evaluation of pleural mesothelioma and pulmonary adenocarcinoma. A biinstitutional study of 47 cases. Am J Surg Pathol 11(6):445, 1987.

912. Churg A: Immunohistochemical staining for vimentin and keratin in malignant mesothelioma. Am J Surg Pathol 9:360, 1985.

913. Jasani B, Edwards RE, Thomas ND, et al: The use of vimentin antibodies in the diagnosis of malignant mesothelioma. Virchows Arch (Pathol Anat) 406:441, 1985.

914. Corson JM, Pinkus GS: Mesothelioma: Profile of keratin proteins and carcinoembryonic antigen. An immunoperoxidase study of 20 cases and comparison with pulmonary adenocarcinomas. Am J Pathol 108:80, 1982.

915. Battifora H, Kopinski MI: Distinction of mesothelioma from adenocarcinoma. An immunohistochemical approach. Cancer 55:1679, 1985.

916. Holden J, Churg A: Immunohistochemical staining for keratin and carcinoembryonic antigen in the diagnosis of malignant mesothelioma. Am J Surg Pathol 8:277, 1984.

917. Montag AG, Pinkus GS, Corson JM: Keratin protein immunoreactivity of sarcomatoid and mixed types of diffuse malignant mesothelioma: An immunoperoxidase study of 30 cases. Hum Pathol 19:336, 1988.

918. Noguchii M, Nakajima T, Hirohashi S, et al: Immunohistochemical distinction of malignant mesothelioma from pulmonary adenocarcinoma with anti-surfactant apoprotein, anti-Lewis[a], and anti-Tn antibodies. Hum Pathol 20:53, 1989.

919. Walts AE, Said JW, Banks-Schlegel S: Keratin and carcinoembryonic antigen in exfoliated mesothelial and malignant cells: An immunoperoxidase study. Am J Clin Pathol 80:671, 1983.

920. Walts AE, Said JW, Shintaku P, et al: Keratins of different molecular weight in exfoliated mesothelial and adenocarcinoma cells—An aid to cell identification. Am J Clin Pathol 81:442, 1984.

921. van der Kwast TH, Versnel MA, Delahaye M, et al: Expression of epithelial membrane antigen on malignant mesothelioma cells. An immunocytochemical and immunoelectron microscopic study. Acta Cytol 32:169, 1988.

922. Guzman J, Bross KJ, Würtemberger G, et al: Immunocytology in malignant pleural mesothelioma. Expression of tumor markers and distribution of lymphocyte subsets. Chest 95:590, 1989.

923. Duggan MA, Masters CB, Alexander F: Immunohistochemical differentiation of malignant mesothelioma, mesothelial hyperplasia and metastatic adenocarcinoma in serous effusions, utilizing staining for carcinoembryonic antigen, keratin and vimentin. Acta Cytol 31:807, 1987.

924. Kahn HJ, Thorner PS, Yeger H, et al: Distinct keratin patterns demonstrated by immunoperoxidase staining of adenocarcinomas, carcinoids, and mesotheliomas using polyclonal and monoclonal antikeratin antibodies. Am J Clin Pathol 86:566, 1986.

925. Sheibani K, Battifora H, Burke JS: Antigenic phenotype of malignant mesotheliomas and pulmonary adenocarcinomas. An immunohistologic analysis demonstrating the value of Leu-M1 antigen. Am J Pathol 123:212, 1986.

926. Rasmussen OØ, Larsen KE: S-100 protein in malignant mesotheliomas. Acta Path Microbiol Immunol Scand (A)93:199, 1985.

927. Ghosil AK, Butler PB: Immunocytological staining reactions of anticarcinoembryonic antigen, Ca, and anti-human milk fat globule monoclonal antibodies on benign and malignant exfoliated mesothelial cells. J Clin Pathol 40:1424, 1987.

928. Jordon D, Jagirdar J, Kaneko M: Blood group antigens, Lewis[x] and Lewis[y] in the diagnostic discrimination of malignant mesothelioma versus adenocarcinoma. Am J Pathol 135:931, 1989.

929. Donna A, Betta PG, Bellingeri D, et al: New marker for mesothelioma: An immunoperoxidase study. J Clin Pathol 39:961, 1986.

930. Lee I, Radosevich JA, Chejfec G, et al: Malignant mesotheliomas. Improved differential diagnosis from lung adenocarcinomas using monoclonal antibodies 44–3A6 and 624A12. Am J Pathol 123:497, 1986.

931. Szpak CA, Johnston WW, Roggli V, et al: The diagnostic distinction between malignant mesothelioma of the pleura and adenocarcinoma of the lung as defined by a monoclonal antibody (B72.3). Am J Pathol 122:252, 1986.

932. Donna A, Betta P-G, Jones SP: Verification of the histologic diagnosis of malignant mesothelioma in relation to the binding of an antimesothelial cell antibody. Cancer 63:1331, 1989.

933. Coleman M, Henderson DW, Mukherjee TM: The ultrastructural pathology of malignant pleural mesothelioma. Pathol Ann 24:303, 1989.

934. Warhol MJ, Corson JM: An ultrastructural comparison of mesotheliomas with adenocarcinomas of the lung and breast. Hum Pathol 16:50, 1985.

935. Dardick I, Al-Jabi M, McCaughey WTE: Ultrastructure of poorly differentiated diffuse epithelial mesotheliomas. Ultrastruct Pathol 7:151, 1984.

936. Waxler B, Eisenstein R, Battifora H: Electrophoresis of tissue glycosaminoglycans as an aid in the diagnosis of mesotheliomas. Cancer 44:221, 1979.

937. Nakano T, Fujii J, Tamura S, et al: Glycosaminoglycan in malignant pleural mesothelioma. Cancer 57:106, 1986.

938. Kawai T, Suzuki M, Shinmei M, et al: Glycosaminoglycans in malignant diffuse mesothelioma. Cancer 56:567, 1985.

939. Iozzo RV, Goldes JA, Chen W-J, et al: Glycosaminoglycans of pleural mesothelioma: A possible biochemical variant containing chondroitin sulfate. Cancer 48:89, 1981.

940. Kawai T, Greenberg SD, Truong LD, et al: Differences in lectin binding of malignant pleural mesothelioma and adenocarcinoma of the lung. Am J Pathol 130:401, 1988.

941. Alexander E, Clark RA, Colley DP, et al: CT of malignant pleural mesothelioma. Am J Roentgenol 137:287, 1981.

942. Rabinowitz JG, Efremidis SG, Cohen B, et al: A comparative study of mesothelioma and asbestosis using computed tomography and conventional chest radiography. Radiology 144:453, 1982.

943. Solomon A: A comparative study of mesothelioma and asbestosis using computed tomography and conventional chest radiography. (Letter to the editor.) Radiology 148:316, 1983.

944. Nichols DM, Johnson MA: Calcification in a pleural mesothelioma. J Can Assoc Radiol 34:311, 1983.

945. Campbell GD, Greenburg SD: Pleural mesothelioma with calcified liver metastases. Chest 79:229, 1981.

946. Wolk RB: Gallium-67 scanning in the evaluation of mesothelioma. J Nucl Med 19:808, 1978.

947. Jones DK, Earis JE, Pearson MG, et al: Pleural mesothelioma presenting as apparent recurrent pulmonary embolism. Br J Dis Chest 75:403, 1981.

948. Harrison RN, Hibberd SC, Dadds JH: Malignant pleural mesothelioma at St. Mary's Hospital. Postgrad Med J 59:712, 1983.

949. Pillgram-Larsen J, Urdal L, Smith-Meyer R, et al: Malignant pleural mesothelioma. A clinical review of 19 patients. Scand J Thorac Cardiovasc Surg 18:69, 1984.

950. Wadler S, Chahinian P, Slater W, et al: Cardiac abnormalities in patients with diffuse malignant pleural mesothelioma. Cancer 58:2744, 1986.

951. Walters LL, Taxy JB: Malignant mesothelioma of the pleura with extensive cardiac invasion and tricuspid orifice occlusion. Cancer 52:1736, 1983.

952. Krumhaar D, Lange S, Hartmann C, et al: Follow-up study of 100 malignant pleural mesotheliomas. J Thorac Cardiovasc Surg 33:272, 1985.

953. Antman KH: Current concepts: Malignant mesothelioma. N Engl J Med 303:200, 1980.

954. Kim SB, Varkey B, Choi H: Diagnosis of malignant pleural mesothelioma by axillary lymph node biopsy. Chest 91:279, 1987.

955. Kaye JA, Wang AM, Joachim CL, et al: Malignant mesothelioma with brain metastases. Am J Med 80:95, 1986.

956. Harrison RN: Sarcomatous pleural mesothelioma and cerebral metastases: Case report and a review of eight cases. Eur J Respir Dis 65:185, 1984.

957. Machin T, Mashiyama ET, Henderson JAM, et al: Bony metastases in desmoplastic pleural mesothelioma. Thorax 43:155, 1988.

958. Ragalie GF, Varkey B, Chai H: Malignant pleural mesothelioma presenting as superior vena cava syndrome. Can Med Assoc J 128:689, 1983.

959. Parks WH, Crow JC, Green M: Mesothelioma associated with the syndrome of inappropriate secretion of antidiuretic hormone. Am Rev Respir Dis 117:789, 1978.

960. Siafakas NM, Tsirogiannis K, Filaditaki B, et al: Pleural mesothelioma and the syndrome of inappropriate secretion of antidiuretic hormone. Thorax 39:872, 1984.

961. Finkelstein MM: Asbestosis in long-term employees of an Ontario asbestos-cement factory. Am Rev Respir Dis 125:496, 1982.

962. Whitaker D, Shilkin KB, Stuckey M, et al: Pleural fluid CEA levels in the diagnosis of malignant mesothelioma. Pathology 18:328, 1986.

963. Faravelli B, D'Amore E, Nosenzo M, et al: Carcinoembryonic antigen in pleural effusions. Cancer 53:1194, 1984.

964. Martinez-Vea A, Gatell JM, Segura F, et al: Diagnostic value of tumoral markers in serous effusions. Carcinoembryonic antigen, alpha₁-acid-glycoprotein, alpha-fetoprotein, phosphohexose isomerase, and beta₂-microglobulin. Cancer 50:1783, 1982.

965. Triol JH, Conston AS, Chandler SV: Malignant mesothelioma. Cytopathology of 75 cases seen in a New Jersey community hospital. Acta Cytol 28:37, 1984.

966. Tao L-C: The cytopathology of mesothelioma. Acta Cytol 23:209, 1979.

967. Boon ME, Veldhuizen RW, Ruinaard C, et al: Qualitative distinctive differences between the vacuoles of mesothelioma cells and of cells from metastatic carcinoma exfoliated in pleural fluid. Acta Cytol 28:443, 1984.

968. Dardick I, Butler EB, Dardick AM: Quantitative ultrastructural study of nuclei from exfoliated benign and malignant mesothelial cells and metastatic adenocarcinoma cells. Acta Cytol 30:379, 1986.

969. Law MR, Hodson ME, Turner-Warwick M: Malignant mesothelioma of the pleura: Clinical aspects and symptomatic treatment. Eur J Respir Dis 65:162, 1984.

970. Martensson G, Hagmar B, Zettergren L: Diagnosis and prognosis in malignant pleural mesothelioma: A prospective study. Eur J Respir Dis 65:169, 1984.

971. Chailleux E, Dabouis G, Pioche D, et al: Prognostic factors in diffuse malignant pleural mesothelioma. A study of 167 patients. Chest 93:159, 1988.

972. DaValle MJ, Faber P, Kittle CF, et al: Extrapleural pneumonectomy for diffuse, malignant mesothelioma. Ann Thorac Surg 42:612, 1986.

973. Rüttner JR, Heinzl S: Squamous-cell carcinoma of the pleura. Thorax 32:497, 1977.

974. Rüttner JR, Heinzl S: Squamous-cell carcinoma of the pleura. Thorax 32:497, 1977.

975. Willén R, Bruce T, Dahlström G, et al: Squamous epithelial cancer in metaplastic pleura following extrapleural pneumothorax for pulmonary tuberculosis. Virchows Arch A Pathol Anat and Histol 370:225, 1976.

976. Smith S, Opipari MI: Primary pleural melanoma. A first reported case and literature review. J Thorac Cardiovasc Surg 75:827, 1978.

977. Ten Eyck EA: Subpleural lipoma. Radiology 74:295, 1960.

978. Gramiak R, Koerner HJ: A roentgen diagnostic observation in subpleural lipoma. Am J Roentgenol 98:465, 1966.

979. Britt K, Kaneko M, Chuang MT: Hemangioleiomyosarcoma of the pleura: A case report and review of the literature. MT Sinai J Med 50:64, 1983.

980. Dubig JT: Solitary rhabdomyosarcoma of the pleura. Report of a case with a note on the nomenclature of pleural tumors. J Thorac Surg 37:236, 1959.

981. Yang H-Y, Weaver LL, Foti PR: Primary malignant fibrous histiocytoma of the pleura. A case report. Acta Cytol 27:683, 1983.

982. Evans AR, Wolstenholme RJ, Shettar SP, et al: Primary pleural liposarcoma. Thorax 40:554, 1985.

983. Knapp MJ, Roggli VL, Kim J, et al: Pleural amyloidosis. Arch Pathol Lab Med 112:57, 1988.

984. Lundin P, Simonsson B, Winberg T: Pneumonopleural amyloid tumour. Report of a case. Acta Radiol 55:139, 1961.

985. Hutton L: Oleothorax: Expanding pleural lesion. Am J Roentgenol 142:1107, 1984.

986. Jariwalla AG, Al-Nasiri NK: Splenosis pleurae. Thorax 34:123, 1979.

987. Yousem SA: Thoracic splenosis. Ann Thorac Surg 44:411, 1987.

988. Carlson BR, McQueen S, Kimbrell F, et al: Thoracic splenosis. Diagnosis of a case by fine needle aspiration cytology. Acta Cytol 32:91, 1988.

989. Roche G, Delanoe Y, Genevrier R: Opacités pseudo-tumorales après pleurésies séro-fibrineuses de la grande cavité. (Pseudotumoral opacities after serofibrinous effusions of the pleural cavity.) J Fr Med Chir Thorac 19:789, 1965.

990. Bumgarner JR, Gahwyler M, Ward DE: Persistent fibrin bodies presenting as coin lesions. Am Rev Tuberc 72:659, 1955.

18

19

Diseases of the Mediastinum

Conditions that predominantly or solely affect the mediastinum constitute only a small proportion of diseases that occur in the thorax; however, their differential diagnosis is often difficult because of a common roentgenographic manifestation—widening of the mediastinal silhouette. The majority have an insidious onset and may be present for a long time without occasioning symptoms or signs. In a small number of cases, symptoms may be abrupt in onset and alarming in acuity, an example being the acute mediastinitis that follows esophageal rupture. Between these two extremes of clinical presentation are those patients who complain of a mild sensation of pressure in the retrosternal area or who seek medical aid because of symptoms resulting from compression of the air-, blood-, or food-conducting passages within this narrow space. Although a history of such symptoms is of differential diagnostic value, knowledge of the location of a lesion within a mediastinal compartment is possibly of greater importance. The reader is urged to refresh his or her memory about the anatomic boundaries of the three compartments by referring to the appropriate section in Chapter 1 (see page 204).

Methods for the investigation of mediastinal abnormalities are described in detail in Chapter 2. Briefly, although investigative algorithms will vary somewhat from institution to institution, it can be stated with some conviction that once a mediastinal abnormality is identified on conventional roentgenograms and the cause is not immediately apparent, the most productive procedure to conduct next is computed tomography (CT).[1-5] As an example of the successful results that have been obtained by various authors, the study by Baron and his colleagues is representative:[1] CT was employed in the study of 71 patients for the assessment of a widened mediastinum; it permitted correct identification of a normal variant, soft tissue mass, or vascular abnormality as the cause of the mediastinal widening in 92 per cent of the patients. In 58 per cent, a specific and correct diagnosis was made that obviated further, more invasive diagnostic procedures. The recommendation made by these authors is one with which we are in complete agreement: invasive diagnostic procedures should be reserved for the minority of cases in which CT is indeterminate or

in which additional information is required prior to surgery. Conclusions similar to those of Baron and his colleagues were reached by a group from Washington University, St. Louis, from a CT study of 23 pediatric patients:[6] CT provided additional diagnostic information in 82 per cent of the patients, and in 65 per cent the CT findings contributed to a change in clinical management.

Although at the time of writing, the impact that magnetic resonance imaging (MRI) will have on the study of the mediastinum has not been firmly established, a number of preliminary studies suggest that it will prove exceedingly useful, particularly because of its ability to distinguish different tissues and its excellent demonstration of vascular structures.[7-17] The relative contributions made by CT and MRI are discussed in greater detail in Chapter 2 (see pages 331 and 336).

For those readers interested in delving more deeply into diseases of the mediastinum, particularly with regard to radiologic correlations with anatomy and pathology, the monograph by Heitzman is highly recommended.[18]

MEDIASTINITIS

Infections of the mediastinum can be acute or chronic. The former are usually caused by bacteria and sometimes progress to abscess formation; they are often associated with signs and symptoms (especially retrosternal pain and fever), and many are fulminating and lethal. By contrast, the chronic form is most often the result of tuberculous or fungal infection but is occasionally idiopathic; it is characteristically insidious in onset and often does not give rise to symptoms. The presence of mediastinal abnormality in the chronic form may become apparent only on a screening chest roentgenogram, although some patients seek medical aid because of the development of symptoms or signs related to obstruction or compression of one or more of the mediastinal structures. In addition to cases of chronic mediastinitis of infectious origin, there is a group of mediastinopathies of unknown cause characterized by the accumulation of dense fibrous tissue, sometimes associated with similar deposits elsewhere in the body, notably the retroperitoneal space.[19, 20]

A monograph dealing with "purulent and fibrous mediastinitis," with emphasis on radiologic diagnosis, was published in 1972.[21] This exhaustive review of these two relatively uncommon disease entities was based on a study of 58 cases of "fibrous mediastinitis"; it is recommended to those interested in a more comprehensive coverage of these topics.

ACUTE MEDIASTINITIS

Acute infections of the mediastinum are rare and in the majority of patients result from esophageal perforation. Such perforation can have a variety of causes, the most common of which is erosion or perforation from a primary carcinoma, an impacted foreign body, or a diagnostic or therapeutic instrument (particularly as a complication of esophagoscopy, balloon dilatation,[22] or insertion of an esophageal prosthesis).[27] Spontaneous perforation (Boerhaave's syndrome) occurs most frequently secondary to episodes of severe vomiting,[23–26] but it can also develop during labor, a severe asthmatic attack, or strenuous exercise. The usual site of rupture is the lower 8 cm of the esophagus, particularly adjacent to the gastroesophageal junction; typically, the tear is vertical and involves the left posterolateral wall.[26, 28] Mediastinitis can also develop following surgery involving mediastinal structures, especially cardiac surgery[29, 30] and colonic interposition (the latter due to either anastomotic leak or ischemic colitis).[31] Rare causes of acute mediastinitis include direct extension of infection from adjacent tissues such as the retropharyngeal space,[32] pericardium, lungs, pleura, or lymph nodes (the last-named particularly in association with *Bacillus anthracis* infection [*see* page 842]) and as a complication of bronchoscopy.[33–35]

The main roentgenographic manifestation of acute mediastinitis is widening of the mediastinum, usually more evident superiorly and typically possessing a smooth, sharply defined margin. When the mediastinitis has resulted from esophageal rupture, air may be visible within the mediastinum as well as in the soft tissues of the neck (Fig. 19–1).[36] There may be an associated pneumothorax or hydropneumothorax; in a study of 24 patients with esophageal perforation, Han and his colleagues[37] showed that when the perforation was in the distal esophagus, hydrothorax or hydropneumothorax occurred on the left, whereas midesophageal perforation tended to cause pleural changes on the right. In a review of the roentgenologic features in 28 patients with esophageal perforation, Appleton and associates[38] found detectable abnormalities on the chest roentgenogram in 25 (89 per cent); the most common were visible gas in the mediastinal or cervical soft tissues and gas or fluid (or both) in the pleural cavity. Multiple abscesses may develop (Fig.

19–2). The diagnosis is readily confirmed roentgenologically by demonstration of extravasation of ingested contrast material into the mediastinum or pleural space (Fig. 19–3).[36] Although we recommend barium sulfate as the medium of choice in this examination, others[39] believe that water-soluble contrast medium should be administered first, followed by barium sulfate ingestion if the water-soluble medium does not demonstrate a perforation and the clinical picture is highly suggestive. Regardless of the contrast substance employed, it is important that the examination be performed as soon as possible after the suspected perforation: in the Appleton and associates series referred to above,[38] of 26 patients who had a barium swallow, a leak was demonstrated in 21 (81 per cent); in the 5 patients in whom no leak was demonstrated, the examination was performed more than 24 hours after the perforation.

The diagnosis should be suspected clinically in any patient in whom severe retrosternal pain develops abruptly and radiates to the neck and whose history points to one of the etiologies described. Chills and high fever are common, and the effects of obstruction of the superior vena cava may be apparent. Physical examination of a patient whose esophagus has perforated commonly reveals subcutaneous emphysema in the soft tissues of the neck or a loud crunching or clicking sound synchronous with the heart beat on auscultation over the apex of the heart (Hamman's sign). Although suggestive of pneumomediastinum, the latter sign is not pathognomonic, being heard in some cases of pneumothorax and occasionally in patients with moderate elevation of the left hemidiaphragm associated with gaseous distention of the fundus of the stomach or the splenic flexure of the colon.

When the diagnosis of mediastinitis is not suspected initially and treatment not instituted promptly, the infection can progress to an abscess that in turn can rupture into the esophagus, a lung, a bronchus, or the pleural cavity. The presence of such a fistula usually can be confirmed by contrast roentgenographic examination or by microscopic examination of the pleural fluid.[40] However, seven patients have been reported[41] in whom iatrogenic esophageal perforation was followed by the development of an esophagopleural fistula without roentgenographic or other evidence of mediastinitis.

The prognosis in cases of acute mediastinitis resulting from esophageal rupture is poor; in one series of 39 patients, 15 died.[25]

CHRONIC SCLEROSING MEDIASTINITIS

Chronic sclerosing mediastinitis (fibrosing mediastinitis, granulomatous mediastinitis, or idiopathic mediastinal fibrosis) is a rare condition characterized by chronic inflammation and fibrosis of mediastinal soft tissues. The process is often pro-

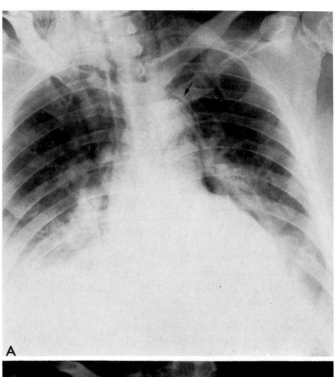

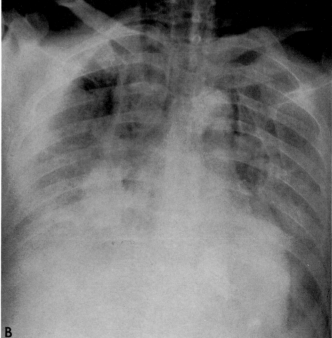

Figure 19–1. Acute Mediastinitis Secondary to Esophageal Rupture. Several hours before the roentgenogram illustrated in *(A)*, this 41-year-old man had had a surgical repair of a hiatus hernia through an abdominal approach. Postoperatively, he complained of dyspnea and retrosternal pain. An anteroposterior roentgenogram exposed in the supine position demonstrated lateral displacement of the left mediastinal pleura *(arrows)* due to an accumulation of gas in the mediastinum. Bilateral basal opacity suggested pleural effusion; there was subcutaneous emphysema in the neck. Twelve hours later *(B)*, the opacity of both lungs had increased greatly, chiefly as a result of pleural effusion. The mediastinal gas had decreased slightly, but there was still considerable subcutaneous emphysema in the neck. These changes were caused by spillage of esophageal contents into the mediastinum and pleural spaces through a tear in the esophagus near the esophagogastric junction.

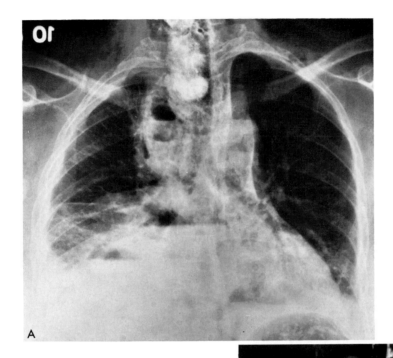

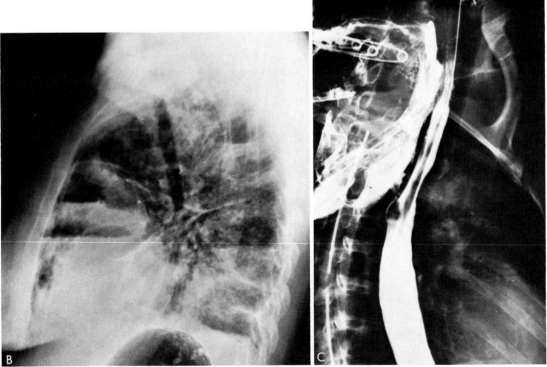

Figure 19–2. Acute Perforation of the Esophagus with Acute Mediastinitis and Mediastinal Abscesses. Three days before the roentgenograms illustrated, this 41-year-old woman swallowed a fork and shortly thereafter developed severe retrosternal pain and fever. Posteroanterior *(A)* and lateral *(B)* roentgenograms in the erect position reveal an irregularly widened upper mediastinum and multiple air fluid levels within the mediastinum anteriorly and posteriorly. There are bilateral pleural effusions and probable bilateral lower lobe pneumonia. Several days later, barium administered by mouth opacified the whole of the esophagus but showed a large sinus tract extending into the mediastinum posteriorly *(C)*. Recovery was prolonged but complete.

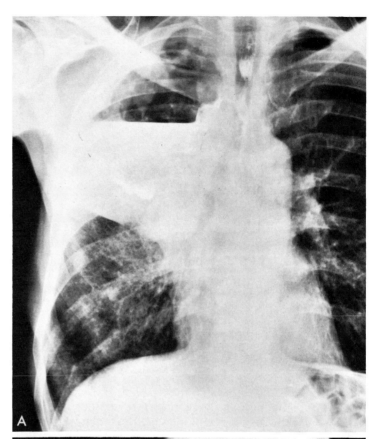

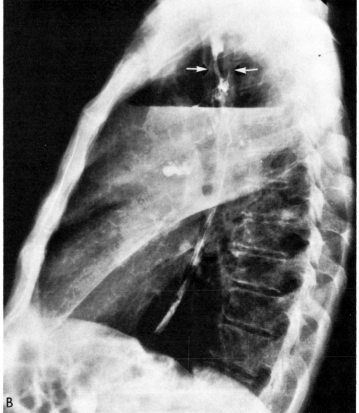

Figure 19–3. Primary Carcinoma of the Esophagus with Perforation into the Right Lung and Abscess Formation. Posteroanterior *(A)* and lateral *(B)* roentgenograms reveal a huge ragged cavity in the upper half of the right lung. Barium administered by mouth reveals deformity of the esophageal lumen characteristic of primary carcinoma *(arrows* in *B)*. Barium has passed from the esophagus into the large lung abscess.

gressive and can occur either focally or more or less diffusely throughout the mediastinum. It can cause compression and sometimes obliteration of vessels, airways, and the esophagus and result in a variety of functional and roentgenographic manifestations and occasionally death.

Etiology and Pathogenesis

A consideration of the etiology and pathogenesis of chronic sclerosing mediastinitis is complicated to some extent by the use of the term "granulomatous mediastinitis" to designate two apparently different conditions: (1) more or less diffuse involvement of mediastinal tissues by a granulomatous inflammatory infiltrate and fibrous tissue (corresponding to the concept of chronic sclerosing mediastinitis as defined above), and (2) more focal involvement in which the inflammatory reaction is relatively localized. The latter condition is most often the result of infection by fungi or *Mycobacterium tuberculosis*, with the disease being confined to one or several matted lymph nodes, usually in the right paratracheal region; these cases often present in an asymptomatic individual as a relatively well-circumscribed mass (*see* farther on).[42, 43] It is not always clear in published articles which cases represent this localized form of mediastinal granulomatous inflammation and which the diffuse fibrosing type;[44] thus, statements about the relative importance of specific infectious organisms in the etiology of chronic sclerosing mediastinitis are sometimes difficult to interpret. Despite this, infection (as evidenced by either positive culture of mediastinal tissue or the identification of organisms within granulomatous inflammation on histologic examination) is probably the most common cause of chronic sclerosing mediastinitis. In the majority of cases the etiology is *Histoplasma capsulatum*,[45, 46] although *M. tuberculosis*,[45] *Aspergillus* species,[47, 48] and the *Phycomycetes*[49] have also been implicated occasionally.

The precise pathogenesis of the progressive mediastinal fibrosis in these cases is not clear. It has been hypothesized[50] that spillage of necrotic material from infected mediastinal lymph nodes into the adjacent mediastinal tissues is an important event, implying progressive infection of the mediastinum and resultant secondary fibrosis. This process is possibly responsible in some cases, but in a review of the literature in 1988 Loyd and colleagues[45] failed to find evidence of such progression and suggested that the majority of cases, especially those caused by *H. capsulatum* infection, represent an idiosyncratic hypersensitivity reaction to the presence of organisms or associated degenerated material.

A second group of cases (sometimes designated idiopathic mediastinal fibrosis) shows no cultural and little histologic evidence of an infectious etiology. This group can be substantial; for example, in one review of 77 cases of chronic sclerosing medi-

astinitis,[44] an infectious etiology was positively established in only three (histoplasmosis in two and tuberculosis in one). Although some of these cases (perhaps the majority) likely represent the end stage of chronic infection in which the organism is difficult to identify, in others the etiology and pathogenesis are undoubtably noninfectious. Evidence for this derives from the occasional patient in whom a similar fibrotic process can be identified elsewhere,[19] including the retroperitoneal space (retroperitoneal fibrosis), the orbit ("pseudotumor of the orbit"), the thyroid (Riedel's struma), and the cecum (ligneous perityphlitis). The number of reported cases with combinations of these sclerosing lesions is sufficient to indicate that the association is more than coincidental[19, 51–55] and has led Comings and associates[20] to propose the term "multifocal fibrosclerosis." The pathogenesis of this condition is probably multifactorial. A genetic effect is suggested by one report of two brothers (the offspring of a cosanguineous marriage) who showed various combinations of sclerosing lesions.[20] Immunologic factors seem to be involved in some cases as evidenced by the reports of both mediastinal and retroperitoneal fibrosis in isolated cases of systemic lupus erythematosus, rheumatoid disease, and in association with Raynaud's phenomenon.[19] Methysergide, a drug used for the alleviation of headache, also has been clearly associated with development of the abnormality.[52, 56]

Pathologic Characteristics

Pathologically, disease tends to affect the upper half of the mediastinum, predominantly anterior to the trachea and around the hilum; more extensive lesions can extend from the brachiocephalic veins to the base of a lung.[44] Grossly, the affected tissue is typically ill-defined and yellowish-grey; compression of vessels (especially the superior vena cava and pulmonary veins), airways, and occasionally the esophagus may be apparent. Histologically, the "mass" varies in appearance depending on the etiology. In some cases, particularly those in which an infectious organism is identified, there is clear-cut necrotizing granulomatous inflammation. In other cases, the granulomatous component is relatively minimal in extent or absent altogether, the abnormal tissue being composed predominantly of lamellae of mature fibrous tissue containing scattered lymphocytes, sometimes with foci of necrotic tissue resembling those in the center of remote granulomas.[45]

Because the fibrosing process tends to compress vessels and airways in the hilar region, secondary effects on the lung itself are relatively common. In lobes in which the draining veins are affected, parenchymal interstitial fibrosis and pneumonitis, intra-alveolar aggregates of hemosiderin-laden macrophages, and vascular changes consistent with pulmonary hypertension may be seen.[57, 58] Occasionally, venous or arterial thrombi (or both) in various stages of organization can be identified,[59] sometimes accompanied by parenchymal infarcts. In one case, multifocal infarcts were centered about interlobular septa;[58] this suggested the cause to be pulmonary venous rather than arterial obstruction.

Roentgenographic Manifestations

The most common roentgenographic manifestation is general widening of the upper half of the mediastinum caused by a somewhat lobulated paratracheal mass that usually projects more to the right than to the left (Fig. 19–4).[60, 61] Calcification occurs in some cases. In a minority of patients, parenchymal disease or bronchopulmonary lymph node enlargement indicates the pulmonary origin of the mediastinal disease. In some cases, the mediastinal silhouette is normal, and the roentgenographic manifestations result from narrowing of the trachea or major bronchi (Fig. 19-5), obstruction of pulmonary veins or arteries, or narrowing of the esophagus. Wieder and his associates[62] have described 5 patients in whom there was complete or partial occlusion of a pulmonary artery secondary to compression or intraluminal granuloma formation (Fig. 19–6). We have seen a similar case in which there was a combination of total occlusion of the left interlobar artery and compression of multiple pulmonary veins leading to interstitial pulmonary edema in all regions except the left lower lobe (Fig. 19–7). Several cases have been reported in which involvement of a pulmonary vein resulted in pulmonary infarction.[58, 63] Feigin and associates[61] have described esophageal obstruction in 4 of 29 patients with sclerosing mediastinitis; in all cases the roentgenographic appearance could be distinguished from carcinoma by the smooth tapering and funnel-shaped upper and lower borders on barium swallow.

Weinstein and his colleagues[64] have described the CT manifestations of chronic sclerosing mediastinitis in seven patients with pathologically proven disease: findings included a mediastinal or hilar mass (in all patients), calcifications within the mass or in associated lymph nodes (in six patients), narrowing of the tracheobronchial tree (in five), and pulmonary infiltrates (*sic*) (in four). In six of the seven patients, CT demonstrated abnormalities that were not evident on conventional roentgenograms. A case has been described recently[65] in which sclerosing mediastinitis presented initially as a predominantly posterior mediastinal mass that subsequently extended into contiguous lung parenchyma and retroperitoneal space. Although CT has been shown to be an excellent method of demonstrating enlarged nodes (with or without calcification) and can sometimes reveal changes suggesting a tuberculous etiology,[66] MRI is superior in assessing vascular patency without the need for contrast media.[67, 68]

When mediastinal and retroperitoneal fibrosis coexist, the two are remote anatomically, the latter being situated in the lower abdomen and pelvis in the region of the common iliac vessels. Such disease is evidenced by medial displacement of the ureters and unilateral or bilateral hydronephrosis.[51, 54] When the fibrosis is methysergide-induced, the roentgenographic abnormalities may disappear following withdrawal of the drug.[69]

Clinical Manifestations

Symptoms and signs of chronic sclerosing mediastinitis are quite variable depending on the extent of the fibrosis and the particular structures within the mediastinum that are affected. Involvement of the superior vena cava is probably the most common cause of clinical abnormalities[44] and results in the typical manifestations of the superior vena caval syndrome—giddiness, tinnitus, headache, epistaxis, hemoptysis, cyanosis, and puffiness of the face, neck, and arms. The severity of these symptoms can lessen with time as collateral venous channels are developed. Obstruction of large central pulmonary veins can cause signs of pulmonary venous hypertension and edema, sometimes with associated pulmonary arterial hypertension; however, the latter can be caused also by direct encroachment on central pulmonary arteries.[70] Such encroachment can also result in recurrent, sometimes copious, hemoptysis.[71–73] Other complications result from involvement of the thoracic duct (chylothorax) and the recurrent laryngeal nerve (hoarseness).[44] Patients with retroperitoneal fibrosis can manifest peripheral edema as a result of obstruction of the inferior vena cava or intermittent claudication secondary to aortic compression. Despite the observation that some of these cases are of infectious origin, patients are rarely febrile.

The diagnosis may be suspected from the roentgenographic appearance in patients with a positive complement fixation or skin test to *H. capsulatum* or in association with fibrotic lesions affecting the orbit, thyroid gland, or retroperitoneal space. Precise diagnosis usually requires histologic examination of tissue removed at mediastinoscopy or thoracotomy; in one series of four patients,[46] *H. capsulatum* was positively established as the etiology in all cases by the histologic identification of organisms in lymph nodes biopsied at mediastinoscopy or in tissue obtained at open thoracotomy. In addition to routine morphologic examination, such tissue should be cultured for mycobacteria and other organisms.

PNEUMOMEDIASTINUM

Pneumomediastinum (mediastinal emphysema) connotes the presence of gas in the mediastinal space. It is rare in adults and undoubtedly is most common in newborn infants in whom it has been

Text continued on page 2809

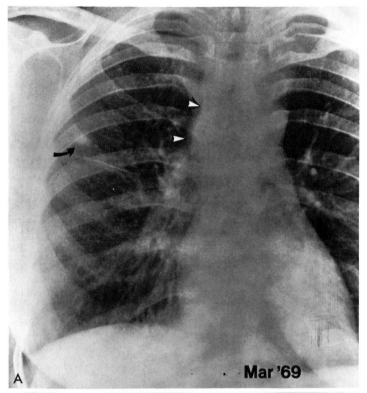

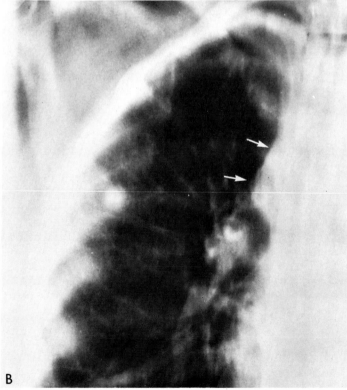

Figure 19–4. Chronic Sclerosing Mediastinitis and Superior Vena Cava Obstruction Secondary to Tuberculosis. This 38-year-old woman presented with a typical superior vena cava syndrome whose severity had been increasing over the past several months. A posteroanterior roentgenogram *(A)* revealed an indistinctly defined soft tissue mass in the region of the right tracheobronchial angle *(arrowheads)* and a 1.0-cm nodular opacity in the axillary portion of the right upper lobe *(curved arrow).* The right hilum was somewhat enlarged and indistinct in outline. A tomogram in anteroposterior projection *(B)* revealed an irregular lobulated mass in the right tracheobronchial angle and immediately above *(arrows).* The pulmonary nodule was seen to be densely calcified.

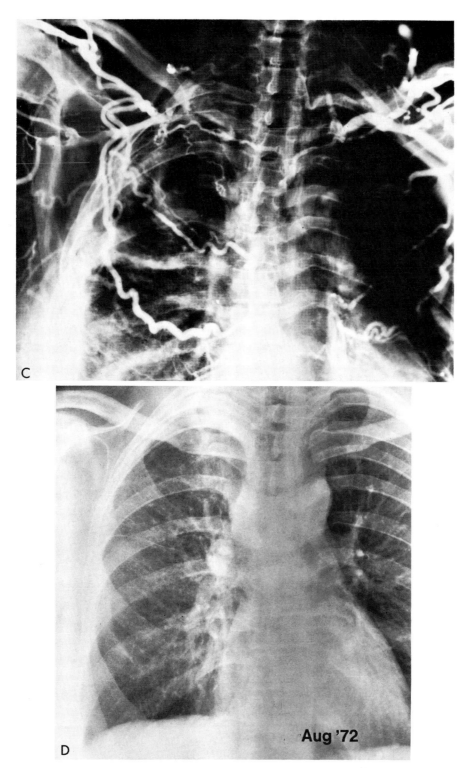

Figure 19–4 *Continued* Contrast medium was injected into both arm veins simultaneously and serial roentgenograms obtained. One of these *(C)* showed total absence of opacification of both innominate veins and the superior vena cava, there being extensive collateral circulation over the anterior and lateral chest wall. At thoracotomy, the right upper lobe was resected. Biopsy of right tracheobronchial lymph nodes revealed caseating granulomas. A posteroanterior roentgenogram obtained 3 years later *(D)* shows persistent widening of the superior mediastinum, although symptoms of superior vena caval obstruction had abated.

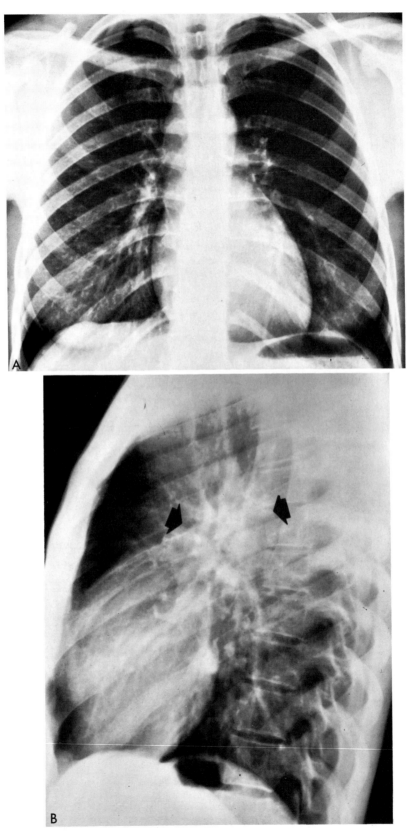

Figure 19–5 *See legend on opposite page.*

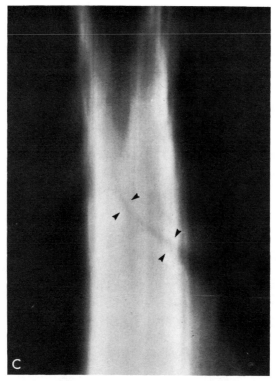

Figure 19–5. Chronic Sclerosing Mediastinitis with Involvement of Major Airways. Five months prior to the roentgenograms illustrated, this 19-year-old girl, a medium-distance runner on her university team, had noted the onset of shortness of breath on exertion, nonproductive cough, and recurrent wheezing episodes precipitated by physical exertion or exposure to cold air. Pulmonary function studies revealed a significant impairment of flow rates. The clinical diagnosis was bronchial asthma. Roentgenograms of her chest in posteroanterior *(A)* and lateral *(B)* projections reveal a normal appearance of her lungs. A smooth, well-defined, homogeneous mass is seen in the right tracheobronchial angle, obscuring the shadow of the azygos vein. In lateral projection, the aortic window is not visualized and has apparently been obliterated. In addition, there is a suggestion of narrowing of the air column of the main bronchi. A tomogram of the carinal region in anteroposterior projection *(C)* reveals a severe degree of stenosis of the whole length of the left main bronchus *(arrowheads).* The lower 2 cm of the trachea and right main bronchus are similarly, but less severely, affected. Biopsies of mediastinal tissue and lymph node obtained at mediastinoscopy revealed findings consistent with fibrosing mediastinitis. At right thoracotomy, a diffuse mass with ill-defined edges was found extending from the posterior wall of the superior vena cava over the trachea, into the mediastinum behind the trachea, and downward around the right upper lobe bronchus and into the mediastinum. Only partial resection of the mass was possible because of technical problems. The region of the left main bronchus could not be explored. Histologically, the tissue was composed of collagenous fibrosis with slight focal lymphocytic infiltration. The etiology was not established and the final diagnosis was idiopathic sclerosing mediastinitis. (Courtesy of St. Boniface General Hospital, St. Boniface, Manitoba.)

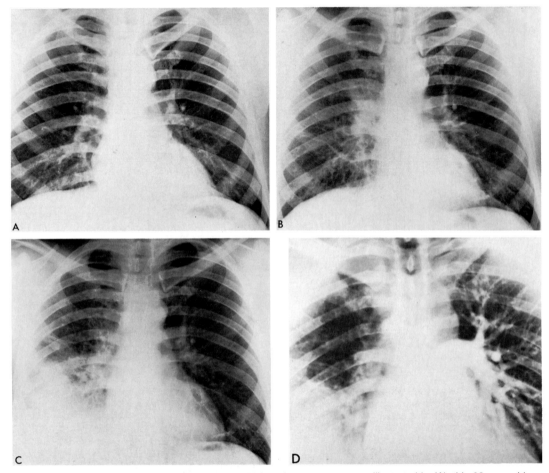

Figure 19–6. Chronic Sclerosing Mediastinitis. Shortly before the roentgenogram illustrated in *(A)*, this 33-year-old man noted the onset of episodic pain in the right chest, hemoptysis, and shortness of breath. The roentgenogram showed no significant abnormalities. Following a similar episode approximately 1 year later, a posteroanterior roentgenogram *(B)* revealed a poorly defined shadow of homogeneous density extending outward from the right hilum. The right hemithorax generally was of greater density than the left. The upper mediastinum was not widened. One year later *(C)*, the shadow in the right parahilar area had disappeared but there was now extensive opacification of the lower portion of the right lung by a shadow that underwent little change on serial examinations. In view of the history suggestive of recurrent episodes of pulmonary infarction, pulmonary angiography was performed *(D)* and demonstrated complete obstruction of the main right pulmonary artery, the total right ventricular output passing to the left lung. The point of obstruction of the right pulmonary artery was not clearly identified.

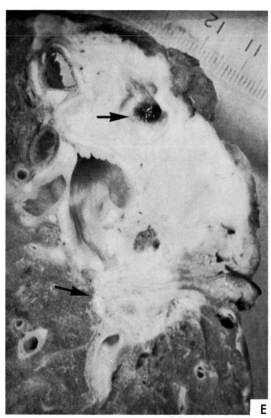

E

Figure 19–6 *Continued* At thoracotomy, a huge, whitish mass was identified on the right side of the mediastinum *(E)*, incorporating the pulmonary arteries and veins in an extensive fibrotic and granulomatous process. The superior vena cava was compressed but not obstructed; the pulmonary arteries *(upper arrow)* and veins *(lower arrow)* were partly or completely obstructed. Both the mass and the right lung were resected with considerable difficulty. Skin tests were negative for histoplasmosis and tuberculosis; the causative organism was not identified pathologically. (Roentgenogram *A* courtesy of St. Mary's Hospital, Montreal; roentgenogram *B* courtesy of Toronto Western Hospital.)

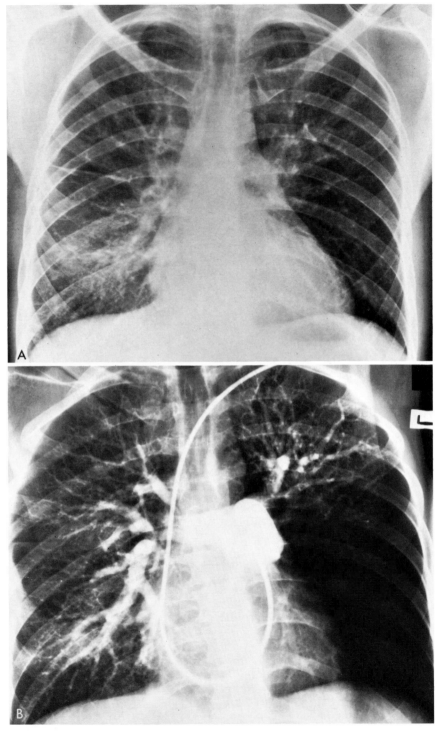

Figure 19–7. Chronic Sclerosing Mediastinitis Due to Histoplasmosis with Encasement of Pulmonary Arteries and Veins. A posteroanterior roentgenogram *(A)* reveals interstitial edema throughout the right lung and left upper zone. Septal lines are present in the right costophrenic angle. A striking disparity in density of the lower half of the two lungs is observed, the left being relatively radiolucent and, in fact, markedly oligemic. A pulmonary arteriogram *(B)* shows almost complete occlusion of the left interlobar artery with virtually no perfusion of the left lower lobe and lingula. Although there appears to be good opacification of the arteries of the right lung, the truncus anterior and interlobar arteries show concentric narrowing medial to the hilum. The venous phase of the angiogram is not available, but it is almost certain that the pulmonary veins are affected in the same manner, resulting in venous hypertension and the interstitial edema apparent on the plain roentgenogram. (Courtesy of Dr. M.J. Palayew, Jewish General Hospital, Montreal.)

variously reported as occurring in 1 per cent,[74] 0.5 per cent,[75] and 0.04 per cent.[76] In adults it occurs predominantly in males during the second and third decades of life.[77]

Etiology and Pathogenesis

Gas within the mediastinum can originate from five sites—the lung, the mediastinal airways, the esophagus, the neck, and the abdominal cavity. Although there is some overlap, the etiology and pathogenesis of pneumomediastinum related to each of these sites are sufficiently distinctive that they can be discussed separately. This subject has been reviewed by Cyrlak and colleagues.[78]

LUNG PARENCHYMA

Extension of gas from the airspaces of the pulmonary parenchyma into the interstitial tissues and thence into the mediastinum is undoubtably the most common mechanism of pneumomediastinum in both neonates and adults. In most patients the initial event is probably similar and is related to an incident that causes an abrupt rise in alveolar pressure, often accompanied by airway narrowing; this results in rupture of marginally situated alveoli whose bases relate to airways or to pulmonary arteries or veins. Gas then passes into the perivascular interstitium and tracks through the interstitial space to the hilum and the mediastinum.[79, 80] Experimental evidence supporting this mechanism has been derived from studies in rabbits, in which the magnitude of tracheal pressure applied by artificial ventilation correlated directly with the frequency of development of perivascular interstitial emphysema;[81] binding the thorax of these animals decreased the incidence of interstitial emphysema, possibly by limiting the increase in lung volume. As well as tracking proximally, gas can also extend peripherally in the interstitial tissue toward the visceral pleura and rupture into the pleural space to cause pneumothorax. This is particularly common in neonates and was identified in 25 of 40 cases in one series.[82] Pneumothorax can also result directly from rupture of the mediastinal pleura when sufficient gas accumulates in this compartment.

Although many patients who develop pneumomediastinum have no convincing evidence of pulmonary disease, an underlying abnormality is clearly present in some patients and probably constitutes an important contributory factor in the pathogenesis of the condition. For example, alveolar walls can be destroyed as a result of an associated pneumonia,[83–85] thus facilitating the passage of gas from parenchyma to interstitial tissue. Similarly, the bronchiolitis that occurs in some conditions such as aspiration pneumonia[86] and measles[87, 88] may cause alveolar rupture as a result of check-valve bronchiolar obstruction and a local increase in airspace pressure. A similar mechanism may be responsible

for the mediastinal emphysema reported to occur following inhalation of chlorine gas[89] and as a complication of bone marrow transplantation.[90]

In some patients a precipitating event for pneumomediastinum cannot be identified, the diagnosis being made following the discovery of subcutaneous emphysema in the soft tissues of the neck or from a chest roentgenogram obtained because of retrosternal discomfort;[91] however, in most patients the development of pneumomediastinum can be clearly related to an incident that results in a sudden rise in alveolar pressure or to a disease process in which such an incident is likely to occur. Such incidents or diseases include:

1. *Deep respiratory maneuvers*, such as those that occur during strenuous exercise[83, 92] or while performing forced vital capacity breaths.[93]

2. *Valsalva maneuvers*, such as those that occur during parturition[94, 95]—a particularly common event leading to pneumomediastinum—or during the smoking of marijuana.[92, 96]

3. *Asthma*, particularly in children[91, 97, 98] but also in adults.[98–101]

4. *Vomiting* of any cause; for example, the association of pneumomediastinum with diabetic acidosis has been well documented and in most cases is probably related to severe and protracted vomiting.[84, 85, 102–104] These patients are particularly susceptible to a rise in intra-alveolar pressure because of the simultaneous occurrence of vomiting and vigorous respiratory effort.[105]

5. *Artificial ventilation*, particularly in patients with obstructive pulmonary disease[106] and in those being maintained on positive end-expiratory pressure (PEEP).[107]

6. *Closed chest trauma*, in which shearing forces directly disrupt alveolar walls.

7. A sudden drop in atmospheric pressure, such as occurs during the rapid ascent of a scuba diver or pilot. In this situation, the mechanism probably involves the sudden expansion of thoracic air-containing spaces such as blebs or bullae that communicate poorly with the conducting system.[108]

MEDIASTINAL AIRWAYS

Rupture of the trachea or proximal mainstem bronchi inevitably results in pneumomediastinum. Such rupture is most often caused by trauma, usually accidental but occasionally following diagnostic instrumentation such as bronchoscopic biopsy; bronchoscopy can also result in pneumomediastinum by inducing fits of paroxysmal coughing.[34, 35] Two cases have been reported in which pneumomediastinum was associated with tracheal neoplasms.[109]

THE ESOPHAGUS

As discussed previously, rupture of the esophagus occurs most frequently during episodes of severe vomiting[23, 24, 26] but can also develop as a result of trauma or during labor, a severe asthmatic attack, or strenuous exercise. It must be remembered that each of these latter events can cause pneumomediastinum in the absence of esophageal injury; because of the almost inevitable development of mediastinitis following esophageal rupture, it is obviously vital to distinguish pneumomediastinum secondary to this injury from that caused by less ominous abnormalities. This has been the subject of an excellent review by Rogers and his colleagues.[26] An esophageal neoplasm can occasionally perforate into the mediastinum with resulting pneumomediastinum.

THE NECK

Air can track into the mediastinum along deep fascial planes as a result of trauma to the neck or following surgical procedures or dental extraction;[110, 111] in one patient,[111] dental extraction was complicated not only by pneumomediastinum but also by pneumopericardium and pneumoperitoneum.

THE ABDOMINAL CAVITY

A rare cause of pneumomediastinum is extension of gas from below the diaphragm, most commonly from the retroperitoneal space following perforation of a hollow abdominal viscus.[112] However, it is important to recognize that the development of pneumomediastinum in association with free abdominal gas need not reflect a retroperitoneal location but can occur in association with an intraperitoneal accumulation as well, as exemplified by the cases of anterior wall perforation of a duodenal ulcer reported by Stahl and associates.[113] The reverse can also be true: as pointed out by Campbell and his colleagues,[114] pneumoperitoneum can occur in the early neonatal period as a result of progressive massive tension pneumomediastinum, the latter characteristically located both anterior and posterior to the heart. Although formerly it was thought that this gas reached the extraperitoneal space via vascular sheaths posteriorly, Kleinman and his colleagues[115] have shown that the route is anterior rather than posterior, and that dissection occurs along internal mammary vessels enclosed between the sternocostal origins of the diaphragm.

Whatever the cause of pneumomediastinum, when sufficient gas accumulates in the mediastinal compartments, pressure can build up and impede blood flow, particularly in low-pressure veins. Respiratory embarrassment can also occur from the presence of large amounts of gas in the pulmonary interstitial space with resulting stiff lungs. Either or both of these mechanisms can lead to the syndrome of mediastinal air block.[79, 80] Such a buildup of pressure occurs only when gas is prevented from passing into the neck, a situation particularly prone to occur in the neonatal period. More frequently—and almost invariably in adults—air escapes from the mediastinum by way of the fascial planes of the great vessels into the neck and anterior chest wall, thus producing subcutaneous emphysema.

Of some interest is the observation that air within the mediastinum engenders an inflammatory reaction associated with relatively numerous eosinophils, similar to that seen in the pleura in association with pneumothorax.[116]

Roentgenographic Manifestations

Roentgenographic signs of pneumomediastinum are usually easy to detect, especially in infants. In posteroanterior projection, the mediastinal pleura is displaced laterally, creating a longitudinal line shadow parallel to the heart border and separated from the heart by gas. This shadow is usually more evident on the left side (Fig. 19–8). Also, a longitudinal gas shadow may be identified adjacent to the thoracic aorta and sometimes around the pulmonary artery ("ring-around-the-artery" sign) (Fig. 19–9).[117] Friedman and his coworkers[118] have pointed out that a thin line of radiolucency can be frequently identified along the border of the heart and aortic knob and that it should not be confused with pneumomediastinum: the lateral margin of this radiolucency consists of pulmonary parenchyma rather than the thin linear opacity characteristic of displaced pleura; it thus represents a Mach band rather than true pneumomediastinum.

In infants with a large accumulation of gas, the thymus may be well outlined and may be displaced upward. In many cases the mediastinal pleural reflection is markedly displaced laterally (Fig. 19–10).[82, 119] Dissection of air into the neck and over the thoracic wall is much less common in infants than in adults. The consequent buildup in pressure in such infants often gives rise to unilateral or bilateral pneumothorax, a less common complication in adolescents and adults. Lillard and Allen[74] described an "extrapleural air sign" in pneumomediastinum consisting of a collection of gas between the parietal pleura and the diaphragm. It is possible that this collection of gas could be confused with pneumothorax, but as pointed out by Felson[119] such an accumulation in pneumomediastinum should not shift with change in body position. When gas becomes interposed between the heart and diaphragm, it permits identification of the central portion of the diaphragm in continuity with the lateral portions by creating what Levin has termed "the continuous diaphragm sign."[120] Gas within the pericardial sac should also conceivably permit visualization of the central portion of the diaphragm. However, as pointed out by Levin,[120] pneumopericardium is almost always associated with fluid within the pericardial cavity, thus leading to obliteration of the central portion of the diaphragm, at least on roentgenograms exposed in the erect position.

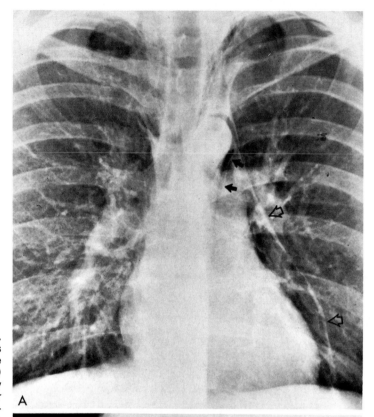

Figure 19–8. Spontaneous Pneumomediastinum.
Shortly before these roentgenograms were obtained, this 20-year-old man had noted an abrupt onset of fairly severe retrosternal pain. Views of the chest in posteroanterior *(A)* and lateral *(B)* projections reveal a long linear opacity roughly paralleling the left heart border in posteroanterior projection *(open arrows),* representing the laterally displaced mediastinal pleura. In addition, considerable gas is present around the aortic arch and proximal descending thoracic aorta *(solid arrows* in both projections). In lateral projection, note the gas outlining the anterior surface of the heart and the brachiocephalic vessels.

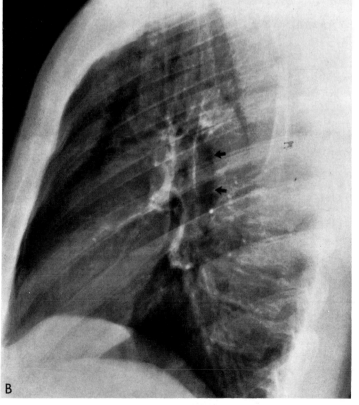

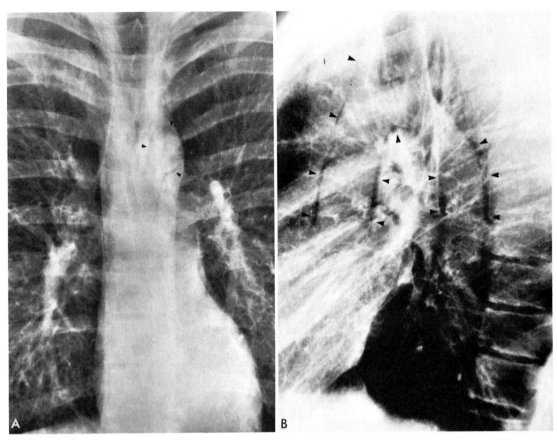

Figure 19–9. Spontaneous Pneumomediastinum. Posteroanterior *(A)* and lateral *(B)* roentgenograms reveal linear and curvilinear shadows of air density outlining almost all portions of the aortic arch in both projections *(arrowheads)*. In lateral projection, the gas outlining the anterior wall of the ascending aorta extends superiorly and relates to the right innominate artery. The patient is a 20-year-old man; roentgenograms were exposed shortly after the abrupt onset of retrosternal chest pain. Etiology was not established.

When it is not certain whether a collection of gas is within the pericardial sac or the mediastinal space, differentiation is readily established by demonstrating a change in the position of pericardial gas on roentgenograms exposed in different body positions.[119]

Sometimes air within the interstitial tissues of the lung ("interstitial emphysema") can be detected roentgenographically. Since gas in the interstitial tissues of otherwise normal lung should not be apparent because of lack of contrast, its identification requires the presence of disease in contiguous parenchyma, a feature of particular note in neonates with respiratory distress syndrome[121–125] and in adults with severe adult respiratory distress syndrome (ARDS).

Pneumomediastinum resulting from either traumatic or spontaneous rupture of the esophagus is associated in many cases with hydrothorax or hydropneumothorax, usually on the left[28] but sometimes bilaterally.[36]

Clinical Manifestations

The symptoms and signs resulting from pneumomediastinum depend largely on the amount of air in the mediastinal space and on the presence or absence of associated infection. In infants, mediastinal emphysema is usually benign[126] and only rarely is associated with respiratory failure or cardiovascular collapse.[127, 128] In the adult, the diagnosis may be suggested by a history of abrupt onset of retrosternal pain radiating to the shoulders and down both arms, usually preceded by some occurrence, such as a spasm of coughing, sneezing, or vomiting that resulted in excessive increase in intrathoracic pressure. The pain usually is aggravated by respiration and sometimes by swallowing. Dyspnea may be severe. Physical examination generally reveals the presence of air in the subcutaneous tissues of the neck or over the thoracic wall. Hamman's sign may be detected on auscultation over the apex of the heart. This sign, consisting of a crunching or clicking noise synchronous with the heartbeat, has been estimated to occur in approximately 50 per cent of cases; it is heard best when the patient is in the left lateral decubitus position.[28] As previously discussed (*see* page 2796), it is not pathognomonic of pneumomediastinum.

Patients in whom air does not freely escape from the mediastinum into the neck, notably neonates, may have engorged neck veins, a rapid, thready pulse, and significant systemic hypotension.

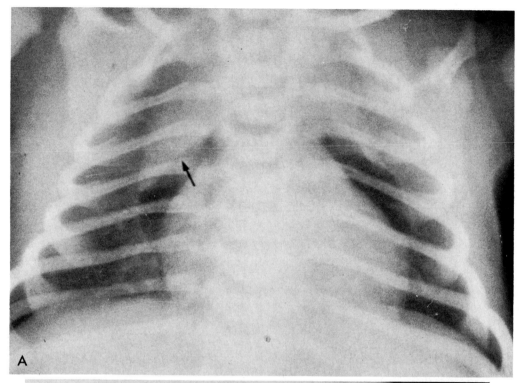

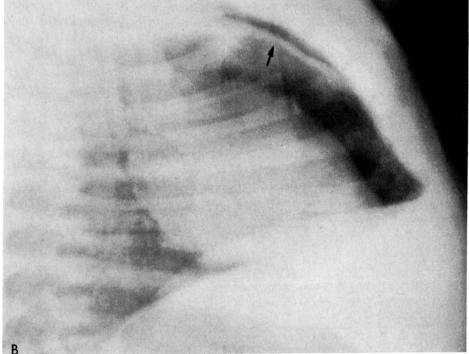

Figure 19–10. Pneumomediastinum. This infant male was born at full term with a difficult midforceps delivery. At birth there was mild to moderate retraction, a forced expiratory cry, and decreased air entry bilaterally. Anteroposterior *(A)* and lateral *(B)* roentgenograms reveal a large accumulation of gas in the mediastinal space, chiefly anteriorly, The mediastinal pleura is displaced far laterally on both sides and the thymus gland is elevated *(arrows).*

MEDIASTINAL HEMORRHAGE

The majority of cases of mediastinal hemorrhage result from trauma, usually of a severe nature such as that associated with an automobile accident[129, 130] or vigorous cardiopulmonary resuscitation. Less common causes include rupture of an aortic aneurysm,[131, 132] perforation of a vein by faulty insertion of a central venous line, extension of blood from the retropharyngeal soft tissues secondary to trauma or to spontaneous hemorrhage associated with coagulation disorders, and a complication of intracoronary infusion of streptokinase for coronary thrombosis.[133] Undoubtedly the majority of cases of mediastinal hemorrhage are unrecognized, the amount of bleeding being insufficient to produce symptoms and signs.

Roentgenologically, hemorrhage typically results in uniform, symmetric widening of the mediastinum in any of its compartments. Local accumulation of blood in the form of a hematoma is manifested by a homogeneous mass that can project to one or both sides of the mediastinum and may be situated in any compartment (Fig. 19–11).[132, 134, 135] Extensive dissection of blood from the mediastinum along the bronchovascular sheaths has been described, resulting in a roentgenographic pattern that simulated interstitial edema.[136] When mediastinal hemorrhage is caused by a ruptured aorta, the blood may extend into a pleural space, usually the left but sometimes the right as well.[137]

Symptoms and signs of mediastinal hemorrhage seldom are striking. Suspicion may be aroused when retrosternal pain radiating into the back develops in a patient who has recently suffered chest trauma. Mediastinal hemorrhage from a coagulation disorder may be suspected if local symptoms are associated with evidence of bleeding elsewhere, such as into the skin or retropharyngeal space. Rarely, these two inciting causes can coexist, as in the case of a hemophiliac who received minor chest injury.[138] A hematoma arising from a dissecting aneurysm may be associated with decreased pulsation in the arteries of the extremities. A hematoma of sufficient size and appropriate location can compress the superior vena cava.[129, 131]

MEDIASTINAL MASSES

The diseases of the mediastinum that have been described to this point show little or no predilection for a specific anatomic zone within the mediastinum. By contrast, a wide variety of lesions that present as tumors or "masses" show a strong predilection for one of the three mediastinal compartments. Thus it is logical to classify these masses on the basis of anatomic location. Despite the usefulness of such a classification, it should be clear that overlap is bound to occur and all that the classification implies is that lesions occur *predominantly* in one or another compartment; in fact, it is difficult if not impossible to classify some lesions anatomically. For example, aortic aneurysms may be situated in any of the three compartments, as may certain rare neoplasms such as leiomyoma and fibrous histiocytoma. Lymph node involvement in lymphoma occurs almost as frequently in the anterior as in the middle compartment; dilatation of the azygos and hemiazygos veins occupies both the middle and posterior com-

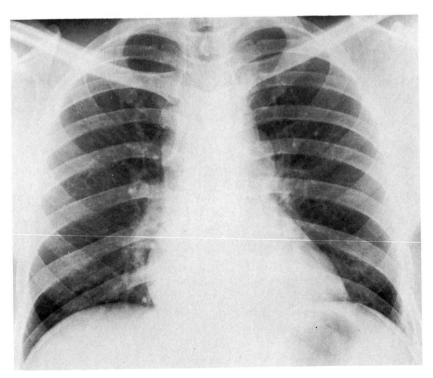

Figure 19–11. Spontaneous Mediastinal Hemorrhage. This 35-year-old hemophiliac was admitted to the hospital with evidence of a fresh hemorrhage in a remote area of the body. He had no symptoms referable to his thorax. A posteroanterior roentgenogram demonstrated bilateral widening of the mediastinum by a process whose lateral margins are somewhat lobulated. Involvement appears to be chiefly of the mid-mediastinal compartment. (A lateral roentgenogram was not helpful in localizing the abnormality.) This spontaneous mediastinal hematoma resolved completely in 10 days without residua.

partments. Such examples of overlap are obvious, since the anatomic structures in which the abnormalities arise are situated in more than one compartment.

It may be recalled that in Chapter 1 (see page 203), the normal anatomy of the mediastinum was described in detail according to the Heitzman classification.[18] This method was employed because we felt that it provides a logical subdivision of spaces within the midmediastinum that emphasizes the importance of major vascular channels to an understanding of mediastinal anatomy; however, we feel that this classification is not particularly appropriate for a logical analysis of mediastinal masses. Other schemes have been proposed for approaching differential diagnosis. For example, Feigin and Padua[139] have described a system for the diagnosis of mediastinal masses based on CT assessment of location and density following bolus injection of contrast medium; their schema seems to possess considerable merit judging from the increased specificity of differential diagnosis they have achieved. Although these and other exceptions must be always borne in mind, there can be little doubt of the overall benefit to differential diagnosis of a classification of mediastinal masses based on the predominant compartment affected—anterior, middle, or posterior—and the following discussion follows this principle.

The wide variety of tissues within the mediastinum is reflected in the many forms of neoplastic, developmental, and inflammatory masses that are seen. A 1971 review of the literature documented 34 previous reports of mediastinal tumors, totaling 3,364 patients.[639] Excluding metastatic pulmonary carcinoma and inflammatory conditions, the frequency of tumors was as follows: neurogenic neoplasms, 19.4 per cent; lymphoma, 15.8 per cent; bronchial and pericardial cysts, 14.2 per cent; germ cell ("teratodermoid") tumors, 12.8 per cent; thymoma, 11.5 per cent; and thyroid tumors, 6 per cent; a variety of miscellaneous tumors comprised the remaining 16 per cent. In another 1971 review of tumors seen over a 40-year period at the Mayo Clinic,[140] the findings were similar: of 1,064 cases, neurogenic neoplasms, thymomas, and benign cysts constituted 60 per cent; malignant lymphomas, teratomas, granulomas, and intrathoracic goiters comprised 30 per cent; and miscellaneous types of benign or malignant mesenchymal tumors, 10 per cent. In this series, the great majority of patients were adults, only 8 per cent being under 15 years of age at the time of diagnosis; there was no sex predominance. Most of the malignant lesions in children were of neurogenic, teratomatous, or vascular origin.[140] Excluding intrinsic neoplasms of the trachea and esophagus, cardiovascular abnormalities, diaphragmatic defects, and granulomatous diseases, most studies have found 25 to 50 per cent of mediastinal masses to be malignant neoplasms.[140-149] The majority of these cancers are located in the

anterior and middle mediastinal compartments. Almost half of all patients with mediastinal masses are asymptomatic, the abnormality being discovered on a screening chest roentgenogram.[140, 142, 146, 148, 150, 151]

The following sections represent little more than a brief outline of a very broad topic. The interested reader is directed to more comprehensive works by Leigh and his coworkers[134, 152] and to the accumulated experience of the Mayo[140, 147] and Cleveland[146] clinics.

MEDIASTINAL MASSES SITUATED PREDOMINANTLY IN THE ANTERIOR COMPARTMENT

This mediastinal compartment is bounded anteriorly by the sternum and posteriorly by the pericardium, aorta, and brachiocephalic vessels. It is the site of thymomas and a variety of other thymic abnormalities as well as almost all mediastinal germ cell tumors and hyperplastic and neoplastic abnormalities of thyroid and ectopic parathyroid tissue.

TUMORS AND TUMOR-LIKE CONDITIONS OF THE THYMUS

Thymic Hyperplasia

True thymic hyperplasia, as opposed to the lymphoid hyperplasia that is associated with myasthenia gravis (see farther on), is distinctly uncommon. It can be defined as an increase in the size of the thymus gland associated with a more or less intact gross architecture and a normal histologic appearance. In practice, the diagnosis can be confirmed either by noting a significant increase in the weight of the thymus compared to that expected for age or by detecting an increase in the size of a histologically normal gland on serial roentgenograms (Fig. 19–12). Although rare, several well-documented cases fulfilling these criteria have been reported.[153-156] In most cases the cause of the hyperplasia is unknown; occasionally, there has been a history of a previous stressful event[154] although the significance of this is unclear. Cases also have been reported in association with Beckwith-Wiedemann syndrome,[153] Graves' disease,[157] and prior chemotherapy for malignant neoplasms.[155, 156, 158-160] In the last-named situation, it has been suggested that the hyperplasia represents a rebound phenomenon secondary to the effects of chemotherapy.[158] Most patients in whom true thymic hyperplasia has been diagnosed are infants or children: of eight cases of massive hyperplasia reviewed by Judd,[154] ages ranged from newborn to 14 years. Symptoms are usually absent, although respiratory distress and dysphagia can occur.

The term "thymic hyperplasia" also has been used to describe a distinctive histologic reaction in

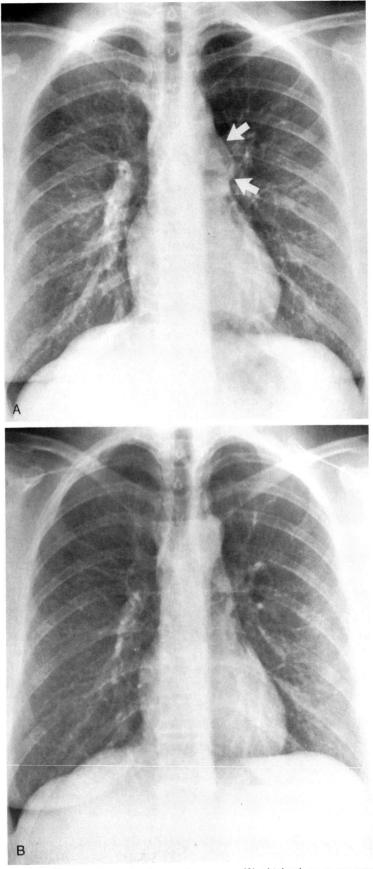

Figure 19–12. Thymic Hyperplasia. A posteroanterior roentgenogram *(A)* obtained as a pre-employment examination of this asymptomatic 25-year-old nurse reveals a sharply defined opacity protruding to the left at the level of the aortopulmonary window *(arrows)*. A film obtained several years previously *(B)* was normal.

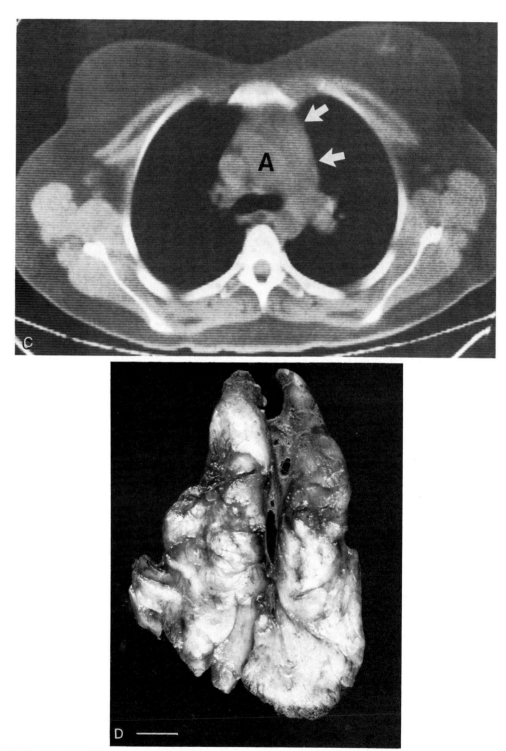

Figure 19–12 *Continued* A CT scan at the level of the carina *(C)* reveals a homogeneous mass *(arrows)* situated in the anterior mediastinum contiguous with the ascending aorta *(A)* and main pulmonary artery. The resected specimen *(D)* resembles a normal thymus gland except for size; histologic examination showed normal thymic tissue. (Bar = 1 cm.)

the thymus of patients with myasthenia gravis. In approximately two thirds of individuals with myasthenia, the thymic cortex is the site of multiple well-defined lymphoid follicles, many containing germinal centers (Fig. 19–13). Since the weight of the thymus gland in these cases is usually within normal limits,[157, 161] the designation thymic hyperplasia is strictly speaking incorrect; in fact, as Levine and Rosai have suggested,[157] the term lymphoid or follicular hyperplasia might be more appropriate to describe the abnormality. Occasionally, lymphoid follicles can be seen in thymus glands of apparently normal individuals; however, in patients with myasthenia gravis they are usually larger and much more numerous. This observation, as well as the large number of cases of myasthenia gravis associated with thymic "hyperplasia" and the favorable response to thymectomy in many patients, suggests a pathogenetic association between the two conditions.[162] However, the details of this relationship remain unclear.

Thymolipoma

Thymolipomas are uncommon anterior mediastinal tumors consisting of an admixture of fat and thymic epithelial and lymphoid tissue. They are said to constitute 2 to 9 per cent of all thymic tumors;[163] by 1973, approximately 50 cases had been reported.[163] No sex predilection is evident and the tumor can occur at any age, although young males appear to be particularly susceptible.[164]

The precise nature of thymolipoma is uncertain.[161] It has been considered to represent no more than a lipoma occurring within the thymus gland; however, since the thymic tissue itself appears to be increased in amount[161] this hypothesis appears unlikely. It also has been suggested that the tumor is a mixed lipoma and thymoma, the predominance of fat perhaps reflecting normal involution of the thymus; however, the normal appearance of the thymic tissue makes this interpretation improbable. A final theory proposes that the tumor begins as a true thymic hyperplasia (i.e., an increase in the amount of normal thymic tissue) that subsequently regresses and is replaced by adipose tissue.[161]

Grossly, thymolipomas are typically yellow, soft, and roughly bilobed in shape, somewhat resembling the normal thymus gland. They are often large and can grow to huge proportions. In 68 per cent of reported cases they have weighed more than 500 gm and in 23 per cent of cases more than 2,000 gm; one reported tumor weighed over 12,000 gm.[163] Histologically, the tumor consists of adult adipose tissue interspersed with areas of normal thymic tissue.[161, 163] Germinal centers such as occur in thymic hyperplasia are typically absent.

When small, thymolipomas present no roentgenographic features that distinguish them from other anterior mediastinal masses. However, as discussed above, they often grow very large and as a result of their soft pliable consistency tend to slump toward the diaphragm. They thus adapt themselves to the diaphragmatic contour by becoming largely inferior in position and leaving the superior mediastinal space relatively clear (Fig. 19–14).[163] Their fat content sometimes helps to distinguish them from other mediastinal masses because of their relative radiolucency, a feature that sometimes can be appreciated roentgenographically but should be readily apparent on a CT scan.[165]

Thymolipomas characteristically cause few or no symptoms even when very large; thus, the lesion is usually discovered on a screening roentgenogram. Rare cases have been reported in association with myasthenia gravis,[166, 167] aplastic anemia,[168] Graves'

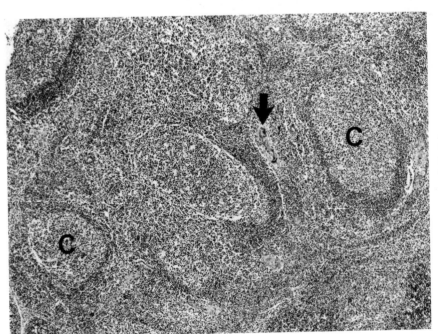

Figure 19–13. Thymic 'Hyperplasia' Associated with Myasthenia Gravis. A histologic section of a grossly normal thymus gland removed from a patient with myasthenia gravis shows several irregularly shaped germinal centers *(C)* that cause considerable distortion of normal thymic architecture. Occasional Hassall's corpuscles are evident *(arrow).* (× 48.)

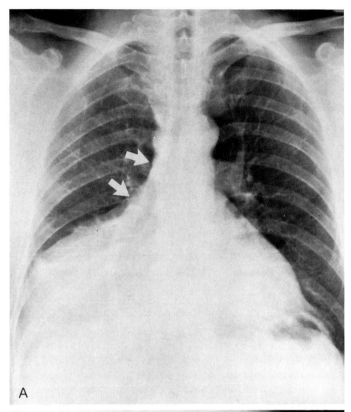

A

Figure 19–14. Thymolipoma. Posteroanterior *(A)* and lateral *(B)* roentgenograms demonstrate a large mass situated in the lower half of the right hemithorax. The obtuse angle the mass creates with the mediastinum (*arrows* in *A*) indicates its origin from that structure. In lateral projection, note that the mass extends almost the whole anteroposterior depth of the thorax, obscuring most of the right hemidiaphragm (the posterior margin of the mass is indicated by *open arrows* in *B*). The anterior mediastinum looks "empty." (Courtesy of Dr. R. Hedvigi, Montreal Chest Hospital.)

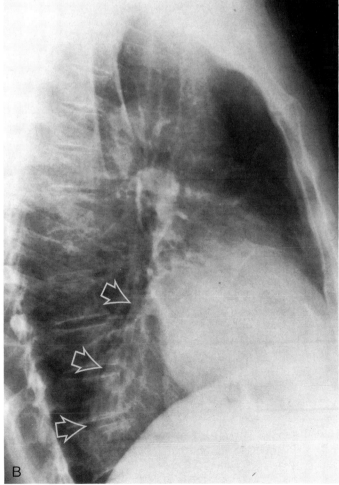

B

disease, red cell hypoplasia, and hypogammaglobulinemia.[167] The behavior is typically benign, no recurrences having been documented following resection; however, an unusual case has been reported of apparent thymic liposarcoma, possibly derived from a thymolipoma.[169]

Thymic Cysts

Thymic cysts are uncommon mediastinal lesions that account for only 1 to 2 per cent of all tumors in the anterior compartment;[170] a review of the literature up to 1964 yielded only 32 cases.[171] Although it has been suggested that they represent degeneration and enlargement of Hassall's corpuscles,[172] it is probable that most are derived from remnants of the fetal thymopharyngeal duct. However, 3 cases of thymic cyst have been reported recently[173] in which the abnormality was discovered some time after thoracic surgery, suggesting a possible relationship to surgical trauma.

Pathologically,[172] the cysts are unilocular or multilocular and range in size from microscopic to 18 cm in maximum diameter. They can contain straw-colored fluid or, if hemorrhage has occurred, brown-green gelatinous or grumous material (Fig. 19–15). Histologically, the cyst wall is lined by squamous, transitional, or simple cuboidal or columnar epithelium; ulceration with underlying fibrosis and chronic inflammation is fairly common as is evidence of remote hemorrhage (hemosiderin-laden macrophages and cholesterol clefts). Thymic tissue can be identified focally in the cyst wall (Fig. 19–15), and in fact its presence is necessary to make the diagnosis.

The appearance of thymic cysts on conventional roentgenograms is in no way characteristic or diagnostic,[170, 171] although their cystic nature should be readily apparent on CT or MR images (Fig. 19–15). Most patients are asymptomatic. In one patient, obstruction of the pulmonary artery by the cyst resulted in chest pain, dyspnea, and a systolic thrill and murmur on physical examination; the patient was originally misdiagnosed as having stenosis of the pulmonary valve.[174]

An important point in the pathologic differential diagnosis is the observation that some malignant tumors, particularly thymoma, Hodgkin's disease, and seminoma, can show prominent cystic change, occasionally associated with neoplastic tissue that is relatively small in amount; consequently thorough sampling of every "thymic cyst" must be carried out to exclude the possibility of neoplasia, especially if the "cyst" wall is thickened by fibrous tissue. In addition to such degenerative changes in a primary neoplasm, it has been suggested that Hodgkin's disease can occasionally develop in the wall of a true thymic cyst.[175] Although rare, carcinoma also has been reported to arise from cyst epithelium.[176]

Inflammatory Conditions Causing Thymic Enlargement

Enlargement of the thymus gland is occasionally caused by an inflammatory process. Reported examples include allergic granulomatosis,[177] hydatid disease, tuberculosis,[178] eosinophilic granuloma (histiocytosis X),[179] and idiopathic (inflammatory "pseudotumor").[180]

Thymoma

Thymomas are neoplasms of thymic epithelium that can behave in either a benign or malignant fashion and that characteristically consist of rather uniform cells with a variable amount of admixed lymphocytes. Thymic epithelial neoplasms composed of cells with significant cytologic atypia and a high mitotic rate are more appropriately termed thymic carcinoma and are discussed separately below. The tendency in former years to use terms such as "seminomatous" or "granulomatous" thymoma to refer to neoplasms of germ cell or lymphoid origin that arise within the thymus[161, 181] has now been abandoned.

Thymoma is probably the second most common primary neoplasm (after lymphoma) to affect the mediastinum; in Ingels and colleagues' 1971 review of the literature on mediastinal tumors,[182] this neoplasm comprised 11.5 per cent of all cases. Of a total of 789 cases in five relatively recent reviews from Sweden,[183] France,[184] Italy,[185] the United States,[186] and Germany,[187] there was a slight female predominance (427 to 362, or 1.2 to 1). Most tumors are discovered in middle-aged adults, the average age at diagnosis in the series cited above being 51, 48, 46, 52, and 45 years, respectively; they occur rarely in individuals under 20 years of age.[188] The etiology and pathogenesis are unknown; one study from Hong Kong suggested an association with Epstein-Barr virus.[189]

PATHOLOGIC CHARACTERISTICS

As might be expected, the vast majority of thymomas arise in the upper portion of the anterior mediastinum, corresponding to the position of the normal thymus gland. Rarely, they are discovered in an unusual location such as the posterior mediastinum,[150, 190] perihilar tissues, or lung parenchyma (see page 1608) or can extend as a continuum from the anterior mediastinum to the posterior chest wall.[38]

Grossly, the majority of tumors present as well-encapsulated, round or slightly lobulated masses. They usually range from 5 to 15 cm in diameter,[161, 186] although they tend to be somewhat smaller in individuals with myasthenia gravis, presumably because of the presence of symptoms at an earlier stage. Cut sections reveal the tumor to be firm, pale

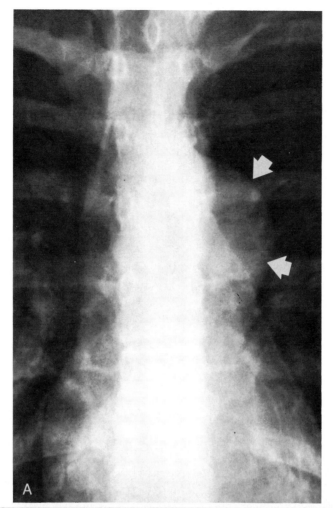

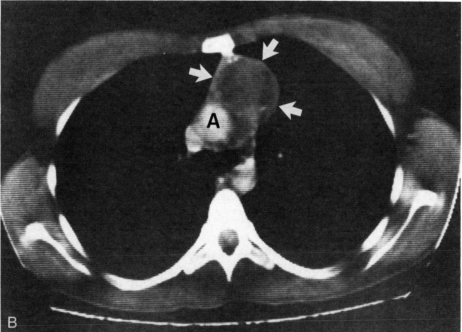

Figure 19–15. Thymic Cyst. A detail view of the mediastinum from a posteroanterior roentgenogram *(A)* reveals a sharply defined homogeneous opacity extending to the left at the level of the aortopulmonary window *(arrows)*. A CT scan at the same level *(B)* shows the lesion to be a fluid-filled cyst *(arrows)* relating to the anterior aspect and left side of the ascending aorta *(A)*.

Illustration continued on following page

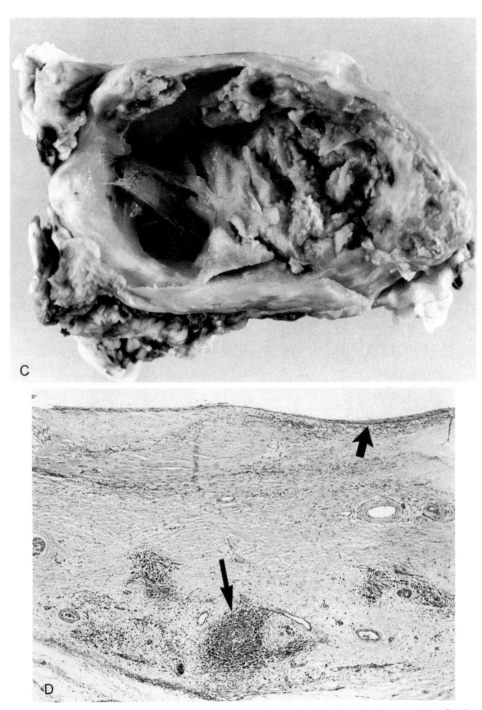

Figure 19–15 *Continued* The excised specimen *(C)* shows the cyst to contain abundant friable material, reflecting prior hemorrhage. A histologic section through the cyst wall *(D)* reveals a flattened squamous epithelium *(short arrow)*, fibrous tissue, and a small amount of residual thymic tissue *(long arrow)*. (× 60.)

gray or tan in color, and frequently subdivided into numerous lobules by variably thick fibrous bands (Fig. 19–16). One or more cysts are not infrequent and are sometimes large, comprising most of the tumor volume. Foci of calcification, hemorrhage, and necrosis also may be seen. Infiltration of adjacent structures, particularly the pleura and lung and less commonly the pericardium, chest wall, diaphragm, and mediastinal vessels, occurs in 10 to 15 per cent of cases, but it is important to recognize

that the tumor can be adherent to adjacent structures without actually invading them (Fig. 19–16).[186] Since the natural history of thymoma can be at least partly predicted by the presence or absence of local extracapsular invasion (*see* farther on), this must be clearly confirmed histologically.

The lobulation noted grossly in many tumors is easily identified histologically, especially in lymphocyte predominant forms (Fig. 19–17); occasionally, there is marked thickening of fibrous intralob-

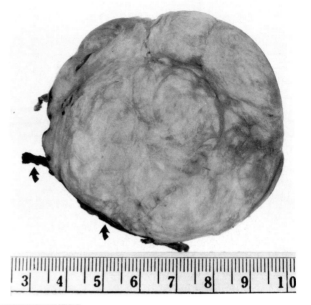

Figure 19–16. Thymoma. A cut section of an anterior mediastinal mass shows a well-circumscribed tumor possessing a distinctly lobulated appearance. There is no necrosis or hemorrhage. A small amount of compressed lung is adherent to the tumor *(arrows)* but is not invaded.

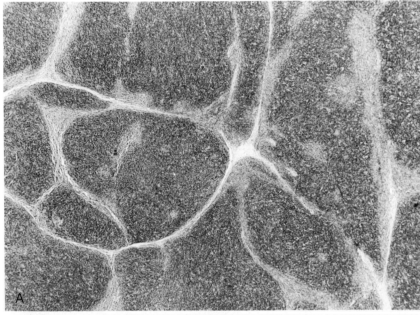

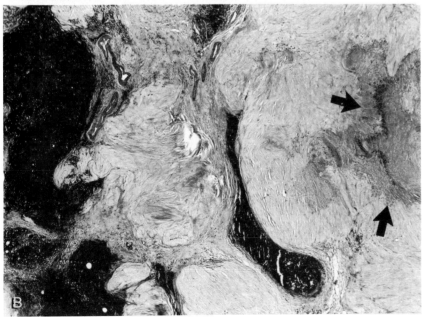

Figure 19–17. Thymoma: Microscopic Lobulation. A low-power view of a predominantly lymphocytic thymoma *(A)* shows the tumor to be divided by thin fibrous bands into numerous lobules of variable size and shape. A section from another tumor *(B)* shows marked thickening of fibrous septa with focal calcification *(arrows).*

Illustration continued on following page

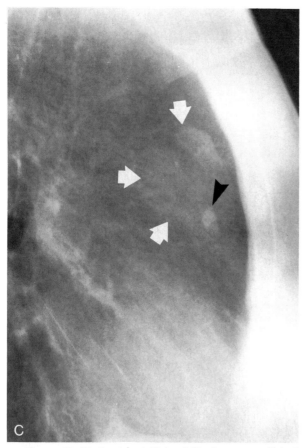

Figure 19–17 *Continued* The calcification was sufficiently extensive to be visible on a laterial roentgenogram of the chest *(C)* (the tumor is indicated by *arrows* and the calcification by an *arrowhead*).

ular bands associated with hyalinization and dystrophic calcification (Fig. 19–17), a process that sometimes can be identified roentgenographically. The cellular composition of thymoma and the appearance of the tumor cells are highly variable, both within a single tumor and between different tumors. The neoplastic epithelial cells vary from polygonal to distinctly spindled in shape, and the associated lymphocytic infiltrate can be absent or can be so marked as to obscure almost completely the presence of the epithelial cells themselves.[161, 184, 186, 187] Such histologic variability has given rise to several morphologic "subtypes" of thymoma, the most common classification consisting of predominantly lymphocytic, mixed lymphoepithelial, and predominantly epithelial forms; the last named is itself sometimes divided into polygonal and spindle cell varieties. In four of the reviews cited above comprising a total of 589 cases,[183, 185–187] the incidence of the subtypes was epithelial, 30 per cent; mixed, 47 per cent; and lymphocytic, 22 per cent. This classification is useful for descriptive and occasionally for diagnostic purposes, but it should be borne in mind that there is a histologic continuum between each of these categories; thus, although there is some evidence of a different clinical behavior in

some variants (*see* farther on), it is unlikely that any one represents a specific entity in itself.

Classification of thymomas based solely on epithelial cell morphology also has been proposed;[191] according to this schema, tumors are divided into cortical, medullary, and mixed forms depending on the shape of the neoplastic epithelial cells, without consideration for the number of admixed lymphocytes. Since there are morphologic, immunohistochemical, and perhaps functional differences[191, 192] between the cortical and medullary regions of the normal thymus, such a classification has some theoretical merit; however, its usefulness in predicting clinical behavior has not been established (*see* farther on).

As the name implies, lymphocytic tumors are composed of an abundance of lymphocytes with scattered admixed epithelial cells (Fig. 19–18). The latter are usually fairly evenly distributed among the lymphocytes and are polygonal in shape; nuclei are round or oval and possess relatively small, uniform nucleoli. In some cases, tumor cells are so infrequent that a diagnosis of lymphoma may be considered, especially if the amount of tissue is small or is obtained from a site other than the anterior mediastinum;[193] this diagnostic difficulty is compounded in some tumors by the presence of reactive changes in the lymphocytes including nuclear pleomorphism and prominent nucleoli (Fig. 19–18). Hassall's corpuscles are relatively common in the epithelial form, as are foci of "medullary differentiation" in which the density of lymphocytes is less than that of the surrounding tissue, resulting in distinct areas of relative pallor at low magnification (Fig. 19–19).

In mixed lymphoepithelial tumors, the epithelial cells tend to occur as well-defined sheets or trabeculae separated by clusters of lymphocytes (Fig. 19–20). Predominantly epithelial tumors possess little or no lymphocytic component (Fig. 19–21). In both the mixed lymphoepithelial and epithelial varieties, the neoplastic thymic cells can be polygonal or distinctly spindled in shape; the cells of the epithelial type may be arranged in nests or in a storiform or fascicular pattern, simulating carcinoid tumor or mesenchymal neoplasms such as hemangiopericytoma. A characteristic histologic feature of all three varieties of thymoma is the presence of perivascular spaces (Fig. 19–22). These spaces are centered about small blood vessels and contain proteinaceous fluid and scattered lymphocytes; the reason for this formation in thymoma is unclear.

ROENTGENOGRAPHIC MANIFESTATIONS

The roentgenographic appearance of the normal thymus gland has been thoroughly reviewed by Baron and associates[194] and by Heiberg and colleagues.[195] Although these authors have recorded some differences in the maximum size of the thymus gland in patients under the age of 20, accurate

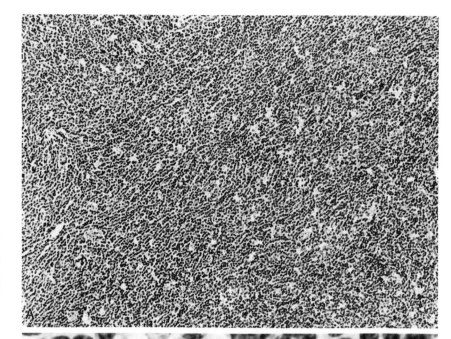

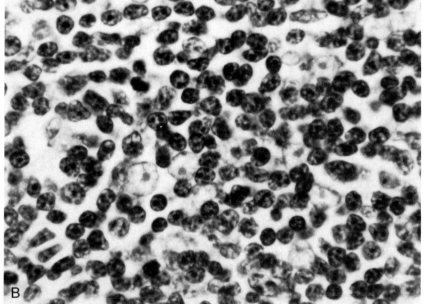

Figure 19–18. Thymoma: Lymphocyte Predominant. A histologic section *(A)* reveals a fairly monotonous infiltrate of lymphocytes in which numerous, evenly distributed pale cells can be identified. The overall pattern results in a "starry sky" appearance. A section at high magnification *(B)* shows the pale areas to consist of neoplastic thymic epithelial cells; nuclei are vesicular with uniform nucleoli, and the cytoplasm is indistinct. Note the mild pleomorphism and prominent nucleoli of lymphocyte nuclei.

Illustration continued on following page

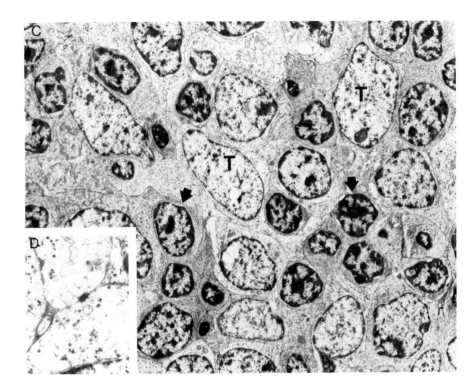

Figure 19–18 *Continued* A transmission electron micrograph *(C)* confirms the presence of lymphocytes *(arrows)* and epithelial cells *(T)*, the latter focally connected by desmosomes (magnified further in the insert, *D*). (*A*, × 120; *B*, × 1,000; *C*, × 5,300; *D*, × 29,100.)

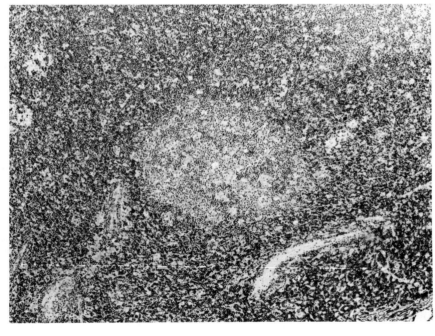

Figure 19–19. Thymoma: Medullary Differentiation. A histologic section of a lymphocyte-predominant thymoma shows a distinct focus of relative pallor caused by a reduced concentration of lymphocytes. This appearance corresponds to the difference between cortical and medullary regions of the normal thymus. (× 70.)

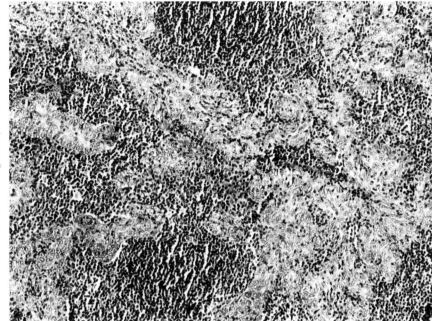

Figure 19–20. Thymoma: Mixed Lymphoepithelial. In this histologic section, well-defined trabeculae and sheets of epithelial cells are separated by clusters of lymphocytes. (× 120.)

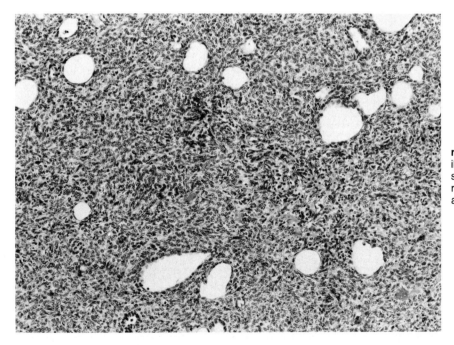

Figure 19–21. Thymoma: Predominantly Epithelial. In contrast to the pattern illustrated in Figure 19–20, this tumor consists almost entirely of uniform polygonal to round epithelial cells with only occasional admixed lymphocytes. (× 120.)

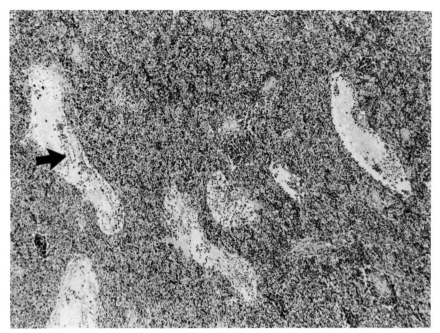

Figure 19–22. Thymoma: Perivascular Spaces. A histologic section of a mixed lymphoepithelial tumor shows several irregularly shaped clear spaces, in all of which proteinaceous fluid and a few lymphocytes can be identified; a small vessel is present in some *(arrow).* (× 60.)

figures are perhaps not of vital importance since thymomas occur so infrequently in patients in that age group.

Most thymomas are situated near the junction of the heart and great vessels. Roentgenologically, they are round or oval and their margins smooth or lobulated (Fig. 19–23).[196] They can protrude to one or both sides of the mediastinum and if of sufficient size can displace the heart and great vessels posteriorly. In some cases, calcification is apparent at the periphery of the lesion or throughout its substance (*see* Fig. 19–17). Occasionally, thymic tumors can simulate massive cardiomegaly[197, 198] or pericardial effusion.[199] When very large in size, their site of origin can be exceedingly difficult to establish short of arteriography (Fig. 19–24).

A spate of articles has appeared in recent years in which an attempt has been made to define the most appropriate roentgenographic techniques for the diagnosis of thymomas, and all are agreed that CT is the examination of choice.[200–203] In a Mayo Clinic study of 69 cases,[200] although CT did not reveal any lesions that were not suspected from other roentgenographic studies (including conventional roentgenography in posteroanterior, oblique, and lateral projections and lateral tomography), it clarified significant anatomic relationships and, perhaps more importantly, demonstrated adherence and invasion to best advantage; however, none of the imaging techniques was accurate in predicting malignancy. In another study of 16 patients with pathologically proven thymoma,[202] CT demonstrated the lesion clearly in all cases; except for two cases in which invasive thymoma showed a markedly irregular and infiltrative pattern on CT. However, the examination failed to discriminate benign from malignant lesions. Baron and his colleagues,[203] in their study of 25 patients with thymic pathology,

found that CT was useful in suggesting or excluding a diagnosis of thymoma and in distinguishing thymic hyperplasia from thymoma in patients with myasthenia gravis (*see* farther on). Smith and her colleagues[204] have described a case of invasive thymoma and superior vena caval obstruction in which the invasive nature of the neoplasm was clearly shown by CT.

CT is also the examination of choice in the investigation of patients with myasthenia gravis.[205–208] For example, in a radiologic/pathologic correlative study by Fon and his colleagues,[206] conventional roentgenograms of the chest and CT scans of the mediastinum were correlated with pathologic findings of the thymus following thymectomy in 57 patients with myasthenia gravis: 14 of 16 cases of thymoma were either suspected or definitely diagnosed on CT evidence; the conclusion that thymoma could be confidently diagnosed by CT bore some relationship to age. These observers concluded that thymoma cannot be predicted with a high level of confidence in patients younger than 40 years of age because of the difficulty in differentiating normal thymus or hyperplasia from thymoma; by contrast, the diagnosis can be made with confidence in patients 40 years of age and older. In another study of 19 patients with myasthenia gravis[208] who subsequently underwent thymectomy, CT was accurate in detecting the nine true thymic masses but could not distinguish thymomas from nonthymomatous masses, including thymic cysts. In eight cases in this series, glands that revealed histologic evidence of lymphoid hyperplasia and those that were histologically normal possessed a similar appearance and could not be differentiated by CT. From a study of 154 consecutive patients who were subjected to thymectomy for myasthenia gravis, Ellis and his colleagues[209] concluded that for patients

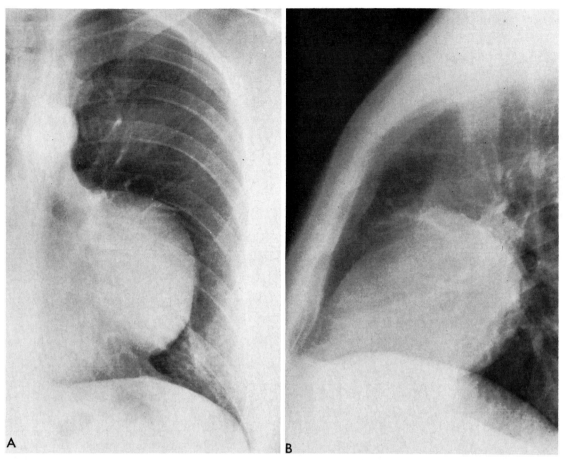

Figure 19–23. Thymoma. A view of the left hemithorax from posteroanterior *(A)* and lateral *(B)* roentgenograms of a 39-year-old asymptomatic man reveals a large, well-defined, homogeneous mass projecting to the left of the mediastinum contiguous to the heart. No calcification is visible.

under 21 years of age CT should be employed only when local symptoms, signs, or conventional roentgenographic findings suggest the presence of thymic abnormality; for patients 21 years of age and older CT should be used routinely.

CLINICAL MANIFESTATIONS

Although some patients with thymoma are asymptomatic when the tumor is discovered, the majority manifest symptoms related to local compression or invasion of thoracic structures or to systemic autoimmune disease, or to both. Hematologic abnormalities, especially pure red cell hypoplasia[640] and less commonly aplastic anemia, are also present in some patients. The effects of local compression or invasion are seen in about one third of patients. For example, of the 283 patients in the 1987 report from the Mayo Clinic,[186] 100 patients presented with symptoms related directly to the tumor, the most frequent being chest pain, shortness of breath, and cough; hoarseness and the superior vena cava syndrome were seen occasionally.

Myasthenia gravis is by far the most common autoimmune disease associated with thymoma. Ap-

proximately 15 per cent of patients with myasthenia have this tumor,[144,186,210] and about 35 per cent (range, 7 to 54 per cent) of patients with thymoma have myasthenia.[140, 146, 186, 211, 212] The tumor is sometimes occult; for example, in their review of 165 patients with thymoma, Maggi and colleagues[185] found 12 patients with myasthenia gravis whose resected thymus was of normal size or was only minimally enlarged. Rarely, myasthenia gravis occurs concomitantly with other disorders such as red cell hypoplasia.[213, 640]

Other autoimmune conditions occasionally associated with thymoma include hypogammaglobulinemia (sometimes associated with persistent candidiasis),[212] systemic lupus erythematosus, rheumatoid disease, polymyositis, Graves' disease, inflammatory bowel disease (including both Crohn's disease and ulcerative colitis), pernicious anemia, Sjögren's syndrome, pemphigus vulgaris, and alopecia areata.[184, 186, 187]

PROGNOSIS

The majority of thymomas are slow-growing encapsulated neoplasms, and their surgical excision results in cure; some, however, are locally aggressive

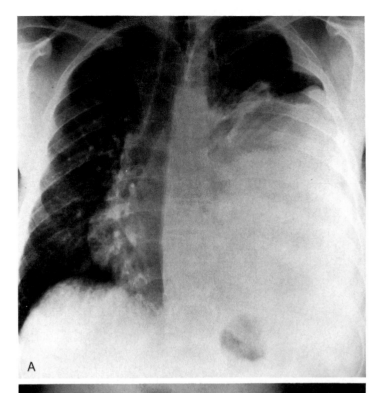

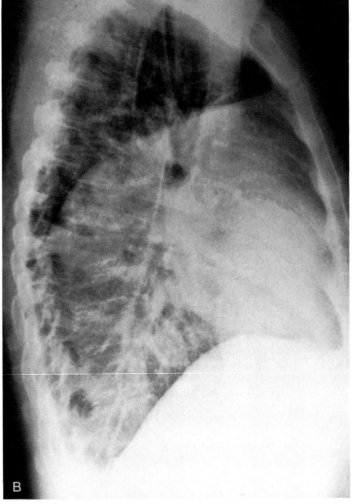

Figure 19–24. Huge Thymoma of the Mediastinum.
Posteroanterior *(A)* and lateral *(B)* roentgenograms reveal
a large homogeneous mass occupying much of the left
hemithorax, displacing the mediastinum markedly to the
right and depressing the left hemidiaphragm (note the
position of the gastric air bubble).

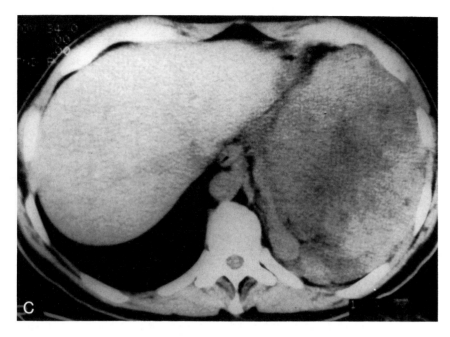

Figure 19–24 *Continued* A CT scan *(C)* through the base of the thorax shows the left hemithorax to be filled with a mass of inhomogeneous density. At this stage, the precise origin of the mass was disputed, and a left internal mammary arteriogram was performed in an attempt to discover the tissue of origin.

Illustration continued on following page

neoplasms that are unresectable or that recur following apparent complete excision. Histologic features are not predictive of the behavior of any one tumor. Thus, local invasion, recurrence after excision, and intrathoracic metastases can occur with different tumors possessing the same histologic appearance. Morphometric studies[214, 215] have suggested that the presence of invasion is more likely in tumors containing cells with increased nuclear area; however, there is substantial overlap between groups of invasive and noninvasive tumors,[214] and this parameter is not useful in the individual patient. Measurement of nuclear DNA content also has been found not to be of predictive value.[214] A number of studies[186] have reported that predominantly epithelial tumors tend to be more aggressive; the exception may be the spindle cell variant which some authors have found to have a relatively indolent course.[186] An association between the spindle cell form and pure red cell hypoplasia has also been proposed.[640] Although a number of studies have shown that the cortical type of thymoma is more likely to be associated with invasion than the medullary form,[191, 192, 216] one relatively large investigation showed no predictive difference between the two with respect to relapse-free survival.[217]

Despite these pathologic observations, there is little question that the best criterion of malignancy or benignancy is the presence or absence of local invasion, a state that is usually established by the surgeon at the time of thoracotomy. The percentage of thymomas that are reported to show such invasion varies widely in different series, ranging from 7 to 50 per cent;[161] our personal experience is more consistent with the former figure. Recurrence is the rule in individuals with these tumors, because complete resection is usually impossible; however, since such tumors can be slow growing, residual disease can be associated with prolonged survival. The

presence of invasion is the most important predictor of prognosis, but it should be remembered that even well-encapsulated tumors that apparently have been completely excised can recur, as was the case in 12 per cent of tumors in the series reported by Lewis and colleagues.[186]

Although thymoma can spread within the thorax by direct extension and by implantation within the pleural space, extrathoracic metastases are very uncommon;[165] in a review of the literature in 1976,[218] only 29 cases were identified and it is possible that some of these represented thymic carcinomas. In their review of 283 patients from the Mayo Clinic, Lewis and colleagues[186] found only 8 patients (3 per cent) with distant metastases. Of 19 cases of "invasive thymoma" reviewed by Scatarige and associates,[219] 6 showed CT evidence of transdiaphragmatic extension, chiefly to the retroperitoneal space, thus suggesting to these authors that the upper abdomen should be included in any CT examination in which a thymic malignancy is considered a possibility.

Thymic Neuroendocrine Neoplasms

This term encompasses several varieties of thymic neoplasm, all of which have in common histologic, ultrastructural, immunohistochemical, and, occasionally, clinical features of neuroendocrine function. Although specific names have been given to the several histologic varieties, it is probable that as with primary neuroendocrine neoplasms of the lung, they represent a spectrum of differentiation rather than specific entities. The etiology and pathogenesis are unknown. The tumors are believed to be derived from neuroendocrine cells analogous to either intestinal Kulchitsky's cells or thyroid C cells (or both) whose presence has been documented in normal thymus.[220] These tumors are

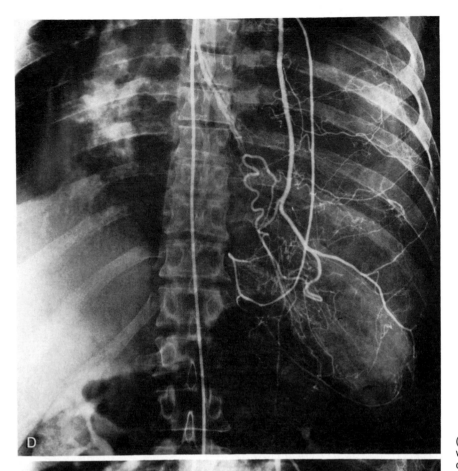

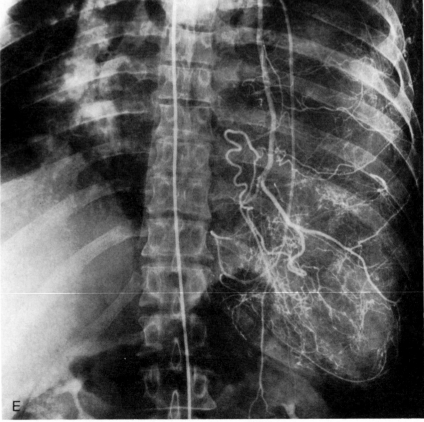

Figure 19–24 *Continued* This study (*D* and *E*) showed that much of the mass was supplied by this vessel, indicating its origin from either the mediastinum or chest wall.

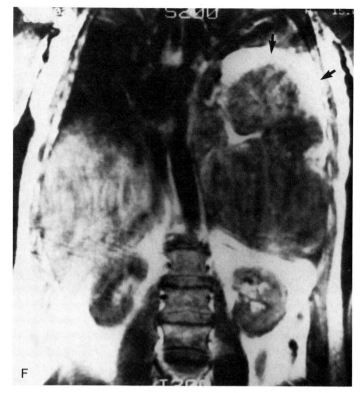

Figure 19–24 *Continued* A T1-weighted coronal reconstruction magnetic resonance image *(F)* shows the mass to be situated above the left hemidiaphragm and to be relatively inhomogeneous in density. A considerable amount of fat relates to the mass superiorly *(arrows)*.

uncommon; according to Viebahn and associates,[221] approximately 100 cases had been reported by 1984. Most occur in young adult males.

Pathologically, the most common histologic subtype of thymic neuroendocrine neoplasm is carcinoid tumor; as with their pulmonary counterparts, these may be well differentiated (so-called "typical" carcinoid tumor) or show features suggestive of a more aggressive nature (moderately differentiated or "atypical" carcinoid tumor). In their 1976 review, Rosai and colleagues[220] found the latter to be the more common form. Grossly, the tumors are usually bulky and somewhat lobulated; about half are encapsulated, the remainder showing invasion of adjacent pleura, pericardium, diaphragm, or mediastinum.[220] The cut surface is solid, gray to tan in color, and soft in consistency; foci of necrosis and hemorrhage are frequent and calcification may be evident.[220–222] The histologic pattern is variable but most commonly consists of nests and trabeculae of fairly uniform cells separated by a delicate fibrovascular stroma. Variants include a spindle cell pattern similar to that of some peripheral pulmonary carcinoid tumors and an appearance resembling thyroid medullary carcinoma (sometimes associated with amyloid).[220] Necrosis, cytologic atypia, and numerous mitotic figures are present in many cases.

As with carcinoid tumors in other locations, silver stains show intracytoplasmic argyrophilic granules in some cases; ultrastructural examination reveals the presence of neurosecretory granules in virtually all.[220, 222] Immunohistochemical examination[222, 223] frequently shows a positive reaction to cholecystokinin, neurotensin, and ACTH; a positive reaction is also common[224] but not invariable[223] for neuron-specific enolase.

In addition to neoplasms with the characteristic histologic appearance of carcinoid tumor, rare cases have been reported of tumors composed predominantly of cells with hyperchromatic nuclei and scanty cytoplasm that resemble small cell (oat cell) carcinoma of the lung.[220, 225, 226] In some cases, an apparent transition between the two histologic patterns can be identified.[225, 226] As with pulmonary carcinoma, occasional tumors have a mixed appearance (usually squamous cell/small cell) at either the light[227] or electron microscopic[226, 227] level. From a practical point of view, metastasis from a primary small cell carcinoma of the lung must be seriously considered in the diagnosis of any anterior mediastinal mass possessing this appearance; nevertheless, it is clear that the neoplasm is occasionally primary at this site.

Roentgenographic features of thymic neuroendocrine neoplasms are nonspecific, generally consisting of a lobulated anterior mediastinal mass; calcification can be identified in some cases.[222] The tumors associated with Cushing's syndrome tend to be smaller and may be identifiable only with CT.[222] As with metastatic carcinoid tumors from other sites, bony metastases tend to be osteoblastic.[222]

Clinically, many mediastinal carcinoid tumors occasion no symptoms and are discovered on screening chest roentgenograms. Signs and symptoms caused by compression or invasion of mediastinal structures may be present and include chest or shoulder pain, dyspnea, cough, and superior vena cava syndrome.[220] Clinical findings of paraneoplastic disease are also present in some patients and reflect the neuroendocrine nature of these neoplasms. Cushing's syndrome is the most common of these:[228, 229] according to Viebahn and associates,[221] it was present in 14 of 70 patients (23 per cent) documented in the literature by 1984. Less common manifestations include inappropriate secretion of ADH,[220] carcinoid syndrome,[230, 231] and hyperparathyroidism[232] (the last named possibly caused by intrinsic parathyroid disease rather than the carcinoid tumor itself). Of the 70 cases reviewed by Viebahn and associates,[221] 8 (13 per cent) were associated with the syndrome of multiple endocrine neoplasia.[220, 233] In this condition, endocrine and neuroendocrine tumors arise in a variety of other locations, including the gastrointestinal tract; thyroid, adrenal, and parathyroid glands; and pancreatic islets.

As might be expected, complete excision of well-differentiated, encapsulated carcinoid tumors of the thymus is associated with a good prognosis,[220] even in the few patients in whom regional lymph node metastases are present. However, the prognosis of patients with "atypical" forms in which mediastinal structures are often directly invaded must be guarded, death being caused in many individuals by local extension of disease or metastases.[220, 222] The overall 5-year survival rate is said to be 65 per cent.[221] Small cell (oat cell) carcinomas are so rare that it is difficult to predict behavior on the basis of published reports, but there is some evidence that they may be somewhat less aggressive than their pulmonary counterparts.[226]

Thymic Carcinoma

As discussed above, a proportion of thymomas that show histologic features suggestive of a benign neoplasm will invade adjacent mediastinal tissues and lung and will occasionally metastasize. Although this behavior indicates that such tumors are malignant and hence might be called carcinomas, this term is usually reserved for neoplasms that possess the traditional histologic and cytologic features of malignancy. These latter tumors are rare; for example, within a 75-year period only 20 cases were identified at the Mayo Clinic. As with other thymic neoplasms, the etiology is unknown. In one case there was a history of prior mediastinal radiotherapy;[226] some cases may be derived from a thymic cyst[227] or thymoma.[234]

Pathologically, thymic carcinomas are usually bulky masses that range from 5 to 15 cm in diameter;[226, 227] they have often invaded adjacent structures at the time of diagnosis. Histologically, a remarkable variety of patterns has been reported, the most common being squamous cell carcinoma (many of which resemble so-called lymphoepithelioma of the nasopharynx) (Fig 19–25).[226, 227] Other variants include small cell carcinoma (discussed above in the section on neuroendocrine tumors), mixed small cell/squamous cell carcinoma, mucoepidermoid carcinoma, adenoid cystic carcinoma, clear cell carcinoma (that resembles renal cell carcinoma), and poorly differentiated spindle cell or "sarcomatoid" carcinoma.[226, 227, 235]

Clinically, most patients are symptomatic at the time of diagnosis, the most common complaints being chest pain and cough; systemic findings such as fever, weight loss, fatigue, and night sweats are fairly common.[226] Unlike thymomas, an association with myasthenia gravis and other autoimmune disorders has not been described. Conventional roentgenographic features are nonspecific, although CT or MR scans should be capable of revealing invasion of the mediastinum or lung.

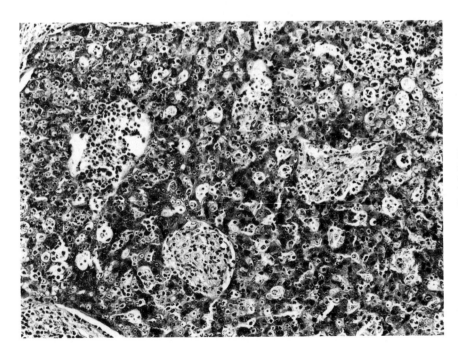

Figure 19–25. Thymic Carcinoma. A histologic section of a well-circumscribed anterior mediastinal mass shows sheets of cytologically atypical cells associated with focal necrosis and an extensive infiltrate of polymorphonuclear leukocytes. (× 170.)

The prognosis of thymic carcinoma is poor; local intrathoracic growth and extrathoracic metastases develop in the majority of patients. In the series described by Wick and colleagues from the Mayo Clinic,[226] 15 of the 18 patients who survived surgery died of the tumor in an average period of only 20.3 months.

Thymic Lymphoma

The thymus is a fairly frequent site of involvement by lymphoma, particularly Hodgkin's disease; for example, in one review of 44 patients with the latter condition in which disease was apparently limited to the mediastinum, the thymus was affected in half of the patients.[236] The histologic type of Hodgkin's disease is almost always nodular sclerosis. The tumor has a tendency to cystic degeneration, particularly following radiation therapy.[237] Lymphoblastic lymphoma, a neoplasm that frequently shows features of T-cell lineage, also commonly affects the thymus and, in fact, is believed by many investigators to be derived from thymic lymphocytes.[238] Other forms of lymphoma affect the thymus less commonly, especially in isolation.[169, 239–241]

The roentgenographic features of lymphoma confined to the thymus gland are not in any way specific; however, should mediastinal or hilar lymph nodes be enlarged in addition to a mass appearing in the region of the thymus the diagnosis should be seriously considered.

GERM CELL NEOPLASMS

This term encompasses a group of tumors histologically identical to certain testicular and ovarian neoplasms, all of which are believed to be derived from primitive germ cell elements. It includes benign and malignant teratoma, seminoma, endodermal sinus tumors, choriocarcinoma, and embryonal carcinoma. In the majority of cases, the neoplasm becomes manifest in adolescence or early adulthood, the mean age at diagnosis in two series that totaled 76 cases being 29 and 32 years;[242, 243] the age incidence of benign and malignant tumors is similar.[140] For unexplained reasons, benign lesions are more common in females and malignant tumors in males. For example, of 86 benign neoplasms reported from the Mayo Clinic in 1971,[140] 52 (60 per cent) occurred in females and 34 (40 per cent) in males; by contrast, of 56 cases of malignant tumors reported from the same institution in 1985,[243] 48 cases (86 per cent) involved males and only 8 (14 per cent) involved females.

The vast majority of mediastinal germ cell neoplasms are located in the anterior compartment: in the 1971 Mayo Clinic review of 86 benign and 20 malignant tumors,[140] 100 (94 per cent) were located at this site; the remaining 6 tumors (4 benign and 2 malignant) were found in the posterior media-stinum. A review of 27 germ cell tumors from the Cleveland Clinic in 1972[146] revealed a similar anatomic predominance; except for a mature cystic teratoma that was situated in the middle mediastinum and a seminoma in the posterior mediastinum, all tumors were located anteriorly.

The most common form of mediastinal germ cell tumor is benign teratoma, particularly the cystic form: 19 of the 27 tumors (70 per cent) reviewed at the Cleveland Clinic[146] and 80 of the 106 neoplasms (75 per cent) studied at the Mayo Clinic[140] were of this type. The most common malignant tumor is seminoma: of three combined series with a total of 103 malignant neoplasms,[140, 242, 243] 29 (28 per cent) had this diagnosis; the remainder included 14 embryonal carcinomas (13.5 per cent), 10 malignant teratomas (9.7 per cent), 5 choriocarcinomas, and 3 endodermal sinus tumors. As an analysis of these figures indicates, many malignant tumors (41 per cent of cases in the three series) have a mixed histologic appearance.

Mediastinal germ cell tumors are generally considered to arise from cell rests whose journey along the urogenital ridge to the primitive gonad is interrupted in the mediastinum.[244–246] Occasionally, clinical or pathological examination of a testicle reveals either viable tumor or focal scarring consistent with regressed tumor,[242, 247] indicating that the mediastinal neoplasm represents a metastasis. Although careful clinical examination must be performed in every case of mediastinal germ cell tumor to exclude this possibility, the relatively large number of negative pathologic examinations at autopsy[242] and the usual lack of emergence of a gonadal primary during prolonged clinical follow-up indicate that this is in fact a rare event. From a diagnostic point of view, metastatic testicular cancer usually involves the retroperitoneal lymph nodes first and can bypass the mediastinum to affect the supraclavicular nodes; when the mediastinum is involved, it is seldom in the anterior compartment.

A relationship between mediastinal germ cell neoplasms and Klinefelter's syndrome was recognized in 1979[251] and has been confirmed since then by other reports;[250, 252,] in one review of the literature, Lachman and associates[250] found that 21 of 272 tumors (7.7 per cent) showed this association. The reason for the increased risk of germ cell neoplasia in these patients is unclear but may be related to the abnormal androgen and gonadotropin secretion that is characteristic of the syndrome or to intrinsically abnormal germ cell tissue in patients with Klinefelter's syndrome (or to both).

Because mediastinal germ cell neoplasms have a varied histologic appearance, pathologic diagnosis can be difficult, especially when the amount of tissue submitted for examination is limited, such as may be obtained by mediastinoscopy or TTNA.[253] Although this diagnostic problem may not be very important in relation to specific typing of the tumors, particularly since many of the neoplasms are of mixed histology in any event, current advances in chemotherapy make the distinction from metastatic carcinoma of some importance. It seems reasonable to suggest, therefore, that the possibility of a primary germ cell neoplasm be considered in any young patient with an anterior mediastinal mass in whom a diagnosis of metastatic carcinoma is made in the absence of an obvious primary focus. In this situation, review of histologic material and testing for the presence of serum and tissue alpha-fetoprotein may alter the diagnosis; if the results of these investigations are equivocal, it is possible that a chemotherapeutic trial for presumed germ cell neoplasm may be advisable in some cases.

The CT features of malignant primary germ cell neoplasms of the mediastinum have been recently reviewed.[254]

Teratoma

A teratoma is a neoplasm consisting of one or several different types of tissue, usually derived from more than one germ cell layer, and at least some of which are not native to the area in which the tumor arises. In the mediastinum, the majority of lesions are cystic and benign; the relatively uncommon solid neoplasms are usually malignant.[255, 256] The tumor is recognized most often in adolescence or early adulthood, although occasional series comprising older individuals have been reported.[43]

PATHOLOGIC CHARACTERISTICS

Pathologically, mediastinal teratomas can be divided into three types, mature, immature, and teratomas with malignant transformation. The term "dermoid cyst" is often used to denote a tumor composed solely of ectodermal elements, specifically epidermis and its appendages, that line a keratin-filled cavity. Although not an uncommon variety of teratoma in the ovary, its occurrence in the mediastinum is rare since almost all tumors that grossly resemble a dermoid cyst are, in fact, associated with foci of endodermal and mesodermal tissue in their walls.[256, 257]

Mature teratomas, the most common form, are usually well delimited from surrounding mediastinal structures and are unicystic or multicystic; solid forms occur occasionally (Fig. 19–26). Although an average diameter of 8 cm is cited in the older literature,[257, 258] it is likely that many tumors removed nowadays are smaller than this because of earlier detection by modern imaging techniques. Histologically, the tumors are composed of irregularly arranged but well-differentiated adult tissues (Fig. 19–26); ectodermal elements, particularly epidermis and skin appendages, predominate.[256, 258] Other relatively common tissues include cartilage, fat, smooth muscle, and respiratory mucosa. Bone, glial tissue, and enteric mucosa are less frequently encountered. Schlumberger[256] documented a high

incidence of pancreatic tissue in his cases, a finding that has been confirmed by others;[259] such tissue may be functionally immature, particularly the endocrine component.[260]

Immature teratomas consist of the same adult tissues as the mature variety but in addition contain foci of primitive, less well-organized tissue resembling that seen in the developing fetus (Fig. 19–27). The behavior of this variety is somewhat dependent on the age of the patient: tumors that present in infancy or early childhood are often treated successfully by surgical excision while those that present later frequently follow a highly malignant course.[261, 262] In immature teratomas, the most common forms of malignancy are soft tissue sarcomas, most often angio- or rhabdomyosarcomas;[263, 264] these are probably derived from foci of immature mesenchymal tissue,[263] and the frankly malignant elements may become predominant following chemotherapy-induced destruction of the relatively sensitive germ cell portion of the tumor.[264]

Teratomas with malignant transformation contain areas of frankly malignant neoplasm in addition to the fetal and well-differentiated adult tissues that are found in the immature and mature varieties. Adenocarcinoma is the most common type of neoplasm, squamous cell and undifferentiated carcinomas occurring less frequently (Fig. 19–28). Teratomas with malignant transformation tend to be larger than their benign counterparts[256, 258] and not infrequently show invasion of contiguous structures at the time of diagnosis. They are usually highly aggressive and cause death within a few months of diagnosis as a result of local spread or metastases, or both.

ROENTGENOGRAPHIC MANIFESTATIONS

Roentgenologically, the majority of mediastinal teratomas occur in the anterior compartment close to the origin of the major vessels from the heart (Fig. 19–29). Benign lesions are round or oval in shape and smooth in contour whereas the malignant forms tend to be lobulated[255] and to extend superiorly, inferiorly, and laterally, often in an asymmetric fashion; on average they are considerably larger than thymomas. Calcification may be present in the periphery of the lesion, particularly in mature cystic teratomas, but since such calcification also occurs in thymomas this finding is of no differential diagnostic value. The diagnosis of mature teratoma can be made with a reasonable degree of confidence on a standard roentgenogram in the occasional case in which mature bone or a tooth is demonstrated within the lesion (however, *see* Fig. 19–17, page 2823). Occasionally a cystic teratoma contains fat that may be apparent roentgenographically as a zone of relative radiolucency that creates a fat-fluid level within the cystic mass; this manifestation can be exquisitely demonstrated by CT (Fig. 19–30).[265, 266] The latter technique is undoubtedly superior to

Text continued on page 2842

Figure 19–26. Mature Teratoma. A section through this well-circumscribed mediastinal tumor *(A)* shows mostly solid tissue containing several small cystic spaces. In addition to the relatively non-descript fleshy areas of tumor, there are scattered foci that possess specific differentiation, including hair *(long straight arrows)*, skin *(short straight arrow)*, mucus *(arrowhead)*, and bone *(curved arrow)*. A histologic section *(B)* shows multiple foci of cytologically mature, but architecturally disorganized, tissue including fat *(F)*, cartilage *(C)*, sebaceous glands *(short arrow)*, salivary or bronchial type glands *(long arrow)*, and squamous *(arrowheads)* and respiratory *(curved arrows)* epithelium. (× 25.)

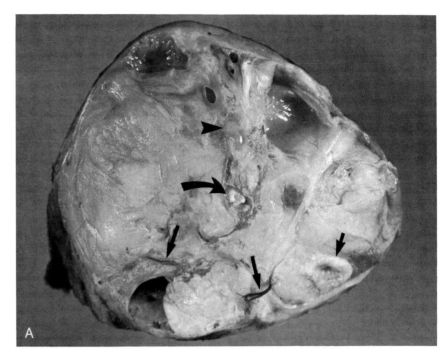

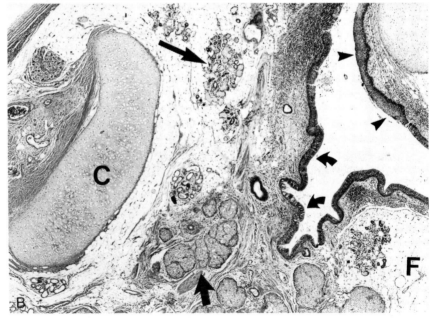

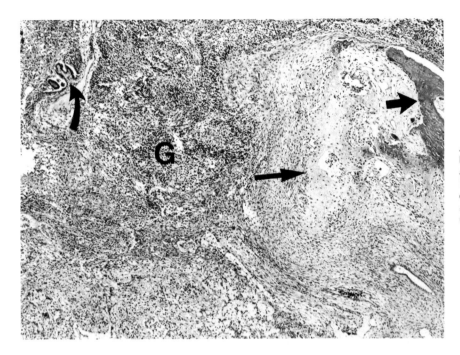

Figure 19–27. Immature Teratoma. A histologic section shows foci of mature bone *(short arrow)*, cartilage *(long arrow)*, and pigmented epithelium *(curved arrow)*. In addition, there is a large focus of disorganized cells with hyperchromatic nuclei *(G)* that represent immature neuroglial elements. (× 48.)

Figure 19–28. Teratoma with Malignant Transformation. A histologic section through a grossly benign, predominantly cystic teratoma shows respiratory type epithelium on the right overlying mature neuroglial tissue *(G)*. On the left are several irregularly shaped sheets of cytologically malignant squamous cells *(arrows)*. (× 50.)

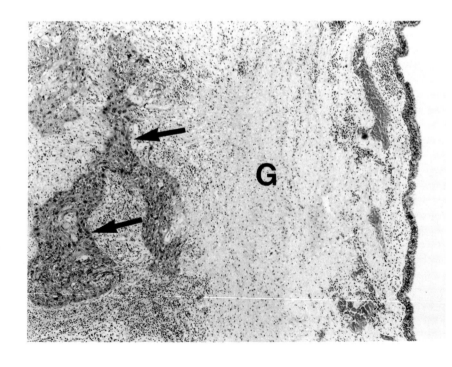

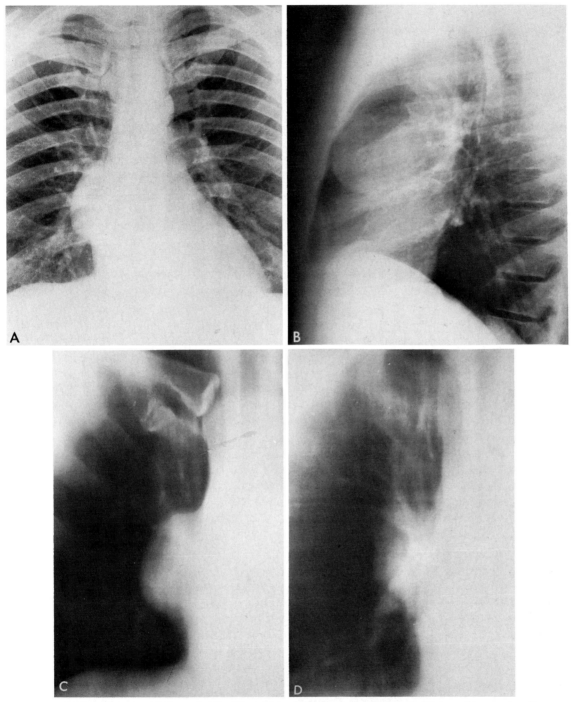

Figure 19–29. Mature Teratoma. Posteroanterior *(A)* and lateral *(B)* roentgenograms of a 33-year-old asymptomatic man reveal a smooth, sharply circumscribed, homogeneous mass projected to the right of the mediastinum and lying predominantly in the anterior compartment. Tomographic cuts at two different levels *(C* and *D)* show the homogeneity of the mass. Note the obtuse angle the mass makes with the mediastinum above and below, indicating its origin inside the mediastinal pleura. In *(D)*, a normal right hilum is clearly visualized, indicating the anterior relationship of the mass to the hilum.

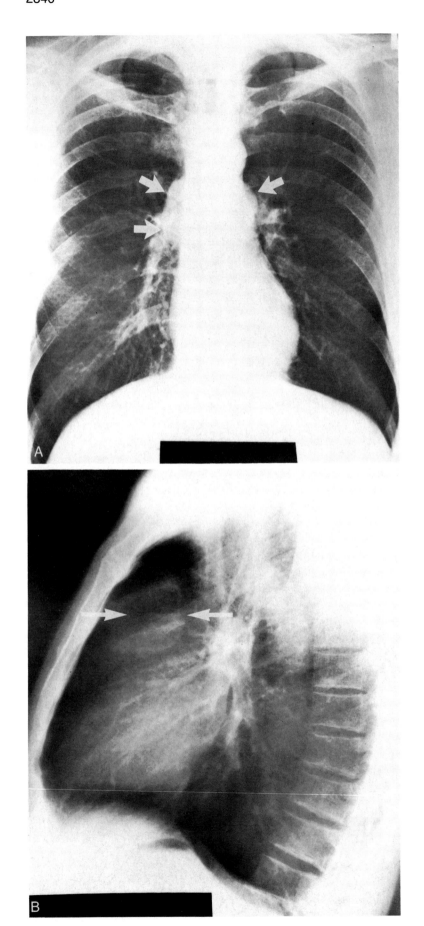

Figure 19–30. Cystic Teratoma of the Anterior Mediastinum Containing a Fat-Fluid Level. Posteroanterior *(A)* and lateral *(B)* roentgenograms reveal a mass of moderate size situated in the anterior mediastinum. The mass is somewhat lobulated and projects to both sides of the mediastinum *(arrows in A)*. In lateral projection, a fluid level is suggested within the mass *(arrows in B)*.

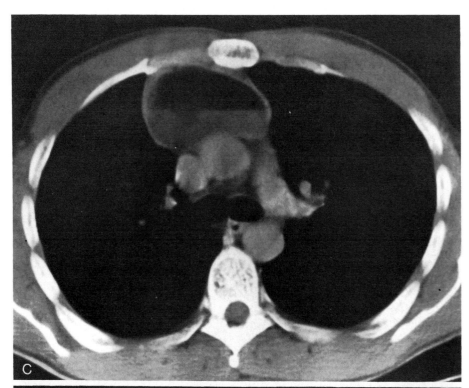

Figure 19–30 *Continued* A CT scan at the level of the left pulmonary artery *(C)* reveals the mass to excellent advantage, its posterior aspect being indented by the ascending aorta. A prominent fluid level is visible in the center of the mass, the surface of the level being deformed slightly just to the left of its center by a small addition defect. A CT scan at the same level *(D)* for measurement of attenuation coefficients revealed the following determinations of Hounsfield units: *1* = 16; *2* = −78; and *3* = −139. The conclusion that can be reached from these measurements is as follows: the material at the bottom of the cyst represents soft tissue detritus of unknown nature; the supernatant represents liquid fat; and the small nubbin (number *2* in *D*) represents a fatty globule presumably composed of an admixture of fat and soft tissue components. The patient is an asymptomatic middle-aged man. (Reprinted with permission slightly modified from Fulcher AS, Proto AV, and Jolles H: Cystic teratoma of the mediastinum: Demonstration of fat/fluid level. AJR *154*:259, 1990.)

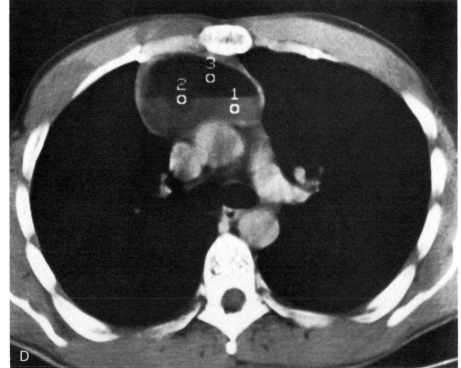

other imaging methods in establishing a diagnosis;[267] in addition to the demonstration of fat, it indicates the presence of globular calcification, bone, or teeth within a solid protuberance in the cystic cavity.

Although these tumors can grow rapidly,[268] it is important to recognize that a rapid increase in size does not necessarily indicate malignancy: hemorrhage into the cyst of a mature teratoma can also result in an abrupt increase in size and can cause severe retrosternal pain or discomfort. An unusual case has been reported of a gastric teratoma that herniated through the diaphragm and presented as a mediastinal mass.[269]

CLINICAL MANIFESTATIONS

Teratomas of the mediastinum usually do not produce symptoms but are discovered on a screening chest roentgenogram. Those that grow to a large size can cause shortness of breath, cough, and a sensation of pressure or pain in the retrosternal area. Large lesions, particularly the malignant forms, may obstruct the superior vena cava or can grow to such a size as to present in the supersternal notch.[270] Rarely, bronchial compression results in obstructive pneumonitis and atelectasis.[271] Compression of the pulmonary artery or right ventricular outflow tract can cause signs of pulmonic stenosis.[272]

Occasionally, a cystic tumor ruptures and spills its contents into the mediastinum or pleural cavity, with resultant mediastinitis or empyema, respectively; similarly, a fistula can develop with adjacent structures including the pericardium (occasionally causing tamponade),[273] aorta, superior vena cava, esophagus, tracheobronchial tree, or externally through the neck. When communication occurs with the airways, the contents of the cyst may be expectorated. If this material contains hair (trichoptysis), the diagnosis of cystic teratoma can be made clinically with certainty. The pathogenesis of cyst rupture is not always clear; although in some cases it may be caused by infection, the possibility has been suggested that it can result from erosion by locally produced pancreatic enzymes.[273, 274] Support for this hypothesis is provided by the relatively common presence of pancreatic tissue in mature teratomas and by the occasional patients in whom high levels of amylase have been found in fluid from a fistulous tract or adjacent lung.[273, 275] Pancreatic islet tissue is rarely functioning but can be so, as exemplified by a patient with a mature teratoma who presented with hypoglycemia and hyperinsulinemia.[276]

Hematologic malignancies, most commonly nonlymphocytic leukemia and occasionally malignant histiocytosis, have been associated with mediastinal germ cell neoplasms, particularly immature teratomas.[277, 278] Some of these have developed following the institution of chemotherapy or radio-

therapy (or both), raising the possibility of therapeutically induced neoplasia. In some cases, however, the teratoma and hematological malignancy have been recognized synchronously, suggesting the possibility of a common pathogenesis. Three hypotheses have been invoked to explain this association:[277] (1) the hematologic neoplasm represents an intrinsic malignant component of the teratoma, an explanation supported by occasional case reports;[279] (2) the teratoma secretes substances that induce the hematologic malignancy; and (3) aberrant intrauterine migration of both primordial germ cells and hematopoietic stem cells occurs, with subsequent independent neoplastic transformation of both cell types. The pros and cons of each of these theories have been discussed in detail by Ladanyi and Roy.[277]

Seminoma

Seminoma is the next most frequent mediastinal germ cell neoplasm after teratoma. As with the malignant form of the latter neoplasm, it occurs almost exclusively in men although at least 6 cases have been reported in women.[280] The average age at presentation is 29 years (range, 11 to 63 years).[280] In their review of the English literature up to 1979, Polansky and his colleagues[280] found 103 recorded cases.

Histologically, mediastinal seminoma is typically composed of nests of cells separated by a variably thick fibrovascular stroma containing numerous lymphocytes (Fig. 19–31). Cell nuclei are round and contain coarsely clumped chromatin and prominent nucleoli; the cytoplasm is usually clear and contains glycogen. In addition to lymphocytes, loosely formed, non-necrotizing granulomas or germinal centers (or both) are found in the stroma of many cases and are a helpful feature in differentiating these neoplasms from lymphoma, thymoma, and thymic cysts.[157, 281] Ultrastructural features are also characteristic and can be useful in differential diagnosis.[282]

Roentgenographically, seminoma usually appears as a lobulated noncalcified mass that cannot be distinguished from other malignant germ cell tumors. It can protrude from one or both sides of the mediastinum.[245, 283, 284]

Clinically, approximately 30 per cent of patients are asymptomatic at the time of initial diagnosis. When present, symptoms usually derive from pressure or invasion of vascular structures within the mediastinum. One of the four cases described by Polanski and associates was a woman who had signs and symptoms of superior vena caval obstruction,[280] an association that these authors state occurs in roughly 10 per cent of patients. The prognosis of patients with pure seminomas is considerably better than that of patients with mixed or nonseminomatous germ cell tumors; the 5-year survival rate is variously reported to range from 50 to 75 percent.[280, 285–288] In one study of 17 pure seminomas

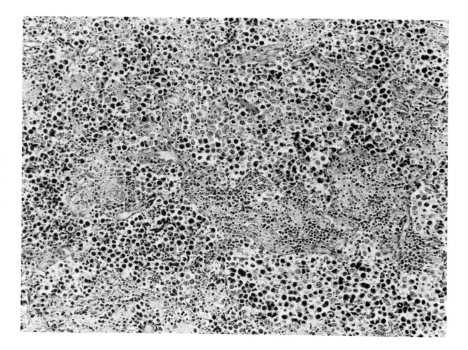

Figure 19–31. Mediastinal Seminoma. A histologic section of an anterior mediastinal tumor from a 23-year-old man shows interconnecting sheets of cells with abundant cytoplasm and fairly uniform, more or less round nuclei; the intervening stroma contains a moderate number of lymphocytes. (× 120.)

and 4 mixed germ cell tumors,[287] features associated with a bad prognosis included age over 35 years, pyrexia, superior vena cava syndrome, supraclavicular or cervical lymph node enlargement, and roentgenographic evidence of hilar abnormality. Characteristically, seminomas are exquisitely radiosensitive.[285, 286, 288]

Endodermal Sinus Tumor

Endodermal sinus tumors are highly malignant germ cell neoplasms believed to show differentiation toward yolk sac endoderm. The mediastinal form is rare, only 38 cases of the pure form having

been reported in the English language literature by 1986.[289] The tumor also occurs occasionally in association with other germ cell neoplasms.[289]

Histologically, this neoplasm is quite variable in appearance, showing reticular, tubulopapillary, cystic, and solid patterns (Fig. 19–32). Perivascular structures resembling the rat endodermal sinus (Shiller-Duval bodies) and small intra- and extracellular globules of PAS-positive material are characteristic features. Immunohistochemical studies have shown a positive reaction in most cases for alpha-fetoprotein and alpha1-antitrypsin;[289] occasional tumors also show CEA and keratin positivity. Extracellular basement membrane-like material is often present on ultrastructural examination.[289, 290]

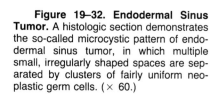

Figure 19–32. Endodermal Sinus Tumor. A histologic section demonstrates the so-called microcystic pattern of endodermal sinus tumor, in which multiple small, irregularly shaped spaces are separated by clusters of fairly uniform neoplastic germ cells. (× 60.)

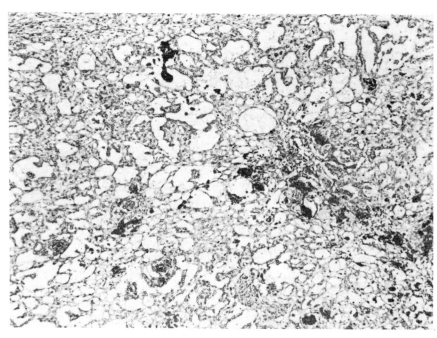

Most endodermal sinus tumors present in young adults, the mean age in Truong and colleagues' review being 22.6 years;[289] the majority occur in males. Roentgenographic findings are non-specific, consisting of an anterior mediastinal mass. Symptoms related to local mediastinal compression or invasion are present in most patients at the time of diagnosis; systemic symptoms (anorexia, weight loss, and fever) are often present as are those related to metastases.[289] Serum levels of alpha-fetoprotein are elevated in virtually all patients and can be a useful indicator of disease progression or remission with therapy. Although the prognosis is generally poor, prolonged survival and even cure have been documented in some patients treated aggressively.[291-293]

Choriocarcinoma

Choriocarcinoma is a rare variety of mediastinal germ cell neoplasm that is usually seen in combination with other forms, especially embryonal carcinoma.[248, 249, 294] By 1975, a total of 23 examples had been reported.[295] The peak age incidence is between 20 and 30 years and, as with other malignant germ cell tumors, most occur in males.

Pathologically, choriocarcinoma is typically a bulky lobulated mass associated with prominent necrosis and hemorrhage. Histologically, sheets of cells with vesicular nuclei and abundant eosinophilic cytoplasm (cytotrophoblasts) are located adjacent to large multinucleated giant cells (syncytiotrophoblasts). The latter show a positive immunohistochemical reaction for beta-HCG.

The roentgenographic appearance is not distinctive, consisting of an anterior mediastinal mass with a somewhat lobulated contour expanding the mediastinum to one or both sides. In comparison with other germ cell tumors, growth tends to be extremely rapid.[244]

At the time of presentation, mediastinal choriocarcinoma is usually associated with signs and symptoms, including dyspnea, hemoptysis, hoarseness, stridor, dysphagia, and Horner's syndrome.[246] Gynecomastia is reported to occur in about two thirds of cases[296] and is invariably associated with elevated serum levels of human chorionic gonadotropin (HCG). In the past, the prognosis was extremely poor, death occurring in most patients within 4 to 6 weeks following diagnosis;[244] with modern therapy, however, remission and even cure may be expected in some patients.

TUMORS OF THYROID TISSUE

Although extension of thyroid tissue into the thorax is seen in only 1 to 3 per cent of patients subjected to thyroidectomy,[141, 297, 298] such tissue nevertheless constitutes a significant percentage of anterior mediastinal masses. The most frequent patho-logic finding is nodular goiter,[299] an abnormality most commonly seen in patients in the fifth decade; there is a female-to-male predominance of 3 or 4 to 1.[300] Occasionally there is acute[301, 302] or chronic[303] thyroiditis or carcinoma.[300] This subject has been reviewed by Katlic and associates.[300]

Seventy-five to 80 per cent of mediastinal thyroid tumors arise from a lower pole or the isthmus and extend into the anterior mediastinum in front of the trachea. Most of the remainder arise from the posterior aspect of either thyroid lobe and extend into the posterior mediastinum behind the trachea, innominant vein, and innominate or subclavian arteries;[304-306] in the latter location, they are situated almost exclusively on the right, as was the situation with all 12 of the cases reported by Rietz and Werner.[305] In a small number of cases (probably less than 1 per cent), there is no evident connection between the cervical and intrathoracic thyroid tissue;[300] in these, it is assumed that the intrathoracic tumor arises from ectopic thyroid tissue displaced during fetal development. As might be expected from this discussion, in the majority of patients the abnormal thyroid tissue is located in the uppermost portion of the mediastinum; occasionally, however, growth may be so massive as to extend to the diaphragm.[300]

Pathologically, most tumors are multinodular goiters that measure 6 to 10 cm in diameter and often show areas of hemorrhage, fibrosis, cyst formation, and calcification (Fig. 19–33). Carcinoma occurs in 2 to 3 per cent.[300] The rare case of intrathoracic oncocytoma may have its origin in ectopic mediastinal thyroid tissue.[307]

Roentgenographically, the appearance is that of a sharply defined, smooth or lobulated mass of homogeneous density (Fig. 19–34.)[134] Anterior me-

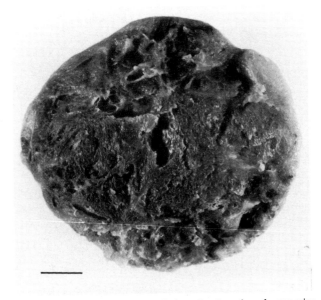

Figure 19–33. Mediastinal Goiter. A cut section of a superior mediastinal tumor shows a well-circumscribed mass that grossly resembles mature thyroid tissue. (Bar = 1 cm.)

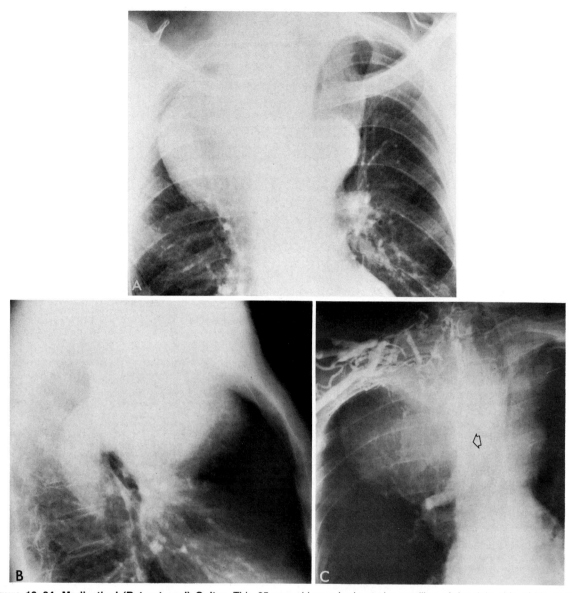

Figure 19–34. Mediastinal (Retrosternal) Goiter. This 65-year-old man had noted a swelling of the right side of his neck for 15 years. He had never noted either dysphagia or dyspnea, nor were there manifestations of either hyperthyroidism or hypothyroidism. Posteroanterior *(A)* and lateral *(B)* roentgenograms demonstrate a huge mass situated in the upper mediastinum, projected chiefly to the right of the midline. It is homogeneous and sharply circumscribed and shows no evidence of calcification. It displaces the trachea markedly to the left and slightly posteriorly. Scanning revealed no evidence of iodine uptake. A venous angiogram *(C)* demonstrates complete obstruction of the subclavian vein, opacification of the superior vena cava *(arrow)* being obtained by numerous collateral channels in the lower portion of the neck (there were no symptoms of venous obstruction). Following removal, the mass weighed 830 g and measured 17 × 12 × 6 cm.

diastinal goiters displace the trachea posteriorly and laterally, whereas those in the posterior mediastinum displace the trachea anteriorly and the esophagus posteriorly and laterally. Calcification within the mass is fairly common. Displacement and obstruction of the brachiocephalic vessels may be demonstrated by arteriography or venography, procedures that also permit differentiation of the mass from a vascular aneurysm (Fig. 19–34).

Radioactive isotopic studies are usually diagnostic and should constitute the first line of investigation once the possibility of a thyroid origin of a mediastinal mass is considered on the basis of con-

ventional roentgenographic studies. However, false-negative radionuclide examinations do occur, in which circumstance computed tomography should be performed as the next most definitive procedure in diagnosis. According to Glazer and his associates,[308] characteristic features of retrosternal thyroid include (1) continuity with the cervical thyroid, (2) focal calcifications, (3) relatively high CT number, (4) a rise in CT number after bolus administration of iodinated contrast material, and (5) prolonged enhancement after contrast administration. More recently, a review of the CT characteristics of 10 patients with intrathoracic goiters[309] listed six signs that are only slightly at variance with those listed above. They are (1) clear continuity with the cervical thyroid gland (8/10 cases); (2) well-defined borders (9/10); (3) punctate, coarse, or ring-like calcifications (8/10); (4) inhomogeneity (9/10), often with discrete, nonenhancing, low-density areas (6/10); (5) precontrast attenuation values at least 15 H greater than adjacent muscles (4/10) and more than 25 H after contrast enhancement (8/8); and (6) characteristic patterns of goiter extension into the mediastinum. CT also can be of value when a goiter is situated in the posterior mediastinum: when radionuclide examinations are negative or inconclusive, CT can provide evidence that a posterior mediastinal mass is directly connected to the posterior aspect of the cervical thyroid or to a retrosternal thyroid gland.[310]

Many patients with intrathoracic goiters are asymptomatic,[140, 146, 300] the abnormalities being discovered on a screening chest roentgenogram. When present, symptoms include respiratory distress (which can be worsened by certain movements of the neck) and hoarseness. Hoarseness is usually caused by compression of the recurrent laryngeal nerve and does not necessarily indicate invasion;[304] however, its presence should raise the possibility of malignancy. Posterior mediastinal goiters can cause dysphagia whereas those in the anterior and middle compartment can cause a superior vena cava syndrome as a result of obstruction of brachiocephalic vessels.[146, 306, 311, 312] Physical examination usually reveals evidence of a goiter ascending into the neck when the patient swallows; inspiratory and expiratory stridor may be apparent. Thyrotoxicosis is present in some patients.[313, 314] An unusual case has been reported in which a huge retrosternal goiter was associated with systemic hypertension (blood pressure 230/130 mm Hg);[315] following removal of the goiter, blood pressure returned to normal and remained so without further medical treatment.

TUMORS OF PARATHYROID TISSUE

Parathyroid tumors constitute a rare cause of an anterior mediastinal mass. Their presence within the mediastinum is best explained on the basis of the normal migration of parathyroid glands with the thymus during embryonic development; although they usually separate and remain in the neck, occasionally they proceed distally, usually in direct continuity with thymic tissue. In one autopsy study[316] of 312 lower parathyroid glands, six (2 per cent) were located in the mediastinum. The tumors are usually situated in the upper or mid portion of the anterior mediastinum;[317] most are adenomas or are hyperplastic, but occasionally they are malignant (parathyroid carcinoma).[318]

Roentgenographically, parathyroid tumors occasionally are sufficiently large to widen the mediastinal silhouette, usually unilaterally.[196, 319–321] In the majority of patients, however, they are so small

as to be invisible. They rarely calcify.[322] In cases of known hyperparathyroidism, if neither standard roentgenography nor tomography reveals a mass and the barium-filled esophagus is not displaced, evidence to date would indicate that selective arteriography is the procedure of choice for identifying mediastinal glands;[323, 324] in fact, opacification of the whole gland with contrast medium can result in eventual ablation (Fig. 19–35). Neither CT nor nonselective digital arteriography has proven to be effective in the identification of these elusive glands.[324, 325] However, for reasons that are unclear, CT can be very useful in patients with previously failed explorations.[323]

Unlike most other mediastinal masses, parathyroid tumors usually can be diagnosed on the basis of clinical and laboratory findings. Since most of these tumors are functioning, patients present with signs and symptoms of hyperparathyroidism, including anorexia, weakness, fatigue, nausea, vomiting, constipation, and hypotonicity of muscles. The typical skeletal roentgenographic appearances of hyperparathyroidism may be seen. Laboratory studies reveal hypercalcemia, hypophosphatemia, elevation of serum alkaline phosphatase levels, and hypercalciuria. The masses are seldom large enough to cause symptoms or signs of local compression.

SOFT TISSUE TUMORS AND TUMOR-LIKE CONDITIONS

Soft tissue tumors account for about 6 per cent of all mediastinal masses[326] and include benign and malignant neoplasms of fat, fibrous tissue, smooth and striated muscle, blood and lymphatic vessels, bone, and neural tissue. In addition, several developmental and acquired abnormalities composed predominantly of mesenchymal tissue (such as hemangioma and lipomatosis) can present as mediastinal masses. Each of these can occur in any mediastinal compartment, but tumors of neural tissue are most common posteriorly (and are described on page 2898) whereas the others are usually located anteriorly.

Tumors of Adipose Tissue

Although uncommon compared with other neoplasms, extrathymic lipoma is probably the most common mesenchymal tumor to occur in the mediastinum;[327] in one series of 396 mediastinal neoplasms, it constituted 2.3 per cent of the total.[327] By contrast, liposarcomas are rare, only 53 cases having been reported by 1981.[328]

Certain roentgenographic features of mediastinal lipomas can aid in their diagnosis. Since the density of fat is lower than that of other soft tissues, the roentgenographic density of lipomas is often—but not always—less than that of other mediastinal masses. This is particularly true if the mass

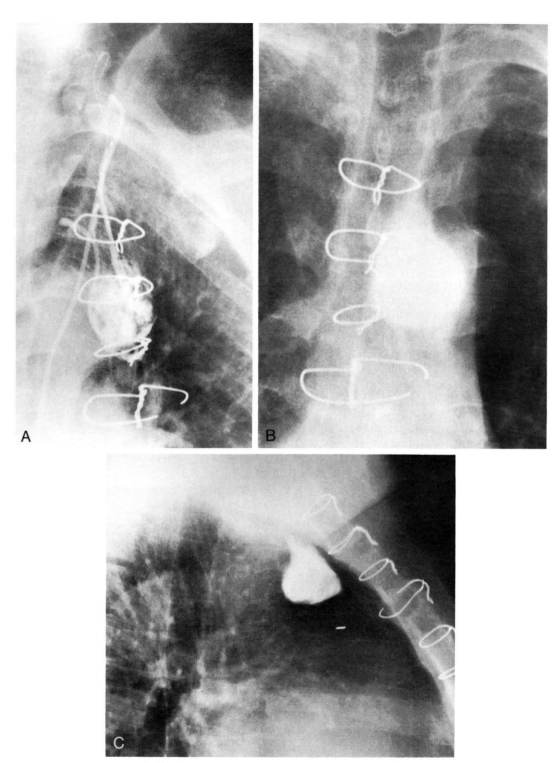

Figure 19–35. Solitary Mediastinal Parathyroid Gland: Opacification and Subsequent Ablation by Arteriography. This middle-aged man had severe secondary hyperparathyroidism as a result of end-stage renal disease. Exploration of the neck resulted in removal of three parathyroid glands but the fourth was not evident. Conventional roentgenograms revealed no abnormality although a contrast-enhanced CT scan showed a mass adjacent to the aortic arch (not reproduced). The patient was referred for arteriography. Injection of the left internal mammary artery with 76 per cent Renografin *(A)* resulted in extensive opacification of a mediastinal gland situated contiguous with the arch of the aorta. Twenty-four hours later, detail views of the upper half of the mediastinum from posteroanterior *(B)* and lateral *(C)* roentgenograms reveal persistent dense opacification of the gland.

Illustration continued on following page

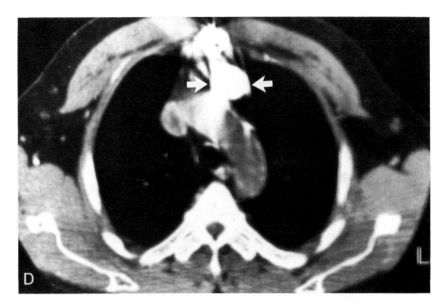

Figure 19–35 *Continued* A CT scan at the level of the aortic arch *(D)* also shows the uniformly opacified parathyroid gland *(arrows)*. Subsequent follow-up revealed reversal of the severe secondary hyperparathyroidism.

happens to be surrounded by mediastinal tissue of unit density, as in the case reported by Wilson.[330] In some patients the masses present in an hourglass configuration, part of the lesion being extrathoracic in either the neck or the chest wall.[143, 150] Usually they project from only one side of the mediastinum.[196] Leigh and Weens[196] described three cases with an identical roentgenographic appearance of a mass which, when the patients were erect, rested on the right hemidiaphragm. This appearance, which may be mistaken for elevation of a hemidiaphragm, is caused by the effect of gravity on the soft, pliable, fatty tissue.[134] When doubt exists as to the true nature of a mediastinal mass of this type, CT will be diagnostic in the majority of patients. As pointed out by Mendez and associates,[331] when the CT number of a fatty lesion is approximately −45 EMI units, intervention is usually unnecessary; however, when the CT numbers range from −10 to −20 EMI units, intervention may be necessary in order to exclude the possibility of liposarcoma.

Perhaps because of their pliability, mediastinal lipomas usually do not cause symptoms, even when massive.[327] By contrast, liposarcomas are often locally invasive at the time of diagnosis, resulting in dyspnea, wheezing, chest pain, or cough;[328, 329] superior venal cava syndrome is a rare manifestation.[329]

The prognosis of mediastinal lipoma is excellent, surgical excision being curative in virtually all cases. The behavior of liposarcomas is variable depending on the histologic grade and the extent of local invasion at the time of attempted excision. In low-grade encapsulated forms cure usually can be expected, whereas in locally invasive or high-grade forms recurrence and death are common. Remote metastases are seldom observed.[327]

Lipomatosis

Lipomatosis is an unusual non-neoplastic abnormality of mediastinal adipose tissue character-
ized by the excessive accumulation of fat in its normal locations. It is most commonly seen in conditions associated with hypercortisolism, such as Cushing's syndrome,[333, 334] ectopic ACTH production,[332] and long term corticosteroid therapy.[334–338] In these situations corticosteriods mobilize and redistribute reserve fatty tissue, resulting in the excessive deposition of fat in the upper mediastinum and in both pleuropericardial angles (Fig. 19–36). Histologically proved mediastinal lipomatosis also has been described in a young man in whom the cause appeared to be excessive weight gain without corticosteroid therapy.[339] We have seen a similar case in an obese patient whose widened mediastinum returned to normal following a 40-pound weight loss (Fig. 19–37).

Roentgenographically, mediastinal widening tends to be smooth and symmetric although margins can be lobulated if the accumulation is very large. The widening usually extends from the thoracic inlet to the hila bilaterally (Fig. 19–37); however, in the three cases reported by Streiter and his associates[340] the accumulation was predominantly paraspinal and symmetrical (Fig. 19–38). Increasing size of the pleuropericardial fat pads may be evident on serial roentgenographic studies.[335, 336, 338] In all cases of mediastinal lipomatosis, should doubt exist on evidence provided by conventional roentgenograms, CT almost invariably will be diagnostic.[340, 343]

Patients with mediastinal lipomatosis do not have symptoms from the fat deposits. It is important that the abnormality be correctly identified in order to avoid subjecting patients to unwarranted investigation or surgery.

Tumors of Vascular Tissue

Vascular tumors of the mediastinum are uncommon and include hemangioma, angiosarcoma (hemangioendothelioma), hemangiopericytoma, and lymphangioma. The first of these is the most com-

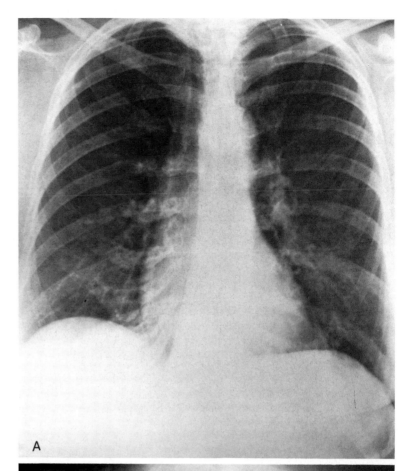

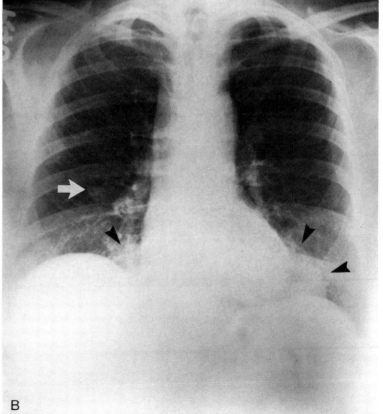

Figure 19–36. Mediastinal Lipomatosis Secondary to Paraneoplastic Cushing's Syndrome. A posteroanterior roentgenogram *(A)* of this 68-year-old woman is normal. Two years later, during which time the patient had gained a great deal of weight, a repeat posteroanterior roentgenogram *(B)* reveals considerable widening of the upper half of the mediastinum and appreciable enlargement of the pleuropericardial fat pads bilaterally *(arrowheads)*. In addition, a solitary pulmonary nodule measuring 12 mm in diameter had appeared in the lower portion of the right lung *(arrow)*.

Illustration continued on following page

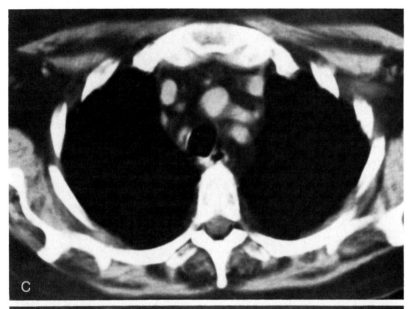

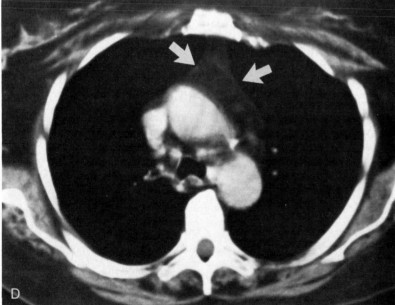

Figure 19–36 *Continued* CT scans through the upper half of the mediastinum (*C* and *D*) reveal the presence of a large amount of fat separating the numerous vessels in the upper mediastinum *(C)* and anterior to the aorta (*arrows* in *D*). Following resection, the solitary pulmonary nodule proved to be a carcinoid tumor. (Courtesy of Dr. Anthony Proto, Virginia Commonwealth University, Medical College of Virginia, Richmond, Virginia).

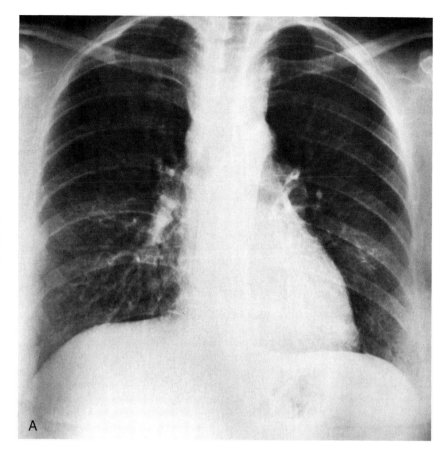

Figure 19–37. Mediastinal Lipomatosis. A posteroanterior roentgenogram *(A)* reveals widening of the upper mediastinum to an equal extent on both sides. The contour is smooth. No other abnormalities are apparent other than thickening of bronchial walls consistent with chronic bronchitis.

Illustration continued on following page

mon, 103 cases having been reported by 1987.[344] The remainder are rare.[345]

HEMANGIOMA

Hemangiomas have been estimated to comprise about 0.5 per cent of all mediastinal tumors.[346] They have been identified in patients ranging in age from newborn to the elderly,[344] but the majority have been discovered in young individuals.[346, 347] They can be isolated or can occur as part of a multifocal hemangiomatous malformation affecting several organs (Osler-Weber-Rendu syndrome).[346, 348] As with their pulmonary counterparts *(see* page 1622), many if not all probably represent developmental malformations rather than true neoplasms. Their occasional association with teratoma[347] has also suggested that they might represent unidirectional development in this neoplasm; however, such an event must be very rare.

Pathologically, hemangiomas are often encapsulated; they are red-brown to tan-gray in color and possess a spongy appearance on cut section.[346, 347] Occasionally the vascular proliferation is nonencapsulated and extends into adjacent tissues,[344, 347] making surgical excision difficult. Histologically, the tumors are composed of thin- or thick-walled vessels of large, small, or mixed size, corresponding to cavernous, capillary, or mixed hemangiomas, respectively.

Roentgenographically, hemangiomas tend to be smooth in outline but are sometimes lobulated; most are located in the upper portion of the anterior mediastinum. Phleboliths may be identified within them,[196, 345] a virtually diagnostic sign. CT may be helpful in delineating the extent of local tissue infiltration. [344, 346] The spinal canal is involved in some cases and may require myelography for proper evaluation. Adjacent ribs may become hypertrophied[134] or eroded.[349]

Clinically, many patients are symptomatic at the time of presentation,[347] the chief complaints being chest pain and dyspnea. Superior vena cava and Horner's syndromes have been reported.[347] Occasionally, a tumor projects superiorly from the upper portion of the mediastinum and can be appreciated as a fullness in the neck.[347]

ANGIOSARCOMA

Angiosarcoma (hemangioendothelioma) is a very rare mediastinal tumor. In a 1963 review of the literature, Pachter and Lattes[347] found only eight well-documented cases, and few have been reported since that time.[326, 350] Most occur in the anterior mediastinum and have no obvious source; a single case has been reported that apparently arose in the superior vena cava.[350] These tumors are aggressive and are usually associated with chest pain at the

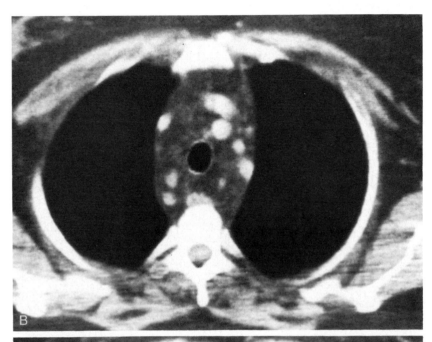

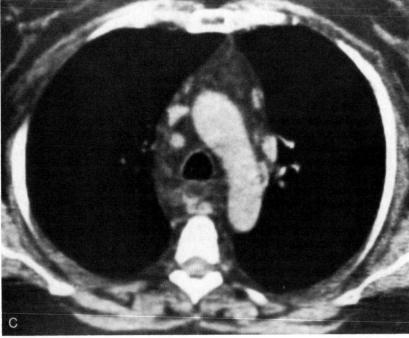

Figure 19–37 *Continued* CT scans at the level of the left brachiocephalic vein *(B)* and the aortic arch *(C)* demonstrate wide separation of vessels as a result of an accumulation of a large amount of fat. This 58-year-old woman was receiving no therapy nor did she have any underlying condition to which the lipomatosis could be attributed: she was simply obese. The widened mediastinum returned to normal following a 40-pound weight loss.

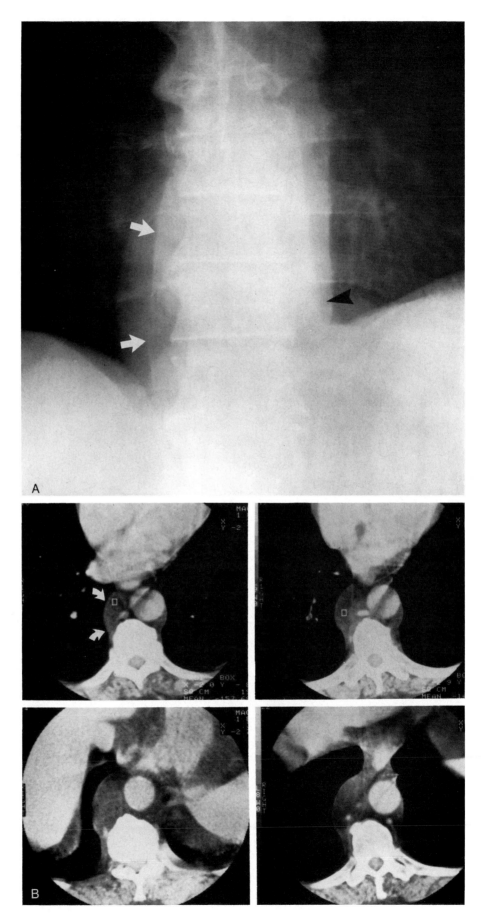

Figure 19–38. Posterior Mediastinal Lipomatosis. An overexposed roentgenogram of the lower thoracic spine in anteroposterior projection *(A)* reveals widening of the paraspinal soft tissues, more marked on the right *(arrows)*. The left paraspinal line is wider than normal in its lower portion *(arrowhead)*. Serial CT scans through the lower mediastinum *(B)* reveal a sharply defined, homogeneous opacity projecting from the right side of the posterior mediastinum and bearing an intimate relationship to the descending aorta and vertebral bodies *(arrows)*. This tissue also extends to the left side of the mediastinum where it relates to the posterolateral aspect of the aorta and vertebral bodies. The mean attenuation of the abnormal tissue in Hounsfield units was −150. Although this mass could conceivably represent a lipoma, it was felt to be more consistent with an unusual localization of lipomatosis.

time of diagnosis; most patients die within 3 years of diagnosis.

HEMANGIOPERICYTOMA

Like its pulmonary counterpart (*see* page 1583), hemangiopericytoma of the mediastinum is believed to be derived from the vascular pericyte. It is very rare: although Pachter and Lattes[347] documented seven cases, they were able to discover only three in the English literature prior to 1963. The tumor can be locally infiltrative and aggressive or can be encapsulated and apparently benign; histologic features of the two varieties are virtually identical. Roentgenographic and clinical manifestations are nonspecific.

LYMPHANGIOMA

Mediastinal lymphangiomas occur in two forms: (1) a cavernous or cystic variety that typically extends from the neck into the mediastinum and usually occurs in infants but occasionally in adults (cystic hygroma) (Fig. 19–39),[265, 352–354] and (2) a more or less well-circumscribed variety that occurs later in life and is usually located in the lower anterior mediastinum remote from the neck;[355, 356]

occasionally they are located more posteriorly (Fig. 19–40). The latter tumors are uncommon, only 40 surgically treated cases having been documented in the literature to 1960.[355] As with hemangiomas, these tumors probably represent developmental anomalies rather than true neoplasms.

Pathologically, both forms consist of thin-walled, usually multilocular cysts lined by endothelial cells and containing clear yellow fluid. The wall is composed of connective tissue with a variable amount of smooth muscle, fat, blood vessels, nerves, and lymphoid tissue.[140] Pachter and Lattes[355] have described two unusual cases that possessed a prominent perivascular cellular component that they labeled "lymphangiopericytoma."

In two cases of cystic mediastinal lymphangioma, CT examination revealed a well-defined lesion of low attenuation that molded to the mediastinal contours and enveloped the great vessels; the diagnosis was suggested in both cases.[357] We have seen one case in which an extensive lymphangioma of the upper half of the mediastinum extended toward the left hilum and thence into the left lung, presumably via the interstitium.

Because of their soft, yielding consistency, these lesions seldom cause symptoms even when large;[352] occasionally, they encroach on the tracheobronchial

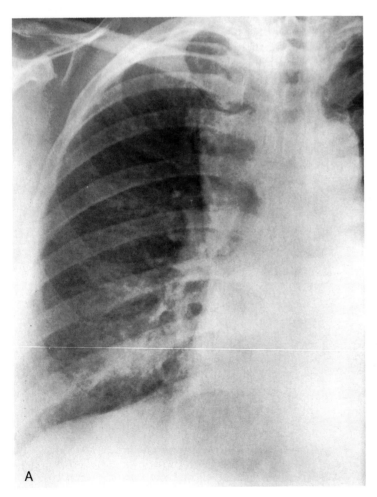

A

Figure 19–39. Cystic Hygroma of the Anterior Mediastinum. A view of the right lung and mediastinum (A) of this asymptomatic 48-year-old woman reveals an opacity in the paramediastinal region, extending superiorly from the upper portion of the right hilum.

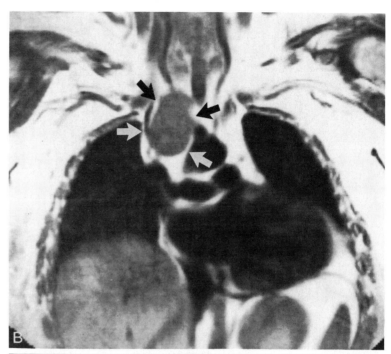

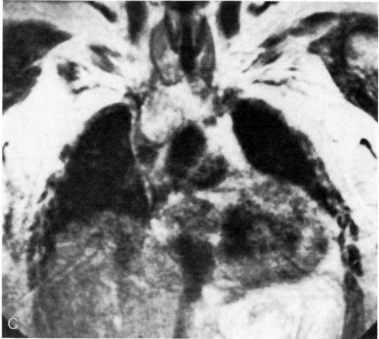

Figure 19–39 *Continued* A T1-weighted magnetic resonance scan *(B)* reveals a sharply defined, homogeneous opacity extending from just above the thoracic inlet downward into the right side of the mediastinum *(arrows)*. A T2-weighted image *(C)* shows an alteration in the density of the mass consistent with the presence of fluid.

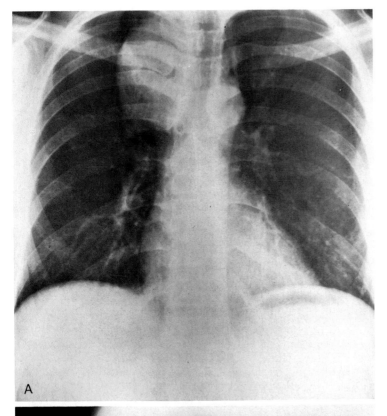

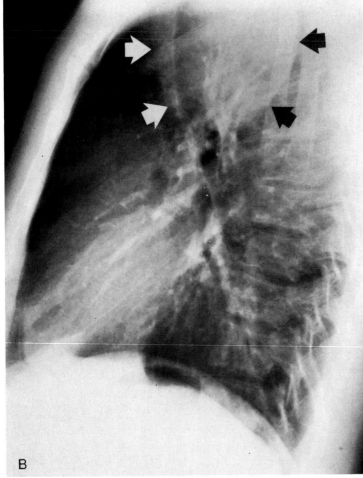

Figure 19–40. Cystic Lymphangioma of the Mediastinum. Posteroanterior *(A)* and lateral *(B)* roentgenograms reveal a large homogeneous opacity situated in the right superior paramediastinal area, extending from a point near the thoracic inlet down to the right tracheobronchial angle. The right tracheal stripe is effaced. The lateral projection shows that the mass is situated in both the middle and posterior mediastinal compartments *(arrows)*. The tracheal air column is displaced slightly to the left and anteriorly but is not narrowed. Note that the conventional roentgenograms reveal the mass to extend down to the level of the azygos arch beyond which it cannot pass.

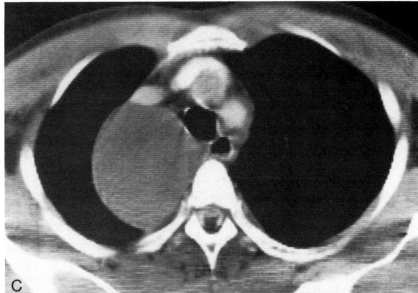

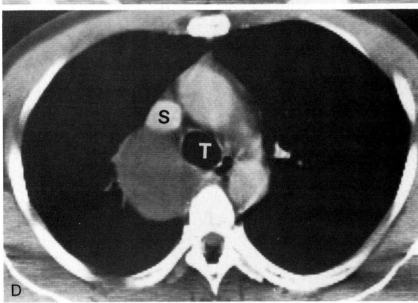

Figure 19–40 *Continued* CT scans at the level of the left brachiocephalic vein *(C)* and aortopulmonary window *(D)* show that the mass is of water density and that it possesses a sharp interface with contiguous lung parenchyma. It relates intimately to the posterior surface of the superior vena cava *(S)* and the right posterolateral wall of the trachea *(T)* which is slightly indented. On other CT scans, the mass was seen to begin just below the level of the thoracic inlet, thus possessing no communication with the neck. This 37-year-old man was asymptomatic.

tree[140] or cause symptomatic compression of the superior vena cava or its major tributaries.[358] A soft tissue mass may be visible in the neck. Chylothorax develops in some cases.[355]

Tumors of Muscle

LEIOMYOMA AND LEIOMYOSARCOMA

Smooth muscle neoplasms, other than those that arise in the esophagus (*see* page 2903), are rare mediastinal neoplasms; in a review of the literature in 1975, Rasaretnam and Panabokke[359] found only nine examples, seven benign and two malignant. Since most of these were located in the posterior mediastinum and since smooth muscle differentiation was not confirmed immunohistochemically or

ultrastructurally in all cases, it is possible that some in fact represented neurogenic neoplasms. The origin of these tumors is often not clear. Although it has been suggested that they represent unidirectional differentiation in a teratoma,[327, 360] it seems more likely that the majority are derived from the walls of small mediastinal blood vessels; apparent origin in the superior vena cava,[361] pulmonary artery, and the wall of a mediastinal bronchial cyst[360] also has been reported. It is also possible that some of the cases in which a definite origin cannot be determined have arisen in the trachea or esophagus. A possible association between leiomyosarcoma and prior radiotherapy has been documented in one case.[363] Pathologic findings are those of a spindle cell neoplasm with varying degrees of nuclear atypia and mitotic rate. Roentgenographic and clinical features are nonspecific.

RHABDOMYOSARCOMA

Primary mediastinal rhabdomyosarcoma is exceedingly rare; although Pachter and Lattes[327] reported three such tumors in their 1963 series, they could find no previous cases in the literature. Only occasional examples have been documented since that time.[364] Again, the origin of these tumors is unclear, although the well-documented occurrence of rhabdomyosarcoma in association with immature teratoma[263, 264] suggests that at least some are derived from this neoplasm.

Fibrous and Fibrohistiocytic Tumors

As Pachter and Lattes have pointed out,[327] the precise incidence of primary mediastinal *fibromas* and *fibrosarcomas* is difficult to determine because of the relative rarity of well-documented cases. For example, it is possible that some neoplasms reported as fibroma or fibrosarcoma may instead represent neurogenic neoplasms or pleural tumors that have extended into the mediastinum. In fact, some of these tumors are histologically identical to fibrous tumor of the pleura (*see* page 2755).[365] Of the reported cases, fibromas are said to be more common anteriorly and fibrosarcomas posteriorly.[196] There are no distinctive roentgenographic features. The majority of patients are asymptomatic even when the tumors are very large.[366] Pleural effusion can occur, not only with fibrosarcoma but with benign lesions also.[134]

Benign fibrous histiocytoma (xanthogranuloma) of the mediastinum is a rare tumor of which approximately 20 cases had been reported by 1963.[327] As with their pulmonary counterparts (*see* page 1617), the precise nature of these tumors is uncertain, particularly with respect to their inflammatory or neoplastic character; further, if neoplastic, it is not certain whether they are derived from a fibroblast, a histiocyte, or a common stem cell. Pathologically, the tumors are usually well encapsulated[327] and are composed of a variable number of intermingled fibroblasts, histiocytes, and multinucleated giant cells. Nuclear atypia, mitotic activity, and necrosis are absent or minimal.

Malignant fibrous histiocytoma of the mediastinum is exceedingly rare, only five cases having been documented by 1986.[367, 368]

Mesenchymoma

Benign[369, 370] and malignant[327] mediastinal mesenchymomas are rare tumors composed of a mixture of two or more mesodermal tissues. Their precise nature is debated, some authors considering them to represent hamartomas (at least the benign forms) and others true neoplasms. It is possible that some represent predominant mesodermal differentiation in a teratoma.

Miscellaneous Mesenchymal Tumors

Other rare varieties of mesenchymal neoplasm that can arise in the mediastinum include *osteosarcoma*[371] (in one case possibly related to previous radiotherapy[372]), *granulocytic sarcoma*,[373] *synovial sarcoma*,[374] and *pleomorphic adenoma* (possibly derived from ectopic tracheobronchial gland tissue within a mediastinal lymph node).[351]

MEDIASTINAL MASSES SITUATED PREDOMINANTLY IN THE MIDDLE COMPARTMENT

The middle mediastinal compartment contains the heart, pericardium, all the major vessels leaving and entering this organ, plus the trachea and main bronchi, paratracheal and tracheobronchial lymph nodes, the phrenic nerves, and the upper portions of the vagus nerves.

LYMPH NODE ENLARGEMENT

Lymph node enlargement is undoubtedly the most common mediastinal abnormality and is caused most often by lymphomas, metastatic carcinoma (Fig. 19–41), sarcoidosis, and infection (particularly due to *H. capsulatum* and *M. tuberculosis*). Uncommon causes include angio-immunoblastic lymphadenopathy (*see* page 1570), infectious mononucleosis (*see* page 1071), drug toxicity (e.g., by diphenylhydantoin—*see* page 2441), and amyloidosis (*see* page 2578).[375, 376] Most of these conditions are discussed elsewhere in the book; only three—primary mediastinal lymphoma, angiofollicular lymph node hyperplasia (Castleman's disease), and granulomatous mediastinitis—are considered in any detail here. With the exception of Hodgkin's disease in which the anterior mediastinal and retrosternal nodes are most often affected, the anatomic distribution of lymph node enlargement in all these diseases is predominantly midmediastinal. In this situation, airway obstruction may be a life-threatening complication, particularly in children.[377] Pulmonic stenosis may develop, frequently in association with chest pain, dyspnea, and a pulmonic ejection murmur.[378]

Primary Mediastinal Lymphoma

Lymphomas are one of the most common causes of mediastinal abnormality: it has been estimated that they comprise 20 per cent of all mediastinal neoplasms in adults and 50 per cent in children.[379] Most often, mediastinal node enlargement occurs in association with clinical or roentgenographic evidence of extrathoracic disease. Occasionally, however, the mediastinum is the sole site of

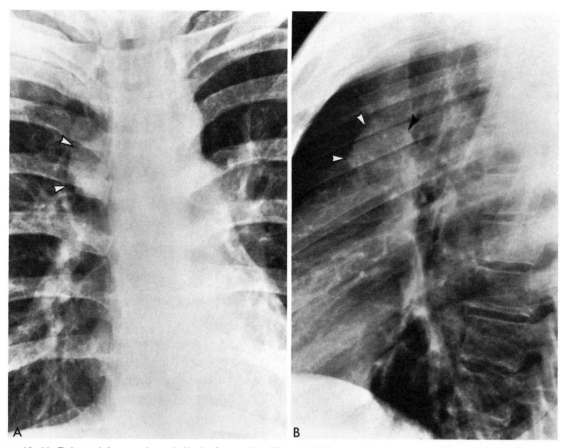

Figure 19–41. Enlarged Azygos Lymph Node Caused by Metastatic Cancer. Posteroanterior *(A)* and lateral *(B)* roentgenograms reveal a well-defined homogeneous mass *(arrowheads)* situated just anterior to the right tracheobronchial angle. This is the anatomic location of both the azygos vein and the azygos lymph node, and an opacity such as is visualized in this patient can be due either to distention of the vein or to enlargement of the node. In this case, it was caused by metastatic carcinoma of the adrenal gland.

abnormality, in which case differentiation from other mediastinal abnormalities can be difficult. For example, disease localized to the mediastinum and adjacent structures was found in 12 of 215 patients (6 per cent) with non-Hodgkin's lymphoma seen at the Massachusetts General Hospital between 1975 and 1979.[380]

Hodgkin's disease is undoubtedly the most common lymphoma to present in the mediastinum, lymph node enlargement being evident on the initial roentgenogram of approximately 50 per cent of patients.[381, 382] Nodular sclerosis is by far the most common histologic subtype (Fig. 19–42). An anterior mediastinal mass involving the thymus is also common.[236] Further details of the roentgenographic and clinical features are provided on page 1508.

About 60 per cent of primary mediastinal non-Hodgkin's lymphomas are classified as lymphoblastic,[379] and approximately 50 per cent of patients with this neoplasm have a prominent mass in the mediastinum at the time of presentation (Fig. 19–43).[383] The majority of patients are either children or young adults; immunologic studies show that most tumors have features of immature T cells. Prognosis is poor, widespread dissemination (especially to bone marrow and the central nervous system) and leukemic transformation occurring in many individuals.

The remaining 40 per cent of primary mediastinal non-Hodgkin's lymphomas are composed of different histologic subtypes, the most common of which is the diffuse large cell (histiocytic) variety. Reports from several centers have documented the clinicopathologic features of these neoplasms, and a fairly characteristic picture has emerged.[238, 241, 379, 383–387] Grossly, the tumors are large, averaging 11.7 cm in diameter in the 31 cases reviewed by Perrone and colleagues.[384] Invasion of contiguous mediastinal structures, chest wall, and lung is common at the time of presentation.[384] Histologically, the majority of the neoplasms are diffuse in type and composed of large cleaved or noncleaved ("histiocytic") cells. The pattern of immunoblastic sarcoma is present in some cases.[384] Most tumors appear to be of B-cell origin. Sclerosis, manifested by either diffuse increase in reticulin or relatively broad bands of fibrous tissue, is a prominent feature in many cases. Pathologic differentiation from other mediastinal neoplasms, particularly thymoma and germ cell tumors, can be difficult, especially with small tissue samples.

The majority of non-Hodgkin's lymphomas oc-

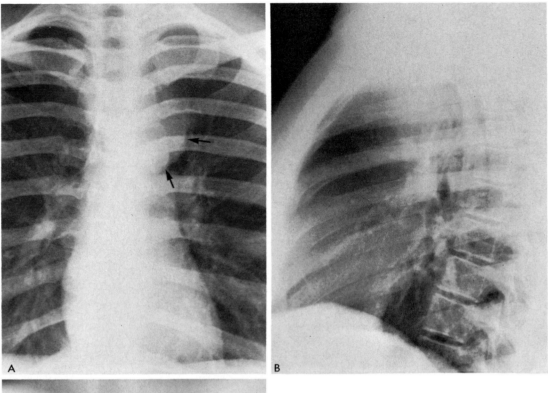

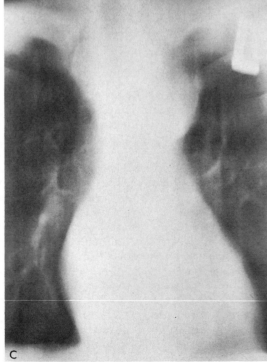

Figure 19–42. Hodgkin's Disease: Solitary Anterior Mediastinal Mass. Posteroanterior *(A)* and lateral *(B)* roentgenograms of a 15-year-old girl reveal a smooth, homogeneous mass projecting to the left of the upper mediastinum *(arrows)*. Although the mass cannot be clearly outlined in lateral projection, its position in the anterior mediastinum is clearly established by the fact that it fades out superiorly as a result of contiguity with the soft tissues of the neck at the thoracic inlet. (If the mass were posteriorly situated, its superior border would be clearly outlined because of contiguity with air-containing lung.) A tomographic cut *(C)* clearly establishes the anterior position of the mass and its loss of definition superiorly (note simultaneous visualization of the manubrium and the medial ends of the clavicles). This mass was the only intrathoracic abnormality visualized. Biopsy revealed Hodgkin's disease of nodular sclerosing type.

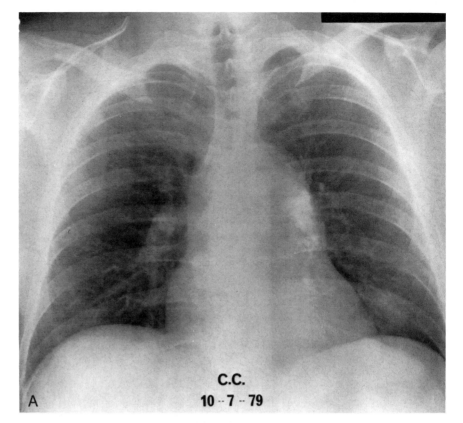

Figure 19–43. Mediastinal Lymph Node Enlargement Secondary to Non-Hodgkin's Lymphoma. A posteroanterior roentgenogram *(A)* reveals widening of the mid mediastinum by a mass that extends from the region of the aortic arch down to just below the left hilum. The lungs are clear.

Illustration continued on following page

C.C.
10 - 7 - 79

A

cur in young adults; in most series, the sex incidence is about equal although in some[384, 385] there is a predominance of females. Symptoms referable to the thorax, particularly dyspnea and pain, are present in the majority of patients; superior vena cava syndrome also occurs in many individuals (in 21 of 63 patients in two series).[380, 384] With aggressive chemotherapy and radiation therapy, a 50 to 60 per cent 5-year survival can be expected.

Giant Lymph Node Hyperplasia

Giant lymph node hyperplasia (Castleman's disease, angiofollicular lymph node hyperplasia) is an unusual condition of unknown etiology and pathogenesis originally described by Castleman in 1954[388] and elaborated upon in greater detail by Keller and his colleagues in 1972.[389] In the latter report, the authors described two distinct histologic types of the condition:

1. The more common (74 of 81 cases in this study), termed the *hyaline vascular type*, was characterized histologically by the presence of multiple germinal centers separated by a polymorphous lymphoreticular infiltrate containing numerous capillaries (Fig. 19–44); some of the capillaries, often with distinctly hyalinized walls, extended into the germinal centers themselves. This form of disease was usually unassociated with symptoms and was discovered as a mass in the mediastinum or perihilar region on a screening chest roentgenogram.

2. The second histologic variant, termed the *plasma cell type*, showed sheets of numerous cytologically mature plasma cells between the germinal centers, there being relatively few capillaries. In contrast to the hyaline vascular type, patients with the plasma cell variant tended to have systemic manifestations of disease, including fever, anemia, weight loss, and hypergammaglobulinemia. (Since the appearance of this report by Keller and colleagues,[389] a variety of other clinical manifestations have been reported,[390] including a syndrome of growth failure and hyperchromic anemia in children,[391, 392] nephrotic syndrome, myelofibrosis,[393] peripheral neuropathy,[394] and thrombotic thrombocytopenic purpura.[395])

Both histologic types of this localized form of the disease tend to occur in young adults and are associated with a good prognosis following surgical excision;[392] systemic manifestations usually resolve and there is typically no tendency to recurrence or the development of new disease.

The lesions described by Castleman and his colleagues[388, 389] were usually solitary and in the majority of patients (70 of 81) affected the mediastinum or hilum. More recently, patients have been described in whom histologically similar tumors have been multifocal and have tended to affect superficial lymph node groups rather than the mediastinum. Sometimes termed *multicentric Castleman's disease* or multicentric lymph node hyperplasia,[390, 396] this condition tends to affect individuals older than

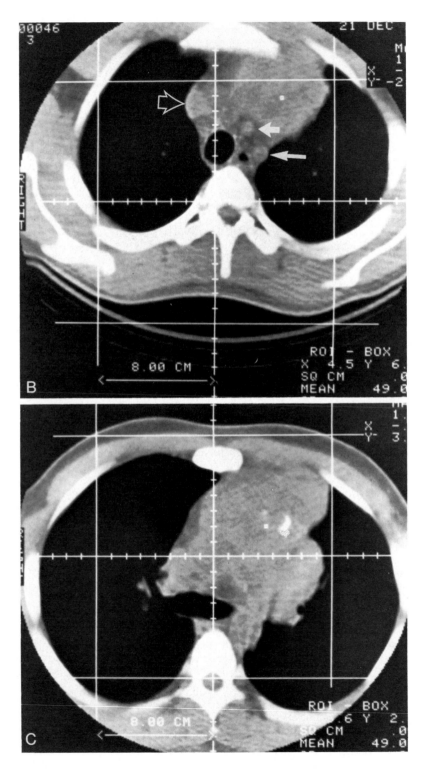

Figure 19–43 *Continued* CT scans at the level of the left brachiocephalic vein *(B)* and tracheal carina *(C)* reveal a large homogeneous mass extending to the left and anteriorly to the thoracic wall. In *C*, normal anatomic structures within the mediastinum are largely effaced, although the left subclavian artery *(long arrow)* and left carotid artery *(short arrow)* can be clearly identified in *B;* however, note the effacement of the left side of the superior vena cava *(open arrow)*. Note the calcified foci on both CT scans; since lymphoma seldom calcifies unless radiation therapy has been performed, it is probable that these foci represent calcified lymph nodes incorporated into the mass. Biopsy of this 32-year-old asymptomatic man revealed lymphoblastic lymphoma.

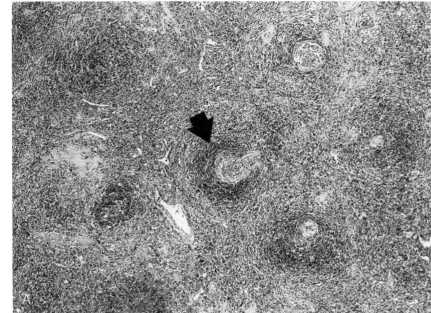

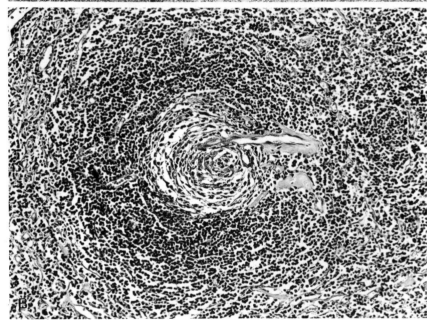

Figure 19–44. Giant Lymph Node Hyperplasia. A histologic section from a large lobulated anterior mediastinal mass *(A)* reveals an extensive infiltrate of lymphoid cells admixed with numerous vessels and several germinal centers *(arrow).* Although this appearance superficially resembles a lymph node, the absence of sinusoids and the configuration of the germinal centers indicate that this is not normal nodal structure. A magnified view of one germinal center *(B)* shows a small vessel with a thickened, hyalinized wall extending into its mid portion. *(A,* × 40; *B,* × 150.)

those with the solitary form and to be associated with signs and symptoms of systemic disease such as hepatosplenomegaly, anemia, hypergammaglobulinemia, altered liver function tests, renal disease, skin rash, and central nervous system manifestations.[390] Some patients have concomitant human immunodeficiency virus (HIV) infection[397] or Kaposi's sarcoma; an association with the POEMS syndrome (polyneuropathy, organomegaly, endocrinopathy, M protein, and skin changes) also has been reported.[398] The prognosis is distinctly poorer than that of the solitary form, there being a tendency in many patients to progression of the lymphoreticular proliferation, the development of serious infectious complications, or evolution to frank lymphoma.

The fundamental nature of giant lymph node hyperplasia and the relationship, if any, between the solitary and multicentric forms are uncertain.[390] It has been suggested that the solitary form might represent a hamartoma of lymphoid tissue, a focus of lymphoid hyperplasia, or an infectious lymphadenitis.[390] The diffuse nature of the multicentric form, its association with conditions known to be accompanied by an abnormal immune reaction such as HIV infection, the relatively frequent progression to lymphoma, and the occasional documentation of altered helper-suppressor T-cell ratios in some individuals[399] suggest a generalized underlying immune abnormality.

The roentgenographic appearance of the localized form of giant lymph node hyperplasia is one

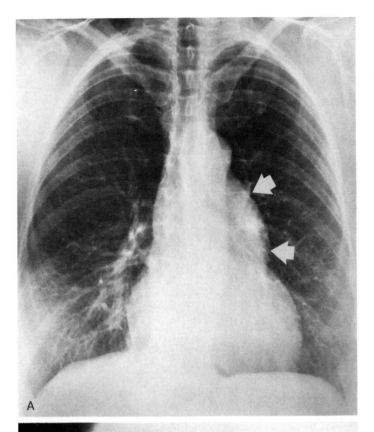

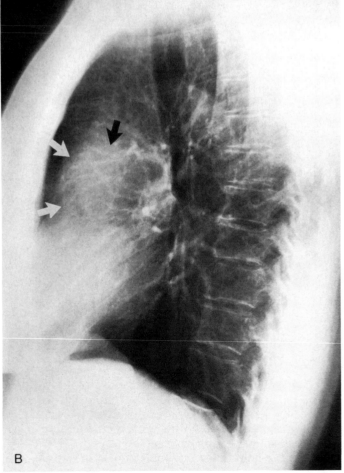

Figure 19–45. Giant Lymph Node Hyperplasia (Castleman's Disease). Posteroanterior *(A)* and lateral *(B)* roentgenograms reveal a well-defined opacity protruding to the left from the region of the main pulmonary artery *(arrows in A)*. In lateral projection, an ill-defined opacity can be identified in the anterior mediastinum *(arrows)*.

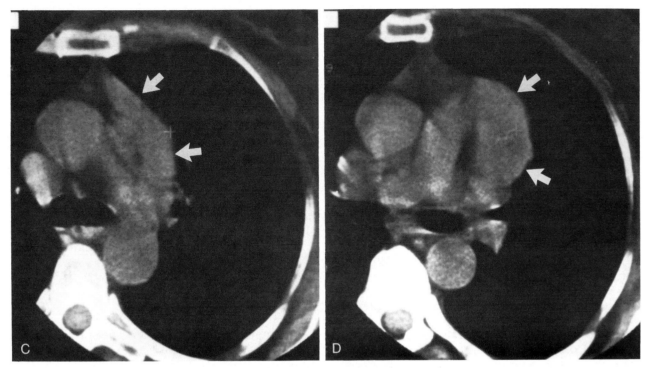

Figure 19–45 *Continued* CT scans at the level of the aortopulmonary window *(C)* and main pulmonary artery *(D)* reveal a well-defined, homogeneous mass *(arrows)* contiguous with the left side of the mediastinum and protruding into the left hemithorax. Following resection, the mass showed histologic features characteristic of giant follicular hyperplasia. The patient is a 63-year-old woman who had no symptoms referable to her chest.

of a solitary mass, with a smooth or lobulated contour (Fig. 19–45), in any of the three mediastinal compartments but most commonly in the middle and posterior ones.[140, 400] In the latter location, the major differential diagnosis is neurogenic tumor, from which lymph node hyperplasia may be indistinguishable, even angiographically.[401] CT can be expected to clarify the precise anatomic location of these masses but cannot clarify their nature; however, in one patient in whom a large lymph node mass was located atypically in a cardiophrenic angle, CT served to rule out the initial diagnosis of pericardial cyst.[402] Calcification is uncommon, but when it does occur it tends to be punctate and discrete rather than curvilinear as in most cystic lesions.[403] Both angiography and contrast-enhanced CT scans characteristically reveal hypervascularity.[403, 404]

Lymph Node Involvement In Granulomatous Mediastinitis

This category includes not only chronic granulomatous mediastinitis attributable to a specific etiology such as tuberculosis or histoplasmosis but also sarcoidosis. In both forms, paratracheal and tracheobronchial lymph node enlargement may be the predominant finding, and in the absence of roentgenographic evidence of pulmonary disease, the differential diagnostic possibilites of mediastinal widening are limited to diseases causing node enlargement.

In the infectious granulomas, node enlargement tends to be predominantly unilateral (*see* Fig. 19–4, page 2802); in sarcoidosis, node enlargement tends to be bilateral and symmetric and, in contrast to the lymphomas, is almost invariably associated with bronchopulmonary node enlargement. Calcification within enlarged nodes suggests an infectious etiology, although calcification also occurs occasionally in the nodes of sarcoidosis in which it can be of the "eggshell" variety. Such calcification within paratracheal or tracheobronchial lymph nodes may be associated with erosion of these airways and the extrusion of calcified masses into their lumina (broncholithiasis) and the expectoration of calcified material (broncholithoptysis).[405–407] Storer and Smith[406] noted that the chronic cough associated with calcified mediastinal nodes may occur only when the head is in certain positions. This subject is discussed in greater detail on page 2220.

Granulomatous involvement of posterior mediastinal nodes can exert local effects on the esophagus, including traction diverticula and esophagobronchial fistula.

MISCELLANEOUS MIDDLE MEDIASTINAL TUMORS

Primary Tracheal Neoplasms

Although pulmonary carcinoma is usually manifested in the mediastinum in the form of metastases to lymph nodes from a primary lesion in the lung, rarely the carcinoma arises in the trachea or main bronchi just distal to the carina and thus is situated within the middle mediastinum. If the neoplasm extends outward into the paratracheal space, it may widen the mediastinum to one or the other side. An irregular shaggy mass is usually evident within the tracheal air column on standard roentgenograms or on conventional or computed tomograms.

Symptoms include cough, hemoptysis, and sometimes severe dyspnea and wheezing; stridor may be apparent.

Aorticopulmonary Paraganglioma (Chemodectoma)

Paragangliomas are neoplasms of the extra-adrenal paraganglionic system; the latter comprises minute macroscopic or microscopic collections of neuroendocrine-like cells in intimate association with the autonomic nervous system.[408] In the thorax, paraganglia occur in two distinct locations:[408] (1) the perivascular adventitial tissue bounded by the aorta superiorly, the pulmonary artery inferiorly, and the ligamentum arteriosum and right pulmonary artery on either side (aorticopulmonary paraganglia); and (2) in association with the segmental ganglia of the sympathetic chain in the posterior mediastinum (aorticosympathetic paraganglia). Paragangliomas derived from the first group thus occur in the middle mediastinum in relation to the aorta and pulmonary artery whereas those in the second arise in the posterior mediastinum in a paravertebral location (see page 2901).

Paragangliomas of the aorticopulmonary region are uncommon, approximately 40 cases having been reported in the English language literature by 1979.[409] The mean age at the time of diagnosis is 49 years and there is a slight female predominance.[409] Tumors, both within and outside the thorax, are occasionally multiple.

Pathologically,[408] these tumors can be either discrete, encapsulated nodules or more diffusely spreading growths encompassing adjacent vascular structures. Histologic features are characteristic and consist of multiple loosely arranged cellular nests ("Zellballen") separated by a prominent fibrovascular stroma. Nuclear atypia may be present but does not predict aggressive behavior. Argyrophilic intracytoplasmic granules can be identified with appropriate silver stains, and electron microscopic examination reveals numerous dense core intracytoplasmic granules.

Roentgenographic features are those of a mass in the middle mediastinum in close relation to the base of the heart and aortic arch.[409] The precise localization of the tumors is aided by the use of angiography,[409, 410] [131]I scintigraphy, two-dimensional echocardiography,[411] and of course CT.

Clinically,[409] most aorticopulmonary paragangliomas do not occasion symptoms and are discovered on a screening chest roentgenogram; however, they can sometimes compress or invade local structures and cause symptoms such as cough, chest pain, hoarseness, dysphagia, and (occasionally) superior vena cava syndrome. Some patients, especially young females, also develop gastric leiomyoblastomas and pulmonary chondromas, either synchronously or metachronously (Carney's triad, see page 1591). Rare cases are hormonally active and secrete catecholamines.

The prognosis of aorticopulmonary paragangliomas must be somewhat guarded. Because of their location and intrinsic vascularity, the operative mortality is high (9 per cent of patients in the review by Lack and colleagues[409]); in addition, complete excision frequently cannot be achieved.[409] Although recurrence is the rule in these patients, the growth rate is often slow. Metastases have been documented in about 13 per cent of reported patients.[409]

Bronchial Cyst

Congenital bronchial cysts of the mediastinum are described in detail in Chapter 5 (see page 714) and are reviewed only briefly here. These cysts usually are discovered in childhood or early adult life. Although it is generally accepted that the majority are situated in the vicinity of the carina in relation to one of the major airways, of the 54 mediastinal bronchial cysts reported from the Mayo Clinic[140] and the 11 studied at the Cleveland Clinic,[146] the majority were located in the midportion of the posterior mediastinum. Almost all have only a single cavity. They rarely communicate with the tracheobronchial tree. Although these cysts may grow very large without occasioning symptoms, even small ones may cause tracheobronchial obstruction in infants and children.[134] They can undergo an abrupt increase in size as a result of hemorrhage or infection. At the other end of the spectrum are cysts that undergo spontaneous disappearance.[412]

MASSES SITUATED IN THE ANTERIOR CARDIOPHRENIC ANGLE

Masses in the vicinity of the cardiophrenic angle on either side, although anteriorly situated, relate to the heart and therefore are truly in the middle mediastinum. The differential diagnosis of such masses is extensive and includes lesions arising within the lung parenchyma, in the visceral or parietal pleural membranes or pleural space, within the space between the pericardium and the mediastinal pleura (usually but not invariably fat), within the pericardium or contiguous myocardium (e.g., cardiac aneurysm), within the diaphragm, from beneath the diaphragm (hernia), and finally tumors such as teratomas or thymomas that much more frequently occupy anatomic sites elsewhere in the mediastinum. Lesions arising in any of these anatomic regions can conceivably produce roentgenographic shadows of a similar nature, although CT can be employed to advantage in their differential diagnosis.[413] Only four are considered here—pleuropericardial fat, mesothelial cysts, hernia through the foramen of Morgagni, and enlargement of diaphragmatic lymph nodes.

Pleuropericardial Fat

Accumulations of fat that normally occupy the cardiophrenic angles can attain a considerable size. Pleuropericardial fat pads are always bilateral but may be asymmetric, that on the right usually being the larger (Fig. 19–46). They can increase considerably in size over time, either from simple obesity or from hyperadrenocorticism (e.g., Cushing's syndrome), and as such can cause a potentially confusing roentgenographic opacity. Variations in the CT appearance of these fat pads have been recently reviewed.[414]

Rarely, pleuropericardial fat pads are the site of fat necrosis, an event associated with the abrupt onset of severe retrosternal pain, sometimes resembling that caused by pulmonary embolism or myocardial infarction. Only seven cases of this unusual abnormality had been reported by 1969.[415] Affected patients are very obese; the only roentgenographic sign of note is a large pleuropericardial fat pad. Microscopic examination of resected tissue reveals the typical changes of fat necrosis, consisting of lipid-filled macrophages, necrotic adipose tissue, and a variable degree of acute and chronic inflammatory cellular reaction.

Mesothelial Cysts

The vast majority of mesothelial cysts (pericardial or pleuropericardial) are probably congenital and result from aberrations in the formation of the coelomic cavities. Rarely, an otherwise typical cyst has developed years after an attack of acute pericarditis,[416] suggesting that some may be acquired. They show no sex predominance.

Grossly, the cysts are spherical or oval in shape, thin-walled, and often translucent; the vast majority are unilocular[140] and contain clear or straw-colored fluid. Microscopically, the cyst wall is composed of a thin layer of fibrous tissue lined by a single layer of flattened or cuboidal cells resembling mesothelial cells (Fig. 19–47). Of the 72 cysts reviewed by a Mayo Clinic group,[140] 54 were in the cardiophrenic angles and 18 arose at a higher level; 11 of the latter cysts extended into the superior mediastinum (Fig. 19–48). Fifty-three were on the right side, a predominance also reported by other workers.[417] Roentgenographically, the great majority of mesothelial cysts are smooth in contour and round or oval. Lateral projection may reveal a teardrop con-

figuration caused by insertion of the cyst into the interlobar fissure between the middle and lower lobes (Fig. 19–49). In most cases they range in diameter from 3 to 8 cm but rarely have been reported to be as small as 1 cm or as large as 28 cm.[265, 418, 419] The cystic nature of these masses can be confirmed by CT[420] or ultrasonography,[416, 419, 421] even when their location is atypical such as the superior mediastinum,[422, 423] thus obviating needless thoracotomy. A case has been reported in which a pathologically proven mesothelial cyst manifested CT numbers in the range of 30 to 40, suggesting the possibility of a solid neoplasm;[424] the lesion was resected and was proven to be a pericardial cyst containing viscous, mucoid material that was undoubtedly responsible for the elevated CT numbers. A similar finding has been reported by others.[417] A case has been reported in which the wall of a pericardial cyst was calcified.[425]

Symptoms are almost invariably absent, most cysts being discovered on a screening chest roentgenogram. Occasionally, a very large cyst can give rise to a sensation of retrosternal pressure or to dyspnea.[142] Very rarely, a pericardial cyst becomes infected.[150]

Hernia Through the Foramen of Morgagni

The foramina of Morgagni are small triangular deficiencies in the diaphragm, a few centimeters from the midline on each side, between muscle fibers originating from the xiphisternum and seventh rib (see Fig. 20–1, page 2922). When larger than normal they can permit herniation of abdominal contents into the thorax. Herniation is almost invariably right-sided since the left foramen is protected by the pericardium; of 50 cases in one series,[426] 4 were bilateral and only 1 case was solely left-sided. Hernial contents include omentum, liver, and small or large bowel. When the hernial sac is filled with liver, the roentgenographic shadow is homogeneous and usually indistinguishable from a large pleuropericardial fat pad (Fig. 19–50). When the hernial sac contains omentum, the density of the mass on conventional roentgenograms seldom indicates its fatty nature although CT can do so convincingly. In such circumstances the transverse colon occupies a high position within the abdomen, peaking anteriorly and superiorly in the vicinity of the hernia. Thus, barium examination of the colon is virtually diagnostic (Fig. 19–51). When the hernial sac contains small or large bowel, the presence of gas-containing loops usually permits ready diagnosis that can be confirmed, if necessary, by barium examination (Figs. 19–52 and 19–53). An interesting sign, termed "the sign of the cane," has been described by Lanuza as a means of recognizing small Morgagni hernias.[427] Since a hernia through a foramen of Morgagni carries peritoneum ahead of it, properitoneal fat also should be present and

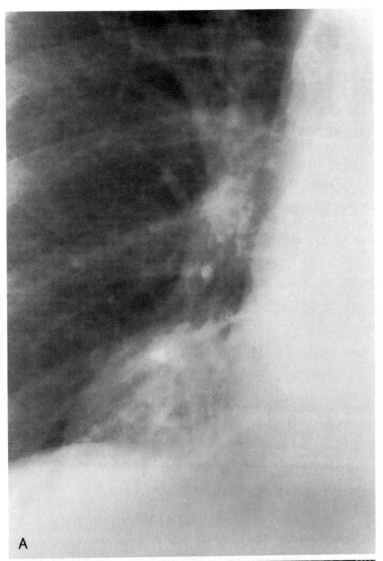

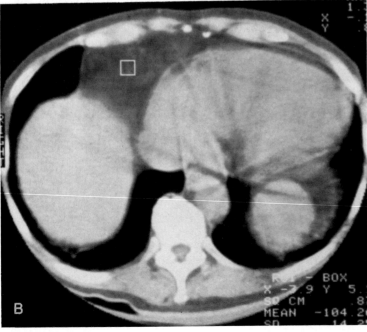

Figure 19–46. Right Cardiophrenic Angle Mass: Fat Pad. A view of the lower portion of the right hemithorax from a posteroanterior roentgenogram (A) reveals a sharply defined opacity of homogeneous density obscuring the medial portion of the right hemidiaphragm and the right border of the heart. The density of the mass is roughly equivalent to that of the pulmonary artery several centimeters above. A CT scan at the level of the right hemidiaphragm (B) reveals the mass to be of fat density, possessing a mean attenuation of – 105 Hounsfield units. The patient is an asymptomatic 64-year-old man.

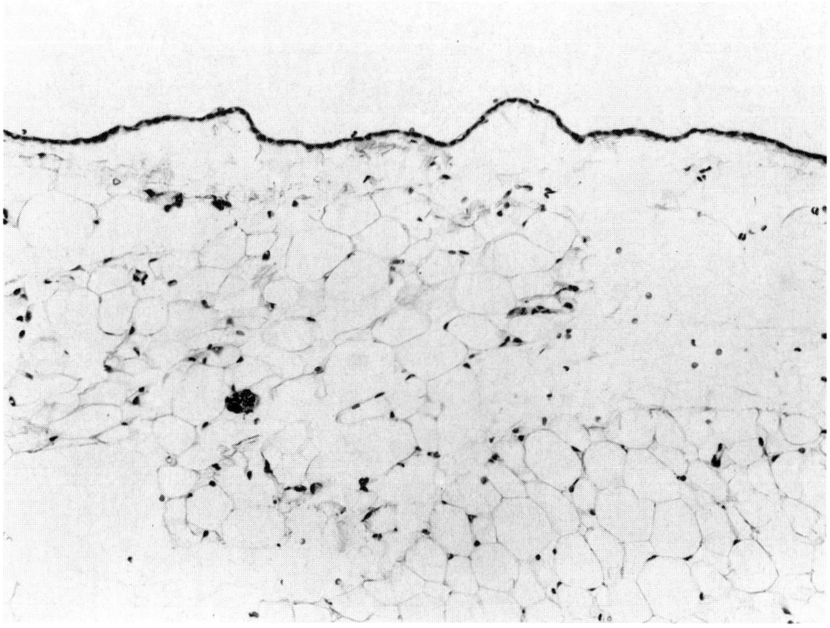

Figure 19–47. Mesothelial Cyst. A histologic section through the wall of a smooth-walled cyst that was situated contiguous with the pericardium shows adipose tissue lined by a layer of flattened mesothelial cells. This appearance is characteristic of a pericardial mesothelial cyst. ($\times$ 150.)

should be visualized external to the hernial contents on lateral roentgenograms of the chest. The "sign of the cane" refers to the curvilinear accumulation of fat in continuity with the properitoneal fat line of the anterior abdominal wall.

Patients usually are asymptomatic but occasionally complain of retrosternal pain or gastrointestinal or respiratory symptoms.[428] Strangulation of hernial contents occurs rarely.

Enlargement of Diaphragmatic Lymph Nodes

The diaphragmatic group of parietal lymph nodes is normally not visualized on chest roentgenograms because of their small size and their investment with fat and other connective tissue adjacent to the pleura. However, when enlarged these lymph nodes displace the pleura laterally and produce a smooth or lobulated mass projecting out of the cardiophrenic angle. In patients with Hodgkin's disease particularly, enlargement of these nodes causes opacities that simulate pleuropericardial fat pads (see Fig. 8–96, page 1517). Although such enlargement may be apparent on conventional roentgenograms, CT is obviously a superior method of assessment: Cho and his colleagues[429] reviewed 274 CT scans of the thorax obtained on 209 patients with malignant lymphoma (153 Hodgkin's disease and 56 non-Hodgkin's lymphoma) and found evidence of enlargement of cardiophrenic angle lymph nodes in 14 patients (6.6 per cent); in only 3 of these was node enlargement clearly evident on conventional roentgenograms. Such node enlargement can occur as the initial presentation in patients with Hodgkin's disease,[430, 431] although Castellino and

Blank[430] have identified it more often during relapse of the disease. Thus, it is important to compare the cardiophrenic angles on serial chest roentgenograms, since this area is a potential site of recurrent disease; when doubt exists, CT examination should be performed. A reduction in the size of nodes can constitute convincing evidence of effective therapy.

DILATATION OF THE MAIN PULMONARY ARTERY

Dilatation of the main pulmonary artery may be of sufficient degree to suggest a mediastinal mass.[432] Although the great majority of cases are associated with either pulmonary arterial hypertension or left-to-right shunt (Fig. 19–54), some are poststenotic and related to pulmonary valve stenosis.[432, 433] A few cases are idiopathic. Rare causes include aneurysms (considered in detail on page 1883), direct communication between the pulmonary artery and left atrium (see page 742),[434] and complications of banding.[435] A case has been reported of a false aneurysm of the pulmonary artery that developed as a result of erosion of fabric subsequent to banding of the left pulmonary artery for tricuspid atresia;[436] the true nature of the abnormality was not apparent on conventional chest roentgenography or angiography but was accurately recognized on enhanced CT.

Roentgenographic manifestations depend upon the cause of dilatation. Differentiation of the idiopathic and poststenotic varieties may be difficult, although fluoroscopic examination usually reveals increased amplitude of arterial pulsation in the latter condition and not in the former.

Text continued on page 2879

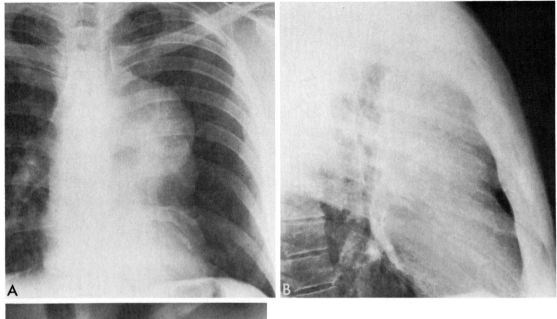

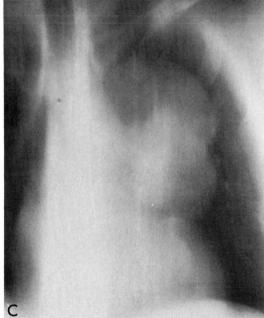

Figure 19–48. Anterior Mediastinal Mesothelial Cyst. Posteroanterior *(A)* and lateral *(B)* roentgenograms of a 34-year-old asymptomatic man reveal a large lobulated mass of homogeneous density projecting to the left of the mediastinum and situated anteriorly in the crotch between the heart and the ascending aorta. It contains no calcium. Its sharp definition and homogeneous density are revealed to advantage on an anteroposterior tomogram *(C)*. At thoracotomy, the mass was found to be a multiloculated cyst containing clear watery fluid. (Tomogram courtesy of St. Mary's Hospital, Montreal.)

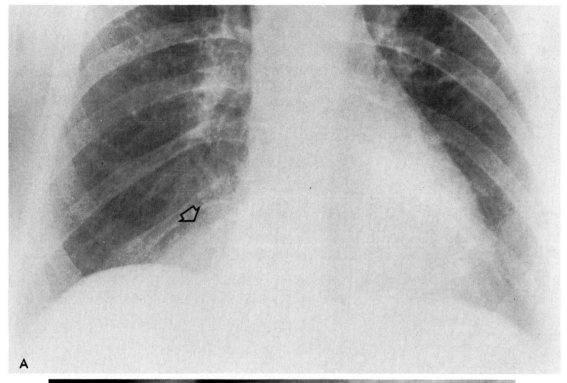

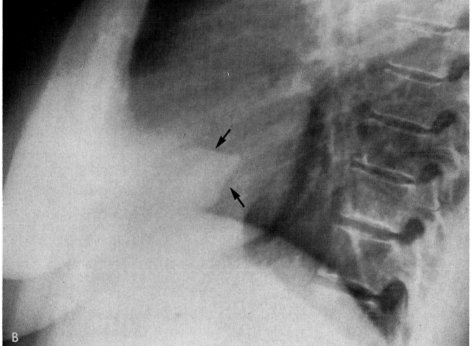

Figure 19–49. Mesothelial Cyst in the Right Cardiophrenic Angle. Views of the lower half of the thorax from posteroanterior *(A)* and lateral *(B)* roentgenograms of a 50-year-old asymptomatic woman reveal a smooth, fairly well-defined, homogeneous mass lying in the right cardiophrenic angle *(arrows)*. In lateral projection, the mass is elliptical. This configuration should suggest the diagnosis of pleuropericardial cyst.

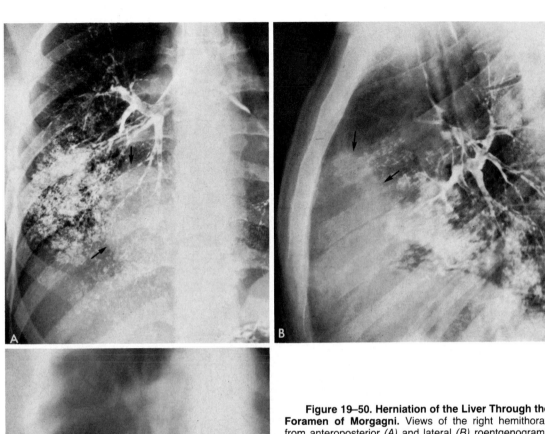

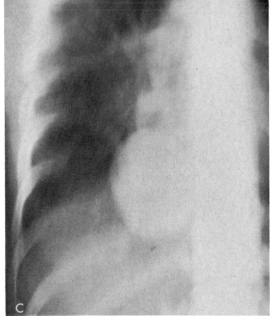

Figure 19–50. Herniation of the Liver Through the Foramen of Morgagni. Views of the right hemithorax from anteroposterior *(A)* and lateral *(B)* roentgenograms following bronchography reveal a smooth, well-defined soft tissue mass occupying the anterior cardiophrenic sulcus *(arrows* in both projections); the bronchial tree is displaced. Numerous anomalies of bronchial distribution are evident. An anteroposterior tomogram *(C)* reveals the sharp definition and homogeneous density of the mass. The fact that all margins can be identified indicates that it is surrounded by air-containing lung, at least at the level of this tomographic cut. At thoracotomy, the mass was found to be an accessory lobe of the liver (histologically normal) that had herniated through a large foramen of Morgagni. The patient was a 24-year-old asymptomatic woman.

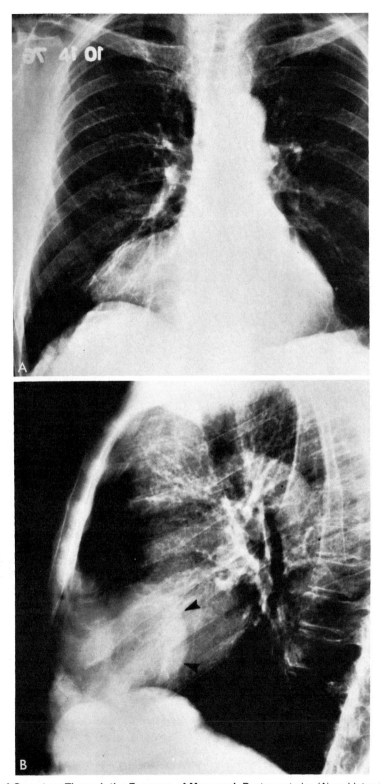

Figure 19–51. Hernia of Omentum Through the Foramen of Morgagni. Posteroanterior *(A)* and lateral *(B)* roentgenograms of this 73-year-old asymptomatic man reveal a large, fairly sharply circumscribed mass in the right cardiophrenic angle *(arrows* in *B)*. In posteroanterior projection the mass appears homogeneous in density, but in lateral projection it is somewhat inhomogeneous. Its central portion is slightly more radiolucent, suggesting tissue of fat density.

Illustration continued on following page

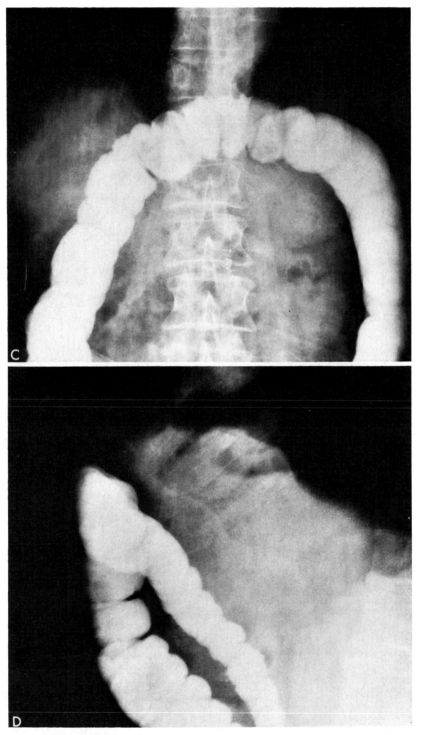

Figure 19–51 *Continued* Anteroposterior *(C)* and lateral *(D)* projections of the abdomen following barium enema reveal moderate elevation of the transverse colon, whose superior aspect lies contiguous to the diaphragm anteriorly. This deformity of the colon is characteristic of herniation of omentum through the foramen of Morgagni, which was proved at thoracotomy.

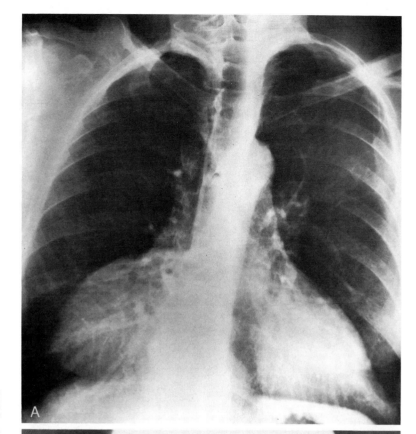

Figure 19–52. Morgagni Hernia Containing Bowel and Omentum. Posteroanterior (A) and lateral (B) roentgenograms reveal a large, sharply defined opacity in the right cardiophrenic angle. The mass is homogeneous in density except for the presence within it of multiple radiolucencies that represent gas-containing loops of bowel, some containing fluid levels. The bowel loops can be seen to best advantage in lateral projection. The patient was a 50-year-old asymptomatic man.

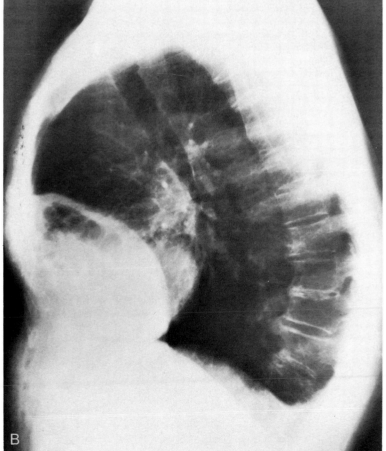

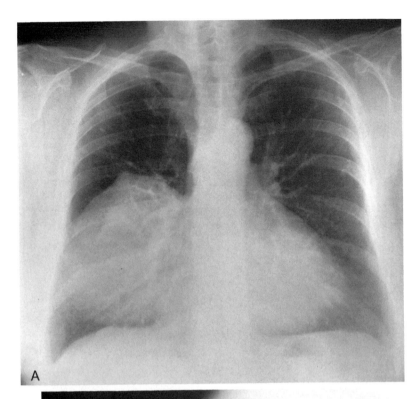

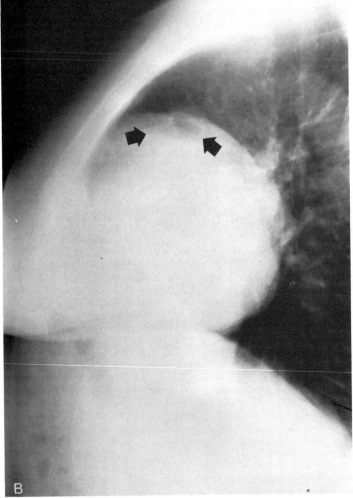

Figure 19–53. Herniation of Omentum and Bowel Through the Foramen of Morgagni. Posteroanterior *(A)* and lateral *(B)* roentgenograms reveal a large mass situated in the inferior portion of the right hemithorax, lying chiefly anteriorly and obliterating the right border of the heart. Its density is homogeneous except for a small radiolucency situated in its most superior portion (*arrows* in *B*).

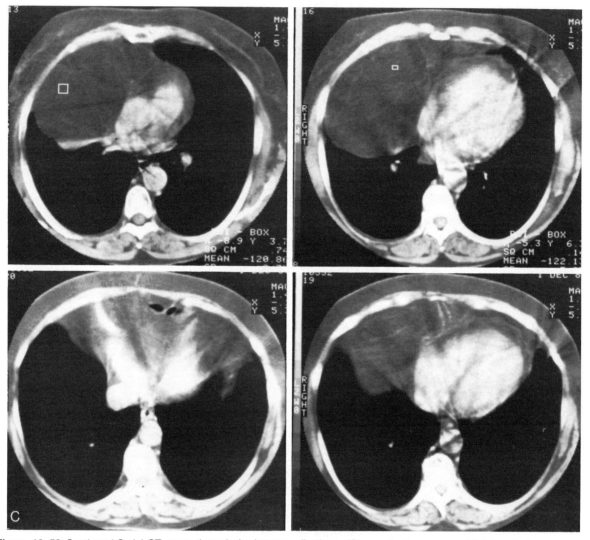

Figure 19–53 *Continued* Serial CT scans through the lower mediastinum *(C)* reveal a large mass of fat density (mean attenuation, −120 Hounsfield units) situated in the region of the right cardiophrenic angle and extending around the anterior aspect of the heart. In the lower left scan, two small loops of bowel can be readily identified. The patient is an asymptomatic 67-year-old man; the hernia was surgically corrected.

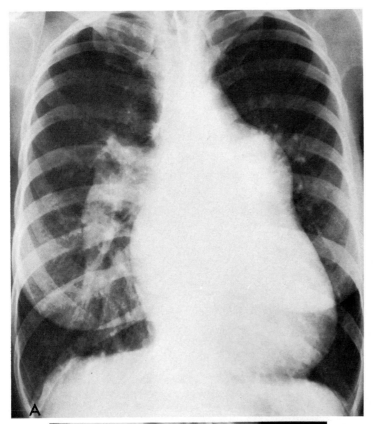

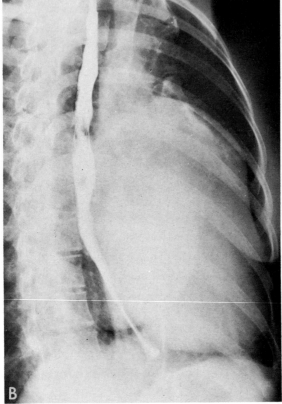

Figure 19–54. Dilatation of the Main Pulmonary Artery. Posteroanterior *(A)* and right anterior oblique *(B)* roentgenograms of the chest reveal marked dilatation of the hilar and peripheral pulmonary arteries, indicating pulmonary pleonemia. The main pulmonary artery is greatly dilated, creating a smooth protruberance of the left border of the cardiovascular silhouette in posteroanterior projection and of the anterior surface in oblique projection. Configuration of the enlarged heart is compatible with patent ductus arteriosus; a duct was successfully corrected surgically.

Idiopathic dilatation invariably does not give rise to symptoms and is unassociated with evidence of hemodynamic abnormality roentgenologically or during cardiac catheterization.[432, 433, 437] Physical examination of a patient with a severe degree of dilatation may reveal a widely split second heart sound, varying little with respiration. The ostensible reason for this sign is a delay in impulse rebound caused by loss of compliance of the dilated pulmonary trunk.[438] With this degree of dilatation, an echocardiogram may reveal increased distance of the pulmonic valve from the chest wall and a fine fluttering of the valve, presumably caused by turbulence.[439]

DILATATION OF THE MAJOR MEDIASTINAL VEINS

Superior and Inferior Vena Cava

The great majority of cases of dilatation of the superior vena cava (SVC) are the result of raised central venous pressure, commonly from cardiac decompensation, and less often from tricuspid valvular stenosis or cardiac tamponade secondary to pericardial effusion or constrictive pericarditis. The roentgenographic appearance is distinctive—a smooth, well-defined widening of the right side of the mediastinum (Fig. 19–55). The width of the vein (and therefore of the mediastinum itself) varies considerably with the phase of respiration and particularly with the marked change in intrathoracic pressure that accompanies the Valsalva and Mueller maneuvers. The azygos vein is almost always dilated as well, and this is a more dependable sign of systemic hypertension because the diameter of the vein in the right tracheobronchial angle can be precisely measured. (The azygos is dilated if its diameter is greater than 10 mm when the patient is erect or 14 mm when the patient is recumbent.)

Occasionally, a right superior mediastinal opacity can be caused by a nondilated but laterally displaced superior vena cava. In the case reported by Drasin and his colleagues,[440] the superior vena cava was displaced laterally by an atherosclerotic ascending aorta. Rarely, the SVC has an aneurysmal dilatation, presumably congenital in origin;[196, 441–443] the aneurysm may be fusiform or saccular in type.[444–446] In either case, the diagnosis should be readily apparent by CT or radionuclide scan and can be confirmed if necessary by angiography. Occasionally the inferior vena cava (IVC) can also undergo localized aneurysmal dilatation and be visible as a smooth, sharply circumscribed opacity in the right cardiophrenic angle.[447] All other anomalies of the IVC occur within the abdomen and possess no intrathoracic manifestations other than those associated with azygos continuation (see farther on).[448–450]

Persistence of a left SVC is an uncommon anomaly that occurs in 0.3 per cent of normal subjects and in 4.4 per cent of patients with congenital heart disease;[451] in 82 to 90 per cent of cases, the right SVC is also present.[451] The right SVC develops partly from the right anterior cardinal vein while the left anterior cardinal vein normally regresses; persistence of the latter results in a left SVC. In such circumstances, a straight-edged shadow is present on the left side of the mediastinum that overlies the aortic arch and proximal descending aorta;[452] drainage is via the coronary sinus. Although the diagnosis of this anomalous vessel may be suggested from plain roentgenographic findings, CT is virtually diagnostic[451] and angiography should not be necessary for confirmation. The shadow created by an anomalous left-sided SVC can be simulated by that caused by anomalous venous drainage of the left upper lobe.[453] A superb treatise on the CT manifestations of vena caval anomalies with embryologic correlation has recently been published.[454]

The clinical findings in patients with dilatation of the SVC are those of the condition responsible for raised central venous pressure.

Azygos and Hemiazygos Veins

The normal anatomy of the azygos vein and its pleural reflections has been described in great detail by Heitzman and his colleagues.[455] In addition, the roentgenographic anatomy of the azygos arch, first described by Stauffer and his colleagues in 1951,[456] has been amplified in an excellent review by Smathers and his colleagues on the basis of CT studies;[457] the course and dimensions of the normal vein are described in detail in Chapter 1 (see page 239).

There are many causes of dilatation of the azygos and hemiazygos veins: intrahepatic and extrahepatic portal vein obstruction,[458] anomalous pulmonary venous drainage, acquired occlusion of the inferior or superior vena cava,[459] azygos continuation (infrahepatic interruption) of the inferior vena cava,[460,461] persistence of the left superior vena cava, hepatic vein obstruction (Budd-Chiari syndrome or veno-occlusive disease of the liver), and elevated central venous pressure of any etiology.[462–465] The last is by far the most common cause and results from cardiac decompensation, tricuspid valvular lesions, acute pericardial tamponade, or constrictive pericarditis. Rarely, dilatation of either venous system is present without discernible cause.[466–468]

Roentgenographically, dilatation of the azygos vein is evidenced by a round or oval shadow in the right tracheobronchial angle more than 10 mm in diameter on standard roentgenograms exposed with patients in the erect position.[469] In a correlative study of 54 adult patients ranging in age from 23 to 77, Preger and his colleagues[470] related the width of the azygos vein to central venous pressure. They found that when the diameter of the vein was greater than 15 mm as measured on an anteroposterior chest roentgenogram obtained in the supine position, the central venous pressure was greater

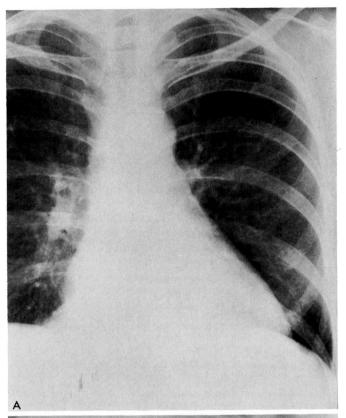

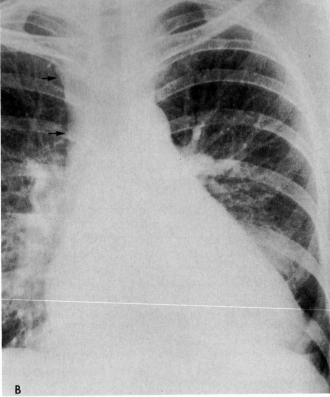

Figure 19–55. Dilatation of the Superior Vena Cava. During a remission, the chest roentgenogram *(A)* of this 35-year-old woman with proved systemic lupus erythematosus revealed no significant abnormalities. On the occasion of an exacerbation several months later (at which time the patient had clinical evidence of cardiac decompensation), a chest roentgenogram *(B)* demonstrated moderate cardiac enlargement (due predominantly to pericardial effusion) and generalized interstitial pulmonary edema. Note the widening of the superior mediastinum caused by dilatation of the superior vena cava *(arrows).*

than 10 cm of water. In a tomographic study of 48 patients in the supine position, none of whom had any lesion known to cause azygos vein enlargement, Doyle and colleagues[462] found the mean diameter of the vein (corrected to a standard patient weight of 140 lb) to be 14.2 mm. Measurements exceeding 10 mm on roentgenograms obtained in the erect position or 14 mm on tomograms obtained in the supine position indicate increase in either pressure or flow.

A dilated azygos vein can be differentiated from an enlarged azygos lymph node fairly easily by comparing the diameter of the shadow on roentgenograms exposed in the erect and supine positions: when the vein is responsible, there is a noticeable difference in size. This technique was employed to advantage by Pomeranz and Proto[471] in a patient in whom a dilated azygos vein was situated in an anomalous azygos fissure; the dilatation was subsequently shown to be caused by azygos continuation of the inferior vena cava (Fig. 19–56). When the nature of such a shadow is in doubt, CT provides definitive information. Dilatation of the posterior portions of the azygos or hemiazygos veins may result in widening and irregularity of the paraspinal line, on the right and left side, respectively (Fig. 19–57).[464, 472, 473] Extreme tortuosity of a dilated azygos arch may simulate a pulmonary mass on a lateral chest roentgenogram.[474]

A spate of articles has appeared in recent years describing the CT appearance of azygos and hemiazygos continuation of the inferior vena cava;[475–478] all express enthusiasm for the ability of CT to establish a positive diagnosis without recourse to angiography, although in some cases angiography was employed for confirmation. It also has been pointed out[479] that the diagnosis can be established by ultrasonographic examination with the same degree of confidence as by CT. Heller and his colleagues[480] have described a sign that they consider useful in the recognition of azygos continuation of the inferior vena cava—absence of the shadow of the inferior vena cava on a lateral chest roentgenogram. We agree that when the azygos vein is obviously distended and the shadow of the inferior vena cava is not visualized, the combination should arouse suspicion of azygos continuation of the IVC. However, as Vidal pointed out to us in

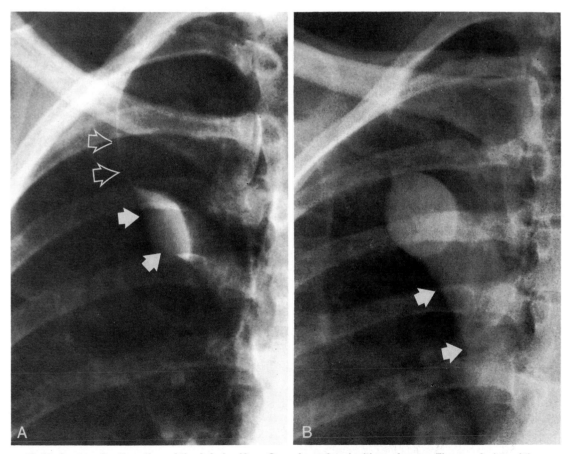

Figure 19–56. Azygos Continuation of the Inferior Vena Cava Associated with an Azygos Fissure. A view of the upper portion of the right hemithorax from a posteroanterior roentgenogram *(A)* reveals a large oval opacity *(solid arrows)* situated at the lower end of a curvilinear opacity representing an azygos fissure *(open arrows)*. In order to prove that this actually represented a dilated azygos vein, the patient was placed in a supine position and the roentgenogram repeated *(B)*. By this procedure the vein has undergone a remarkable degree of dilatation and now can be seen to extend inferiorly to the right side of the mediastinum *(arrows)*. (Courtesy of Dr. Anthony Proto, Virginia Commonwealth University, Medical College of Virginia, Richmond.)

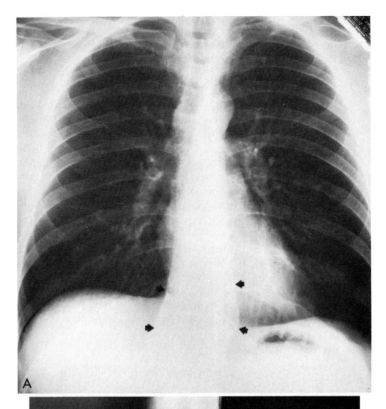

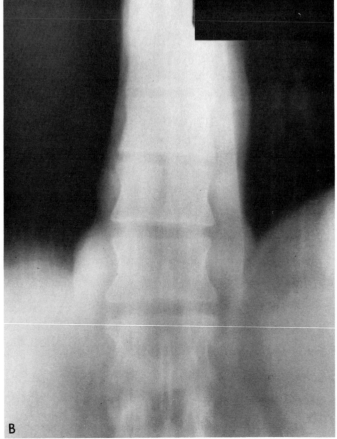

Figure 19–57. Proximal Interruption (Azygos and Hemiazygos Continuation) of the Inferior Vena Cava. A screening chest roentgenogram *(A)* of this 31-year-old asymptomatic man revealed an increased width of the paraspinal soft tissues in the lower thoracic region bilaterally *(arrows).* The shadow of the azygos vein in the right tracheobronchial angle measured 10 mm, the upper limits of normal. An anteroposterior tomogram of the lower thoracic spine in the supine position *(B)* shows the bilateral opacities to be greater in width than on the erect study and to be somewhat lobulated in contour. In the recumbent position, the diameter of the azygos vein had increased to 24 mm, a marked degree of dilatation.

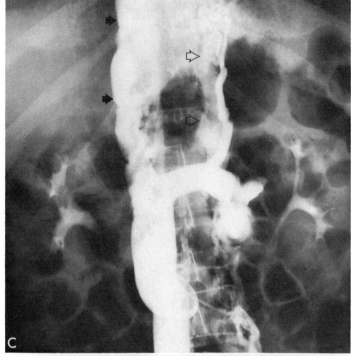

Figure 19–57 *Continued* Following insertion of a catheter into the inferior vena cava, contrast medium was injected *(C)*. Excellent opacification of the inferior vena cava was observed up to the level of the renal veins, but flow proximal to that point was by way of markedly dilated azygos *(solid arrows)* and hemiazygos *(open arrows)* veins. Within the thorax *(D)*, the hemiazygos vein *(open arrows)* passed across the midline to join the azygos *(solid arrows)* at the level of T-8 *(curved arrow)*. The markedly dilated azygos then continued cephalad to terminate in the superior vena cava at its familiar location in the right tracheobronchial angle.

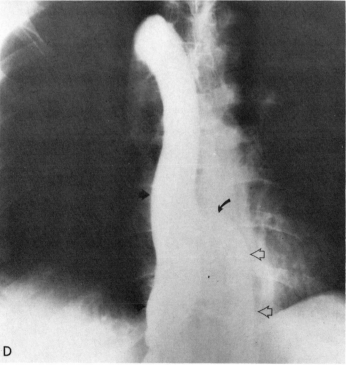

personal communication, the hepatic vein is always preserved in such cases and can cast a shadow in both posteroanterior and lateral projections that is indistinguishable from that of the IVC.

The symptoms and signs of azygos and hemiazygos vein dilatation depend entirely on the cause. Azygos continuation of the inferior vena cava is often associated with a congenital cardiac malformation (Fig. 19–58),[481, 482] with errors in abdominal situs,[483] or with asplenia or polysplenia.[484] Most patients are asymptomatic, but some have symptoms or signs attributable to the associated heart disease.

Left Superior Intercostal Vein

Dilatation of the left superior intercostal vein generally possesses the same etiological significance as dilatation of the azygos vein, although visibility of this vein roentgenographically is not nearly as frequent as that of the azygos. It will be recalled from the description in Chapter 1 (*see* page 218) that the normal left superior intercostal vein originates from a confluence of the second, third, and fourth left intercostal veins. As it passes anteriorly from the spine it relates intimately to some portion of the aortic arch and in this location is seen end-on as the "aortic nipple," a local protuberance in the contour of the arch that is identifiable in 9.5 per cent of normal subjects.[485] On erect posteroanterior chest roentgenograms, the maximum diameter of the aortic nipple in normal subjects is 4.5 mm.[486] A diameter greater than this is a useful sign of circulatory abnormalities, the most common of which are azygos continuation of the inferior vena

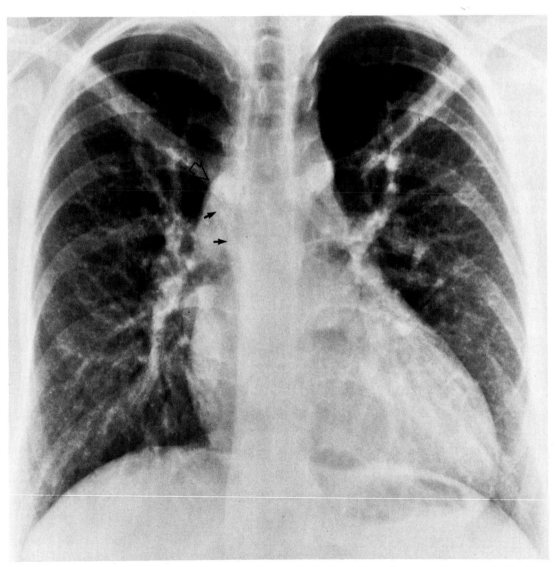

Figure 19–58. Azygos Continuation (Proximal Interruption) of the Inferior Vena Cava Associated with Ventricular Septal Defect. A roentgenogram of the chest in posteroanterior projection of this 20-year-old asymptomatic woman reveals a smooth, well-defined opacity in the right tracheobronchial angle *(open arrow)*. This represents a moderately dilated azygos vein (width 20 mm). In its course superiorly, the dilated vein has displaced the right mediastinal pleura laterally, thus creating a right paraspinal interface *(solid arrows)* analogous to the left paraspinal interface caused by the aorta. In addition, this roentgenogram reveals moderate pulmonary pleonemia and mild ventricular enlargement attributable to a ventricular septal defect.

cava, hypoplasia of the left innominate vein, cardiac decompensation, portal hypertension, Budd-Chiari syndrome, obstruction of the superior or inferior vena cava,[486] and congenital absence of the azygos vein.[487]

SUPERIOR VENA CAVA SYNDROME

The superior vena cava syndrome is characterized by edema of the face, neck, upper extremities, and thorax and is associated with prominent dilated chest wall veins. It is caused by obstruction of the vena cava, either by external compression or, more commonly, by intraluminal thrombosis or neoplastic infiltration; not infrequently, a combination of all three processes is involved. In most published series, the etiology is malignancy in 95 per cent or more of cases.[488-493] Pulmonary carcinoma is the cause in 80 to 85 per cent, and lymphoma and metastatic carcinoma of nonpulmonary origin in 5 to 10 per cent. Of the pulmonary carcinomas, small cell carcinoma is the most common cell type;[494] in one series of 366 cases of this neoplasm,[493] 10 per cent presented with superior vena cava syndrome at the time of diagnosis. The most common benign lesion is chronic sclerosing mediastinitis,[490, 495] although individual examples of a great variety of diseases also have been documented, including tuberculosis,[496] syphilitic aortic aneurysm,[497] goiter,[312] and filarial mediastinal lymphadenitis.[498]

The most common symptoms are dyspnea and a feeling of fullness in the head. Physical findings include dilatation of the veins of the neck and chest wall; although such dilatation is usually bilateral, in the rare case where obstruction is limited to one or the other brachiocephalic vein it may be unilateral.[499] The diagnosis is usually apparent clinically, but has been made by CT in some patients with an upper mediastinal mass before the characteristic clinical signs were manifested.[500] Venography is not required in most instances but is a safe procedure that can establish the diagnosis in doubtful cases.[491] In most cases a mass can be readily detected roentgenographically, widening the mediastinum to the right.

The concept that this complication represents a medical emergency[488] is no longer generally accepted.[490, 501] There is no doubt, however, that the prognosis is poor: most patients whose superior vena cava syndrome is caused by a malignant neoplasm will be dead within months[489] and over 80 per cent will have succumbed within 1 year.[491]

DILATATION OF THE AORTA OR ITS BRANCHES

Aneurysms of the Thoracic Aorta

Aneurysms of the *ascending aorta* may be saccular or fusiform, the former usually extending anteriorly and to the right (Fig. 19–59). When large enough, such an aneurysm can erode the sternum and give rise to a prominent thumping pulsation over the anterior chest wall—thus the designation "aneurysm of signs." Aneurysms of the *transverse arch* tend to compress contiguous structures, resulting in a brassy cough, hemoptysis, hoarseness, and cyanosis of the face and upper extremities, and thus are sometimes referred to as the "aneurysm of symptoms." They produce a mass in the mid mediastinum that characteristically obliterates the aortic window. Aneurysms of the *descending aorta* can become large without occasioning symptoms but may erode the vertebral column. They are most often arteriosclerotic in origin.[502] In a study of 12 patients, Higgins and his coworkers[503] found that localized descending thoracic aortic aneurysms characteristically project from the posterolateral aspect of the aorta on its left side. Rim calcification and vertebral erosion were not encountered. During aortography only a small portion of the aneurysm may be outlined with contrast medium because of partial obliteration of the aneurysmal cavity by a thrombus. In one study of 71 cases of arteriosclerotic or dissecting aneurysms of the aorta, mural thrombus was identified on CT in 86 per cent of the cases.[504] The pattern of thrombus formation was classified by these authors into three types, the most common being a ring shape followed in order of frequency by a left crescent thrombus and left posterior crescent thrombus.

Calcification of the walls of thoracic aneurysms is relatively common (Fig. 19–59). At one time, the presence of calcification in the supravalvular portion of the ascending arch was highly suggestive of syphilis, but this view is no longer valid. In a study of 20 patients with ascending aortic calcification, Higgins and Reinke[505] found venereal disease research laboratory (VDRL) and fluorescent treponemal antibody absorption (FTA-ABS) tests to be reactive in only 5 patients. Nowadays, such calcification is much more frequently associated with advanced atherosclerosis and with aortic valve disease. Even in cases in which such calcification is associated with syphilitic aortitis, it is secondary to atherosclerosis; the syphilitic involvement of the aorta apparently predisposes to the development of atherosclerotic calcification in this region. In the absence of calcification, it has been suggested by Szamosi[506] that an aneurysm of even small size may be recognized by the presence of a periaortic fat layer; this occurred in 19 of 25 successive cases of aneurysm of the ascending aorta studied by this author.

Aortic aneurysms may be classified as arteriosclerotic, syphilitic, traumatic, dissecting, poststenotic (coarctation of the aorta), and mycotic. *Traumatic* aneurysms of the thoracic aorta typically involve the posterior portion of the descending arch just beyond the origin of the left subclavian artery (Fig. 19–60). They tend to project to the left. Early recognition of aortic laceration is imperative in view

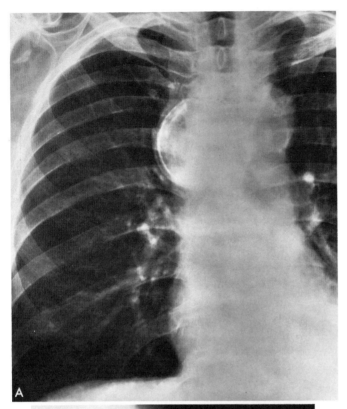

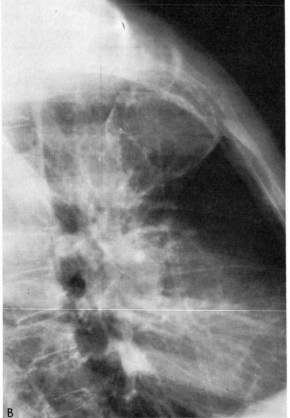

Figure 19–59. Saccular Aneurysm of the Ascending Thoracic Aorta. Posteroanterior *(A)* and lateral *(B)* roentgenograms of this 52-year-old asymptomatic man reveal a well-circumscribed mass situated in the anterior mediastinum and projecting entirely to the right. Its wall is densely calcified. The etiology of the aneurysm was not established.

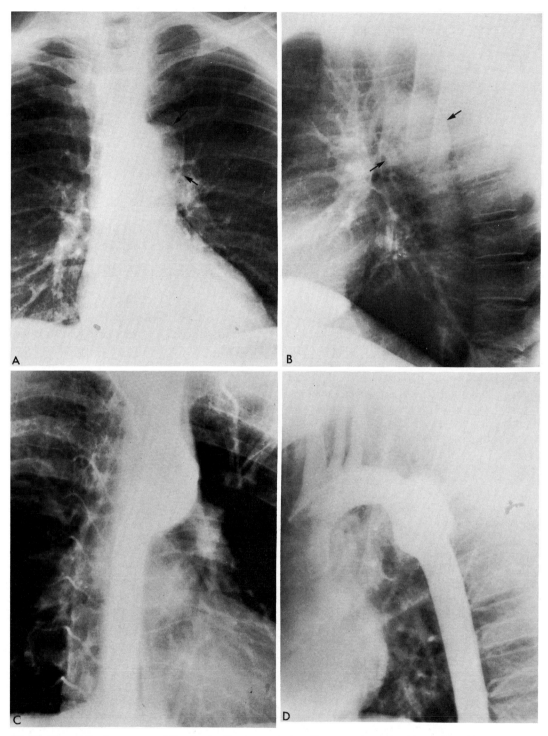

Figure 19–60. Traumatic Aneurysm of the Aorta. Two years before these roentgenographic studies, this 43-year-old airline pilot was involved in a serious car accident in which he suffered severe trauma to his chest and multiple rib fractures. A chest roentgenogram (not illustrated) shortly before the accident was reported as being normal. Roentgenograms of the chest in posteroanterior *(A)* and lateral *(B)* projections 2 years after the accident (at which time the patient was asymptomatic) demonstrated a smooth, well-defined soft tissue mass situated in relation to the posterior portion of the arch of the aorta *(arrows* in both projections). Aortography in anteroposterior *(C)* and lateral *(D)* projections shows the mass to opacify with contrast medium and to be situated approximately 3 cm beyond the origin of the left subclavian artery. The aneurysm is symmetric, involving the whole circumference of the aorta. At thoracotomy, there was found to be a complete tear of the intima and media of the aorta, the continuity of the vessel being maintained by adventitial coats only. The segment was resected and a Teflon graft successfully inserted.

of the poor survival rates of undiagnosed patients with this type of injury.[507] Diagnosis rests with the use of appropriate imaging techniques, because there are no presenting symptoms or physical findings to help distinguish patients with aortic rupture from those without it.[508] Approximately 20 per cent of patients with aortic rupture survive the initial trauma, although the majority of survivors have a thin-walled aneurysm that, if untreated, will rupture within 2 weeks in approximately 60 per cent of these patients and within 10 weeks in 90 per cent.[509] Despite these dismal statistics, many aneurysms of traumatic origin are unrecognized at the time and may remain so for many years until screening chest roentgenograms of asymptomatic patients reveal the abnormality.[509, 510] This subject is discussed in greater detail on page 2499.

Dissecting aneurysms can occur at any site in the thoracic aorta but originate most often in the ascending arch. Their highest incidence is in patients with Marfan's syndrome, aortic coarctation, or hypertension, or during pregnancy (Fig. 19–61); so-called cystic medial necrosis is identifiable histologically in the aortic wall in many cases. Because of the age of most of these patients arteriosclerosis also may be present, but it is more likely a coincidental finding than a significant contributing factor in the dissection. As pointed out by Beachley and his colleagues,[511] dissecting aneurysms are most common in the ascending aorta where arteriosclerosis is relatively mild in severity, and dissections rarely begin in the lower abdominal aorta where arteriosclerosis is very common and often severe.

Hemorrhage into the tissues surrounding a dissection may be revealed by widening or obliteration of the paraspinal shadow at any point along the descending aorta. Figiel and associates[512] regard this sign as highly suggestive of dissecting aneurysm. However, whereas CT with bolus injection of contrast medium was formerly considered the procedure of choice in the initial investigation of most patients with suspected aortic dissection (Fig. 19–62),[513–519] experience with MRI in recent years strongly suggests that this procedure is superior to CT (Fig. 19–63).[520–524] Findings with the two techniques include localized increase in aortic caliber, displaced intimal calcifications, intimal flaps, differential time density between the two lumens, and false channels (Fig. 19–64). Aortography should be performed if there is a strong clinical suspicion of a type I or type II dissection and if MRI or CT examination shows a dilated aorta or a pericardial effusion. However, when CT either shows convincing evidence of dissection or is normal, angiography can be avoided in many cases.[519, 525] Digital subtraction angiography is said to be an efficient method of examination in some cases, particularly in the evaluation of the aortic lumen following dissection repair.[526]

In a necropsy study of 196 cases of dissecting aneurysms, Talbot[527] concluded that 91 per cent of patients die within 1 week of the dissection and that most of these never reach the hospital. It is apparent that dissecting aneurysms that develop in the community are predominantly proximal in site and suggest a diagnosis of myocardial infarction or pulmonary embolism. They usually have a fatal outcome. The majority of patients who reach the hospital have distal aortic dissections that tend to be confused clinically with renal colic or pancreatitis.[527] In a review of 50 patients seen over a period of 15 years,[528] it was concluded that those with either proximal or complex dissection had a better prognosis when managed surgically, whereas those with a distal dissection were offered a better chance of survival when treated medically.

The clinical manifestations of aortic aneurysms vary according to the size and location of the dilatation. Many patients are asymptomatic. Symptoms caused by aneurysms of the transverse arch are particularly notable and result from compression of the superior vena cava, recurrent laryngeal nerve, or tracheobronchial tree. Aneurysms of the descending aorta at times cause bone erosion that may occasion severe pain. They can also cause dysphagia as a result of esophageal compression.[529] Respiratory insufficiency has been reported to result from tracheobronchial compression by a large calcified aneurysm of the descending aorta;[530] and an anterior spinal artery syndrome has been described as a result of compression from an aneurysm of the descending aorta years after trauma.[531] Dissecting aneurysms usually cause severe retrosternal pain that radiates through to the back; sometimes there is syncope. Physical examination may reveal evidence of acute peripheral arterial occlusion, aortic insufficiency, or bruits over the affected portion of aorta.[532]

An unusual form of aortic aneurysm is that involving an aortic sinus, almost invariably the posterior or right anterior sinus. The former can rupture into the right atrium and the latter into the infundibular area of the right ventricle, producing a clinical picture of aortic regurgitation and left-to-right shunt. Roentgenography of the chest before rupture occurs may reveal a mediastinal mass in the region of the root of the aorta. Cooperberg and his colleagues[533] have reported the successful preoperative diagnosis by echocardiography of an aneurysm of the right coronary sinus of Valsalva with rupture into the right ventricle.

Rarely, the descending thoracic aorta may be so elongated that it assumes a horizontal position just above the diaphragm and curves sharply to the right and anteriorly, sometimes crossing the midline. This orientation is such that a posterior mediastinal mass may be simulated roentgenologically (Fig. 19–65).

Buckling and Aneurysm of the Innominate Artery

Both of these conditions are evident roentgenographically as a smooth, well-defined opacity in

Text continued on page 2895

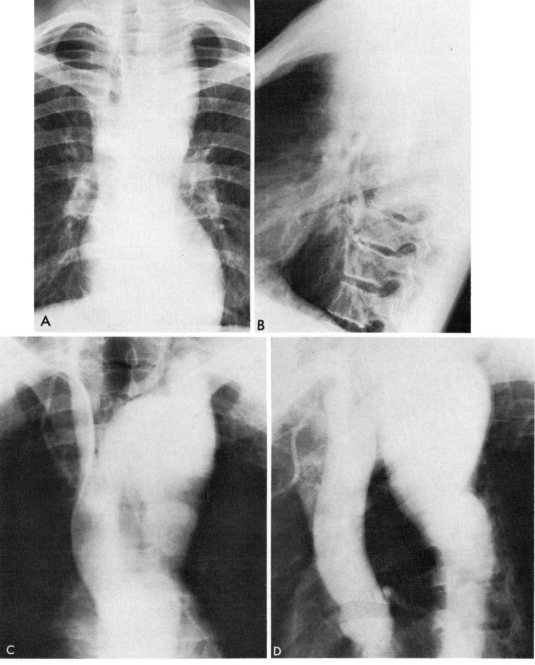

Figure 19–61. Dissecting Aneurysm of the Aorta. The night before these roentgenograms, this 22-year-old man was awakened by a severe pain in the right anterior chest, extending into the infrascapular area on the left. One hour later he noted numbness of his left hand, which persisted for approximately 2 hours. Roentgenograms of the chest in posteroanterior *(A)* and lateral *(B)* projections demonstrated uniform widening of the upper mediastinum, slightly more to the left than to the right. The trachea was deviated to the right, and the mass extended to the thoracic inlet posteriorly. (Its posterior position is indicated by the fact that it relates to air-containing lung up to the level of the second rib.) Note the smooth, well-defined "knob" at the lower portion of the mass on the left side, resembling the aortic knob but on a slightly lower level. An aortogram in anteroposterior *(C)* and left anterior oblique *(D)* projections revealed a severe aneurysmal dilatation of the descending portion of the arch of the aorta, involving the left subclavian artery to the origin of the vertebral artery. Note the buckling of the descending aorta immediately beyond the aneurysm; it was this deformity (pseudocoarctation) that created the shadow of the "knob" on the plain roentgenogram. At thoracotomy, the involved aorta and a portion of the left subclavian artery were resected, no more than 1 1/2 inches of Teflon graft being required for anastomosis. The specimen showed a dissecting aneurysm associated with "cystic medial necrosis." Recovery was uneventful.

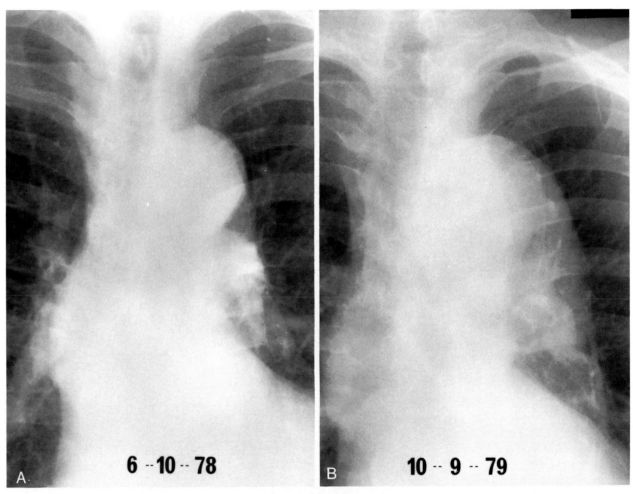

Figure 19–62. Dissecting Aneurysm of the Descending Thoracic Aorta. A view of the upper mediastinum from a posteroanterior roentgenogram *(A)* reveals marked elongation of the thoracic aorta consistent with atherosclerosis. Approximately 1 year later shortly following the abrupt onset of severe pain in the back, a repeat roentgenogram *(B)* of this elderly man reveals a marked widening of the mediastinum in the region of the aorta that possesses a configuration consistent with acute dissection.

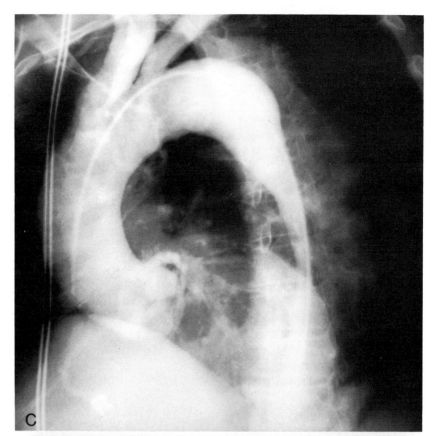

Figure 19–62 *Continued* An aortogram in left anterior oblique projection *(C)* shows an abrupt narrowing of the lumen of the aorta at the beginning of the descending arch. The false lumen of this dissection did not opacify. A CT scan through the arch *(D)* reveals the nonopacified false channel situated posterolaterally *(arrows).*

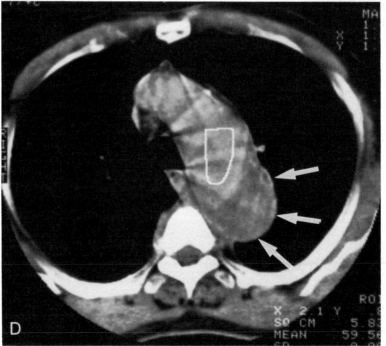

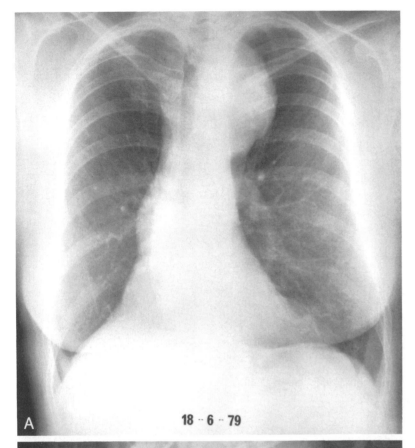

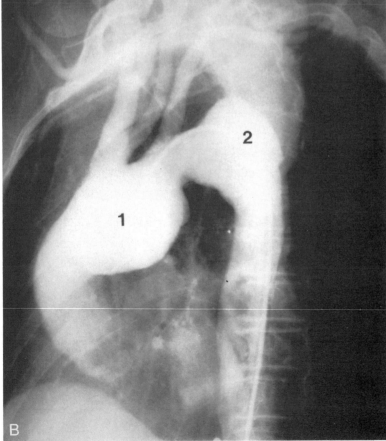

Figure 19–63. Saccular Aneurysms of the Thoracic Aorta. A posteroanterior roentgenogram *(A)* reveals a rather large, well-defined, slightly lobulated opacity projecting to the left of the superior mediastinum suggestive of a large aortic aneurysm. No other abnormalities are apparent. An aortogram in left anterior oblique projection *(B)* reveals a double aneurysm of the aortic arch, one situated at the level of the origin of the brachiocephalic artery (number *1*) and the other in the distal transverse portion of the arch distal to the takeoff of the left subclavian artery (number *2*).

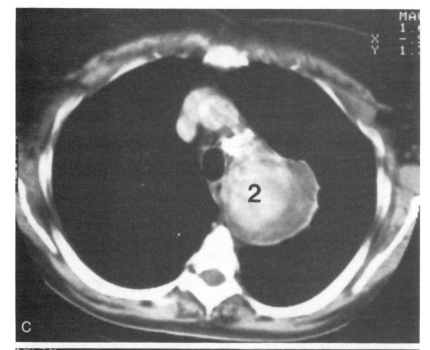

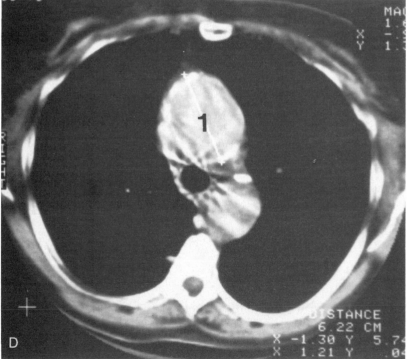

Figure 19–63 *Continued* A CT scan at the level of the junction of the right innominate vein and superior vena cava *(C)* reveals a marked degree of dilatation of the aorta in the distal portion of the arch, corresponding to aneurysm 2 in *(B);* note the presence of a broad curvilinear radiolucency in the left side of the aneurysm that represents thrombus. A CT scan 3 cm distally *(D)* shows the aneurysm of the ascending aorta, corresponding to aneurysm 1 in *(B)*.

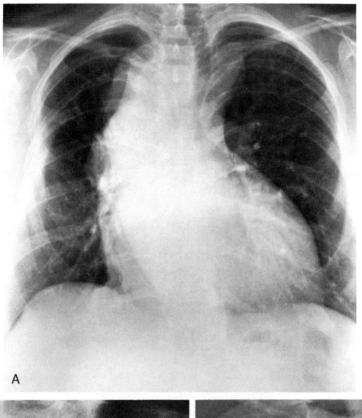

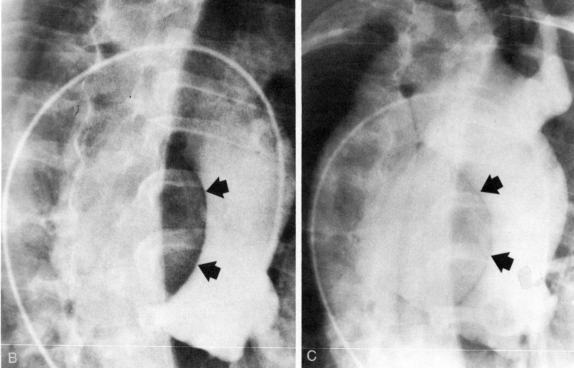

Figure 19–64. Dissecting Aneurysm of the Ascending Aorta in a Patient with a Right Aortic Arch. A posteroanterior roentgenogram *(A)* reveals evidence of a former right thoracotomy that had been performed many years previously for repair of a coarctation and aortic valvotomy. The trachea is deviated markedly to the left by a right-sided aortic arch. The width of the aorta at the point of maximal tracheal displacement is obviously wider than normal. Because of the concern over the possibility of a dissecting aneurysm in this 27-year-old woman with Turner's syndrome, an aortogram was performed: an early phase following injection of contrast medium *(B)* reveals opacification of the true aortic lumen; two or three seconds later *(C)*, there has occurred opacification of a structure situated posteromedial to the true arch *(arrows)*, indicating partial opacification of a false channel. (Compare the density indicated by *arrows* in *[B]* with that indicated by *arrows* in *[C]*.)

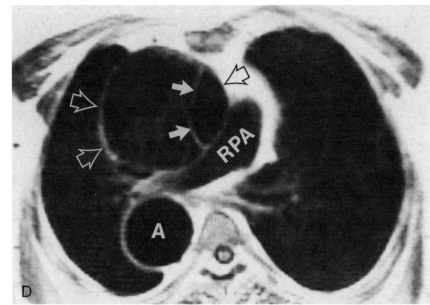

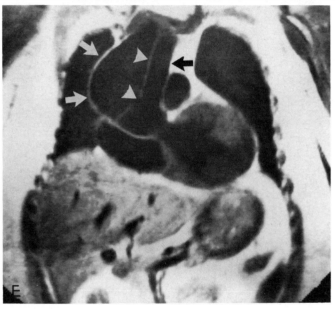

Figure 19–64 *Continued* A T1-weighted magnetic resonance scan in transverse section *(D)* at the level of the right pulmonary artery *(RPA)* shows a markedly dilated ascending aorta *(open arrows);* situated within it is a curvilinear shadow *(arrows)* representing the intimal flap, the smaller area to the left of the flap representing the true lumen and the larger area to the right representing the false lumen of the dissection. Note that the descending aorta *(A)* at this level is still on the right side. A coronal reconstruction *(E)* again reveals the markedly dilated ascending aorta *(arrows)* containing the intimal flap *(arrowheads);* again the true lumen is on the left and the false lumen on the right.

the right superior paramediastinal area, extending upward from the aortic arch. Buckling is a relatively common condition that occurs in an estimated 17 per cent of patients with hypertension or atherosclerosis or both.[534] Aneurysms are much less common. Schneider and Felson[535] postulated the following explanation for buckling: the innominate artery is about 5 cm long and is firmly fixed proximally at its origin from the aorta and distally by the subclavian and carotid arteries. When the thoracic aorta elongates and dilates as a result of atherosclerosis, the arch moves cephalad, carrying with it the origin of the innominate artery. Because of its fixation superiorly, the innominate artery buckles to the right. Occasionally the artery buckles posteriorly and laterally, in these circumstances it impresses deeply into the lung and becomes almost completely surrounded by lung parenchyma, thus simulating a mass.[536, 537] This complication, however, is uncommon; Christensen and associates[538] surveyed 200 randomly selected patients over 50 years of age and found only one with an innominate artery that presented as an apparent pulmonary mass. Occasionally, a similar appearance can be caused by an aneurysm or pseudoaneurysm of the right carotid artery, in one reported case simulating a Pancoast tumor;[539] buckling of the left common carotid artery can similarly simulate a mediastinal neoplasm.[540] Rarely, an aneurysm of the innominate artery is of syphilitic origin and can simulate a mediastinal mass on conventional chest roentgenograms.[541]

Aneurysms can cause pain, cough, dyspnea, hoarseness, dysphagia, Horner's syndrome, and clubbing of the fingers of the right hand. They may

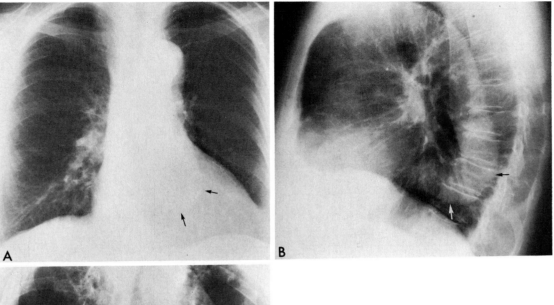

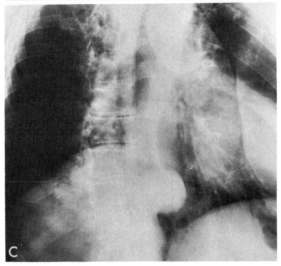

Figure 19–65. Mediastinal Mass Caused by Severe Elongation of the Descending Thoracic Aorta. Roentgenograms of the chest in posteroanterior *(A)* and lateral *(B)* projections reveal marked elongation of the descending thoracic aorta, its distal portion turning sharply to the right and anteriorly just above the level of the diaphragm *(arrows* in both projections). This sharp angulation creates the appearance of a soft-tissue mass in the posterior mediastinum, particularly when the horizontal segment is visualized in profile, as in right anterior oblique projection *(C).* The patient is a 73-year-old asymptomatic man.

be evidenced by a pulsatile mass at the base of the neck.[534] Although buckling seldom occasions symptoms, it may give rise to a small, palpable, pulsatile mass in the right supraclavicular fossa and thereby indicate that the common carotid artery also is affected.[534, 535] Buckling occurs most often in middle-aged or older obese females who have clinical evidence of atherosclerosis and hypertension. Its presence in patients under the age of 30 years should suggest the possibility of coarctation of the aorta.[535]

Congenital Anomalies of the Aorta

The majority of cases of congenital malformations of the aortic arch become manifest during the first year of life[542] but occasionally are not recognized until adulthood.[543, 544] A congenital aortic vascular ring results from persistence of the two aortic arches or of the right aortic arch and left ductus arteriosus; in a minority of patients the right subclavian artery, also of anomalous origin, arises from the descending aorta.[545] The roentgeno-graphic diagnosis may be made by the demonstration of a double aortic knob and of a vessel posterior to the esophagus. Symptoms result from compression of the trachea or esophagus and include frequent respiratory infections, shortness of breath, and, in some cases, dysphagia.

Other congenital anomalies that result in abnormalities of mediastinal contour include (1) *pseudocoarctation* of the aorta (Fig. 19–66), in which a left paramediastinal "mass" is visible just above the aortic knob, caused by simple elongation and buckling of the aorta;[546, 547] (2) the *cervical aortic arch,* a rare congenital anomaly in which the aortic arch extends into the soft tissues of the neck before turning downward on itself to become the descending aorta;[548, 549] (3) the three types of *aortic diverticula;*[550] and (4) by far the most common, the three types of *right aortic arch.*[551] A right aortic arch can occasionally compress the trachea sufficiently to cause a clinical picture suggesting exercise-induced asthma.[552] M. Cosio has informed us in personal communication that at the pulmonary function laboratory of the Royal Victoria Hospital, Montreal,

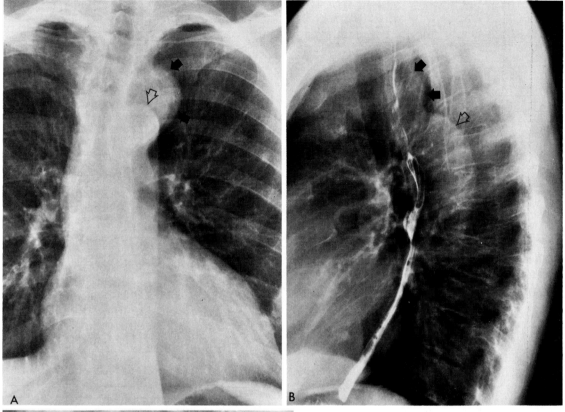

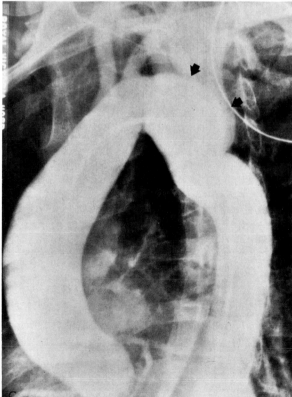

Figure 19–66. Pseudocoarctation of the Aorta.
A posteroanterior view *(A)* of the chest of this 63-year-old asymptomatic woman reveals a homogeneous soft tissue opacity *(solid arrows)* projected above the shadow of the aortic knob *(open arrow)*. In lateral projection *(B)*, the posterior aspect of the "mass" is again identified by *solid arrows* and the posterior portion of the aortic arch by an *open arrow*. Although on the basis of this plain film evidence the findings were thought to be compatible with pseudocoarctation of the aorta, an aortogram was performed for confirmation. This study in oblique projection *(C)* confirms the fact that the abnormal opacity observed on the plain roentgenogram is due to an unusually high aortic arch *(solid arrows)* that buckled in its descending portion so as to produce a prominent notch on its posterior and left lateral aspects.

abnormalities in the expiratory loop of the flow-volume curve have been detected in patients with right-sided aortic arch.

Magnetic resonance imaging has been indicated as a valuable substitute for other techniques in effective, noninvasive evaluation of congenital aortic arch anomalies.[553]

MEDIASTINAL MASSES SITUATED PREDOMINANTLY IN THE POSTERIOR COMPARTMENT

The posterior mediastinal compartment lies between the pericardium and anterior aspect of the vertebral column. It contains the descending thoracic aorta, the esophagus, the thoracic duct, the lower portion of the vagus nerves, and the posterior group of mediastinal lymph nodes. Since by definition the posterior limit of the mediastinum is formed by the anterior surface of the vertebral column, the paravertebral zones and posterior gutters are anatomically excluded. However, since these areas contain structures of importance in the histogenesis of posterior mediastinal masses, including the sympathetic nerve chains and peripheral nerves, these zones customarily are included in a discussion of masses in the posterior mediastinum.

Approximately 30 per cent of posterior mediastinal tumors are malignant neoplasms.[142, 554]

TUMORS AND TUMOR-LIKE CONDITIONS OF NEURAL TISSUE

Neoplasms of neural tissue have been said to comprise almost 20 per cent of mediastinal tumors.[182] There are two basic types, those arising from the peripheral nerves and those originating from sympathetic ganglia.

Tumors Arising from Peripheral Nerves

This group includes neurofibroma, neurilemoma (schwannoma), and neurogenic sarcoma (malignant schwannoma). The vast majority of these tumors arise in the posterior mediastinum from one of the intercostal nerves. Neoplasms arising from other nerves are rare; for example, only 21 cases of vagal neurofibroma had been reported by 1971.[555]

Pathologically, most tumors are encapsulated, roughly spherical masses projecting from the chest wall into the paravertebral space; occasionally, a tumor extends through a spinal foramen and grows in a dumbbell fashion in both spinal canal and mediastinum. Although malignant tumors (numbering about one tenth of the benign form)[182] can show invasion of contiguous structures at the time of diagnosis, they also can be encapsulated. Histologically, neurofibromas are somewhat variable in

appearance and consist of a mixture of spindle cells, myxoid stroma, and mature collagen. Neurilemomas are composed of spindle cells arranged in either a relatively compact and orderly architecture (so-called Antoni A pattern) or more haphazardly in a loose myxomatous stroma (Antoni B pattern). Malignant schwannomas are usually more cellular than the benign form and show nuclear atypia and mitotic activity.

Roentgenographic features of the three forms of tumor are similar and consist of a sharply defined, round or oval shadow of homogeneous density in the paravertebral zone on one or the other side. Tumors that originate in a nerve root within the spinal canal can expand the intervertebral foramen. Neurofibromas or neurilemomas originating elsewhere in the thorax can sometimes have unusual manifestations; for example, in one patient a neurilemoma of the left vagus nerve simulated an aortic aneurysm.[556] Special procedures that may be helpful in certain cases include CT, MRI, myelography (to determine whether a neurofibroma is of intraspinal origin), and angiography (to distinguish a neural tumor from an aortic aneurysm). Neurilemomas have been shown to have a mixed attenuation on CT, attributable according to Cohen and his colleagues[557] to confluent areas of hypocellularity adjacent to densely cellular or collagenous regions, xanthomatous change, or regions of cystic degeneration.

Clinically, these tumors occur most commonly in young adults; they usually do not cause symptoms and are discovered on a screening chest roentgenogram.[142] Of the 49 patients with a neurogenic neoplasm in a Cleveland Clinic series,[146] 32 (65 per cent) were asymptomatic. In a minority of patients, compression of intercostal nerves or tracheobronchial airways gives rise to pain or dyspnea, respectively. Mediastinal neurofibromas can be associated with neurofibromas and other neoplasms elsewhere in the body (usually in the setting of von Recklinghausen's neurofibromatosis).

Provided complete surgical excision can be achieved, the prognosis of benign peripheral nerve tumors of the mediastinum is excellent. By contrast, the malignant neoplasms are usually aggressive; of 40 cases of malignant schwannoma reviewed by Ingels and colleagues,[182] 29 (72.5 per cent) were fatal, the average survival time from the time of diagnosis being only 2 years.

Tumors Arising from Sympathetic Ganglia

The principal tumors in this category are ganglioneuroma, ganglioneuroblastoma, and neuroblastoma. Paragangliomas arise from paraganglionic tissue related to the sympathetic ganglia and are discussed farther on. In addition, a rare form of pigmented tumor believed to originate in sympathetic ganglia (melanocytic schwannoma) has been reported.[558, 559]

Pathologically, ganglioneuroma, ganglioneuroblastoma, and neuroblastoma represent a continuum of histologic changes from mature, fully differentiated tissue in the first-named to immature tissue in the last. Because of this, distinction between these neoplasms is to some extent arbitrary[560] and sometimes can be difficult. Ganglioneuromas are composed of an intimate admixture of mature Schwann cells, collagen, and ganglion cells, whereas neuroblastomas consist of primitive cells, usually with scanty cytoplasm and pleomorphic, hyperchromatic nuclei; rosette formation is common in the latter neoplasm. Ganglioneuroblastomas show features of both tumors in varying degrees.[560]

The roentgenographic appearance of these tumors is similar to that of the peripheral nerve tumors described above, consisting of a sharply defined homogeneous opacity in the paravertebral zone. Wychulis and associates[140] have stated that ganglioneuromas may have an elongated, flattened, or triangular configuration with a broad base toward the mediastinum, thus possessing somewhat less definition than nerve sheath tumors, especially in lateral projection (Fig. 19–67). This observation was confirmed by Reed and his colleagues in their review of 160 tumors of neural origin.[561] However, Bar-Ziv and Nogrady[562] regard these neoplasms as

being "obvious" compared with primary neuroblastomas that tend to be ill-defined and "ghost-like." Calcification is relatively common in these neoplasms; Schweisguth and associates[563] found evidence of it in 10 of 40 cases (7 cases of neuroblastoma and 3 of ganglioneuroma) (Fig. 19–68). This can be an important aid in the differentiation of these from other mediastinal tumors, particularly from metastases in which calcification is rare.[562] The presence of calcification is also helpful in distinguishing a neoplasm from a cyst; however, it is not a reliable indicator of the benignity or malignancy of a neoplasm.[561] The ribs or vertebrae are eroded in some cases, just as often by benign as by malignant forms; rib erosions can be striking in neuroblastoma but tend to be more subtle in ganglioneuroma.[562]

Neuroblastomas and ganglioneuroblastomas occur most commonly in infants and children whereas ganglioneuromas tend to occur in adolescents and young adults.[560] About half the patients are asymptomatic, the remainder having nonspecific respiratory symptoms. Relatively uncommon clinical manifestations include paraplegia, Horner's syndrome, chronic diarrhea, and pain.[560] Urinary catecholamines are elevated in some patients.[560]

Ganglioneuromas are benign neoplasms; com-

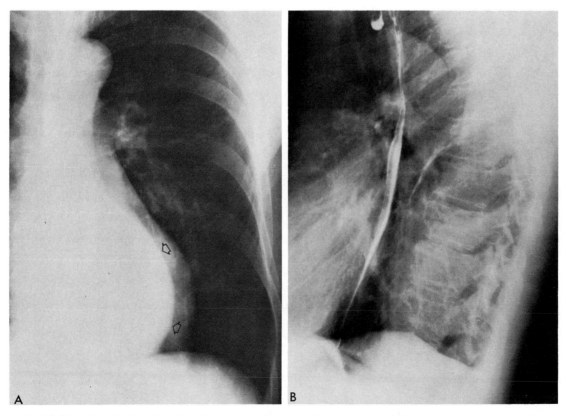

Figure 19–67. Posterior Mediastinal Ganglioneuroma. Views of the left hemithorax from posteroanterior (A) and lateral (B) roentgenograms of a 42-year-old asymptomatic man show a smooth, well-defined, homogeneous mass in the posterior mediastinum (arrows). The mass creates an obtuse angle with the mediastinal soft tissues, indicating its origin from the mediastinum (it is this obtuse angle that leads to such poor visibility of the mass in lateral projection). It contains no visible calcium. The thoracic spine showed no abnormality. This was a proved ganglioneuroma.

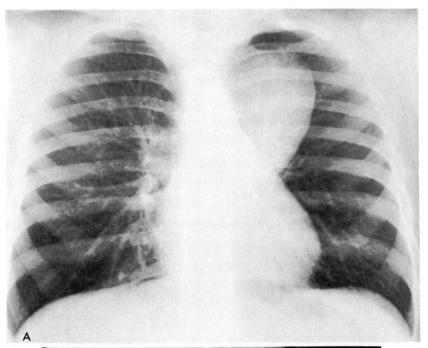

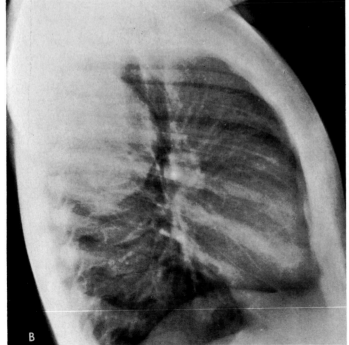

Figure 19–68. Posterior Mediastinal Ganglioneuroma. Roentgenograms of the thorax in posteroanterior *(A)* and lateral *(B)* projections reveal a smooth, sharply circumscribed mass situated in the left paravertebral gutter superiorly. The mass contains numerous speckled deposits of calcium throughout its substance, better visualized in an anteroposterior roentgenogram of the thoracic spine *(C)*. The spine itself was normal. Histologically, the mass proved to be a ganglioneuroma. The patient was an asymptomatic 5-year-old boy. (Courtesy of Montreal Children's Hospital.)

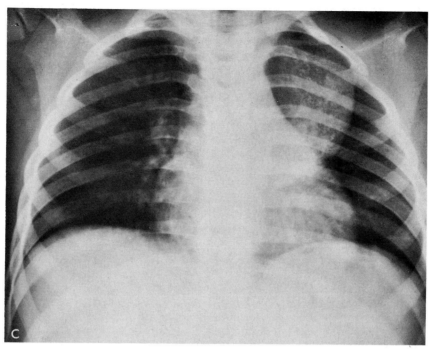

Figure 19–68 *Continued*

plete excision should result in cure. By contrast, neuroblastomas are aggressive neoplasms for which a 2-year survival rate of between 45 and 50 per cent is usual.[560] The prognosis of ganglioneuroblastoma is less predictable and depends to some extent on the age at diagnosis (a younger age being associated with a better outcome), stage, and the histologic growth pattern;[560] in the 1981 AFIP review of 55 patients covering a period of 2 to 23 years, the 5-year actuarial survival rate was 88 per cent.[560]

Aorticosympathetic (Paravertebral) Paraganglioma

As discussed previously (*see* page 2866), intra-thoracic paragangliomas usually occur in either the middle mediastinum in relation to the aorticopulmonary paraganglia or in the posterior mediastinum in relation to the aorticosympathetic paraganglia. As with tumors arising in the former location, those in the posterior mediastinum are uncommon; Odze and Bégin documented 47 cases in the literature by 1990.[641] The average age at the time of diagnosis is 29 years and there is a male-to-female predominance of 2 to 1. Histologic features are identical to those in an aorticopulmonary location.

Roentgenographically, most aorticosympathetic paragangliomas are sharply defined, round or oval masses in the paravertebral area and are indistinguishable from other neurogenic neoplasms. The majority are located in the mid-thoracic region adjacent to the fifth, sixth, or seventh ribs, and there is a right-sided predominance of 2 to 1.[565]

Clinically, about 50 per cent of patients are asymptomatic or complain of chest pain;[565] rare manifestations include Horner's syndrome and lower extremity weakness secondary to spinal cord compression. Unlike aorticopulmonary paragliomas that are rarely biochemically functional, about half of the reported patients with the aorticosympathetic variety have shown signs and symptoms related to excess catecholamine production, including headache, sweating, tachycardia, palpitations, dyspnea, and nausea. Hypertension is present in most, as are increased levels of plasma and urinary catecholamines.[566, 567] Many patients have adrenal and other extrathoracic paraganglionic tumors that can present either synchronously or metachronously.[565]

The prognosis of aorticosympathetic paragangliomas is better than the prognosis of those in the aorticopulmonary region.[565] In many cases, complete surgical excision and cure are possible, but in a few patients local invasion or extensive hemorrhage during surgery precludes complete excision. In the latter patients, the neoplasm usually recurs, although sometimes after a prolonged interval. Metastases were documented in only 7 per cent of the cases reviewed by Gallivan and colleagues.[565]

Meningocele and Meningomyelocele

These rare anomalies of the intrathoracic spinal canal consist of herniation of the leptomeninges through an intervertebral foramen. Of the 70 cases reported in the literature by 1969,[568] the lesion was single in 62 patients and multiple in the remainder. They occur slightly more often on the right side than on the left and can be situated anywhere between the thoracic inlet and the diaphragm. They are usually detected in middle age, approximately 75 per cent of patients presenting between the ages of 30 and 60 years.[568] A meningocele contains cerebrospinal fluid only; a meningomyelocele also contains nerve elements.

On conventional roentgenograms, these lesions show no specific features that distinguish them from solid neurogenic neoplasms. However, CT examination should prove diagnostic, especially if associated with metrizamide myelography which usually reveals passage of contrast medium into the meningocele.[134] An associated kyphoscoliosis is frequent, being observed in 47 of the 70 cases reviewed by Miles and associates;[568] the meningocele was usually situated at the apex of the curvature on its convex side. Enlargement of the intervertebral foramen is a very common finding but was specifically absent in 5 of the 70 cases in the Miles and associates series. An association with vertebral and rib anomalies is also fairly frequent and should suggest the diagnosis.[140, 570] Similarly, the association with generalized neurofibromatosis is common, being recorded in 46 of 70 cases.[568] This association is of little differential value, however, since posterior mediastinal neurofibroma and neurogenic sarcoma can also be part of von Recklinghausen's disease.

A rare lesion has been described in a 19-year-old male following trauma that resulted in a fracture of the right first rib, separation of the lateral aspect of the C7 to T1 intervertebral disk, and a dural tear at that level.[571] Termed "pseudomeningocele" by the authors, the lesion consisted of a collection of cerebrospinal fluid in the extrapleural space overlying the lung apex. Contrast medium entered and exited the cavity freely.

POSTERIOR MEDIASTINAL CYSTS

Gastroenteric (Neurenteric) Cyst

Although there are several theories of the origin of gastroenteric (neurenteric) cysts, according to Salyer and colleagues[572] the most likely is that they result from incomplete separation of endoderm from the notochord during early fetal life. (The embryology of the neurenteric canal and the cysts derived therefrom have been described in some detail by Madewell and his colleagues,[573] and the interested reader is directed to this discussion for more information.) Histologically, the cysts are lined by a variety of epithelial types, including gastric, small intestinal, duodenal, and ciliated columnar.[572] The first-named can be functional and associated with peptic ulceration.

The roentgenographic appearance is that of a sharply defined, lobulated opacity of homogeneous density situated in a paravertebral location. Because of their fluid content, they tend to mold themselves to surrounding structures. The cysts are often connected by a stalk to the meninges and commonly also to a portion of the gastrointestinal tract. If attachment is to the esophagus within the thorax, communication is rare; however, if it is to the gastrointestinal tract within the abdomen, in most cases there is communication, permitting gas to enter the cyst. In fact, the cyst may opacify with barium during examination of the upper gastrointestinal tract. Some cases (termed neurenteric cysts[573]) are associated with congenital defects of the thoracic spine;[134, 265] in these cases, myelography occasionally reveals a patent stalk communicating with the spinal subarachnoid space.[265] Very large cysts may be associated with scoliosis.[150]

Gastroenteric cysts typically produce symptoms and therefore become manifest early in life;[574] they are said to be more common in males.[150] They can grow very large and cause compression atelectasis, thereby leading to respiratory distress. Peptic ulceration can cause pain.[150]

Esophageal Cyst

Esophageal (esophageal duplication) cysts[575] are believed to represent a failure of complete vacuolation of the originally solid esophagus to produce a hollow tube.[572] They are lined by nonkeratinizing squamous or ciliated columnar epithelium; a double layer of smooth muscle in their walls and a lack of cartilage are necessary findings to exclude a diagnosis of bronchial cyst. The cysts are usually located within or adjacent to the wall of the esophagus. Many patients are asymptomatic, although esophageal compression can cause dysphagia;[572] chronic cough, misinterpreted as a symptom of asthma and bronchitis, also has been attributed to an esophageal cyst.[576]

Thoracic Duct Cyst

This is an extremely rare type of posterior mediastinal mass of which only 10 cases had been reported by 1978.[577–579] The cysts can occur anywhere from the thoracic inlet to the diaphragm and can communicate with the thoracic duct either superiorly or inferiorly. They may be large enough to displace the mediastinum to the opposite side. It has been shown that lymphangiography can occasionally opacify such cysts.[580, 581] Patients are most often asymptomatic but sometimes complain of dysphagia or back pain;[577–579] tracheal compression may result in acute respiratory insufficiency.[582] The diagnosis has been made by fluoroscopically guided needle aspiration.[583]

DISEASES OF THE ESOPHAGUS

Esophageal lesions that may present roentgenographically as mediastinal masses or as diffuse mediastinal widening include neoplasm, diverticulum, esophageal hiatus hernia, and megaesophagus.

Neoplasms

Although barium examination and esophagoscopy are the two definitive procedures in the diagnosis of primary carcinoma of the esophagus, conventional roentgenograms of the chest can provide clues to its presence and computed tomography is an essential procedure in staging. In a review of the conventional posteroanterior and lateral chest roentgenograms of 103 patients with proven carcinoma of the esophagus, Lindell and his colleagues[584] found significant abnormalities in 49 patients: the most frequent of these included an abnormal azygoesophageal recess interface (27 per cent), a widened mediastinum (18 per cent), posterior tracheal indentation or mass (16 per cent), widened retrotracheal stripe (11 per cent), and tracheal deviation (10 per cent) (Fig. 19–69); less common abnormalities included deformity of the gastric air bubble, a retrocardiac mass, an esophageal fluid level, and a retrohilar mass.

In another plain film study of 102 patients with carcinoma of the middle third of the esophagus,[585] 63 (62 per cent) revealed thickening of the retrotracheal stripe, anterior bowing of the posterior wall of the trachea, or a combination of these findings; of considerable importance was the observation that prognosis was not significantly different in patients with or without retrotracheal abnormalities. Progressive thickening of the posterior tracheal band also has been shown to be a useful sign of recurrent esophageal carcinoma following surgery or radiation therapy.[586] Although there exists some variation in the maximum width accepted by different authors for the posterior tracheal band or stripe, the figures provided by Palayew seem to us to be most reliable.[587] This author states that the upper limit of normal for a posterior tracheal band (the posterior wall of the trachea plus contiguous connective tissue) should be 2.5 to 3 mm, and that for the tracheoesophageal stripe (the posterior tracheal wall plus the esophagus) should be 3 mm or slightly more.

CT of the esophagus has received considerable attention in recent years and the accumulated experience would suggest that this procedure is of great value in the staging of esophageal carcinoma. In their study of 52 patients with histologically proved carcinoma, Picus and his colleagues[588] found CT to be highly accurate in predicting tumor size and in assessing invasion of the tracheobronchial tree and spread to the liver, adrenals, and upper abdominal lymph nodes. By quantifying the contact between the tumor and the aorta, these authors found that the CT appearance correctly predicted the presence or absence of aortic invasion in 24 of 25 cases. In this series,[588] proved metastases to local periesophageal nodes were seldom associated with nodal enlargement, so that CT was insensitive in detecting this type of spread. In their CT study of 76 patients with carcinoma of either the esophagus or the gastroesophageal junction, Thompson and his associates[589] found that CT correctly identified 40 of 44 patients with mediastinal invasion and 11 of 15 patients without invasion (accuracy 88 per cent); in this series, CT correctly staged 46 of 49 patients (94 per cent) with esophageal carcinoma but only 5 of 12 patients (42 per cent) with neoplasms at the gastroesophageal junction. Despite the foregoing, in a study of 33 patients with esophageal carcinoma, Quint and associates[590] found that CT correctly staged the carcinoma in only 13 patients and was not useful in assessing resectability. The tracheobronchial tree is frequently involved in patients with carcinoma of the esophagus: in one study of 525 patients with esophageal carcinoma who were bronchoscoped, impingement was identified in 91 and invasion in 87 patients;[591, 592] the incidence was highest for lesions arising in the cervical and upper thoracic esophagus. The prognosis for the patients with impingement was considerably better than for those with invasion.

Although thickening of the esophageal wall is the earliest CT manifestation of esophageal carcinoma, it is by no means diagnostic of that condition. In a study of 200 consecutive CT examinations of the thorax, Reinig and his coworkers[593] found thickened esophageal walls (over 3 mm) in 35 per cent; however, in only half of these cases was there esophageal carcinoma. Other causes included reflux and monilial esophagitis, esophageal varices, and postirradiation scarring.

Benign neoplasms of the esophagus (which are rare) can grow large and present as a rounded mass projecting to one or both sides of the posterior mediastinum (Fig. 19–70).[594] Leiomyomas, fibromas, and lipomas constitute the bulk of these benign neoplasms. Of the 81 primary neoplasms of the mediastinum in adults reported by Daniel and associates,[142] 4 were leiomyomas of the esophagus, all originating in the lower third. Although leiomyomas are usually solitary, multiple tumors occur in about 4 per cent of cases.[595] Leiomyosarcoma has been reported.[596]

Diverticula

Diverticula occur in the pharyngeal region (Zenker's), in the mid-thoracic region as a result of cicatricial contraction from healed infected lymph nodes (traction diverticula), and in the lower esophagus as a result of outpouching of the mucosa through defects in the muscular wall at the point of entry of blood vessels (pulsion diverticula). Unlike the other two varieties, traction diverticula seldom if ever are visible on plain roentgenograms.

Zenker's diverticulum originates between the transverse and oblique fibers of the inferior pharyngeal constrictor muscle and thus is a pharyngeal rather than an esophageal diverticulum. It may become large enough to be identified in the superior mediastinum on plain roentgenograms, frequently containing an air-fluid level. Barium studies not only clearly outline the sac but also reveal the degree

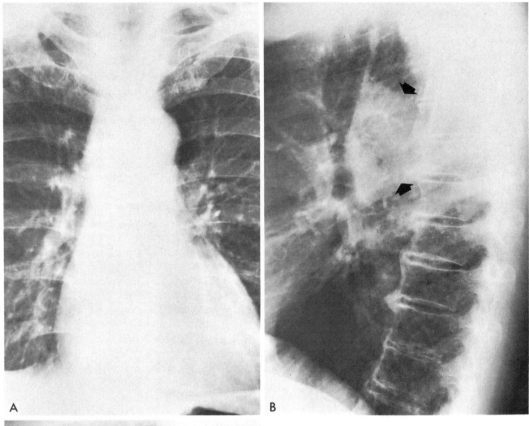

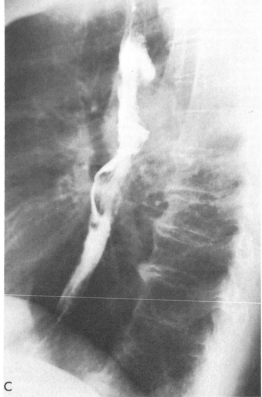

Figure 19–69. Posterior Mediastinal Mass Caused by Carcinoma of the Esophagus. This 56-year-old man presented with a 2-month history of increasing dysphagia. A posteroanterior roentgenogram *(A)* revealed no significant abnormalities of the mediastinal silhouette, but in lateral projection *(B),* there was evidence of a poorly defined increase in density in the posterior mediastinum, obliterating the aortic window and causing slight anterior displacement of the trachea *(arrows).* In the absence of significant pulmonary abnormality, such an appearance is highly suggestive of a primary esophageal neoplasm (a similar appearance could be produced by posterior mediastinal lymph node metastases from a primary bronchogenic carcinoma). A lateral view of the thorax following ingestion of barium *(C)* reveals severe deformity of the esophageal contour characteristic of primary esophageal cancer. The neoplasm had invaded the adjacent mediastinal soft tissues and had metastasized to regional posterior mediastinal nodes.

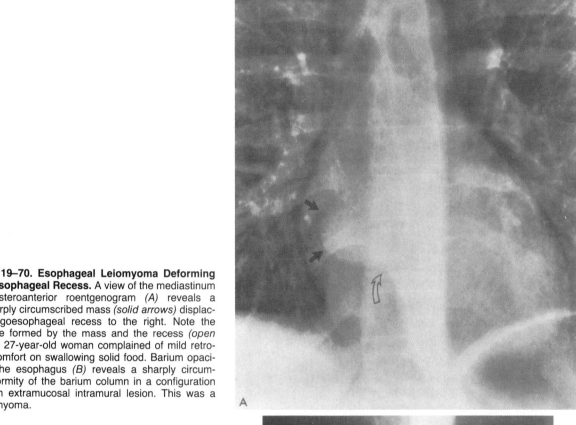

Figure 19–70. Esophageal Leiomyoma Deforming the Azygoesophageal Recess. A view of the mediastinum from a posteroanterior roentgenogram *(A)* reveals a smooth, sharply circumscribed mass *(solid arrows)* displacing the azygoesophageal recess to the right. Note the obtuse angle formed by the mass and the recess *(open arrow).* This 27-year-old woman complained of mild retrosternal discomfort on swallowing solid food. Barium opacification of the esophagus *(B)* reveals a sharply circumscribed deformity of the barium column in a configuration typical of an extramucosal intramural lesion. This was a proved leiomyoma.

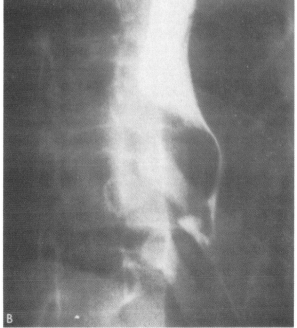

of anterior displacement of the proximal esophagus (*see* Fig. 13–10, page 2397). Symptoms include dysphagia, chronic cough due to aspiration, and in some patients recurrent pneumonia.

Diverticula arising from the lower third of the esophagus are almost always congenital in origin and present as round, cyst-like structures to the right of the midline just above the diaphragm. An air-fluid level is present in most cases. Barium studies are diagnostic.[597] A rare form of multiple pulsion diverticula has been described that closely resembles that seen in the colon; barium studies are required for identification.[598]

Megaesophagus

Of the many causes of dilatation of the esophagus—inflammatory stenosis (secondary to mediastinitis or reflux esophagitis), progressive systemic sclerosis (PSS), carcinoma, and achalasia—the last-named causes the most severe generalized dilatation. Depending on the underlying cause, an air-fluid level may be observed in the dilated esophagus, most frequently in achalasia but seldom in PSS. The dilated esophagus is apparent as a shadow projecting entirely to the right side of the mediastinum. Since it is behind the heart, it does not cause a silhouette sign with that structure. The trachea may be bulged anteriorly (Fig. 19–71). Although a barium study is the diagnostic procedure of choice in these conditions, CT findings should enable one to suggest the diagnosis, even in patients in whom the condition is not suspected.[599] On conventional chest roentgenograms, an air-containing esophagus may be identified in some patients with progressive systemic sclerosis, in some patients postoperatively,[600] and in patients who employ esophageal speech following laryngectomy.[601]

Symptoms of achalasia include dysphagia, pain on swallowing, and in some cases chronic cough and recurrent pneumonia due to aspiration. Stridor is observed occasionally.[602, 603] In patients with achalasia, acute trapping of air within the esophagus distal to the cricopharyngeal sphincter has been described as a cause of tracheal obstruction and vena caval compression.[602] Achalasia secondary to gastrointestinal and nongastrointestinal malignancies is a recognized entity.[604]

TRACHEOESOPHAGEAL AND BRONCHOESOPHAGEAL FISTULAS

Fistulas between the esophagus and the airways can be congenital or acquired. Although usually identified in neonates, the former type may not be recognized until adolescence or adulthood. In most of these cases, there is a long history of cough, often with expectoration of food particles; occasionally, there is associated bronchiectasis.[605, 606] Congenital communication between the esophagus and the respiratory conducting system is considered in greater detail in Chapter 5 (*see* page 727).

The most common cause of acquired fistula between the esophagus and the respiratory tract is carcinoma of the esophagus, in some instances precipitated by irradiation therapy.[607–610] Of 474 patients with carcinoma of the esophagus in one series,[607] 25 (5.3 per cent) developed a fistula. Once this complication has developed, the prognosis is extremely bad, most patients dying within weeks to months.

Acquired nonmalignant tracheoesophageal fistulas can be caused by cuffed tracheal tubes, surgical trauma, blunt injuries, and foreign bodies.[611–613] Although generally diagnosed by endoscopic or barium examination, they have been revealed by computed tomography.[614]

ESOPHAGEAL VARICES

Esophageal varices do not in themselves occasion respiratory symptoms, but complicating hematemesis may be confused with hemoptysis. In addition, transient pleural effusions and mediastinal opacities have been identified roentgenographically following endoscopic injection sclerotherapy;[615] in one patient this form of treatment caused an esophageal-pleural fistula.[616]

MEDIASTINAL MASSES DUE TO TRANSDIAPHRAGMATIC HERNIATION OF ABDOMINAL CONTENTS

Herniation of abdominal contents, most often the stomach, liver or omentum, occurs occasionally through a variety of deficiencies in the diaphragm. These are discussed in some detail in Chapter 20 and only brief mention is made of them here.

Esophageal Hiatus Hernia

Esophageal hiatus hernia is undoubtedly the most common diaphragmatic hernia. In this condition, conventional roentgenograms of the chest often reveal the herniated portion of stomach directly behind the heart and slightly to the right of the midline. A fluid level is present in many cases, although obviously gas cannot be identified when the hernial sac (rarely) contains omentum or liver.[617] When the diagnosis is in doubt on the basis of evidence provided by plain roentgenograms, barium opacification confirms the presence or absence of a hernia. Rarely, a loop of transverse colon rather than the stomach is the herniated structure. An appearance similar to hiatus hernia is created by the Thal procedure performed for repair of distal esophageal stricture.[618] A most unusual cause of a mediastinal mass has been described in which a

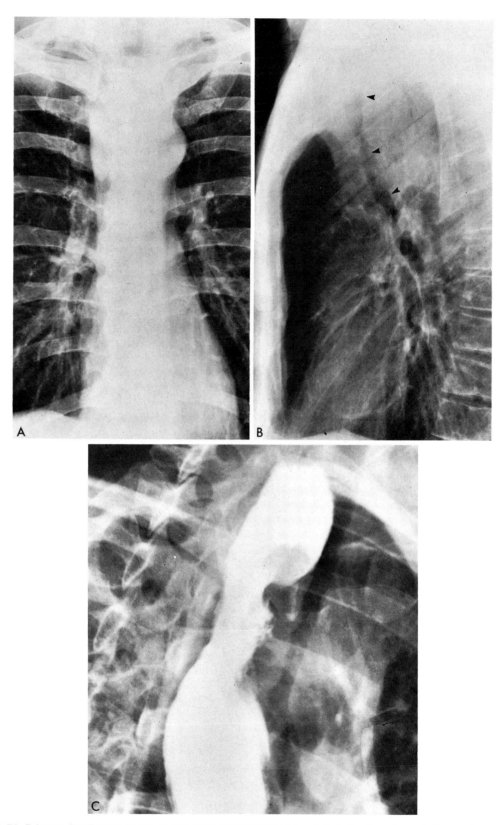

Figure 19–71. Primary Carcinoma of the Esophagus Superimposed on Achalasia. A posteroanterior roentgenogram *(A)* of this 42-year-old woman reveals widening of the superior mediastinum, chiefly to the right. In lateral projection *(B),* the air column of the trachea is displaced slightly anteriorly *(arrowheads)* by a fairly large homogenous mass lying posterior to it. This type of deformity is characteristic (but not diagnostic) of severe esophageal dilatation. Following ingestion of barium *(C),* an oblique view of the esophagus reveals a marked degree of dilatation. In addition, its anterior wall is the site of an irregular fungating mass that proved to be primary esophageal carcinoma superimposed upon achalasia.

large calcified leiomyoma arose from the herniated portion of stomach in a large hiatus hernia.[619]

Occasionally, patients with an incarcerated hiatus hernia complain of severe retrosternal chest pain difficult to distinguish from that of myocardial or pericardial origin. However, pain from esophageal disease is often precipitated by changes in posture, such as lying down or bending over, and there is almost always the additional complaint of dysphagia.

In a 1986 review, Johnston and associates[620] described one case and found 29 previous cases reported in the literature of a *pancreatic pseudocyst* that had extended into the posterior mediastinum, usually through the esophageal or aortic hiatus. They occurred in individuals aged 7 months to 73 years; those in the older age group were commonly associated with alcoholic pancreatitis whereas those in the younger individuals often involved a history of trauma. Roentgenographic findings are those of a mass in the retrocardiac area; pleural effusion is present in about half the cases. In the Johnston and associates review, weight loss occurred in 85 per cent of patients; other complaints included dyspnea, chest pain, nausea, vomiting, and dysphagia. The serum amylase was often elevated. The precise nature and anatomic extent of this abnormality can be exquisitely demonstrated by CT;[621, 622] diagnosis also can be aided by ultrasonography.

Bochdalek Hernia

Herniation of abdominal contents through the foramina of Bochdalek usually occurs into one or the other hemithorax but occasionally into the mediastinum. The contour and density of the mass depend on the contents of the hernial sac which can be virtually any intra-abdominal organ, including omentum, bowel, spleen, or kidney.[623] Diagnosis may be confirmed by barium examination of the gastrointestinal tract or by CT; intravenous pyelography can establish the presence of a kidney within the thorax. Although herniation of a significant nature is usually manifested during the neonatal period, it can be occasionally delayed, sometimes into adolescence.[624]

Rarely, *duplication cysts (or diverticula) of the small intestine* can project through foramina in the diaphragm and present in the mediastinum.[625]

DISEASES OF THE THORACIC SPINE

Neoplasms

A wide variety of primary neoplasms of bone and cartilage can involve the thoracic spine and posterior rib cage, including osteochondroma, aneurysmal bone cyst, chondrosarcoma, osteogenic sarcoma, Ewing's tumor, myeloma, and most commonly, metastatic neoplasm. In a few cases, the major roentgenographic finding is an extraosseous soft tissue mass, and identification of the primary bone lesion requires careful roentgenographic study. The lymphomas, particularly Hodgkin's disease, may be manifested roentgenologically as a fusiform paraspinal soft tissue mass produced by enlargement of the posterior parietal group of lymph nodes; in such cases, contiguous vertebrae may be eroded by extranodal invasion.

Infectious Spondylitis

Tuberculous and nontuberculous spondylitis is often associated with a paraspinal mass caused by inflammation and abscess formation in contiguous soft tissues. Commonly, there is a bilateral fusiform mass in the paravertebral zone, with its maximal diameter at the point of major bone destruction (Fig. 19–72).

Fracture with Hematoma Formation

Fractures of thoracic vertebral bodies can result in extraosseous hemorrhage and the development of unilateral or bilateral paraspinal masses. Although the fracture is usually visible roentgenographically, the major evidence of its presence may be deformity of the contiguous paraspinal soft tissues.

EXTRAMEDULLARY HEMATOPOIESIS

Extramedullary hematopoiesis occurs as a compensatory phenomenon in various diseases in which there is inadequate production or excessive destruction of blood cells. The most common sites are the liver and spleen, but foci can also occur in many other organs and tissues[626] including the paravertebral areas of the thorax. Its presence in the latter location is uncommon; by 1980, only 56 cases had been reported.[627]

The origin of extramedullary hematopoiesis in the paravertebral regions is unclear; it has been postulated that it represents extension of hyperplastic marrow from adjacent bone or lymph nodes or that it develops from embryonic nests of primitive hematopoietic tissue.[628] In one study,[629] CT images showed that the bone in the region in which the mass had developed was usually the widest and thinnest, supporting the Ross and Logan[630] thesis that there occurs extrusion of bone marrow through thinned trabeculae of ribs. Long and associates[629] postulated that negative intrathoracic pressure may facilitate such extrusion, perhaps explaining the observation that the proliferation of paravertebral marrow is primarily intrathoracic rather than extrathoracic.

Pathologically, foci of extramedullary hematopoiesis appear as one or more soft, reddish nodules that can resemble hematomas.[627] Histologically, all

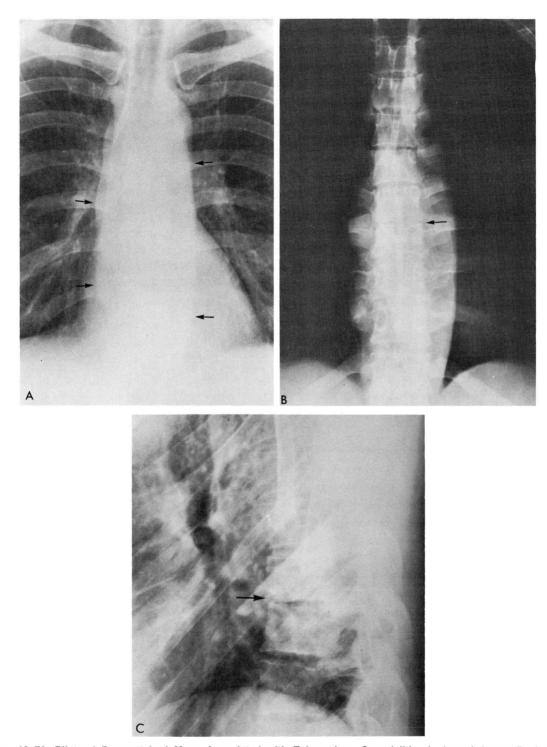

Figure 19–72. Bilateral Paravertebral Mass Associated with Tuberculous Spondylitis. A view of the mediastinum from a posteroanterior roentgenogram *(A)* demonstrates a smooth, sharply circumscribed widening of the posterior mediastinum bilaterally *(arrows),* the shadow on the right side being slightly lobulated. An anteroposterior roentgenogram of the thoracic spine *(B)* demonstrates the paravertebral masses to better advantage. Note that the paravertebral line is obliterated. In the anteroposterior and lateral *(C)* roentgenograms of the spine, an *arrow* points to a narrowed intervertebral disk between T-7 and T-8. Note the small areas of bone destruction in the contiguous surfaces of these vertebral bodies. This case was proved tuberculous spondylitis with bilateral paraspinal abscesses.

marrow elements can be identified, usually with marked erythroid hyperplasia.

The characteristic roentgenographic finding is of multiple masses, smooth or lobulated in contour and of homogeneous density, situated in the paravertebral regions, either unilaterally or bilaterally;[196] they are usually located below the level of the seventh thoracic vertebra. A presumptive diagnosis usually can be made when this roentgenographic finding is present in patients with severe anemia and splenomegaly, and it is supported by the presence of changes in the bony skeleton attributable to a condition that causes marrow abnormalities such as chronic hemolytic anemia or myelofibrosis.[630]

The majority of cases of extramedullary hematopoiesis are associated with congenital hemolytic anemia (usually hereditary spherocytosis) or thalassemia (usually thalassemia major or intermedia);[627] occasional cases also have been reported in association with sickle cell disease.[631] The abnormality was present in 5 of the 45 patients with thalassemia reported by Papavasiliou.[632] One patient has been reported in whom there was no obvious cause.[633] The masses seldom occasion symptoms, although paraplegia occurs occasionally as a result of spinal cord compression.[627]

MISCELLANEOUS POSTERIOR MEDIASTINAL TUMORS

Rare forms of posterior mediastinal neoplasm include *chordoma* (a malignant neoplasm believed to be derived from fetal notochord rests and usually located in the upper posterior mediastinum),[634] *ependymoma*,[635] *plasmacytoma*,[636] and *meningioma*.[637] An unusual non-neoplastic cause of a posterior mediastinal mass is *ectopic kidney*, 16 cases of which had been reported by 1974.[638]

REFERENCES

1. Baron RL, Levitt RG, Sagel SS, et al: Computed tomography in the evaluation of mediastinal widening. Radiology 138:107, 1981.
2. Pugatch RD, Faling LJ, Robbins AH, et al: CT diagnosis of benign mediastinal abnormalities. Am J Roentgenol. 34:685, 1980.
3. Sones PJ Jr, Torres WE, Colvin RS, et al: Effectiveness of CT in evaluating intrathoracic masses. Am J Roentgenol 139:469, 1982.
4. Zylak CJ, Pallie W, Jackson R: Correlative anatomy and computed tomography. A module on the mediastinum. RadioGraphics 2:555, 1982.
5. Shin MS, McElvein RB, Ho KJ: Computed tomography evaluation of pathologic processes in the potential spaces of the mediastinum. J Comput Tomogr 12:230, 1988.
6. Siegel MJ, Sagel SS, Reed K: The value of computed tomography in the diagnosis and management of pediatric mediastinal abnormalities. Radiology 142:149, 1982.
7. Cohen AM, Creviston S, LiPuma JP, et al: Nuclear magnetic resonance imaging of the mediastinum and hili: Early impressions of its efficacy. Am J Roentgenol 141:1163, 1983.
8. Axel L, Kressel HY, Thickman D, et al: NMR imaging of the chest at 0.12 T: Initial clinical experience with a resistive magnet. Am J Roentgenol 141:1157, 1983.
9. Webb WR, Gamsu G, Crooks LE: Multisection sagittal and coronal magnetic resonance imaging of the mediastinum and hila. Radiology 150:475, 1984.
10. Brasch RC, Gooding CA, Lallemand DP, et al: Magnetic resonance imaging of the thorax in childhood. Radiology 150:463, 1984.
11. Gamsu G, Stark DD, Webb WR, et al: Magnetic resonance imaging of benign mediastinal masses. Radiology 151:709, 1984.
12. Webb WR, Gamsu G, Stark DD, et al: Evaluation of magnetic resonance sequences in imaging mediastinal tumors. Am J Roentgenol 153:723, 1984.
13. Cohen AM: Magnetic resonance imaging of the thorax. Radiol Clin North Am 22:829, 1984.
14. Levitt RG, Glazer HS, Roper CL, et al: Magnetic resonance imaging of mediastinal and hilar masses: Comparison with CT. Am J Roentgenol 145:9, 1985.
15. Westcott JL, Henschke CI, Berkmen Y: MR imaging of the hilum and mediastinum: Effects of cardiac gating. J Comput Assist Tomogr 9:1073, 1985.
16. von Schulthess GK, McMurdo K, Tscholakoff D, et al: Mediastinal masses: MR imaging. Radiology 158:289, 1986.
17. Siegel MJ, Nadel SN, Glazer HS, et al: Mediastinal lesions in children: Comparison of CT and MR. Radiology 160:241, 1986.
18. Heitzman ER: The Mediastinum. Radiologic Correlations with Anatomy and Pathology. St. Louis, CV Mosby, 1977.
19. Dozois RR, Bernatz PE, Woolner LB, et al: Sclerosing mediastinitis involving major bronchi. Mayo Clin Proc 43:557, 1968.
20. Comings DE, Skubi K-B, Eyes JV, et al: Familial multifocal fibrosclerosis. Findings suggesting that retroperitoneal fibrosis, mediastinal fibrosis, sclerosing cholangitis, Riedel's thyroiditis, and pseudotumor of the orbit may be different manifestations of a single disease. Ann Intern Med 66:884, 1967.
21. Leszcyński St Z, Pawlicka L (in collaboration): Purulent and Fibrous Mediastinitis. Radiological Diagnosis. Warsaw, PZWL (Polish Medical Publishers), 1972.
22. LaBerge JM, Kerlan RK Jr, Pogany AC, et al: Esophageal rupture: Complication of balloon dilatation. Radiology 157:56, 1985.
23. Härmä RA, Koskinen YO, Suukari SO: Spontaneous rupture of the oesophagus. Endoscopic treatment in the primary stage. Thorax 23:210, 1968.
24. Marston EL, Valk HL: Spontaneous perforation of the esophagus: Review of the literature and report of a case. Ann Intern Med 51:590, 1959.
25. Craddock DR, Logan A, Mayell M: Traumatic rupture of the oesophagus and stomach. Thorax 23:657, 1968.
26. Rogers LF, Puig AW, Dooley BN, et al: Diagnostic considerations in mediastinal emphysema: A pathophysiologic-roentgenologic approach to Boerhaave's syndrome and spontaneous pneumomediastinum. Am J Roentgenol 115:495, 1972.
27. Chavy AL, Rougier M, Pieddeloup C, et al: Esophageal prosthesis for neoplastic stenosis. A prognostic study of 77 cases. Cancer 57:1426, 1986.
28. Gray JM, Hanson GC: Mediastinal emphysema: Aetiology, diagnosis, and treatment. Thorax 21:325, 1966.
29. Sarr MG, Gott VL, Townsend TR: Mediastinal infection after cardiac surgery. Ann Thorac Surg 35:415, 1984.
30. Rutledge R, Applebaum RE, Kim BJ: Mediastinal infection after open heart surgery. Surgery 97:88, 1985.
31. Larson TC III, Shuman LS, Libshitz HI, et al: Complications of colonic interposition. Cancer 56:681, 1985.
32. Hendler BH, Quinn PD: Fatal mediastinitis secondary to odontogenic infection. J Oral Surg 36:308, 1978.
33. Körösj A, Halász G: Acute mediastinitis as a complication of bronchoscopy. Tuberkulózis 14:15, 1961.
34. Tsai SH, Cohen SS, Fenger EPK: Bronchial perforation as a complication of bronchoscopy. Am Rev Tuberc 78:106, 1958.
35. Armen RN, Morrow CS, Sewell S: Mediastinal emphysema: A complication of bronchoscopy. Ann Intern Med 48:1083, 1958.
36. Christoforidis A, Nelson SW: Spontaneous rupture of the esophagus with emphasis on the roentgenologic diagnosis. Am J Roentgenol 78:574, 1957.
37. Han SY, McElvein RB, Aldrete JS, et al: Perforation of the esophagus: Correlation of site and cause with plain film findings. Am J Roentgenol 145:537, 1985.
38. Appleton DS, Sandrasagra FA, Flower CDR: Perforated oesophagus: Review of twenty-eight consecutive cases. Clin Radiol 30:493, 1979.
39. Dodds WJ, Stewart ET, Vlymen WJ: Appropriate contrast media for evaluation of esophageal disruption. Radiology 144:439, 1982.
40. Eriksen KR: Oesophageal fistula diagnosed by microscopic examination of pleural fluid. Acta Chir Scand 128:771, 1964.
41. Wechsler RJ, Steiner RM, Goodman LR, et al: Iatrogenic esophageal-pleural fistula: Subtlety of diagnosis in the absence of mediastinitis. Radiology 144:239, 1982.
42. Vincken W, Vandenbrande P, Roels P, et al: Isolated paratracheal mass of tuberculous origin in an adult patient. Eur J Respir Dis 64:630, 1983.
43. Le Roux BT: Mediastinal teratomata. Thorax 15:333, 1960.
44. Schowengerdt CG, Suyemoto R, Main FB: Granulomatous and fibrous mediastinitis—A review and analysis of 180 cases. J Thorac Cardiovasc Surg 57:365, 1969.
45. Loyd JE, Tillman BF, Atkinson JB, et al: Mediastinal fibrosis complicating histoplasmosis. Medicine 67:295, 1988.
46. Wieder S, Rabinowitz JG: Fibrous mediastinitis: A late manifestation of mediastinal histoplasmosis. Radiology 125:305, 1977
47. Cohen DM, Goggans EA: Sclerosing mediastinitis and terminal valvular endocarditis caused by fungus suggestive of Aspergillus species. Am J Clin Pathol 56:91, 1971.
48. Ahmad M, Weinstein AJ, Hughes JA, et al: Granulomatous mediastinitis due to Aspergillus flavus in a nonimmunosuppressed patient. Am J Med 70:887, 1981.
49. Leong ASY: Granulomatous mediastinitis due to Rhizopus species. Am J Clin Pathol, 70:103, 1978.
50. Dines DE, Payne WS, Bernatz PE, et al: Mediastinal granuloma and fibrosing mediastinitis. Chest 75:320, 1979.
51. Morgan AD, Loughridge LW, Calne, RY: Combined mediastinal and retroperitoneal fibrosis. Lancet 1:67, 1966.
52. DuPont HL, Varco RL, Winchell CP: Chronic fibrous mediastinitis simulating pulmonic stenosis, associated with inflammatory pseudotumor of the orbit. Am J Med 44:447, 1968.
53. Raphael HA, Beahrs OH, Woolner LB, et al: Riedel's struma associated with fibrous mediastinitis: Report of a case. Mayo Clin Proc 41:375, 1966.
54. Salmon HW: Combined mediastinal and retroperitoneal fibrosis. Thorax 23:158, 1968.
55. Cameron DD, Ing ST, Boyle M, et al: Idiopathic mediastinal and retroperitoneal fibrosis. Can Med Assoc J 85:227, 1961.
56. Graham JR, Suby HI, LeCompte PR, et al: Fibrotic disorders associated with methysergide therapy for headache. N Engl J Med 274:359, 1966.
57. Andrews EC Jr: Five cases of an undescribed form of pulmonary interstitial fibrosis caused by obstruction of the pulmonary veins. Bull Johns Hopkins Hosp 100:28, 1957.
58. Katzenstein ALA, Mazur MT: Pulmonary infarct: An unusual manifestation of fibrosing mediastinitis. Chest 77:521, 1980.
59. Sobrinho-Simões MA, Vaz Saleiro J, Wagenvoort CA: Mediastinal and hilar fibrosis. Histopathology 5:53, 1981.
60. Karlson KE, Timmes JJ: Granulomata of the mediastinum surgically treated and followed up to nine years. J Thorac Surg 35:617, 1958.

19

61. Feigin DS, Eggleston JC, Siegelman SS: The multiple roentgen manifestations of sclerosing mediastinitis. Johns Hopkins Med J 144:1, 1979.

62. Wieder S, White TJ III, Salazar J, et al: Pulmonary artery occlusion due to histoplasmosis. Am J Roentgenol. 138:243, 1982.

63. Mendelson EB, Mintzer RA, Hidvegi DF: Veno-occlusive pulmonary infarct: An unusual complication of fibrosing mediastinitis. Am J Roentgenol 141:175, 1983.

64. Weinstein JB, Aronberg DJ, Sagel SS: CT of fibrosing mediastinitis: Findings and their utility Am J Roentgenol 141:247, 1983.

65. Kountz PD, Molina PL, Sagel S: Fibrosing mediastinitis in the posterior thorax. Am J Roentgenol 153:489, 1989.

66. Im J-G, Song KS, Kang HS, et al: Mediastinal tuberculous lymphadenitis: CT manifestations. Radiology 164:115, 1987.

67. Farmer DW, Moore E, Amparo E, et al: Calcific fibrosing mediastinitis: Demonstration of pulmonary vascular obstruction by magnetic resonance imaging. Am J Roentgenol 143:1189, 1984.

68. Rholl KS, Levitt RG, Glazer HS: Magnetic resonance imaging of fibrosing mediastinitis. Am J Roentgenol 145:255, 1985.

69. Morrison G: Retroperitoneal fibrosis associated with methysergide therapy. J Can Assoc Radiol 19:61, 1968.

70. Arnett N, Bacos JM, Macher AM, et al: Fibrosing mediastinitis causing arterial hypertension without pulmonary venous hypertension. Clinical and necropsy observations. Am J Med 63:634, 1977.

71. Dye TE, Saab SB, Almond CH, et al: Sclerosing mediastinitis with occlusion of pulmonary veins. Manifestations and management. J Thorac Cardiovasc Surg 74:137, 1977.

72. Hicks, GL Jr: Fibrosing mediastinitis. Causing pulmonary artery and vein obstruction with hemoptysis. NY State J Med 83:242, 1983.

73. Shin MS, Fulmer JD, Ho KJ: Bilateral hilar enlargement and hypoperfusion of the right lower lobe. Chest 90:120, 1986.

74. Lillard RL, Allen R. P.: The extrapleural air sign in pneumomediastinum. Radiology 85:1093, 1965.

75. Emery JL: Interstitial emphysema, pneumothorax, and "air-block" in the newborn. Lancet 1:405, 1956.

76. Chasler CN: Pneumothorax and pneumomediastinum in the newborn. Am J Roentgenol 91:550, 1964.

77. Bodey GP: Medical mediastinal emphysema. Ann Intern Med 54:46, 1961.

78. Cyrlak D, Milne EN, Imray TJ: Pneumomediastinum: A diagnostic problem. CRC Crit Rev Diagn Imaging 23(1):75–117, 1984.

79. Macklin MT, Macklin CC: Malignant interstitial emphysema of the lungs and mediastinum as an important occult complication in many respiratory diseases and other conditions. An interpretation of the clinical literature in the light of laboratory experiment. Medicine 23:281, 1944.

80. Macklin CC: Pneumothorax with massive collapse from experimental local overinflation of the lung substance. Can Med Assoc J 36:414, 1937.

81. Caldwell EJ, Powell RD Jr Mullooly JP: Interstitial emphysema: A study of physiologic factors involved in the experimental induction of the lesion. Am Rev Respir Dis 102:516, 1970.

82. Rudhe U, Ozonoff MB: Pneumomediastinum and pneumothorax in the newborn. Acta Radiol (Diagn) 4:193, 1966.

83. Millard CE: Pneumomediastinum. Dis Chest 56:297, 1969.

84. Grieve NWT, Bird DRH, Collyer AJ, et al: Pneumomediastinum and diabetic hyperpnoea. Br Med J 1:186, 1969.

85. McNicholl B, Murray JP, Egan B, Pneumomediastinum and diabetic hyperpnoea. Br Med J 4:493, 1968.

86. Wilson RE: Personal communication, 1969.

87. Gilmartin D: Mediastinal emphysema in Melbourne children: With particular reference to measles and giant-cell pneumonia. Australas Radiol 15:27, 1971.

88. Yalaburgi SB: Subcutaneous and mediastinal emphysema following respiratory tract complications in measles. S Afr Med J 58:521, 1980.

89. Gapany-Gapanavicius M, Yellin A, Almog S, et al: Pneumomediastinum: A complication of chlorine exposure from mixing household cleaning agents. JAMA 248:349, 1982.

90. Hill G, Helenglass G, Powles R, et al: Mediastinal emphysema in marrow transplant recipients. Bone Marrow Transplant 2:315, 1987.

91. Munsell WP: Pneumomediastinum: A report of 28 cases and review of the literature. JAMA 202:689, 1967.

92. Morgan EJ, Henderson DA: Pneumomediastinum as a complication of athletic competition. Thorax 36:155, 1981.

93. Varkey B, Kory RC: Mediastinal and subcutaneous emphysema following pulmonary function tests. Am. Rev Respir Dis 108:1393, 1973.

94. Karson EM, Saltzman D, Davis MR: Pneumomediastinum in pregnancy: Two case reports and a review of the literature, pathophysiology, and management. Obstet Gynecol 64(3 Suppl):395, 1984.

95. Dudley DK, Patten DE: Intrapartum pneumomediastinum associated with subcutaneous emphysema. Can Med Assoc J 139:641, 1988.

96. Miller WE, Spiekerman RE, Hepper NG: Pneumomediastinum resulting from performing Valsalva maneuvers during marihuana smoking. Chest 62:233, 1972.

97. Kirsh MM, Orvald TO: Mediastinal and subcutaneous emphysema complicating acute bronchial asthma. Chest 57:580, 1970.

98. Payne TW, Geppert LJ: Mediastinal and subcutaneous emphysema complicating bronchial asthma in a nine-year-old male. J Allergy 32:135, 1961.

99. Dines DE, Peters GA: Mediastinal emphysema complicating acute asthma—Report of two cases. Minn Med 50:341, 1967.

100. Gittelson G, Altman DH: Pneumomediastinum as a complication of acute bronchial asthma. J Fla Med Assoc 52:318, 1965.

101. Dattwyler RJ, Goldman MA, Bloch KJ: Pneumomediastinum as a complication of asthma in teenage and young adult patients. J Allergy Clin Immunol 63:412, 1979.

102. Beigelman PM, Miller LV, Martin HE: Mediastinal and subcutaneous emphysema in diabetic coma with vomiting, report of four cases. JAMA 208:2315, 1969.

103. Tashima CK, Reyes CV, Kerlow A: Letters to the editor. JAMA 209:1720, 1969.

104. Girard DE, Carlson V, Natelson EA, et al: Pneumomediastinum in diabetic ketoacidosis: Comments on mechanism, incidence, and management. Chest 60:455, 1971.

105. Ruttley M, Mills RA: Subcutaneous emphysema and pneumomediastinum in diabetic ketoacidosis. Br J Radiol 44:672, 1971.

106. Rohlfing BM, Webb WR, Schlobohm RM: Ventilator-related extraalveolar air in adults. Radiology 121:25, 1976.

107. Altman AR, Johnson TH: Pneumoperitoneum and pneumoretroperitoneum. Consequences of positive end-expiratory pressure therapy. Arch Surg 114:208, 1979.

108. Norman JC, Rizzolo PJ: Subcutaneous, mediastinal and probable subpericardial emphysema treated with recompression. N Engl J Med 261:269, 1959.

109. Darch GH: Tracheal neoplasms presenting with mediastinal emphysema. Br J Dis Chest 56:212, 1962.

110. Tomsick TA: Dental surgical subcutaneous and mediastinal emphysema: A case report. J Can Assoc Radiol 25:49, 1974.

111. Sandler CM, Libshitz HI, Marks G: Pneumoperitoneum, pneumomediastinum and pneumopericardium following dental extraction. Radiology 115:539, 1975.

112. Thorsøe H: Mediastinal emphysema due to perforation of the intestinal tract. Nord Med 59:286, 1958.

113. Stahl JD, Goldman SM, Minkin SD, et al: Perforated duodenal ulcer and pneumomediastinum. Radiology 124:23, 1977.

114. Campbell RE, Boggs TR, Jr, Kirkpatrick JA: Early neonatal pneumoperitoneum from progressive massive tension pneumomediastinum. Radiology 114:121, 1975.

115. Kleinman PK, Brill PW, Whalen JP: Anterior pathway for transdiaphragmatic extension of pneumomediastinum. Am J Roentgenol 131:271, 1978.

116. Halíček F and Rosai J: Histioeosinophilic granulomas in the thymuses of 29 myasthenic patients. A complication of pneumomediastinum. Hum Pathol 15:1137, 1984.

117. Landay MJ, Cohen DJ, Deaton CW Jr: Another look at the "ring-around-the-artery" in pneumomediastinum. J Can Assoc Radiol 36:343, 1985.

118. Friedman AC, Lautin EM, Rothenberg L: Mach bands and pneumomediastinum. J Can Assoc Radiol 32:232, 1981.

119. Felson B: The mediastinum. Semin Roentgenol 4:40, 1969.

120. Levin B: The continuous diaphragm sign. A newly recognized sign of pneumomediastinum. Clin Radiol 24:337, 1973.

121. Fletcher BD, Outerbridge EW, Dunbar JS: Pulmonary interstitial emphysema in the newborn. J Can Assoc Radiol 21:273, 1970.

122. Campbell RE: Intrapulmonary interstitial emphysema: A complication of hyaline membrane disease. Am J Roentgenol 110:449, 1970.

123. Macpherson RI, Chernick V, Reed M: The complications of respirator therapy in the newborn. J Can Assoc Radiol 23:91, 1972.

124. Magilner AD, Capitanio MA, Wertheimer I, et al: Persistent localized intrapulmonary interstitial emphysema: An observation in three infants. Radiology 111:379, 1974.

125. Swischuk LE: Bubbles in hyaline membrane disease. Differentiation of three types. Radiology 122:417, 1977.

126. Ransome-Kuti O, Veiga-Pires JA, Audu IS: Mediastinal emphysema in infants. Clin Radiol 19:47, 1968.

127. Cooley JC, Gillespie JB: Mediastinal emphysema: Pathogenesis and management. Report of a case. Dis Chest 49:104, 1966.

128. Becker AH, Sablay BA: Mediastinal emphysema. Clin Pediatr 3:335, 1964.

129. Laforet EG: Traumatic hemomediastinum. J Thorac Surg 29:597, 1955.

130. Coté J, Hodgson CH, Ellis FH Jr: Traumatic mediastinal hematoma: Report of unusual case. Mayo Clin Proc 34:264, 1959.

131. Strax TE, Ryvicker MJ, Elguezabal A: Superior vena caval syndrome due to a mediastinal hematoma secondary to dissecting aortic aneurysm. Dis Chest 55:338, 1969.

132. Raphael MJ: Mediastinal haematoma. A description of some radiological appearances. Br J Radiol 36:921, 1963.

133. Singh S, Ptacin MJ, Bamrah VS: Spontaneous mediastinal hemorrhage. A complication of intracoronary streptokinase infusion for coronary thrombosis. Arch Intern Med 143:562, 1983.

134. Leigh TF: Mass lesions of the mediastinum. Radiol Clin North Am 1:377, 1963.

135. Cohen G: Traumatic haemomediastinum: A case report. S Afr Med J 32:298, 1958.

136. Panicek DM, Ewing DK, Markarian B, et al: Interstitial pulmonary hemorrhage from mediastinal hematoma secondary to aortic rupture. Radiology 162(1 Pt 1):165, 1987.

137. Kucich VA, Vogelzang RL, Hartz RS, et al: Ruptured thoracic aneurysm: Unusual manifestation and early diagnosis using CT. Radiology 160:87, 1986.

138. Jivani SKM, Mann JR: Haemomediastinum in a haemophiliac after minor trauma. Thorax 25:372, 1970.

139. Feigin DS, Padua EM: Mediastinal masses: A system for diagnosis based on computed tomography. CT: J Comput Tomogr 10:11, 1986.

140. Wychulis AR, Payne WS, Clagett OT, et al: Surgical treatment of mediastinal tumors. A 40-year experience. J Thorac Cardiovasc Surg 62:379, 1971.

141. Derra E, Imer W: Über mittelfellgeschwülste, ihre klinik und therapie. (Clinical features and treatment of mediastinal tumors.) Deutsch Med Wochenschr 86:569, 1961.

142. Daniel RA Jr, Diveley WL, Edwards WH, et al: Mediastinal tumors. Ann Surg 151:783, 1960.

143. Hodge J, Aponte G, McLaughlin E: Primary mediastinal tumors. J Thorac Surg 37:730, 1959.

144. Joseph WL, Murray JF, Mulder DG: Mediastinal tumors—Problems in diagnosis and treatment. Dis Chest 50:150, 1966.

145. Al-Naaman YD, Al-Ani MS, Al-Omeri MM: Primary mediastinal tumours. Thorax 29:475, 1974.

146. Benjamin SP, McCormack LJ, Effler DB, et al: Critical review—"Primary tumours of the mediastinum." Chest 62:297, 1972.

147. Boyd DP, Midell AI: Mediastinal cysts and tumors. An analysis of 86 cases. Surg Clin North Am 48:493, 1968.

148. Sabiston DC Jr, Spencer FC: Gibbon's Surgery of the Chest. Philadelphia, WB Saunders, 1976.

149. Hallgrimsson JG: Primary mediastinal tumors in Iceland. Thorax 27:468, 1972.

150. Lyons HA, Calvy GL, Sammons BP: The diagnosis and classification of mediastinal masses. I. A Study of 782 cases. Ann Intern Med 51:897, 1959.

151. Streete BG, Thomas DE: Mediastinal masses. Analysis of seventy-two surgical cases. AMA Arch Surg 77:105, 1958.

152. Leigh TF, Weens HS: The Mediastinum. Springfield, Ill, Charles C Thomas, 1959.

153. Balcom RJ, Hakanson DO, Werner A, et al: Massive thymic hyperplasia in an infant with Beckwith-Wiedemann syndrome. Arch Pathol Lab Med 109:153, 1985.

154. Judd RL: Massive thymic hyperplasia with myoid cell differentiation. Hum Pathol 18:1180, 1987.

155. Carmosino L, DiBenedetto A, Feffer S: Thymic hyperplasia following successful chemotherapy. Cancer 56:1526, 1985.

156. Shin MS, Ho K-J: Diffuse thymic hyperplasia following chemotherapy for nodular sclerosing Hodgkin's disease. Cancer 51:30, 1983.

157. Levine GD, Rosai J: Thymic hyperplasia and neoplasia: A review of current concepts. Hum Pathol 9:495, 1978.

158. Düe W, Dieckmann K-P, Stein H: Thymic hyperplasia following chemotherapy of a testicular germ cell tumor. Immunohistological evidence for a simple rebound phenomenon. Cancer 63:446, 1989.

159. Choyke PL, Zeman RK, Gootenberg JE, et al: Thymic atrophy and regrowth in response to chemotherapy: CT evaluation. Am J Roentgenol 149:269, 1987.

160. Kissin CM, Husband JE, Nicholas D, et al: Benign thymic enlargement in adults after chemotherapy: CT demonstration. Radiology 163:67, 1987.

161. Rosai J, Levine GD, Atlas of Tumor Pathology: Tumors of the Thymus. Second Series, Fascicle 13. Washington DC, Armed Forces Institute of Pathology, 1976.

162. Clark RE, Marbarger JP, West PN, et al: Thymectomy for myasthenia gravis in the young adult: Long-term results. J Thorac Cardiovasc Surg 80:696, 1980.

163. Teplick JG, Nedwich A, Haskin ME: Roentgenographic features of thymolipoma. Am J Roentgenol 117:873, 1973.

164. Levine S, Labiche H, Chandor S: Thymolipoma. Am Rev Respir Dis 98:875, 1968.

165. Yeh H-C, Gordon A, Kirschner PA, et al: Computed tomography and sonography of thymolipoma. Am J Roentgenol 140:1131, 1983.

166. Reintgen D, Fetter BF, Roses A, et al: Thymolipoma in association with myasthenia gravis. Arch Pathol Lab Med 102:463, 1978.

167. Otto HF, Löning T, Lachenmayer L, et al: Thymolipoma in association with myasthenia gravis. Cancer 50:1623, 1982.

168. Barnes RDS, O'Gorman P: Two cases of aplastic anaemia associated with tumours of the thymus. J Clin Pathol 15:264, 1962.

169. Havlíček F, Rosai J: A sarcoma of thymic stroma with features of liposarcoma. Am J Clin Pathol 82:217, 1984.

170. McCafferty MH, Bahnson HT: Thymic cyst extending into the pericardium: A case report and review of thymic cysts. Ann Thorac Surg 33:503, 1982.

171. Indeglia RA, Shea MA, Grage TB: Congenital cysts of the thymus gland. Arch Surg 94:149, 1967.

172. Bieger RC, McAdams AJ: Thymic cysts. Arch Pathol 82:535, 1966.

173. Jaramillo D, Perez-Atayde A, Griscom NT: Apparent association between thymic cysts and prior thoracotomy. Radiology 172:207, 1989.

174. Soorae AS, Stevenson HM: Cystic thymoma simulating pulmonary stenosis. Br J Dis Chest 74:193, 1980.

175. Smith PLC, Jobling C, Rees A: Hodgkin's disease in a large thymic cyst in a child. Thorax 38:392, 1983.

176. Leong AS-Y, Brown JH: Malignant transformation in a thymic cyst. Am J Surg Pathol 8:471, 1984.

177. Jessurun J, Azevedo M, Saldana M: Allergic angiitis and granulomatosis (Churg-Strauss syndrome): Report of a case with massive thymic involvement in a nonasthmatic patient. Hum Pathol 17:637, 1986.

178. Duprez A, Cordier R, Schmitz P: Tuberculoma of the thymus. First case of surgical excision. J Thorac Cardiovasc Surg 44:445, 1962.

179. Siegal GP, Dehner LP, Rosai J: Histiocytosis X (Langerhans' cell granulomatosis) of the thymus. A clinicopathologic study of four childhood cases. Am J Surg Pathol 9:117, 1985.

180. Harpaz N, Gribetz AR, Krellenstein DJ, et al: Inflammatory pseudotumor of the thymus. Ann Thorac Surg 42:331, 1986.

181. Keller AR, Castleman B: Hodgkin's diseases of the thymus gland. Cancer 33:1615, 1974.

182. Ingels GW, Campbell DC, Giampetro AM, et al: Malignant schwannomas of the mediastinum. Cancer 27:1190, 1971.

183. Bergh NP, Gatzinsky P, Larsson S, et al: Tumors of the thymus and thymic region: I. Clinicopathological studies on thymomas. Ann Thorac Surg 25:91, 1978.

184. Verley JM, Hollmann KH: Thymoma. A comparative study of clinical stages, histologic features, and survival in 200 cases. Cancer 55:1074, 1985.

185. Maggi G, Giaccone G, Donadio M, et al: Thymomas. A review of 169 cases, with particular reference to results of surgical treatment. Cancer 58:765, 1986.

186. Lewis JE, Wick MR, Scheithauer BW, et al: Thymoma. A clinicopathologic review. Cancer 60:2727, 1987.

187. Hofmann W, Möller P, Manke H-G, et al: Thymoma. A clinicopathologic study of 98 cases with special reference to three unusual cases. Pathol Res Pract 179:337, 1985.

188. Furman WL, Buckley PJ, Green AA, et al: Thymoma and myasthenia gravis in a 4-year-old child. Cancer 56:2703, 1985.

189. McGuire LJ, Huang DP, Teoh R, et al: Epstein-Barr virus genome in thymoma and thymic lymphoid hyperplasia. Am J Pathol 131:385, 1988.

190. Cooper GN Jr, Narodick BG: Posterior mediastinal thymoma. Case report. J Thorac Cardiovasc Surg 63:561, 1972.

191. Marino M, Müller-Hermelink HK: Thymoma and thymic carcinoma. Relation of thymoma epithelial cells to the cortical and medullary differentiation of thymus. Virchows Arch (Pathol Anat) 407:119, 1985.

192. Lee D, Wright DH: Immunohistochemical study of 22 cases of thymoma. J Clin Pathol 41:1297, 1988.

193. Salter DM, Krajewski AS: Metastatic thymoma: A case report and immunohistological analysis. J Clin Pathol 39:275, 1986.

194. Baron RL, Lee JKT, Sagel SS, et al: Computed tomography of the normal thymus. Radiology 142:121, 1982.

195. Heiberg E, Wolverson JK, Sundaram M, et al: Normal thymus: CT characteristics in subjects under age 20. Am J Roentgenol 138:491, 1982.

196. Leigh TF, Weens HS: Roentgen aspects of mediastinal lesions. Semin Roentgenol 4:59, 1969.

197. Schluger J, Scarpa WJ, Rosenblum DJ, et al: Thymic cyst simulating massive cardiomegaly. Report of a case and review of the literature. Dis Chest 53:365, 1968.

198. Almog Ch, Weissberg D, Herczeg E, et al: Thymolipoma simulating cardiomegaly: A clinicopathological rarity. Thorax 32:116, 1977.

199. Greipp PR, Gau GT, Dockerty MB, et al: Thymic cyst presenting as an acute mediastinal mass. Chest 64:125, 1973.

200. Brown LR, Muhm JR, Gray JE: Radiographic detection of thymoma. Am J Roentgenol 134:1181, 1980.

201. Dixon AK, Hilton CJ, Williams GT: Computed tomography and histological correlation of the thymic remnant. Clin Radiol 32:255, 1981.

19

202. Machida K, Tasaka A, Yoshitake T: Computed tomography in the evaluation of benign and malignant thymoma. Nippon J Tomogr 9(2):56, 1982.
203. Baron RL, Lee JKT, Sagel SS, et al: Computed tomography of the abnormal thymus. Radiology 142:127, 1982.
204. Smith SH, Shin MS, Tishler JM, et al: Computed tomography of invasive thymoma. Comput Radiol 7:189, 1983.
205. Mink JH, Bein ME, Sukov R, et al: Computed tomography of the anterior mediastinum in patients with myasthenia gravis and suspected thymoma. Am J Roentgenol 130:239, 1978.
206. Fon GT, Bein ME, Mancuso AA, et al: Computed tomography of the anterior mediastinum in myasthenia gravis. A radiologic-pathologic correlative study. Radiology 142:135, 1982.
207. Moore AV, Korobkin M, Powers B, et al: Thymoma detection by mediastinal CT: Patients with myasthenia gravis. Am J Roentgenol 138:217, 1982.
208. Brown LR, Muhm JR, Sheedy PF II, et al: The value of computed tomography in myasthenia gravis. Am J Roentgenol 140:31, 1983.
209. Ellis K, Austin JHM, Ill AJ: Radiologic detection of thymoma in patients with myasthenia gravis. Am J Roentgenol 151:873, 1988.
210. Seybold WD, McDonald JR, Clagett OT, et al: Tumors of the thymus. J Thorac Surg 20:195, 1950.
211. Bertelsen S, Malmstrøm J, Heerfordt J, et al: Tumours of the thymic region. Thorax 30:19, 1975.
212. Rosenthal T, Hertz M, Samra Y, et al: Thymoma: Clinical and additional radiologic signs. Chest 65:428, 1974.
213. Bailey RO, Dunn HG, Rubin AM, et al: Myasthenia gravis with thymoma and pure red blood cell aplasia. Am J Clin Pathol 89:687, 1988.
214. Asamura H, Nakajima T, Mukai K, et al: Degree of malignancy of thymic epithelial tumors in terms of nuclear DNA content and nuclear area. An analysis of 39 cases. Am J Pathol 133:615, 1988.
215. Nomori H, Horinouchi H, Kaseda S, et al: Evaluation of the malignant grade of thymoma by morphometric analysis. Cancer 61:982, 1988.
216. Nomori H, Ishihara T, Torikata C: Malignant grading of cortical and medullary differentiated thymoma by morphometric analysis. Cancer 64:1694, 1989.
217. Kornsstein MJ, Curran WJ Jr, Turrisi AT, et al: Cortical versus medullary thymomas: A useful morphologic distinction? Hum Pathol 19:1335, 1988.
218. Nickels J, Franssila K: Thymoma metastasizing to extrathoracic sites. Acta Pathol Microbiol Scand Sect A 84:331, 1976.
219. Scatarige JC, Fishman EK, Zerhouni EA, et al: Transdiaphragmatic extension of invasive thymoma. Am J Roentgenol 144:31, 1985.
220. Rosai J, Levine G, Weber WR, et al: Carcinoid tumors and oat cell carcinomas of the thymus. Pathol Ann 11:201, 1976.
221. Viebahn R, Hiddemann W, Klinke F, et al: Thymus carcinoid. Pathol Res Pract 180:445, 1985.
222. Wick MR, Bernatz PE, Carney JA, et al: Primary mediastinal carcinoid tumors. Am J Surg Pathol 6:195, 1982.
223. Herbst WM, Kummer W, Hofmann W, et al: Carcinoid tumors of the thymus. An immunohistochemical study. Cancer 60:2465, 1987.
224. Wick MR, Scheithauer BW, Kovacs K: Neuron-specific enolase in neuroendocrine tumors of the thymus, bronchus, and skin. Am J Clin Pathol 79:703, 1983.
225. Wick MR, Scheithauer BW: Oat-cell carcinoma of the thymus. Cancer 49:1652, 1982.
226. Wick MR, Weiland LH, Scheithauer BW, et al: Primary thymic carcinomas. Am J Surg Pathol 6:613, 1982.
227. Snover DC, Levine GD, Rosai J: Thymic carcinoma. Five distinctive histological variants. Am J Surg Pathol 6:451, 1982.
228. Felson B, Castleman B, Levinsohn EM, et al: Cushing syndrome associated with mediastinal mass. Radiologic-pathologic correlation conference. SUNY Upstate Medical Center. Am J Roentgenol 138:815, 1982.
229. Brown LR, Aughenbaugh GL, Wick MR, et al: Roentgenologic diagnosis of primary corticotropin-producing carcinoid tumors of the mediastinum. Radiology 142:143, 1982.
230. Hughes JP, Ancalmo N, Leonard GL, et al: Carcinoid tumour of the thymus gland: Report of a case. Thorax 30:470, 1975.
231. Lowenthal RM, Gumpel JM, Kreel L, et al: Carcinoid tumour of the thymus with systemic manifestations: A radiological and pathological study. Thorax 29:553, 1974.
232. Birnberg FA, Webb WR, Selch MT, et al: Thymic carcinoid tumors with hyperparathyroidism. Am J Roentgenol 139:1001, 1982.
233. Rosai J, Higa E, Davie J: Mediastinal endocrine neoplasm in patients with multiple endocrine adenomatosis. Cancer 29:1075, 1971.
234. Herezea E, Kahn LB: Primary thymic carcinoma. An unusual case originating in a lymphocytic rich thymoma. Virchows Arch (Pathol Anat) 409:163, 1986.
235. Ibrahim NBN, Briggs JC, Jeyasingham K, et al: Metastasizing thymoma. Thorax 37:771, 1982.
236. Keller AR, Castleman B: Hodgkin's disease of the thymus gland. Cancer 33:1615, 1974.
237. Kim HC, Nosher J, Haas A, et al: Cystic degeneration of thymic Hodgkin's disease following radiation therapy. Cancer 55:354, 1985.
238. Yousem SA, Weiss LM, Warnke RA: Primary mediastinal non-Hodgkin's lymphomas: A morphologic and immunologic study of 19 cases. Am J Clin Pathol 83:676, 1985.
239. Suematsu N, Watanabe S, Shimosato Y: A Case of large "thymic granuloma." Neoplasm of T-zone histiocyte. Cancer 54:2480, 1984.
240. Szporn AH, Dikman S, Jagirdar J: True histiocytic lymphoma of the thymus. Report of a case and a study of the distribution of histiocytic cells in the fetal and adult thymus. Am J Clin Pathol 82:734, 1984.
241. Lamarre L, Jacobson JO, Aisenberg AC, et al: Primary large cell lymphoma of the mediastinum. A histologic and immunophenotypic study of 29 cases. Am J Surg Pathol 13(9):730, 1989.
242. Luna MA, Valenzuela-Tamariz J: Germ-cell tumors of the mediastinum, postmortem findings. Am J Clin Pathol 65:450, 1976.
243. Knapp RH, Hurt RD, Payne WS, et al: Malignant germ cell tumors of the mediastinum. J Thorac Cardiovasc Surg 89:82, 1985.
244. Yurick BS, Ottoman RE: Primary mediastinal choriocarcinoma. Radiology 75:901, 1960.
245. Steinmetz WH, Hays RA: Primary seminoma of the mediastinum. Report of a case with an unusual site of metastasis and review of the literature. Am J Roentgenol 86:669, 1961.
246. Wenger ME, Dines DE, Ahmann DL, et al: Primary mediastinal choriocarcinoma. Mayo Clin Proc 43:570, 1968.
247. Aliotta PJ, Castillo J, Englander LS, et al: Primary mediastinal germ cell tumors. Histologic patterns of treatment failures at autopsy. Cancer 62:982, 1988.
248. Sandhaus L, Strom RL, Mukai K: Primary embryonal-choriocarcinoma of the mediastinum in a woman. A case report with immunohistochemical study. Am J Clin Pathol 75:573, 1981.
249. Knapp RH, Fritz SR, Reiman HM: Primary embryonal carcinoma and choriocarcinoma of the mediastinum. Arch Pathol Lab Med 106:507, 1982.
250. Lachman MF, Kim K, Koo B-C: Mediastinal teratoma associated with Klinefelter's syndrome. Arch Pathol Lab Med 110:1067, 1986.
251. Sogge MR, McDonald SD, Cofard PB: The malignant potential of the dysgenetic germ cell in Klinefelter's syndrome. Am J Med 66:515, 1979.
252. McNeil MM, Leong A S-Y, Sage RE: Primary mediastinal embryonal carcinoma in association with Klinefelter's syndrome. Cancer 47:343, 1981.
253. Richardson RL, Schoumacher BS, Fer MF, et al: The unrecognized extragonadal germ cell cancer syndrome. Ann Intern Med 94:181, 1981.
254. Lee KS, Im J-G, Han CH, et al: Malignant primary germ cell tumors of the mediastinum: CT features. Am J Roentgenol 153:947, 1989.
255. Templeton AW: Malignant mediastinal teratoma with bone metastases. A case report. Radiology 76:245, 1961.
256. Schlumberger HG: Teratoma of the anterior mediastinum in the group of military age. Arch Pathol 41:398, 1946.
257. Inada K, Nakano A: Structure and genesis of the mediastinal teratoma. AMA Arch Pathol 66:183, 1958.
258. Pachter MR, Lattes R: "Germinal" tumors of the mediastinum: A clinicopathologic study of adult teratomas, teratocarcinomas, choriocarcinomas and seminomas. Dis Chest 45:301, 1964.
259. Bordi C, De Viia O, Pollice L: Full pancreatic endocrine differentiation in a mediastinal teratoma. Hum Pathol 16:961, 1985.
260. Dunn PJS: Pancreatic endocrine tissue in benign mediastinal teratoma. J Clin Pathol 37:1105, 1984.
261. Carter D, Bibro M, Touloukian RJ: Benign clinical behavior of immature mediastinal teratoma in infancy and childhood: Report of two cases and review of the literature. Cancer 49:398, 1982.
262. Harms D, Jänig U: Immature teratomas of childhood. Report of 21 cases. Pathol Res Pract 179:388, 1985.
263. Ulbright TM, Loehrer PJ, Roth LM, et al: The development of non-germ cell malignancies within germ cell tumors. Cancer 54:1824, 1984.
264. Manivel C, Wick, MR, Abenoza P, et al: The occurrence of sarcomatous components in primary mediastinal germ cell tumors. Am J Surg Pathol 10:711, 1986.
265. Ochsner JL, Ochsner SF: Congenital cysts of the mediastinum: 20-year experience with 42 cases. Ann Surg 163:909, 1966.
266. Weinberg JM, Rose JS, Stavros C, et al: Posterior mediastinal teratoma (cystic dermoid): Diagnosis by computerized tomography. Chest 77:694, 1980.
267. Friedman AC, Pyatt RS, Hartman DS, et al: CT of benign cystic teratomas. Am J Roentgenol 138:659, 1982.
268. Hirshaut Y, Reagan RL, Perry S, et al: The search for a viral agent in Hodgkin's disease. Cancer 34:1080, 1974.
269. Chiba T, Suzuki H, Hebiguchi T, et al: Gastric teratoma extending into the mediastinum. J Pediatr Surg 15:191, 1980.

270. Rusby NL: Dermoid cysts and teratomata of the mediastinum. A review. J Thorac Surg 13:169, 1944.
271. Clagett OT, Woolner LB: Clinicopathologic Conference—Recurrent chest infection in a teen-ager. Mayo Clin Proc 43:134, 1968.
272. Marshall ME, Trump DL: Acquired extrinsic pulmonic stenosis caused by mediastinal tumors. Cancer 49:1496, 1982.
273. Southgate J, Slade PR: Teratodermoid cyst of the mediastinum with pancreatic enzyme secretion. Thorax 37:476, 1982.
274. Sommerlad BC, Cleland WP, Yong NK: Physiological activity in mediastinal teratomata. Thorax 30:510, 1975.
275. Suda K, Mizuguchi K, Hebisawa A, et al: Pancreatic tissue in teratoma. Arch Pathol Lab Med 108:835, 1984.
276. Honicky RE, dePapp EW: Mediastinal teratoma with endocrine function. Am J Dis Child 126:650, 1973.
277. Landanyi M, Roy I: Mediastinal germ cell tumors and histiocytosis. Hum Pathol 19:586, 1988.
278. DeMent SH, Eggleston JC, Spivak JL: Association between mediastinal germ cell tumors and hematologic malignancies. Report of two cases and review of the literature. Am J Surg Pathol 9:23, 1985.
279. Larsen M, Evans WK, Shepherd FA, et al: Acute lymphoblastic leukemia. Possible origin from a mediastinal germ cell tumor. Cancer 53:441, 1984.
280. Polansky SM, Barwick KW, Ravin CE: Primary mediastinal seminoma. Am J Roentgenol 132:17, 1979.
281. Burns, BF McCaughey WTE: Unusual thymic seminomas. Arch Pathol Lab Med 110:539, 1986.
282. Levine GD: Primary thymic seminoma—A neoplasm ultrastructurally similar to testicular seminoma and distinct from epithelial thymoma. Cancer 31:729, 1973.
283. Hochholzer L, Theros EG, Rosen SH: Some unusual lesions of the mediastinum: Roentgenologic and pathologic features. Semin Roentgenol 4:74, 1969.
284. Shin MS, Ho KJ: Computed tomography of primary mediastinal seminomas. J Comput Assist Tomogr 7:990, 1983.
285. Vogelzang NJ, Raghavan D, Anderson RW, et al: Mediastinal nonseminomatous germ cell tumors: The role of combined modality therapy.
286. Economou JS, Trump DL, Holmes EC, et al: Management of primary germ cell tumors of the mediastinum. J Thorac Cardiovasc Surg 83:643, 1982.
287. Hurt RD, Bruckman JE, Farrow GM, et al: Primary anterior mediastinal seminoma. Cancer 49:1658, 1982.
288. Raghavan D, Barrett A: Mediastinal seminomas. Cancer 46:1187, 1980.
289. Truong LD, Harris L, Mattioli C, et al: Endodermal sinus tumor of the mediastinum. A report of seven cases and review of the literature. Cancer 58:730, 1986.
290. Mukai K, Adams WR: Yolk sac tumor of the anterior mediastinum. Case report with light- and electron-microscopic examination and immunohistochemical study of alpha-fetoprotein. Am J Surg Pathol 3:77, 1979.
291. Kuzur ME, Cobleigh MA, Greco A, et al: Endodermal sinus tumor of the mediastinum. Cancer 50:766, 1982.
292. Rusch VW, Logothetis C, Samuels M: Endodermal sinus tumor of the mediastinum. Report of apparent cure in two patients with extensive disease. Chest 86:745, 1984.
293. Sham JST, Fu KH, Chiu CSW, et al: Experience with the management of primary endodermal sinus tumor of the mediastinum. Cancer 64:756, 1989.
294. Fine G, Smith RW Jr, Pachter MR: Primary extragenital choriocarcinoma in the male subject. Case report and review of the literature. Am J Med 32:776, 1962.
295. Cohen BA, Needle MA: Primary mediastinal choriocarcinoma in a man. Chest 67:106, 1975.
296. Leading article. Primary mediastinal choriocarcinoma. Br Med J 2:135, 1969.
297. Crile G Jr: Intrathoracic goiter. Cleve Clin Q 6:313, 1939.
298. Lahey FH: Intrathoracic goiters. Surg Clin North Am 25:609, 1945.
299. Nielsen VM, Løvgreen NA, Elbrønd O: Intrathoracic goitre. Surgical treatment in an ENT department. J Laryngol Otol 97:1039, 1983.
300. Katlic MR, Wang C, Grillo HC: Substernal goiter. Ann Thorac Surg 39:391, 1985.
301. Karadeniz A, Hacihanefioglu U: Abscess formation in an intrathoracic goiter. Thorax 37:556, 1982.
302. Irwin RS, Pratter MR, Hamolsky MW: Chronic persistent cough: An uncommon presenting complaint of thyroiditis. Chest 81:386, 1982.
303. Ward MJ, Davies D: Riedel's thyroiditis with invasion of the lungs. Thorax 36:956, 1981.
304. Dontas NS: Intrathoracic goitre. Br J Tuberc 52:154, 1958.
305. Rietz K-A, Werner B: Intrathoracic goiter. Acta Chir Scand 119:379, 1960.
306. Fragomeni LS, Ceratti de Zambuja P: Intrathoracic goitre in the posterior mediastinum. Thorax 35:638, 1980.
307. Meijer S, Hoitsma FW: Malignant intrathoracic oncocytoma. Cancer 49:97, 1982.
308. Glazer GM, Axel L, Moss AA: CT diagnosis of mediastinal thyroid. Am J Roentgenol 138:495, 1982.
309. Bashist B, Ellis K, Gold RP: Computed tomography of intrathoracic goiters. Am J Roentgenol 140:455, 1983.
310. Binder RE, Pugatch RD, Faling LJ, et al: Diagnosis of posterior mediastinal goiter by computed tomography. Case report. J Comput Assist Tomogr 4:550, 1980.
311. Silverstein GE, Burke G, Goldberg D, et al: Superior vena caval system obstruction caused by benign endothoracic goiter. Dis Chest 56:519, 1969.
312. Hershey CO, McVeigh RC, Miller RP: Transient superior vena cava syndrome due to propylthiouracil therapy in intrathoracic goiter. Chest 79:356, 1981.
313. Owen WJ, Gleeson MJ, McColl I: Thyroid crisis and tracheal compression in patient with retrosternal goitre. Br Med J 2:997, 1978.
314. Samanta A, Jones GR, Burden AC, et al: Thoracic inlet compression due to amiodarone induced goitre. Postgrad Med J 61:249, 1985.
315. Holden MP, Wooler GH, Ionescu MI: Massive retrosternal goitre presenting with hypertension. Thorax 27:772, 1972.
316. Wang C-A: The anatomic basis of parathyroid surgery. Ann Surg 183:271, 1976.
317. Hardy JD, Snaveley JR, Langford HG: Low intrathoracic parathyroid adenoma. Large functioning tumor representing fifth parathyroid, opposite eighth dorsal vertebra with independent arterial supply and opacified at operation with arteriogram. Ann Surg 159:310, 1965.
318. Murphy MN, Glennon PG, Diocee MS, et al: Nonsecretory parathyroid carcinoma of the mediastinum. Light microscopic, immunocytochemical, and ultrastructural features of a case, and review of the literature. Cancer 58:2468, 1986.
319. Lee YT, Hutcheson JK: Mediastinal parathyroid carcinoma detected on routine chest film. Chest 65:354, 1974.
320. Becker FO, Tausk K: Radiologically evident functioning mediastinal parathyroid adenoma. Chest 58:79, 1970.
321. Braxel C, Haemers S, van der Straeten M: Mediastinal parathyroid adenoma detected on a routine chest X-ray. Scand J Respir Dis 60:367, 1979.
322. Hanson DJ Jr: Unusual radiographic manifestations of parathyroid adenoma. Report of a case. N Engl J Med 267:1080, 1962.
323. Krudy AG, Doppman JL, Brennan MF, et al: The detection of mediastinal parathyroid glands by computed tomography, selective arteriography and venous sampling. An analysis of 17 cases. Radiology 140:739, 1981.
324. Krudy AG, Doppman JL, Miller DL, et al: Detection of mediastinal parathyroid glands by nonselective digital arteriography. Am J Roentgenol 142:693, 1984.
325. Adams E, Adams PH, Mamtora H, et al: Computed tomography and the localisation of parathyroid tumours. Clin Radiol 32:251, 1981.
326. Gibbs AR, Johnson NF, Giddings JC, et al: Primary angiosarcoma of the mediastinum: Light and electron microscopic demonstration of factor VIII-related antigen in neoplastic cells. Hum Pathol 15:687, 1984.
327. Pachter MR, Lattes R: Mesenchymal tumors of the mediastinum. I. Tumors of fibrous tissue, adipose tissue, smooth muscle, and striated muscle. Cancer 16:1963.
328. Standerfer RJ, Armistead SH, Paneth M: Liposarcoma of the mediastinum: Report of two cases and review of the literature. Thorax 36:693, 1981.
329. Schweitzer DL, Aguam AS: Primary liposarcoma of the mediastinum. J Thorac Cardiovasc Surg 74:83, 1977.
330. Wilson ES: Radiolucent mediastinal lipoma. Radiology 118:44, 1976.
331. Mendez G Jr, Isikoff MB, Isikoff SK: et al: Fatty tumors of the thorax demonstrated by CT. Am J Roentgenol 133:207, 1979.
332. Drasin GF, Lynch T, Temes GP: Ectopic ACTH production and mediastinal lipomatosis. Radiology 127:610, 1978.
333. Santini LC, Williams JL: Mediastinal widening (presumably lipomatosis) in Cushing's syndrome. N Engl J Med 284:1357, 1971.
334. Price JE, Rigler LG: Widening of the mediastinum resulting from fat accumulation. Radiology 96:497, 1970.
335. Koerner HJ, Sun DI-C: Mediastinal lipomatosis secondary to steroid therapy. Am J Roentgenol 98:461, 1966.
336. Bodman SF, Condemi JJ: Mediastinal widening in iatrogenic Cushing's syndrome. Ann Intern Med 67:399, 1967.
337. Teates CD: Steroid-induced mediastinal lipomatosis. Radiology 96:501, 1970.
338. van de Putte LBA, Wagenaar JPM, San KH: Paracardiac lipomatosis in exogenous Cushing's syndrome. Thorax 28:653, 1973.
339. Lee WJ, Fattal G: Mediastinal lipomatosis in simple obesity. Chest 70:308, 1976.

19

340. Streiter ML, Schneider HJ, Proto AV: Steroid-induced thoracic lipomatosis: Paraspinal involvement. Am J Roentgenol 139:679, 1982.
341. Bein ME, Mancuso AA, Mink JH, et al: Computed tomography in the evaluation of mediastinal lipomatosis. J Comput Assist Tomogr 2:379, 1978.
342. Homer MJ, Wechsler RJ, Carter BL: Mediastinal lipomatosis. CT confirmation of a normal variant. Radiology 128:657, 1978.
343. Chalaoui J, Sylvestre J, Dussault RG, et al: Thoracic fatty lesions: some usual and unusual appearances. J Can Assoc Radiol 32:197, 1981.
344. Cohen AJ, Sbaschnig RJ, Hochholzer L, et al: Mediastinal hemangiomas. Ann Thorac Surg 43:656, 1987.
345. Davis JM, Mark GJ, Greene R: Benign blood vascular tumors of the mediastinum. Radiology 126:581, 1978.
346. Gindhart TD, Tucker WY, Choy SH: Cavernous hemangioma of the superior mediastinum. Report of a case with electron microscopy and computerized tomography. Am J Surg Pathol 3:353, 1979.
347. Pachter MR, Lattes R: Mesenchymal tumors of the mediastinum. II. Tumors of blood vascular origin. Cancer 16:95, 1963.
348. Kings GLM: Multifocal haemangiomatous malformation. A case report. Thorax 30:485, 1975.
349. Leibovici D, Oner V: Hemangioma of the posterior mediastinum. Review of the literature and report of a case. Am Rev Respir Dis 86:415, 1962.
350. Abratt RP, Williams M, Raff M, et al: Angiosarcoma of the superior vena cava. Cancer 52:740, 1983.
351. Feigin GA, Robinson B, Marchevsky A: Mixed tumor of the mediastinum. Arch Pathol Lab Med 110:80, 1986.
352. Khoury GH, Demong CV: Mediastinal cystic hygroma in childhood. J Pediatr 62:432, 1963.
353. Divertie MB, Lim RA, Harrison EG, et al: Mediastinal cystic hygroma: Report of two cases. Mayo Clin Proc 35:460, 1960.
354. Woods D, Young JEM, Filice R, et al: Late-onset cystic hygromas: The role of CT. J Can Assoc Radiol 40:159, 1989.
355. Pachter MR, Lattes R: Mesenchymal tumors of the mediastinum. III. Tumors of lymph vascular origin. Cancer 16:108, 1963.
356. Feng Y-F, Masterson JB, Riddell RH: Lymphangioma of the middle mediastinum as an incidental finding on a chest radiograph. Thorax 35:955, 1980.
357. Pilla TJ, Wolverson MK, Sundaram M, et al: CT evaluation of cystic lymphangiomas of the mediastinum. Radiology 144:841, 1982.
358. Daniel TM, Staub EW, Clark DE: Symptomatic venous compression from a mediastinal cystic lymphangioma. Chest 63:834, 1973.
359. Rasaretnam R, Panabokke RG: Leiomyosarcoma of the mediastinum. Brit J Dis Chest 69:63, 1975.
360. Bernheim J, Griffel B, Versano S, et al: Mediastinal leiomyosarcoma in the wall of a bronchial cyst. Letter to the editor. Arch Pathol Lab Med 104:221, 1980.
361. Sunderrajan EV, Luger AM, Rosenholtz MJ, et al: Leiomyosarcoma in the mediastinum presenting as superior vena cava syndrome. Cancer 53:2553, 1984.
362. Baldwin R, Drigo R, Schiraldi C, et al: Antemortem diagnosis of primary leiomyosarcoma of the pulmonary artery. Respiration 49:307, 1986.
363. Weiss KS, Zidar BL, Wang S, et al: Radiation-induced leiomyosarcoma of the great vessels presenting as superior vena cava syndrome. Cancer 60:1238, 1987.
364. Lloyd RV, Hajdu SI, Knapper WH: Embryonal rhabdomyosarcoma in adults. Cancer 51:557, 1983.
365. Witkin GB, Rosai J: Solitary fibrous tumor of the mediastinum. A report of 14 cases. Am J Surg Pathol 13(7):547, 1989.
366. Laustela E: Mediastinal fibroma. Ann Chir Gynaecol Fenn 48:505, 1959.
367. Natsuaki M, Yoshikawa Y, Itoh T, et al: Xanthogranulomatous malignant fibrous histiocytoma arising from posterior mediastinum. Thorax 41:322, 1986.
368. Chen W, Chan CW, Mok CK: Malignant fibrous histiocytoma of the mediastinum. Cancer 50:797, 1982.
369. Majeski JA, Paxton ES, Wirman JA, et al: A thoracic benign mesenchymoma in association with hemihypertrophy. Am J Clin Pathol 76:827, 1981.
370. Pachter MR: Benign mesenchymoma of the mediastinum. A case with extramedullary hematopoiesis within the tumor and vascular malformations in the lungs. Arch Pathol 74:179, 1962.
371. Greenwood SM, Meschter SC: Extraskeletal osteogenic sarcoma of the mediastinum. Arch Pathol Lab Med 113:430, 1989.
372. Catanese J, Dutcher JP, Dorfman HD, et al: Mediastinal osteosarcoma with extension to lungs in a patient treated for Hodgkin's disease. Cancer 62:2252, 1988.
373. Kubonishi I, Ohtsuki Y, Machida K-I, et al: Granulocytic sarcoma presenting as a mediastinal tumor. Am J Clin Pathol 82:730, 1984.
374. Witkin GB, Miettinen M, Rosai J: A biphasic tumor of the mediastinum with features of synovial sarcoma. A report of four cases. Am J Surg Pathol 13(6):490, 1989.
375. Naschitz JE, Yeshurun D, Pick AI: Intrathoracic amyloid lymphadenopathy. Respiration 49:73, 1986.
376. Shaw P, Grossman R, Fernandes BJ: Nodular mediastinal amyloidosis. Hum Pathol 15:1183, 1984.
377. Azizkhan RG, Dudgeon DL, Buck JR, et al: Life-threatening airway obstruction as a complication in the management of mediastinal masses in children. J Pediatr Surg 20:816, 1985.
378. Marshall ME, Trump DL: Acquired extrinsic pulmonic stenosis caused by mediastinal tumors. Cancer 49:1496, 1982.
379. Waldron JA Jr, Dohring EJ, Farber LR: Primary large cell lymphomas of the mediastinum: An analysis of 20 cases. Semin Diagn Pathol 2:281, 1985.
380. Levitt LJ, Aisenberg AC, Harris NL, et al: Primary non-Hodgkin's lymphoma of the mediastinum. Cancer 50:2486, 1982.
381. Martin JJ: The Nisbet Symposium: Hodgkin's disease. Radiological aspects of the disease. Australas Radiol 11:206, 1967.
382. Fisher AMH, Kendall B, Van Leuven BD: Hodgkin's disease. A radiological survey. Clin Radiol 13:115, 1962.
383. Trump DL, Mann RB: Diffuse large cell and undifferentiated lymphomas with prominent mediastinal involvement. A poor prognostic subset of patients with non-Hodgkin's lymphoma. Cancer 50:277, 1982.
384. Perrone T, Frizzera G, Rosai J: Mediastinal diffuse large-cell lymphoma with sclerosis. A clinicopathologic study of 60 cases. Am J Surg Pathol 10(3):176, 1986.
385. Möller P, Lämmler B, Eberlein-Gonska M, et al: Primary mediastinal clear cell lymphoma of B-cell type. Virchows Arch (Pathol Anat) 409:79, 1986.
386. Menestrina F, Chilosi M, Bonetti F, et al: Mediastinal large-cell lymphoma of B-type, with sclerosis: Histopathological and immunohistochemical study of eight cases. Histopathology 10:589, 1986.
387. Addis BJ, Isaacson PG: Large cell lymphoma of the mediastinum: A B-cell tumour of probable thymic origin. Histopathology 10:379, 1986.
388. Castleman B (ed): Case Records of the Massachusetts General Hospital, Case 40011. N Engl J Med 250:26, 1954.
389. Keller AR, Hochholzer L, Castleman B: Hyaline-vascular and plasma-cell types of giant lymph node hyperplasia of the mediastinum and other locations. Cancer 29:670, 1972.
390. Frizzera G: Castleman's disease: More questions than answers. Hum Pathol 16:202, 1985.
391. Neerhout RC, Larson W, Mansur P: Mesenteric lymphoid hamartoma associated with chronic hypoferremia, anemia, growth failure and hyperglobulinemia. N Engl J Med 280:922, 1969.
392. Maier HC, Sommers SC: Mediastinal lymph node hyperplasia, hypergammaglobulinemia, and anemia. J Thorac Cardiovasc Surg 79:860, 1980.
393. Karcher DS, Pearson CE, Butler WM, et al: Giant lymph node hyperplasia involving the thymus with associated nephrotic syndrome and myelofibrosis. Am J Clin Pathol 77:100, 1982.
394. Yu GSM, Carson JW: Giant lymph-node hyperplasia, plasma-cell type, of the mediastinum, with peripheral neuropathy. Am J Clin Pathol 66:46, 1976.
395. Couch WD: Giant lymph node hyperplasia associated with thrombotic thrombocytopenic purpura. Am J Clin Pathol 74:340, 1980.
396. Weisenburger DD, Nathwani BN, Winberg CD, et al: Multicentric angiofollicular lymph node hyperplasia, Hum Pathol 16:162, 1985.
397. Lowenthal DA, Filippa DA, Richardson ME, et al: Generalized lymphadenopathy with morphologic features of Castleman's disease in an HIV-positive man. Cancer 60:2454, 1987.
398. Bitter MA, Komaiko W, Franklin WA: Giant lymph node hyperplasia with osteoblastic bone lesions and the POEMS (Takatsuki's) syndrome. Cancer 56:188, 1985.
399. Carbone A, Manconi R, Volpe R, et al: Immunohistochemical, enzyme histochemical, and immunologic features of giant lymph node hyperplasia of the hyaline-vascular type. Cancer 58:908, 1986.
400. Culver GJ, Choi BK: Benign lymphoid hyperplasia (Castleman's tumor) mimicking a posterior mediastinal neurogenic tumor. Chest 62:516, 1972.
401. Hammond DI: Giant lymph node hyperplasia of the posterior mediastinum. J Can Assoc Radiol 30:256, 1979.
402. Gibbons JA, Rosencrantz H, Posey DJ, et al: Angiofollicular lymphoid hyperplasia (Castleman's tumor) resembling a pericardial cyst: Differentiation by computerized tomography. Ann Thorac Surg 32:193, 1981.
403. Breatnach E, Myers JD, McElvein RB, et al: Unusual cause of a calcified anterior mediastinal mass. Chest 89:113, 1986.
404. Walter JF, Rottenberg RW, Cannon WB, et al: Giant mediastinal lymph node hyperplasia (Castleman's disease): Angiographic and clinical features. Am J Roentgenol 130:447, 1978.
405. Moersch HJ, Schmidt HW: Broncholithiasis. Ann Otol 68:548, 1959.

406. Storer J, Smith RC: The calcified hilar node: Its significance and management. A review. Am Rev Respir Dis 81:858, 1960.
407. Unfug HV: Vocal cord paralysis from calcified hilar lymph node cured by spontaneous broncholithoptysis. N Engl J Med 272:527, 1965.
408. Glenner GG, Grimley PM: Atlas of Tumor Pathology: Second Series, Fascicle 9. Tumors of the extra-adrenal paraganglion system (including chemoreceptors). Washington, DC, Armed Forces Institute of Pathology, 1974.
409. Lack EE, Stillinger RA, Colvin DB, et al: Aorticopulmonary paraganglioma. Report of a case with ultrastructural study and review of the literature. Cancer 43:269, 1979.
410. Drucker EA, McLoud TC, Dedrick CG, et al: Mediastinal paraganglioma: Radiologic evaluation of an unusual vascular tumor. Am J Roentgenol 148:521, 1987.
411. Sheps SG, Brown ML: Localization of mediastinal paragangliomas (pheochromocytoma). Chest 87:807, 1985.
412. Sanders DE: Asymptomatic resorption of mediastinal cysts: A further report of two cases. J Can Assoc Radiol 20:239, 1969.
413. Modic MT, Janicki PC: Computed tomography of mass lesions of the right cardiophrenic angle. J Comput Assist Tomogr 4:521, 1980.
414. Paling MR, Williamson BRJ: Epipericardial fat pad: CT findings. Radiology 165:335, 1987.
415. Behrendt DM, Scannell JG: Pericardial fat necrosis. An unusual cause of severe chest pain and thoracic "tumor." N Engl J Med 279:473, 1968.
416. Peterson DT, Katz LM, Popp RL: Pericardial cyst 10 years after acute pericarditis. Chest 67:719, 1975.
417. Stoller JK, Shaw C, Matthay RA: Enlarging, atypically located pericardial cyst. Recent experience and literature review. Chest 89:402, 1986.
418. Pader E, Kirschner PA: Pericardial diverticulum. Dis Chest 55:344, 1969.
419. Snyder SN: Massive pericardial coelomic cyst: Diagnostic features and unusual presentation. Chest 71:100, 1977.
420. Pugatch RD, Braver JH, Robbins AH, et al: CT diagnosis of pericardial cysts. Am J Roentgenol 131:515, 1978.
421. Felner JM, Fleming WH, Franch RH: Echocardiographic identification of a pericardial cyst. Chest 68:386, 1975.
422. Rogers CI, Seymour EQ, Brock JG: Atypical pericardial cyst location: The value of computed tomography. Case report. J Comput Assist Tomogr 4:683, 1980.
423. Stoller JK, Shaw C, Matthay RA: Enlarging, atypically located pericardial cyst. Recent experience and literature review. Chest 89:402, 1986.
424. Brunner DR, Whitley NO: A pericardial cyst with high CT numbers. Am J Roentgenol 142:279, 1984.
425. Zhao F, Wang C, Song XL: Calcified pericardial cyst—A case report and the roentgenologic and pathologic differentiation from other calcified mediastinal cysts. J Thorac Cardiovasc Surg 32:193, 1984.
426. Comer TP, Clagett OT: Surgical treatment of hernia of the foramen of Morgagni. J Thorac Cardiovasc Surg 52:461, 1966.
427. Lanuza A: The sign of the cane. A new radiological sign for the diagnosis of small Morgagni hernias. Radiology 101:293, 1971.
428. Paris F, Tarazona V, Casillas M, et al: Hernia of Morgagni. Thorax 28:631, 1973.
429. Cho CS, Blank N, Castellino RA: CT evaluation of cardiophrenic angle lymph nodes in patients with malignant lymphoma. Am J Roentgenol 143:719, 1984.
430. Castellino RA, Blank N: Adenopathy of the cardiophrenic angle (diaphragmatic) lymph nodes. Am J Roentgenol 114:509, 1972.
431. Fayos JV, Lampe I: Cardiac apical mass in Hodgkin's disease. Radiology 99:15, 1971.
432. Buckingham WB, Sutton GC, Meszaros WT: Abnormalities of the pulmonary artery resembling intrathoracic neoplasms. Dis Chest 40:698, 1961.
433. Bock K, Richter H, Trenckmann H, et al: Über die ektasie und das aneurysma der arteria pulmonalis. (Dilatation and aneurysm of the pulmonary artery.) Fortschr Roentgenstr 99:639, 1963.
434. Lucas RV Jr, Lund GW, Edwards JE: Direct communication of a left pulmonary artery with the left atrium. An unusual variant of pulmonary arteriovenous fistula. Circulation 24:1409, 1961.
435. Hoeffel JC, Pernot C, Worms AM, et al: Calcified aneurysm of the main pulmonary artery: A complication of banding. Radiology 113:167, 1974.
436. Shin MS, Ceballos R, Bini RM, et al: CT diagnosis of false aneurysm of the pulmonary artery not demonstrated by angiography. Case report. J Comput Assist Tomogr 7:524, 1983.
437. Befeler, MacLeod CA, Baum GL, et al: Idiopathic dilatation of the pulmonary artery. Am J Med Sci 254:667, 1967.
438. Kumar S, Murthy KV, Brandfonbrener M: Possible mechanism of wide splitting of second sound in idiopathic dilatation of the pulmonary artery. Chest 68:739, 1975.
439. Asayama J, Matsunra T, Endo N, et al: Echocardiographic findings of idiopathic dilatation of pulmonary artery. Chest 71:671, 1977.
440. Drasin E, Sayre RW, Castellino RA: Non-dilated superior vena cava presenting as a superior mediastinal mass. J Can Assoc Radiol 23:273, 1972.
441. Farr JE, Anderson WT, Brundage, BH: Congenital aneurysm of the superior vena cava. Chest 65:566, 1974.
442. Okay NH, Bryk D, Kroop IG: Phlebectasia of the jugular and great mediastinal veins. Radiology 95:6291, 1970.
443. Bell MJ, Gutierrez JR, DuBois JJ: Aneurysm of the superior vena cava. Radiology 95:317, 1970.
444. Hidvegi RS, Modry DL, LaFléche L: Congenital saccular aneurysm of the superior vena cava: Radiographic features. Am J Roentgenol 133:924, 1979.
445. Mok CK, Chan CW, Clarke RT, et al: Coexisting congenital primary superior vena cava aneurysm and rheumatic mitral stenosis. Thorax 36:638, 1981.
446. Modry DL, Hidvegi RS, Lafléche LR: Congenital saccular aneurysm of the superior vena cava. Ann Thorac Surg 29:258, 1980.
447. Oh KS, Dorst JP, Haroutunian LM: Inferior vena caval varix. Radiology 109:161, 1973.
448. Mayo J, Gray R, St Louis E, et al: Anomalies of the inferior vena cava. Am J Roentgenol 140:339, 1983.
449. Jasinski RW, Yang C-F, Rubin JM: Vena cava anomalies simulating adenopathy on computed tomography. Case report. J Comput Assist Tomogr 5:921, 1981.
450. Alexander ES, Clark RA, Gross BH, et al: CT of congenital anomalies of the inferior vena cava. Comput Radiol 6:219, 1982.
451. Webb WR, Gamsu G, Speckman JM, et al: Computed tomographic demonstration of mediastinal venous anomalies. Am J Roentgenol 139:157, 1982.
452. Fleming JS, Gibson RV: Absent right superior vena cava as an isolated anomaly. Br J Radiol 37:696, 1964.
453. Adler SC, Silverman JF: Anomalous venous drainage of the left upper lobe. A radiographic diagnosis. Radiology 108:563, 1973.
454. Kellman GM, Alpern MB, Sandler MA, et al: Computed tomography of vena caval anomalies with embryologic correlation. RadioGraphics 8:533, 1988.
455. Heitzman ER, Scrivani JV, Martino J, et al: The azygos vein and its pleural reflections. II. Applications in the radiological diagnosis of mediastinal abnormality. Radiology 101:259, 1971.
456. Stauffer HM, LaBree J, Adams FH: The normally situated arch of the azygos vein: Its roentgenologic identification and catheterization. Am J Roentgenol 66:353, 1951.
457. Smathers RL, Buschi AJ, Pope Jr, et al: The azygous arch: Normal and pathologic CT appearance. Am J Roentgenol 139:477, 1982.
458. Blendis LM, Laws JW, Williams R, et al: Calcified collateral veins and gross dilatation of the azygos vein in cirrhosis. Br J Radiol 41:909, 1968.
459. Milner LB, Marchan R: Complete absence of the inferior vena cava presenting as a paraspinous mass. Thorax 35:798, 1980.
460. Schneeweiss A, Bleiden LC, Deutsch V, et al: Uninterrupted inferior vena cava with azygos continuation. Chest 80:114, 1981.
461. van der Horst RL, Hastreiter AR: Congenital interruption of the inferior vena cava. Chest 80:638, 1981.
462. Doyle FH, Read AE, Evans KT: The mediastinum in portal hypertension. Clin Radiol 12:114, 1961.
463. Castellino RA, Blank N, Adams DF: Dilated azygos and hemiazygos veins presenting as paravertebral intrathoracic masses. N Engl J Med 278:1087, 1968.
464. Campbell HE, Baruch RJ: Aneurysm of hemiazygos vein associated with portal hypertension. Am J Roentgenol 83:1024, 1960.
465. Bernal-Ramirez M, Hatch HB Jr, Bower PJ: Interruption of the inferior vena cava with azygos continuation. Chest 65:469, 1974.
466. Stern WZ, Bloomberg AE: Idiopathic azygos phlebectasia simulating mediastinal tumor. Radiology 77:622, 1961.
467. Magbitang MH, Hayford FC, Blake JM: Dilated azygos vein simulating a mediastinal tumor. Report of a case. N Engl J Med 263:598, 1960.
468. Hoffman GH, Larson VO, Shipman GA, et al: Venous anomaly of the hemiazygos system. Radiology 77:626, 1961.
469. Felson B: Chest Roentgenology. Philadelphia, WB Saunders, 1973.
470. Preger L, Hooper TI, Steinbach HL, et al: Width of azygos vein related to central venous pressures. Radiology 93:521, 1969.
471. Pomeranz SJ, Proto AV: Tubular shadow in the lung. Chest 89:447, 1986.
472. Steinberg I: Dilatation of the hemiazygos veins in superior vena caval occlusion simulating mediastinal tumor. Am J Roentgenol 87:248, 1962.
473. Floyd GD, Nelson WP: Developmental interruption of the inferior vena cava with azygos and hemiazygos substitution. Unusual radiographic features. Radiology 119:55, 1976.
474. Rockoff SD, Druy EM: Tortuous azygos arch simulating a pulmonary lesion. Am J Roentgenol 138:577, 1982.

19

475. Allen HA, Haney PJ: Left-sided inferior vena cava with hemiazygos continuation. Case report. J Comput Assist Tomogr 5:917, 1981.

476. Ginaldi S, Chuang VP, Wallace S: Absence of hepatic segment of the inferior vena cava with azygous continuation. Case report. J Comput Assist Tomogr 4:112, 1980.

477. Churchill RJ, Wesby G III, Marsan RE, et al: Computed tomographic demonstration of anomalous inferior vena cava with azygos continuation. Case report. J Comput Assist Tomogr 4:398, 1980.

478. Breckenridge JW, Kinlaw WB: Azygos continuation of inferior vena cava: CT appearance. J Comput Assist Tomogr 4:392, 1980.

479. Garris JB, Kangarloo H, Sample WF: Ultrasonic diagnosis of infrahepatic interruption of the inferior vena cava with azygos (hemiazygos) continuation. Radiology 134:179, 1980.

480. Heller RM, Dorst JP, James AE Jr, et al: A useful sign in the recognition of azygos continuation of the inferior vena cava. Radiology 101:519, 1971.

481. Petersen RW: Infrahepatic interruption of the inferior vena cava with azygos continuation (persistent right cardinal vein). Radiology 84:304, 1965.

482. Milledge RD: Absence of the inferior vena cava. Radiology 85:860, 1965.

483. Pacofsky KB, Wolfel DA: Azygos continuation of the inferior vena cava. Am J Roentgenol 113:362, 1971.

484. Berdon WE, Baker DH: Plain film findings in azygos continuation of the inferior vena cava. Am J Roentgenol 104:452, 1968.

485. Ball JB Jr, Proto AV: The variable appearance of the left superior intercostal vein. Radiology 144:445, 1982.

486. Friedman AC, Chambers E, Sprayregen S: The normal and abnormal left superior intercostal vein. Am J Roentgenol 131:599, 1978.

487. Hatfield MK, Vyborny CJ, MacMahon H, et al: Congenital absence of the azygos vein: A cause for "aortic nipple" enlargement. Am J Roentgenol 149:273, 1987.

488. Perez CA, Presant CA, Van Amburg AL III: Management of superior vena cava syndrome. Semin Oncol 5:123, 1978.

489. Lochridge SK, Knibbe WP, Doty DB: Obstruction of the superior vena cava. Surgery 85:14, 1979.

490. Schraufnagel DE, Hill R, Leech JA, at al: Superior vena caval obstruction: Is it a medical emergency? Am J Med 70:1169, 1981.

491. Davies PF, Shevland JE: Superior vena caval obstruction: An analysis of seventy-six cases, with comments on the safety of venography. Angiology 36:354, 1985.

492. Armstrong BA, Perez CA, Simpson JR, et al: Role of irradiation in the management of superior vena cava syndrome. Int J Radiol Oncol Biol Phys 13:531, 1987.

493. Spiro SG, Shah S, Harper PG, et al: Treatment of obstruction of the superior vena cava by combination chemotherapy with and without irradiation in small-cell carcinoma of the bronchus. Thorax 38:501, 1983.

494. Shimm DS, Logue GL, Rigsby LC: Evaluating the superior vena cava syndrome. JAMA 245:951, 1981.

495. Doty DB: Bypass of superior vena cava: 6 years experience with spiral vein graft for obstruction of superior vena cava due to benign and malignant disease. J Thorac Cardiovasc Surg 83:326, 1982.

496. Harbecke RG, Schlueter DP, Rosenzweig DY: Reversible superior vena caval syndrome due to tuberculosis. Thorax 34:410, 1979.

497. Phillips PL, Amberson JB, Libby DM: Syphilitic aortic aneurysm presenting with the superior vena cava syndrome. Am J Med 71:171, 1981.

498. Seetharaman ML, Bahadur P, Shrinivas V, et al: Filarial mediastinal lymphadenitis. Another cause of superior vena caval syndrome. Chest 94:871, 1988.

499. Forman JW, Unger KM: Unilateral superior vena caval syndrome. Thorax 35:314, 1980.

500. Bechtold RE, Wolfman NT, Karstaedt N, et al: Superior vena caval obstruction: Detection using CT. Radiology 157:485, 1985.

501. Bell DR, Woods RL, Levi JA: Superior vena caval obstruction: A 10-year experience. Med J Aust 145:566, 1986.

502. Davis JG, Winsor P: Roentgen findings in aneurysm of the descending thoracic aorta. Am J Roentgenol 81:819, 1959.

503. Higgins CB, Silverman NR, Harris RD, et al: Localised aneurysm of the descending thoracic aorta. Clin Radiol 26:475, 1975.

504. Machida K, Tasaka A: CT patterns of mural thrombus in aortic aneurysms. J Comput Assist Tomogr 4:840, 1980.

505. Higgins CB, Reinke RT: Nonsyphilitic etiology of linear calcification of the ascending aorta. Radiology 113:609, 1974.

506. Szamosi A: Radiological detection of aneurysms involving the aortic root. Radiology 138:551, 1981.

507. Freed TA, Neal MP Jr, Vinik M: Roentgenographic findings in extracardiac injury secondary to blunt chest automobile trauma. Am J Roentgenol 104:424, 1968.

508. Sturm JT, Perry JF Jr, Olson FR, et al: Significance of symptoms and signs in patients with traumatic aortic rupture. Ann Emerg Med 13:876, 1984.

509. Parmley LF, Mattingly TW, Manion WC, et al: Nonpenetrating traumatic injury of the aorta. Circulation 17:1086, 1958.

510. Langbein IE, Brandt PWT: Traumatic rupture of the aorta. Australas Radiol 12:102, 1968.

511. Beachley MC, Ranniger K, Roth FJ: Roentgenographic evaluation of dissecting aneurysms of the aorta. Am J Roentgenol 121:617, 1974.

512. Figiel SJ, Figiel LS, Rush DK: Changes in the linear thoracic paraspinal shadow due to para-aortic hemorrhage: A new sign of dissecting aortic aneurysm. Dis Chest 49:379, 1966.

513. Godwin JD, Herfkens RL, Sklödebrand CG: et al: Evaluation of dissections and aneurysms of the thoracic aorta by conventional and dynamic CT scanning. Radiology 136:125, 1980.

514. Lardé D, Belloir C, Vasile N, et al: Computed tomography of aortic dissection. Radiology 136:147, 1980.

515. Gross SC, Barr I, Eyler WR, et al: Computed tomography in dissection of the thoracic aorta. Radiology 136:135, 1980.

516. Egan TJ, Neiman HL, Herman RJ, et al: Computed tomography in the diagnosis of aortic aneurysm dissection or traumatic injury. Radiology 136:141, 1980.

517. Heiberg E, Wolverson M, Sundaram M, et al: CT findings in thoracic aortic dissection. Am J Roentgenol 136:13, 1981.

518. Oudkerk M, Overbosch E, Dee P: CT recognition of acute aortic dissection. Am J Roentgenol 141:671, 1983.

519. Thorsen MK, San Dretto MA, Lawson TL, et al: Dissecting aortic aneurysm accuracy of computed tomographic diagnosis. Radiology 148:773, 1983.

520. Geisinger MA, Risius B, O'Donnell JA, et al: Thoracic aortic dissections: Magnetic resonance imaging. Radiology 155:407, 1985.

521. Amparo EG, Higgins CB, Hricak H, et al: Aortic dissection: Magnetic resonance imaging. Radiology 155:399, 1985.

522. Dinsmore RE, Liberthson RR, Wismer GL, et al: Magnetic resonance imaging of thoracic aortic aneurysms: Comparison with other imaging methods. Am J Roentgenol 146:309, 1986.

523. White RD, Dooms GC, Higgins CB: Advances in imaging thoracic aortic disease. Invest Radiol 21:761, 1986.

524. Kersting-Sommerhoff BA, Higgins CB, White RD, et al: Aortic dissection: Sensitivity and specificity of MR imaging. Radiology 166:651, 1988.

525. Moncada R, Salinas M, Churchill R, et al: Diagnosis of dissecting aortic aneurysm by computed tomography. Lancet 1:238, 1981.

526. Guthaner DF, Miller DC: Digital subtraction angiography of aortic dissection. Am J Roentgenol 141:157, 1983.

527. Talbot S: Clinical features and prognosis of dissecting aneurysms and ruptured saccular aneurysms. Chest 66:252, 1974.

528. Vecht RJ, Besterman EMM, Bromley LL, et al: Acute dissection of the aorta: Long-term review and management. Lancet 1:109, 1980.

529. Birnholz JC, Ferrucci JT, Wyman SM: Roentgen features of dysphagia aortica. Radiology 111:93, 1974.

530. Charrette EJ, Winton TL, Salerno TA: Acute respiratory insufficiency from an aneurysm of the descending thoracic aorta. J Thorac Cardiovasc Surg 85:467, 1983.

531. Conti VR, Calverley J, Safley WL, et al: Anterior spinal artery syndrome with chronic traumatic thoracic aortic aneurysm. Ann Thorac Surg 33:81, 1982.

532. O'Donovan TPB, Osmundson PJ, Payne WS: Painless dissecting aneurysm of the aorta. Report of a case. Circulation 29:782, 1964.

533. Cooperberg P, Mercer EN, Mulder DS, et al: Rupture of a sinus Valsalva aneurysm. Report of a case diagnosed preoperatively by echocardiography. Radiology 113:171, 1974.

534. Green RA: Enlargement of the innominate and subclavian arteries simulating mediastinal neoplasm. Am Rev Tuberc 79:790, 1959.

535. Schneider HJ, Felson B: Buckling of the innominate artery simulating aneurysm and tumor. Am J Roentgenol 85:1106, 1961.

536. Christensen EE, Landay MJ, Dietz GW, et al: Buckling of the innominate artery simulating a right apical lung mass. Am J Roentgenol 131:119, 1978.

537. Tamaki M, Tanabe M, Kamiuchi H, et al: Buckling of the distal innominate artery simulating a nodular lung mass. Chest 83:829, 1983.

538. Christensen EE, Landay MJ, Dietz GW, et al: Buckling of the innominate artery simulating a right apical lung mass. Am J Roentgenol 131:119, 1978.

539. Rong SH: Carotid pseudoaneurysm simulating Pancoast's tumor. Am J Roentgenol 142:349, 1984.

540. Sandler CM, Toombs BD, Lester RG: Buckling of the left common carotid artery simulating mediastinal neoplasm. Am J Roentgenol 133:312, 1979.

541. Tadavarthy SM, Castaneda-Zuniga WR, Klugman J, et al: Syphilitic aneurysms of the innominate artery. Radiology 139:31, 1981.

542. Hallman GL, Cooley DA: Congenital aortic vascular ring. Surgical considerations. Arch Surg 88:666, 1964.

543. Lam CR, Kabbani S, Arciniegas E: Symptomatic anomalies of the aortic arch. Surg Gynecol Obstet 147:673, 1978.

544. Idbeis B, Levinsky L, Srinivasan V, et al: Vascular rings: Management and a proposed nomenclature. Ann Thorac Surg 31:255, 1981.

545. Engelman RM, Madayag M: Aberrant right subclavian artery aneurysm: A rare cause of a superior mediastinal tumor. Chest 62:45, 1972.

546. Soto B, Shin MS, Papapietro SE: Nonobstructive coarctation. Cardiovasc Radiol 2:231, 1979.

547. Gaupp RJ, Fagan CJ, Davis M, et al: Pseudocoarctation of the aorta. Case report. J Comput Assist Tomogr 5:571, 1981.

548. Moncada R, Shannon M, Miller R, et al: The cervical aortic arch. Am J Roentgenol 125:591, 1975.

549. Kennard DR, Spigos DG, Tan WS: Cervical aortic arch: CT correlation with conventional radiologic studies. Am J Roentgenol 141:295, 1983.

550. Salomonowitz E, Edwards JE, Hunter DW, et al: The three types of aortic diverticula. Am J Roentgenol 142:673, 1984.

551. Shuford WH, Sybers RG, Edwards FK: The three types of right aortic arch. Am J Roentgenol 109:67, 1970.

552. Bevelaqua F, Schicchi JS, Haas F, et al: Aortic arch anomaly presenting as exercise-induced asthma. Am Rev Respir Dis 140:805, 1989.

553. Kersting-Sommerhoff BA, Sechtem UP, Fisher MR, et al: MR imaging of congenital anomalies of the aortic arch. Am J Roentgenol 149:9, 1987.

554. Kent EM, Blades B, Valle AR, et al: Intrathoracic neurogenic tumors. J Thorac Surg 13:116, 1944.

555. Newman A, So SK: Bilateral neurofibroma of the intrathoracic vagus associated with von Recklinghausen's disease. Am J Roentgenol 112:389, 1971.

556. Hutton L: Unusual presentations of benign intrathoracic neurogenic tumors. J Can Assoc Radiol 34:26, 1983.

557. Cohen LM, Schwartz AM, Rockoff SD: Benign schwannomas: Pathologic basis for CT inhomogeneities. Am J Roentgenol 147:141, 1986.

558. Krausz T, Azzopardi JG, Pearse E: Malignant melanoma of the sympathetic chain: With a consideration of pigmented nerve sheath tumours. Histopathology 8:881, 1984.

559. Kayano H, Katayama I: Melanotic schwannoma arising in the sympathetic ganglion. Hum Pathol 19:1355, 1988.

560. Adam A, Hochholzer L: Ganglioneuroblastoma of the posterior mediastinum. A clinicopathologic review of 80 cases. Cancer 47:373, 1981.

561. Reed JC, Hallet KK, Feigin DS: Neural tumors of the thorax: Subject review from the AFIP. Radiology 126:9, 1978.

562. Bar-Ziv J, Nogrady MB: Mediastinal neuroblastoma and ganglioneuroma. The differentiation between primary and secondary involvement on the chest roentgenogram. Am J Roentgenol 125:380, 1975.

563. Schweisguth O, Mathey J, Renault P, et al: Intrathoracic neurogenic tumors in infants and children: A study of forty cases. Ann Surg 150:29, 1959.

564. Adam A, Hochholzer L: Ganglioneuroblastoma of the posterior mediastinum: Clinicopathologic review of 80 cases. Cancer 47:373, 1981.

565. Gallivan MVE, Chun B, Rowden G, et al: Intrathoracic paravertebral malignant paraganglioma. Arch Pathol Lab Med 104:46, 1980.

566. Nigam BK, Hyer SL, Taylor EJ, et al: Intrathoracic chemodectoma with noradrenaline secretion. Thorax 36:66, 1981.

567. Ogawa J, Inoue H, Koide S, et al: Functioning paraganglioma in the posterior mediastinum. Ann Thorac Surg 33:507, 1982.

568. Miles J, Pennybacker J, Sheldon P: Intrathoracic meningocele. Its development and association with neurofibromatosis. J Neurol Neurosurg Psychiatry, 32:99, 1969.

569. Dische MR: Mediastinal lymphangioma with chylothorax in infancy. Am J Clin Pathol 49:392, 1968.

570. Cabooter M, Bogaerts Y, Javaheri S, et al: Intrathoracic meningocele. Eur J Respir Dis 63:347, 1982.

571. Epstein BS, Epstein JA: Extrapleural intrathoracic apical traumatic pseudomeningocele. Am J Roentgenol 120:887, 1974.

572. Salyer DC, Salyer WR, Eggleston JC: Benign developmental cysts of the mediastinum. Arch Pathol Lab Med 101:136, 1977.

573. Madewell JE, Sobonya RE, Reed JC: Neurenteric cyst. RPC from the AFIP. Radiology 109:707, 1973.

574. Benton C, Silverman FN: Some mediastinal lesions in children. Semin Roentgenol 4:91, 1969.

575. Kirwan WO, Walbaum PR, McCormack RJM: Cystic intrathoracic derivatives of the foregut and their complications. Thorax 28:424, 1973.

576. Bowton DL, Katz PO: Esophageal cyst as a cause of chronic cough. Chest 86:150, 1984.

577. Sambrook Gowar FJ: Mediastinal thoracic duct cyst. Thorax 33:800, 1978.

578. Hori S, Harada K, Morimoto S, et al: Lymphangiographic demonstration of thoracic duct cyst. Chest 789:652, 1980.

579. Tsuchiya R, Sugiura Y, Ogata T, et al: Thoracic duct cyst of the mediastinum. J Thorac Cardiovasc Surg 79:856, 1980.

580. Tsuchiya R, Sugiura Y, Ogata T, et al: Thoracic duct cyst of the mediastinum. J Thorac Cardiovasc Surg 79:856, 1980.

581. Hori S, Harada K, Morimota S, et al: Lymphangiographic demonstration of thoracic duct cyst. Chest 78:652, 1980.

582. Fromang DR, Seltzer MB, Tobias JA: Thoracic duct cyst causing mediastinal compression and acute respiratory insufficiency. Chest 67:725, 1975.

583. Morettin LB, Allen TE: Thoracic duct cyst: Diagnosis with needle aspiration. Radiology 161:437, 1986.

584. Lindell MM Jr, Hill CA, Libshitz HI: Esophageal cancer: Radiographic chest findings and their prognostic significance. Am J Roentgenol 133:461, 1979.

585. Daffner RH, Postlethwait RW, Putman CE: Retrotracheal abnormalities in esophageal carcinoma: Prognostic implications. Am J Roentgenol 130:719, 1978.

586. Yrjana J: The posterior tracheal band and recurrent esophageal carcinoma. Radiology 146:433, 1983.

587. Palayew MJ: The tracheoesophageal stripe and the posterior tracheal band. Radiology 132:11, 1979.

588. Picus D Balfe DM, Koehler RE, et al: Computed tomography in the staging of esophageal carcinoma. Radiology 146:433, 1983.

589. Thompson WM, Halvorsen RA, Foster WL Jr, et al: Computed tomography for staging esophageal and gastroesophageal cancer: Reevaluation. Am J Roentgenol 141:951, 1983.

590. Quint LE, Glazer GM, Orringer MB, et al: Esophageal carcinoma: CT findings. Radiology 155:171, 1985.

591. Choi TK, Siu KF, Lam KH, et al: Bronchoscopy and carcinoma of the esophagus I. Findings of bronchoscopy in carcinoma of the esophagus. Am J Surg 147:757, 1984.

592. Choi TK, Siu KF, Lam KH, et al: Bronchoscopy and carcinoma of the esophagus II. Carcinoma of the esophagus with tracheobronchial involvement. Am J Surg 147:760, 1984.

593. Reinig JW, Stanley JH, Schabel SI: CT evaluation of thickened esophageal walls. Am J Roentgenol 140:931, 1983.

594. Cohen AM, Cunat JS: Giant esophageal leiomyoma as a mediastinal mass. J Can Assoc Radiol 32:129, 1981.

595. Godard JE, McCranie D: Multiple leiomyomas of the esophagus. Am J Roentgenol 117:259, 1973.

596. Almeida JMM: Leiomyosarcoma of the esophagus. Chest 81:761, 1982.

597. Jalundhwala JM, Shah RC: Epiphrenic esophageal diverticulum. Chest 57:97, 1970.

598. Montgomery RD, Mendl K, Stephenson SF: Intramural diverticulosis of the oesophagus. Thorax 30:278, 1975.

599. Tishler JM, Shin MS, Stanley RJ, et al: CT of the thorax in patients with achalasia. Dig Dis Sci 28:692, 1983.

600. Blomquist G, Mahoney PS: Noncollapsing air-filled esophagus in diseased and postoperative chests. Acta Radiol 55:32, 1961.

601. Schabel SI, Stanley JH: Air esophagram after laryngectomy. Am J Roentgenol 136:19, 1981.

602. McLean RDW, Stewart CJ, Whyte DGC: Acute thoracic inlet obstruction in achalasia of the oesophagus. Thorax 31:456, 1976.

603. Giustra PE, Killoran PJ, Wasgatt WN: Acute stridor in achalasia of the esophagus (cardiospasm). Am J Gastroenterol 60:160, 1973.

604. Feczko PJ, Halpert RD: Achalasia secondary to nongastrointestinal malignancies. Gastrointest Radiol 10:273, 1985.

605. Grant DM, Thompson GE: Diagnosis of congenital tracheoesophageal fistula in the adolescent and adult. Anesthesiology 49:139, 1978.

606. Osinowo O, Harley HR, Janigan D: Congenital broncho-oesophageal fistula in the adult. Thorax 38:138, 1983.

607. Fitzgerald RH, Bartles DM, Parker EF: Tracheoesophageal fistulas secondary to carcinoma of the esophagus. J Thorac Cardiovasc Surg 82:194, 1981.

608. Dunn EK, Man AC, Lin K, et al: Scintigraphic demonstration of tracheoesophageal fistula. J Nucl Med 24:1151, 1983.

609. Little AG, Ferguson MK, DeMeester TR, et al: Esophageal carcinoma with respiratory tract fistula. Cancer 53:1322, 1984.

610. Symbas PN, McKeown PP, Hatcher CR Jr, et al: Tracheoesophageal fistula from carcinoma of the esophagus. Ann Thorac Surg 38:382, 1984.

611. Keszler P, Buzna E: Surgical and conservative management of esophageal perforation. Chest 80:158, 1981.

612. Hjelms E, Jensen H, Lindewald H: Nonmalignant oesophagobronchial fistula. Eur J Respir Dis 63:351, 1982.

613. Hilgenberg AD, Grillo MC: Acquired nonmalignant tracheoesophageal fistula. J Thorac Cardiovasc Surg 85:492, 1983.

614. Leeds WM, Morley TF, Zappasodi SJ, et al: Computed tomography for diagnosis of tracheoesophageal fistula. Crit Care Med 14:591, 1986.

615. Saks BJ, Kilbey AE, Dietrich PA, et al: Pleural and mediastinal changes following endoscopic injection sclerotherapy of esophageal varices. Radiology 149:639, 1983.

616. Reddy SC: Esophagopleural fistula. J Comput Assist Tomogr 7:376, 1983.

19

617. Poe RG, Schowengerdt CG: Two cases of atraumatic herniation of the liver. Am Rev Respir Dis 105:959, 1972.
618. Maulsby GO, Fontenelle LJ, Dalinka MK, et al: Radiographic appearance of the chest following the Thal procedure. Radiology 100:293, 1971.
619. Graham JC Jr, Blanchard IT, Scatliff JH: Calcified gastric leiomyoma presenting as a mediastinal mass. Am J Roentgenol 114:529, 1972.
620. Johnston RH Jr, Owensby LC, Vargas GM, et al: Pancreatic pseudocyst of the mediastinum. Ann Thorac Surg 41:210, 1986.
621. Owens GR, Arger PH, Mulhern CB Jr, et al: Case report. CT evaluation of mediastinal pseudocyst. J Comput Assist Tomogr 4:256, 1980.
622. Pear BL: Pancreatic pseudocyst of the mediastinum. Case of the day. Am J Roentgenol 134:1284, 1980.
623. deNoronha LL, deCosta MF, Godinho MTM: Thoracic kidney. Am Rev Respir Dis 109:678, 1974.
624. Kraus RA, Mann CI: Delayed presentation of a Bochdalek hernia in a child. J Can Assoc Radiol 40:176, 1989.
625. Gross RE: The Surgery of Infancy and Childhood. Its Principles and Techniques. Philadelphia, WB Saunders, 1953, p. 221.
626. Seidler RC, Becker JA: Intrathoracic extramedullary hematopoiesis. Radiology 83:1057, 1964.
627. Verani R, Olson J, Moake JL: Intrathoracic extramedullary hematopoiesis. Report of a case in a patient with sickle cell disease–β-thalassemia. Am J Clin Pathol 73:133, 1980.
628. Da Costa JL, Loh YS, Hanam E: Extramedullary hemopoiesis with multiple tumor-simulating mediastinal masses in hemoglobin E-thalassemia disease. Chest 65:210, 1974.
629. Long JA Jr, Doppman JL, Nienhuis AW: Computed tomographic studies of thoracic extramedullary hematopoiesis. J Comput Assist Tomogr 4:67, 1980.
630. Ross P, Logan W: Roentgen findings in extramedullary hematopoiesis. Am J Roentgenol 106:604, 1969.
631. Gumbs RV, Higginbotham-Ford EA, Teal JS, et al: Thoracic extramedullary hematopoiesis in sickle cell disease. Am J Roentgenol 149:889, 1987.
632. Papavasiliou CG: Tumor simulating intrathoracic extramedullary hemopoiesis. Clinical and roentgenologic considerations. Am J Roentgenol 93:695, 1965.
633. Elbers H, Stadt JVD, Wagenaar SSC: Tumor-simulating thoracic extramedullary hematopoiesis. Ann Thorac Surg 30:584, 1980.
634. Maesen F, Baur C, Lamers J, et al: Chordoma of the thorax. Eur J Respir Dis 68:68, 1986.
635. Doglioni C, Bontempini L, Iuzzolino P, et al: Ependymoma of the mediastinum. Arch Pathol Lab Med 112:194, 1988.
636. Childress WG, Adie GC: Plasma cell tumors of the mediastinum and lung. J Thorac Surg 19:794, 1950.
637. Wilson AJ, Ratliff JL, Lagios MD, et al: Mediastinal meningioma. Am J Surg Pathol 3:557, 1979.
638. Leite de Noronha L, Freitas E Costa M, Magalhães Godinho MT: Thoracic kidney. Am Rev Respir Dis 109:678, 1974.
639. Ingels GW, Campbell DC, Giampetro AM, et al: Malignant schwannomas of the mediastinum. Report of two cases and review of the literature. Cancer 27:1190, 1971.
640. Masaoka A, Hashimoto T, Shibata K, et al: Thymomas associated with pure red cell aplasia. Histologic and follow-up studies. Cancer 64:1872, 1989.
641. Odze R, Bégin LR: Malignant paraganglioma of the posterior mediastinum. A case report and review of the literature. Cancer 65:564, 1990.

20

Diseases of the Diaphragm and Chest Wall

The thoracic cage, including the chest wall and diaphragm, serves the dual purpose of enclosing and protecting the contents of the thorax and of producing the movements that result in the changes in pleural pressure necessary for respiration. A multitude of diseases and anomalies involve these structures, and whether primary or secondary they can affect either or both major functions of the thoracic cage. The logical subdivision of diseases of the thoracic cage into those involving the diaphragm and those affecting the chest wall is used in this chapter. Traumatic abnormalities of the thoracic cage are not considered. (The effects of trauma on the thorax are discussed in Chapter 15.)

THE DIAPHRAGM

The normal embryology, anatomy, physiology, and roentgenology of the diaphragm are described in detail in Chapter 1 (*see* page 262). Briefly, in review, the diaphragm consists of a musculotendi-nous sheet that separates the thoracic and abdominal contents (Fig. 20–1). It can be divided into three components: (1) a *sternal* portion that originates from the xiphoid process of the sternum, (2) a *costal* portion that arises from the lower six ribs, and (3) a *crural* portion that originates from the anterolateral aspects of the first three lumbar vertebrae on the right and the first two lumbar vertebrae on the left. A portion of the crural (or lumbar) diaphragm arises from the medial and lateral arcuate ligaments, and the thickening of the thoracolumbar fascia overlying the anterior surfaces of the psoas and quadratus lumborum muscles. The muscle fibers from all three components insert into the boomer-ang-shaped central tendon.

Three major openings in the normal diaphragm allow passage of the aorta, esophagus, inferior vena cava, and accompanying nerves and vascular and lymphatic channels. The aortic aperture is located posterior to the left median arcuate ligament at the level of the 12th thoracic vertebra; in addition to the aorta, it transmits the thoracic

FORAMINA OF MORGAGNI

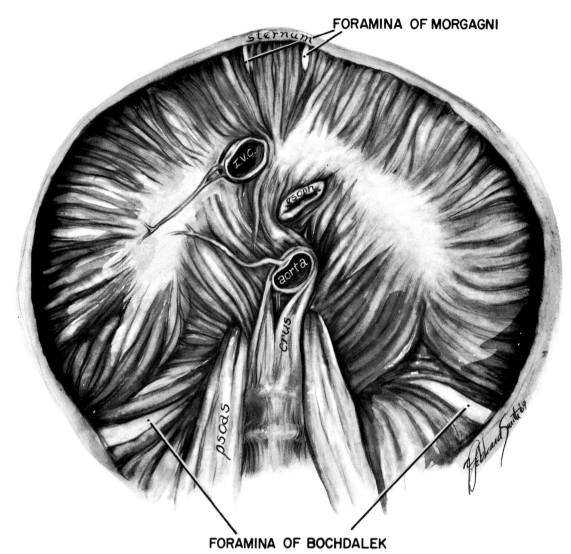

FORAMINA OF BOCHDALEK

Figure 20–1. Anatomy of the Normal Diaphragm Viewed from Below.

duct, lymphatic vessels, and the azygos and hemi-azygos veins. The esophageal aperture consists of a splitting of the medial fibers of the right crus of the lumbar diaphragm; in addition to the esophagus, this aperture allows passage of the vagal nerves and the gastric vessels. The inferior vena cava passes through the most anterior opening, which lies at the level of T-8 between the costal portion of the right hemidiaphragm and the central tendon. In addition to these normal openings, there are two symmetric "weak areas" known eponymously as the foramina of Morgagni and Bochdalek. The former is located anteriorly and the latter posterolaterally; they are sometimes the sites of herniation of abdominal contents.

The roentgenographic appearances of the normal and diseased diaphragm have been the subject of three excellent recent reviews.[1–3] In 94 per cent of normal subjects, posteroanterior roentgenograms show the cupola or dome of the right hemidiaphragm to project into a plane ranging from the anterior end of the fifth rib to the sixth anterior interspace.[4] In the 500 normal subjects studied by Lennon and Simon,[4] the right hemidiaphragm projected at the level of the sixth rib anteriorly in 41 per cent and at or below the level of the seventh rib in only 4 per cent. In the great majority of normal subjects, the right hemidiaphragm projects half an interspace higher than the left, being at the same level as or lower than the left hemidiaphragm in only 9 per cent.[5] The discrepancy in position of the two hemidiaphragms is the result of the position of the ventricular mass of the heart rather than that of the liver, as is commonly believed: in patients with dextrocardia without dextroversion of the abdominal viscera, the right hemidiaphragm is on a plane lower than the left, despite the right-sided position of the liver.[6] Variations in diaphragmatic contour such as scalloping[5] and prominence of the costophrenic muscle slips are fairly frequent and must not be interpreted as evidence of disease.

Excursion of the diaphragm is estimated to account for 60 to 75 per cent of vital capacity,[7] with the remainder being the result of intercostal and accessory muscle contraction. Simon[8] compared the range of excursion of the two hemidiaphragms from full inspiration to full expiration in 204 patients. In 23 per cent excursion was equal and symmetric, in 50 per cent the right hemidiaphragm made a greater excursion than the left (mean difference, 0.75 cm), and in 27 per cent the reverse occurred (mean difference, 0.94 cm). The mean excursion was measured in 188 of these patients. It was 3 to 6 cm in 128 (77 per cent), less than 3 cm in 44 (23 per cent), and greater than 6 cm in only 4 patients. These figures of Simon's are at some variance with those reported by Alexander,[9] who studied 127 patients undergoing upper gastrointestinal examinations who had no detectable significant intrathoracic or gastrointestinal abnormality. This investigator found the mean excursion of the left hemidiaphragm to be 3.15 cm and that of the right 2.75 cm. The two hemidiaphragms moved equally in only 16 patients (12 per cent), the left hemidiaphragm showing a greater excursion in 78 patients and the right in 33 patients.

Roentgenologic assessment of diaphragmatic motion is best accomplished fluoroscopically, particularly when subtle changes are sought—for example, the relatively minor degrees of restriction of motion that may be associated with acute subphrenic disease. Although major asymmetry of diaphragmatic excursion may be evidenced on roentgenograms exposed at total lung capacity (TLC) and residual volume (RV) (for example, in the assessment of air trapping from obstructing endobronchial lesions or in unilateral emphysema), minor degrees of asymmetry may become evident only when the motion of both hemidiaphragms is observed simultaneously. Fluoroscopic examination should be carried out not only in posteroanterior projection but also in various degrees of obliquity to reveal any disturbance in motion of portions of the diaphragm that may not be present in other portions. For example, a subphrenic abscess localized to the posterior subphrenic space on the right side may produce local restriction of motion of the posterior portion of the hemidiaphragm without concomitant disturbance in the excursion of the anterior portion. Diaphragmatic motion should be observed during breathing at tidal volume, while the patient breathes deeply and preferably rapidly, and while he or she sniffs. In many cases, sniffing reveals restriction or paradoxical motion not clearly apparent during either tidal or deep breathing. Of some importance is the observation made by Alexander[9] that sniffing by normal subjects may produce paradoxical excursion of one hemidiaphragm. He concluded that such a finding can be regarded as pathologic only if paradoxical excursion exceeds 2 cm and if it involves the whole hemidiaphragm as seen in oblique or lateral projection.

Other aspects of the physiology of the diaphragm are described in Chapter 21 with reference to paralysis of both hemidiaphragms and alveolar hypoventilation.

ABNORMALITIES OF DIAPHRAGMATIC POSITION OR MOTION

Unilateral Diaphragmatic Paralysis

Paralysis of a hemidiaphragm usually results from interruption of transmission of the nerve impulses through the phrenic nerve. The most common causes of unilateral diaphragmatic paralysis are listed in Table 20–1. Although invasion of the nerve by a neoplasm, usually of pulmonary origin, is the most frequent etiology, a wide variety of benign conditions can be responsible.[10] The second most common category is paralysis of unknown etiology; in these idiopathic cases, the paralysis is almost invariably right-sided and usually occurs in males. Riley[10] has suggested that so-called idiopathic paralysis may result from an episode of acute infectious neuritis or may be caused by viral neurotoxin. Unilateral diaphragmatic paralysis can be a manifestation of herpes zoster, presumably as a result of extension of the infection from the dorsal root to adjacent posterior and lateral portions of the spinal cord and anterior horn cells.[11]

Unilateral diaphragmatic paralysis can occur as a complication of radical neck[12] or thoracic[13] surgery, especially coronary artery bypass surgery.[14–18] In the latter circumstance, the mechanism by which the hemidiaphragm is paralyzed has not been positively established, but the use of cold topical cardioplegia has been suggested as a possible etiology. It has been shown that cooling of the phrenic nerves in experimental animals causes reversible diaphragmatic paralysis.[19] During cardiopulmonary bypass and aortocoronary bypass grafting, ice slush cooled to subfreezing temperatures by the addition of salt is packed into the pericardial cavity around the heart. Since the left phrenic nerve runs immediately within the posterior pericardium on the left side, a cold-induced injury can occur.[20, 21] It also has been suggested that left lower lobe atelectasis may be attributable to left phrenic nerve palsy and that it can be alleviated to some extent by the use of a

Table 20–1. Causes of Unilateral Diaphragmatic Paralysis

Neoplasms
Idiopathic
Surgical section or stretch[26]
Phrenic thermal injury[17]
Cervical manipulation[26]
Cervical spondylosis[30]
Cervical venipuncture[29]
Birth injury[13]
Brachial neuritis[351]
Neuralgic amyotrophy[352]
Mediastinal lymph node enlargement[353]
Aortic aneurysm
Substernal thyroid
Herpes zoster[354]
Vasculitis (mononeuritis multiplex)
Multiple sclerosis[32]
Diabetes mellitus

pericardial insulation technique.[22, 23] Despite the foregoing, Wilcox and associates[17] recently studied the incidence of left hemidiaphragmatic paralysis in 57 patients undergoing coronary artery bypass grafting in whom cold topical cardioplegia was employed: they found that only 10 per cent of the patients demonstrated unequivocal evidence of phrenic nerve damage, whereas the vast majority had significant atelectasis of the left lower lobe. The results of this study suggest that although phrenic nerve damage and hemidiaphragmatic paralysis can occur following the use of cold topical cardioplegia, this cannot be the sole explanation of the almost invariable left lower lobe atelectasis. Rarely, cold topical cardioplegia can be associated with bilateral phrenic nerve damage.[24, 25]

Phrenic nerve damage can also result from chiropractic manipulation of the cervical spine[26] and from catheterization of the large cervical veins.[27–29] Abnormalities of the nerve roots from C-3 to C-5 can also cause diaphragmatic paralysis as a result of severe cervical spondylosis[30, 31] or as a consequence of rhizotomy.[366] Unilateral upper motor neuron phrenic palsy has been reported in a patient with multiple sclerosis,[32] and transient hemidiaphragmatic elevation can occur on the side contralateral to a supratentorial stroke.[33]

In a review of the roentgenologic manifestations of unilateral diaphragmatic paralysis, Alexander[9] described four cardinal signs: (1) elevation of a hemidiaphragm above the normal range; (2) diminished, absent, or paradoxical motion during respiration; (3) paradoxical motion under conditions of augmented load such as sniffing; and (4) mediastinal swing during respiration. Roentgenologically, an elevated, paralyzed hemidiaphragm presents an accentuated dome configuration in both posteroanterior and lateral projections (Fig. 20–2). Since the peripheral points of attachment of the diaphragm are fixed, costophrenic and costovertebral sulci tend to be deepened, narrowed, and sharpened (Fig. 20–3). If the paralysis is left-sided, the stomach and splenic flexure of the colon relate to the inferior surface of the elevated hemidiaphragm and usually contain more gas than normal (Fig. 20–4). In many cases, the stomach undergoes mesenterioaxial volvulus so that its greater curvature faces upward; in such circumstances, two fluid levels are apparent within the stomach, one in the inverted fundus and the other in the body or antrum. This broad relationship of distended stomach and colon to the inferior surface of the diaphragm has been stressed by Felson[5] as a valuable sign in the differentiation of eventration or diaphragmatic paralysis from traumatic diaphragmatic hernia (see page 2511). Rarely, paralysis or eventration of the right hemidiaphragm is associated with inversion of the liver and a suprahepatic position of the gallbladder.[34]

The most reliable roentgenographic maneuver to detect hemidiaphragmatic paralysis is the sniff test. The test is accomplished by having the subject produce a rapid inspiration, usually through the nostrils since this represents an easily accomplished respiratory maneuver for even the most naive subject; diaphragmatic position and movement are observed fluoroscopically. Normally, both hemidiaphragms descend sharply during a sniff, but with unilateral diaphragmatic paralysis there is paradoxical upward motion of the affected side. Although significant paradoxical motion provides strong evidence for diaphragmatic paralysis or eventration, Alexander[9] has pointed out that the incidence of false-positive results is approximately 6 per cent and that false-negative results also can be recorded if the subject uses the abdominal musculature to elevate the diaphragm during the expiratory phase of breathing (see farther on).

Alexander[9] has stressed the fallibility of the roentgenologic signs of diaphragmatic paralysis: (1) assessment of abnormal elevation may be erroneous because of the considerable variation in the height of the hemidiaphragms normally; (2) mediastinal swing during respiration is a totally unreliable sign in the presence of bronchial obstruction or atelectasis; (3) motion may be absent or paradoxical during respiration in various pulmonary, pleural, and subphrenic diseases, which makes this sign unreliable unless such diseases can be excluded; and (4) sniffing can cause paradoxical motion of one hemidiaphragm in some normal subjects, and in order for it to be considered pathologic it should consist of a reverse excursion of at least 2 cm. Although we agree that these exceptions are valid, we feel that with reasonable care in excluding these variables the diagnosis of unilateral diaphragmatic paralysis can be made roentgenologically in the majority of cases. Invasion or compression of the phrenic nerve by such abnormalities as pulmonary carcinoma or calcified lymph nodes can be clarified by CT should the nature of the abnormalities be unclear from conventional roentgenographic studies.[35]

Patients with a paralyzed hemidiaphragm are usually asymptomatic, although some patients may complain of dyspnea on effort.[11] The severity of symptoms relates to the rapidity of development of the diaphragmatic paralysis and to the presence or absence of underlying pulmonary disease. Physical examination may reveal an elevated hemidiaphragm and decreased breath sounds over the affected side. Diaphragmatic excursion as assessed by percussion is decreased. Examination of the anterior abdominal wall of some individuals in the supine position may reveal paradoxical inward movement of the ipsilateral abdominal wall.

Pulmonary function tests typically show mild restrictive insufficiency. Total lung capacity is usually 85 per cent of predicted, whereas vital capacity is reduced to 75 per cent of predicted; functional residual capacity and the ratio of FEV_1 to forced vital capacity are usually normal.[36–38] Maximal inspiratory pressures, measured either at the mouth (PI Max) or across the diaphragm (Pdi Max), are

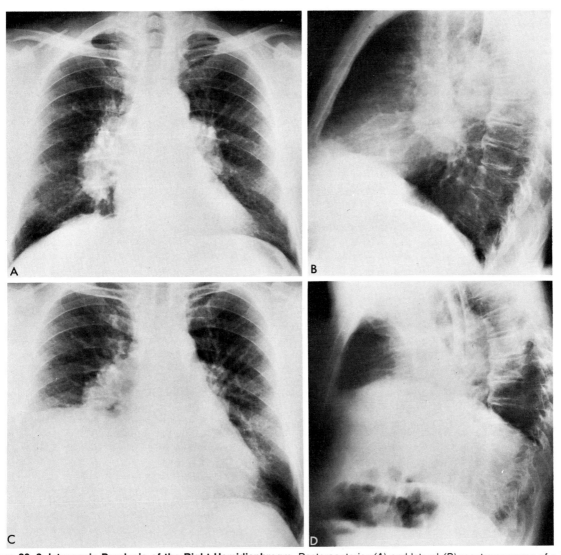

Figure 20–2. Iatrogenic Paralysis of the Right Hemidiaphragm. Posteroanterior *(A)* and lateral *(B)* roentgenograms of a 49-year-old native of Greece reveal marked enlargement of the hilar lymph nodes bilaterally. No other intrathoracic abnormality is evident. Note the normal position of both hemidiaphragms. As part of the investigation, a right scalene node biopsy was performed, during which the right phrenic nerve was accidentally severed. Ten days later roentgenograms of the chest in posteroanterior *(C)* and lateral *(D)* projections demonstrate marked elevation of the right hemidiaphragm. The contour of the hemidiaphragm is smooth and arcuate but does not present the sharp costophrenic angles that usually characterize diaphragmatic paralysis. The scalene node biopsy revealed multiple, small, round spores compatible with *Histoplasma capsulatum*. It was reasonably assumed that the massive hilar lymph node enlargement was the result of histoplasmosis. (Courtesy of Montreal Chest Hospital Center.)

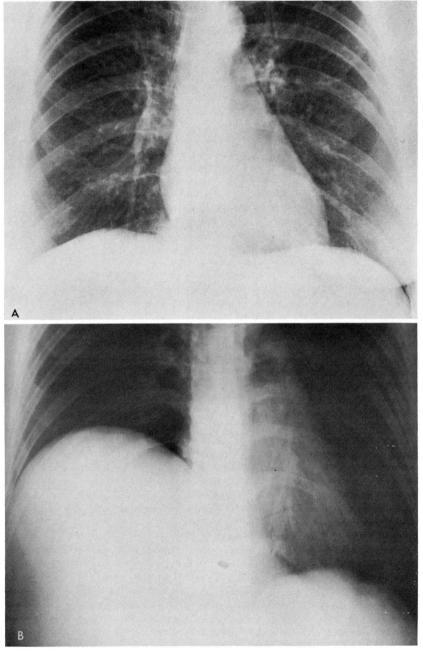

Figure 20–3. Iatrogenic Paralysis of the Right Hemidiaphragm (Temporary). This 33-year-old woman was admitted to the hospital for repair of a lacerated finger tendon. A view of the lower half of the thorax from a preoperative roentgenogram *(A)* revealed a normal position of both hemidiaphragms. Anesthesia was established by brachial plexus block, 45 ml of 1 per cent Carbocaine with Adrenalin being injected by way of a supraclavicular approach. One hour after the anesthesia, the patient complained of mild dyspnea, and roentgenography of the chest *(B)* revealed marked elevation of the right hemidiaphragm in a contour typical of diaphragmatic paralysis. The patient received supportive therapy only, and a roentgenogram exposed 12 hours after anesthesia *(C)* demonstrated return of the right hemidiaphragm to its normal level. The dyspnea had disappeared.

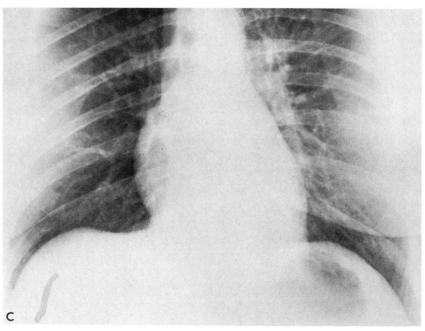

Figure 20-3 *Continued*

only mildly reduced, and values are similar whether the paralysis is right-sided or left-sided.[39, 40] Lower values for vital capacity, PI Max, and Pdi Max are observed in patients with concomitant cardiopulmonary disease.[39] The decrease in lung volumes is greater when measured in the supine, rather than in the upright, position.[41, 42] The average decrease in vital capacity when normal subjects move from the erect to the supine posture is 7.5 ± 6.0 per cent; a decrease of 20 per cent or greater indicates the need for a study of diaphragmatic function.[43]

Hypoxemia is usually absent or mild, although hypoxia may develop when patients assume a supine position.[2, 41] Regional ventilation is decreased, particularly of the lung base on the side of the paralyzed hemidiaphragm.[11] Plication of the paralyzed hemidiaphragm can improve lung volumes and arterial blood gases, presumably by stiffening the paralyzed side and preventing paradoxical motion.[44, 45]

Patients with unilateral hemidiaphragmatic paralysis can manifest an abnormal pattern of gastric pressure swings in relation to pleural or esophageal pressure swings. Normally, gastric pressure becomes more positive as esophageal pressure becomes more negative during inspiration. In 12 of the 15 patients with unilateral diaphragmatic paralysis studied by Lisboa and colleagues,[39] an abnormal pattern of gastric pressure swings occurred during quiet tidal breathing: gastric pressure became more *negative* during inspiration although to a lesser extent than the negative swing in esophageal pressure. In patients with bilateral diaphragmatic paralysis (*see* farther on), gastric pressure decreases to the same extent as esophageal pressure during tidal breathing so that no active transdiaphragmatic pres-

sure is generated.[42] This pattern of pressure swings could be caused by either an upward movement of the paralyzed hemidiaphragm that was greater than the downward movement of the functioning hemidiaphragm, or by recruitment of expiratory muscles and a sudden relaxation of these muscles at the onset of inspiration.

A definitive diagnosis of phrenic nerve dysfunction as the cause of hemidiaphragmatic paralysis can be obtained by employing the technique of phrenic nerve stimulation in the neck and the measurement of phrenic nerve latency.[17, 40, 46] Felt-tipped electrodes are placed over the phrenic nerve in the neck, and the stimulation voltage is increased in a step-wise fashion while the compound action potential of the ipsilateral hemidiaphragm is recorded using surface electrodes placed on the anterolateral aspect of the chest in the eighth and ninth intercostal spaces. Phrenic nerve latency is the time from stimulation of the nerve to the first detection of the compound action potential; in normal subjects it ranges from 7 to 9 milliseconds with an upper limit of 9.75 milliseconds.[47] When the phrenic nerve is completely interrupted or is significantly demyelinated, the compound action potential of the hemidiaphragm will be absent or will show prolonged latency. Although this technique can be useful in detecting complete phrenic nerve interruption, it may not be sensitive in identifying partial axonal degeneration since latency may be normal if only a portion of the phrenic nerve axons are conducting. Unfortunately, measurements of the magnitude of the compound action potential from surface electrodes do not accurately reflect the extent of activation of the underlying diaphragm. A useful maneuver may be to combine phrenic nerve

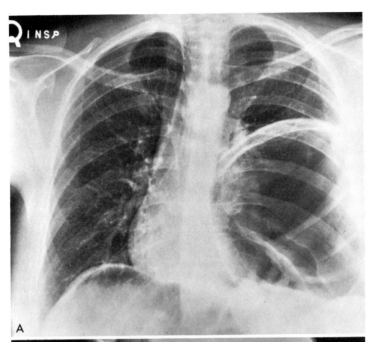

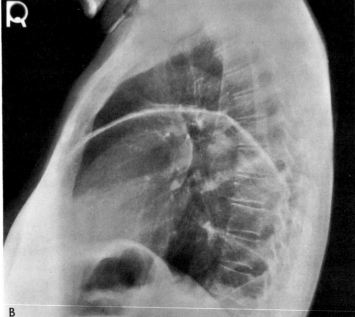

Figure 20–4. Paralysis or Eventration of the Left Hemidiaphragm Associated with Severe Colonic Dilatation Secondary to Sigmoid Volvulus. Posteroanterior (A) and lateral (B) roentgenograms reveal a remarkable degree of elevation of the left hemidiaphragm. Severely dilated loops of colon are situated beneath this hemidiaphragm and to a lesser extent beneath the right one. The mediastinum is displaced considerably into the right hemithorax.

stimulation with fluoroscopic examination of diaphragmatic motion.

End-to-end anastomosis of surgically transected phrenic nerves has been reported to result in eventual recovery of diaphragmatic function.[48]

Bilateral Diaphragmatic Paralysis

In contrast to patients with unilateral diaphragmatic paralysis, those with bilateral paralysis have profound respiratory symptoms and functional derangement.[49] Bilateral diaphragmatic weakness, rather than paralysis, causes less severe symptoms, but it can be recognized when dyspnea is exaggerated in the supine position.[50] The causes of bilateral diaphragmatic paralysis are in some respects similar to those of unilateral paralysis (Table 20–2). Severe diaphragmatic weakness may be the principal manifestation of a generalized disorder such as myopathy[49, 51] or muscular dystrophy.[52] A rare genetic form of bilateral diaphragmatic paralysis has been described in homozygous twins.[53]

The roentgenographic appearance of bilateral diaphragmatic paralysis consists of elevated hemidiaphragms in both posteroanterior and lateral projections.[9] Horizontal linear opacities, possibly caused by plate-like atelectasis, may be present at the lung bases. Paradoxical upward motion of both hemidiaphragms during an inspiratory effort or sniff is usually observed on fluoroscopic examination, although recruitment of abdominal expiratory muscles can cause a false-negative sniff test.[49, 54] Some patients with bilateral diaphragmatic paralysis actively expire to a lung volume below the true resting functional residual capacity and then use the elastic recoil forces of the abdominothoracic structures to assist the next inspiration passively. The sudden downward motion of the diaphragm coincident with abdominal muscle relaxation may be misinterpreted as diaphragmatic contraction when viewed fluoroscopically. Diaphragmatic motion also can be monitored by ultrasonography.[55, 56]

Most patients with bilateral diaphragmatic paralysis or significant weakness eventually develop ventilatory respiratory failure and hypercapnia; some present with evidence of cor pulmonale and

Table 20–2. Causes of Bilateral Diaphragmatic Paralysis

Birth injury[355]
Infantile spinomuscular atrophy[58, 356]
Neuralgic amyotrophy[352]
Arnold-Chiari malformation[357]
Syringomyelia[358]
Peripheral neuropathy[359]
Brachial neuritis[360]
Multiple sclerosis[361]
Cervical disc surgery[362]
Paraneoplastic neuritis[363]
Blunt chest trauma[364]
Topical cardiac hypothermia[25]
Idiopathic[365]

right ventricular failure. Dyspnea on exertion and on assuming the supine position is a characteristic complaint. Dyspnea during recumbency is particularly distressing; it can interfere with adequate sleep and result in daytime hypersomnolence. We have seen patients who were able to sleep only when on their hands and knees. The inadequate inspiratory effort predisposes to atelectasis and respiratory tract infections.

On physical examination, percussion reveals dullness at both bases and decreased or absent diaphragmatic excursion owing to the elevated resting position of the diaphragm. Patients are usually tachypneic and are clearly using the accessory inspiratory muscles. The characteristic physical finding, readily detectable in the supine position, is a paradoxical inward motion of the anterior abdominal wall on inspiration (see Fig. 21–5, page 2993). The paradoxical motion is caused by an upward movement of the flaccid diaphragm during inspiration as a result of the negative intrathoracic pressure generated by the normally contracting external intercostal and accessory muscles. Just as activation of abdominal expiratory muscles can cause a false-negative fluoroscopic sniff test, it can mask the physical finding of paradoxical motion. However, abdominal muscle activation during expiration can be detected by gentle palpation of the abdominal wall during the breathing cycle. In addition, a biphasic abdominal motion may be appreciated—an outward motion at the beginning of inspiration due to the sudden relaxation of the abdominal muscles and a later inward motion as the relaxed abdominal wall follows the paradoxical upward movement of the paralyzed diaphragm. The paradoxical motion of the abdomen can be quantified by using magnetometry.[57]

The presence of bilateral diaphragmatic paralysis can be confirmed by measuring transdiaphragmatic pressure swings during tidal breathing and maximal inspiratory efforts.[49, 54, 57] Transdiaphragmatic pressure is measured by recording gastric and esophageal pressures: during inspiration, gastric pressure normally becomes positive and esophageal pressure negative. In the presence of diaphragmatic paralysis, weakness, or fatigue, the diaphragm acts as a flaccid membrane with the result that the negative intrathoracic pressure is transmitted to the abdominal cavity so that transdiaphragmatic pressure does not change. Even with maximal inspiratory effort, no transdiaphragmatic pressure develops, although maximal expiration may be associated with some transdiaphragmatic pressure as the diaphragm is passively stretched near residual volume.[57]

Bilateral diaphragmatic paralysis causes quite severe lung restriction. Total lung capacity and functional residual capacity are between 55 and 65 per cent predicted, and vital capacity is in the range of 45 to 50 per cent predicted.[53, 58] The FEV_1 is usually decreased in proportion to the forced vital capacity (FVC) so that the ratio of FEV_1/FVC is normal. Maximal inspiratory mouth pressure is reduced to well below the normal range and maximal transdiaphragmatic pressure is characteristically zero in the presence of complete paralysis. Blood gas measurements show arterial hypoxemia and, in some cases, hypercarbia. The hypoxemia is related to ventilation-perfusion mismatching at the lung bases and is exacerbated in the supine position.[59]

Eventration

Eventration is a congenital anomaly consisting of failure of muscular development of part or all of one or both hemidiaphragms.[60–62] In some cases it may be difficult or impossible to distinguish eventration from diaphragmatic paralysis; in fact, there is a tendency to use the terms synonymously.[63, 64] When marked diaphragmatic elevation can be attributed to a specific cause (for example, interruption of the phrenic nerve by invasive neoplasm or surgical section), it is clearly possible to employ specific terminology in describing the situation. In many cases, however, there is no way of knowing whether elevation is caused by congenital absence of muscle or by phrenic paralysis. In infants, for example, hemidiaphragmatic elevation may be attributed just as logically to birth injury as to congenital absence or deficiency of diaphragmatic muscle, and the only method of distinguishing the two short of visual inspection is by faradic stimulation of the phrenic nerve.[60] In an extensive roentgenographic survey of individuals older than nursery school age, a group of Japanese investigators[65] showed that the incidence of partial eventration of the right hemidiaphragm increased with age, particularly among women over the age of 60 years; the authors concluded that the majority of right-sided eventrations are acquired and may be attributable to dietary and dressing habits!

Pathologically, a totally eventrated hemidiaphragm consists of a thin membranous sheet attached peripherally to normal muscle at points of origin from the rib cage. Originally described by Petit early in the eighteenth century and sometimes referred to as Petit's eventration, it occurs almost exclusively on the left side, a point that may be of value in its differentiation from diaphragmatic paralysis. The latter has an approximately equal incidence on the two sides, except in idiopathic cases in which it occurs almost invariably on the right side.[10] Bilateral eventration has been described but is extremely rare.[66]

Partial eventration is somewhat more common than total eventration and is usually present in the anteromedial portion of the right hemidiaphragm;[60, 67, 68] it occurs with equal frequency in men and women.[1, 69] Campbell[70] feels that it has not been established whether these local elevations are normal variants or pathologic entities. Local elevation occurs rarely on the left and occasionally in the central portion of either cupola.

The roentgenologic signs of eventration are identical to those described for diaphragmatic paralysis. Although seldom performed now, pneumoperitoneum may be diagnostic in cases of local eventration, not only by demonstrating descent into the abdomen of the viscus occupying the space but also by revealing thinning of the leaf in the region of the weakness.[71–73] A confident diagnosis can be established by liver scan,[74, 75] or in questionable cases by CT.[76] A localized eventration can be mistaken for a pleural mass, and CT may be required for the differentiation.[3]

Characteristically, eventration of the diaphragm does not give rise to symptoms and is discovered on a screening chest roentgenogram. The major exception occurs in neonates, in whom hemidiaphragmatic elevation and mediastinal shift may be severe enough to result in ventilatory, cardiovascular, and gastrointestinal embarrassment. Surgical correction in these cases may be lifesaving.[60, 64] In the adult, symptoms may develop with increasing obesity and consequent raised intra-abdominal pressure. They are usually gastrointestinal in type, but respiratory embarrassment and, rarely, cardiac distress have been attributed to this anomaly.[60, 77]

Restriction of Diaphragmatic Motion

A great variety of diseases of the lungs, pleura, intra-abdominal organs, and of the diaphragm itself may lead to restriction of diaphragmatic motion. In some the limitation of motion is imposed by the character of the disease itself—for example, the severe pulmonary overinflation and air trapping that categorize diffuse emphysema or spasmodic asthma prevent normal ascent of the diaphragm during expiration. In other diseases, local irritation causes "splinting" of a hemidiaphragm that is manifested not only by reduced excursion but also by elevation; such splinting can be caused by acute lower lobe pneumonia or infarction, acute pleuritis, rib fractures, and acute intra-abdominal processes such as subphrenic abscess, cholecystitis, and peritonitis. It has been stated that acute intra-abdominal processes are much more likely to limit diaphragmatic excursion than are intrathoracic diseases.[78, 79]

While other skeletal muscle groups react to irritation or injury by spasm, the diaphragm appears to react by relaxation; this is the only way to explain the elevation that characteristically accompanies local inflammation. The mechanism by which the diaphragm "splints" in the postoperative period is thought to be neural inhibition of diaphragmatic activation,[80–82] possibly caused by stimulation of diaphragmatic or splanchnic afferents. By employing diaphragmatic electromyograms and measuring transdiaphragmatic pressure following upper abdominal surgery in dogs, Road and colleagues[81] demonstrated a localized decrease in neural activation. Easton and associates found similar diaphragmatic dysfunction following laparotomy by measuring diaphragmatic muscle shortening with sonomicrometry crystals;[83] general anesthesia alone and lower abdominal surgery did not produce similar results. Following upper abdominal surgery, diaphragmatic dysfunction is maximal in patients 8 hours after surgery, with function improving over the subsequent 2 to 7 days.[80] The decreased diaphragmatic activation is not directly related to pain; in one study[82] narcotic analgesia did not improve the deficit in transdiaphragmatic pressure generation. Similarly, postoperative diaphragmatic dysfunction is not caused by a decrease in diaphragmatic contractility, since direct stimulation of the phrenic nerve can result in a normal transdiaphragmatic pressure.[84]

Incidental Causes of Disturbance in Diaphragmatic Motion

Several conditions other than restriction or paradox may be associated with abnormal movements of the diaphragm. *Tonic contraction* may occur in tetany, tetanus, rabies, strychnine poisoning, and in the pleurodynia that accompanies Coxsackie B virus infection. *Diaphragmatic "flutter"* (respiratory myoclonus) was originally described in 1723 by Antonj van Leeuwenhoek when he recognized that he was having abnormal contractions of his diaphragm.[85] Some cases appear to develop peripherally and possibly are precipitated by emotional tension or excitement.[86, 87] Other patients appear to suffer from a central epileptic focus, with involvement of all muscles of respiration, including the accessory muscles.[85] This disorder may present as part of a symptom complex including palatal, oropharyngeal, eye, and facial muscle myoclonus. These rapid diaphragmatic contractions may occasion pain and dyspnea. In one patient, diaphragmatic flutter was documented and followed by respiratory inductive plethysmography.[88] In *persistent hiccups,* a form of chronic contraction of the diaphragm that occurs at a much lower frequency than "flutter," an inspiratory sound is created as air is drawn into the thorax through a partially closed glottis. We have seen one patient who manifested periodic irregular, sudden diaphragmatic contractions late in the expiratory phase of respiration that seemed analogous to a premature heart beat but caused the patient considerably more discomfort.

DIAPHRAGMATIC HERNIAS

Herniation of abdominal or retroperitoneal organs or tissues into the thorax may occur through congenital or acquired weak areas in the diaphragm or through rents resulting from traumatic rupture. Traumatic diaphragmatic hernias are discussed in detail in Chapter 15 (*see* page 2509) and are not considered here. By far the most common diaphrag-

matic hernia is that which occurs through the esophageal hiatus. Although these hernias may be associated with considerable morbidity, the associated mortality is much lower than with congenital hernias through the pleuroperitoneal hiatus (the foramen of Bochdalek). Hernias through the retrosternal or parasternal hiatus (the foramen of Morgagni) are the rarest form of congenital hernia and constitute less than 10 per cent of most series.[89–91]

Hernia Through the Esophageal Hiatus

Although hiatus hernia is the most common form of diaphragmatic hernia in the adult, its effects relate almost entirely to the gastrointestinal tract and only seldom is its presence manifested by changes in the chest roentgenogram. Although a congenital weakness of the esophageal hiatus may be partly responsible for the development of hernia in adults, there is little doubt that acquired factors play a significant role, the most important being obesity and pregnancy. In infants, esophageal hiatus hernia is less common than hernias through the foramen of Bochdalek but more common than those through the foramen of Morgagni. Of 48 cases of diaphragmatic hernia reported by Reed and Lang,[91] 12 (25 per cent) involved the esophageal hiatus. In infants, this type of hernia may be associated with a congenitally short esophagus.

The diagnosis of hiatus hernia requires barium study of the esophagogastric junction. Plain roentgenograms of the chest may show a mass in the posteroinferior mediastinum, usually containing an air-fluid level (Fig. 20–5). Hiatus hernias also can be detected with CT[92] and two-dimensional echocardiography,[93, 94] although with the latter technique they can be confused with a cardiac mass. In cases in which most of the stomach has herniated through the hiatus, the stomach may undergo volvulus within the mediastinum and present as a large mass, sometimes containing a double air-filled level (Fig. 20–6). Incarceration of such hernial contents is frequent, and although earlier reports suggested that strangulation was much less common in hiatal than in congenital or traumatic hernias,[95, 96] more recent studies have indicated that the incidence of strangulation is about equal. In addition, a number of cases have been reported of strangulation of contents that have herniated through the diaphragmatic incision made for repair of hiatus hernia.[97] Menuck[98] has pointed out that the development of acute upper gastrointestinal tract symptoms in a patient with a herniated stomach that has undergone volvulus should immediately raise the suspicion of acute strangulation, caused by torsion greater than 180 degrees with resultant impairment of gastric blood supply. This complication is life-threatening and necessitates immediate surgical intervention. It is noteworthy that many cases of acute volvulus of this type occur in patients with chronic or recurring gastric volvulus of the organoaxial type.

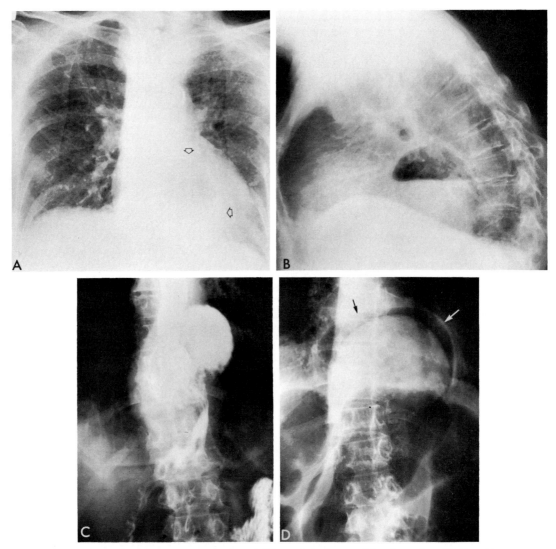

Figure 20–5. Hiatus Hernia. Posteroanterior *(A)* and lateral *(B)* roentgenograms of the chest of an 87-year-old woman reveal a large soft tissue mass containing a prominent air-fluid level occupying the posteroinferior portion of the mediastinum *(arrows in A)*. An anteroposterior roentgenogram of the lower mediastinum and upper abdomen following the ingestion of barium *(C)* confirms the presence of herniation of a large portion of stomach into the posterior mediastinum. The patient had no symptoms referable to this hernia. Somewhat later, the patient developed an acute abdomen, with severe abdominal distention and signs of peritonitis. An anteroposterior roentgenogram *(D)* revealed a double density in the posterior mediastinum, the hernial sac being outlined by gas *(arrows)* and the central portion of the sac containing a homogeneous mass representing a fluid-filled gastric fundus. A hollow abdominal viscus had perforated, releasing gas into the peritoneal space; some of the gas had passed through the esophageal hiatus, outlining the sac.

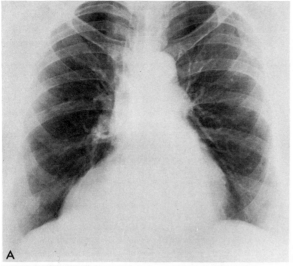

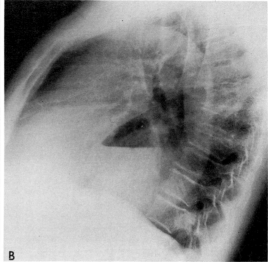

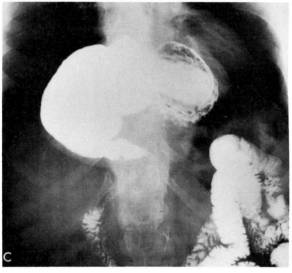

Figure 20–6. Hiatus Hernia. Posteroanterior *(A)* and lateral *(B)* roentgenograms reveal a large soft tissue mass in the posterior mediastinum, projecting to the right as a smooth, well-defined shadow in the plane of the cardiophrenic angle. A prominent air-fluid level is present within it. Note the downward displacement of the right hemidiaphragm. Roentgenography following ingestion of barium *(C)* shows herniation of the whole stomach through the esophageal hiatus into the posterior mediastinum; in the process the stomach has undergone complete organoaxial volvulus. The shadow projected in the plane of the right cardiophrenic angle on the posteroanterior roentgenogram is caused by the rotated greater curvature of the stomach. The patient is a 65-year-old woman who had no definite symptoms referable to the hernia.

Occasionally, the transverse colon herniates through the esophageal hiatus. In addition, ascitic fluid can extend from the peritoneal cavity into the posterior mediastinum via the esophageal hiatus, an occurrence that can be demonstrated to excellent advantage on CT scans.[99]

The majority of patients with esophageal hiatus hernias are asymptomatic, the abnormality being discovered on a screening examination of the upper gastrointestinal tract or during examination because of unrelated complaints. When present, symptoms consist of retrosternal "burning" and pain, typically occurring after meals and accentuated when the patient lies down; they are relieved by the ingestion of antacid. Symptoms of anemia caused by blood loss may be predominant. Of 267 cases reported by Felder and associates,[100] 61 (23 per cent) evidenced blood loss attributable to the hernia; 27 (10 per cent) of these patients presented with hematemesis, 19 (7 per cent) with melena or a history thereof, and 16 (6 per cent) with established blood loss anemia and only a trace of blood or none in the

stool. Sixty-two per cent of the 61 patients were over 60 years of age.

Hernia Through the Foramen of Bochdalek

In infants, herniation through the pleuroperitoneal hiatus is not only the most common form of diaphragmatic hernia but also by far the most serious. When large, it is associated with a high death rate unless surgically corrected. In a study of selected congenital anomalies in Pennsylvania, Boch and Zimmerman[101] found an incidence of Bochdalek hernias of 4.8 per 10,000 live births. Between 80 and 90 per cent of Bochdalek hernias detected on conventional roentgenograms occur on the left side,[91, 102] partly because defects in the right hemidiaphragm are protected by the liver. The incidence of Bochdalek hernias is much higher on CT scans than on conventional roentgenograms. In a recent study, Gale found an incidence of 6 per cent in 940 adults who had chest and abdominal CT examinations;[103] left-sided hernias showed a preponderance

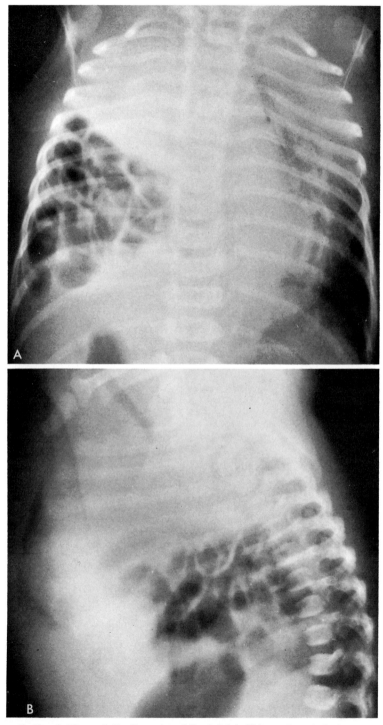

Figure 20–7. Diaphragmatic Hernia Through the Foramen of Bochdalek. This newborn baby boy was referred for roentgenography of the chest when it was noted in the nursery that he was cyanotic and showed chest retraction, subcostal indrawing, and grunting respiration. These roentgenograms in anteroposterior *(A)* and lateral *(B)* projections demonstrate numerous loops of air-filled bowel in the posteroinferior portion of the right hemithorax. The right lung above the hernia contents is airless, and the mediastinum is displaced considerably to the left. Only the lower portion of the left lung appears to be air-containing. At thoracotomy, the right hemithorax was found to contain the liver, stomach, small intestine, kidneys, and adrenal gland; the right lung was severely hypoplastic. The hernial contents were returned to the abdomen and a large right pleuroperitoneal foramen was closed. The infant died 2 days later.

of only 2:1 over right-sided hernias in contrast to the reported preponderance of 9:1 on conventional roentgenograms.

Closure of the posterolateral portion of the diaphragm by fusion of the pleuroperitoneal membrane with the septum transversum normally occurs by the 7th week of fetal life. Since the intestines return from the yolk stalk to the abdominal cavity during the 10th week, herniation through the pleuroperitoneal hiatus may occur if the intestines return prematurely before the 7th week or if there is delayed or incomplete closure of the pleuroperitoneal membrane.[104]

The size of the defect ranges widely. When large, as with complete, or almost complete, absence of a hemidiaphragm, almost the entire abdominal contents, including the stomach, may be in the left hemithorax, thereby interfering with normal lung development and resulting in hypoplasia.[105] In the rare instance in which herniation is bilateral, pulmonary hypoplasia may be incompatible with life. Following repair of a unilateral defect, the ipsilateral lung may reinflate and develop normally or may have suffered permanent damage, particularly of the lower lobe.[106, 107] In most cases of large hernia there is no peritoneal sac, and communication between the pleural and peritoneal cavities is wide open. When the defect is small, a sac lined by pleura and containing retroperitoneal fat, a portion of the spleen or kidney,[117] or omentum may be the only discernible abnormality.[108, 109] The latter form of limited herniation is the type found by chance in asymptomatic adults, either roentgenographically or at necropsy.

The roentgenographic manifestations depend almost entirely on hernial contents and thus on the size of the defect. In infants in whom the defect is large, the roentgenographic appearance is characteristic (Fig. 20–7). The ipsilateral hemidiaphragm is partly or completely obscured, multiple radiolucencies representing gas-containing loops of intestine—some containing fluid levels—are seen within the hemithorax, the heart and mediastinum are shifted into the opposite hemithorax and the ipsilateral lung is compressed and airless, and there is partial or complete absence of intestinal gas within the abdomen.[91, 110]

In some infants the presentation may be delayed: in one report of seven infants ranging in age from 2 to 20 months,[111] the roentgenographic findings were classic in only one patient; in two patients, acute pneumonia was simulated; in three, gastric volvulus; and in one, pneumothorax. Congenital diaphragmatic hernia can be diagnosed by fetal ultrasonography, as in four of seven cases described in one series;[112] diagnosis relied upon the demonstration of abdominal organs within the thorax. Fetal ultrasonography performed as early as 17 weeks of gestational age has been reported capable of detecting bilateral diaphragmatic aplasia and associated defects of the thoracic and abdominal walls.[113]

Although it might be anticipated that prenatal diagnosis of diaphragmatic hernia would aid in preventing postnatal complications, the results of one study suggest that this is not the case. Nakayama and associates found that 15 of 20 patients in whom a prenatal diagnosis of congenital diaphragmatic hernia was made died in the immediate postnatal period, either before or after corrective surgery.[114] Contralateral pneumothorax has been described as a complication in infants receiving artificial ventilation before surgery.[102] In one series of 21 neonates with congenital diaphragmatic hernia,[115] none of the 14 infants with pre- or postoperative contralateral pneumothorax survived, whereas nearly half the remaining neonates did well. Kelvin and Starer[116] have drawn attention to the frequency with which congenital diaphragmatic hernia is associated with 13 pairs of ribs; 3 of 13 cases studied by these authors were so affected.

Although Bochdalek defects are most commonly situated posterolaterally, they may occur anywhere along the posterior aspect of the diaphragm, even in the vicinity of the costovertebral junction. In adults suspected of having a Bochdalek hernia from the roentgenographic demonstration of a "bump" on the superior aspect of the diaphragm posteriorly, CT and ultrasonography can be useful in establishing the diagnosis.[118, 119]

Large left-sided Bochdalek hernias are a rare cause of acute respiratory distress in neonates and are usually fatal unless surgical correction is performed promptly. If infants survive without surgical correction, there is the added danger of strangulation of herniated bowel.[91] The diagnosis of hernias that present later in the postnatal period or in childhood can be difficult;[120, 121] Berman and associates[120] identified 26 such patients during a 20-year period and recommended barium studies and conventional roentgenography after nasogastric intubation as useful investigations.

The roentgenographic presentation of congenital right diaphragmatic hernia may be delayed for several days after birth; the hernial content is usually liver.[122] Radionuclide scintigraphy using technetium 99m sulphur colloid to outline the liver can aid in diagnosis.[123]

Hernia Through the Foramen of Morgagni

Morgagni (retrosternal or parasternal) hernia is an uncommon form of diaphragmatic hernia, constituting fewer than 10 per cent in most series.[89–91] The foramina of Morgagni are small clefts bounded by diaphragmatic muscle fibers originating from the sternum medially and from the seventh costal cartilages laterally. They are triangular, the base being formed by the anterior thoracic wall and the apex being directed posteriorly. The clefts contain the mammary vessels and normally are filled with loose areolar connective tissue and fat. Since the left foramen relates to the heart, the majority of herniations occur on the right.

Although these defects are developmental in origin, it is probable that herniation requires the additional presence of obesity, at least in adults.[89] In contrast to Bochdalek hernias, a peritoneal sac is present in most cases. The content of the hernial sac is usually omentum,[89] but sometimes liver or bowel. Even a stone-filled gallbladder[124] and a congenital hepatic cyst[125] have been reported as herniating through the foramen of Morgagni. In the rare instances in which a portion of stomach is herniated, it has been stated that considerable trouble can be expected,[126] presumably from strangulation. Cases have been reported in which the defect in the diaphragm extends into the pericardial sac and permits displacement of abdominal contents into this area.[127, 128] A complex syndrome has been described in a small number of infants that consisted of cardiac malrotation (dextroposition), intracardiac defects (including ventricular septal defect), deficient development of the lower sternum, a defect in the anterior portion of the diaphragm (Morgagni), and a midline abdominal defect with diastasis recti and umbilical hernia or omphalocele.[70, 129]

Roentgenographically, the typical appearance is that of a smooth, well-defined opacity in the right cardiophrenic angle. In the majority of patients the shadow is of homogeneous density. Occasionally it is inhomogeneous as a result of either an air-containing loop of bowel or the predominantly fatty nature of the hernial contents. In the latter situation the hernia is likely to contain omentum, and a barium enema study will reveal the transverse colon to be situated high in the abdomen with a peak situated anteriorly and superiorly, a finding that is virtually diagnostic (see Fig. 19–51, page 2873). Bilateral anteromedial defects in the diaphragm produce a characteristic roentgenographic pattern when abdominal organs herniate through a single midline opening.[130] In infants and children, the usually solid herniated structures elevate the heart and thymus to produce a three-tiered snowman appearance; the high incidence of liver herniation permits the confirmation of the diagnosis by radionuclide scanning. Lanuza[131] has described a roentgenologic sign for the diagnosis of small Morgagni hernias consisting of a curvilinear extension of the properitoneal fat line into the thorax anteriorly. Termed "the sign of the cane," it represents a thin layer of abdominal fat surrounding the hernial contents. In the rare case in which the hernia penetrates into the pericardial sac, many loops of air-containing bowel may be identified anterior to the cardiac shadow.[127, 128] Ultrasonography can be a valuable addition to roentgenography in the characterization of anteromedial diaphragmatic defects and helps to define accurately the size of the defect and the contents of the hernial sac.[132]

The majority of hernias through the foramen of Morgagni do not give rise to symptoms, although of nine patients in one highly selected series,[133] four had gastrointestinal symptoms, two had respiratory symptoms, and one had retrosternal pain; only two patients were asymptomatic. When the sac contains portions of the gastrointestinal tract, strangulation and obstruction may occur; these complications have been reported in 10 to 15 per cent of cases.[89] Extension of the defect into the pericardial sac may produce severe cardiorespiratory symptoms and necessitate prompt corrective surgery, particularly in infants. Because of the association of congenital cardiac anomalies, angiocardiography should be performed for clarification of the presence and type of such an anomaly. The minority of adults who have symptoms complain of epigastric or lower sternal pressure and discomfort[89] and sometimes cardiorespiratory and gastrointestinal symptoms.[134] Affected patients are usually overweight, middle-aged females; the hernias presumably result from rapid changes in intra-abdominal pressure engendered by coughing and straining.[89, 134] Abrupt enlargement of a previously existing diaphragmatic hernia with subsequent strangulation has been reported as a complication of pregnancy and labor.[135]

SUBPHRENIC ABSCESS

Formerly, subphrenic abscess occurred predominantly in young patients after such incidents as perforation of the appendix and developed chiefly in the posterior subphrenic space of the right hemidiaphragm. Recent reports, however, suggest that subphrenic infection now occurs as frequently after abdominal surgery, that its incidence on the two sides is approximately equal,[136] and that it involves the anterior and posterior subphrenic spaces equally as often. The pathogenesis of abscess formation differs somewhat depending on whether it occurs on the right or left side of the abdomen. Meyers[137] has shown that the main pathway by which infection spreads to and from the upper and lower peritoneal compartments is the right paracolic gutter. Further, he states that it is probable that the hydrostatic pressure differences between the lower and upper abdomen are capable of helping to convey infected peritoneal fluid from the lower abdomen to the subhepatic and subphrenic regions, even in the erect position. Superiorly, the right paracolic gutter is continuous with the subhepatic space and its posterosuperior extension, Morison's pouch, and from there with the right subphrenic space.[137] Thus, an abscess in the right subhepatic space often spreads to the right subphrenic space.

Abdominal abscesses located in the left upper quadrant can occur in two major anatomic locations, the subphrenic space and the lesser sac. Both the lesser sac and left anterior subphrenic space extend to the right of midline,[138] the latter compartment being bounded on the right by the falciform ligament while the lesser sac extends to the right coronary ligament and foramen of Winslow. Therefore, abscesses arising in either of these locations can extend across the midline into the right upper quadrant. Abscesses in the left anterior subphrenic space and in the lesser sac can be differentiated by the fact that the former is immediately subdiaphragmatic whereas the latter usually is not contiguous with the diaphragm.[138] Subphrenic abscesses on the left side usually result from perforated gastric or duodenal ulcers[137] and tend to cause a characteristic CT appearance.[139]

Roentgenologic signs of subphrenic abscess include abnormalities within the lung, the pleural space, the subphrenic space, and the diaphragm itself (Figs. 20–8 and 20–9). In an analysis of the signs in 48 cases of subphrenic abscess, Miller and Talman[140] reported the following findings:

Elevation of the ipsilateral hemidiaphragm	44/47	(95%)
Restriction of diaphragmatic motion	33/36	(92%)
Fixation of the hemidiaphragm	19/36	(53%)
Pleural effusion	37/47	(79%)
Basal pulmonary opacity (pneumonitis or atelectasis or both)	33/47	(70%)

Gas in the abscess cavity was identified in 30 per cent of the 48 patients and displacement of intra-abdominal viscera in 35 per cent. The gas may have one of several causes, including gas-forming organisms, a residuum of "air" after laparotomy or perforation of a hollow abdominal viscus, and, rarely, a bronchohepatic fistula. The most frequent early roentgenologic findings in 36 patients with subphrenic abscess reported by Johnson[141] were elevation of a hemidiaphragm (observed in 100 per cent of cases) and blunting of the costophrenic angle (noted in 91 per cent of cases). Less frequent and

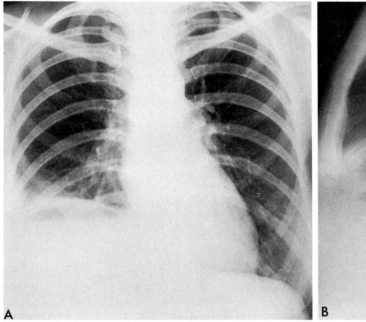

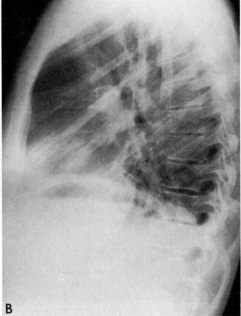

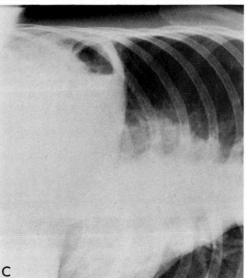

Figure 20–8. Subphrenic Abscess. Two weeks prior to this roentgenographic examination, this 34-year-old woman had had an appendectomy for acute, gangrenous appendicitis. Her only complaint on admission was a vague discomfort in the upper right abdomen. Posteroanterior (A), lateral (B), and lateral decubitus (C) roentgenograms revealed a large accumulation of gas and fluid beneath a moderately elevated right hemidiaphragm; there was a small right pleural effusion. Focal areas of increased density in the right lung base represent inflammatory reaction in the contiguous lung.

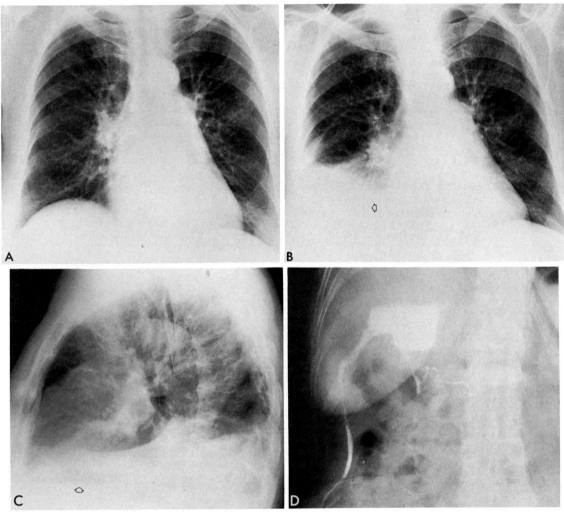

Figure 20–9. Subphrenic Abscess. Following the normal preoperative roentgenogram illustrated in *(A)*, this 65-year-old woman had a cholecystectomy; recovery was uneventful, and she was discharged. Seven weeks later, she was readmitted to the hospital because of the discovery of increased dullness over the right lung base on routine postoperative follow-up examination; she was completely asymptomatic. Shortly after admission, pus was seen to be draining from her upper abdominal incision. Roentgenograms of the chest in posteroanterior *(B)* and lateral *(C)* projections revealed moderate elevation of the right hemidiaphragm associated with right pleural effusion and basal pulmonary opacity. A small collection of gas and fluid could be identified beneath the right hemidiaphragm anteriorly *(arrow* in both projections). Contrast material was injected through a catheter inserted into the incision; a roentgenogram exposed in the erect position *(D)* demonstrated a large pocket in the right subphrenic space containing contrast medium, fluid, and gas. Of some note is the fact that such a large subphrenic abscess could be present in the absence of clinical symptoms.

generally later findings were pleural effusion and basal atelectasis. Subphrenic gas (with or without fluid) was present in 42 per cent of the patients in that series.

In one retrospective study of the roentgenographic findings in 82 patients with proven subphrenic abscess,[142] conventional roentgenograms revealed extraluminal gas or a soft-tissue mass in 58 patients (71 per cent), the diagnosis being suggested in the majority. It is probable that conventional roentgenograms of the abdomen represent the most important diagnostic modality in the diagnosis of these abscesses, as in 65 per cent of 55 subphrenic abscesses in one series.[143] Procedures of value in confirming the diagnosis include barium examination of the gastrointestinal tract (particularly in abscesses situated on the left), CT, gallium scanning,[144] and ultrasonic examination (the last procedure is particularly useful for confirmation of subphrenic abscesses on the right).[143]

An occasional diagnostic problem is the differentiation of pleural effusion and subphrenic abscess. In a study of 66 patients with pleural effusion or subphrenic abscess or both, Alexander and associates[145] found that CT was both sensitive and specific in separating the entities. Of the 66 patients, 38 had proven subphrenic abscess with or without pleural effusion and 28 had proven pleural effusion without abscess. As might be anticipated, accurate differentiation requires correct identification of the diaphragmatic position. Alexander and associates found that in 26 per cent of cases the diaphragm could be clearly identified on CT as a radiopaque stripe and that in 71 per cent diaphragmatic position was identified indirectly by the contour formed by juxtaposition of thoracic and abdominal contents. The distinction between subphrenic abscess and pleural effusion was correct in 95 per cent of cases. The differentiation of subpulmonic pleural effusions from subphrenic collections is sometimes difficult but usually can be clarified by lateral decubitus roentgenography or, if necessary, by CT.[146] Similarly, differentiation between subphrenic abscess and hepatic abscess can be difficult and may require CT examination.

A subphrenic abscess should be suspected in any patient with chronic fever, vague upper abdominal pain, loss of weight, and sometimes chills and anemia.[136, 147] It is probable that in many patients postoperative antibiotic therapy prevents the development of subphrenic suppuration, although in some patients it may only suppress the acute symptoms and thus permit the development of chronic low-grade infection that is difficult to recognize.[136] In fact, several months may elapse between the episode resulting in the development of subphrenic infection and the appearance of symptoms produced by the accumulation of pus; symptoms sometimes may be absent altogether (see Fig. 20–9). We have seen one patient in whom a subphrenic abscess evolved over a period of years into a large calcified mass (Fig. 20–10). Physical findings include elevation and fixation of the affected hemidiaphragm and tenderness on pressure over the 12th rib posteriorly (if the abscess is in the posterior space) or along the lateral and anterior costal margin (if the abscess is anteriorly situated).

NEOPLASMS OF THE DIAPHRAGM

Primary neoplasms of the diaphragm, a subject reviewed by Anderson and Forrest,[148] are very uncommon; in a review of the literature from 1868 to 1968, Olafsson and coworkers[149] found only 84 acceptable cases. Most develop from the tendinous or anterior muscular portion. Benign and malignant forms occur with relatively equal frequency.[150, 151] The former include lipoma (the most common),[152, 153] angiofibroma, neurofibroma, neurilemoma,[154] leiomyoma, teratoma (Fig. 20–11),[155, 156] and tumors with various mesenchymal admixtures.[150] Malignant neoplasms include fibrosarcoma (the most common), malignant fibrous histiocytoma,[157] hemangiopericytoma,[158] endodermal sinus tumor,[159] and leiomyosarcoma.[160] Various non-neoplastic abnormalities that form localized tumors, such as "leioangioma," lymphangioma, and endometriosis,[148] are also occasionally found in the diaphragm.

Roentgenographically, most diaphragmatic tumors present as smooth or lobulated soft tissue masses protruding into the inferior portion of the lung. Benign neoplasms may calcify. In many cases, malignant tumors involve much of one hemidiaphragm and thus simulate diaphragmatic elevation; associated pleural effusion is common. The presence of an intradiaphragmatic mass can be established most easily by CT,[153, 154, 155] although more complicated procedures such as pneumothorax or pneumoperitoneum (or both) may be required to differentiate primary diaphragmatic lesions from masses arising above or below the diaphragm.[151, 161] Variations in diaphragmatic thickness on CT can occasionally mimic an intradiaphragmatic mass or a tumor in an adjacent organ.[146]

Characteristically, benign neoplasms occasion no symptoms; by contrast, the majority of patients with primary malignant neoplasms complain of epigastric or lower chest pain, cough, dyspnea, and gastrointestinal discomfort.[148, 149]

Secondary neoplastic involvement of the diaphragm is not uncommon. It occurs most frequently by direct extension of neoplasm from the basal pleura in cases of pulmonary carcinoma or mesothelioma (see Fig. 18–22, page 2765); however, any neoplasm that metastasizes to the pleura or that involves the basal lung, liver, or subphrenic peritoneum can involve the diaphragm. Discrete diaphragmatic metastases, derived from either lymphatic or hematogenous spread, are rare. Roentgenographic features and clinical manifestations are usually related to the presence of neoplasm in contiguous structures or elsewhere, rather than in the diaphragm itself.

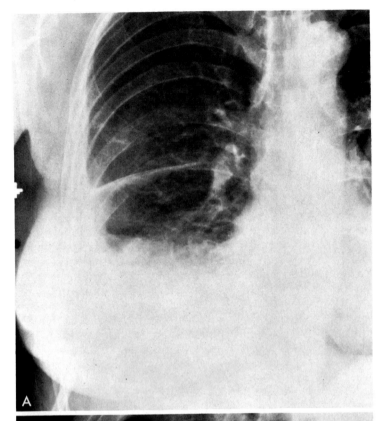

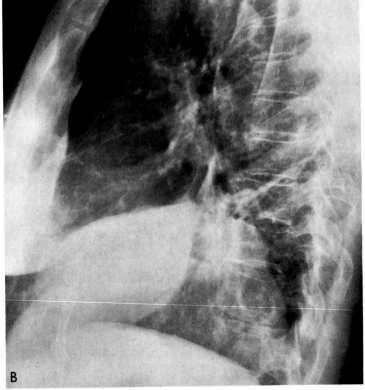

Figure 20–10. Acute Subphrenic Abscess Evolving Over Many Years into a Large Calcified Mass. Several days prior to the roentgenograms illustrated in *(A)* and *(B)*, this middle-aged woman had had a cholecystectomy. These views reveal moderate elevation of the right hemidiaphragm, a right pleural effusion, and poorly defined parenchymal opacities in the right lower lobe. This picture is highly suggestive of an acute subphrenic abscess. Management was conservative and there was uneventful recovery.

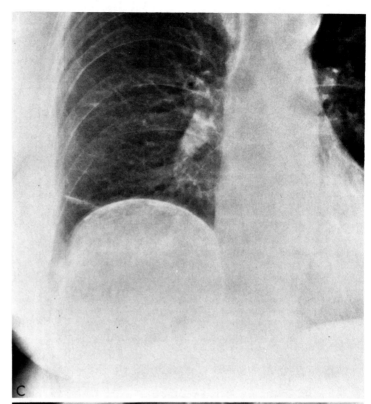

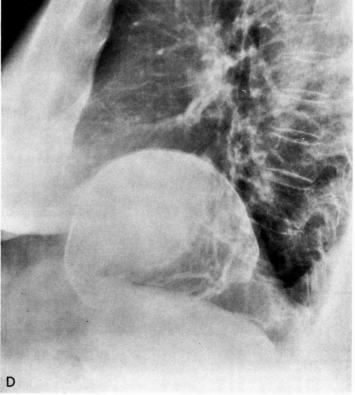

Figure 20–10 *Continued* Twelve years later, roentgenograms in posteroanterior *(C)* and lateral *(D)* projections reveal a large, irregular calcified mass in the right subphrenic space, presumed to be calcification of the wall of a large cyst that was the residuum of the previous subphrenic abscess. Since the patient was asymptomatic, further intervention was not indicated. (Courtesy of Montreal Chest Hospital Center.)

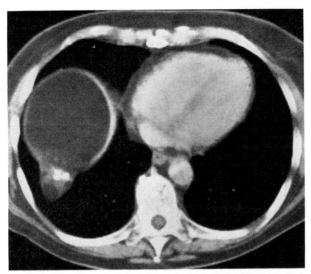

Figure 20–11. Cystic Teratoma of the Right Hemidiaphragm. A CT scan at the level of the right hemidiaphragm shows a mass containing fat (CT attenuation, – 70 HU), a small amount of soft tissue posteriorly, and two small areas of calcification. The mass was resected and proved to be a cystic teratoma of the diaphragm. Pathologically, the mass was also shown to contain a tooth. This 65-year-old woman presented with a 1-year history of right upper quadrant pain and nausea. (From Müller NL: J Comput. Assist. Tomogr. *10*:325, 1986.)

MISCELLANEOUS ABNORMALITIES OF THE DIAPHRAGM

Accessory diaphragm is a rare anomaly in which the right hemithorax is partitioned into two compartments by a musculotendinous membrane resembling a diaphragm.[70, 162, 163] The accessory leaf usually is situated within the oblique fissure, separating the lower lobe from the remainder of the right lung. It is attached medially to the pericardium, inferiorly and anteriorly to the diaphragm, and laterally and posteriorly to the chest wall. Roentgenographically, it may be mistaken for a somewhat thickened major fissure. The anomaly has been reported as a cause for neonatal respiratory distress[163] but usually does not give rise to symptoms.

Diaphragmatic defects, too small to allow passage of a hernial sac, may explain in part the pleural effusions that develop in patients with conditions such as Meigs' syndrome or cirrhosis and ascites.[164, 165] Such defects may be congenital or acquired and can be demonstrated either directly at autopsy or indirectly by the development of pneumothorax following intraperitoneal administration of gas.[165] Similar small defects have been postulated as the entry sites for tissue or air in some cases of pleural endometriosis (*see* page 2744) and catamenial pneumothorax,[166] the hypothesized route being via the fallopian tube to the peritoneal cavity and via the diaphragmatic defects to the pleural space.

Intradiaphragmatic cysts are very rare and usually can be categorized as extralobar sequestration. The abnormality is presumably caused by entrapment of the accessory lung bud within the diaphragm during its development. In the majority of cases the cyst receives its blood supply from the abdominal aorta or one of its branches[167] and characteristically drains by way of the systemic veins. The anomaly relates to the left hemidiaphragm in 90 per cent of cases[168] and is usually associated with diaphragmatic eventration (*see* page 709). Rarely, cystic lesions of the liver such as amebic or hydatid cysts can simulate a diaphragmatic cyst (Fig. 20–12).

THE CHEST WALL

This section describes briefly the more common abnormalities affecting the soft tissues and bones of the thoracic wall. Traumatic abnormalities of the ribs and spine are described in Chapter 15 (*see* page 2513) and are not discussed here.

ABNORMALITIES OF THE PECTORAL GIRDLE AND ADJACENT STRUCTURES

Several congenital anomalies affect the pectoral girdle. With few exceptions, they occasion no serious disabilities, but their recognition is important, particularly for the roentgenologist. This subject was thoroughly reviewed by Goldenberg and Brogdon in 1967.[169] The most important anomaly of the clavicle is *cleidocranial dysostosis,* a syndrome characterized by incomplete ossification of the clavicle and defective development of the pubic bones, vertebral column, and long bones. A case has been described of bilateral retrosternal subluxation of the medial ends of the clavicles that was considered by the author to be congenital in origin;[170] the posterior position of the medial ends of the clavicles suggested a retrosternal mass on a lateral roentgenogram.

The chief anomaly of the scapula is *Sprengel's deformity,* in which the scapula fails to descend normally so that its superior angle lies on a plane higher than the neck of the first rib. This is frequently associated with fusion of two or more cervical vertebrae, resulting in a short, wide neck with considerably limited movement (Klippel-Feil deformity). Other anomalies of the scapula include *ununited apophyses,* frequently bilateral and symmetric, which may simulate fractures, and *pseudoforamen,* in which the supraspinatous and infraspinatous fossae are formed by fibrous tissue rather than bone and create the roentgenographic appearance of lytic lesions. Finally, a "foramen" may be formed at the superior border of the scapula by calcification of the superior transverse ligament.

Poland's syndrome is a congenital anomaly consisting of hypoplasia or aplasia of the pectoralis major muscle and ipsilateral syndactyly.[171] Other anomalies that may be associated include absence of the pectoralis minor muscle, absence or atrophy of ipsilateral ribs two to five, aplasia of the ipsilateral

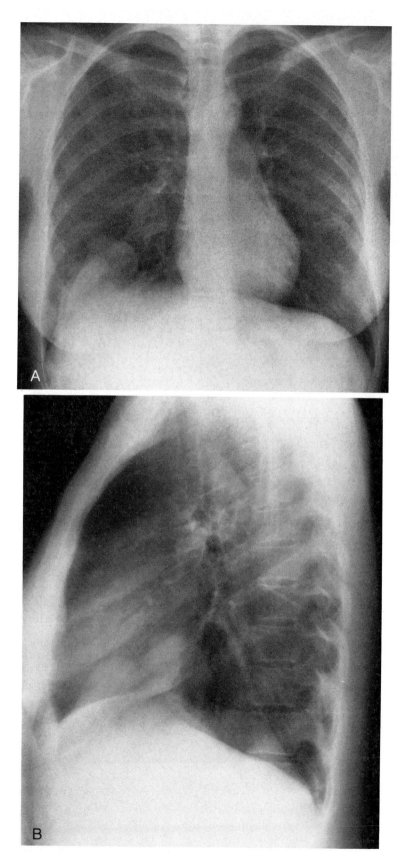

Figure 20–12. Hydatid Cyst Involving the Right Hemidiaphragm. Posteroanterior *(A)* and lateral *(B)* chest roentgenograms reveal a lobulated mass extending from the right hemidiaphragm into the inferior aspect of the right middle lobe.

Illustration continued on following page

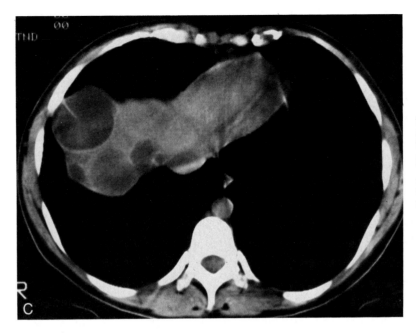

Figure 20–12 *Continued* A CT scan through the dome of the right hemidiaphragm *(C)* shows several cystic lesions. At surgery, the patient was found to have hydatid disease of the liver that extended through the diaphragm and into the lung. This 30-year-old woman presented with right upper quadrant pain. (Courtesy of Dr. Nestor Müller, Vancouver General Hospital, Vancouver, British Columbia.)

breast or nipple, and simian crease of the affected extremity.[171] Absence of the pectoralis muscles results in unilateral hypertranslucency on the chest roentgenogram, not to be confused with the Swyer-James syndrome (however, see Fig. 11–88, page 2178). Poland's syndrome has been reported to be associated with an increased incidence of leukemia and perhaps also of non-Hodgkin's lymphoma.[172, 173]

It has been postulated that Sprengel's deformity, Klippel-Feil deformity, and Poland's syndrome may be the result of an interruption of the early embryonic blood supply provided by the subclavian or vertebral arteries or their branches.[174]

The roentgenologic appearance of the chest following *radical neck dissection* reveals a number of abnormalities that may not be anticipated ordinarily, as noted in the study carried out by Mueller and Moseley.[175] In their review of 30 cases, these authors found the following abnormalities, in decreasing order of frequency: hyperlucent supraclavicular fossa (in 28 cases), absent sternocleidomastoid muscle (23 cases), a drooping shoulder (20 cases), medial continuation of the ipsilateral companion shadow (19 cases), and sternoclavicular subluxation (8 cases). The last-named appears to occur as a later complication of the drooping pectoral girdle, which in turn is a result of muscle resection and interruption of the spinal accessory nerve.

Cervical lung hernia results from excessive excursion of the dome of the pleura, which permits protrusion of the apex of the lung into the cervical region during periods of increased intrathoracic pressure. The herniation usually occurs between the anterior scalene and sternocleidomastoid muscles. Usually it follows severe trauma but in some cases is associated with chronic obstructive pulmonary disease (COPD).[139] Rarely, such hernias appear to be secondary to a congenital defect in Sibson's fascia, as was the case in a child whose mother had a hernia through the foramen of Morgagni.[176]

ABNORMALITIES OF THE RIBS

Congenital Anomalies

Congenital anomalies of the ribs, including *fusion of two or more ribs,* and various types of *bifid ribs,* are relatively common and are of little or no significance. Of potentially greater importance is an anomalous *accessory rib* ("Eve's rib," cervical rib) that usually arises from the seventh cervical vertebra. According to Fisher,[177] this abnormality occurs in about 0.5 per cent of the population; both the anomaly and symptoms that derive therefrom are said to be more common in women in a ratio of approximately 2.5.[177] In about 90 per cent of cases, cervical ribs do not cause symptoms; however, when they compress subclavian vessels or the brachial plexus, symptoms may be present and are sometimes disabling.

The diagnosis of *cervical rib syndrome* is certain when there is roentgenographic evidence of a cervical rib associated with the typical symptoms and signs of pain and weakness of the arm, swelling of the hand, and variation in the intensity of the pulses in the two arms when the affected extremity is in certain positions. This syndrome may be mimicked by other syndromes in which structures at the cervicothoracic inlet are compressed, including the scalenus anticus, costoclavicular, hyperabduction, subcoracoid, pectoralis minor, and first thoracic rib syndromes.[178–180] A brachiocephalic vascular syndrome has been described in which pressure exerted by a cervical rib results in subclavian artery thrombosis that extends to the ipsilateral carotid artery and produces symptoms of cerebrovascular insufficiency.[181] Bilateral thoracic outlet obstruction caused by bone deformity and compression of the main arterial vessels has been described in one patient[182] who experienced episodes of tetany of the hands that were relieved by resection of the first ribs. In most of these situations, arteriography can be of considerable assistance in evaluation and is essential in some patients for diagnosis and preoperative assessment.[183]

Intrathoracic rib is a rare congenital anomaly. According to Kelleher and associates,[184] 15 cases had been documented in the literature since the anomaly was first described in 1947; these authors described 2 additional cases. This anomaly, which is an innocuous intrathoracic structure, consists of an accessory rib that arises within the bony thorax, more commonly on the right, either from the anterior surface of a rib or from a contiguous vertebral body; it usually extends downward and slightly laterally to end at or near the diaphragm. The pattern may vary. For example, in one patient the supernumerary rib originated from the posterior portion of the left third rib and extended through lung substance to join the anterior portion of the left second rib;[185] this "transthoracic rib" occasioned no symptoms. An even rarer irregularity is an anomalous rib arising from the right side of the last sacral vertebra—a pelvic rib.[186]

A rare congenital anomaly of the ribs characterizes so-called *asphyxiating thoracic dystrophy of the newborn*,[187] an osteochondrodystrophy, generally fatal, in which the ribs are very short and stubby and extend no further than the midaxilla. The anomaly results in poor respiratory mobility and frequent respiratory infections.

Another rare hereditary condition that can cause severe chest wall restriction is *fibrodysplasia ossificans progressiva*. Connor and associates[188] have described 21 patients with this inherited disorder that is characterized by progressive ossification of voluntary muscles and ligaments associated with a characteristic skeletal malformation consisting of short big toes containing only a single phalanx. Affected patients are usually infertile and die of pneumonia in their third or fourth decade. Since ventilatory capacity is maintained by relatively preserved diaphragmatic function, respiratory failure is unusual except in the terminal stages.

King and associates[189] have described a middle-aged man with long-standing *polyostotic fibrous dysplasia*, in whom extensive involvement of the rib cage resulted in severe progressive restrictive lung disease, pulmonary hypertension, and heart failure. Despite the presence of extraosseous proliferation of the abnormal tissue, subtotal resection of the benign tissue mass improved respiratory efficiency and decreased signs of pulmonary hypertension and right-sided heart failure.

Notching and Erosion

Pathologic notching of ribs may occur on the inferior or superior aspect; it is most frequent in the former location and has many causes (Table 20–3).[190] By far the most common cause, coarctation of the aorta, typically produces notching several centimeters lateral to the costovertebral junction on the inferior aspect of ribs three to nine (Fig. 20–13). The notches result from erosion by pulsating, dilated intercostal arteries taking part in collateral arterial flow. These arteries may become extremely tortuous and may even extend to and erode the superior aspects of contiguous ribs. Rib notching secondary to coarctation of the aorta seldom is seen in patients before the age of 6 or 7 years and usually is not well developed until the early teens.[191] However, it can be present in infancy and early childhood, as evidenced by the six cases that have been reported in infants under the age of 1 year.[191]

Rib notching can also occur in the presence of aortic obstruction other than that caused by coarctation. For example, Takayasu's arteritis causing obstruction of the abdominal aorta has been reported to be associated with notching of ribs 9 and 10 bilaterally.[192] Rib notching also may occur in other conditions, particularly the tetralogy of Fallot; in one study,[193] 19 of 245 patients with this condition had rib notching that was unilateral on the left side in most cases. Of considerable interest is the authors' observation that the notching occurred not only after Blalock-Taussig anastomosis (Fig. 20–14) but

Table 20–3. Causes of Inferior Rib Notching

ARTERIAL
A. Aortic obstruction
    1. Coarctation of the aortic arch
    2. Thrombosis of the abdominal aorta
B. Subclavian artery obstruction
    1. Blalock-Taussig operation
    2. "Pulseless disease"
C. Widened arterial pulse pressure
D. Decreased pulmonary blood flow
    1. Tetralogy of Fallot
    2. Pulmonary atresia (pseudotruncus)
    3. Ebstein's malformation
    4. Pulmonary valve stenosis
    5. Unilateral absence of the pulmonary artery
    6. Pulmonary emphysema

VENOUS
A. Superior vena cava obstruction

ARTERIOVENOUS
A. Pulmonary arteriovenous fistula
B. Intercostal arteriovenous fistula

NEUROGENIC
A. Intercostal neurinoma

OSSEOUS
A. Hyperparathyroidism

IDIOPATHIC

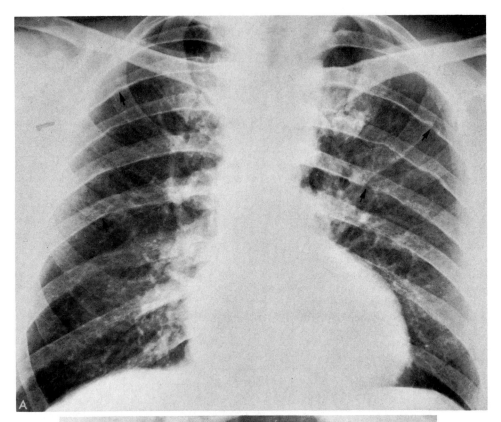

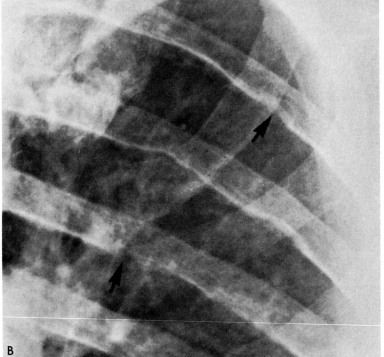

Figure 20–13. Rib Notching: Coarctation of the Aorta. A posteroanterior roentgenogram *(A)* and a magnified view of the left upper ribs *(B)* demonstrate numerous defects of the inferior surfaces of ribs 4 to 8 bilaterally (several are indicated by *arrows*). The configuration of vascular shadows in the region of the aortic knob is strongly suggestive of aortic coarctation. This is a proven case in a 58-year-old man.

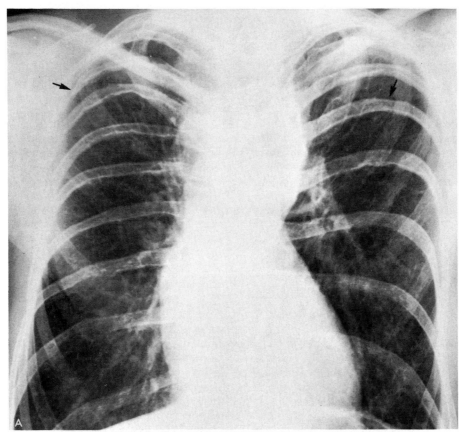

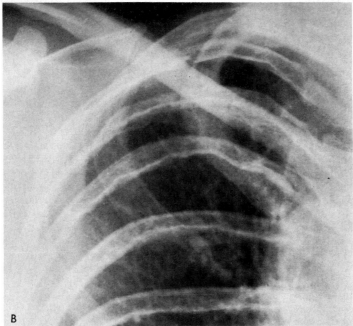

Figure 20–14. Rib Notching: Postoperative Bilateral Blalock-Taussig Anastomosis for Tetralogy of Fallot. A posteroanterior roentgenogram *(A)* reveals extensive notching of ribs 3 to 7 bilaterally, affecting not only the inferior surface of the ribs (as in Figure 20–13) but in some areas the superior surface as well *(arrows)*. The erosions are seen to advantage on a magnified view of the right upper ribs *(B)*. Such notching is the result of hypertrophy of intercostal arteries to provide anastomotic circulation to the upper extremities. The patient is a 25-year-old man.

also after thoracotomy without vascular anastomosis.

Notching or erosion of the *superior* aspects of the ribs is considerably less common than that of the inferior aspects, but we suspect that it may be present more often than is generally recognized because of its more subtle roentgenologic appearance. This subject has been reviewed by Sargent and colleagues,[194] who classified superior marginal rib defects into three main etiologic groups (Table 20–4): (1) disturbance of osteoblastic activity (decreased or deficient bone formation); (2) disturbance of osteoclastic activity (increased bone resorption); and (3) idiopathic (no demonstrable associated etiology). As pointed out by these authors, bone is laid down throughout life by the activity of osteoblasts and is absorbed by osteoclasts, the two processes occurring simultaneously and in reasonable dynamic equilibrium. They postulate that the causes of superior marginal rib erosion may be related to an imbalance of osteoblastic-osteoclastic activity.

Formerly, the most common cause of notching or erosion of the superior aspects of the ribs undoubtedly was chronic paralytic poliomyelitis.[194–196] However, the rarity with which this disease is now seen places it far down on the list of differential diagnoses; since the same mechanism is in effect in patients who are quadriplegic as a result of cervical cord injury, it is possible that this condition will replace poliomyelitis as one of the more common causes of superior rib erosion.[197] Consisting of localized shallow indentations ranging from 1 to 4 cm in length on the superior margins of ribs three to nine posterolaterally, the erosions were considered at one time to result from continued pressure of the medial margins of the scapulae. However, for a variety of reasons, this mechanism appears most unlikely.[194] A more reasonable explanation is the absence of the "stress stimulus" provided by repetitive contraction of the intercostal muscles as a result of atrophy.[194] The cause of superior rib erosions in the autoimmune connective tissue diseases, particularly rheumatoid arthritis and progressive systemic

sclerosis, is unknown but conceivably could be related to intercostal muscle atrophy in association with restrictive lung disease, as suggested by Keats.[198] However, we have not seen similar erosions in patients with chronic idiopathic interstitial pulmonary fibrosis and suspect that it is not the restrictive lung disease *per se* that leads to this unusual osseous manifestation.

Inflammatory Diseases

Primary *osteomyelitis* of the ribs is rare and may be difficult to appreciate roentgenologically until bone destruction is advanced. More commonly, osteomyelitis is secondary to infectious processes in the lung (usually of tuberculous or fungal etiology) or to empyema (empyema necessitatis). Of 16 patients from Ibadan who had pyogenic osteomyelitis of the ribs, 9 had pre-existing empyema and 14 presented with discharging chest wall sinuses; *Staphylococcus aureus* was the causative organism in 8 of the 16 cases.[199] *Tuberculous osteitis* was formerly the most common inflammatory lesion of a rib and occasionally was the first manifestation of the disease.[200] It may begin as a chondritis or osteitis;[200] according to Wolstein and colleagues,[200] the roentgenographic manifestations of these two forms evolve somewhat differently but eventually are characterized by destructive lesions associated with a periosteal reaction and a soft tissue mass. However, either form may be associated with little or no superficial abscess formation and can be confused with malignancy.[201] Rib lesions of this and other types often can be detected by bone scanning before they are apparent on chest roentgenograms.[202] Primary costal *echinococcosis* is rare; only 38 cases had been reported in the Western medical literature by 1973.[203] In its early form, it presents as a solitary expanding osteolytic lesion within a rib and is unassociated with layering of periosteal new bone. In the more advanced forms, the disease tends to affect the posterior portions of the ribs and the vertebrae and is usually associated with soft tissue masses. Sometimes, extraosseous lesions, such as pleural hydatid cysts, cause pressure atrophy of the ribs.[203]

Costochondral osteochondritis (Tietze's syndrome) is characterized by painful, nonsuppurative swelling of one or more costochondral or sternochondral joints.[204–208] By 1983, reports of 316 cases had appeared in the world literature;[209] in the majority of these, sternocostal joint involvement was an isolated finding, although in some patients it was associated with a systemic arthritic disorder or psoriasis. The etiology of this rare, benign, self-limited process is unknown, although Dunlop[210] has invoked chronic postural stress that is exacerbated by coughing or trauma. Involved cartilage is said to be histologically normal.[205, 206] The condition shows no sex predominance.[208] It almost invariably becomes manifest in the second to fourth decades of life, with the very young and very old being immune.[210] An epidemic of Tietze's syndrome has been described in six

Table 20–4. Causes of Superior Rib Notching

DISTURBANCE OF OSTEOBLASTIC ACTIVITY (DECREASED OR DEFICIENT BONE FORMATION)
1. Paralytic poliomyelitis (bulbar or spinal)
2. Collagen diseases (rheumatoid arthritis, scleroderma, lupus erythematosus, Sjögren's syndrome)
3. Localized pressure (rib retractors, chest tubes, multiple hereditary exostoses, neurofibromatosis, thoracic neuroblastoma, and coarctation of the aorta with superior and inferior rib erosion)
4. Osteogenesis imperfecta
5. Marfan's syndrome
6. Radiation damage

DISTURBANCE OF OSTEOCLASTIC ACTIVITY (INCREASED BONE RESORPTION)
1. Hyperparathyroidism
2. Hypervitaminosis D

IDIOPATHIC

employees of a copper mine; this led the author to postulate that the disease may be caused by a virus.[211]

Although the majority of affected patients undoubtedly manifest no roentgenologic changes, a variety of abnormalities occasionally can be identified. Skorneck[208] described hypertrophy and excess calcification of the costal cartilages, best demonstrated by tangential roentgenography. The second ribs are the most commonly involved. The affected ribs may show evidence of periosteal reaction and increased size and density anteriorly. When subperiosteal new bone formation develops, it tends to occur along the superior aspects of the affected ribs. In addition there may be enlargement and alteration of the trabecular pattern of the anterior portion of the first ribs, which may become extremely dense. CT can sometimes help to distinguish the swelling of Tietze's syndrome from more sinister causes of chest wall masses:[212, 213] of six patients with Tietze's syndrome in one series,[213] CT showed no abnormality in two, ventral angulation of the involved costal cartilage in two, and enlargement of the costal cartilage at the site of the complaint in two.[213]

The clinical picture consists of painful, nonsuppurative swelling of one or more upper rib cartilages, without apparent cause; in some cases, it alternates between remission and exacerbation. The pain may antedate or coincide with the swelling and is accentuated by movement, deep respiration, and cough. Multiple sites are involved in approximately one third of cases.[208] Weeks or months may elapse before the swelling and pain disappear, and slight chest deformity may remain. Symptomatic improvement has been reported following treatment with anti-inflammatory agents and calcitonin.[214]

A variant of Tietze's syndrome has been termed "costosternal chondrodynia." It is characterized by local pain and tenderness in the upper or middle costal cartilages without associated swelling.[215]

ABNORMALITIES OF THE STERNUM

Pectus Excavatum

This common deformity of the sternum, also known as "funnel chest," consists of the sternum being depressed so that the ribs on each side protrude anteriorly more than the sternum itself. It is generally believed that the deformity results from a genetically determined abnormality of the sternum and related portions of the diaphragm and that it can occur either sporadically or as a dominant pattern of inheritance.[216, 217] Several mechanisms have been proposed for its development: (1) an overstimulation of the anterior fibers of the diaphragm; (2) an anomalous position of the heart to the left of the midline, leaving the retrosternal area "empty" and permitting the sternum and costal cartilages to be sucked in to fill the empty space;[218]

and (3) an inherent defect in connective tissue affecting the skeleton itself. The last possibility is supported by the frequent association of the deformity with congenital connective tissue disorders, such as Marfan's syndrome, Poland's syndrome, scoliosis, and Pierre Robin syndrome.[219] For example, of the 54 patients reported by Guller and Hable,[216] 6 patients had connective tissue disorders; 15 per cent of the remaining patients had one or more relatives with a funnel chest compared with an incidence in the general population ranging from 0.13 to 0.4 per cent. Occasionally, multiple congenital defects may be associated with the deformity.[220]

The roentgenographic manifestations are easily recognized (Fig. 20–15). In posteroanterior projection, the heart is seen to be displaced to the left[221] and rotated in a way suggestive of a "mitral configuration." The parasternal soft tissues of the anterior chest wall, which are seen in profile rather than en face, are apparent as increased density over the inferomedial portion of the right hemithorax and should not be mistaken for disease of the right middle lobe, even though the right heart border is obscured by a silhouetting effect (see Fig. 20–15). The degree of sternal depression is easily seen on lateral roentgenograms. Mosetitsch[222] observed exaggerated respiratory movements of the diaphragm in his series of 16 patients. Inspiratory-expiratory roentgenograms have been said to show a paradoxical increase in heart size on inspiration.[223] Possibly as a result of upward compression deformity of the heart and great vessels, pectus excavatum occasionally can be associated with an unusual mediastinal configuration that can simulate a mediastinal mass;[224] usually the true nature of the configuration can be readily clarified by CT. By altering the normal anatomic position of the adjacent structures, pectus excavatum can also cause false-positive scintigraphic studies by mimicking a mass in the liver or lungs.[225, 226]

The severity of the defect is best quantified by CT. The "pectus index" can be derived by dividing the transverse diameter of the chest by the anteroposterior diameter. Haller and associates[227] found the normal value of this index to be 2.56 ($\pm$ 0.35 SD) and suggested that patients with a ratio of 3.25 or greater required surgical correction. Similar indices derived from CT have been employed to assess the results of surgical repair.[228]

The vast majority of patients with pectus excavatum are symptom-free except for the anxiety occasioned by the physical deformity.[216, 229] However, cardiac[230, 231] or respiratory[232] symptoms are occasionally attributed to the abnormality. A heart murmur is also fairly common; for example, in their study of 54 children with pectus excavatum, Guller and Hable[216] identified a murmur in 44 per cent, the most common simulating pulmonic stenosis and probably resulting from kinking of the pulmonary artery. Increased splitting of the second

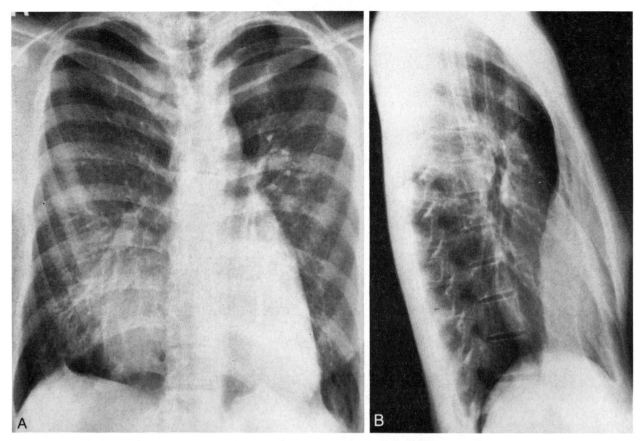

Figure 20–15. Severe Pectus Excavatum. Posteroanterior *(A)* and lateral *(B)* roentgenograms of the chest reveal a fairly large opacity projected over the lower portion of the right hemithorax contiguous with the shadow of the thoracic spine. The pulmonary arteries to the right lower lobe are displaced laterally and the heart is displaced to the left. The severe deformity of the sternum can be readily identified in lateral projection and is of sufficient degree to displace the heart posteriorly such that the contour of the left ventricle is projected over the thoracic vertebral bodies. The patient is a young woman who had no symptoms other than those of a cosmetic nature.

heart sound was frequently observed and, in association with the pulmonic murmur, suggested atrial septal defect. The electrocardiogram usually showed increased left-sided potentials, presumably as a result of leftward displacement of the heart. Although auscultatory, electrocardiographic, and roentgenographic abnormalities suggestive of significant heart disease were frequent in this series, the authors considered that all 54 children had normal hearts. Only two were symptomatic, both experiencing infrequent episodes of mild syncope. In some individuals a murmur can be caused by mitral valve prolapse; this incidence is reported to be increased in patients with pectus excavatum.[233] The incidence of Wolff-Parkinson-White syndrome is increased in children with pectus excavatum.[234] Results of pulmonary function tests are usually normal or reveal only slight decreases in vital capacity (VC) and MBC; however, occasional patients manifest severe lung restriction.

Considerable controversy surrounds the usefulness and advisability of surgical correction of pectus excavatum. Although the majority of studies have found little or no functional benefit from surgical correction,[232, 235] the occasional patient with lung restriction can show considerable improvement.[219, 236] In one careful study of 14 patients with pectus excavatum on whom preoperative and postoperative pulmonary function tests were performed and progressive exercise performance was assessed, a slight but significant improvement was observed in total lung capacity, maximum voluntary ventilation, and total exercise time and maximum oxygen consumption during exercise.[237] In another study of 13 patients,[238] no improvement was demonstrated in maximal exercise capacity following surgical repair; however, radionuclide scintigraphy performed during rest and bicycle exercise in the erect position showed an increase in right and left ventricular end-diastolic volumes, suggesting that the depressed sternum may have been exerting some cardiac compression. One investigator[231] has described 2 patients with pectus excavatum in whom anginoid pain and abnormal electrocardiograms were considered to be caused by a cartilaginous protrusion of the xiphoid; both patients benefited from surgery. A review of the literature suggests that surgical correction is seldom indicated for functional impairment, although repair may be important in preventing psychological upset due to cosmetic deformity.[229]

Pectus Carinatum

The reverse of pectus excavatum is pectus carinatum or "pigeon breast," a congenital or acquired deformity in which the sternum protrudes anteriorly more than normal. It occurs more often in boys than in girls; it is associated with a family history of chest wall deformity in 26 per cent and of scoliosis in 12 per cent of affected individuals.[239] The most common variety of congenital pectus carinatum consists of simple anterior protrusion of the sternum and costal cartilages that develops with growth.[240] A rare variety is associated with premature ossification of the sternal suture lines that results in forward angulation of the body of the sternum.[241]

The most common cause of acquired pectus carinatum is congenital atrial or ventricular septal defect;[242] the character of the deformity is slightly different in these two anomalies. In the former, the forward bulging tends to be predominantly unilateral and directly over the right ventricle, whereas in the latter the protuberance is symmetric and affects chiefly the upper portion of the sternum. Approximately 50 per cent of patients with atrial and ventricular septal defects have a pigeon breast deformity.[242] Another acquired cause of pectus carinatum is prolonged and severe asthma dating from early childhood.[243]

The great majority of patients with congenital pectus carinatum are asymptomatic, although it has been suggested that children with the deformity are more subject to respiratory infections.[240] Surgery can satisfactorily correct the cosmetic deformity but is rarely indicated for functional abnormalities.[239] Pulmonary hypertension develops in most patients in whom ventricular septal defect is associated with pigeon breast deformity, but it is undoubtedly caused by the heart disease rather than by the sternal abnormality.[242]

Inflammatory Diseases

Inflammatory diseases affecting the sternum and sternal articulations are uncommon and nowadays occur most frequently in patients whose sternum has been "split" for surgical procedures on the mediastinum. *Osteomyelitis* causes localized pain, swelling, and redness and may be detectable on a lateral chest roentgenogram[244] or on conventional or computed tomograms. Heroin addicts are unusually prone to develop *septic arthritis* of the sternoclavicular and sternochondral joints, the most common causative organisms being *Pseudomonas aeruginosa* and *Staphylococcus aureus*;[245] occasionally, *Candida albicans* is the etiology.[246]

Sternocostoclavicular hyperostosis is a disease of unknown etiology consisting of club-like, symmetric enlargement of the clavicles associated with venous congestion of the upper half of the body as a result of bilateral subclavian vein occlusion. Roentgenographically, patients with this condition reveal symmetric hyperostosis of the sternal and midportions of the clavicles; synostosis of the sternoclavicular joints; a widened, thickened sternum; and varying degrees of similar involvement of the upper ribs.[247]

ABNORMALITIES OF THE THORACIC SPINE

Abnormalities of Curvature (Kyphoscoliosis)

Abnormalities of curvature of the thoracic spine may be predominantly lateral (scoliosis), predominantly posterior (kyphosis), or a combination of the two (kyphoscoliosis). Although such abnormalities are common, particularly scoliosis, deformity of sufficient degree to cause symptoms and signs of cardiac or pulmonary disease is rare. In the United States, the incidence of scoliosis in which the Cobb angle (*see* farther on) is less than 35 degrees is 1:1,000; the incidence of the deformity with an angle greater than 70 degrees is 1:10,000.[248] Respiratory or cardiovascular embarrassment seldom occurs in patients with simple scoliosis or kyphosis and almost invariably indicates a severe degree of kyphoscoliosis.

The etiology of abnormalities of curvature can be divided into three groups: (1) *congenital*, including anomalies of the thoracic spine such as hemivertebrae, and various hereditary disorders in which spinal deformity constitutes only a part of the clinical picture—neurofibromatosis, Friedreich's ataxia, muscular dystrophy, Morquio's syndrome, and Marfan's syndrome;[243, 249] (2) *paralytic*, the majority of cases being secondary to poliomyelitis, muscular dystrophy, or cerebral palsy; and (3) *idiopathic*, which includes approximately 80 per cent of patients with severe kyphoscoliosis. Patients in the third group do not have congenital defects or other diseases to which the abnormal curvature may be ascribed (Fig. 20–16). This variety shows a female sex predominance of 4 to 1.

The major pathophysiologic effect of severe kyphoscoliosis is restrictive lung disease that results in chronic alveolar hypoventilation, hypoxic vasoconstriction, and eventually pulmonary arterial hypertension and cor pulmonale. Pathologic examination reveals small lungs with a reduction in both functioning parenchyma and the pulmonary vascular bed.[250] Histologic features consist of alveolar dilatation in some regions and partial collapse in others.[251, 252] Muscular hypertrophy of pulmonary arteries is common. The major influence in its development is probably chronic hypoxic vasoconstriction, although mechanical factors such as com-

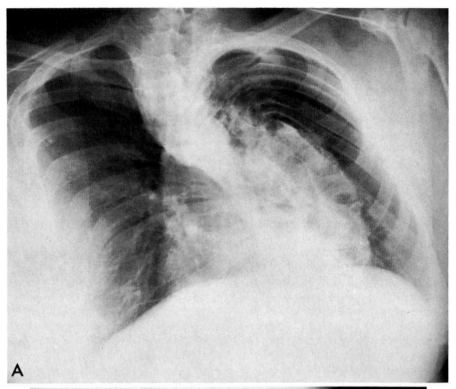

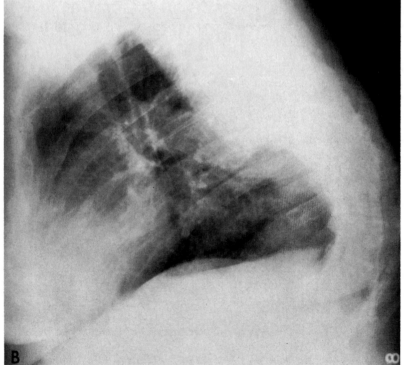

Figure 20–16. Kyphoscoliosis. Posteroanterior *(A)* and lateral *(B)* roentgenograms reveal severe deformity of the thoracic skeleton, the spine possessing a marked scoliosis to the left in the midthoracic region and a severe kyphos in the mid and lower regions. Deformity of the rib cage is as might be anticipated from the thoracic curvature. The 48-year-old woman had no significant complaints referable to her respiratory tract; her thoracic deformity was the result of a remote poliomyelitis. Pulmonary function tests revealed remarkably normal values, there being only a slight reduction in VC and FRC.

pression of small intraparenchymal vessels due to low lung volumes may also contribute. In addition, pulmonary vessels may fail to develop fully when the deformity occurs during the growth period of childhood.[251, 253]

Apart from the spinal curvature itself, the roentgenographic changes in severe kyphoscoliotic cardiopulmonary disease can be extremely difficult to assess. In the great majority of cases, the scoliosis is convex to the right, and there is generally good correlation between the degree of curvature and the presence and severity of cardiopulmonary disease. The angle of scoliosis is best determined by the Cobb method:[254] lines are drawn parallel to the upper border of the highest and the lower border of the lowest vertebral bodies of the curvature as seen on an anteroposterior roentgenogram of the spine, and the angle is measured at the intersection point of lines drawn perpendicular to these. The angle also can be measured simply by drawing lines parallel to the upper and lower borders of the vertebral bodies encompassing the curvature and calculating the angle at the intersection. Assessment of cardiac size and the state of the pulmonary parenchyma and vasculature can be exceedingly difficult because of the severe deformity of the thoracic cage. Occasionally, regional areas of oligemia may be detected; they suggest a local reduction in perfusion, presumably resulting from hypoxic vasoconstriction secondary to hypoventilation.

Most children with kyphoscoliosis are asymptomatic,[255] and the presence of cardiac abnormalities in these individuals should suggest primary heart disease independent of the kyphoscoliosis. There is a tendency for disability to relate to an increasing angle of scoliosis and to age.[256] Bergofsky and associates[251] suggest that it is the combination of the kyphotic and scoliotic defects that determines the severity of symptoms and the likelihood of developing ventilatory respiratory failure. Lesser degrees of scoliosis cause more severe impairment in the presence of severe kyphosis and vice versa.

In general, adults whose scoliotic angle is 100 degrees or more will develop respiratory failure. Symptoms and signs of respiratory and cardiac failure usually do not appear until the fourth or fifth decade. Once failure has become manifest, the clinical course is usually rapidly downhill and is characterized by repeated episodes of respiratory and cardiac failure, often precipitated by pulmonary infection. Despite the foregoing, even adults with severe kyphoscoliosis can remain asymptomatic; in a study of 500 patients, Godfrey[257] found that cardiorespiratory failure did not develop if VC remained more than 40 per cent of predicted.

Tests of pulmonary function characteristically reveal a decrease in VC and TLC and normal or increased values of RV.[255, 258] In patients with cor pulmonale, TLC may be reduced to as low as 2 liters.[259–261] Predicted values for lung volumes are based at least partly on height, however, and it has been suggested that it is more accurate to use arm span in predicting values in patients with kyphoscoliosis.[262] Flow is reduced only in proportion to the reduction in VC, and direct measurement of airway resistance reveals normal values.[259] In patients with mild or moderate lung restriction, measurement of steady-state diffusing capacity with oxygen[263] reveals relatively normal values for gas transfer corrected for the reduction in alveolar volume, although in patients who are hypercapnic and in heart failure the values are decreased out of proportion to the reduced lung volumes. Mixing efficiency may[264] or may not[255] be impaired, perhaps depending on the degree of scoliosis.

Arterial blood gas values are almost invariably abnormal in adults and occasionally in adolescents.[251, 255, 260, 261, 264] In the more advanced cases, it is common to find both hypoxemia and hypercarbia, a combined form of respiratory failure that can be attributed to alveolar hypoventilation secondary to shallow respiration[251, 261] and to a ventilation-perfusion (V̇/Q̇) imbalance.[258, 264] Studies with radioactive xenon have shown defects in both ventilation and perfusion:[265, 266] employing a bolus method of xenon injection, Bake and associates[266] found no consistent difference in perfusion of the lungs on the convex and concave sides of the curvature; although the lung bases were more severely affected than the apices, perfusion and ventilation were reduced equally and progressively with increasing spinal deformity. In this study,[266] the defect in gas exchange was thought to result from regional inhomogeneity of ventilation and perfusion, a finding that is seen more often in older patients. In one series of 40 patients with idiopathic scoliosis,[256] 17 showed evidence of airway closure at lung volumes greater than functional residual capacity (FRC), whereas in another study of 19 patients whose average age was younger, closing volumes were all below FRC.[255] This discrepancy almost certainly can be explained by the age of the patients and the degree of scoliosis.

Although the arterial hypoxemia associated with severe kyphoscoliosis can be ascribed to both gas exchange impairment and hypoventilation, the relative contribution of gas exchange abnormalities is much less than in patients who have similar degrees of alveolar hypoventilation secondary to COPD.[263] In patients with mild or moderate kyphoscoliosis, the alveolar-arterial oxygen tension gradient may be in the normal range. In fact, even in the presence of advanced disease associated with arterial hypertension and cor pulmonale, the majority of the arterial hypoxemia is caused by alveolar hypoxia rather than V̇/Q̇ mismatch or shunt. The relative preservation of the lung's ability to function as a gas-exchanging organ, if adequately ventilated, is also evidenced by the normal or low values for dead space in patients with kyphoscoliosis.[267] In contrast to patients with COPD in whom hypoventilation develops because of increased dead space despite normal or increased levels of minute ventilation, patients with kyphoscoliosis develop alveolar hypoventilation as a result primarily of a decrease in minute ventilation secondary to small tidal volumes.

Compliance of both the chest wall and lung is decreased in kyphoscoliosis. The decrease in chest wall compliance may be profound and correlates significantly with the angle of scoliosis.[268] The mechanism by which lung compliance is reduced is unclear, but it could be caused by either microatelectasis or an increase in the surface tension resulting from failure of the lung to inflate because of the chest wall restriction (or both). In a study of six kyphoscoliotic patients with combined cardiorespiratory failure, Sinha and Bergofsky[269] found a highly significant increase in compliance after 5 minutes of positive pressure breathing, an improvement that they attributed to a decrease in alveolar surface forces, although they could not exclude expansion of collapsed air spaces as a contributory factor.

Kafer[258] has pointed out that the abnormalities of pulmonary function in patients with paralytic scoliosis are somewhat different from those in patients with the idiopathic variety, probably because of the additional component of respiratory muscle dysfunction. However, a decrease in respiratory muscle and diaphragmatic function also has been reported in patients with advanced idiopathic kyphoscoliosis; it is probably attributable to altered muscle length and inefficiency related to the deformed thorax.[270] Respiratory muscle performance can be improved in patients with kyphoscoliosis by specific muscle training programs and can be accompanied by an increase in lung volumes and a reduction in dyspnea.[271]

Patients with kyphoscoliosis can be particularly susceptible to ventilatory depression and oxygen desaturation during sleep;[272-274] desaturation is particularly profound during rapid eye movement sleep.[273] A reasonable pathophysiologic mechanism of the development of ventilatory respiratory failure in patients with kyphoscoliosis is the increased work of breathing caused by stiffness of the respiratory system. In the presence of increased work of breathing and decreased respiratory muscle performance, the normal ventilatory depression that occurs during sleep results in progressive alveolar hypoventilation.

Although the development of respiratory failure in patients with kyphoscoliosis was formerly associated with a relatively rapid downhill course, recent studies[275-277] suggest that the prognosis may be considerably improved by the use of intermittent mechanical ventilation. Either cuirass-type or positive-pressure ventilation applied during the nocturnal hours can result in a prolonged interim improvement in pulmonary gas exchange and lung mechanics and a reduction in pulmonary artery pressures and the severity of symptoms. It is unclear

whether these benefits are the consequence of a simple improvement in respiratory system mechanics resulting from the maintenance of larger tidal volumes, or if they are related to an improvement in respiratory drive or alleviation of chronic respiratory muscle fatigue.

Severe skeletal deformity and resultant respiratory failure can also occur in Hurler's syndrome[278] and Morquio's disease.[279] These rare disorders of mucopolysaccharide metabolism are associated with spinal and other skeletal deformities, corneal opacities, and deafness. We have seen a 21-year-old man with Hurler's syndrome who required repeated hospitalization for respiratory failure. Similarly, two siblings with Morquio's disease have been reported, aged 34 and 35 years, whose pattern of pulmonary dysfunction closely resembled that of kyphoscoliosis.[279]

Miscellaneous Anomalies of the Thoracic Spine

A developmental anomaly that seldom, if ever, results in disturbed cardiorespiratory function or in symptoms and signs is characterized by deep paraspinal gutters and a position of the thoracic spine within the thorax that is much more anterior than normal.[280] Since the distance between the sternum and the spine is reduced, the heart may be displaced into the left hemithorax, as in pectus excavatum. A similar and perhaps identical deformity is the absence of physiologic thoracic kyphosis known as the "straight back syndrome"; extensive pulmonary function assessment, both at rest and on exercise, has shown that despite some decrease in TLC, affected individuals manifest no significant impairment of pulmonary function.[281]

Ankylosing Spondylitis

Involvement of the thoracic spine by ankylosing spondylitis results in fixation of the chest cage in an inspiratory position and leads to the paradoxical combination of hyperinflation (increased FRC) and lung restriction (decreased TLC and VC) on pulmonary function testing. The disorder develops in approximately 1 in 2,000 persons in the general population. It is strongly associated with the histocompatibility antigen HLA-B27.[282-284] Twenty per cent of HLA-B27–positive subjects will develop the disease[285] and approximately 88 per cent of patients with ankylosing spondylitis have this histocompatibility antigen.[283] Although the disease has been reported to occur four to eight times more frequently in males than in females, Calin and Fries[286] have shown that the distribution of HLA-B27–positive individuals is approximately equal in the two sexes; they explain the discrepancy in sex incidence by the fact that the disease in women tends to be milder and therefore is diagnosed less often. In any event, the typical patient with ankylosing spondylitis who is seen by the physician is a young male with a history of onset of symptoms early in the third decade of life. Although peripheral joint involvement develops eventually in about 18 to 25 per cent of cases, there is little question that ankylosing spondylitis is an entity distinct from rheumatoid arthritis,[287] although both diseases probably have an autoimmune pathogenesis in common.

Pathologically, ankylosing spondylitis consists of synovitis, chondritis, and juxta-articular osteitis of the sacroiliac, apophyseal, and costovertebral articulations. Progression of the disease is marked by erosion of subchondral bone, destruction of cartilage, and eventual bony ankylosis. Calcification and ossification deep to the paraspinal ligaments are late changes. Aortic valvulitis develops in approximately 4 per cent of patients,[287, 288] an incidence that increases to 10 per cent in patients who have had the disease for 30 years.[288]

In addition to the characteristic changes in the thoracic skeleton, approximately 1 to 2 per cent of patients develop pleuropulmonary manifestations,[289, 290] most commonly in the form of upper lobe fibrotic and bullous disease (see page 1208).[291, 292] These fibrobullous lesions sometimes contain mycetomas and occasionally are the result of atypical mycobacterial infection. From a review of the literature, Rosenow and colleagues[289] found approximately 100 cases of upper lobe fibrobullous disease in ankylosing spondylitis; 8 of these patients developed spontaneous pneumothorax, an incidence well above that expected in the population at large. Bronchocentric granulomatosis confined to the upper lobes also has been described.[293] Computed tomography is useful in characterizing the extent and nature of the upper lobe changes as well as detecting or excluding an intracavitary mycetoma.[294] In the Mayo Clinic series of 2,080 patients with ankylosing spondylitis,[289] an unexpected number manifested evidence of pleuritis and pleurisy with effusion. Bilateral pleural effusions have been reported in a patient with quiescent joint disease.[295]

The clinical picture is characterized by intermittent or continuous low back pain, sometimes associated with constitutional symptoms such as fatigue, weight loss, anorexia, and low-grade fever. The back pain of ankylosing spondylitis can be distinguished from that of a mechanical or nonspecific type by its insidious onset, its duration (usually more than 3 months before the patient seeks medical help), its association with morning stiffness, and its improvement with exercise.[285] As the disease progresses upward and involves the thoracic spine, the patient may complain of chest pain that is sometimes accentuated during respiration.[296] As the spine fuses, the kyphotic curvature gradually increases and chest expansion progressively diminishes. Few patients complain of dyspnea.

In an investigation of age-specific death rates of 836 patients with ankylosing spondylitis, Radford and coworkers[297] found a high mortality in men for those diseases known to be associated with spondy-litis, including ulcerative colitis, nephritis, and tuberculosis or other respiratory disease.

The pattern of pulmonary function is one of restriction and overinflation, the result of fixation of the thorax in an expanded position. VC is reduced, often to 70 per cent or less of predicted values; RV and FRC are usually, but not always, increased.[298–301] In one study, maximal exercise capacity was only mildly reduced in six patients with moderate ankylosing spondylitis (TLC 85 ± 5 per cent predicted) and ventilatory impairment was not the factor that limited exercise.[302] Mixing efficiency and flow resistance are normal. Maximal static inspiratory transpulmonary pressure is diminished, as in emphysema. Although ventilation-perfusion relationships are usually normal,[298] Renzetti and associates[303] found evidence in some patients of inequality that gave rise to mild arterial hypoxemia and increase in the physiologic dead space. This they attributed to underventilation of upper lobes in contrast to relative hyperventilation of lower lobes as a consequence of maintenance of diaphragmatic movement. Employing xenon 133, Stewart and associates[304] also showed an overall diminution in lung volume and a reduced proportion of inhaled xenon reaching the lung apices. However, distribution of injected xenon was normal. These investigators postulated that diminished apical ventilation may be a contributing factor in the development of fibrobullous disease.

NEOPLASMS OF THE CHEST WALL

Detailed discussion of neoplasms of the chest wall is outside the scope of this work. The interested reader is directed to the excellent reviews of the subject by Ochsner and Ochsner,[305] by Ochsner and associates,[306] and to a number of more recent reports.[307–311] The CT characteristics of chest wall masses have been described in considerable detail by Jafri and colleagues.[312]

The etiology of most primary chest wall neoplasms is unknown. An exception is the group of individuals who have received prior chest wall radiation, in whom the risk of developing sarcoma is clearly increased (Fig. 20–17).[157, 313, 314] A history of breast carcinoma or, less commonly, Hodgkin's disease is present in most of these patients. In one series, the latency between radiation and the appearance of the sarcoma ranged from 5 to 28 years (mean, 13 years).[313] The most common soft tissue neoplasms that develop in these circumstances are malignant fibrohistiocytoma and fibrosarcoma, and the usual bone tumor is osteogenic sarcoma; other histologic types are rare.[315]

Neoplasms of Soft Tissues

Primary neoplasms of the soft tissues of the chest wall are rare. In adults, the most common benign lesion is lipoma and the most common

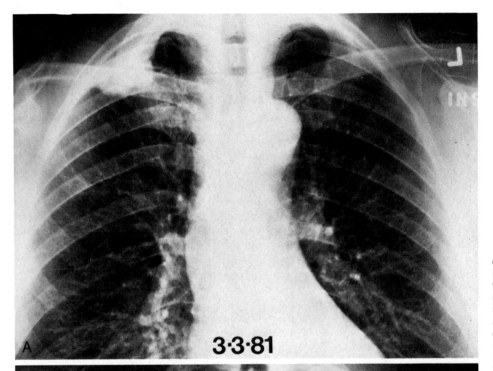

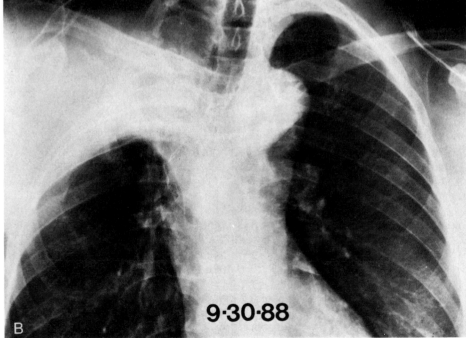

Figure 20–17. Fibrosarcoma of the Chest Wall Following Radiation Therapy. A posteroanterior roentgenogram of the upper half of the chest *(A)* of this 52-year-old man in 1981 reveals a homogeneous mass at the apex of the right lung. Biopsy revealed squamous cell carcinoma and a right upper lobectomy was performed. At thoracotomy, there was evidence of chest wall invasion, and postoperative irradiation therapy was administered. Seven years later *(B)*, there had developed a large opacity in the right apical region associated with extensive destruction of ribs.

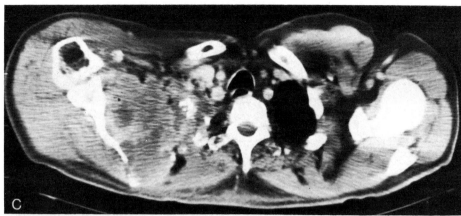

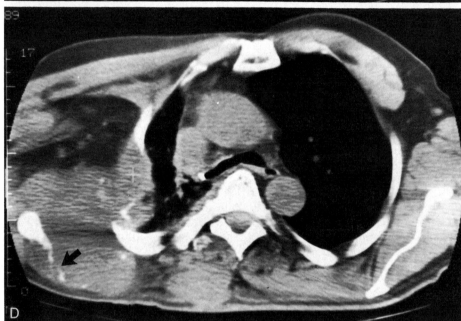

Figure 20–17 *Continued* CT scans just below the thoracic inlet *(C)* and at the level of the main bronchi *(D)* reveal an almost complete absence of ribs in the apical region and extensive invasion of the soft tissues of the chest wall. The scapula has been partly destroyed, seen to best advantage in *D (arrow)*. (Courtesy of Dr. Jim Wilson, Montreal Chest Hospital.)

malignant neoplasms are fibrosarcoma and malignant fibrohistiocytoma. The histologic types of malignant neoplasm that occur in children are different. The most common of these are primitive neuroectodermal tumor,[316, 317] rhabdomyosarcoma, extraosseous Ewing's sarcoma,[318] and "malignant small cell tumor of thoracopulmonary region" (Askin's tumor);[319] the last two are sometimes considered the same entity and labeled "malignant small round cell tumor."[320]

The point of origin of a lipoma in the chest wall establishes its mode of presentation. When it originates adjacent to the parietal pleura, it causes a soft tissue mass that indents the lung and possesses a contour characteristic of its extrapulmonary origin. When it arises outside the rib cage, it presents as a palpable soft tissue mass that may be visualized roentgenographically if viewed in profile or, if of sufficient size, even *en face*. Most lipomas that arise between the ribs have a dumbbell or hourglass configuration, part projecting inside and part out-

side the thoracic cage. The density of lipomas is intermediate between that of air and soft tissue. Therefore, when a lipoma relates to lung parenchyma it may not be readily distinguishable roentgenographically from other soft tissue masses, whereas when it relates to the soft tissues of the chest wall the contrast with contiguous soft tissues usually permits its identification as of fat origin.[321–323] As a result of the specificity of CT in identifying fat-containing structures, this technique is especially valuable in the diagnosis of chest wall and diaphragmatic lipomas.[324]

An uncommon benign tumor of the chest wall that may be confused with fibrosarcoma is *desmoid tumor*. This bony-hard fibrous tissue tumor arises most commonly from the aponeurosis of the abdominal wall musculature in multiparous females, although several cases have been reported in which it originated in the chest wall, usually after trauma.[325–327] The roentgenographic appearance is not distinctive, but the physical detection of a bony-hard intercostal mass should suggest the possibility of this tumor. Although most pathologists consider desmoid tumors to be a form of benign fibromatosis, others interpret them as low-grade fibrosarcomas and recommend wide surgical excision.[328]

Other benign tumors of the soft tissues of the chest wall include neurogenic neoplasms of the intercostal nerves (neurofibroma, ganglioneuroma, and schwannoma), fibromas and angiofibromas of the intercostal muscles and diaphragm, and fibromas of the parietal pleura.[329] Non-neoplastic tumors, such as elastofibromas, abscesses, various granulomas, and, in Mediterranean countries, echinococcal cysts, also must be considered in the differential diagnosis of a chest wall mass.[329–332]

Chest wall involvement occasionally can be the presenting manifestation of Hodgkin's disease, in which it probably represents direct spread from internal mammary lymph nodes.[333]

CT scanning has been shown to be a sensitive method of evaluating possible chest wall involvement by lymphoma[334, 335] and of assessing the extent of primary neoplasms of the chest wall.[336] However, its accuracy in the evaluation of chest wall invasion by intrapulmonary lesions is open to question.[337, 338] Pearlberg and colleagues[338] identified 20 patients in whom chest wall involvement was suggested by CT scans on the basis of apparent extension of the mass into fat or muscle of the chest wall or around ribs or on the definite presence of bone destruction. Chest wall invasion was proven in 11 of the 20 cases at surgery or autopsy, but in 6 of the 9 remaining cases it was shown to be not present. These authors suggest that only destruction of bone can be used as a definite indication of chest wall involvement on CT.

A soft tissue neoplasm of the chest wall may be identified roentgenographically in asymptomatic subjects or may become evident clinically as a soft tissue mass outside the chest wall. The tumor is likely to be malignant if it occasions pain. Rarely, both benign and malignant neoplasms of the chest wall may be associated with hypertrophic osteoarthropathy.[339]

Neoplasms and Non-neoplastic Tumors of Bone

Neoplasms of the thoracic skeleton are uncommon. Ochsner and colleagues[306] reported 134 such cases from the Mary S. Sherman Laboratory of Bone and Joint Pathology. The cases represented only 5 per cent of all neoplasms of bones and joints studied from 1953 to 1956. Of the 134 cases, 84 (63 per cent) were primary (48 benign and 36 malignant) and the remainder metastatic. The majority of the latter were from primaries in the lung and breast. The average age of the patients with malignant neoplasms was 48 years and of those with benign neoplasms, 26 years.

The majority of osseous neoplasms occur in the ribs. In the 100 patients reported by Pairolero and Arnold,[308] tumor was localized to the ribs in 78 and to the sternum in 22. Of the 134 cases reported by Ochsner and coworkers,[306] 72 involved the ribs, 26 the scapulae, 15 the thoracic vertebrae, 14 the clavicles, and 7 the sternum. The following characteristics were noted: (1) *rib* lesions were most commonly metastatic, chiefly from the lung and breast; (2) the majority of lesions arising in the *sternum* were malignant, most often chondrosarcoma; (3) involvement of the *clavicles* was most often by metastatic neoplasm, with benign neoplasms the next most common; (4) primary neoplasms in the *scapulae* were more numerous than metastatic ones, with the majority benign; (5) involvement of the *thoracic vertebrae* was almost invariably metastatic in origin.

Sternal metastases most frequently originate in the breast, thyroid, or lung and may be associated with pathologic fractures.[340] Hodgkin's disease can also involve the sternum and parasternal chest wall as a result of contiguous spread from retrosternal lymph nodes.[341]

Of the cartilaginous and osteogenic neoplasms and non-neoplastic tumors, osteochondroma is the most common benign type, rarer varieties being enchondroma, osteoblastoma[342] and endostoma ("bone islands"). The most common malignant neoplasm is chondrosarcoma;[342] osteogenic sarcoma, malignant fibrohistiocytoma, hemangiopericytoma, and fibrosarcoma are less frequent (Figs. 20–18 and 20–19).[306, 309–311, 343] As with neoplasms of soft tissue, those of the osseous skeleton are different in children than in adults; small-cell tumors (Ewing's sarcoma or "Askin's tumor") are much more common.[320] In infants, a rare form of chest wall tumor called benign mesenchymoma or mesenchymal hamartoma has been described.[344, 345] Gorham's syndrome is an unusual disorder consisting of an intraosseous proliferation of vascular or lymphatic channels that can involve the chest wall diffusely and that can prove fatal.[346]

The most common non-neoplastic tumor of the thoracic skeleton is fibrous dysplasia (Fig. 20–20), although eosinophilic granuloma, hemangioma, and aneurysmal bone cyst also occur.[306, 347, 348] Involvement of the rib cage by Paget's disease represents a typical roentgenographic appearance similar to that in any other bone (Fig. 20–21). Myeloma and (occasionally) solitary plasmacytoma are the most frequent malignant neoplasms of reticuloendothelial origin, followed by Hodgkin's disease and large-cell lymphoma.[306, 349] In older patients, particularly males, the association of a destructive lesion of one or more ribs with a soft tissue mass that protrudes into the thorax and indents the lung is highly suggestive of myeloma (Fig. 20–22).[350] However, a similar appearance can be created by primary lung carcinoma invading the chest wall and by other primary chest wall neoplasms. Advanced

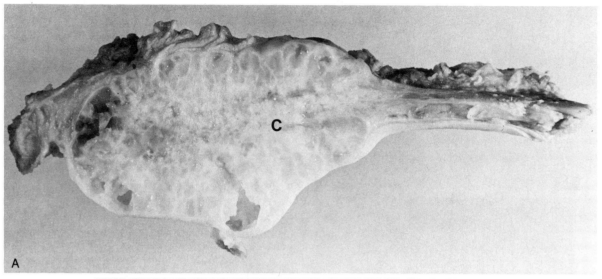

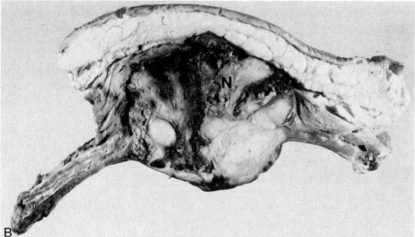

Figure 20–18. Sarcoma of a Rib. A gross specimen of rib *(A)* shows a segment to be expanded and partly destroyed by a lobulated, well-circumscribed mass composed of gelatinous, somewhat translucent tissue and more solid white areas resembling mature cartilage (C). Histologic examination showed a well-differentiated chondrosarcoma. A segment of rib from another patient *(B)* is similarly expanded and destroyed by a well-defined mass, in this case with focal necrosis (N) and hemorrhage. Fat and skin of the chest wall are present above the mass. Histologic examination showed a malignant fibrous histiocytoma.

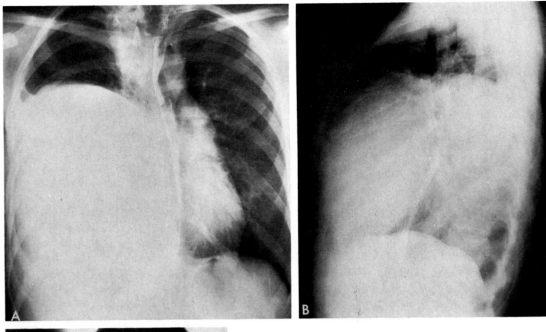

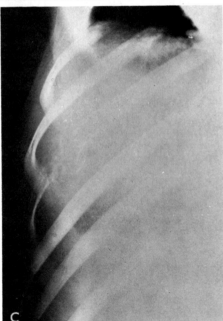

Figure 20–19. Hemangiopericytoma Arising from the Right Rib Cage. This 12-year-old girl was admitted to the hospital with an 8-week history of pain in the right side of her chest and a 12-pound weight loss. Physical examination revealed a smooth, nonfluctuant soft tissue mass in the lower axilla, fixed to the underlying thoracic wall. Posteroanterior *(A)* and lateral *(B)* roentgenograms demonstrate a huge mass in the lower portion of the right hemithorax displacing the mediastinum to the left. The mass is homogeneous in density and slightly lobulated in contour. An oblique view of the lower right ribs *(C)* reveals a destructive lesion of the sixth rib. The mass was resected, along with a considerable portion of the right chest wall. The histologic diagnosis was hemangiopericytoma.

myelomatosis of the rib cage may be associated with expansion of bone (Fig. 20–23). Pathologic fractures, particularly of the sternum (Fig. 20–24), may result in severe deformity of the chest wall.

The majority of benign neoplasms of the thoracic skeleton occasion no symptoms and usually are detected in asymptomatic subjects on a screening chest roentgenogram. A pathologic fracture will occasionally cause a patient to seek medical advice. Malignant neoplasms may cause pain and, if extensive, respiratory insufficiency (Fig. 20–25). Roentgenologic assessment may be of value in suggesting the diagnosis, but definitive diagnosis requires close correlation between the histologic and roentgenologic appearances of the neoplasm.

Text continued on page 2968

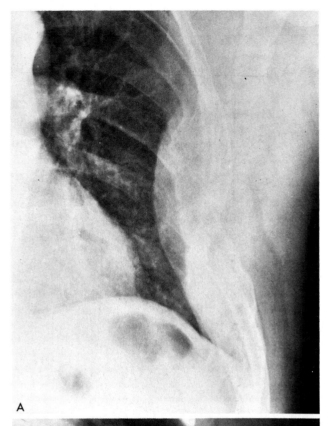

Figure 20–20. Polyostotic Fibrous Dysplasia of the Left Rib Cage. Posteroanterior (A) and oblique (B) views of the left rib cage reveal considerable expansion and distortion of ribs along the lower axillary lung zone (one rib has been removed). The left innominate bone and left tibia were affected in a similar manner. Bone involvement is thus unilateral, representing the osseous manifestation of Albright's syndrome.

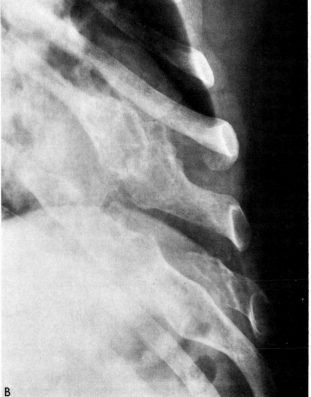

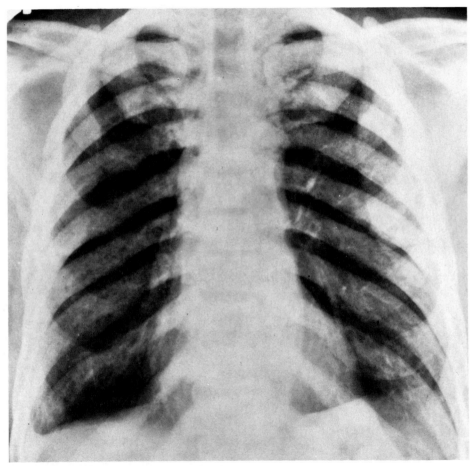

Figure 20–21. Paget's Disease of the Rib Cage. A posteroanterior roentgenogram reveals a marked increase in density and uniform expansion of all ribs bilaterally. The clavicles are involved in a similar process.

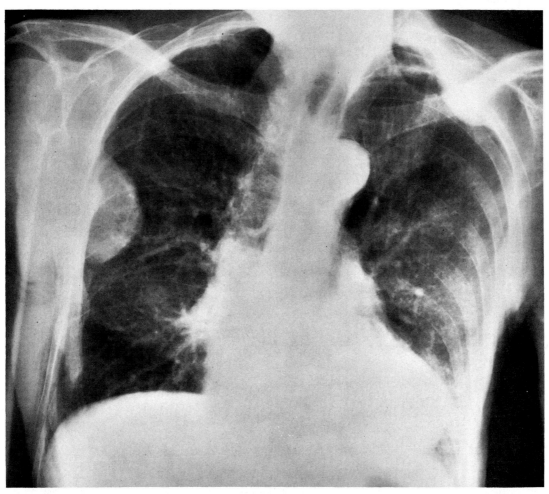

Figure 20–22. Multiple Myeloma of the Rib Cage. A posteroanterior roentgenogram reveals large homogeneous masses protruding into the thorax along the right axillary lung zone and left apex. The obtuse angle that these masses create with the pleura indicates their origin from either the pleura or the chest wall. Such an appearance is highly suggestive of multiple myeloma affecting the rib cage but also can be produced by metastatic carcinoma.

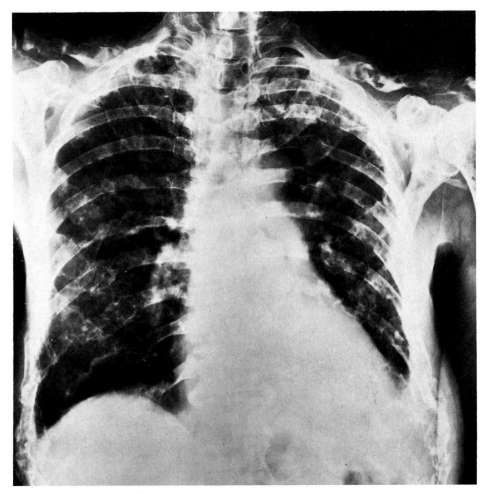

Figure 20–23. Multiple Myeloma of the Rib Cage. A posteroanterior roentgenogram reveals extensive destruction of virtually all ribs bilaterally. Note that several of the ribs have been expanded, a common feature in multiple myeloma of ribs.

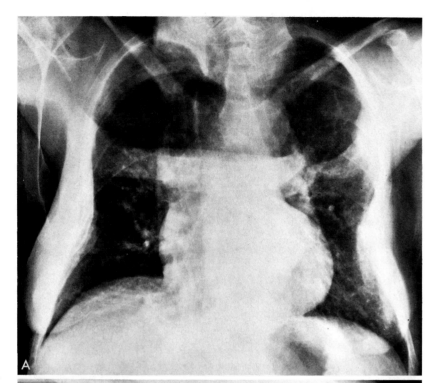

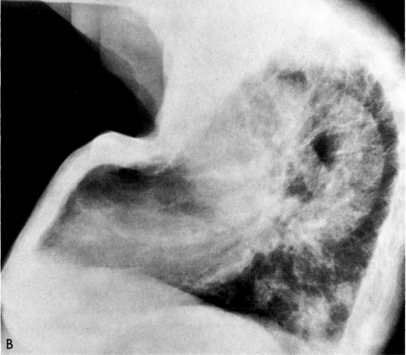

Figure 20–24. Collapse of the Anterior Chest Wall Caused by Involvement of the Sternum in Multiple Myeloma. In postero-anterior projection *(A)*, a rather unusual broad opacity can be identified passing across the whole of the chest from side to side. This opacity obviously cannot arise from *within* the thorax. In lateral projection *(B)*, the upper portion of the anterior chest wall has collapsed inward, thus creating a horizontal "shelf" that casts the unusual shadow in posteroanterior projection. The patient is a 63-year-old woman with widespread multiple myeloma. Note the extensive involvement of the rib cage.

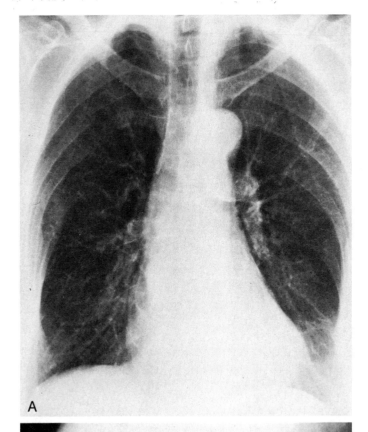

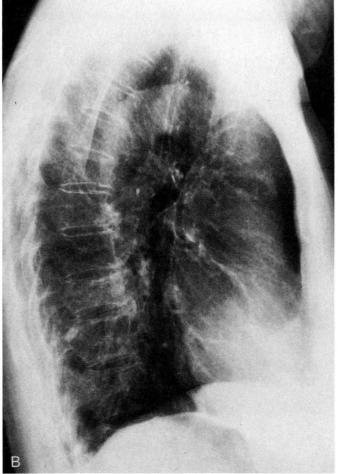

Figure 20–25. Thoracic Bony Metastases from Cervical Carcinoma. Posteroanterior *(A)* and lateral *(B)* chest roentgenograms show a normal skeleton except for several vertebral osteophytes.

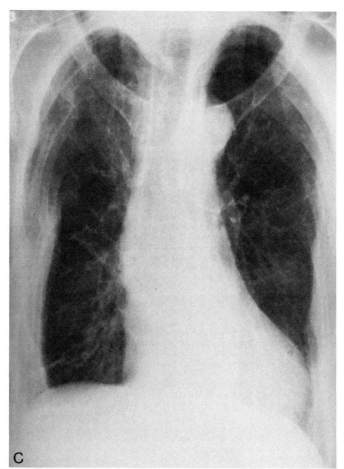

C

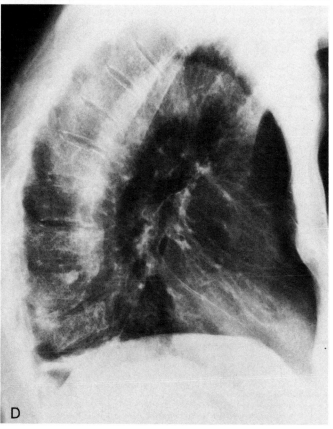

D

Figure 20–25 *Continued* Five months later, similar examinations *(C* and *D)* reveal fractures of the ribs bilaterally and of the sternum; these were associated clinically with a flail sternum and collapse of virtually the entire chest wall that resulted in respiratory failure. The patient is an elderly woman with squamous cell carcinoma of cervix and biopsy-proven skeletal metastases. (Courtesy of Dr. Jim Gruber, Montreal General Hospital.)

REFERENCES

1. Tarver RD, Godwin JD, Putman CE: The diaphragm. Radiol Clin North Am 22:615, 1984.
2. Panicek DM, Benson CB, Gottlieb RH, et al: The diaphragm: Anatomic, pathologic, and radiologic considerations. Radiographics 8:385, 1988.
3. Naidich DP, Zerhouni FA, Siegelman SS: Diaphragm. In Computed Tomography of the Thorax. New York, Raven Press, 1984.
4. Lennon EA, Simon G: The height of the diaphragm in the chest radiograph of normal adults. Br J Radiol 38:937, 1965.
5. Felson B: Chest Roentgenology. Philadelphia, WB Saunders, 1973.
6. Wittenborg MH, Aviad I: Organ influence on the normal posture of the diaphragm: A radiological study of inversions and heterotaxies. Br J Radiol 36:280, 1963.
7. Lasser EC: Some aspects of pulmonary dynamics revealed by concurrent roentgen kymography of spirometric movements and diaphragmatic excursions. Radiology 77:434, 1961.
8. Simon G: Personal communication, 1967.
9. Alexander C: Diaphragm movements and the diagnosis of diaphragmatic paralysis. Clin Radiol 17:79, 1966.
10. Riley EA: Idiopathic diaphragmatic paralysis. A report of eight cases. Am J Med 32:404, 1962.
11. Ridyard JB, Stewart RM: Regional lung function in unilateral diaphragmatic paralysis. Thorax 31:438, 1976.
12. Moorthy SS, Gibbs PS, Losasso AM, et al: Transient paralysis of the diaphragm following radical neck surgery. Laryngoscope 93:642, 1983.
13. Smith CD, Sade RM, Crawford FA, et al: Diaphragmatic paralysis and eventration in infants. J Thorac Cardiovasc Surg 91:490, 1986.
14. Markand ON, Moorthy S, Mahomed Y, et al: Postoperative phrenic nerve palsy in patients with open heart surgery. Ann Thorac Surg 39:68, 1985.
15. Large FR, Heywood LJ, Flower CD, et al: Incidence and aetiology of a raised hemidiaphragm after cardiopulmonary bypass. Thorax 40:444, 1985.
16. Estenne N, Yernault JC, De Smett JN, et al: Phrenic and diaphragm function after coronary artery bypass grafting. Thorax 40:293, 1985.
17. Wilcox P, Baile EM, Hards J, et al: Phrenic nerve function and its relationship to atelectasis after coronary artery bypass surgery. Chest 93:693, 1988.
18. Gould L, Kaplan S, McElhinney AJ: A method for the production of hemidiaphragmatic paralysis. Am Rev Respir Dis 96:812, 1967.
19. Nochomovitz ML, Goldman M, Mitra J, et al: Respiratory responses in reversible diaphragm paralysis. J Appl Physiol 51:1150, 1981.
20. Benjamin JJ, Cascade PN, Reubenfire N, et al: Left lower atelectasis and consolidation following cardiac surgery: The effect of topical cooling on the phrenic nerve. Radiology 142:11, 1982.
21. Rousou JA, Parker T, Angelman RM, et al: Phrenic nerve paresis associated with the use of iced slush and the cooling jacket for topical hypothermia. J Thorac Cardiovasc Surg 89:921, 1985.
22. Esposito RA, Spencer FC: The effect of pericardial insulation on hypothermic phrenic nerve injury during open heart surgery. Ann Thorac Surg 43:303, 1987.
23. Wheeler WE, Rubis LJ, Jones CW, et al: Etiology and prevention of topical cardiac hypothermia-induced phrenic nerve injury and left lower lobe atelectasis during cardiac surgery. Chest 88:680, 1985.
24. Kohorst WR, Schonfeld SA, Altman M: Bilateral diaphragmatic paralysis following topical cardiac hypothermia. Chest 85:65, 1984.
25. Cabrera MR, Edsall JR: Bilateral diaphragm paralysis associated with topical cardiac hypothermia. NY State J Med 87:514, 1987.
26. Heffner JE: Diaphragmatic paralysis following chiropractic manipulation of the cervical spine. Arch Intern Med 145:562, 1985.
27. Drachler DH, Koepke GW, Weg G: Phrenic nerve injury from subclavian vein catheterization: Diagnosis by electromyography. JAMA 236:2280, 1976.
28. Best JB, Pereira M, Senior RM: Phrenic nerve injury associated with the venopuncture of the internal jugular vein. Chest 28:777, 1980.
29. Hadeed HA, Braun TW: Paralysis of the hemidiaphragm as a complication of internal jugular vein cannulation: Report of a case. J Oral Maxillofac Surg 46:409, 1988.
30. Buszek MC, Szymke TE, Honet JC, et al: Hemidiaphragmatic paralysis: An unusual complication of cervical spondylosis. Arch Phys Med Rehab 64:601, 1983.
31. Mellem H, Johansen B, Nakstad P, et al: Unilateral phrenic nerve paralysis caused by osteoarthritis of the cervical spine. Eur J Respir Dis 71:56, 1987.
32. Balbierz JM, Ellenberg M, Honet JC: Complete hemidiaphragmatic paralysis in a patient with multiple sclerosis. Am J Phys Med Rehabil 67:161, 1988.
33. Santamaria J, Ruiz C: Diaphragmatic elevation in stroke. Eur Neurol 28:81, 1988.
34. Anderson RD, Connell TH, Lowman RM: Inversion of the liver and suprahepatic gallbladder associated with eventration of the diaphragm. Radiology 97:87, 1970.
35. Shin MS, Ho K-J: Computed tomographic evaluation of the pathologic lesion for the idiopathic diaphragmatic paralysis. J Comput Tomogr 6:257, 1982.
36. Arborelius M, Lilja B, Senyk J: Regional and total lung function studies in patients with hemidiaphragmatic paralysis. Respiration 32:253, 1975.
37. Ridyard JB, Stewart RM: Regional lung function in unilateral diaphragmatic paralysis. Thorax 31:438, 1976.
38. Easton PA, Fleetham JA, De la Rocha A, et al: Respiratory function after paralysis of the right hemidiaphragm. Am Rev Respir Dis 127:1125, 1983.
39. Lisboa C, Paré PD, Pertuze J, et al: Inspiratory muscle function in unilateral diaphragmatic paralysis. Am Rev Respir Dis 134:488, 1986.
40. LaRoche CM, Mier AK, Mixham J, et al: Diaphragm strength in patients with recent hemidiaphragm paralysis. Thorax 43:170, 1988.
41. Clague HW, Hall DR: Effect of posture on lung volume, airway closure and gas exchange in hemidiaphragmatic paralysis. Thorax 34:523, 1979.
42. Newsom Davis J, Goldman M, Loh L, et al: Diaphragm function and alveolar hypoventilation. Q J Med 45:87, 1976.
43. Allen SM, Hunt B, Green M: Fall in vital capacity with posture. Br J Dis Chest 79:267, 1985.
44. Wright CD, Williams JG, Ogilvie CM, et al: Results of diaphragmatic plication for unilateral diaphragmatic paralysis. J Thorac Cardiovasc Surg 90:195, 1985.
45. Schonfeld T, O'Neal MH, Platzker ACG, et al: Function of the diaphragm before and after plication. Thorax 35:631, 1980.
46. Shochina M, Ferber I, Wolf E: Evaluation of the phrenic nerve in patients with neuromuscular disorders. Int J Rehabil Res 6:455, 1983.
47. Newsom Davis J: Phrenic nerve conduction in man. J Neurol Neurosurg Psychiatry 30:420, 1967.
48. Brouillette RT, Hahn YS, Noah ZL, et al: Successful reinnervation of the diaphragm after phrenic nerve transection. J Pediatr Surg 21:63, 1986.
49. Newsom Davis J, Goldman M, Loh L, et al: Diaphragm function and alveolar hypoventilation. Q J Med 45:87, 1976.
50. Mier A, Brophy C, Green M: Diaphragm weakness. J Royal Soc Med 80:315, 1987.
51. Schiani EA, Roncoroni AJ, Duy RJM: Isolated bilateral diaphragmatic paralysis with interstitial lung disease. Am Rev Respir Dis 129:337, 1984.
52. Skatrud J, Iber C, McHugh W, et al: Determinants of hypoventilation during wakefulness and sleep in diaphragmatic paralysis. Am Rev Respir Dis 121:580, 1980.
53. Molho M, Katz I, Schwartz E, et al: Familial bilateral paralysis of the diaphragm. Chest 91:464, 1987.
54. Loh L, Goldman M, Newsom Davis J: The assessment of diaphragm function. Medicine 56:165, 1977.
55. Ambler R, Gruenewald SJ: Ultrasound monitoring of diaphragm activity in bilateral diaphragmatic paralysis. Arch Dis Child 60:170, 1985.
56. Diament MJ, Boechat MI, Kangarloo H: Real-time sector ultrasound in the evaluation of suspected abnormalities of diaphragmatic motion. J Clin Ultrasound 13:539, 1985.
57. Kreitzer SM, Feldman NT, Saunders NA, et al: Bilateral diaphragmatic paralysis with hypercapnic respiratory failure. Am J Med 65:89, 1978.
58. Bove KE, Iannaccone ST: Atypical infantile spinomuscular atrophy presenting as acute diaphragmatic paralysis. Pediatr Pathol 8:95, 1988.
59. Loh L, Hughes JBM, Newsom Davis J: Gas exchange problems in bilateral diaphragm paralysis. Bull Eur Physiopathol Respir 15:137, 1979.
60. Chin EF, Lynn RB: Surgery of eventration of the diaphragm. J Thorac Surg 32:6, 1956.

61. Prasad R, Nath J, Mukerji PK: Eventration of diaphragm. J Indian Med 84:187, 1986.
62. Bhattacharya SK, Singh NK, Lahiri TK: Eventration of diaphragm. J Indian Med 84:15, 1986.
63. Tamas A, Dunbar JS: Eventration of the diaphragm. J Can Assoc Radiol 8:1, 1957.
64. Paris F, Blasco E, Canto A, et al: Diaphragmatic eventration in infants. Thorax 28:66, 1973.
65. Okuda K, Nomura F, Kawai M, et al: Age-related gross changes of the liver and right diaphragm, with special reference to partial eventration. Br J Radiol 52:870, 1979.
66. Avnet NL: Roentgenologic features of congenital bilateral anterior diaphragmatic eventration. Am J Roentgenol 88:743, 1962.
67. Laustela E: Partial eventration of the left diaphragm. An unusual case. Ann Chir Gynaecol Fenn 48:218, 1959.
68. Vogl A, Small A: Partial eventration of the right diaphragm (congenital diaphragmatic herniation of the liver). Ann Intern Med 43:61, 1955.
69. Hesselink JR, Chung KJ, Peters ME, et al: Congenital partial eventration of the left diaphragm. Am J Roentgenol 131:417, 1978.
70. Campbell JA: The diaphragm in roentgenology of the chest. Radiol Clin North Am 1:395, 1963.
71. Baker DH, Maisel B, Goldberg HP: Use of pneumoperitoneum in differential diagnosis of paracardiac masses in children. Arch Surg 79:63, 1959.
72. Lavender JP, Potts DG: Differential diagnosis of elevated right diaphragmatic dome. Br J Radiol 32:56, 1959.
73. Vaughn CC: Pneumoperitoneum for diagnosis of localized eventration of the diaphragm with liver hernia. Dis Chest 54:467, 1968.
74. Spencer RP, Spackman TJ, Pearson HA: Diagnosis of right diaphragmatic eventration by means of liver scan. Radiology 99:375, 1971.
75. Hesselink JR, Chung KJ, Peters ME, et al: Congenital partial eventration of the left diaphragm. Am J Roentgenol 131:417, 1978.
76. Rubinstein ZJ, Solomon A: CT findings in partial eventration of the right diaphragm. J Comput Assist Tomogr 5:719, 1981.
77. Larson RK, Evans BH: Eventration of the diaphragm. Am Rev Respir Dis 87:753, 1963.
78. Schmidt S: Respiratory kymography in acute abdominal conditions. Acta Radiol 54:49, 1960.
79. Epstein BS: Roentgen kymography of the diaphragm. Am J Roentgenol 74:70, 1955.
80. Ford GT, Whitelaw WA, Rosenal TW, et al: Diaphragm function after upper abdominal surgery in humans. Am Rev Respir Dis 127:431, 1983.
81. Road JD, Burgess KR, Whitelaw WA, et al: Diaphragm function and respiratory response after upper abdominal surgery in dogs. J Appl Physiol 57:576, 1984.
82. Simonneau G, Vivien A, Sartene R, et al: Diaphragm dysfunction induced by upper abdominal surgery—Role of postoperative pain. Am Rev Respir Dis 128:899, 1983.
83. Easton PA, Fitting JW, Arnoux R, et al: Recovery of diaphragm function after laparotomy and chronic sonomicrometer implantation. J Appl Physiol 66:613, 1989.
84. Bertrand D, Viires N, Cantineau J-P, et al: Diaphragmatic contractility after upper abdominal surgery. J Appl Physiol 61:1775, 1986.
85. Phillips JR, Eldridge FL: Respiratory myoclonus (Leeuwenhoek's disease). N Engl J Med 289:1390, 1973.
86. Ting EY, Karliner JS, Williams MH Jr: Diaphragmatic flutter associated with apneustic respiration: A case report with pulmonary function studies. Am Rev Respir Dis 88:833, 1963.
87. Rigatto M, De Medieros NP: Diaphragmatic flutter. Report of a case and review of literature. Am J Med 32:103, 1962.
88. Barrio JL, Feinerman D, Hesla PE, et al: Diaphragmatic flutter in a patient with lymphoma. Mt Sinai J Med 54:188, 1987.
89. Betts RA: Subcostosternal diaphragmatic hernia, with report of five cases. Am J Roentgenol 75:269, 1956.
90. Harrington SW: Various types of diaphragmatic hernia treated surgically. Surg Gynecol Obstet 86:735, 1948.
91. Reed JO, Lang EF: Diaphragmatic hernia in infancy. Am J Roentgenol 82:437, 1959.
92. Pupols A, Ruzicka FF: Hiatal hernia causing a cardia pseudomass on computed tomography. J Comput Assist Tomogr 8:699, 1984.
93. Nishimura RA, Tajik AJ, Schattenberg TT, et al: Diaphragmatic hernia mimicking an atrial mass: A two dimensional echocardiographic pitfall. J Am College Cardiol 5:992, 1985.
94. Baerman JM, Hogan L, Swiryn S: Diaphragmatic hernia producing symptoms and signs of a left atrial mass. Am Heart J 116:198, 1988.
95. Carter BN, Giuseffi J: Strangulated diaphragmatic hernia. Ann Surg 128:210, 1948.
96. Pearson S: Strangulated diaphragmatic hernia: Report of four cases. Arch Surg 66:155, 1953.
97. Hoffman E: Strangulated diaphragmatic hernia. Thorax 23:541, 1968.
98. Menuck L: Plain film findings of gastric volvulus herniating into the chest. Am J Roentgenol 126:1169, 1976.
99. Godwin JD, MacGregor JM: Extension of ascites into the chest with hiatal hernia: Visualization on CT. Am J Roentgenol 148:31, 1987.
100. Felder SL, Masley PM, Wolff WI: Anemia as a presenting symptom of esophageal hiatal hernia of the diaphragm. AMA Arch Intern Med 105:873, 1960.
101. Boch HB, Zimmerman JH: Study of selected congenital anomalies in Pennsylvania. Public Health Rep 82:446, 1967.
102. Young DG: Contralateral pneumothorax with congenital diaphragmatic hernia. Br Med J 4:433, 1968.
103. Gale ME: Bochdalek hernia: Prevalence and CT characteristics. Radiology 156:449, 1985.
104. Whittaker LD Jr, Lynn HB, Dawson B, et al: Hernias of foramen of Bochdalek in children. Mayo Clin Proc 43:580, 1958.
105. Page DV, Stocker JT: Anomalies associated with pulmonary hypoplasia. Am Rev Respir Dis 125:216, 1982.
106. Berdon WE, Baker DH, Amoury R: The role of pulmonary hypoplasia in the prognosis of newborn infants with diaphragmatic hernia and eventration. Am J Roentgenol 103:413, 1968.
107. Morris JJ, Black FO, Stephenson HE Jr: The fate of the unexpanded lung in congenital diaphragmatic hernia. Report of a case. Dis Chest 48:649, 1965.
108. Le Roux BT: Supraphrenic herniation of perinephric fat. Thorax 20:376, 1965.
109. Israël-Asselain R, Uzzan D, Dérrida J: Image pseudo-tumorale par hernie diaphragmatique de graisse supra-rénale. (Transdiaphragmatic herniation of suprarenal fat simulating a tumor mass.) J Franc Med Chir Thorac 20:567, 1966.
110. Bingham JAW: Herniation through congenital diaphragmatic defects. J Surg 47:1, 1959.
111. Siegel MJ, Shackelford GD, McAlister WH: Left-sided congenital diaphragmatic hernia: delayed presentation. Am J Roentgenol 137:43, 1981.
112. Chinn DH, Filly RA, Callen PW, et al: Congenital diaphragmatic hernia diagnosed prenatally by ultrasound. Radiology 148:119, 1983.
113. Seeds JW, Cefalo RC, Lies SC, et al: Early prenatal sonographic appearance of rare thoraco-abdominal eventration. Prenatal Diag 4:437, 1984.
114. Nakayama DK, Harrison MR, Chinn DH, et al: Prenatal diagnosis and natural history of the fetus with a congenital diaphragmatic hernia: Initial clinical experience. J Pediatr Surg 20:118, 1985.
115. Fliegel CP, Kaufmann HJ: Problems caused by pneumothorax in congenital diaphragmatic hernia. Ann Radiol (Paris) 15:159, 1972.
116. Kelvin FM, Starer F: Congenital diaphragmatic hernia and 13 pairs of ribs. Letter to the editor. Br J Radiol 48:152, 1975.
117. Lundius B: Intrathoracic kidney. Am J Roentgenol 125:678, 1975.
118. Khan AN, Gould DA: Sonographic diagnosis of right renal herniation through the canal of Bochdalek. J Clin Ultrasound 12:237, 1984.
119. Curley FJ, Hubmayr RD, Raptopoulos V: Bilateral diaphragmatic densities in a 72-year-old woman. Chest 86:915, 1986.
120. Berman L, Stringer DA, Ein S, et al: Childhood diaphragmatic hernias presenting after the neonatal period. Clin Radiol 39:237, 1988.
121. Singer JI: Herniation of abdominal contents simulating status asthmaticus. Pediatr Emerg Care 3:250, 1987.
122. Kirchner SG, Burko H, O'Neill JA, et al: Delayed radiographic presentation of congenital right diaphragmatic hernia. Radiology 115:155, 1975.
123. Yeung SC, Park C, Kramer N: Diaphragmatic herniation of the liver in a newborn demonstrated by liver scan. Clin Nuclear Med 9:729, 1984.
124. Fischel RE, Joel EM: Herniation of a stone-filled gallbladder through the diaphragm. Acta Radiol (Diagn) 2:172, 1964.
125. Chu DY, Olson AL, Mishaalany HG: Congenital liver cyst presenting as congenital diaphragmatic hernia. J Pediatr Surg 21:897, 1986.
126. Vaughan BF: Diaphragmatic hernia as a finding in the chest radiograph. Proc Coll Radiol Aust 3:42, 1959.
127. Smith L, Lippert KM: Peritoneopericardial diaphragmatic hernia. Ann Surg 148:798, 1958.
128. Wallace DB: Intrapericardial diaphragmatic hernia. Radiology 122:596, 1977.
129. Crittenden IH, Adams FH, Mulder DG: A syndrome featuring defects of the heart, sternum, diaphragm, and anterior abdominal wall. Circulation 20:396, 1959.
130. Robinson AE, Gooneratne NS, Blackburn WR, et al: Bilateral anteromedial defect of the diaphragm in children. Am J Roentgenol 135:301, 1980.
131. Lanuza A: The sign of the cane. A new radiological sign for the diagnosis of small Morgagni hernias. Radiology 101:293, 1971.
132. Merten DF, Bowie JD, Kirks DR, et al: Anteromedial diaphragmatic defects in infancy: Current approaches to diagnostic imaging. Radiology 142:361, 1982.

20

133. Paris F, Tarazona V, Casillas M, et al: Hernia of Morgagni. Thorax 28:631, 1973.
134. Boyd DP, Wooldridge BF: Diaphragmatic hernia through the foramen of Morgagni. Surg Gynecol Obstet 104:727, 1957.
135. Reed MWR, de Silva PHP, Mostafa SM, et al: Diaphragmatic hernia in pregnancy. Br J Surg 74:435, 1987.
136. Rosenberg M: Chronic subphrenic abscess. Lancet 2:379, 1968.
137. Meyers MA: The spread and localization of acute intraperitoneal effusions. Radiology 95:547, 1970.
138. Halvorsen RA, Jones MA, Rice RP, et al: Anterior left subphrenic abscess: Characteristic plain film and CT appearance. Am J Roentgenol 139:283, 1982.
139. Lightwood RG, Cleland WP: Cervical lung hernia. Thorax 29:349, 1974.
140. Miller WT, Talman EA: Subphrenic abscess. Am J Roentgenol 101:961, 1967.
141. Johnson TH Jr: Chest roentgen findings of subdiaphragmatic abscess with antibiotic therapy. Am J Roentgenol 104:584, 1968.
142. Connell TR, Stephens DH, Carlson HC, et al: Upper abdominal abscess: A continuing and deadly problem. Am J Roentgenol 134:759, 1980.
143. Fataar S, Schulman A: Subphrenic abscess: The radiological approach. Clin Radiol 32:147, 1981.
144. Briggs RC: Combined liver-lung scanning in detecting subdiaphragmatic abscess. Semin Nucl Med 2:150, 1972.
145. Alexander ES, Proto AV, Clark RA: CT differentiation of subphrenic abscess and pleural effusion. Am J Roentgenol 140:47, 1983.
146. Federle MP, Mark AS, Guillaumin ES: CT of subpulmonic pleural effusions and atelectasis. Criteria for differentiation from subphrenic fluid. Am J Roentgenol 146:685, 1986.
147. Warraki SE, Mishad MM, Youssef HH, et al: Subdiaphragmatic infection. Dis Chest 52:166, 1967.
148. Anderson LS, Forrest JV: Tumors of the diaphragm. Am J Roentgenol 119:259, 1973.
149. Olafsson G, Rausing A, Holen O: Primary tumors of the diaphragm. Chest 59:568, 1971.
150. Ochsner A, Ochsner A Jr: Tumors of the diaphragm. In Spain D (ed): Diagnosis and Treatment of Tumors of the Chest. New York, Grune & Stratton, 1960, p 240.
151. Stanty P, Galy P, Chassard A: Les tumeurs conjonctives primitive du diaphragme. (Primary connective tissue tumors of the diaphragm.) J Franc Med Chir Thorac 18:745, 1964.
152. Ferguson DD, Westcott JL: Lipoma of the diaphragm. Report of a case. Radiology 118:527, 1976.
153. Tihansky DP, Lopez G: Bilateral lipomas of the diaphragm. NY State J Med, March: 151, 1988.
154. McHenry CR, Pickleman J, Winters G, et al: Diaphragmatic neurilemoma. J Surg Oncology 37:198, 1988.
155. Müller NL: CT features of cystic teratoma of the diaphragm. J Comput Assist Tomogr 10:325, 1986.
156. Müller NL: CT features of cystic teratoma of the diaphragm. J Comput Assist Tomogr 10:325, 1986.
157. Tanaka F, Sawada K, Ishida I, et al: Prosthetic replacement of entire left hemidiaphragm in malignant fibrous histiocytoma of the diaphragm. J Thorac Cardiovasc Surg 83:278, 1982.
158. Seaton D: Primary diaphragmatic haemangiopericytoma. Thorax 29:595, 1974.
159. Kekomaki M, Ekfors TO, Nikkanen V, et al: Intrapleural endodermal sinus tumor arising from the diaphragm. J Pediatr Surg 19:312, 1984.
160. Parker MC: Leiomyosarcoma of the diaphragm—A case report. Eur J Surg Oncology 11:171, 1985.
161. Weilgoni M: Zwerchfell-Lipom. Ubersicht und Bericht über 7 verifizierte Fälle. (Lipoma of the diaphragm. Review and report of 7 proved cases.) Radiologe 3:401, 1963.
162. Nigogosyan G, Ozarda A: Accessory diaphragm. A case report. Am J Roentgenol 85:309, 1961.
163. Hashida Y, Sherman FE: Accessory diaphragm associated with neonatal respiratory distress. J Pediatr 59:529, 1961.
164. Lieberman FL, Hidemura R, Peters RL, et al: Pathogenesis and treatment of hydrothorax complicating cirrhosis with ascites. Ann Int Med 64:341, 1966.
165. Lieberman FL, Peters RL: Cirrhotic hydrothorax. Further evidence that an acquired diaphragmatic defect is at fault. Arch Intern Med 125:114, 1970.
166. Slasky BS, Siewers RD, Lecky JW, et al: Catamenial pneumothorax: The roles of diaphragmatic defects and endometriosis. Am J Roentgenol 138:639, 1982.
167. Ranniger K, Valvassori GE: Angiographic diagnosis of intralobar pulmonary sequestration. Am J Roentgenol 92:540, 1964.
168. Wier JA: Congenital anomalies of the lung. Ann Intern Med 52:330, 1960.
169. Goldenberg DB, Brogdon BG: Congenital anomalies of the pectoral girdle demonstrated by chest radiography. J Can Assoc Radiol 18:472, 1967.
170. Newlin NS: Congenital retrosternal subluxation of the clavicle simulating an intrathoracic mass. Am J Roentgenol 130:1184, 1978.
171. Pearl M, Chow TF, Friedman E: Poland's syndrome. Radiology 101:619, 1976.
172. Esquembre C, Ferris J, Verdeguer A, et al: Poland syndrome and leukaemia. Eur J Pediatr 146:444, 1987.
173. Sackey K, Odone V, Geroge S, et al: Poland's syndrome associated with childhood non-Hodgkin's lymphoma. Am J Dis Child 138:600, 1984.
174. Bavinck JNB, Weaver DD: Subclavian artery supply disruption sequence: Hypothesis of a vascular etiology for Poland, Klippel-Feil, and Möbius anomalies. Am J Med Genetics 23:903, 1986.
175. Mueller CF, Moseley RD Jr: Roentgenologic appearance of the chest following radical neck dissection. Am J Roentgenol 117:840, 1973.
176. Catalona WJ, Crowder WL, Chretien PB: Occurrence of hernia of Morgagni with filial cervical lung hernia: A hereditary defect of the cervical mesenchyme? Chest 62:340, 1972.
177. Fisher MS: Eve's rib. Letters to the editor. Radiology 140:841, 1981.
178. Siegel RS, Steichen FM: Cervicothoracic outlet syndrome. Vascular compression caused by congenital abnormality of thoracic ribs: A case report. J Bone Joint Surg 49A:1187, 1967.
179. Rasmussen P, Simonsen NG: The scalenus anticus syndrome. I Nord Med 62:1569, 1959.
180. Rasmussen P, Simonsen NG: The scalenus anticus syndrome. II. Results of operative treatment in 20 cases, including 16 with costa cervicalis syndrome. Nord Med 62:1572, 1959.
181. De Villiers JC: A brachiocephalic vascular syndrome associated with cervical rib. Br Med J 2:140, 1966.
182. Lagerquist LG, Tyler FH: Thoracic outlet syndrome with tetany of the hands. Am J Med 59:281, 1975.
183. Dick R: Arteriography in neurovascular compression at the thoracic outlet, with special reference to embolic patterns. Am J Roentgenol 110:141, 1970.
184. Kelleher J, O'Connell DJ, MacMahon H: Intrathoracic rib: Radiographic features of two cases. Br J Radiol 52:181, 1979.
185. Shoop JD: Transthoracic rib. Radiology 93:1335, 1969.
186. Sullivan D, Cornwell WS: Pelvic rib: Report of a case. Radiology 110:355, 1974.
187. Pirnar T, Neuhauser EBD: Asphyxiating thoracic dystrophy of the newborn. Am J Roentgenol 98:358, 1966.
188. Connor JM, Evans CC, Evans DAP: Cardiopulmonary function in fibrodysplasia ossificans progressiva. Thorax 36:419, 1981.
189. King RM, Payne WS, Olafsson S, et al: Surgical palliation of respiratory insufficiency secondary to massive exuberant polyostotic fibrous dysplasia of the ribs. Ann Thorac Surg 39:185, 1985.
190. Boone ML, Swenson BE, Felson B: Rib notching: Its many causes. Am J Roentgenol 91:1075, 1964.
191. Ferris RA, LoPresti JM: Rib notching due to coarctation of the aorta: Report of a case initially observed at less than one year of age. Br J Radiol 47:357, 1974.
192. Chinitz LA, Kronzon I, Trehan N, et al: Total occlusion of the abdominal aorta in a patient with Takayasu's arteritis: The importance of lower rib notching in the differential diagnosis. Cath Cardiovasc Diagn 12:405, 1986.
193. Sturm A Jr, Loogen F: Rippenusuren ohne Aortenisthrusstenose, unter besonderer Berücksichtigung der Fallotschen Tetralogie und Pentalogie. (Notching of the ribs in the absence of coarctation of the aorta, with particular consideration to Fallot's tetralogy and pentalogy.) Fortschr Roentgenstr 97:464, 1962.
194. Sargent EN, Turner AF, Jacobson G: Superior marginal rib defects. An etiologic classification. Am J Roentgenol 106:491, 1969.
195. Gilmartin D: Cartilage calcification and rib erosion in chronic respiratory poliomyelitis. Clin Radiol 17:115, 1966.
196. Bernstein C, Loeser WD, Manning LG: Erosive rib lesions in paralytic poliomyelitis. Radiology 70:368, 1958.
197. Wignall BK, Williamson BRJ: The chest x-ray in quadriplegia: A review of 119 patients. Clin Radiol 31:81, 1980.
198. Keats TE: Superior marginal rib defects in restrictive lung disease. Am J Roentgenol 124:449, 1975.
199. Osinowo O, Adebo OA, Okubanjo AO: Osteomyelitis of the ribs in Ibadan. Thorax 41:58, 1986.
200. Wolstein D, Rabinowitz JG, Twersky J: Tuberculosis of the rib. J Can Assoc Radiol 25:307, 1974.
201. Ip M, Chen NK, So SY, et al: Unusual rib destruction in pleuropulmonary tuberculosis. Chest 95:242, 1989.
202. Fogelman I: Lesions in the ribs detected by bone scanning. Clin Radiol 31:317, 1980.
203. Bonakdarpour A, Zadeh YFA, Maghssoudi H, et al: Costal echinococcosis. Report of six cases and review of the literature. Am J Roentgenol 118:371, 1973.

204. Kennedy AC: Tietze's syndrome: An unusual cause of chest wall swelling. Scott Med J 2:363, 1957.
205. Pohl R: Zur Aetiologie des Tietze-Syndrome. (Etiology of Tietze's syndrome.) Wien Klin Wochenschr 69:370, 1957.
206. Ausubel H, Cohen BD, LaDue JS: Tietze's disease of eight years' duration. N Engl J Med 261:190, 1959.
207. Karon EH, Achor RWP, Janes JM: Painful nonsuppurative swelling of costochondral cartilages (Tietze's syndrome). Mayo Clin Proc 33:45, 1958.
208. Skorneck AB: Roentgen aspects of Tietze's syndrome. Painful hypertrophy of costal cartilage and bone—Osteochondritis? Am J Roentgenol 83:748, 1960.
209. Jurik AG, Graudal H: Sternocostal joint swelling—Clinical Tietze's syndrome. Scand J Rheumatol 17:33, 1988.
210. Dunlop RF: Tietze revisited. Letter to the editor. Clin Orthop 62:223, 1969.
211. Gill GV: Epidemic of Tietze's syndrome. Br Med J 2:499, 1977.
212. Edelstein G, Levitt RG, Slaker DP, et al: CT observation of rib abnormalities: Spectrum of findings. J Comput Assist Tomogr 9:65, 1985.
213. Edelstein G, Levitt RG, Slaker DP, et al: Computed tomography of Tietze syndrome. J Comput Assist Tomogr 8:20, 1984.
214. Ricevuti G: Effects of human calcitonin on pain in the treatment of Tietze's syndrome. Clin Ther 7:669, 1985.
215. Carabasi RK, Christian JJ, Brindley HH: Costosternal chondrodynia: A variant of Tietze's syndrome? Dis Chest 41:559, 1962.
216. Guller B, Hable K: Cardiac findings in pectus excavatum in children: Review and differential diagnosis. Chest 66:165, 1974.
217. Leung AKC, Hoo JJ: Familial congenital funnel chest. Am J Med Genet 26:887, 1987.
218. Wooler GH, Mashhour YAS, Garcia JB, et al: Pectus excavatum. Thorax 24:557, 1969.
219. Shamberger RC, Welch KJ: Surgical repair of pectus excavatum. J Pediatr Surg 23:615, 1988.
220. Ravitch MM, Matzen RN: Pulmonary insufficiency in pectus excavatum associated with left pulmonary agenesis, congenital clubbed feet and extromelia. Dis Chest 54:58, 1968.
221. Backer Ole G, Brünner S, Larsen V: Radiologic evaluation of funnel chest. Acta Radiol 55:249, 1961.
222. Mosetitsch W: Pectus excavatum. Fortschr Roentgenstr 100:31, 1964.
223. Ben-Menachem Y, O'Hara AE, Kane HA: Paradoxical cardiac enlargement during inspiration in children with pectus excavatum: A new observation. Br J Radiol 46:38, 1973.
224. Soteropoulos GC, Cigtay OS, Schellinger D: Pectus excavatum deformities simulating mediastinal masses. J Comput Assist Tomogr 3:596, 1979.
225. Moreno AJ, Parker AL, Fredericks P, et al: Pectus excavatum defect on liver-spleen scintigraphy. Eur J Nucl Med 12:309, 1986.
226. Muherji S, Zeissman HA, Earll JM, et al: False-positive iodine-131 whole body scan due to pectus excavatum. Clin Nucl Med 13:207, 1988.
227. Haller JA, Kramer SS, Lietman SA: Use of CT scans in selection of patients for pectus excavatum surgery: A preliminary report. J Pediatr Surg 22:904, 1987.
228. Nakahara K, Ohno K, Shinichiro M, et al: An evaluation of operative outcome in patients with funnel chest diagnosed by means of the computed tomogram. J Thorac Cardiovasc Surg 93:577, 1987.
229. Clark JB, Grenville-Mathers R: Pectus excavatum. Br J Dis Chest 56:202, 1962.
230. Wachtel FW, Ravitch MM, Grishman A: The relation of pectus excavatum to heart disease. Am Heart J 52:121, 1956.
231. Skinner EF: Xiphoid horn in pectus excavatum. Thorax 24:750, 1969.
232. Fink A, Rivin A, Murray JF: Pectus excavatum. An analysis of twenty-seven cases. Arch Intern Med 108:427, 1961.
233. Shamberger RC, Welch K, Sanders SP: Mitral valve prolapse associated with pectus excavatum. J Pediatr 111:404, 1987.
234. Park JM, Farmer AR: Wolff-Parkinson-White syndrome in children with pectus excavatum. J Pediatr 112:926, 1988.
235. Orzalesi MM, Cook CD: Pulmonary function in children with pectus excavatum. J Pediatr 66:898, 1965.
236. Moore RA, McNicholas K, Murphy DMF, et al: Cardiorespiratory failure due to recurrent pectus excavatum deformity. J Med Soc NJ 82:44, 1985.
237. Cahill JL, Lees GM, Robertson HT: A summary of preoperative and postoperative cardiorespiratory performance in patients undergoing pectus excavatum and carinatum repair. J Pediatr Surg 19:430, 1984.
238. Peterson RJ, Young WG, Godwin JD, et al: Noninvasive assessment of exercise cardiac function before and after pectus excavatum repair. J Thorac Cardiovasc Surg 90:251, 1985.
239. Schamberger RC, Welch KJ: Surgical correction of pectus carinatum. J Pediatr Surg 22:48, 1987.
240. Lester CW: Pectus carinatum, pigeon breast and related deformities of the sternum and costal cartilages. Arch Paediatr 77:399, 1960.
241. Currarino G, Silverman FN: Premature obliteration of the sternal sutures and pigeon-breast deformity. Radiology 70:532, 1958.
242. Davies H: Chest deformities in congenital heart disease. Br J Dis Chest 53:151, 1959.
243. Zorab PA: Chest deformities. Br Med J 1:1155, 1966.
244. Biesecker GL, Aaron BL, Mullen JT: Primary sternal osteomyelitis. Chest 63:236, 1973.
245. Goldin RH, Chow AW, Edwards JE Jr, et al: Sternoarticular septic arthritis in heroin users. N Engl J Med 289:616, 1973.
246. Gimferrer J-M, Callejas M-A, Sánchez-Lloret J, et al: Candida albicans costochondritis in heroin addicts. Ann Thorac Surg 41:89, 1986.
247. Kohler H, Uehlinger E, Kutzner J, et al: Sternocostoclavicular hyperostosis: Painful swelling of the sternum, clavicles, and upper ribs. Ann Intern Med 87:192, 1977.
248. Kane WJ: Prevalence of scoliosis. Clin Orthop 126:43, 1977.
249. Loop JW, Akeson WH, Clawson DK: Acquired thoracic abnormalities in neurofibromatosis. Am J Roentgenol 93:416, 1965.
250. Naeye RL: Kyphoscoliosis and cor pulmonale. A study of the pulmonary vascular bed. Am J Pathol 38:561, 1961.
251. Bergofsky EH, Turino GM, Fishman AP: Cardiorespiratory failure in kyphoscoliosis. Medicine 38:263, 1959.
252. Reid L: Pathological changes in the lungs in scoliosis. In Zorab PA (ed): Symposium on Scoliosis, 2nd ed. New York, Longman, Inc, 1969.
253. Reid L: Autopsy studies of the lungs in kyphoscoliosis. In Zorab PA (ed): Proceedings of a symposium on scoliosis. London, National Fund for Research in Poliomyelitis and Other Crippling Diseases, 1966, p 71.
254. James JIP: Scoliosis. Baltimore, Williams & Wilkins, 1968.
255. Weber B, Smith JP, Briscoe WA, et al: Pulmonary function in asymptomatic adolescents with idiopathic scoliosis. Am Rev Respir Dis 111:389, 1975.
256. Bjure J, Grimby G, Kasalicky J, et al: Respiratory impairment and airway closure in patients with untreated idiopathic scoliosis. Thorax 25:451, 1970.
257. Godfrey S: Respiratory and cardiovascular consequences of scoliosis. Respiration 27(suppl):67, 1970.
258. Kafer ER: Respiratory function in paralytic scoliosis. Am Rev Respir Dis 110:450, 1974.
259. Bates DV, Macklem PT, Christie RV: Respiratory Function in Disease; an Introduction to the Integrated Study of the Lung, 2nd ed. Philadelphia, WB Saunders, 1971.
260. Bühlmann A, Gierhake W: Die Lungenfunktion bei der jugendlichen Kyphoskoliose. (Pulmonary function in adolescents with kyphoscoliosis.) Schweiz Med Wochenschr 90:1153, 1960.
261. Bruderman I, Stein M: Physiologic evaluation and treatment of kyphoscoliotic patients. Ann Intern Med 55:94, 1961.
262. Hepper NGG, Black LF, Fowler WS: Relationships of lung volume to height and arm span in normal subjects and in patients with spinal deformity. Am Rev Respir Dis 91:356, 1965.
263. Bergofsky EH: Respiratory failure in disorders of the thoracic cage. Am Rev Respir Dis 119:643, 1979.
264. Shaw DB, Read J: Hypoxia and thoracic scoliosis. Br Med J 2:1486, 1960.
265. Dollery CT, Gillam PMS, Hugh-Jones P, et al: Regional lung function in kyphoscoliosis. Thorax 20:175, 1965.
266. Bake B, Bjure J, Kasalichy J, et al: Regional pulmonary ventilation and perfusion distribution in patients with untreated idiopathic scoliosis. Thorax 27:703, 1972.
267. Kafer E: Idiopathic scoliosis. Gas exchange and the age dependence of arterial blood gases. J Clin Invest 58:825, 1976.
268. Kafer E: Idiopathic scoliosis. Mechanical properties of the respiratory system and the ventilatory response to carbon dioxide. J Clin Invest 55:1153, 1975.
269. Sinha R, Bergofsky EH: Prolonged alteration of lung mechanics in kyphoscoliosis by positive pressure hyperinflation. Am Rev Respir Dis 106:47, 1972.
270. Lisboa C, Moreno R, Fava M, et al: Inspiratory muscle function in patients with severe kyphoscoliosis. Am Rev Respir Dis 132:48, 1985.
271. Hornstein S, Inman V, Ledsome JR: Ventilatory muscle training in kyphoscoliosis. Spine 12:859, 1987.
272. Kryger MH: Sleep in restrictive lung disorders. Clin Chest Med 6:675, 1985.
273. Sawicka EH, Branthwaite MA: Respiration during sleep in kyphoscoliosis. Thorax 42:801, 1987.
274. George CF, Kryger MH: Sleep in restrictive lung disease. Sleep 10:409, 1987.
275. Garay S, Turino G, Goldring R: Sustained reversal of chronic

20

hypercapnia in patients with alveolar hypoventilation syndromes. Am J Med 70:269, 1981.

276. Hoeppner V, Cockcroft D, Dosman J, et al: Nighttime ventilation improves respiratory failure in secondary kyphoscoliosis. Am Rev Respir Dis 129:240, 1984.

277. Wiers W, LeCoulture R, Dallinga O, et al: Cuirass respiratory treatment of chronic respiratory failure in scoliotic patients. Thorax 32:221, 1977.

278. Murray JF: Pulmonary disability in the Hurler syndrome (lipochondrodystrophy). A study of two cases. N Engl J Med 261:378, 1959.

279. Buhain WJ, Rammohan G, Berger HW: Pulmonary function in Morquio's disease—A study of two siblings. Chest 68:41, 1975.

280. Cimmino CV: The paraspinal-thoracic ratio in chest teleroentgenograms. Radiology 69:251, 1957.

281. Gould KG, Cooper KH, Harkleroad LE: Pulmonary function and work capacity in the absence of physiologic dorsal kyphosis of the spine. Dis Chest 55:405, 1969.

282. Brewerton DA, Caffrey M, Hart FD, et al: Ankylosing spondylitis and HLA 27. Lancet 1:904, 1973.

283. Schlosstein L, Terasaki PI, Bluestone R, et al: High association of an HLA antigen, W27, with ankylosing spondylitis. N Engl J Med 288:704, 1973.

284. Danilevicius Z: HLA system and rheumatic disease. JAMA 231:283, 1975.

285. Calin A, Porta J, Fried JF, et al: Clinical history as a screening test for ankylosing spondylitis. JAMA 237:2613, 1977.

286. Calin A, Fries JF: Striking prevalence of ankylosing spondylitis in "healthy" W27 positive males and females. A controlled study. N Engl J Med 293:835, 1975.

287. Boland EW: Ankylosing spondylitis. In Hollander JL (ed): Arthritis and Allied Conditions, 7th ed. Philadelphia, Lea & Febiger, 1966, pp 633–655.

288. Graham DC, Smythe HA: The carditis and aortitis of ankylosing spondylitis. Bull Rheum Dis 9:171, 1958.

289. Rosenow EC III, Strimlan CV, Muhm JR, et al: Pleuropulmonary manifestations of ankylosing spondylitis. Mayo Clin Proc 52:641, 1977.

290. Luthra HS: Extra-articular manifestations of ankylosing spondylitis. Mayo Clin Proc 52:655, 1977.

291. Jessamine AG: Upper lobe fibrosis in ankylosing spondylitis. Can Med Assoc J 98:25, 1968.

292. Campbell AH, MacDonald CB: Upper lobe fibrosis associated with ankylosing spondylitis. Br J Dis Chest 59:90, 1965.

293. Rohatgi PK, Turrisi BC: Bronchocentric granulomatosis and ankylosing spondylitis. Thorax 39:317, 1984.

294. Rumancik WM, Firooznia H, Davis MS, et al: Fibrobullous disease of the upper lobes: An extraskeletal manifestation of ankylosing spondylitis. J Comput Tomogr 8:225, 1984.

295. Kinnear WJ, Shneerson JM: Acute pleural effusions in inactive ankylosing spondylitis. Thorax 40:150, 1985.

296. Good AE: The chest pain of ankylosing spondylitis. Its place in the differential diagnosis of heart pain. Ann Intern Med 58:926, 1963.

297. Radford EP, Doll R, Smith PG: Mortality among patients with ankylosing spondylitis not given x-ray therapy. N Engl J Med 297:572, 1977.

298. Travis DM, Cook CD, Julian DG, et al: The lungs in rheumatoid spondylitis. Gas exchange and lung mechanics in a form of restrictive pulmonary disease. J Clin Invest 29:623, 1960.

299. Miller JM, Sproule BJ: Pulmonary function in ankylosing spondylitis. Am Rev Respir Dis 90:376, 1964.

300. Feltelius N, Hedenstrom H, Hillerdal G, et al: Pulmonary involvement in ankylosing spondylitis. Ann Rheum Dis 45:736, 1986.

301. Franssen MJ, van Herwaarden CL, van de Putte LB: Lung function in patients with ankylosing spondylitis. A study of the influence of disease activity and treatment with nonsteroidal anti-inflammatory drugs. J Rheumatol 13:936, 1986.

302. Elliott CG, Hill TE, Crapo RO, et al: Exercise performance of subjects with ankylosing spondylitis and limited chest expansion. Bull Eur Physiopathol Respir 21:363, 1985.

303. Renzetti AD Jr, Nicholas W, Dutton RE Jr, et al: Some effects of ankylosing spondylitis on pulmonary gas exchange. N Engl J Med 262:215, 1960.

304. Stewart RM, Ridyard JB, Pearson JD: Regional lung function in ankylosing spondylitis. Thorax 31:433, 1976.

305. Ochsner A, Ochsner A Jr: Tumors of the thoracic wall. In Spain D (ed): Diagnosis and Treatment of Tumors of the Chest. New York, Grune & Stratton, 1960, p 209.

306. Ochsner A Jr, Lucas GL, McFarland GB Jr: Tumors of the thoracic skeleton. Review of 134 cases. J Thorac Cardiovasc Surg 52:311, 1966.

307. Omell GH, Anderson LS, Bramson RT: Chest wall tumors. Radiol Clin North Am 11:197, 1973.

308. Pairolero PC, Arnold PG: Chest wall tumors: Experience with 100 consecutive patients. J Thorac Cardiovasc Surg 90:367, 1985.

309. Greager JA, Patel MK, Briele HA, et al: Soft tissue sarcomas of the adult thoracic wall. Cancer 59:370, 1987.

310. Graeber GM, Snyder RJ, Fleming AW, et al: Initial and long-term results in the management of primary chest wall neoplasms. Ann Thorac Surg 34:664, 1982.

311. King RM, Pairolero PC, Trastek VF, et al: Primary chest wall tumors: Factors affecting survival. Ann Thorac Surg 41:597, 1986.

312. Jafri SZH, Roberts JL, Bree RL, et al: Computed tomography of chest wall masses. RadioGraphics 9:51, 1989.

313. Souba WW, McKenna RJ Jr, Meis J, et al: Radiation-induced sarcomas of the chest wall. Cancer 57:610, 1986.

314. Huvos AG, Woodard HQ, Cahan WG, et al: Postradiation osteogenic sarcoma of bone and soft tissues. A clinicopathologic study of 66 patients. Cancer 55:1244, 1985.

315. Lo TCM, Silverman ML, Edelstein A: Postirradiation hemangiosarcoma of the chest wall. Report of a case. Acta Radiol Oncol 24:237, 1985.

316. Stefanko J, Turnbull AD, Nelson L, et al: Primitive neuroectodermal tumors of the chest wall. J Surg Oncol 37:33, 1988.

317. Gonzalez-Crussi F, Wolfson SL, Misugi K, et al: Peripheral neuroectodermal tumors of the chest wall in childhood. Cancer 54:2519, 1984.

318. Raney RB Jr, Ragab AH, Ruymann FB, et al: Soft-tissue sarcoma of the trunk in childhood. Results of the intergroup rhabdomyosarcoma study. Cancer 49:2612, 1982.

319. Linnoila RI, Tsokos M, Triche TJ, et al: Evidence for neural origin and PAS-positive variants of the malignant small cell tumor of thoracopulmonary region ("Askin tumor"). Am J Surg Pathol 10:124, 1986.

320. Shamberger RC, Grier HE, Weinstein HJ, et al: Chest wall tumors in infancy and childhood. Cancer 63:774, 1989.

321. Seltzer RA: Subpleural lipoma. Lancet 84:100, 1964.

322. Doubleday LC, Durham ME Jr, Durham ME Sr: Lipoma of a chest wall. Report of a case. Texas State J Med 59:24, 1963.

323. Rosenberg RF, Rubinstein BM, Messinger NH: Intrathoracic lipomas. Chest 60:507, 1971.

324. Castillo M, Shirkhoda A: Computed tomography of diaphragmatic lipoma. J Comput Assist Tomogr 9:167, 1985.

325. Jones ER, Golebiowski A: Desmoid tumour of chest wall. Br Med J 2:1134, 1960.

326. Nickell WK, Kittle CF, Boley JO: Desmoid tumour of the chest. Thorax 13:218, 1958.

327. Klein DL, Gamsu G, Gant TD: Intrathoracic desmoid tumor of the chest wall. Am J Roentgenol 129:524, 1977.

328. King RM, Pairolero PC, Trastek VF, et al: Primary chest wall tumors: Factors affecting survival. Ann Thorac Surg 41:597, 1986.

329. Rami-Porta R, Bravo-Bravo JL, Aroca-Gonzalez MJ, et al: Tumours and pseudotumours of the chest wall. Scand J Thorac Cardiovasc Surg 19:97, 1985.

330. Sabanathan S, Salama FD, Morgan WE, et al: Primary chest wall tumors. Ann Thorac Surg 39:4, 1985.

331. Berthoty DP, Shulman SN, Miller HAB: Elastofibroma: Chest wall pseudotumor. Radiology 160:341, 1986.

332. Alvarez-Sala R, Gomez de Terreros FJ, Caballero P: Echinococcus cyst as a cause of chest wall tumor. Ann Thorac Surg 43:689, 1987.

333. Meis JM, Butler JJ, Osborne BM: Hodgkin's disease involving the breast and chest wall. Cancer 57:1859, 1986.

334. Cho CS, Blank N, Castellino RA: Computerized tomography evaluation of chest wall involvement in lymphoma. Cancer 55:1892, 1985.

335. Frija J, Bellin M-F, Laval-Jeantet M, et al: Role of CT in the study of recurrences of Hodgkin's disease on the chest wall. Eur J Radiol 7:229, 1987.

336. Gouliamos AD, Carter BL, Emami B: Computed tomography of the chest wall. Radiology 134:433, 1980.

337. Shin MS, Anderson SD, Myers J, et al: Pitfalls in CT evaluation of chest wall invasion by lung cancer. Case report. J Comput Assist Tomogr 10:136, 1986.

338. Pearlberg JL, Sandler MA, Beute GH, et al: Limitations of CT in evaluation of neoplasms involving chest wall. J Comput Assist Tomogr 11:290, 1987.

339. Trivedi SA: Neurilemmoma of the diaphragm causing severe hypertrophic pulmonary osteoarthropathy. Br J Tuberc 52:214, 1958.

340. Urovitz EPM, Fornasier VL, Czitrom AA: Sternal metastases and associated pathological fractures. Thorax 32:444, 1977.

341. Goldman JM: Parasternal chest wall involvement in Hodgkin's disease. Chest 59:133, 1971.

342. Marcove RC, Huvos AG: Cartilaginous tumors of the ribs. Cancer 27:794, 1971.

343. Joffe N: Malignant synovioma of the chest wall. Br J Radiol 32:619, 1959.
344. Oakley RH, Carty H, Cudmore RE: Multiple benign mesenchymomata of the chest wall. Pediatr Radiol 15:58, 1985.
345. Odell JM, Benjamin DR: Mesenchymal hamartoma of chest wall in infancy: Natural history of two cases. Pediatr Pathol 5:135, 1986.
346. Choma ND, Biscotti CV, Bauer TW, et al: Gorham's syndrome: A case report and review of the literature. Am J Med 83:1151, 1987.
347. Robinson AE, Thomas RL, Monson DM: Aneurysmal bone cyst of the rib. A report of two unusual cases. Am J Roentgenol 100:526, 1967.
348. Mendl K, Evans CJ: Cyst-like and cystic lesions of the rib with special reference to their radiological differential diagnosis based on the discussion of five cases. Br J Radiol 31:146, 1958.
349. Eygelaar A, Homan Van Der Heide JN: Diagnosis and treatment of primary malignant costal and sternal tumors. Dis Chest 52:683, 1967.
350. Wolfel DA, Dennis JM: Multiple myeloma of the chest wall. Am J Roentgenol 89:1241, 1963.
351. Biberstein MP, Eisenberg H: Unilateral diaphragmatic paralysis in association with Erb's palsy. Chest 75:209, 1979.
352. Graham AN, Martin PD, Haas LF: Neuralgic amyotrophy with bilateral diaphragmatic palsy. Thorax 40:635, 1985.
353. Shin MS, Ho K-J: Computed tomographic evaluation of the pathologic lesion for the idiopathic diaphragmatic paralysis. J Comput Assist Tomogr 6:257, 1982.
354. Dervaux L, Lacquet LM: Hemidiaphragmatic paralysis after cervical herpes zoster. Thorax 37:870, 1982.
355. Bowman ED, Murton LJ: A case of neonatal bilateral diaphragmatic paralysis requiring surgery. Aust Paediatr J 20:331, 1984.
356. McWilliam RC, Gardner-Medwyn D, Doyle D, et al: Diaphragmatic paralysis due to spinal muscular atrophy. Arch Dis Child 60:145, 1985.
357. Montserrat JM, Picado CF, Agusti-Vidal A: Arnold-Chiari malformation and paralysis of the diaphragm. Respiration 53:128, 1988.
358. Mier A, Brophy C, Green M: Diaphragm weakness and syringomyelia. J R Soc Med 81:59, 1988.
359. Goldstein RL, Hyde RW, Lapham LW, et al: Peripheral neuropathy presenting with respiratory insufficiency as the primary complaint. Am J Med 56:443, 1974.
360. Walsh NE, Dumitru D, Kalantri A, et al: Brachial neuritis involving the bilateral phrenic nerves. Arch Phys Med Rehabil 68:46, 1987.
361. Cooper CB, Trend PJ, Wiles CM: Severe diaphragm weakness in multiple sclerosis. Thorax 40:633, 1985.
362. Spiteri MA, Mier AK, Brophy CJ, et al: Bilateral diaphragm weakness. Thorax 40:631, 1985.
363. Thomas NE, Passamonte PM, Sunderrajan EV, et al: Bilateral diaphragmatic paralysis as a possible paraneoplastic syndrome from renal cell carcinoma. Am Rev Respir Dis 129:507, 1984.
364. Sandham JD, Shaw DT, Guenter CA: Acute supine respiratory failure due to bilateral diaphragmatic paralysis. Chest 72:97, 1977.
365. Camfferman F, Bogaard JM, van der Meche FGA, et al: Idiopathic bilateral diaphragmatic paralysis. Eur J Respir Dis 66:65, 1985.
366. Lenz H, Rohr H: Zur radikulären Genese der sogenannten Relaxatio diaphragmatis. (Radicular genesis of so-called relaxatio diaphragmatis.) Fortschr Roentgenstr 103:540, 1965.

20

21

Respiratory Disease Associated with a Normal Chest Roentgenogram

There is considerable experimental and clinical evidence to support the observation that significant pulmonary and pleural disease, sometimes of life-threatening severity, can exist in the presence of a normal chest roentgenogram (*see* page 291). This limitation of roentgenographic visibility exists not only in the early stages of various alveolar and interstitial diseases but also during the healing stage when acute inflammatory changes have been re-placed by organization tissue or mature fibrous tissue. In many cases, this finding constitutes a significant, positive diagnostic feature and excludes those diseases in which respiratory symptoms and signs are commonly associated with roentgenographic abnormalities.

In addition to cases in which the roentgenogram is undoubtedly normal, from time to time a roentgenographic pattern is encountered in the "gray area"—at the outer range of normal but not unequivocally abnormal. An example of such a situation is encountered in deciding whether one or both hemidiaphragms are elevated beyond the normal range; although a high diaphragm is often a reflection of suboptimal inspiration (not necessarily the result of poor patient effort as is sometimes implied), it can be an important indication of small lung volume.

Both the equivocal and unequivocal situations are most easily discussed in terms of whether disease is localized or generalized. In each instance, a repeat roentgenogram may resolve the problem, or comparison with previous roentgenograms may establish whether the film in question represents a deviation from the normal pattern.

In this chapter the local and diffuse diseases of the lung parenchyma, pleura, and airways that may be associated with a normal chest roentgenogram are discussed. In addition, the broad spectrum of conditions that can cause alveolar hypoventilation and hyperventilation (usually associated with a normal chest roentgenogram) is described in some detail. Finally, we will review the anatomic and biochemical abnormalities that can cause decreased oxygen-carrying capacity of the blood and the development of pulmonary symptoms, despite a normal chest roentgenogram and normal conventional pulmonary function tests.

DISEASES OF THE LUNG PARENCHYMA

In Chapter 1 (see page 295) the limitations of roentgenographic visibility in alveolar and interstitial pulmonary disease are discussed. Even in ideal circumstances, with technically perfect roentgenograms interpreted carefully by experienced observers, lesions may be so minute as to be imperceptible or may be hidden behind or juxtaposed to skeletal or vascular shadows. A solitary uncalcified lesion less than 6 mm in diameter is rarely appreciated and then usually only in retrospect when the lesion has grown and is detected on subsequent roentgenograms. In fact, nodules as large as 2 cm in diameter may be overlooked, particularly if they are situated over the convexity of the lung or in the paramediastinal area where the rib cage, large vessels, and mediastinal contents tend to obscure their image. In contrast, multiple micronodular opacities measuring no more than 1 or 2 mm in diameter are usually appreciated, possibly because of the effect of superimposition. Reference is made throughout this book to those diseases that at some stage of their development or regression fail to cast detectable roentgenographic shadows. No attempt is made in this chapter to review all of these conditions, but attention is directed to those in which a normal chest roentgenogram is more than an occasional finding.

LOCAL DISEASES

Acute airspace disease such as that caused by bacterial infection or alveolar hemorrhage characteristically produces roentgenographic shadows at a very early stage. By contrast, acute local disease confined largely to the interstitium of the lung (e.g., viral or mycoplasma pneumonia) can cause symptoms that precede roentgenographic signs by 48 hours or longer.[1] Localized abnormalities of the pulmonary vascular system, particularly acute pulmonary embolism, also frequently show no roentgenographic abnormalities in the chest. Even in patients in whom embolism results in an infarct, an opacity is seldom visible until 12 to 24 hours following the embolic episode. This clinical observation is supported by experimental investigations; for example, Liebow and colleagues[2] reported a delay of 1 to 7 days before the appearance of pulmonary hemorrhage after the occlusion of a pulmonary artery.

Chronic pulmonary disease also may be present and active for months or even years before it becomes roentgenographically visible. It has been estimated, for example, that a focus of active tuberculosis is not roentgenologically detectable until 2 or 3 months after initial infection.[1] Similarly, most pulmonary carcinomas are present for years before they become visible; studies of the growth rate of primary lung neoplasms and back-extrapolation of the doubling time indicate that these tumors are invisible during two thirds to three quarters of their existence (see page 1407). Although the majority of such tumors do not occasion symptoms during this time, occasionally there are signs and symptoms related to intra- or extrathoracic metastases or to the secretion of a variety of biologically active substances (paraneoplastic syndromes).

GENERAL DISEASES

Diffuse granulomatous and fibrotic diseases of the lungs may be present with a normal chest roentgenogram. In contrast to primary or secondary localized pulmonary *tuberculosis* in which symptoms and signs may not appear for many weeks after the chest roentgenogram has become abnormal, in miliary tuberculosis fever, general malaise, and headaches may develop some weeks before roentgenologic abnormality; in some instances the minute pulmonary lesions are not detected before death. In one very unusual case seen by the authors a patient who had fever and hematuria was subjected to nephrectomy for suspected carcinoma of the kidney. Not only was a hypernephroma found, but miliary tuberculous lesions measuring 1 to 2 mm in diameter dotted the kidney substance, although at that time the chest roentgenogram was normal. Antituberculosis therapy was started at once, and 10 days after the operation a chest roentgenogram showed minute miliary lesions; these disappeared completely with continued treatment.

In diseases such as *sarcoidosis, eosinophilic granuloma,* and *progressive systemic sclerosis,* no lesions may be roentgenographically visible even when symptoms and disturbances of pulmonary function indicate involvement of the lung interstitium. Cases of *sarcoidosis* have been reported in which chest roentgenograms were normal despite abnormal findings in biopsy specimens[3, 4] or pulmonary function abnormalities, the latter consisting of a reduction in compliance,[5] vital capacity, and diffusing capacity.[4, 6, 7] Patients with *fibrosing alveolitis*[8, 9] and *allergic alveolitis* have been shown pathologically to have interstitial fibrosis despite normal chest roentgenograms. Among the connective tissue (collagen) diseases, *progressive systemic sclerosis* is frequently associated with a lowered diffusing capacity and arterial blood P_{O_2} despite a normal chest roentgenogram.[6, 10, 11] By contrast, pulmonary involvement in rheumatoid disease typically is detectable roentgenologically before pulmonary function becomes impaired.[12] In *systemic lupus erythematosus,* pulmonary function may be distinctly abnormal (reduction in vital capacity) despite a normal chest roentgenogram. However, when serial roentgenographic studies are available, in some cases a progressive loss of lung volume may be evidenced by diaphragmatic elevation.[12–15]

In addition to these more common interstitial diseases in which morphologic evidence of parenchymal infiltration may be present despite normal chest roentgenograms, there are occasional diseases of pathologic interest, such as *pulmonary tumorlets* (*see* page 1494) and *chemodectomas* (*see* page 1602), in which the lesions rarely become large enough to be visible roentgenographically or to produce symptoms. Normal pulmonary function tests and chest roentgenograms also have been reported in cases of diffuse interstitial *leukemic infiltration* of the lungs. In patients who die of leukemia, parenchymal infiltration is commonly observed pathologically (in approximately 25 per cent of cases[16–18]) but seldom roentgenographically. It has been estimated that infiltration with leukemic cells is sufficiently extensive to produce symptoms and disturb pulmonary function in less than 3 per cent of cases.[17]

Pulmonary vascular disease may be of significant degree without roentgenographic manifestation—for example, the extensive obstruction of the vasculature in *thromboembolic disease* and the prehypertensive vasculopathy of *progressive systemic sclerosis, rheumatoid disease,* and *polymyositis.*[19]

DISEASES OF THE PLEURA

The chest roentgenogram may be normal in cases of acute pleuritis. However, "dry pleurisy" often is associated with diaphragmatic elevation and reduction in diaphragmatic excursion. As discussed in Chapter 4 (*see* page 663), effusions as large as 300 ml may not be visible on standard posteroanterior and lateral chest roentgenograms exposed in the erect position.[1] However, films exposed in the lateral decubitus position can reveal effusions of 100 ml or less, and special roentgenographic techniques may show as little as 10 to 15 ml, an amount that may be visible even in healthy subjects.[20, 21]

DISEASES OF THE AIRWAYS

Many patients with diseases of the conducting airways have normal chest roentgenograms. In fact, in simple *chronic bronchitis* characterized by a history of cough and expectoration, this is the rule rather than the exception. Although the majority of patients who experience *acute asthmatic attacks* show evidence of pulmonary overinflation on pulmonary function testing, roentgenographic evidence of its presence is seldom convincing except in children and adolescents with early-onset asthma. However, the presence of overinflation during an attack can sometimes be appreciated by comparison with films obtained during remission. Using a roentgenographic technique, Blackie and associates[22] recently measured total lung capacity (TLC) in a group of 10 asthmatic subjects at the time of an acute attack when mean forced expiratory volume in one second (FEV_1) was 1.44 ± 0.43 and compared this to similar measurements obtained at the time of recovery (mean FEV_1, 2.76 ± 0.58). In 9 of the 10 subjects TLC decreased between exacerbation and recovery (mean values were 6.21 during exacerbation and 5.51 at recovery). A chest radiologist was able to detect the hyperinflation in most patients when comparing the acute and recovery roentgenograms but was unable to appreciate its presence on the exacerbation films alone.[22]

Approximately 7 per cent of patients with *bronchiectasis* fail to show evidence of this disease on standard chest roentgenograms.[23] Patients with *emphysema,* particularly in the advanced stages of the disease, show distinctly abnormal roentgenograms. However, pathologic-roentgenologic correlative studies have shown that patients with mild to moderate emphysema may have completely normal films.[24] In one study of 696 patients in which the accuracy of the roentgenologic diagnosis of emphysema was assessed on the basis of paper-mounted whole lung sections made following necropsy,[25] only 41 per cent of the patients with moderately severe emphysema were correctly diagnosed radiologically, although two thirds of the patients with the most severe grades were recognized. It is of considerable interest that for a given grade of emphysema, the roentgenologic diagnosis was made more frequently in patients who manifested severe chronic airflow obstruction.[25] (We are of the opinion that the results of this study were somewhat skewed by the fact that the major roentgenologic sign of emphysema employed was oligemia rather than overinflation.) Several studies have shown that computed tomography (CT) is much more sensitive than conventional roentgenograms in detecting emphysema.[26–29]

Patients with various types of *endobronchial tumors* that only partly obstruct an airway can have normal chest roentgenograms (Fig. 21–1), at least when films are exposed at full inspiration. For example, normal chest roentgenograms have been described in patients with bronchial carcinoid tumor,[36] bronchogenic carcinoma,[30–35] papillomatosis of the trachea and bronchi,[37, 38] and leiomyoma and lipoma of the trachea.[39, 40] More commonly, the volume of lung parenchyma distal to the partial obstruction is *smaller* than normal; obviously in such circumstances a roentgenogram exposed following full expiration, preferably forced, will reveal air trapping distal to the partial obstruction. When the obstruction is in the trachea or a major bronchus, dyspnea and generalized wheezing may suggest the diagnosis of asthma. As pointed out by Sanders and Carnes,[39] lesions arising within the trachea or compressing the trachea from outside should be suspected when wheezing (sometimes relieved by a change in position) is more pronounced during inspiration than expiration, when there is hemoptysis, and when the patient's symptoms fail to respond to the usual therapy for asthma. In such cases the true diagnosis may be suspected from careful clinical and roentgenographic examination and can be confirmed by bronchoscopy. A particularly difficult problem is presented by cases of pulmonary carcinoma in which the diagnosis is made cytologically but a lesion is not apparent either bronchoscopically or roentgenographically. These patients sometimes present with hemoptysis, although a number are now being identified in screening studies of heavy smokers who are more than 45 years of age.[41–43]

ALVEOLAR HYPOVENTILATION

The term alveolar hypoventilation (ventilatory respiratory failure) is used to designate a deficiency in ventilation that is sufficient to raise the arterial level of carbon dioxide (CO_2) to greater than 45 mm Hg. The diagnosis cannot be made by clinical examination or by measurement of minute ventilation. In patients breathing room air, alveolar hypoventilation is necessarily accompanied by a degree of alveolar hypoxia and therefore arterial hypoxemia. Although regional underventilation can contribute to ventilation-perfusion mismatch and arterial hypoxemia without causing hypercapnia, the term hypoventilation should be reserved for a generalized decrease in ventilation that is characterized by the presence of hypercapnia.

A circumstance in which a marked decrease in alveolar ventilation can exist without an elevated carbon dioxide tension is when there is an additional method for removal of CO_2 from the blood. Martin[44] has described the development of "alveolar hypoventilation" and a decrease in arterial Po_2 during renal hemodialysis: CO_2 was removed in the dialysate; this lowered mixed venous and alveolar CO_2 and resulted in "hypoventilation" relative to metabolic CO_2 production despite a normal arterial Pco_2.

It is obvious that in circumstances in which ventilation-perfusion inequality results in regional underventilation and hypoxemia, an absence of hypercapnia indicates that overall ventilation is adequate. This occurs because ventilation to certain areas of the lung is relatively increased to compensate for the regional carbon dioxide retention that is occurring in areas of reduced ventilation. As discussed in Chapter 1 (*see* page 134), the shapes of the dissociation curves for carbon dioxide and oxygen are the explanation for the respiratory system's ability to compensate for regional hypercapnia and its inability to compensate for regional hypoxia; the relatively overventilated areas of lung cannot compensate for the underventilated areas with regard to oxygen because of the curvilinear nature of the oxygen dissociation curve.

Pulmonary diseases that cause ventilation-perfusion mismatch and intrapulmonary shunt resulting in hypoxemia and a normal or low arterial Pco_2 are discussed elsewhere in various sections of this book. Acute hypoxemic respiratory failure of this type is seen most commonly in the adult respiratory distress syndrome, cardiogenic pulmonary edema, and acute bacterial pneumonia, whereas chronic hypoxemic respiratory failure occurs predominantly in interstitial granulomatous and fibrotic disorders. Respiratory failure associated with hypercapnia occurs in two broad groups of disorders, those of pulmonary origin (Table 21–1) and those of nonpulmonary origin (Table 21–2). The latter disorders are dealt with more extensively in this chapter, since they are frequently associated with a normal chest roentgenogram.

Disorders of the mechanisms that drive the chest bellows may result in either acute or chronic respiratory failure, pathophysiologic states that vary not only in their management but also in clinical presentation. For purposes of clarity, these disorders are considered under two headings—those that result from defective ventilatory control and those caused by an inadequate respiratory pump (Table 21–2). Included under the heading of ventilatory control are disorders of cerebral and brain stem respiratory center functions and abnormalities of the efferent outputs from the upper motor neurons that drive the respiratory muscles and of the afferent inputs into the central nervous system from peripheral receptors. Disorders of the respiratory pump include abnormalities of the anterior horn cells, the myoneural junction, the respiratory muscles, the phrenic and intercostal nerves that innervate those muscles, and the chest cage itself.

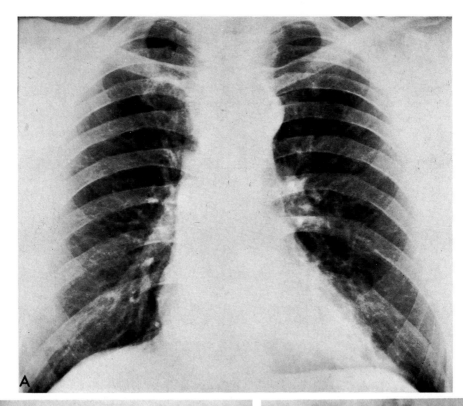

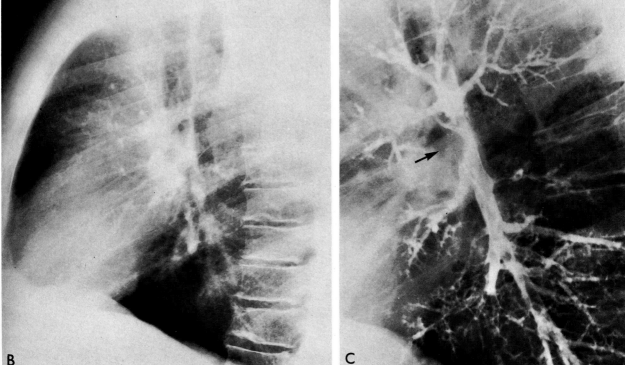

Figure 21–1. Bronchogenic Carcinoma with a Normal Chest Roentgenogram. This 56-year-old man was admitted to the hospital with a 2-month history of right-sided wheeze; he had had one episode of hemoptysis. Posteroanterior (*A*) and lateral (*B*) roentgenograms reveal a normal appearance of the lungs and mediastinum. In view of abnormal findings on bronchoscopy, a right bronchogram was performed (*C*) and showed an irregular mass arising from the anterior wall of the intermediate stem bronchus (*arrow*). It is probable that roentgenography of the chest in expiration would have shown evidence of air trapping in the right middle and lower lobes. This was proved squamous-cell carcinoma.

Table 21–1. Pulmonary Causes of Respiratory Failure with Hypercapnia

UPPER AIRWAY OBSTRUCTION

Acute: Infection (pharyngitis, tonsillitis, epiglottitis, laryngotracheitis)
               Edema (irritant gases, angioneurotic edema)
               Retropharyngeal hemorrhage (trauma, postoperative, hemophilia, acute leukemia)
               Foreign bodies

Chronic: Postintubation stenosis (fibrosis, granulation tissue)
               Neoplasm (squamous cell carcinoma, adenoid cystic carcinoma)
               Vocal cord paralysis
               Hypertrophied tonsils and adenoids
               Macroglossia
               Micrognathia
               Obstructive sleep apnea

LOWER AIRWAY OBSTRUCTION

Acute: Infection (acute bronchiolitis)
               Edema (pulmonary venous hypertension, capillary leakage)
               Bronchospasm (asthma, anaphylactoid reactions)

Chronic: Chronic obstructive pulmonary disease
               Bronchiolitis
               Extensive idiopathic bronchiectasis
               Cystic fibrosis
               Familial dysautonomia

The chest roentgenogram is within normal limits in most cases of hypoventilation resulting from central nevous system disturbances or neuromuscular disease. In those instances in which hypoventilation is caused by respiratory muscle weakness or paralysis, the diaphragm is often elevated, but this finding is frequently ignored on the supposition that the chest roentgenogram was exposed at a position of incomplete inspiration. Although initially the chest roentgenogram may be normal in patients who hypoventilate, the complications and consequences of prolonged alveolar underventilation may become apparent over time. Patients who hypoventilate, particularly those with a raised diaphragm, are subject to atelectasis and pneumonia,[45] and in fact such complications may be responsible for bringing the primary disease to the attention of the physician. In severe, prolonged states of hypoventilation, cor pulmonale also may develop; this may be reflected in the chest roentgenogram by diminution of the peripheral vasculture and enlargement of the cardiac silhouette.

DISORDERS OF VENTILATORY CONTROL

Some basic knowledge of normal ventilatory control is required in order to comprehend the various disorders of this system that result in alveolar hypoventilation. The subject is extensively reviewed in Chapter 1 (*see* page 252), and the interested reader is also directed to excellent reviews in the literature.[46–49] The main components of central ventilatory control and the neurologic inputs and outputs from the central nervous system are only summarized here.

Central control of ventilation resides in two anatomically and functionally separate systems that subserve voluntary and automatic breathing. Neurons in the cerebral cortex control voluntary ventilation and can also influence brainstem output or can completely bypass it to accomplish behavior-related respiratory activities such as speech, defecation, micturition, and so on (Fig. 21–2). Automatic breathing originates from a highly complex accumulation of interconnected nerve cell groups situated in the brainstem. The most rostral of these centers is the pneumotaxic center (PNC) situated within the pons; it is believed to be responsible for the fine tuning of the respiratory pattern rather than the generation of primary respiratory rhythm. Caudal to the PNC near the pontomedullary border lies the apneustic center (APC), the site of projection of the various inputs that can terminate an inspiration. Damage to this area inactivates the inspiratory cutoff switch and results in the phenomenon of apneusis (prolonged respiratory pause at end inspiration). Transsection of the brainstem between the medulla and pons does not abolish respiratory rhythmicity, and it is the current view that the medulla alone is capable of generating a primary respiratory pattern and that the PNC and the APC are modulators of that primary pattern.

Within the medulla, respiratory neurons are grouped into two distinct areas, the dorsal respiratory group (DRG) consisting almost entirely of inspiratory cells and the ventral respiratory group (VRG) containing both inspiratory and expiratory cells. The DRG is the site of primary projection of numerous afferent fibers that constitute the afferent inputs into the respiratory center. These include afferents that originate in the upper airways, lungs, and peripheral chemoreceptors and travel in the cranial nerves, as well as afferents from the respiratory muscles themselves. It is thought that the DRG is the primary site of rhythm generation; the axons of cells from this area descend in the contra-

Table 21–2. *Nonpulmonary Causes of Respiratory Failure with Hypercapnia*

DISORDERS OF VENTILATORY CONTROL

CEREBRAL DYSFUNCTION

Infection (encephalitis), trauma, vascular accident
Status epilepticus
Narcotic and sedative overdose
Respiratory dyskinesia

RESPIRATORY CENTER DYSFUNCTION

Impaired brain stem controller
  Primary alveolar hypoventilation (Ondine's curse)
  Obesity hypoventilation syndrome
  Myxedema
  Metabolic alkalosis (compensatory)
  Sudden infant death syndrome
  Parkinson's syndrome
  Tetanus
Ablation of afferent and efferent spinal pathways:
  Bilateral high cervical cordotomy
  Cervical spinal cord trauma
  Transverse myelitis
  Multiple sclerosis
  Parkinson's disease

PERIPHERAL RECEPTOR DYSFUNCTION

Carotid body destruction (bilateral carotid endarterectomy and carotid body resection for asthma)
Bilateral damage to afferent nerves (Arnold-Chiari syndrome with syringomyelia)
  Familial dysautonomia
  Diabetic neuropathy
  Tetanus

DISORDERS OF THE RESPIRATORY PUMP

NEUROMUSCULAR DISEASE

Anterior horn cells
  Poliomyelitis
  Amyotrophic lateral sclerosis
Peripheral nerves
  Landry–Guillain-Barré syndrome
  Acute intermittent porphyria
  Toxic dinoflagellate poisoning
    Neurotoxic shellfish poisoning *(Ptychodiscus brevis)*
    Paralytic shellfish poisoning *(Protogonyaulyx cantenella* and *P. tamarensis)*
    Ciguatera fish poisoning *(Gambierdiscus toxicus)*
  Puffer fish poisoning (Tetrodotoxin)
Myoneural junction
  Myasthenia gravis
  Myasthenia-like syndromes (medications, particularly antibiotics, and associated neoplasm)
  Clostridium botulinum poisoning
Respiratory muscles
  Muscular dystrophies
  Acid maltase deficiency
  Nemaline myopathy
  Polymyositis
  Hypokalemia (in treatment of diabetes with insulin, renal tubular acidosis)
  Hypophosphatemia
  Hypermagnesemia
  Idiopathic rhabdomyolysis (myoglobinuria)

CHEST CAGE DISORDERS

Flail chest
Kyphoscoliosis
Thoracoplasty

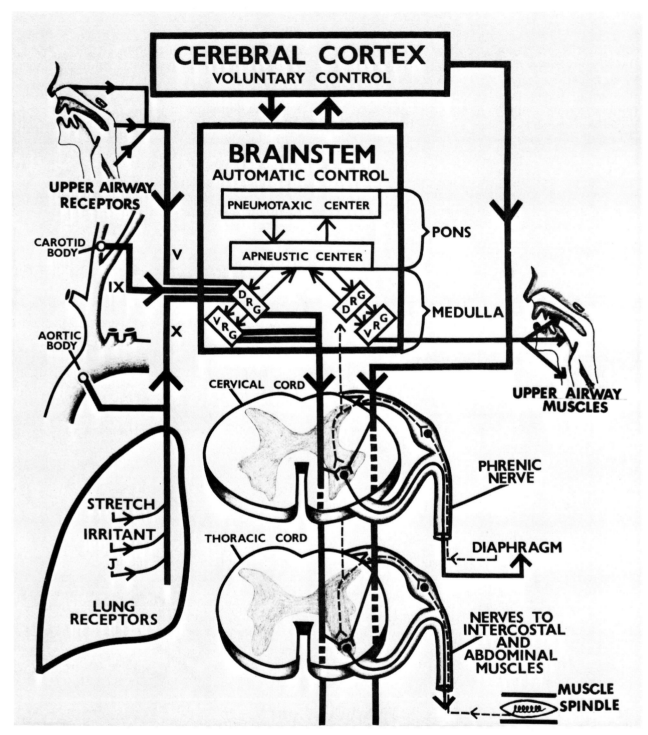

Figure 21–2. The Respiratory Control System. The central respiratory control is shared by voluntary (cerebral) and automatic (brainstem) centers. The efferent fibers from each run in distinct spinal cord pathways, as depicted on the left side of the coronally sectioned spinal cord (right side of drawing). A variety of interconnections exist between the cortex and the different components of the brainstem. Afferent fibers ascending the fifth (V), ninth (IX), and tenth (X) cranial nerves from upper airway receptors, peripheral chemoreceptors, and lung receptors connect with the ipsilateral dorsal respiratory group of neurons (DRG). In addition, afferents from Golgi tendon organs in the diaphragm and intercostal muscle spindles travel in the phrenic and intercostal nerves and reach the anterior horn cells as well as ascending to the DRG via the dorsal columns. Respiratory neurons in the DRG are connected with those in the ventral respiratory group (VRG) from which the descending neural output originates. The efferent fibers cross in the brainstem and supply the upper airway muscles via cranial nerves as well as descending in the cord to supply the diaphragm, intercostal, accessory, and expiratory muscles.

lateral spinal cord to innervate the diaphragm and inspiratory intercostals. The VRG does not appear to have primary respiratory rhythmicity or sensory input but receives input from the DRG and sends projections down the contralateral spinal cord to innervate the anterior horn cells of the cervical and thoracic cord; these in turn project to the intercostal inspiratory and expiratory muscles and the accessory muscles of inspiration. In addition, neurons from the DRG project to the lower motor neurons subserving the abdominal expiratory muscles and to the muscles of the larynx and upper airway that serve to maintain airway patency.

Sensory input, both chemical and neurogenic, plays a major role in the regulation of respiration. This originates in several sites including the peripheral chemoreceptors located in the carotid and aortic bodies, the central chemoreceptors that are believed to lie near the ventrolateral surface of the medulla, receptors situated in the upper airways and lungs, and the muscle spindles and tendon organs that are located in the respiratory muscles themselves.

The carotid and aortic bodies respond to increased arterial Pco_2 and decreased arterial Po_2. The pertinent stimulus for the central chemoreceptors is the hydrogen ion concentration of the brain's extracelluar fluid. The various respiratory tract and lung receptors that influence breathing have been discussed previously (see page 255). Briefly, receptors in the nose, oropharynx, larynx, and tracheobronchial tree can influence the intensity of respiratory center neural output and the timing of respiration. Tracheobronchial receptors are subclassified into irritant, stretch, and J-receptors. The main striated muscle receptors are Golgi tendon organs and muscle spindles. In the diaphragm there are abundant Golgi tendon organs but only rare muscle spindles, the latter being more frequent in intercostal and accessory muscles. Finally, it has been suggested that splanchnic receptors in abdominal organs can also influence respiratory control.[50]

Axons from the automatic (involuntary) controller in the brainstem descend in the ventro-lateral spinal white matter, whereas fibers involved in voluntary respiration originate in the cortex and travel separately in the dorsolateral columns of the spinal cord. Impulses from cortical and brainstem centers are integrated at the level of the spinal respiratory motor neurons in the anterior horns, the site of transmission of local spinal reflexes. Newsom Davis[51] has described a patient with partial transverse cervical myelitis and paralysis of limb and trunk muscles who possessed rhythmic respiratory movement but could not voluntarily alter his respiration. The converse of this situation, impaired automatic control with maintenance of normal voluntary breathing, can occur following bilateral cordotomy performed for the relief of pain. This procedure interrupts the spinothalamic tracts and results in ablation of respiratory axons, including those that both ascend and descend in the ventrolateral spinal cord. In the resulting syndrome (Ondine's curse) the patient breathes relatively normally during the day but experiences long periods of apnea at night when respiratory control is automatic (see farther on).

Various techniques have been devised to determine the output of the respiratory center (see page 439). These tests consist of the measurement of ventilatory responses to altered inspired oxygen and carbon dioxide tension, added inspiratory and expiratory loads, and exercise. Since a subject's lung mechanics can profoundly influence the ventilator response to these challenges, a measurement of mouth occlusion pressure (PO.1) has been used as a more specific estimate of respiratory drive. Ultimately, electromyographic or electroneurographic recordings of diaphragmatic and phrenic activation provide the most accurate assessment of the output of the respiratory center.

Disorders of the Central Nervous System

CEREBRAL DYSFUNCTION

Many disorders that affect cerebral function are associated with respiratory depression. In some, the depression is a direct effect of cerebral dysfunction while in others it is secondary to the effects on the brainstem of increased intracranial pressure. Narcotic, analgesic, and sedative agents in prescribed amounts frequently produce hypoventilation and respiratory failure in patients with underlying chronic pulmonary disease but only rarely in individuals with normal lungs; in the latter group, drug-induced hypoventilation usually occurs in adults following suicide attempts and in children following accidental ingestion. Drugs that result in respiratory depression in adults include the barbiturates,[52–55] glutethimide,[56] the phenothiazines and benzodiazepines,[54, 57–60] the tricyclic antidepressants,[57, 61] ethchlorvynol,[54, 62] diphenhydramine,[57, 63] and meprobamate.[54, 64]

Cerebral damage resulting from infection, trauma, or vascular accidents can cause hypoventilation that usually follows an initial period of hyperventilation. In many patients with these abnormalities, it is probable that increased intracranial pressure, caused at least partly by edema, plays a role in the hypoventilation. An unusual cerebrovascular cause of respiratory arrest is familial hemiplegic migraine; one case was reported in which deep microinfarcts were identified in the basal ganglia.[65]

Another group of conditions in which higher centers can influence respiration (but not necessarily cause respiratory depression) consists of the disorders associated with *respiratory dyskinesia*. Dyskinesia of the respiratory muscles is characterized by irregular contraction of inspiratory and expiratory muscles and simultaneous contraction of opposing muscles acting on the rib cage and upper airway. It occurs most often in patients with neuroleptic-induced tardive dyskinesia in association with a generalized choreiform movement disorder.[66–68] A polysomnographic study of one such patient disclosed a varying position of the rib cage and abdomen at end-expiration that indicated variable end-expiratory lung volume; grunting sounds appeared to be caused by simultaneous contraction of anterior abdominal wall muscles and partial closure of the laryngeal airway. During sleep, the respiratory pattern became normal, indicating that the origin of the impulses was in centers above the brainstem respiratory center.[69] A similar ventilatory dyskinesia has been reported in Rett's syndrome, a disorder found in girls that consists of autistic tendency, dementia, ataxia, and loss of purposeful hand movements.[70–73]

PRIMARY ALVEOLAR HYPOVENTILATION (ONDINE'S CURSE)

Alveolar hypoventilation that occurs predominantly as a result of an abnormality of central neurogenic control has been termed primary alveolar hypoventilation of the nonobese—Ondine's curse[74] or central sleep apnea.[75] It is a condition in which gas exchange and lung function are normal or almost so when the patient is awake and operating under voluntary ventilatory control, but in which respiratory failure and even death may ensue during sleep.[76, 77] The disorder can be caused by a specific congenital or hereditary defect in the respiratory center, or it can be acquired as a consequence of a variety of diseases that affect the central nervous system.

The characteristic physiologic feature of patients with Ondine's curse is a decrease in the sensitivity of the central nervous system to CO_2 that results in alveolar hypoventilation, especially during sleep. At least in some patients, a profound decrease in the ventilatory response to hypoxemia also has been seen.[78] Characteristically, these patients can voluntarily increase their ventilation and lower their PCO_2 to within the normal range. Since upper or lower airway obstruction and neuromuscular disorders first must be excluded before the diagnosis is acceptable, primary alveolar hypoventilation represents a diagnosis of exclusion. Suggested criteria for diagnosis include an arterial PCO_2 greater than 45, respiratory arrest or apnea during sleep, normal or near-normal tests of ventilatory capacity, and a marked decrease in the ventilatory response to CO_2.

Although in the vast majority of patients upper airway obstruction is the pathophysiologic mechanism of sleep apnea, it is important to recognize the occasional individuals in whom central neurogenic hypoventilation is the cause of the nocturnal apnea; the management of the two groups of patients is very different. In patients with primary alveolar hypoventilation, the apneic episodes are usually of shorter duration and are associated with less bradycardia than occurs in patients with obstruction. In addition, patients with primary alveolar hypoventilation complain more of insomnia and less of daytime hypersomnolence.[79]

As indicated, primary alveolar hypoventilation can be congenital or can present in adulthood. The congenital form becomes manifest within minutes or hours of birth in the form of cyanosis and respiratory acidosis that require prolonged mechanical ventilation.[80, 81] Two patients suffering from neonatal Ondine's curse have been reported in whom the level of the dopamine metabolite, homovanillic acid, in the cerebrospinal fluid was approximately 2.4 times higher than normal. It was unclear whether this represented a primary defect that induced the central hypoventilation or was a consequence of it. Beckerman and associates[82] described four infants with primary alveolar hypoventilation who also showed generalized hypotonia and hyporeflexia and abnormal brainstem-evoked potentials in response to auditory stimuli. Interestingly, this last abnormality also has been observed in an alcoholic patient with acquired Ondine's curse, presumably secondary to brainstem damage from excess alcohol.[83]

Familial forms of Ondine's curse also have been described.[84, 85] In one family, central apnea was associated with subacute necrotizing encephalomyopathy (Leigh's disease);[84] autopsy showed that lesions were confined to the respiratory center of the lower brainstem. Leigh's disease has been associated also with the development of primary alveolar hypoventilation in the adult.[86] In a second familial aggregation of patients with central sleep apnea, concomitant findings included anosmia, color blindness, seizures, and cognitive dysfunction.[85] Primary alveolar hypoventilation can also occur in association with Leber's disease, a sex-linked recessive disorder associated with hereditary optic atrophy.[87]

In adults, central neurogenic hypoventilation occurs equally as often in association with another primary disease as it does in an isolated fashion. Mellins and colleagues[76] reviewed 31 cases of "primary alveolar hypoventilation" and found that the syndrome was more common in men than in women in a ratio of five to one. The patients' ages ranged from 20 to 50 years and approximately 50 per cent had a history of prior central nervous system disease, usually encephalitis, Parkinson's disease, syringomyelia, or neurosyphilis; the other 50 per cent had no associated neurologic disorder.[76, 88, 89, 90–96] Alveolar hypoventilation during sleep and wakefulness is also a sequela of western equine encephalitis[97, 98] and has been reported following radiation therapy for midline cerebellar hemangioblastoma,[99] following high percutaneous cordotomy for relief of chronic pain,[100] and transiently after bilateral carotid endarterectomy.[101] In the latter two conditions, the apnea and hypoventilation are secondary to an interruption of afferent input into the respiratory center rather than to a disturbance of the respiratory center itself. Primary alveolar hypoventilation has been seen also in association with total colonic aganglionosis (Zuelzer-Wilson syndrome), a rare congenital form of gut immotility related to Hirschsprung's disease.[102]

There is a clinical spectrum of severity in patients with primary alveolar hypoventilation. Hypoventilation occurs only at night in some patients, and arterial blood gas tensions become normal during waking hours. The hypoventilation persists throughout the day in others; as expected, these patients have the worst prognosis.[103] Primary alveolar hypoventilation has been treated with nocturnal oxygen,[104, 105] respiratory stimulants,[104, 106] and phrenic nerve stimulation.[107–109] In some patients, nocturnal oxygen therapy decreases the frequency of apneas and increases nocturnal ventilation, suggesting that hypoxic depression of ventilation may occur.[104, 105, 110] In other patients, although nocturnal oxygen alleviates the hypoxemia, it also exacerbates hypercapnia; headache and lethargy can result.[111]

An unusual neurologic syndrome characterized by an abnormality of ventilatory control virtually opposite to primary alveolar hypoventilation has been described in three girls who showed a major abnormality of breathing pattern consisting of an irregular and inadequate minute ventilation during wakefulness but normal ventilation during sleep.[112]

OBESITY HYPOVENTILATION SYNDROME

The first description of the obesity hypoventilation syndrome probably can be ascribed to Felix Platter (1536–1614), who described a morbidly obese patient "who tended to fall asleep all the time: in the course of talking, even while eating."[113] A constellation of cyanosis, polycythemia, and obesity was described by Kerr and Lagen in 1936,[114] but it was not until 1956 that the syndrome became widely recognized after Burwell and his colleagues[115] designated it the "Pickwickian syndrome" because of the similar appearance and behavior of their patient to the fat boy Joe in the novel *Pickwick Papers* by Charles Dickens.

Although various mechanisms have been proposed to explain the hypoventilation in obese individuals, recent studies of breathing during sleep have allowed the separation of obese hypoventilators into those in whom the primary problem is obstructive sleep apnea and those in whom the problem appears to be primarily one of ventilatory control in the absence of nocturnal obstruction. Considerable confusion exists in the literature as to precisely what the term obesity hypoventilation syndrome means; we suggest that it be reserved for those individuals who hypoventilate but do not fit the criteria for obstructive sleep apnea. In some of these patients, there may be a primary hypothalamic defect that causes both obesity and hypoventilation. Alternatively, affected individuals may be those

whose ventilatory response to CO_2 and hypoxemia are at the low end of the wide normal range. When challenged by the increased work of breathing associated with obesity, these individuals may hypoventilate in much the same way that so-called blue bloaters hypoventilate when faced with the increased work of breathing associated with chronic obstructive pulmonary disease (COPD).[75]

The interrelationships among obesity, obstructive sleep apnea, and depressed central respiratory drive are complex.[116] Although it is likely that differences in central drive to breathe are responsible for the hypoventilation, there is some evidence that patients who hypoventilate have a lower thoracic compliance, an increased work of breathing, an increased VD/VT, and decreased respiratory muscle efficiency compared with equally obese subjects who do not hypoventilate.[117] Patients often have additional respiratory problems because of heavy smoking, asthma, or recurrent pulmonary emboli. In many, it is probable that the combination of cigarette smoke-induced abnormalities of airflow and ventilation-perfusion matching plus the mechanical effects of obesity cause respiratory failure. Obese smokers have significant hypoxemia; nocturnal ventilation is decreased even in normal subjects and such a decrease has a greater effect on arterial PO_2 in obese smokers, since they are on or close to the steep portion of the oxygen dissociation curve.

The term "Pickwickian syndrome" has outlived its usefulness;[118] it is now preferable to refer to patients as having obesity and obstructive sleep apnea or the obesity hypoventilation syndrome. As discussed in Chapter 11, obesity markedly increases the incidence of obstructive sleep apnea, probably because of narrowing of the oropharyngeal airway by increased fat deposition. In addition, obesity exerts profound effects on the static and dynamic mechanical properties of the respiratory system; by altering lung volumes, it influences ventilation-perfusion matching and arterial blood gas tensions.

Despite the foregoing, the vast majority of patients with morbid obesity do not suffer from obstructive sleep apnea or the obesity hypoventilation syndrome. Sugerman and colleagues[119] found that only 12 per cent of their patients who were undergoing gastric surgery for morbid obesity had ventilatory respiratory failure. They considered that one third of these patients had obesity hypoventilation syndrome alone, one third had obstructive sleep apnea alone, and the final third had a combination of the two conditions. In another study of 200 morbidly obese men whose average weight was 144 kg, only 8 were considered to fulfill the criteria for "Pickwickian syndrome."[120]

MYXEDEMA

Although a decrease in central neurogenic drive to breathe can be a contributing factor in the hypoventilation sometimes observed in patients with myxedema,[121, 122] other factors are also involved in some individuals. Obstructive sleep apnea[123, 124] is not uncommon in patients with myxedema and is possibly caused by narrowing of the upper airway by macroglossia secondary to deposition of mucopolysaccharides in the pharynx and tongue.[121] Patients with hypothyroidism also demonstrate significant respiratory muscle weakness that improves following thyroid replacement therapy.[122]

Coma is not uncommon in patients with myxedema and usually occurs in elderly, obese women.[125, 126] In a survey of 77 patients, Forester[125] found 60 to be female and nearly half to be in their seventh decade; hypoventilation appeared to be responsible for coma in one third of the cases. Since most patients are obese, it has been suggested that the hypoventilation may be a consequence of the obesity *per se*. However, this conclusion was not supported by the findings of Massumi and Winnacker[127] or of Domm and Vassalo[128] whose patients had blood gas values that returned to normal on thyroid therapy despite little or no change in body weight.

METABOLIC ALKALOSIS

Another form of central respiratory depression that results in hypoventilation is caused by metabolic alkalosis. We have seen several patients in whom repeated episodes of vomiting, due either to psychological or organic causes, were associated with hypoxemia, carbon dioxide retention, and an increase in serum bicarbonate. This combination also has been reported following gastric resection in a patient with gastrointestinal hemorrhage.[129] These changes appear to represent compensatory mechanisms that permit a rise in serum bicarbonate, thereby enabling the acid-base balance to return toward normal.

SUDDEN INFANT DEATH SYNDROME

Sudden infant death syndrome (SIDS) occurs in about 2 per 100,000 children in the United States. Death usually occurs at night during sleep in male children and during the winter months.[130] Although there is a familial aggregation, there is no clear mendelian inheritance.

Considerable evidence has accumulated recently to suggest that disturbed regulation of ventilation may be responsible for at least some cases of sudden death in infants. Much of this evidence has come from studies of infants who are considered to have had "near misses." These patients show an abnormal breathing pattern characterized by an excessive number of episodes of apnea that may be both central and obstructive; in addition, some infants hypoventilate at rest and show decreased ventilatory responses to hypoxia and hypercapnia.[131] Parents of infants who die of SIDS demonstrate decreased ventilatory responses to CO_2 and

hypoxemia as well as decreased PO.1 responses to added loads.[132, 133] However, in one study[134] the acute response to hypercapnia was normal in 68 parents of SIDS victims.[134] Similarly, in a comparative study of 12 parents of six infants who died of SIDS and 12 age- and weight-matched control subjects,[135] no difference was observed in the incidence of apnea or sleep-disordered breathing.

The basis for the hypothesized disturbance in ventilatory regulation in individuals with SIDS is unclear. Pathologic examination of the brains of infants who have died of the condition has demonstrated glial abnormalities around the brainstem nuclei.[130] The finding of a marked increase in the incidence of SIDS in infants whose mothers use methadone suggests that an alteration in endogenous opiates may also play a role. In a study by Myer and associates,[136] 21 infants at risk for SIDS (by virtue of "near misses," proved apnea, or sibship to patients with SIDS) demonstrated significantly higher CSF beta-endorphin levels than 22 control subjects.

PARKINSON'S SYNDROME

Patients with Parkinson's syndrome can suffer respiratory insufficiency for several reasons.[137, 138] In some individuals, the hypoventilation and hypoxemia appear to be related to central hypoventilation.[139, 140] A familial syndrome also has been described[141] in which patients present with mental depression that progresses to Parkinson's syndrome and primary alveolar hypoventilation. Apps and associates[142] have investigated respiration during sleep in patients with Parkinson's syndrome: they found that those with classic idiopathic Parkinson's disease had little abnormality when compared with an age- and sex-matched control group, whereas those in whom the parkinsonism was associated with autonomic disturbance demonstrated disorganized respiration and frequent episodes of central and obstructive apnea. However, before ascribing ventilatory respiratory failure to brainstem depression in patients with Parkinson's syndrome, it is important to remember that the respiratory muscles may be involved in this condition. Patients demonstrate decreased maximal expiratory flow and oscillatory fluctuations in expiratory flow that are believed to be related to tremor involving the upper airway[143] and expiratory muscles.[144] In one study,[145] pulmonary function tests suggested that subclinical upper airway obstruction and decreased effective muscle strength were responsible for pulmonary insufficiency in a significant number of patients with Parkinson's disease.

Respiratory failure in Parkinson's disease can be caused also by intrinsic pulmonary disease such as aspiration pneumonia and atelectasis, both of which are not infrequent complications in this condition. In a comprehensive pulmonary function study of 31 patients with Parkinson's disease,[146] obstructive ventilatory defects were identified in one third of the patients. Those with obstruction had a history of chronic bronchitis and showed no functional improvement following therapy with 3,4-dihydroxyphenylalanine (L-dopa); however, since significant neurologic improvement was observed, it was concluded that the impairment of pulmonary function was not the result of the Parkinson's disease *per se*. In a similar study of 10 patients,[147] a significant increase in maximal voluntary ventilation was observed following treatment with L-dopa, although there was no direct correlation between clinical and pulmonary functional improvement.

TETANUS

The mechanism of the ventilatory respiratory failure that can accompany tetanus is unclear, although it is probable that the severe, prolonged spasm of the respiratory musculature causes inadequate ventilation in these patients.[148] Tetanus toxin has been shown to cause blockade of inhibitory synapses at both the cortical[149, 150] and spinal cord[151] levels. Tetanus is frequently associated with symptoms and signs of autonomic dysfunction, including hypertension, tachycardia, bradycardia, cardiac arrhythmias, profuse sweating, pyrexia, increased urinary catecholamine excretion, and, in some cases, the development of hypotension indicating that parasympathetic and sympathetic fibers may be affected.[152, 153] Therefore, it is possible that involvement of the afferent inputs to the respiratory center contributes to the respiratory failure. However, the remarkable improvement that occurs in patients with severe tetanus following the administration of muscle-paralyzing agents and the institution of artificial ventilation[148, 154-156] indicates that respiratory failure due to ventilatory muscle dysfunction plays a significant role in this disease. In one study a case fatality rate of 44 per cent was reduced to 15 per cent following establishment of an intensive care unit in which all patients were treated with paralysis and assisted ventilation. In another study of 100 patients with tetanus who were admitted to an intensive care unit, the disease was sufficiently severe to require paralysis and assisted ventilation in 90.[157]

Tetanus is now more often found in developing countries where hygiene is poor and there is increased likelihood of wound contamination on bare feet by animal feces containing *Clostridium tetani*.[158, 159] In the United States, the incidence has decreased considerably;[160] however, in certain large cities such as New York where drug addiction is a major problem, the disease has undergone a resurgence. Puncture wounds and lacerations acquired on the farm or in the garden are common sites of infection, although ulcers due to pressure (decubitus ulcers), venous stasis, and frostbite, tumors, and dental abscesses[160] can also serve as nidi; even an aspirated foreign body has been incriminated.[161] A

common cause of death is cardiac arrest, tending to occur during the second or third week of the illness, that can be caused by either increased catecholamine secretion or respiratory failure secondary to toxin-induced myopathy.[162] Patients with mild tetanus experience trismus (inability to open the mouth) and hypertonicity of the chest wall and abdominal muscles; those with moderate and severe disease also have tetanic spasms. Even patients with mild disease manifest hypoxemia and hyperventilation associated with metabolic acidosis and a restrictive pattern of pulmonary function.[163, 164]

Disorders of the Spinal Cord

Lesions of the cervical and thoracic spinal cord can interfere with both afferent and efferent spinal pathways to and from the respiratory center. An appreciation of the various syndromes that result from spinal cord damage is aided by knowledge of the spinal levels from which innervation of the various respiratory muscles originates. The diaphragm is innervated by the nerve roots from C-3 to C-5, which join to form the phrenic nerve, whereas parasternal and lateral external intercostal muscles are innervated by the nerve roots from T-1 to T-12 via the intercostal nerves. Of the accessory muscles, the scalenes are innervated by nerve roots from C-4 to C-8, while the sternocleidomastoid is innervated by cranial nerve 11 and the cervical nerve roots C-1 and C-2. The expiratory muscles consist of the lateral internal intercostal muscles, which derive innervation from T-1 to T-12 via the intercostal nerves, and the rectus abdominis, external and internal obliques, and transversus abdominis, which are innervated by lumbar nerves originating from nerve roots T-7 to L-1.

Patients who suffer spinal cord injury at the level of C-5 or lower have preserved diaphragmatic function but paralyzed intercostal muscles. In these circumstances, diaphragmatic contraction during inspiration results in exaggerated protrusion of the abdomen and indrawing of the sternum and lower ribs; on expiration the diaphragm relaxes and ascends, with the abdomen flattening and the lower chest expanding as a result of the elasticity of the rib cage.[165] This pattern, termed chest wall paradox, tends to decrease with time following the development of quadriplegia, presumably because the denervated intercostal muscles develop spasticity. As a result, pulmonary function tends to improve during the period of 6 to 12 months after the injury.[153] Ledsome and Sharp[166] made serial measurements of lung volumes at 1, 3, and 5 weeks and at 3 and 5 months after spinal cord injury. They found that patients whose lesions were at the C-5 to C-6 level showed initial reductions in vital capacity to 30 per cent of predicted, although over the ensuing 3 months this doubled to 60 per cent; patients with lesions at levels C-4 and higher showed greater decreases in vital capacity. The investigators[166] found that patients whose vital capacity was 25 per cent of predicted or less tended to develop hypercapnia, whereas hypoxemia was common even in the absence of hypercapnia, presumably as a result of the patients' inability to take deep breaths and reverse microatelectasis.

Although hypoventilation following spinal cord injury is caused mainly by inspiratory muscle dysfunction, involvement of expiratory muscles is of great clinical significance as well since it interferes with effective clearance of pulmonary secretions. This was illustrated in one retrospective study in which 9 of 22 patients with high cervical cord lesions died; in the same study, of 22 patients who were followed prospectively and in whom careful attention was given to tracheal toilet and the need for mechanical ventilation, none of the patients died.[167]

Although there is little doubt that the majority of patients die when cervical cord lesions are above the origin of the phrenic motor neurons, a case has been described[168] of a quadriplegic patient with a spinal cord lesion at the C-2 to C-3 level whose breathing was totally dependent on neck muscles supplied by the upper two spinal nerves and the 11th cranial nerve. He employed "glossopharyngeal breathing," a repetitive maneuver consisting of coordinated movements of the tongue, cheeks, and soft palate to pump a bolus of air into the lungs, using the glottis as a one-way check valve. This form of breathing resulted in a three-fold increase in vital capacity.

As indicated above, cervical cordotomy can interfere with respiratory control and result in sleep-induced apnea and even sudden death. This surgical procedure, used to relieve intractable pain, is accomplished by inserting a stainless steel needle electrode into the ventral quadrant of the cervical spinal cord and applying a radiofrequency current to the electrode. Lesions produced in this way are permanent, and in some cases both afferent and efferent respiratory axons are severed. The result is a reduction in vital capacity, maximal breathing capacity, minute ventilation, and tidal volume, particularly if the operation is bilateral. Although such findings can be attributed to section of efferent pathways to the phrenic nerve nuclei, there is evidence that respiratory control mechanisms are also disturbed, probably as a result of ablation of reticular formation spinal tracts.[169] The major clinical manifestations consist of hypoventilation, diminished CO_2 response, and irregular breathing. In two patients, bilateral cervical cordotomy resulted in sleep-induced apnea and oxygen-induced sudden death.[170] Of 100 patients on whom bilateral percutaneous cervical cordotomy was performed for intractable pain associated with malignant disease, relief of pain was complete in 64 patients; however, 6 patients died as a result of postoperative respiratory dysfunction.[171] A similar physiologic dysfunction has been described in patients with multiple sclerosis, presumably caused by destruction of cer-

vical spinal pathways[172] or midline ventral medullary lesions.[173] Unilateral cervical spinal cord injury can result in hemiplegia and unilateral chest wall paradoxical motion that mimics a flail chest.[174]

Disorders of the Peripheral Chemoreceptors

In humans, peripheral chemoreceptors that are situated chiefly in the carotid bodies account for virtually all the hypoxic drive.[175] Bilateral carotid endarterectomy[176] or removal of both carotid bodies, a "therapeutic procedure" that has been advocated (without proven benefit) for relief of bronchial asthma,[177, 178] can abolish compensatory hyperventilation when patients become hypoxemic. Bilateral (not unilateral) carotid body resection causes a decreased ventilatory response to exercise.[179] Sleep apnea has been reported as a complication following bilateral excision of carotid body tumors.[180]

The syndromes of autonomic dysfunction represent a heterogeneous group of congenital and acquired disorders usually characterized by orthostatic hypotension, hypohidrosis, a relatively fixed heart rate, and bladder and sexual dysfunctions.[181] In patients with such syndromes there may be abnormalities of peripheral chemoreceptor and mechanoreceptor input to the respiratory center resulting in respiratory difficulty. For example, in one large review, 5 per cent of 297 patients with autonomic dysfunction had a history of respiratory arrest.[181] Children with familial dysautonomia (Riley-Day syndrome) are relatively unresponsive to hypoxia and hypercapnia:[182, 183] in a study of 210 children with this syndrome, Brunt and McKusick[184] found 66 per cent to have "breathholding attacks." The breathing of hypoxic mixtures by patients with familial dysautonomia results in a dramatic fall in arterial oxygen saturation. Some workers consider this lack of ventilatory response to hypoxia to be the result of a defect in the carotid body.[182] Others have observed a fleeting hyperventilation followed by profound hypoxia,[185] a phenomenon they attributed to an inordinate central depression consequent upon reduced cerebral blood flow. Unlike normal subjects, patients with dysautonomia become hypotensive while hypoxic.

Diabetics with severe autonomic neuropathy have been reported to have unexplained cardiac arrest that appears to be primarily respiratory in origin.[186, 187] Since this complication occurs following anesthesia, bronchopneumonia, or the administration of depressant drugs, the sequence of events has suggested the possibility that the chemoreceptors are unable to respond to hypoxia.[186] A number of studies have demonstrated depressed ventilatory responses to hypoxia and hypercapnia in diabetic patients, especially those with autonomic neuropathy.[188, 189] Despite these findings, a comparative study of eight diabetic patients with severe autonomic neuropathy and eight age-matched diabetic patients without neuropathy disclosed no increase in the incidence of sleep-disordered breathing or apnea in the former.[190]

Patients with Arnold-Chiari malformation and syringomyelia have been described in whom central respiratory failure was presumably caused by destruction of afferent pathways in the ninth cranial nerve.[191, 192] As discussed above, tetanus toxin has been shown to cause a blockade of inhibitory synapses at both the cortical[149, 150] and spinal cord levels.[151] It is frequently associated with evidence of autonomic dysfunction; this suggests that interference with afferent input to the respiratory center may be a contributing factor to the respiratory depression in this complex disorder.

A patient whose unusual illness may represent a unique disorder of respiratory control has been described by Bradley and associates:[72] an elderly man presented with chronic ventilatory defect. Although ventilatory responses to carbon dioxide were normal, he developed marked hypoventilation associated with rapid shallow breathing during sleep; the hypoventilation was unassociated with obstructive apnea. The abnormal nocturnal ventilatory pattern was corrected by diaphragmatic pacing.

DISORDERS OF THE RESPIRATORY PUMP

For descriptive purposes, it is useful, although somewhat arbitrary, to visualize the central ventilatory control as terminating in the anterior horn cells where impulses that serve voluntary and automatic stimulation of breathing are integrated with spinal reflexes. Thus, for the purposes of this text the respiratory pump includes not only the rib cage and muscles of respiration but also their electrical connections. Disturbances of the respiratory pump can result from disease of the anterior horn cells, the phrenic and intercostal nerves, the myoneuronal junctions, or the respiratory muscles themselves.

The respiratory muscles are divided into three distinct groups that have different mechanisms of action—the diaphragm, the intercostal and accessory muscles, and the abdominal muscles.[193, 194] Although these muscles are involved in both inspiration and expiration, only dysfunction of the inspiratory muscles causes significant ventilatory impairment. Expiration is largely passive, and expiratory flow limitation results from alteration in the mechanical properties of the lungs rather than from muscle failure. However, since the expiratory muscles are important for the generation of an effective cough, and an inadequate cough can result in retained secretions and pulmonary infection, expiratory muscle dysfunction can exacerbate respiratory failure in patients with neuromuscular disease.

Respiratory muscles differ from other skeletal muscles in several respects: (1) they function continuously for a lifetime; (2) they are under both automatic and voluntary control; and (3) unlike most other skeletal muscles that must overcome inertial loads, the respiratory muscles cope primarily with elastic and resistive loads. The diaphragm is the principal muscle of inspiration. It probably acts alone during quiet breathing, the intercostal and accessory muscles being recruited only when the demand for ventilation increases.[195] The abdominal muscles play an important role in augmenting ventilation when exertion increases oxygen requirements; contraction during expiration displaces the abdominal contents inwards and upwards, lengthens the diaphragmatic muscle, and decreases its radius, and thus improves the efficiency of the diaphragm as a pressure generator on the subsequent inspiration.[193]

It is not necessary that respiratory muscle weakness be profound to provoke symptoms and signs. Disability from weakened respiratory muscles can be accentuated or precipitated by an increased load on the respiratory system, such as that occasioned by exercise or concomitant COPD. Respiratory muscles, like other skeletal muscles, may become fatigued. The mechanical aspects of respiratory muscle contraction and the factors that can cause their fatigue are discussed in some detail in Volume I (see pages 268 and 270). However, since fatigue is probably the final common pathway causing respiratory failure in patients with neuromuscular and chest wall abnormalities, a brief review of respiratory muscle fatigue is warranted.

Respiratory Muscle Fatigue

Muscle fatigue is defined as the inability of a muscle to generate a predetermined force continuously. For the inspiratory muscles, force is assessed by measuring pressure generation, either maximal inspiratory pressure at the mouth that gives an overall estimate of inspiratory muscle strength or transdiaphragmatic pressure that provides a specific estimate of the force generated by the diaphragm. Respiratory muscle fatigue can be either central or peripheral. *Central fatigue* is characterized by a diminution in force generation that is greater during voluntary effort than during electrical stimulation. *Peripheral fatigue* is characterized by decreased force generation despite maximal stimulation and can be separated into high- and low-frequency fatigue. High-frequency fatigue is a loss of force-generating ability at very high stimulation frequencies and is thought to be caused by impaired neuromuscular transmission; it is distinguished by a decrease in amplitude of electromyographically recorded muscle action potential. Low-frequency fatigue is a loss of force generation at low stimulation frequencies; it is thought to be caused by impaired excitation contraction coupling and is not associated with a decrease in the size of the action potential. High-frequency fatigue is reversible within minutes, but the low-frequency variety can persist for hours or days. Factors that may be responsible for fatigue include a depletion of nutrient stores in the muscle, the accumulation of metabolic end products that inhibit or reduce muscular contraction, and actual damage to respiratory muscle fibers.

Ultimately, respiratory muscles fatigue when an imbalance exists between the energy demand of the contracting muscle and the energy supply. Adenosine triphosphate (ATP) is the basic fuel for muscular contraction. The factors that determine the energy demand on a respiratory muscle are the work of breathing and the strength and endurance of the muscle; the strength is in turn affected by the length-tension relationship. As with all skeletal muscles, respiratory muscles display distinct length-tension behavior. There is a specific muscle length at which the overlap between actin and myosin filaments is optimal for the generation of pressure. When contracting at this length, the muscle is most efficient in terms of tension generation for a given consumption of ATP. At lengths shorter or longer than optimal length, less tension can be generated despite similar activation and fuel consumption. Chronically, the respiratory muscles can adapt so that optimal length occurs within the operating range of the muscle, but any factor that acutely alters the resting length (such as hyperinflation) will have a profound effect on efficiency. Respiratory muscle strength is also decreased in patients with neuromuscular disease and in those who are malnourished. Malnutrition causes a depletion of energy stores and can result in atrophy of muscle fibers. Respiratory muscles require oxygen and substrate to generate ATP. Oxygen transport is directly related to blood flow and to the oxygen content of the arterial blood; substrate is derived from circulating glucose and free fatty acids and from substrate stores, largely in the form of glycogen.

Respiratory muscles will inevitably fatigue when they are forced to continuously generate greater than 40 to 50 per cent of the maximal pressure of which they are capable.[196–198] The development of respiratory muscle fatigue in response to a load can be predicted if one knows the pressure generated by the muscle as a percentage of the maximal capacity of that muscle and the fraction of the total respiratory cycle time devoted to inspiratory muscle effort. Bellemare and Grassino[199, 200] have shown that this can be best calculated as the "tension-time" index. For example, the tension-time index of the diaphragm (TTdi) is calculated by multiplying the ratio of the mean transdiaphragmatic pressure during inspiration (ΔPdi) over the maximal transdiaphragmatic pressure achieved with voluntary contraction (Pdi Max) by the respiratory duty cycle expressed as the inspiratory time (TI) divided by the total respiratory cycle time (T_{Tot}):

$$TTdi = \frac{\Delta Pdi}{Pdi\ Max} \times \frac{TI}{T_{Tot}}$$

When the tension-time index exceeds 0.15 for an appreciable length of time, respiratory muscle fatigue will inevitably occur. Examination of this relationship illustrates that respiratory muscle fatigue is more likely to occur in the following three situations: (1) when ΔPdi is increased as a result of an increase in the work of breathing, (2) when Pdi Max is decreased secondary to any of the disorders discussed below that result in respiratory muscle weakness, or (3) when both factors are operative. Respiratory muscle fatigability is increased in the presence of respiratory acidosis[201] and hypoxemia.[202]

Although the diagnosis of respiratory muscle fatigue is ultimately made on the basis of a failure of pressure generation, a number of investigators have recommended the use of tests to predict the eventual development of fatigue prior to a decline in force generation. For example, examination of the frequency spectrum of the diaphragmatic or intercostal muscle electromyogram (EMG) signal shows a characteristic decrease in the ratio of high-to-low frequency impulses even before mechanical fatigue can be demonstrated;[203, 204] such a pattern can be detected using either esophageal or surface EMG signals.[205] A more practical approach to predicting fatigue is the measurement of the relaxation rate of respiratory muscles following contraction: fatiguing skeletal muscle shows delayed relaxation, and measurement of the rate of decline in the transdiaphragmatic pressure[206] or mouth pressure[207] (or both) has been shown to predict fatigue.

Clinical Features of Respiratory Muscle Weakness

Respiratory muscle weakness can be suspected from the clinical history and physical examination as well as from characteristic abnormalities on pulmonary function testing. In addition, there are specific tests to assess respiratory muscle strength and endurance and to delineate whether the abnormality is primarily neural or muscular.

Patients with respiratory failure secondary to neuromuscular abnormalities complain of anxiety, lethargy, headache, dyspnea, and sometimes a feeling of suffocation. When ventilation is severely restricted, confusion, coma, and death can ensue rapidly. Cyanosis may or may not be present depending upon the degree of hypoventilation. It is important to remember that, in the presence of a normal hemoglobin concentration, hypoxemia can be detected clinically by a change in color of the nail beds and mucous membranes only when arterial oxygen saturation has dropped to 80 per cent or less. Similarly, appreciation of the degree of alveolar ventilation clinically is unreliable except when apnea has occurred,[208] by which time the patient will be severely cyanotic.

Since the diaphragm is the principal muscle of inspiration, evidence on physical examination of diaphragmatic weakness or paralysis is important in establishing a neuromuscular cause for respiratory failure. When it contracts, the diaphragm not only pushes down on the abdominal viscera and displaces the abdominal wall outward, but it also lifts and expands the rib cage. This latter action results in an increase in the diameter of the chest in both its anteroposterior and lateral axes and is dependent on the acute angle of insertion of diaphragmatic muscle fibers into the ribs. The degree of thoracic expansion depends on the abdominal pressure: if the abdominal muscles are contracted, descent of the diaphragm is restricted and rib cage movement accentuated. At the end of a quiet expiration, the diaphragm is relaxed; pleural pressure and abdominal pressure are almost equal. On inspiration, intrapleural pressure becomes more negative and abdominal pressure more positive; a transdiaphragmatic pressure difference develops (ΔPdi). When the abdominal muscles are relaxed, this increase in intra-abdominal pressure causes the abdominal wall to protrude (Fig. 21–3).

When one hemidiaphragm is paralyzed or weakened, its movement is paradoxical (Fig. 21–4). The development of negative intrapleural pressure secondary to rib cage expansion and the normal descent of the nonparalyzed hemidiaphragm "suck" the paralyzed hemidiaphragm into the thoracic cavity. Although the resulting inward motion of the anterior abdominal wall on the paralyzed side can be detected clinically, paradoxical motion is much more apparent on fluoroscopic examination: on inspiration the paralyzed hemidiaphragm moves upward coincident with expansion of the rib cage and descent of the normal hemidiaphragm, a motion that can be appreciated to better advantage during sniffing.

When both hemidiaphragms are paralyzed, as in bilateral phrenic nerve palsy or when a neuropathic or myopathic disorder causes bilateral diaphragmatic weakness, abdominal paradox is more apparent clinically. With each inspiratory effort of the external intercostal and accessory muscles of respiration, the rib cage expands, which lowers intrapleural pressure and "sucks" the diaphragm into the thorax—a most inefficient form of breathing (Fig. 21–5 A–D). This upward movement of the diaphragm results in an equal reduction of both abdominal and pleural pressures, so that the transdiaphragmatic pressure difference remains zero. The fall in abdominal pressure induces indrawing of the abdominal wall that is readily apparent clinically. In patients who have incipient diaphragmatic fatigue, abdominal paradox can develop during or after a period of increased respiratory muscle activity, for example, when they are being "weaned" from ventilatory support.

The recruitment of abdominal expiratory muscles can mask paradoxical breathing and diaphragmatic weakness.[209] During expiration the abdominal wall muscles contract and force the flaccid diaphragm into the thoracic cavity; at the onset of inspiration the sudden relaxation of these muscles causes rapid diaphragmatic descent and apparent outward movement of the abdomen (Fig. 21–5E, F). Recruitment of expiratory abdominal muscles during tidal breathing can be detected by palpation of the anterior abdominal wall. Abdominal muscle contraction can restore an apparently normal pattern of movement to the anterior abdominal wall (Fig. 21–5 G–J). This pattern of expiratory muscle recruitment may be responsible for the false-negative results of fluoroscopic examination of the diaphragm in some patients with bilateral diaphragmatic paralysis or weakness.[210]

Routine pulmonary function tests may suggest the possibility of respiratory neuromuscular disease. When the lung parenchyma is normal and patient cooperation is complete, a decrease in total lung capacity or an increase in residual volume (thus a decrease in vital capacity) may indicate respiratory muscle weakness.[193] When vital capacity is reduced to 25 per cent or less of that predicted, ventilatory failure is either present or imminent.[211] Flow rates may also reflect neurogenic or myopathic disorders. Most laboratories include flow-time or flow-volume curves as screening procedures: since expiratory flow early in the forced expiratory maneuver is effort-dependent and late flow is effort-independent, a disproportionate decrease in flow in the first part of the forced expiratory vital capacity breath suggests a neuromuscular defect.[212] Thus, a disproportionate reduction in FEV_1 compared to FEF_{25-75} can suggest respiratory muscle weakness; it should be remembered, however, that upper airway obstruction can produce a similar pattern (see page 1980). Abnormalities of arterial blood gas tensions are late findings in patients with primary neuromuscular disease. Initially, patients may hyperventilate,[211] but hyperventilation is inevitably succeeded by hypoventilation as the disease progresses. However, even severe hypoxemia and hypercapnia can be corrected in these patients by voluntary hyperventilation; this is a clear indication that measurements of static and dynamic lung volumes (i.e., flows and pressures that require maximal effort and hence cerebral cortical input) may not truly reflect the degree of dysfunction.

In patients with severe weakness or complete paralysis of the diaphragm, assumption of the supine posture causes further deterioration in gas exchange. The explanation for this lies in a change of gravitational forces. The weight of the abdominal organs displaces the flaccid diaphragm upward into the thoracic cavity, thus further reducing the effectiveness of the remaining inspiratory muscles.[213–215] In addition, a further drop in PaO_2 and a rise in $PaCO_2$ often occur during sleep when breathing control is solely automatic.[215]

Impedance plethysmography or magnetometry measures the anteroposterior and lateral dimensions of the rib cage and abdomen simultaneously and separately during the respiratory cycle. Either

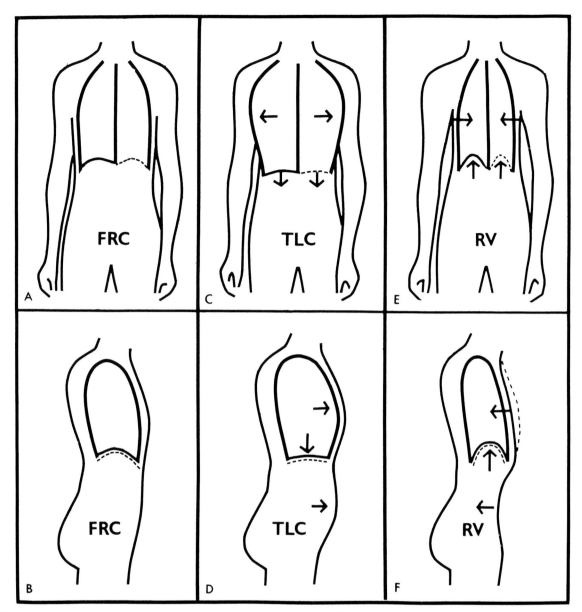

Figure 21–3. Schematic Depiction of Chest Cage and Diaphragmatic Movements Throughout the Respiratory Cycle: Normal. Anteroposterior (*A*) and lateral (*B*) views show the position of the chest wall and diaphragm at resting lung volume (FRC). At full inspiration (*C* and *D*), the diaphragm contracts with resultant expansion of the chest cage, increase in intra-abdominal pressure, and a consequent protrusion of the abdominal wall. At full expiration (*E* and *F*), abdominal muscle contraction causes a rise in intra-abdominal pressure and elevation of the relaxed diaphragm. FRC = functional residual capacity; TLC = total lung capacity; RV = residual volume.

method can be useful in documenting diaphragmatic weakness and paralysis. Normally on inspiration, volume increases in both the abdominal and rib cage compartments. When the diaphragm is nonfunctioning or weak, the diameter of the thorax increases, while that of the abdomen decreases during inspiration.[216]

The measurement of maximal inspiratory and expiratory pressures provides useful indices of respiratory muscle strength; although this is a simple test, its performance requires patient cooperation. There is a wide variation in inspiratory and expiratory pressures among normal subjects, but in any given subject measurement is reasonably reproduc-

ible. Serial measurements of inspiratory and expiratory pressures are useful means of recognizing the development of respiratory muscle weakness or fatigue and of documenting recovery of respiratory muscle strength.[217] Measurement of the pressure-volume curve of the lung may suggest respiratory muscle weakness when lung volumes and pulmonary compliance are decreased, despite a normal or low maximal elastic recoil pressure.[218]

Perhaps the most specific method of identifying weakness or paralysis of the diaphragm is measurement of transdiaphragmatic pressures (Pdi). This is accomplished by recording pressures in balloons placed in both the esophagus (reflecting pleural

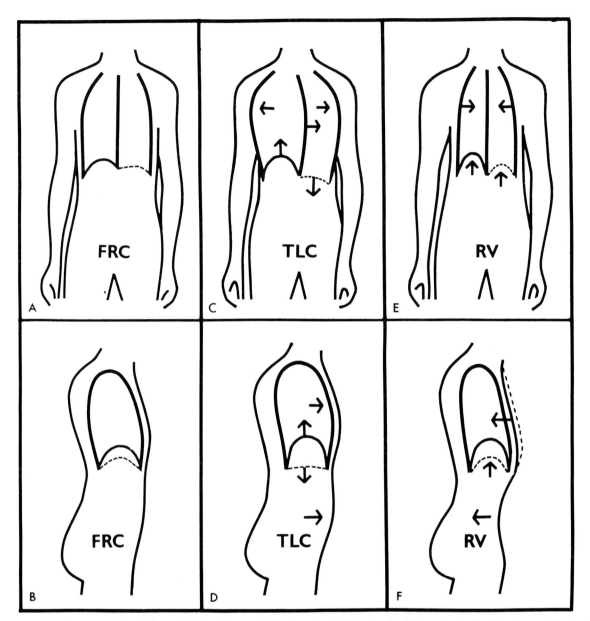

Figure 21–4. Schematic Depiction of Chest Cage and Diaphragmatic Movements Throughout the Respiratory Cycle: Right Hemidiaphragmatic Paralysis. At FRC (*A* and *B*), the right hemidiaphragm is elevated. On full inspiration to TLC (*C* and *D*), the left hemidiaphragm contracts and descends, whereas the flaccid right hemidiaphragm passively elevates in response to the more negative intrapleural pressure. On full expiration to RV (*E* and *F*), a rise in intra-abdominal pressure evokes an even greater elevation of the paralyzed right hemidiaphragm.

pressure) and the stomach (reflecting abdominal pressure). As with maximal inspiratory and expiratory pressures, there is a wide range of normal values, but those below 60 cm H$_2$O are indicative of diaphragmatic weakness. In the presence of complete diaphragmatic paralysis, Pdi does not change during maximal inspiratory effort against a closed airway or during full inspiration. As discussed in Chapter 20 (*see* page 2927), phrenic nerve function can be measured by recording the diaphragmatic muscle action potential with either esophageal[219] or surface[220] electrodes following transcutaneous stimulation of the phrenic nerve in the neck. A positive response in the presence of documented diaphrag-

matic paralysis indicates that the disorder is myopathic rather than neuropathic.[193]

Disorders of the Anterior Horn Cells

A variety of disorders of the anterior horn cells that subserve the respiratory muscles can result in acute or chronic respiratory failure. Although *poliomyelitis* associated with respiratory failure has been almost eradicated in the western world by immunization, occasional cases are still seen and affected patients can develop unexpected life-threatening hypoventilation.[221] Some patients with poliomyelitis develop a state of chronic hypoventilation[222–224] that

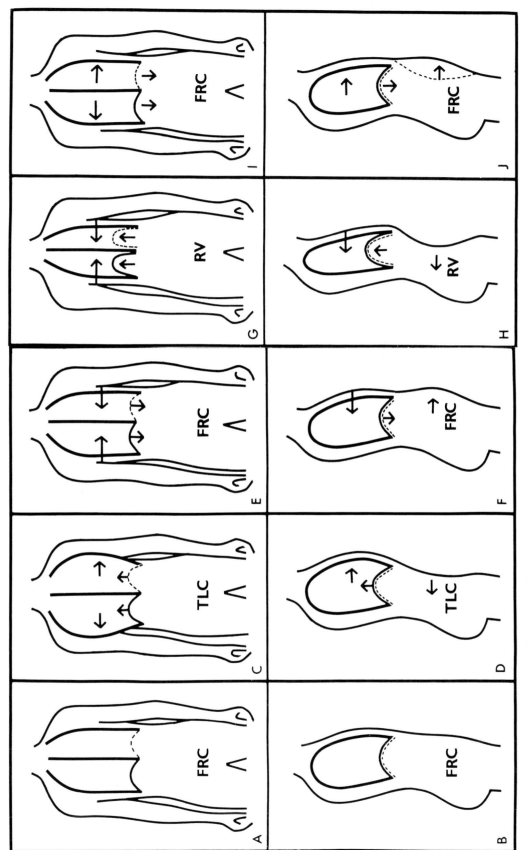

Figure 21–5. Schematic Depiction of Chest Cage and Diaphragmatic Movements Throughout the Respiratory Cycle: Bilateral Diaphragmatic Paralysis. On inspiration to TLC from FRC (*A* to *D*), the increased negative intrapleural pressure "sucks" the diaphragm up and draws the abdominal wall in. On expiration to FRC (*E* and *F*), the diaphragm descends and the abdomen protrudes. With a deeper expiration to RV accompanied by active contraction of the abdominal muscles (*G* and *H*), the diaphragm rises. Subsequently, during the first part of inspiration to FRC (*I* and *J*), abdominal muscle recoil is associated with descent of the flaccid diaphragm, creating the false impression of active contraction.

may result in secondary polycythemia.[224] Other patients develop gas volume and blood volume (V/Q) imbalance secondary to kyphoscoliosis and exhibit late onset respiratory failure. In a follow-up study of 55 patients who had had poliomyelitis, 33 were found to manifest exertional dyspnea and frequent respiratory tract infections;[225] gross kyphoscoliosis (Cobb's angle > 60°) was present in 15 of these patients and fluoroscopic evidence of unilateral diaphragmatic paralysis in 13. Poliomyelitis should be suspected as the cause of acute respiratory failure when symptoms of bulbar palsy are present in an unvaccinated individual.

Amyotrophic lateral sclerosis (motor neuron disease) can also result in ventilatory respiratory failure.[210, 226] Although in most patients resiratory muscle involvement develops after the diagnosis has been well established on the basis of peripheral muscle weakness, respiratory failure in some patients may be the initial mode of presentation, one that can result in a difficult diagnostic problem.[227–230] In addition to ventilatory respiratory failure caused by destruction of the anterior horn cells that innervate the inspiratory muscles, involvement of the neurons supplying the abdominal expiratory muscles and the muscles of the upper airway can result in abnormalities of expiratory flow. Kreitzer and associates[231] have described a characteristic flow-volume curve in which expiratory flow is decreased and residual volume increased, a combination that occurs in patients with predominant expiratory muscle weakness. Selective paralysis of upper airway and oropharyngeal muscles can also influence maximal expiratory flow.[232] An uncommon hereditary and slowly progressive form of anterior horn cell degeneration, Kugelberg-Welander syndrome, can also present with respiratory muscle paralysis and ventilatory respiratory failure.[233]

As in many forms of neuromuscular disease that cause ventilatory respiratory failure, patients with spinal cord degeneration may benefit from intermittent assisted ventilation, particularly at night; such assistance can stabilize or temporarily improve the respiratory status.[234] The exact mechanism by which mechanical ventilation improves interim lung function remains speculative. Possibilities include the reversal of chronic respiratory muscle fatigue, a resetting of central chemoreceptors, or an improvement in pulmonary mechanics.

Disorders of the Peripheral Nerves

Landry–Guillain-Barré Syndrome

Acute polyneuritis (Landry–Guillain-Barré syndrome) is probably the most common of all neuromuscular diseases that cause respiratory failure,[235] and it can be associated with either acute or subacute hypoventilation. Although in some respects it is a diagnosis of exclusion, an accepted clinical presentation includes symmetric ascending paralysis and a lack of cellular response in the cerebrospinal fluid. The disease shows a striking predilection for patients less than 26 years of age of either sex; a second, smaller peak occurs between the ages of 45 and 60 years. Cases tend to show a seasonal clustering, almost half the patients being afflicted during a 4-month period of late summer and autumn.[236]

In several large series, the incidence of respiratory failure has been examined as well as the benefits that are achieved with mechanical ventilation.[237–240] Between 15[237] and 61[240] per cent of patients develop sufficient respiratory muscle paralysis to require mechanical ventilation. In these patients there is a slow but progressive improvement in respiratory muscle strength, although assisted ventilation may be required for a period of 2 months or longer; two patients have been reported who were ventilated for 374 and 396 days, respectively, before being successfully "weaned."[238] The need for assisted ventilation should be assessed by repeated measurements of vital capacity or preferably maximal inspiratory pressure. Serial measurements of phrenic nerve conduction velocity may be a more sensitive method of assessing the severity of the disease and of predicting impending ventilatory failure.[241] Patients sometimes manifest evidence of autonomic dysfunction, including elevated blood pressure, tachycardia, cardiac arrhythmias, and episodes of pyrexia and hyperhidrosis, and may require treatment with alpha- and beta-blocking agents.[235]

Porphyria

The hereditary hepatic porphyrias (acute intermittent porphyria, porphyria variegata, and hereditary coproporphyria) are inborn errors of porphyrin metabolism inherited in an autosomal dominant fashion. Each can be associated with ascending paralysis and respiratory failure. These diseases are characterized by increased excretion of porphyrins and the porphyrin precursors, aminolevulinic acid (ALA) and porphobilinogen (PBG). The basic defect appears to be a partial block along the heme-biosynthetic pathway of the enzyme ALA-synthetase. The peripheral neuropathy is caused by the toxic effect of the accumulated porphyrin precursors ALA and PBG.[242] Some patients also manifest symptoms of bulbar involvement and experience difficulty in clearing bronchial secretions. The diagnosis is supported when it is learned that other members of the family are afflicted, and confirmation can be obtained by the discovery of porphyrin precursors, including ALA and PBG, in the urine.[242] Our experience with two patients has been similar to that of Doll and colleagues;[243] exacerbations of the disease were prolonged and required artificial ventilation. Remissions may be followed by exacerbations that do not necessarily affect the respiratory musculature.

FISH AND SHELLFISH POISONING FROM TOXIC DINOFLAGELLATES

At least four different species of toxic dinoflagellates can cause shellfish and fish poisoning, and in all of these the respiratory muscles can be involved.[244] These microscopic unicellular sea algae are the cause of "red tide," a reddish discoloration of sea water resulting from an extremely high concentration of organisms. The four dinoflagellates that produce toxins for man are *Ptychodiscus brevis* (formerly *Gymnodinium breve*), *Protogonyaulyx cantenella*, *Protogonyaulyx tamarensis*, and *Gambierdiscus toxicus*. Three forms of poisoning occur depending on the species involved.

Neurotoxic Shellfish Poisoning. The syndrome known as neurotoxic shellfish poisoning is caused by the ingestion of clams or oysters contaminated with the toxins of *P. brevis;* the bivalves ingest the algae and concentrate these toxins (brevetoxins), which are the classic "red tide toxins."[245] The syndrome typically causes gastrointestinal symptoms of nausea, diarrhea, and abdominal pain. Neurologic symptoms include circumoral paresthesia; onset can range from a few minutes to three hours after ingestion of the clams or oysters. Paresthesia typically progresses to involve the pharynx, trunk, and extremities. Cerebellar symptoms, vertigo, incoordination, convulsions, bradycardia, and respirtory depression may develop. In addition to the problems associated with ingestion of the toxin, respiratory symptoms can also develop following inhalation of the toxin generated by whitecaps and breaking waves and liberated as an odorless aerosol. People exposed to the toxin on beaches can develop nonproductive cough, shortness of breath, lacrimation, sneezing, and rhinorrhea.[244, 246] *In vitro* studies have shown that the toxin of *P. brevis* contracts both animal[247] and human[248] airway smooth muscle.

Paralytic Shellfish Poisoning. The second major syndrome resulting from the toxins of unicellular sea algae, paralytic shellfish poisoning, is caused by the ingestion of mussels, clams, scallops, and oysters that have concentrated saxitoxin, the neurotoxin present in *Protogonyaulyx cantenella* and *Protogonyaulyx tamarensis*. The symptoms are very similar to those associated with the ingestion of brevetoxins and consist of circumoral paresthesia followed by cerebellar symptoms, dysphonia, dysphagia, and paralysis; the paralysis sometimes affects the respiratory muscles.[249, 250] The case mortality rate ranges from 3 to 23 per cent.[244]

Ciguatera Fish Poisoning. Another form of algae-related neurotoxicity, ciguatera fish poisoning, results from eating a fish contaminated with toxins derived from the organism *Gambierdiscus toxicus*. The toxin is concentrated in the flesh of large fish that feed on the plankton. Symptoms usually develop within 12 hours of ingestion and include gastrointestinal symptoms, cerebellar involvement, sensory disturbances, and motor paralysis; the paralysis can develop up to 1 week after the onset of the illness. In one series of 33 patients,[251] gastrointestinal symptoms developed in 91 per cent of the patients, pain and weakness in 58 per cent, and dysesthesias in 58 per cent; the dysesthesias lasted as long as two months. Of 129 cases reviewed retrospectively in the Miami area, 39 displayed significant muscle weakness but none required mechanical ventilation.[252] Muscle weakness can persist for long periods of time.[244, 253] Between 1970 and 1980, there were 418 cases of ciguatera fish poisoning reported in the United States, mainly from Florida and Hawaii. These occurred in 94 outbreaks and the mortality rate ranged from zero to as high as 20 per cent.[254] Although ciguatera fish poisoning occurs primarily in the tropics, isolated cases have been reported in temperate climates in people who have eaten fish imported from tropical areas.[255]

Miscellaneous Respiratory Muscle Toxins

A recent outbreak of poisoning related to the ingestion of contaminated mussels was reported in Nova Scotia, Canada.[256] The responsible agent, demoic acid, had not been previously recognized as a toxin. Symptoms included memory loss, an increase in bronchial secretions, and neurologic impairment; respiratory failure developed in the patients who died.[256]

Severe neuromuscular paralysis with rapid respiratory failure can occur after ingestion of puffer fish. The responsible neurotoxin, tetrodotoxin, blocks sodium channels in the peripheral nerves. In Japan, where puffer fish are considered a delicacy, specially trained chefs are entrusted with their preparation. The case fatality rate for puffer fish poisoning is approximately 50 per cent; death occurs as a result of respiratory muscle paralysis.[257]

A variety of other toxins and poisons can affect peripheral nerve function and result in respiratory muscle paralysis and ventilatory failure. Walker[258] has reported two cases of survival following respiratory failure induced by envenomation from the blue-ringed octopus, *Hapalochlaena maculosa*. Envenomation by the eastern coral snake, *Micrurus fulvius fulvius;* the krait, *Bungarus;*[259] and the Philippine cobra, *Naja naja philippinensis*[260] can cause respiratory muscle paralysis.[261] Tibballs and Cooper[262] have reported respiratory failure necessitating mechanical ventilation following envenomation from a tick, *Ixodes cornuatus*, that is widely distributed in Victoria, Tasmania, and New South Wales, Australia. Although unusual, acute respiratory muscle paralysis and ventilatory respiratory failure can also occur following accidental or suicidal ingestion of organophosphate insecticide.[263]

DISORDERS OF THE MYONEURAL JUNCTION

Conditions that cause impaired neuromuscular transmission at the myoneural junction with consequent acute or chronic hypoventilation include myasthenia gravis, myasthenia-like syndromes associated with neoplasms, the ingestion of various medications, and infection with or ingestion of toxins from *Clostridium botulinum*.

Myasthenia Gravis

The defect in myasthenia gravis is postsynaptic and is related to autoantibodies of the IgG class that attach to and destroy acetylcholine receptors at the motor end plate.[264-266] Exacerbations of respiratory muscle weakness and the development of respiratory failure in patients with myasthenia gravis can be precipitated by surgery, infection, or the parenteral administration of radiographic contrast media.[267, 268] Prior to the onset of hypoventilation, patients with myasthenia and myasthenia-like syndromes usually manifest paresthesia, diplopia, dysphagia, ptosis, generalized weakness, and dyspnea. In some cases, the diagnosis of myasthenia is brought to a physician's attention only after a surgical procedure in which the effects of sedation and muscle relaxants cause a long period of inadequate ventilation postoperatively.[269] The administration of acetylcholinesterase inhibitors results in an immediate increase in respiratory muscle strength and lung volume,[270, 271] although it can also cause a transient increase in airway resistance and a decrease in maximal expiratory flow, presumably because of an accentuation of cholinergic tone in the airway smooth muscle.[272] Some patients show a remission of symptoms while receiving steroid therapy, and it has been shown that a regime of alternate-day prednisone results in only a small reduction of respiratory function on the day after administration of the drug.[273]

Myasthenic patients who do not respond to more conservative therapy show a dramatic response to plasmapheresis[267, 274] and immunosuppressive drug therapy, an improvement that has been shown to correlate with a marked fall in titers of serum antibody directed against the acetylcholine receptor.[275] In our experience, respiratory failure in patients with myasthenia gravis usually necessitates ventilatory support for days to weeks and sometimes for months; a patient has been reported on whom ventilatory support was maintained for two years![276]

Myasthenia-like syndromes occur in association with neoplasia, the administration of various antibiotics, and antiseizure therapy.[277] In three cases of Eaton-Lambert syndrome, a myasthenia-like syndrome associated with malignancy, plasmapheresis and immunosuppressive therapy improved symptoms, thus suggesting an autoimmune etiology.[278] Neuronal antinuclear antibodies have been described in a patient with Eaton-Lambert syndrome secondary to small cell lung cancer.[279]

Respiratory paralysis caused by antibiotics has been well documented:[280-283] neomycin,[284] streptomycin,[285] dihydrostreptomycin,[286] viomycin,[287] kanamycin,[288] polymyxin B, and colistin (polymyxin E)[280, 289] have been reported to cause neuromuscular blockade, usually in patients with renal disease or myasthenia gravis.[280, 282] Kanamycin and streptomycin are believed to produce a competitive blockade that may be reversed by neostigmine. By contrast, polymyxins produce a noncompetitive blockade that actually can be potentiated by neostigmine.[280] Ventilatory muscle depression can develop within 1 to 24 hours after the administration of these drugs. In most cases, the respiratory failure is of short duration and spontaneous ventilation is resumed within 24 hours.[280] The reaction can occur following administration of these drugs intraperitoneally,[290] intrapleurally, or into pseudocyst cavities.[283] Respiratory depression can be very prolonged following the intraperitoneal administration of neomycin or streptomycin in patients who also have been treated with succinylcholine chloride as a muscle relaxant during abdominal surgery.[281]

Penicillamine, a drug used in the treatment of rheumatoid arthritis and Wilson's disease, can be associated with the development of myasthenia gravis.[291] In the few cases reported, anti-acetylcholine receptor and antistriational antibodies have been found in the serum. Respiratory paralysis has been also identified in four patients being treated for systemic hypertension with trimethaphan camsylate;[292] this drug is a ganglionic blocking agent that probably produces its hypotensive effect by competing for receptor sites at the postsynaptic membranes, thus blocking the action of acetylcholine.

Organophosphate poisoning caused by the insecticides parathion and malathion[293, 294] results from inhibition of acetylcholinesterase at nerve endings (*see* further discussion in Chapter 14). Acetylcholine accumulates at cholinergic synapses, resulting in an initial stimulation and a later inhibition of synaptic transmission, with consequent paralysis of the respiratory muscles.

Clostridium botulinum Poisoning

Although *Clostridium botulinum* types A and B are the organisms most often responsible for acute respiratory failure, it can also develop as a complication of type E botulism following the ingestion of contaminated canned fish.[295, 296] The neurotoxin of botulism acts by causing a presynaptic blockade at the cholinergic neuromuscular junction, possibly by inhibiting calcium-dependent exocytosis and a release of acetylcholine.[297, 298] Respiratory involvement in botulism poisoning can occur after ingestion of food contaminated with the toxin[299] or as a result of wound infection by *Clostridium botulinum*;[300] the latter has been reported to occur in needle-track infections in chronic drug abusers.[301]

Peripheral muscle weakness and bulbar symptoms secondary to cranial nerve involvement usually appear within 18 to 36 hours after ingestion of contaminated food. Patients complain of blurred vision, weakness, dizziness, dysphonia, dysphagia, respiratory difficulty, and urinary retention. The pupils are dilated and nonreactive, and there is marked dryness of the mouth and tongue associated with muscle weakness.[295, 302] Ocular findings may be prominent and early features:[303] in one study of 59 patients, 98 per cent developed a fourth nerve palsy and 51 per cent partial or complete third nerve palsy. The development of full-blown third nerve palsy was predictive of eventual respiratory failure; 8 of the 9 patients who required ventilatory support showed evidence of complete third nerve palsy, whereas only 1 patient with respiratory failure did not have pre-existing complete third nerve palsy. Respiratory failure secondary to ventilatory muscle weakness occurs in 30 to 60 per cent of affected patients and is the primary cause of mortality.[299, 304] Respiratory failure may be very prolonged, but there is usually slow and eventual complete recovery of muscle strength. Despite this, a number of patients continue to complain of fatigability and exertional dyspnea 1[304] or 2[299] years after the initial ingestion of toxin.

DISORDERS OF THE RESPIRATORY MUSCLES

Muscular Dystrophies

The muscular dystrophies are inherited myopathies characterized by progressive weakness of skeletal muscle. They are generally divided into four types: Duchenne type dystrophy, a sex-linked recessive disorder that begins in childhood; facioscapulohumeral dystrophy, an autosomal dominant disorder that begins in adolescence; limb-girdle dystrophy, also autosomal dominant and adolescent in onset; and myotonic dystrophy, an autosomal dominant condition that can begin at any age.

Duchenne type muscular dystrophy causes death from respiratory failure in at least 80 per cent of affected individuals;[305] the respiratory muscle failure typically develops insidiously[306–309] and, as with other forms of respiratory failure related to muscle weakness, is aggravated during sleep.[310, 311] A syndrome of facioscapulohumeral dystrophy associated with sensorineural hearing loss, tortuosity of retinal arterioles, and an early onset of rapid progression of respiratory failure has been recently described.[312] Respiratory failure develops in approximately 10 per cent of patients with myotonic muscular dystrophy;[309, 313] the respiratory difficulties relate not only to weakness but also to an increase in impedance of the respiratory system secondary to myotonia of the abdominal and chest wall muscles.[314, 315] The increased tone is caused by inappropriate electrical activity of the muscles during the respiratory cycle.[316] Of 17 patients with progressive muscular dystrophy reviewed by Kilburn and colleagues,[306] 9 exhibited myotonia; 12 of the 17 patients had dyspnea or other respiratory symptoms. Although impairment of vital capacity and maximal breathing capacity was more severe in the nonmyotonic patients, those with myotonia had reduced minute ventilation, hypoxemia, hypercapnia, and pulmonary hypertension.[306] As in other forms of ventilatory failure related to neuromuscular disease, intermittent ventilatory support can result in an improvement of lung function and a prolongation of useful life.[317]

Acid Maltase Deficiency

Acid maltase deficiency, a recessively inherited disorder, is being recognized with increasing frequency as a cause of neuromuscular respiratory failure.[318, 319] It is a type 2 glycogen storage disease in which glycogen accumulates in intracellular vacuoles in muscle and other organs; it is caused by a deficiency of the enzyme acid maltase.[215, 319–322] The condition occurs in three forms depending on the age of onset: (1) an infantile form in which patients usually die before the age of 2 years and in which hepatic and splenic enlargement is a prominent finding as a result of the accumulation of glycogen; (2) a childhood form characterized by variable muscle and organ involvement and usually by slow progression to respiratory failure; and (3) an adult form in which specific muscle groups can be involved and the course is even more insidiously progressive.[319] The accumulation of glycogen in diaphragmatic muscle cells can occur predominantly in type 1 fibers.[323] In adults, ventilatory respiratory failure may be the presenting feature,[324, 325] as in 3 of 10 patients described by Rosenow and Engel[319] and in 4 of 9 patients described by Keunen and associates.[326] Respiratory failure is an inevitable development in the majority of patients.[324, 325]

Nemaline Myopathy

Nemaline myopathy is a nonprogressive myopathy that usually affects neonates and that has a relatively good prognosis.[325] Although it is very uncommon in adults, it can present as respiratory failure.[327–330] The term nemaline derives from the formation in affected muscle cells of rod-like structures composed of nuclear material.

Myopathy in Connective Tissue Disease

Although the usual cause of pulmonary problems in polymyositis and dermatomyositis is aspiration of gastric contents secondary to pharyngeal muscle paralysis, some patients have sufficient involvement of the diaphragm to cause acute or chronic hypoventilation. Respiratory muscular dysfunction is sometimes not recognized because of undue attention directed to associated interstitial pulmonary disease; in such patients withdrawal of corticosteroid therapy may uncover the underlying respiratory muscle weakness. Some patients with bilateral diaphragmatic paralysis or myopathy appear to have an associated blunting of respiratory drive;[215, 320, 331] the cause of this is not entirely clear, but it may result from a resetting of central sensitivity to carbon dioxide attributable to intermittent hypercapnia during sleep-induced hypoventilation.[215, 331]

Muscular weakness has been postulated as the mechanism that causes "shrinking" of the lungs in patients with systemic lupus erythematosus (SLE).[332] In the "shrinking lung syndrome," serial chest roentgenograms reveal progressive loss of lung volume unassociated with other abnormalities of the lung parenchyma. Although it is clear that patients with SLE often show a decrease in respiratory muscle strength,[333, 334] the pathogenesis of the weakness has not been established. Generalized neuropathic[335] and myopathic[336] processes are known to occur in patients with SLE and either process could involve the diaphragm. However, to date the "shrinking lung syndrome" has been observed mainly in patients without generalized neuromuscular disease. In a recent study,[333] the possibility that the weakness might be caused by a mononeuritis involving the phrenic nerves was directly tested by using measurements of phrenic nerve latency: it was found that despite significant diaphragmatic weakness, there was no abnormality of nerve conduction.

Miscellaneous Myopathic Processes

Respiratory muscle weakness and resulting respiratory failure have been reported in patients with hyperthyroidism,[335] in uremic patients on continuous peritoneal dialysis,[336] and in asthmatics following the parenteral administration of large doses of steroids.[337] A rare muscular disease that causes acute respiratory paralysis and hypoventilation is rhabdomyolysis (myoglobinuria).[338–340] Although the cause of this condition is unknown in most cases, a 23-year-old woman has been described in whom the rhabdomyolysis was associated with a deficiency of muscle carnitine and in whom treatment with d, l-carnitine was followed by dramatic improvement.[341] Acute flaccid paralysis requiring artificial ventilation has been reported in association with hypophosphatemia;[342–344] this condition, whether caused by infection or the use of phosphate-binding antacids, can cause worsening respiratory failure in patients with COPD[345] or in patients with respiratory failure of other cause who are difficult to "wean" from artificial respiration. In one patient with respiratory failure secondary to hypophosphatemia, monitoring of phosphocreatine and pH by nuclear magnetic resonance spectroscopy revealed defective muscle metabolism.[346] Hypokalemia related to familial pe-

riodic paralysis, diabetes, diabetic ketoacidosis,[347, 348] or renal tubular acidosis[349] can rarely result in sufficient muscle weakness to cause respiratory failure. Severe hypermagnesemia caused by irrigation of the renal pelvis, chronic renal failure, or the ingestion of magnesium-containing antacids can also result in hypoventilation and respiratory failure.[350, 351]

VENOARTERIAL SHUNTS

EXTRAPULMONARY VENOARTERIAL SHUNTS

Oxygen transport to the tissues may be inadequate despite normal structure and function of the lung parenchyma, airways, and respiratory pump. In these circumstances, the hypoxemia is caused by shunting of venous blood into arterial channels, and blood gas analysis reveals a reduced Po_2 and a normal or reduced Pco_2. The most common cause of shunting is congenital heart disease, usually manifested by roentgenographic evidence of pulmonary pleonemia or pulmonary hypertension; this subject is considered briefly in Chapter 5 (see page 755). In this section we are concerned primarily with extrapulmonary venoarterial shunts in which chest roentgenograms are normal.

A form of venoarterial shunting that in some cases at least, is extrapulmonary in type may be found in patients with advanced cirrhosis. These patients usually have normal chest roentgenograms, and evidence of shunting lies in the results of arterial blood gas analyses that reveal mild-to-moderate hypoxemia and respiratory alkalosis.[352, 353] The lowered Pco_2 is balanced by a proportional decrease in bicarbonate, indicating that a prolonged state of hyperventilation has resulted in compensation through renal excretion of bicarbonate. Abelmann and colleagues[354] compared arterial blood gas values in 34 patients with cirrhosis with those in a control group of 20 normal subjects. Mean arterial oxygen saturation was 93.2 per cent in the patients and 95.8 per cent in the normal subjects, and the mean Pao_2 in 17 of the patients was 73 mm Hg and in the control group 95 mm Hg.

There is reason to believe that more than one mechanism is responsible for the hypoxemia associated with cirrhosis, the shunt being extrapulmonary in some patients and intrapulmonary in others. In the extrapulmonary form, blood from the portal system reaches the left side of the heart through anastomoses with pulmonary veins. Rodman and associates[355] believed this to be the explanation in a patient in whom 40 per cent of cardiac output was shunted from right to left; careful pathologic examination of the lungs failed to reveal arteriovenous fistulas. Shaldon and associates[356] injected radioactive krypton into the spleen in an attempt to determine the mechanism of hypoxemia in five patients with cirrhosis: definite portopulmonary anastomoses were apparent in one case but none was detected in the other four.

PULMONARY VENOARTERIAL SHUNTS

The intrapulmonary form of shunting that occurs in patients with cirrhosis can also occur in the presence of a normal chest roentgenogram. Using a micropaque gelatin suspension, Berthelot and colleagues[357] demonstrated severe dilatation of fine peripheral branches of the pulmonary artery in 13 patients who had died of cirrhosis; spider nevi were detected on the pleura in 6 patients. The peripheral pulmonary arterial shunts in 1 patient were sufficiently extensive to explain the hypoxemia detected during life. Eight of the 13 patients were considered to show parenchymal abnormalities roentgenologically. In six cases the abnormalities were described as small, rather ill-defined nodular shadows and in two cases as linear shadows; in all cases they were bilateral and predominant in the lower lobes.

Ventilation-perfusion mismatch caused by increased airway closure at the lung bases contributes to the hypoxemia in patients with cirrhosis and hypoproteinemia.[358-363] In addition, $\dot{V}/\dot{Q}$ mismatch can be caused by impaired hypoxic vasoconstriction in some patients with cirrhosis.[364] Studies employing quantitative perfusion scintigraphy[365, 366] have revealed indirect evidence for pulmonary arteriovenous communications that are too small to be detected angiographically. For example, in a study of three patients with cirrhosis and moderate hypoxemia, Wolfe and associates[366] showed that the amount of intravenously injected macroaggregated albumin that traversed the pulmonary vasculature was much larger than in normal subjects. These abnormal vascular channels were considered to be responsible for the hypoxemia; chest roentgenograms were normal. The demonstration of shunts by measuring the passage of macroaggregated albumin through the lung may improve with time. Chen and associates[367] have described a patient whose arterial blood gases worsened as a result of the opening up of intrapulmonary shunts during periods of hepatic functional deterioration, but in whom improvement in clinical status occurred coincident with a reduction in shunt. Intrapulmonary right-to-left shunting also can be demonstrated in patients with cirrhosis by contrast echocardiography.[368] Normally, when ultrasound contrast material (which contains microbubbles) is injected into the peripheral circulation, it is removed during the first pass through the pulmonary circulation and no echogenic material reaches the left side of the heart; in patients with intrapulmonary or extrapulmonary right-to-left shunt, bubbles reach the left heart and can be detected ultrasonographically.

Krowka and Cortese attempted to decrease the blood flow through intrapulmonary arteriovenous (AV) shunts by the administration of almitrine bismesylate;[369] since almitrine enhances hypoxic vasoconstriction, they reasoned that it might decrease blood flow through the dilated intrapulmonary vessels. However, they were able to show improvement in only one of five subjects so treated. Although the severe hypoxemia in patients with cirrhosis is related primarily to intrapulmonary AV shunting through dilated peripheral pulmonary vessels, the response of this "shunt" to the breathing of 100 per cent oxygen is greater than would be expected in a true anatomic shunt. It is probable that the shunt in these cases actually represents a unique form of diffusion impairment in which there is failure of equilibration between alveolar gas and capillary blood as a result of the large diameter of the vessels, the long distances for diffusion to occur, and a very rapid red blood cell transit time through the vessels. Patients with intrapulmonary right-to-left shunt may have lowered carbon monoxide diffusing capacity.[370]

The hypoxemia observed in patients with hepatic cirrhosis is more severe in the erect than in the recumbent position (orthodeoxia),[371] a phenomenon that is attributable to the increased blood flow through the lung bases where most spider nevi are found. When orthodeoxia is severe, the patient may complain of increased dyspnea when in the erect position (platypnea).[372, 373] Most patients with advanced cirrhosis present with symptoms and signs attributable to the liver damage; the hypoxemia and hypocapnia are rarely severe enough to cause symptoms or signs. Secondary polycythemia may occur occasionally and, without the benefit of blood gas analysis, can be confused with the erythrocytosis associated with hepatomas.[374]

In addition to patients with cirrhosis whose hypoxemia is caused by pulmonary arteriovenous shunts, there are some patients in whom blood is shunted from pulmonary artery to pulmonary vein during the postoperative period but whose chest roentgenograms are within normal limits. When hypoxemia persists for several days after surgery, impairment of ventilation-perfusion ratios may be demonstrable.[375, 376] However, Diament and Palmer's study of 23 patients whose arterial blood gases were measured while they breathed 100 per cent oxygen before and after surgery showed a mean true shunt of 12 per cent during the postoperative period.[377] These workers correlated the degree of shunting with roentgenographic appearances postoperatively. Shunting averaged 7 per cent in the 12 patients whose chest roentgenograms showed "plate atelectasis," and 19 per cent in the 6 patients whose roentgenograms revealed segmental atelectasis. The authors[377] ascribed these findings to true pulmonary venoarterial shunting caused by inability of patients to breathe deeply in the immediate postoperative period. They considered that this inability had resulted in loss of surfactant and collapse of acinar units.

METHEMOGLOBINEMIA AND CARBON MONOXIDE POISONING

Oxygen transport to the tissues can be reduced as a result of methemoglobinemia or carbon monoxide poisoning. Methemoglobin is hemoglobin in which the ferrous iron has been oxidized to the ferric form. Blood turns a chocolate brown color when approximately 15 per cent of hemoglobin is oxidized to methemoglobin; the result is cyanosis that is unresponsive to oxygen therapy.[378] Methemoglobinemia can result from exposure to drugs or chemicals that act by increasing the rate of hemoglobin oxidation or by overstimulating the intraerythrocyte mechanisms that protect hemoglobin against oxidation.[379–381] It can also result from impairment of a patient's capacity to reduce hemoglobin, either on an enzymatic or chemical basis.

Methemoglobinemia can be either hereditary or acquired. The latter is most often caused by nitrates that can be introduced into the body in several ways. The condition is reported to follow the ingestion of well water containing a high concentration of nitrate;[382] in fact, what must be a unique event has been reported in which a patient on renal dialysis developed methemoglobinemia as a result of nitrate-contaminated well water being used as a dialysate.[383] This complication has also occurred following the use of topically applied nitrate in the treatment of burns,[384, 385] following the ingestion of meat to which nitrates had been applied as preservatives,[386] and secondary to the use of topical anesthetic containing Cetacaine,[387] benzocaine, and lidocaine.[388] Three cases of methemoglobinemia have been described following absorption of nitrates through skin burned in a chemical explosion of nitrates.[378] Two types of hereditary methemoglobinemia have been described, one caused by enzymatic lack and the other associated with an abnormal type of hemoglobin (hemoglobin M).

Methemoglobinemia causes no alteration in the chest roentgenogram. Patients usually present with symptoms and signs caused by tissue anoxia, including headache, nausea, dizziness, pounding pulse, and listlessness.[380] In most cases a diffuse, persistent, grayish cyanosis is present, although it may not be obvious. The congenital variety of the disease is associated with mental retardation.[379]

Carbon monoxide poisoning can be an acute respiratory emergency or can cause a more chronic presentation characterized by abnormal behavior when lower concentrations of gas have been inhaled over a prolonged period.[389] Carbon monoxide, the product of incomplete combustion, is an odorless, colorless gas. It binds in a reversible manner with hemoglobin and has an affinity for the hemoglobin binding site that is 200 times greater than the affinity for oxygen. In addition, carboxyhemoglobin shifts the oxygen dissociation curve to the left and has a direct toxic effect on the cytochrome enzymes.[390, 391] When carboxyhemoglobin levels reach 20 per cent of total hemoglobin, symptoms develop that include headache, nausea and vomiting, and decreased manual dexterity. When levels reach 50 per cent, convulsions, coma, and death rapidly ensue.[390] Acute poisoning can cause death as a result of either cerebral anoxia[392] or an ARDS-like picture,[393] the pulmonary edema possibly being caused by a direct effect of carbon monoxide on the permeability of the alveolocapillary membrane.[393]

Acute carbon monoxide poisoning usually results from inhalation of exhaust fumes in suicide attempts; less often it occurs in association with defective heating and cooking systems.[394] Fisher and Rubin[391] described 12 patients in New York who developed chronic poisoning (average carboxyhemoglobin level, 18 per cent) caused by defective home heaters during a very cold winter.[391] A patient has been described who developed acute poisoning after inhalation of methylene chloride, which is converted to carbon monoxide in the blood.[391] Carboxyhemoglobin levels of 10 to 15 per cent are found in heavy cigarette and cigar smokers.[395–397]

ALVEOLAR HYPERVENTILATION

Normally, alveolar ventilation is proportional to the metabolic requirements of the tissues. In response to fever, exertion, or thyrotoxicosis the demand for oxygen at the tissue level increases, as does carbon dioxide production. Alveolar ventilation increases, but since the increase is appropriate, arterial P_{CO_2} remains within the normal range. Hyperventilation is ventilation in excess of that required to maintain P_{CO_2} between 35 and 40 mm Hg.

Assessment of the adequacy of ventilation requires either direct analysis of the carbon dioxide tension in the blood, or measurement of the mixed venous P_{CO_2} by the rebreathing technique. Every clinician who has experience in the management of respiratory disease and uses blood gas analysis is aware of the inaccuracy of the clinical appraisal of ventilation. In an observer error study in which students, house staff, and attending staff observed a normal person breathing at different tidal volumes and rates, Mithoefer and associates[208] showed how undependable clinical estimation can be. Not only was the clinical estimate of ventilatory volume grossly inaccurate, but also individual observers could not repeat their original estimates when the subjects breathed at the same tidal volume. Training and experience were of little help in the clinical assessment of the volume of ventilation. This study also showed that gross degrees of overventilation could be recognized with greater accuracy than underventilation, but there was still a definite tendency to overestimate minute volume.

Hyperventilation that causes a reduction in P_{CO_2} to 35 mm Hg or less can result from both pulmonary and extrapulmonary causes. In the majority of patients, excessive ventilation is of psychogenic origin.

ORGANIC PULMONARY DISEASE

Hyperventilation and hypocapnia may occur in patients with bronchial asthma, pneumonia, pulmonary embolism, and diffuse granulomatous or fibrotic interstitial disease. Hypocapnia is usually associated with hypoxemia, although in some patients with diffuse pulmonary fibrosis the PO_2 may be normal at rest and fall only during exercise. Diffuse interstitial disease sometimes engenders dyspnea on exertion, but by itself overventilation at rest seldom causes symptoms.

If the hyperventilation is of recent origin, bicarbonate levels remain relatively elevated in proportion to the PCO_2, and this is reflected in a lower hydrogen ion concentration (elevated pH). If overventilation is of longer standing, renal compensation for the lowered PCO_2 results in increased urinary excretion of bicarbonate and a lowered serum bicarbonate level; the hydrogen ion concentration is maintained within normal limits. In some patients with COPD or asthma, the minute ventilation may be greatly increased over the estimated normal value and yet the PCO_2 may be normal or higher than normal because of severe $\dot{V}/\dot{Q}$ inequality.

EXTRAPULMONARY DISORDERS

Central Nervous System Disorders

Central nervous system (CNS) disorders that can cause hyperventilation include cerebrovascular accidents, brain trauma, meningitis, and encephalitis. The mechanism by which hyperventilation develops has not been established. From a study of patients with cerebral hemorrhage, however, Froman and Smith[398] suggested that some breakdown product in the brain is responsible for a rise in hydrogen ion concentration of cerebrospinal fluid that directly stimulates the respiratory center to cause a state of hyperventilation. In many patients with organic brain disease, hypoxemia and hypercapnia develop as a result of compression of the respiratory center by increasing intracranial pressure. Blood gas analysis during the initial stage in these patients may indicate respiratory alkalosis. Later, when the hydrogen ion concentration begins to rise as a result of hypoventilation and carbon dioxide retention, respiratory acidosis may develop.

Cheyne-Stokes Breathing

Cheyne-Stokes respiration is a form of hyperventilation recognizable clinically by the contrast between periods of hyperventilation and apnea. Tidal volume increases progressively during the phase of hyperpnea and subsequently decreases without change in respiratory rate.[399] This cyclic form of breathing is caused by instability of the ventilatory control system, in which circulation time, controller sensitivity, and the damping characteristics of the oxygen and carbon dioxide stores play an important role.[400] Instability of the automatic control systems occurs when the activity of the controller is excessive, either because of a delay in the feedback signal or because the controller is too sensitive or responds to stimulation in a nonlinear fashion.[401] Contrasted with the change in blood gases that occurs during voluntary hyperventilation and breath-holding, in Cheyne-Stokes respiration the stage of hyperventilation, because of the delay in feedback signal, is associated with a decreased PaO_2 and increased $PaCO_2$. During the apneic phase, PaO_2 and pH are increased and $PaCO_2$ decreased.[402] This form of periodic breathing occurs in patients with left ventricular failure or impaired cerebrovascular circulation. In those with impaired left ventricular function, the Cheyne-Stokes breathing occurs particularly during sleep and its presence is a poor prognostic sign.[403] Although the respiratory centers of such patients are hypersensitive to carbon dioxide,[404] the fluctuations that occur in mental state, electroencephalogram, and neurologic signs probably result primarily from phasic alterations in cerebral circulation.[405] Periodic cardiac dysrhythmia has been noted to occur coincidentally and synchronously with fluctuations in ventilatory pattern.[406]

Psychogenic Hyperventilation

By far the most common cause of hyperventilation is of psychological origin. As defined by Lewis and Howell,[407] "the hyperventilation syndrome is a syndrome characterized by a variety of somatic symptoms induced by physiologically inappropriate hyperventilation and usually reproduced in whole or in part by voluntary hyperventilation." Psychogenic hyperventilation varies in degree and clinical presentation, ranging from patients who complain of dyspnea at rest and who require frequent deep respiratory efforts to the hysterical patient who overbreathes to the extent of inducing coma or tetany. Occasionally, psychogenic hyperventilation is epidemic in type: Moss and McEvedy[408] described its occurrence in one third of 550 girls at a secondary school, 85 of whom required admission to the hospital. Subsequent psychological testing of these schoolchildren revealed an increase in susceptibility to hysteria among those who had reacted most dramatically. The psychogenic hyperventilation syndrome has been closely related to a psychiatric condition termed "panic disorder" that is characterized by the sudden onset of extreme fear for which there is no known cause.[409] At least 50 per cent of these patients suffer from the hyperventilation syndrome that can develop during the attack; in fact, attacks can be precipitated by voluntary hyperventilation.

The symptoms of psychogenic hyperventilation are primarily neurologic and cardiorespiratory. In one study of 78 patients,[409] neurologic symptoms of giddiness or light-headedness were observed in 59 per cent, paresthesias in 36 per cent, loss of consciousness in 31 per cent, and visual disturbances in 28 per cent of the patients; other symptoms included headache, ataxia, tremor, and tinnitus. Of the cardiorespiratory symptoms, dyspnea and palpitations were the most common, the former occurring in 53 per cent and the latter in 33 per cent of patients. The majority of patients described the shortness of breath as an inability to "get enough air down into their lungs" although some complained of a smothering feeling at night just before falling asleep or immediately on wakening.[410] They also complained of an inability to take a satisfying breath.[411] Rice[410] reviewed the records of 107 patients in whom the major diagnosis was hyperventilation syndrome of psychological origin. In his experience, as in ours, dyspnea is usually noted at rest, but when associated with exertion, it characteristically occurs following rather than during effort. Rice[410] described two types of pain suffered by patients with the hyperventilation syndrome. One is a sharp pain that he considers as being caused by distention of the stomach, and the other is a dull, aching tightness in the chest; the latter sensation is the more common of the two and probably results from excessive use of the intercostal muscles.

The mechanism for the neurologic symptoms in the hyperventilation syndrome probably consists of both cerebral hypoxia and metabolic alkalosis. By producing hypocapnia, hyperventilation decreases cerebral blood flow and causes a shift of the O_2 dissociation curve to the left, decreasing unloading of oxygen at the tissue level.[412] Although in many patients the diagnosis of psychogenic hyperventilation is readily made on the basis of the characteristics of psychoneurosis, in some patients the symptoms closely simulate organic disease. For example, Coyle and Sternman[413] described 19 patients who initially presented with focal neurologic symptoms, such as transient ischemic attacks, or with symptoms suggestive of multiple sclerosis or myasthenia gravis. Hyperventilation can also precipitate migraine headaches[414] or seizure disorders.[415] Although most patients who experience numbness and tingling during periods of hyperventilation state that these sensations are bilateral, some describe them in only one extremity. In a study of 90 volunteers who hyperventilated for 3 to 5 minutes, Tavel[416] found that 16 per cent developed symptoms of unilateral numbness, tingling, weakness, pain, and muscle spasm, usually in an upper extremity.

Spirometry often confirms the diagnosis of psychogenic hyperventilation when its presence is suspected on clinical grounds. The characteristic pattern is highly irregular breathing punctuated by deep inspiration. In the majority of cases arterial blood gas analysis shows a reduction in the P_{CO_2}, usually with a proportional reduction in bicarbonate levels. The electrocardiogram may reveal depression of the ST segment and a reduction or inversion of the T waves in any or all leads.[410, 417, 418] Hyperventilation is also associated with junctional tachycardia[418] and has been implicated in the production of angina owing to coronary vasospasm.[358] When hyperventilation is severe, the electroencephalogram may record slowed activity.

Although hyperventilation is usually a benign disturbance readily reversible by suggestion or reassurance, in some patients the overbreathing can have serious consequences. For example, it is probable that maternal hyperventilation during labor can sometimes result in severe fetal hypoxia and metabolic acidosis.[419, 420] The critical level of P_{CO_2} in maternal arterial blood is estimated to be 15 to 17 mm Hg, a level unlikely to develop in most spontaneous deliveries but one that could occur in hysterical mothers or in women being maintained on artificial ventilation during cesarean section.[420]

Occasionally, primary respiratory alkalosis is caused by extrapulmonary organic disease; affected patients develop lactic acidosis, presumably as a "compensatory" mechanism to the alkalotic state.[421–423] Papadopoulos and Keats[424] measured changes in the acid-base balance in 20 patients who were hyperventilated while under anesthesia. Serial arterial blood samples were drawn from 1 to 4 hours after initiation of hyperventilation; in the presence of respiratory alkalosis (Pa_{CO_2} = 15 to 20 mm Hg), the hydrogen ion concentration rose and both total fixed acid and blood lactic acid levels increased. In patients in whom abnormal prolonged hyperventilation is the result of organic disease,[422, 423] "overcompensation" appears to occur and the hydrogen ion concentration can actually exceed normal, with the patient presenting a picture of acidosis rather than alkalosis. The acidosis can be very difficult to control and can hasten death. Death also has been reported after voluntary hyperventilation in a patient with chronic alveolar hypoventilation.[425] This patient had a Pa_{O_2} of 38 mm Hg and a Pa_{CO_2} of 83 mm Hg; he was requested to hyperventilate during which the pH rose from 7.39 to 7.63 and apnea and convulsions promptly ensued. Intensive therapy resulted in the patient becoming alert once again, but apnea recurred and was followed by ventricular fibrillation and death.

MISCELLANEOUS CAUSES OF HYPERVENTILATION

Hyperventilation in primary metabolic acidosis results from stimulation of the respiratory center and carotid bodies by an increase in hydrogen ion concentration. The major causes of this type of hyperventilation are the ketosis associated with uncontrolled diabetes and the metabolic acidosis of renal failure. In contrast to other disorders that cause hyperventilation, blood gas analysis reveals acidosis, the hydrogen ion concentration being increased and the bicarbonate level reduced; PO_2 is within normal limits and PCO_2 reduced. Many patients who overventilate as a result of CNS lesions or metabolic acidosis are semicomatose; the hyperventilation is obviously an inconsequential feature of a much more complex problem.

The ingestion of salicylates in sufficiently large quantities to provoke hyperventilation usually occurs accidentally in children, but sometimes constitutes suicidal attempts by young adults or abuse of prescribed medications by the elderly.[426] Salicylates probably act by increasing the sensitivity of the respiratory center to the existing level of PCO_2. The acid-base disorder usually consists of a mixed respiratory alkalosis and anion gap-type metabolic acidosis, although occasionally it is an uncomplicated respiratory alkalosis or a pure metabolic acidosis.[426] Salicylate intoxication in young individuals is generally considered to be a benign condition with a low mortality rate, but such is not the case in the elderly in whom the clinical presentation is often confusing and may suggest cardiopulmonary disease or encephalopathy.[426] Permeability pulmonary edema (ARDS) is a frequent complication and is associated with a high mortality.

Severe hypoproteinemia in patients with cirrhosis and other diseases is associated with hyperventilation; the lowering of $PaCO_2$ is proportional to the reduction in serum albumin and total protein concentration.[428]

REFERENCES

1. Rigler LG: Roentgen examination of the chest. Its limitations in the diagnosis of disease. JAMA 142:773, 1950.
2. Liebow AA, Hales MR, Bloomer WE, et al: Studies on the lung after ligation of the pulmonary artery. II. Anatomical changes. Am J Pathol 26:177, 1950.
3. Smellie H, Hoyle C: The natural history of pulmonary sarcoidosis. Q J Med 29:539, 1960.
4. Young RL, Krumholz RA, with the technical assistance of Harkleroad LE: A physiologic roentgenographic disparity in sarcoidosis. Dis Chest 50:81, 1966.
5. Snider GL, Doctor L: The mechanics of ventilation in sarcoidosis. Am Rev Respir Dis 89:897, 1964.
6. Adhikari PK, Bianchi F, Boushy SF, et al: Pulmonary function in scleroderma. Its relation to changes in the chest roentgenogram and the skin of the thorax. Am Rev Respir Dis 86:823, 1962.
7. Marshall R, Smellie H, Baylis JH, et al: Pulmonary function in sarcoidosis. Thorax 13:48, 1958.
8. Massaro D, Katz S: Fibrosing alveolitis: Its occurrence, roentgenographic and pathologic features in von Recklinghausen's neurofibromatosis. Am Rev Respir Dis 93:934, 1966.
9. Rubin EH, Lubliner R: The Hamman-Rich syndrome: Review of the literature and analysis of 15 cases. Medicine 36:397, 1957.
10. Wilson RJ, Rodnan GP, Robin ED: An early pulmonary physiologic abnormality in progressive systemic sclerosis (diffuse scleroderma). Am J Med 36:361, 1964.
11. Ritchie B: Pulmonary function in scleroderma. Thorax 19:28, 1964.
12. Huang CT, Lyons HA: Comparison of pulmonary function in patients with systemic lupus erythematosus, scleroderma and rheumatoid arthritis. Am Rev Respir Dis 93:865, 1966.
13. Hoffbrand BI, Beck ER: "Unexplained" dyspnoea and shrinking lungs in systemic lupus erythematosus. Br Med J 1:1273, 1965.
14. Huang CT, Hennigar GR, Lyons HA: Pulmonary dysfunction in systemic lupus erythematosus. N Engl J Med 272:288, 1965.
15. Myhre JR: Pleuropulmonary manifestations in lupus erythematosus disseminatus. Acta Med Scand 165:55, 1959.
16. Green RA, Nichols NJ: Pulmonary involvement in leukemia. Am Rev Respir Dis 80:833, 1959.
17. Resnick ME, Berkowitz RD, Rodman T: Diffuse interstitial leukemic infiltration of the lungs producing the alveolar-capillary block syndrome. Report of a case, with studies of pulmonary function. Am J Med 31:149, 1961.
18. Goudemand M, Leduc M, Savinel E, et al: The lung in the course of leukoses. Lille Med 7:412, 1962.
19. Pace WR Jr, Decker JL, Martin CJ: Polymyositis: Report of two cases with pulmonary function studies suggestive of progressive systemic sclerosis. Am J Med Sci 245:322, 1963.
20. Müller R, Löfstedt S: The reaction of the pleura in primary tuberculosis of the lungs. Acta Med Scand 122:105, 1945.
21. Hessen I: Roentgen examination of pleural fluid: A study of the localization of free effusion, the potentialities of diagnosing minimal quantities of fluid and its existence under physiological conditions. Acta Radiol Suppl 86: 1951.
22. Blackie S, Al-Majed S, Staples C, et al: Acute changes in total lung capacity in asthma. American Thoracic Society Annual Meeting, 1988.
23. Gudbjerg CE: Bronchiectasis; radiological diagnosis and prognosis after operative treatment. Acta Radiol (Suppl)143, 1957.
24. Thurlbeck WM, Henderson JA, Fraser RG, et al: Chronic obstructive lung disease. A comparison between clinical, roentgenologic, functional and morphological criteria in chronic bronchitis, emphysema, asthma and bronchiectasis. Medicine 49:81, 1970.
25. Thurlbeck WM, Simon G: Radiographic appearance of the chest in emphysema. Am J Roentgenol 130:429, 1978.
26. Goddard PR, Nicholson EM, Laszlo G, et al: Computed tomography in pulmonary emphysema. Clin Radiol 33:379, 1982.
27. Bergin C, Muller N, Nichols DN, et al: The diagnosis of emphysema; a computed tomographic-pathologic correlation. Am Rev Respir Dis 133:541, 1986.
28. Hayhurst MD, MacNee W, Flenley DC, et al: Diagnosis of pulmonary emphysema by computerized tomography. Lancet 2(8398):320, 1984.
29. Gould GA, MacNee W, McLean A, et al: CT measurement of lung density in life and quantitated distal air space enlargement—An essential defining feature of human emphysema. Am Rev Respir Dis 137:380, 1988.
30. Lerner MA, Rosbash H, Frank HA, et al: Radiologic localization and management of cytologically discovered bronchial carcinoma. N Engl J Med 264:480, 1961.
31. Woolner LB, Andersen HA, Bernatz PE: "Occult" carcinoma of the bronchus: A study of 15 cases of in situ or early invasive bronchogenic carcinoma. Dis Chest 37:278, 1960.
32. Schneider L: Bronchogenic carcinoma heralded by hemoptysis and ignored because of negative x-ray results. NY State J Med 59:637, 1959.
33. Somner AAR, Hillis BR, Douglas AC, et al: Value of bronchoscopy in clinical practice. A review of 1,109 examinations. Br Med J 1:1079, 1958.
34. Melamed MR, Koss LG, Cliffton EE: Roentgenologically occult lung cancer diagnosed by cytology. Report of 12 cases. Cancer 16:1537, 1963.
35. Holman CW, Okinaka A: Occult carcinoma of the lung. J Thorac Cardiovasc Surg 47:466, 1964.
36. Weisel W, Lepley D Jr, Watson RR: Respiratory tract adenomas: A ten year study. Ann Surg 154:898, 1961.
37. Singer DB, Greenberg SD, Harrison GM: Papillomatosis of the lung. Am Rev Respir Dis 94:777, 1966.
38. Greenfield H, Herman PG: Papillomatosis of the trachea and bronchi. Am J Roentgenol 89:45, 1963.
39. Sanders JS, Carnes VM: Leiomyoma of the trachea. Report of a case, with a note on the diagnosis of partial tracheal obstruction. N Engl J Med 264:277, 1961.
40. Spinka J, Zwetschke O: Tracheal lipoma simulating the picture of severe bronchial asthma. Cas Lek Cesk 101:395, 1962.
41. Fontana RS, Sanderson DR, Taylor WF, et al: Early lung cancer detection: Results of the initial (prevalence) radiologic and cytologic screening in the Mayo Clinic study. Am Rev Respir Dis 130:561, 1984.
42. Frost JK, Ball WC, Levin ML, et al: Early lung cancer detection: Results of the initial (prevalence) radiologic and cytologic screening in the Johns Hopkins study. Am Rev Respir Dis 130:519, 1984.
43. Flehinger BJ, Melamed MR, Zaman MB, et al: Early lung cancer detection: Results of the initial (prevalence) radiologic and cytologic screening in the Memorial Sloan-Kettering study. Am Rev Respir Dis 130:555, 1984.
44. Martin L: Hypoventilation without elevated carbon dioxide tension. Chest 77:720, 1980.
45. Wathen CG, Capewell SJ, Heath JP, et al: Recurrent lobar pneumonia associated with idiopathic Eaton-Lambert syndrome. Thorax 43:574, 1988.
46. Berger AJ, Mitchell RA, Feveringhaus JW: Regulation of respiration (first of three parts). N Engl J Med 297:92, 1977.
47. Berger AJ, Mitchell RA, Feveringhaus JW: Regulation of respiration (second of three parts). N Engl J Med 297:138, 1977.
48. Berger AJ, Mitchell RA, Feveringhaus JW: Regulation of respiration (third of three parts). N Engl J Med 297:194, 1977.
49. Hornbein TF, Lenfant C (eds): Regulation of Breathing, Parts 1 and 2. Lung Biology in Health and Disease. New York, Marcel Dekker, 1981.
50. Ford GT, Whitelaw WA, Rosenal TW, et al: Diaphragm function after upper-abdominal surgery in humans. Am Rev Respir Dis 127:431, 1983.
51. Newsom Davis J: Control of the muscles of respiration. In Widdicombe, JB (ed): Respiratory Physiology (MTP International Review of Science—Physiology Series: Vol. 2). Baltimore, University Park Press, 1974, pp 221–245.
52. Spear PW, Protass LM: Barbiturate poisoning—An endemic disease. Five years' experience in a municipal hospital. Med Clin North Am 57:1471, 1973.
53. Hadden J, Johnson K, Smith S, et al: Acute barbiturate intoxication. Concepts of management. JAMA 209:893, 1969.
54. Jay SJ, Johanson WG Jr, Pierce AK: Respiratory complications of overdose with sedative drugs. Am Rev Respir Dis 112:591, 1975.
55. Johns MW: Self-poisoning with barbiturates in England and Wales during 1959–74. Br Med J 1:1128, 1977.
56. Hansen AR, Kennedy KA, Ambre JJ, et al: Glutethimide poisoning. A metabolite contributes to morbidity and mortality. N Engl J Med 292:250, 1975.
57. Matthew H, Proudfoot AT, Brown SS, et al: Acute poisoning: Organization and work-load of a treatment centre. Br Med J 3:489, 1969.

58. Clark TJH, Collins JV, Tong D: Respiratory depression caused by nitrazepam in patients with respiratory failure. Lancet 2:737, 1971.
59. Hall SC, Ovassapian A: Apnea after intravenous diazepam therapy. JAMA 238:1052, 1977.
60. Varma AJ, Fisher BK, Sarin MK: Diazepam-induced coma with bullae and eccrine sweat gland necrosis. Arch Intern Med 137:1207, 1977.
61. Biggs JT, Spiker DG, Petit JM, et al: Tricyclic antidepressant overdose. Incidence of symptoms. JAMA 238:135, 1977.
62. Teehan BP, Maher JF, Carey JJH, et al: Acute ethchlorvynol (Placidyl) intoxication. Ann Intern Med 72:875, 1970.
63. Leading article: Management of unconscious poisoned patients. Br Med J 2:647, 1969.
64. Maddock RK Jr, Bloomer HA: Meprobamate overdosage. Evaluation of its severity and methods of treatment. JAMA 201:123, 1967.
65. Neligan P, Harriman DGF, Pearce J: Respiratory arrest in familial hemiplegic migraine: A clinical and neuropathological study. Br Med J 2:732, 1977.
66. Weiner WJ, Goetz CG, Nausieda PA, et al: Respiratory dyskinesias: Extrapyramidal dysfunction and dyspnea. Ann Intern Med 88:327, 1978.
67. Goswami U, Channabasavanna SM: On the lethality of acute respiratory component of tardive dyskinesia. Clin Neurol Neurosurg 87:99, 1985.
68. Chiang E, Pitts WM, Rodriguez-Garcia M: Respiratory dyskinesia: Review and case reports. J Clin Psychiatry 46:232, 1985.
69. Kuna ST, Awan R: The irregularly irregular pattern of respiratory dyskinesia. Chest 90:779, 1986.
70. Cirignotta F, Lugaresi E, Montagna P: Breathing impairment in Rett syndrome. Am J Med Genet 24(suppl 1):167, 1986.
71. Lugaresi E, Cirignotta F, Montagna P: Abnormal breathing in the Rett syndrome. Brain Develop 7:329, 1985.
72. Bradley TD, Day A, Hyland RH, et al: Chronic ventilatory failure caused by abnormal respiratory pattern generation during sleep. Am Rev Respir Dis 130:678, 1984.
73. Southall DP, Kerr AM, Tirosh E, et al: Hyperventilation in the awake state: Potentially treatable component of Rett syndrome. Arch Dis Child 63:1039, 1988.
74. Severinghaus JW, Mitchell RA: Ondine's curse—Failure of respiratory center automaticity while awake. Clin Res 10:122, 1962.
75. Ahmad M, Cressman M, Tomashefski JF: Central alveolar hypoventilation syndromes. Arch Intern Med 140:29, 1980.
76. Mellins RB, Balfour HH Jr, Turino GM, et al: Failure of automatic control of ventilation (Ondine's curse): Report of an infant born with this syndrome and review of the literature. Medicine 49:487, 1970.
77. Naughton J, Block R, Welch M: Central alveolar hypoventilation: A case report. Am Rev Respir Dis 103:557, 1971.
78. Farmer WC, Glenn WW, Gee JB: Alveolar hypoventilation syndrome. Studies of ventilatory control in patients selected for diaphragm pacing. Am J Med 64:39, 1978.
79. Kryger MH: Central apnea. Arch Intern Med 142:1793, 1982.
80. Yasuma F, Nomura A, Sotobata I, et al: Congenital central alveolar hypoventilation (Ondine's curse): A case report and review of the literature. Eur J Pediatr 146:81, 1987.
81. Mather SJ: Ondine's curse and the anesthetist. Anaesthesia 42:394, 1987.
82. Beckerman R, Meltzer J, Sola A, et al: Brain-stem auditory response in Ondine's syndrome. Arch Neurol 43:698, 1986.
83. Long KJ, Allen N: Abnormal brain-stem auditory evoked potentials following Ondine's curse. Arch Neurol 41:1109, 1984.
84. Adickes ED, Buehler BA, Sanger WG: Familial lethal sleep apnea. Hum Genet 73:39, 1986.
85. Manon-Espaillat R, Gothe B, Adams N, et al: Familial "sleep apnea plus" syndrome; Report of a family. Neurology 38:190, 1988.
86. Cummiskey J, Guilleminault C, Davis R, et al: Automatic respiratory failure: Sleep studies and Leigh's disease (case report). Neurology 37:1876, 1987.
87. Hunter AR: Idiopathic alveolar hypoventilation in Leber's disease. Unusual sensitivity to mild analgesics and diazepam. Anaesthesia 39:781, 1984.
88. Paré JAP, Lowenstein L: Polycythemia associated with disturbed function of the respiratory center. Blood 2:1077, 1956.
89. Rodman T, Close HP: The primary hypoventilation syndrome. Am J Med 26:808, 1959.
90. Lawrence LT: Idiopathic hypoventilation, polycythemia, and cor pulmonale. Am Rev Respir Dis 80:575, 1959.
91. Rodman TR, Resnick ME, Berkowitz RD, et al: Alveolar hypoventilation due to involvement of the respiratory center by obscure disease of the central nervous system. Am J Med 32:208, 1962.
92. Tsitouris G, Fertakis A: Alveolar hypoventilation due to respiratory center dysfunction of unknown cause. Am J Med 39:173, 1965.
93. Grant JL, Arnold W Jr: Idiopathic hypoventilation. JAMA 194:119, 1965.
94. Richter T, West JR, Fishman AP: The syndrome of alveolar hypoventilation and diminished sensitivity of the respiratory center. N Engl J Med 256:1165, 1957.
95. Paine CJ, Hargrove MD Jr: Primary alveolar hypoventilation in a thin young woman. Chest 63:854, 1973.
96. Sukumalchantra Y, Tongmitr V, Tanphaichitr V, et al: Primary alveolar hypoventilation. A case report with hemodynamic study. Am Rev Respir Dis 98:1037, 1968.
97. Cohn JE, Kuida H: Primary alveolar hypoventilation associated with western equine encephalitis. Ann Intern Med 56:633, 1962.
98. White DP, Miller F, Erickson RW: Sleep apnea and nocturnal hypoventilation after western equine encephalitis. Am Rev Respir Dis 127:132, 1983.
99. Udwadia ZF, Athale S, Misra VP: Radiation necrosis causing failure of automatic ventilation during sleep with central sleep apnea. Chest 92:567, 1987.
100. Polatty RC, Cooper KR: Respiratory failure after percutaneous cordotomy. South Med J 79:897, 1986.
101. Beamish D, Wildsmith JA: Ondine's curse after carotid endarterectomy. Br Med J 2:1607, 1978.
102. O'Dell K, Staren E, Bassuk A: Total colonic aganglionosis (Zuelzer-Wilson syndrome) and congenital failure of automatic control of ventilation (Ondine's curse). J Pediatr Surg 22:1019, 1987.
103. Bradley TD, McNicholas WT, Rutherford R, et al: Clinical and physiologic heterogeneity of the central sleep apnea syndrome. Am Rev Respir Dis 134:217, 1986.
104. Raetzo MA, Junod AF, Kryger MH: Effect of aminophylline and relief from hypoxia on central sleep apnoea due to medullary damage. Bull Eur Physiopathol Respir 23:171, 1987.
105. McNicholas WT, Carter JL, Rutherford R, et al: Beneficial effect of oxygen in primary alveolar hypoventilation with central sleep apnea. Am Rev Respir Dis 125:773, 1982.
106. Hung CE, Inwood RJ, Shannon DC: Respiratory and nonrespiratory effects of doxapram in congenital hypoventilation syndrome. Am Rev Respir Dis 119:263, 1979.
107. Fodstad H, Anderson G, Blom S, et al: Phrenic nerve stimulation (diaphragm pacing) in respiratory paralysis. Appl Neurophysiol 48:351, 1985.
108. Vanderlinden RG, Epstein SW, Hyland RH, et al: Management of chronic ventilatory insufficiency with electrical diaphragm pacing. Can J Neurol Sci 15:63, 1988.
109. Wilcox PG, Paré PD, Fleetham JA: Conditioning of the diaphragm by phrenic nerve pacing in primary alveolar hypoventilation. Thorax 43:1017, 1988.
111. Barlow PB, Bartlett D, Hauri P, et al: Idiopathic hypoventilation syndrome: Importance of preventing nocturnal hypoxemia and hypercapnia. Am Rev Respir Dis 121:141, 1980.
112. Lugaresi E, Cirignotta F, Rossi PG, et al: Infantile behavioural regression and respiratory impairment. Neuropediatrics 15:211, 1984.
113. Schiller J: A note on the Pickwickian syndrome and Felix Platter (1536–1614). J Hist Med 40:66, 1985.
114. Kerr WJ, Lagen JB: The postural syndrome related to obesity leading to postural emphysema and cardiorespiratory failure. Ann Intern Med 10:569, 1936.
115. Burwell CS, Robin ED, Whaley RD, et al: Extreme obesity associated with alveolar hypoventilation—A Pickwickian syndrome. Am J Med 21:811, 1956.
116. Lopata M, Onal E: Mass loading, sleep apnea, and the pathogenesis of obesity hypoventilation. Am Rev Respir Dis 126:640, 1982.
117. Sugerman HJ: Pulmonary function in morbid obesity. Gastroenterol Clin North Am 16:225, 1987.
118. Phillipson EA: Pickwickian, obesity-hypoventilation, or Fee-Fi-Fo-Fum syndrome? Am Rev Respir Dis 121:781, 1980.
119. Sugerman HJ, Baron PL, Fairman RP, et al: Hemodynamic dysfunction in obesity hypoventilation syndrome and the effects of treatment with surgically induced weight loss. Ann Surg 207:604, 1988.
120. Drenick EJ, Baie GS, Seltzer F, et al: Excessive mortality and causes of death in morbidly obese men. JAMA 243:443, 1980.
121. Millman RP, Bevilacqua J, Peterson DD, et al: Central sleep apnea in hypothyroidism. Am Rev Respir Dis 127:504, 1983.
122. Weiner M, Chausow A, Szidon P: Reversible respiratory muscle weakness in hypothyroidism. Br J Dis Chest 80:391, 1986.
123. Skatrud J, Iber C, Ewart R, et al: Disordered breathing during sleep in hypothyroidism. Am Rev Respir Dis 124:325, 1981.
124. McNamara ME, Southwick SM, Fogel BS: Sleep apnea and hypothyroidism presenting as depression in two patients. J Clin Psychiatry 48:164, 1987.
125. Forester CF: Coma in myxedema. Report of a case and review of the world literature. Arch Intern Med 111:734, 1963.
126. Menendez CE, Rivlin RS: Thyrotoxic crisis and myxedema coma. Med Clin North Am 57:1463, 1973.
127. Massumi RA, Winnacker JJ: Severe depression of the respiratory center in myxedema. Am J Med 36:876, 1964.

21

128. Domm BM, Vassalo CL: Myxedema coma with respiratory failure. Am Rev Respir Dis 107:842, 1973.
129. Shear L, Brandman IS: Hypoxia and hypercapnia caused by respiratory compensation for metabolic alkalosis. Am Rev Respir Dis 107:836, 1973.
130. Shannon DC, Kelly DH: SIDS and near-SIDS (first of two parts). N Engl J Med 306:959, 1982.
131. Shannon DC, Kelly DH: SIDS and near-SIDS (second of two parts). N Engl J Med 306:1022, 1982.
132. Schiffman PL, Westlake RE, Santiago TV, et al: Ventilatory control in parents of victims of sudden-infant-death syndrome. N Engl J Med 302:486, 1980.
133. Schiffman PL, Remolina C, Westlake RE, et al: Ventilatory response to isocapnic hypoxia in parents of victims of sudden death syndrome. Chest 81:707, 1982.
134. Couriel JM, Olinsky A: Response to acute hypercapnia in the parents of victims of sudden infant death syndrome. Pediatrics 73:652, 1984.
135. Acres JC, Sweatman P, West P, et al: Breathing during sleep in parents of sudden infant death syndrome victims. Am Rev Respir Dis 125:163, 1982.
136. Myer EC, Morris DL, Adams ML, et al: Increased cerebrospinal fluid beta-endorphin immunoreactivity in infants with apnea and in siblings of victims of sudden infant death syndrome. J Pediatr 111:660, 1987.
137. Nugent CA, Harris HW, Cohn J, et al: Dyspnea as a symptom in Parkinson's syndrome. Am Rev Respir Dis 78:682, 1958.
138. Lilker ES, Woolf CR: Pulmonary function in Parkinson's syndrome: The effect of thalamotomy. Can Med Assoc J 99:752, 1968.
139. Fraser RS, Sproule BJ, Dvorkin J: Hypoventilation, cyanosis and polycythemia in a thin man. Can Med Assoc J 89:1178, 1963.
140. Garland T, Linderholm H: Hypoventilation syndrome in a case of chronic epidemic encephalitis. Acta Med Scand 162:333, 1958.
141. Darwish RY, Fairshter RD, Vaziri ND, et al: Hypoventilation in a case of nonfamilial Parkinson's disease. West J Med 143:383, 1985.
142. Apps MC, Sheaff PC, Ingram DA, et al: Respiration and sleep in Parkinson's disease. J Neurol Neurosurg Psychiatry 48:1240, 1985.
143. Vincken WG, Gauthier FG, Dollfuss RE, et al: Involvement of upper airway muscles in extrapyramidal disorders: A cause of air flow limitation. N Engl J Med 3311:438, 1984.
144. Estenne M, Hubert M, De Troyer A: Respiratory-muscle involvement in Parkinson's disease. N Engl J Med 311:1516, 1984.
145. Hovestadt A, Bogaard JM, Meerwaldt JD, et al: Pulmonary function in Parkinson's disease. J Neurol Neurosurg Psychiatry 52:329, 1989.
146. Obenour WH, Stevens PM, Cohen AA, et al: The causes of abnormal function in Parkinson's disease. Am Rev Respir Dis 105:382, 1972.
147. Langer H, Woolf CR: Changes in pulmonary function in Parkinson's syndrome after treatment with L-dopa. Am Rev Respir Dis 104:440, 1971.
148. Adams EB, Holloway R, Thambiran AK, et al: Usefulness of intermittent positive-pressure respiration in the treatment of tetanus. Lancet 2:1176, 1966.
149. Carrea R, Lanari A: Chronic effect of tetanus toxin applied locally to the cerebral cortex of the dog. Science 137:342, 1962.
150. Brooks VB, Asanuma H: Action of tetanus toxin in the cerebral cortex. Science 137:674, 1962.
151. Brooks VB, Curtis DR, Eccles JC: The action of tetanus toxin on the inhibition of motor-neurones. J Physiol 135:655, 1957.
152. Kerr JH, Corbett JL, Prys-Roberts C, et al: Involvement of the sympathetic nervous system in tetanus. Studies on 82 cases. Lancet 2:236, 1968.
153. Udwadia FE, Lall A, Udwadia ZF, et al: Tetanus and its complications: Intensive care and management experience in 150 Indian patients. Epidemiol Infect 99:675, 1987.
154. Lawrence JR, Sando MJW: Treatment of severe tetanus. Br Med J 2:113, 1959.
155. Wessler S, Avioli LA: Therapeutic grand round—No. 10. Tetanus. JAMA 207:123, 1969.
156. Smythe PM, Bull AB: Treatment of tetanus: With special reference to tracheotomy. Br Med J 2:732, 1961.
157. Edmondson RS, Flowers MW: Intensive care in tetanus: Management, complications, and mortality in 100 cases. Br Med J 1(6175):1401, 1979.
158. MacRae J: A new look at infectious diseases: Tetanus. Br Med J 1:730, 1973.
159. Editorial: Tetanus—Still here? N Engl J Med 280:614, 1969.
160. LaForce FM, Young LS, Bennett JV: Tetanus in the United States (1965–1966): Epidemiologic and clinical features. N Engl J Med 280:569, 1969.
161. Notcutt WG, Ashley D: Tetanus and inhalation of a foreign body. Br Med J 2:1193, 1977.
162. Heurich AE, Brust JCM, Richter RW: Management of urban tetanus. Med Clin North Am 57:1373, 1973.
163. Femi-Pearse D: Blood gas tensions, acid-base status, and spirometry in tetanus. Am Rev Respir Dis 110:390, 1974.
164. Femi-Pearse D, Afonja AO, Elegbeleye OO: Value of determination of oxygen consumption in tetanus. Br Med J 1:74, 1976.
165. Sandor F: Diaphragmatic respiration: A sign of cervical cord lesion in the unconscious patient ("horizontal paradox"). Br Med J 1:465, 1966.
166. Ledsome JR, Sharp JM: Pulmonary function in acute cervical cord injury. Am Rev Respir Dis 124:41, 1981.
167. McMichan JC, Michel L, Westbrook PR: Pulmonary dysfunction following traumatic quadriplegia. JAMA 243:528, 1980.
168. James WS, Minh V-D, Minteer MA, et al: Cervical accessory respiratory muscle function in a patient with a high cervical cord lesion. Chest 71:59, 1977.
169. Kuperman AS, Krieger AJ, Rosomoff HL: Respiratory function after cervical cordotomy. Chest 59:128, 1971.
170. Kuperman AS, Fernandez RB, Rosomoff HL: The potential hazard of oxygen after bilateral cordotomy. Chest 59:232, 1971.
171. Lahuerta J, Lipton S, Wells JC: Percutaneous cervical cordotomy: Results and complications in a recent series of 100 patients. Ann R Coll Surg Engl 67:41, 1985.
172. Rizvi SS, Ishikawa S, Faling LJ, et al: Defect in automatic respiration in a case of multiple sclerosis. Am J Med 56:433, 1974.
173. Yamamoto T, Imai T, Yamasaki M: Acute ventilatory failure in multiple sclerosis. J Neurol Sci 89:313, 1989.
174. Jaspar N, Kruger M, Ectors P, et al: Unilateral chest wall paradoxical motion mimicking a flail chest in a patient with hemilateral C7 spinal injury. Intensive Care Med 12:396, 1986.
175. Swanson GD, Whipp BJ, Kaufman RD, et al: Effect of hypercapnia on hypoxic ventilatory drive in carotid body-resected man. J Appl Physiol 45:971, 1978.
176. Wade JG, Larson CP Jr, Hickey RF, et al: Effect of carotid endarterectomy on carotid chemoreceptor and baroreceptor function in man. N Engl J Med 282:823, 1970.
177. Lugliani R, Whipp BJ, Seard C, et al: Effect of bilateral carotid-body resection on ventilatory control at rest and during exercise in man. N Engl J Med 285:1105, 1971.
178. Holton P, Wood JB: The effects of bilateral removal of the carotid bodies and denervation of the carotid sinuses in two human subjects. J Physiol (Lond) 181:365, 1965.
179. Honda Y, Myojo S, Hasegawa S, et al: Decreased exercise hyperpnea in patients with bilateral carotid chemoreceptor resection. J Appl Physiol 46:908, 1979.
180. Zikk D, Shanon E, Rapoport Y, et al: Sleep apnea following bilateral excision of carotid body tumors. Laryngoscope 93:1470, 1983.
181. Hines S, Houston M, Robertson D: The clinical spectrum of autonomic dysfunction. Am J Med 70:1091, 1981.
182. Bartels J, Mazzia VDB: Familial dysautonomia. JAMA 212:318, 1970.
183. Filler J, Smith AA, Stone S, et al: Respiratory control in familial dysautonomia. J Pediatr 66:509, 1965.
184. Brunt PW, McKusick VA: Familial dysautonomia: A report of genetic and clinical studies, with a review of the literature. Medicine 49:343, 1970.
185. Edelman NH, Cherniack NS, Lahiri S, et al: The effects of abnormal sympathetic nervous function upon the ventilatory response to hypoxia. J Clin Invest 49:1153, 1970.
186. Page MM, Watkins PJ: Cardiorespiratory arrest and diabetic autonomic neuropathy. Lancet 1:14, 1978.
187. Lloyd-Mostyn RH, Watkins PJ: Defective innervation of heart in diabetic autonomic neuropathy. Br J Med 3:15, 1975.
188. Montserrat JM, Cochrane GM, Wolf C, et al: Ventilatory control in diabetes mellitus. Eur J Respir Dis 67:112, 1985.
189. Silverstein D, Michlin B, Sobel HJ, et al: Right ventricular failure in a patient with diabetic neuropathy (myopathy) and central alveolar hypoventilation. Respiration 44:460, 1983.
190. Catterall JR, Calverley PM, Ewing DJ, et al: Breathing, sleep, and diabetic autonomic neuropathy. Diabetes 33:1025, 1984.
191. Bokinsky GE, Hudson LD, Weil JV: Impaired peripheral chemosensitivity and acute respiratory failure in Arnold-Chiari malformation and syringomyelia. N Engl J Med 288:947, 1973.
192. Bullock R, Todd NV, Easton J, et al: Isolated central respiratory failure due to syringomyelia and Arnold-Chiari malformation. Br Med J 297:1448, 1988.
193. Derenne JP, Macklem PT, Roussos CL: The respiratory muscles: Mechanics, control and pathophysiology. I. Am Rev Respir Dis 118:119, 1978. (II and III in press.)
194. Campbell EJM, Agostoni E, Newsom Davis J: The Respiratory Muscles: Mechanics and Neural Control. 2nd ed. Philadelphia, WB Saunders, 1970.
195. Loh L, Goldman M, Davis JN: The assessment of diaphragm function. Medicine 56:165, 1977.
196. Roussos C: The failing ventilatory pump. Lung 160:59, 1982.
197. Roussos C, Macklem PT: Diaphragmatic fatigue in man. J Appl Physiol 43:189, 1977.
198. Roussos C, Fixley M, Gross D, et al: Fatigue of inspiratory muscles and their synergic behavior. J Appl Physiol 46:897, 1979.

199. Bellemare F, Grassino A: Effect of pressure and timing of contraction on human diaphragm fatigue. J Appl Physiol 53:1190, 1982.
200. Bellemare F, Grassino A: Evaluation of human diaphragm fatigue. J Appl Physiol 53:1196, 1982.
201. Juan G, Calverley P, Talamo C, et al: Effect of carbon dioxide on diaphragmatic function in human beings. N Engl J Med 310:874, 1984.
202. Jardim J, Farkas G, Prefaut C, et al: The failing inspiratory muscles under normoxic and hypoxic conditions. Am Rev Respir Dis 124:274, 1981.
203. Cohen CA, Zagelbaum G, Gross E, et al: Clinical manifestations of inspiratory muscle fatigue. Am J Med 73:308, 1982.
204. Roussos C: Respiratory muscle fatigue in the hypercapnic patient. Bull Eur Physiopathol Respir 15:117, 1979.
205. Gross D, Grassino A, Ross WRD, et al: Electromyogram pattern of diaphragmatic fatigue. J Appl Physiol 46:1, 1979.
206. Esau SA, Bye PTP, Pardy RL: Changes in rate of relaxation of sniffs with diaphragmatic fatigue in humans. J Appl Physiol 55:731, 1983.
207. Levy RD, Esau SA, Bye PTP, et al: Relaxation rate of mouth pressure with sniffs at rest and with inspiratory muscle fatigue. Am Rev Respir Dis 130:38, 1984.
208. Mithoefer JC, Bossman OG, Thibault DW, et al: The clinical estimation of alveolar ventilation. Am Rev Respir Dis 98:868, 1968.
209. Grinman S, Whitelaw WA: Pattern of breathing in a case of generalized respiratory muscle weakness. Chest 84:770, 1983.
210. Miller A, Granada M: In-hospital mortality in the Pickwickian syndrome. Am J Med 56:144, 1974.
211. Harrison BDW, Collins JV, Brown KGE, et al: Respiratory failure in neuromuscular disease. Thorax 26:579, 1971.
212. Goldstein RL, Hyde RW, Lapham LW, et al: Peripheral neuropathy presenting with respiratory insufficiency as the primary complaint. Problem of recognizing alveolar hypoventilation due to neuromuscular disorders. Am J Med 56:443, 1974.
213. Spitzer SA, Korczyn AD, Kalaci J: Transient bilateral diaphragmatic paralysis. Chest 64:355, 1973.
214. Sandham JD, Shaw DT, Guenter CA: Acute supine respiratory failure due to bilateral diaphragmatic paralysis. Chest 72:96, 1977.
215. Newsom Davis J, Goldman M, Loh L, et al: Diaphragm function and alveolar hypoventilation. Q J Med 45:87, 1976.
216. Konno K, Mead J: Measurement of the separate volume changes of rib cage and abdomen during breathing. J Appl Physiol 22:407, 1967.
217. Black LF, Hyatt RE: Maximal static respiratory pressures in generalized neuromuscular disease. Am Rev Respir Dis 103:641, 1971.
218. Gibson GJ, Pride NB, Davis JN, et al: Pulmonary mechanics in patients with respiratory muscle weakness. Am Rev Respir Dis 115:389, 1977.
219. Delhez L: Modalités chez l'homme normal de la réponse électrique des piliers du diaphragme à la stimulation électrique des nerfs phréniques par des chocs uniques. Arch Int Physiol 73:832, 1965.
220. Newsom Davis J: Phrenic nerve conduction in man. J Neurol Neurosurg Psychiatry 30:420, 1967.
221. Saxton GA Jr, Rayson GE, Moody E, et al: Alveolar-arterial gas tension relationships in acute anterior poliomyelitis. Am J Med 30:871, 1961.
222. Steinborn KE, Zimdahl WT, Loeser WD: Chronic cor pulmonale in the respiratory poliomyelitis patient. Arch Intern Med 110:249, 1962.
223. Thomson AE: Electrolyte studies in the respiratory paralysis of poliomyelitis. Am J Med 22:549, 1957.
224. Cherniack RM, Ewart WB, Hildes JA: Polycythemia secondary to respiratory disturbances in poliomyelitis. Ann Intern Med 46:720, 1957.
225. Lane DJ, Hazleman B, Nichols PJR: Late onset respiratory failure in patients with previous poliomyelitis. Q J Med 43:551, 1974.
226. Fromm GB, Wisdom PJ, Block AJ: Amyotrophic lateral sclerosis presenting with respiratory failure—Diaphragmatic paralysis and dependence on mechanical ventilation in two patients. Chest 71:612, 1977.
227. Mayrignac C, Poirier J, Degos JD: Amyotrophic lateral sclerosis presenting with respiratory insufficiency as the primary complaint. Clinicopathological study of a case. Eur Neurol 24:115, 1985.
228. Hill R, Martin J, Hakim A: Acute respiratory failure in motor neuron disease. Arch Neurol 40:30, 1983.
229. Parhad IM, Clark AW, Barron KD, et al: Diaphragmatic paralysis in motor neuron disease. Report of two cases and a review of the literature. Neurology 28:18, 1978.
230. Nightingale S, Bates D, Bateman DE, et al: Enigmatic dyspnoea: An unusual presentation of motor-neurone disease. Lancet 1:933, 1982.
231. Kreitzer SM, Saunders NA, Tyler HR, et al: Respiratory muscle function in amyotrophic lateral sclerosis. Am Rev Respir Dis 117:437, 1978.
232. Brach BB: Expiratory flow patterns in amyotrophic lateral sclerosis. Chest 75:648, 1979.
233. Haas H, Johnson LR, Gill TH, et al: Diaphragm paralysis and

ventilatory failure in chronic proximal spinal muscular atrophy. Am Rev Respir Dis 123:465, 1981.
234. Braun SR, Sufit RL, Giovannoni R, et al: Intermittent negative pressure ventilation in the treatment of respiratory failure in progressive neuromuscular disease. Neurology 37:1874, 1987.
235. O'Donohue WJ, Baker JP, Bell GM, et al: Respiratory failure in neuromuscular disease management in a respiratory intensive care unit. JAMA 235:733, 1976.
236. Dowling PC, Menonna JP, Cook SD: Guillain-Barré syndrome in greater New York-New Jersey. JAMA 238:317, 1977.
237. Gracey DR, McMichan JC, Divertie MB, et al: Respiratory failure in Guillain-Barré syndrome: A 6-year experience. Mayo Clin Proc 57:742, 1982.
238. Sunderrajan EV, Davenport J: The Guillain-Barré syndrome: Pulmonary-neurologic correlations. Medicine (Baltimore) 64:333, 1985.
239. Ropper AH, Kehne SM: Guillain-Barré syndrome: Management of respiratory failure. Neurology 35:1662, 1985.
240. Hu-Sheng W, Qi-Fen Y, Tian-Ci L, et al: The treatment of acute polyradiculoneuritis with respiratory paralysis. Brain Develop 10:147, 1988.
241. Gourie-Devi M, Ganapathy GR: Phrenic nerve conduction time in Guillain-Barré syndrome. J Neurol Neurosurg Psychiatry 48:245, 1985.
242. Becker DM, Kramer S: The neurological manifestations of porphyria: A review. Medicine 56:411, 1977.
243. Doll SG, Bower AG, Affeldt JW: Acute intermittent porphyria with respiratory paralysis. JAMA 168:1973, 1958.
244. Sakamoto Y, Lockey RF, Krzanowski JJ: Shellfish and fish poisoning related to the toxic dinoflagellates. South Med J 80:866, 1987.
245. Ellis S: Introduction to symposium—Brevetoxins: Chemistry and pharmacology of "red tide" toxins from Ptychodiscus brevis (formerly Gymnodinium breve). Toxicon 23:469, 1985.
246. Pierce RH: Red tide (Ptychodiscus brevis) toxin aerosols: A review. Toxicon 24:955, 1986.
247. Ishida Y, Shibata S: Brevetoxin-B of Gymnodinium breve toxin-induced contractions of smooth muscles due to the transmitter release from nerves. Pharmacology 31:237, 1985.
248. Shimoda T, Krzanowski J, Nelson R, et al: In vitro red tide toxin effects on human bronchial smooth muscle. J Allergy Clin Immunol 81:1187, 1988.
249. Hughes JM, Merson MH: Fish and shellfish poisoning. N Engl J Med 295:1117, 1976.
250. Paralytic Shellfish Poisoning. Laboratory Center for Disease Control, Ottawa, Ontario. Canada Diseases Weekly Report 4:21, 1978.
251. Morris JG, Lewin P, Hargrett NT, et al: Clinical features of ciguatera fish poisoning—A study of the disease in the United States Virgin Islands. Arch Int Med 142:1090, 1982.
252. Lawrence DN, Enriquez MB, Lumish RM, et al: Ciguatera fish poisoning in Miami. JAMA 244:254, 1980.
253. Withers NW: Ciguatera fish poisoning. Ann Rev Med 33:97, 1982.
254. Morris JG: Ciguatera fish poisoning. JAMA 244:273, 1980.
255. Tatnall FM, Smith HG, Welsby PD, et al: Ciguatera poisoning. Br Med J 281:948, 1980.
256. Gray C: Mussel mystery: "The more you know, the more you don't know." Can Med Assoc J 138:350, 1988.
257. Mills AR, Passmore R: Pelagic paralysis. Lancet 1:161, 1988.
258. Walker DG: Survival after severe envenomation by the blue-ringed octopus (Hepalochlaena maculosa). Med J Aust 2:663, 1983.
259. Karalliedde LD, Sanmuganathan PS: Respiratory failure following envenomation. Anesthesia 43:753, 1988.
260. Watt G, Padre L, Tauzon L, et al: Bites of the Philippine cobra (Naja naja philippinensis): Prominent neurotoxicity with minimal local signs. Am J Trop Med Hyg 39:306, 1988.
261. Kitchens CS, Van Mierop LH: Envenomation by the Eastern coral snake (Micrurus fulvius fulvius). A study of 39 victims. JAMA 258:1615, 1987.
262. Tibballs J, Cooper SJ: Paralysis with Ixodes cornuatus envenomation. Med J Aust 145:37, 1986.
263. Rivett K, Potgieter PD: Diaphragmatic paralysis after organophosphate poisoning. S Afr Med J 72:881, 1987.
264. Engel AG, Lambert EH, Howard FM Jr: Immune complexes (IgG and C3) at the motor end-plate in myasthenia gravis: Ultrastructural and light microscopic localization and electrophysiologic correlations. Mayo Clin Proc 52:267, 1977.
265. Toyka KV, Drachman DB, Griffin DE, et al: Myasthenia gravis: Study of humoral immune mechanisms by passive transfer to mice. N Engl J Med 296:125, 1977.
266. Drachman DB, Adams RN, Josifek LF, et al: Functional activities of autoantibodies to acetylcholine receptors and the clinical severity of myasthenia gravis. N Engl J Med 307:769, 1982.
267. Dua PC: Respiratory failure in myasthenia gravis; use of plasmapheresis. Chest 85:721, 1984.
268. Chagnac Y, Hadani M, Goldhammer Y: Myasthenic crisis after intravenous administration of iodinated contrast agent. Neurology 35:1219, 1985.

21

1

269. Editorial: Suxamethonium apnoea. Lancet 1:246, 1973.
270. De Troyer A, Broestein S: Acute changes in respiratory mechanics after pyridostigmine injection in patients with myasthenia gravis. Am Rev Respir Dis 121:629, 1980.
271. Radwan L, Strugalska M, Koziorowski A: Changes in respiratory muscle function after neostigmine injection in patients with myasthenia gravis. Eur Res J 1:119, 1988.
272. Shale DJ, Lane DJ, David CJF: Air-flow limitation in myasthenia gravis—The effect of acetylcholinesterase inhibitor therapy on air-flow limitation. Am Rev Respir Dis 128:618, 1983.
273. Newball HH, Brahim SA: Effects of alternate-day prednisone therapy on respiratory function in myasthenia gravis. Thorax 31:410, 1976.
274. Gracey DR, Howard FM, Divertie MB: Plasmapheresis in the treatment of ventilator-dependent myasthenia gravis patients. Report of four cases. Chest 85:739, 1984.
275. Dau PC, Lindstrom JM, Cassel CK, et al: Plasmapheresis and immunosuppressive drug therapy in myasthenia gravis. N Engl J Med 297:1134, 1977.
276. Selecky PA, Ziment I: Prolonged respiratory support for the treatment of intractable myasthenia gravis. Chest 65:207, 1974.
277. Booker HE, Chun RWM, Sanguino M: Myasthenia gravis syndrome associated with trimethadione. JAMA 212:2262, 1970.
278. Lang B, Newsom Davis J, Wray D, et al: Autoimmune aetiology for myasthenic (Eaton-Lambert) syndrome. Lancet 2:224, 1981.
279. Dropcho EJ, Stanton C, Oh SJ: Neuronal antinuclear antibodies in a patient with Lambert-Eaton myasthenic syndrome and small-cell lung carcinoma. Neurology 39:249, 1989.
280. Lindesmith LA, Baines D Jr, Bigelow DB, et al: Reversible respiratory paralysis associated with polymyxin therapy. Ann Intern Med 68:318, 1968.
281. Foldes FF, Lunn JN, Benz HG: Prolonged respiratory depression caused by drug combinations. Muscle relaxants and intraperitoneal antibiotics as etiologic agents. JAMA 183:672, 1963.
282. Editorial: Antibiotic-induced myasthenia. JAMA 204:164, 1968.
283. Davidson EW, Modell JH, Moya F, et al: Respiratory depression after antibiotic use in pleural and pseudocyst cavities. JAMA 196:456, 1966.
284. Pridgen JE: Respiratory arrest thought to be due to intraperitoneal neomycin. Surgery 40:571, 1956.
285. Fisk GC: Respiratory paralysis after a large dose of streptomycin. Report of a case. Br Med J 1:556, 1961.
286. Timmerman JC, Long JP, Pittinger CB: Neuromuscular blocking properties of various antibiotic agents. Toxicol Appl Pharmacol 1:299, 1959.
287. Adamson RH, Marshall FN, Long JP: Neuromuscular blocking properties of various polypeptide antibiotics. Proc Soc Exp Biol Med 105:494, 1960.
288. Ream CR: Respiratory and cardiac arrest after intravenous administration of kanamycin with reversal of toxic effects by neostigmine. Ann Intern Med 59:384, 1963.
289. Koch-Weser J, Sidel VW, Federman EB, et al: Adverse effects of sodium colistimethate. Manifestations and specific reaction rates during 317 courses of therapy. Ann Intern Med 72:857, 1970.
290. Emery ERJ: Neuromuscular blocking properties of antibiotics as a cause of post-operative apnoea. Anaesthesia 18:57, 1963.
291. Masters CL, Dawkins RL, Zilko PJ, et al: Penicillamine-associated myasthenia gravis, antiacetylcholine receptor and antistriational antibodies. Am J Med 63:689, 1977.
292. Dale RC, Schroeder ET: Respiratory paralysis during treatment of hypertension with trimethaphan camsylate. Arch Intern Med 136:816, 1976.
293. Namba T, Nolte CT, Jackrel J, et al: Poisoning due to organophosphate insecticides. Acute and chronic manifestations. Am J Med 50:475, 1971.
294. Hunter D: Devices for the protection of the worker against injury and disease. Part II. Br Med J 1:506, 1950.
295. Koenig MG, Spickard A, Cardella MA, et al: Clinical and laboratory observations on type E botulism in man. Medicine 43:517, 1964.
296. Armstrong RW, Stenn F, Dowell VR Jr, et al: Type E botulism from home-canned gefilte fish. JAMA 210:303, 1969.
297. Kao I, Drachman DB, Price DL: Botulinum toxin: Mechanism of a presynaptic blockade. Science 193:1256, 1976.
298. Koenig MG, Drutz DJ, Mushlin AI, et al: Type B botulism in man. Am J Med 42:208, 1967.
299. Wilcox P, Andolfatto G, Fairbarn MS, et al: Long-term follow-up of symptoms, pulmonary function, respiratory muscle strength, and exercise performance after botulism. Chest (in press).
300. Lewis SW, Pierson DJ, Cary JM, et al: Prolonged respiratory paralysis in wound botulism. Chest 75:59, 1979.
301. MacDonald KL, Rutherford GW, Friedman SM, et al: Botulism and botulism-like illness in chronic drug abusers. Ann Intern Med 102:616, 1985.
302. Whittaker RL, Gilbertson RB, Garrett AS: Botulism type E, report of eight simultaneous cases. Ann Intern Med 61:448, 1964.
303. Terranova W, Palumbo JN, Breman JG: Ocular findings in botulism type B. JAMA 241:475, 1979.
304. Schmidt-Nowara WW, Samet JM, Rosario PA: Early and late pulmonary complications of botulism. Arch Intern Med 143:451, 1983.
305. Begin R, Bureau M, Lupien L, et al: Control of breathing in Duchenne's muscular dystrophy. Am J Med 69:227, 1980.
306. Kilburn KH, Eagan JT, Sieker HO, et al: Cardiopulmonary insufficiency in myotonic and progressive muscular dystrophy. N Engl J Med 261:1089, 1959.
307. Kilburn KH, Eagan JT, Heyman A: Cardiopulmonary insufficiency associated with myotonic dystrophy. Am J Med 26:929, 1959.
308. McCormack WM, Spalter HF: Muscular dystrophy, alveolar hypoventilation, and papilledema. JAMA 197:957, 1966.
309. Gillam PMS, Heaf PJD, Kaufman L, et al: Respiration in dystrophia myotonica. Thorax 19:112, 1964.
310. Skatrud J, Iber C, McHugh W, et al: Determinants of hypoventilation during wakefulness and sleep in diaphragmatic paralysis. Am Rev Respir Dis 121:587, 1980.
311. Cirignotta F, Mondini S, Zucconi M, et al: Sleep-related breathing impairment in myotonic dystrophy. J Neurol 235:80, 1987.
312. Yasukohchi S, Yagi Y, Akabane T, et al: Facioscapulohumeral dystrophy associated with sensorineural hearing loss, tortuosity of retinal arterioles, and an early onset and rapid progression of respiratory failure. Brain Develop 10:319, 1988.
313. Cannon PJ: The heart and lungs in myotonic muscular dystrophy. Am J Med 32:765, 1962.
314. Begin R, Bureau MA, Lupien L: Control and modulation of respiration in Steinert's myotonic dystrophy. Am Rev Respir Dis 121:281, 1980.
315. Begin R, Bureau MA, Lupien L, et al: Pathogenesis of respiratory insufficiency in myotonic dystrophy—The mechanical factors. Am Rev Respir Dis 125:312, 1982.
316. Jammes Y, Pouget J, Grimaud C, et al: Pulmonary function and electromyographic study of respiratory muscles in myotonic dystrophy. Muscle Nerve 8:586, 1985.
317. Bach JR, O'Brien J, Krotenberg R, et al: Management of end stage respiratory failure in Duchenne muscular dystrophy. Muscle Nerve 10:177, 1987.
318. Engel AG, Gomez MR, Seybold ME, et al: The spectrum and diagnosis of acid maltase deficiency. Neurology 23:95, 1973.
319. Rosenow EC, Engel AG: Acid maltase deficiency in adults presenting as respiratory failure. Am J Med 64:485, 1978.
320. Bellamy D, Newsom Davis J, Hickey BP, et al: A case of primary alveolar hypoventilation associated with mild proximal myopathy. Am Rev Respir Dis 112:867, 1975.
321. Kolodny EH: Current concepts: Lysosomal storage diseases. N Engl J Med 294:1217, 1976.
322. Lightman NI, Schooley RT: Adult-onset acid maltase deficiency—Case report of an adult with severe respiratory difficulty. Chest 72:250, 1977.
323. Papapetropoulos T, Paschalis C, Manda P: Myopathy due to juvenile acid maltase deficiency affecting exclusively the type I fibres. J Neurol Neurosurg Psychiatry 47:213, 1984.
324. Lenders MB, Martin JJ, de Barsy T, et al: Acid maltase deficiency in adults. A study of five cases. Acta Neurol Belg 86:152, 1986.
325. Trend PS, Wiles CM, Spencer GT, et al: Acid maltase deficiency in adults. Diagnosis and management in five cases. Brain 108:845, 1985.
326. Keunen RW, Lambregts PC, Op de Coul AA, et al: Respiratory failure as initial symptom of acid maltase deficiency. J Neurol Neurosurg Psychiatry 47:549, 1984.
327. Brownwell AKW, Gilbert JJ, Shaw TT, et al: Adult onset nemaline myopathy. Neurology 28:1306, 1978.
328. Harati Y, Niakan E, Bloom K, et al: Adult onset of nemaline myopathy presenting as diaphragmatic paralysis. J Neurol Neurosurg Psychiatry 50:108, 1987.
329. Maayan C, Springer C, Armon Y, et al: Nemaline myopathy as a cause of sleep hypoventilation. Pediatrics 77:390, 1986.
330. Dodson RF, Crisp GO, Nicotra B, et al: Rod myopathy with extensive systemic and respiratory muscular involvement. Ultrastruct Pathol 5:129, 1983.
331. Riley DJ, Santiago TV, Daniele RP, et al: Blunted respiratory drive in congenital myopathy. Am J Med 63:459, 1977.
332. Gibson GJ, Edmonds JP, Hughes GRV: Diaphragm function and lung involvement in systemic lupus erythematosus. Am J Med 63:926, 1977.
333. Wilcox PG, Stein HB, Clarke SD, et al: Phrenic nerve function in patients with diaphragmatic weakness and systemic lupus erythematosus. Chest 93:353, 1988.
334. Worth H, Grahn S, Lakomek HJ, et al: Lung function disturbances versus respiratory muscle fatigue in patients with systemic lupus erythematosus. Respiration 53:81, 1988.
335. Gibson T, Myers AR: Nervous system involvement in systemic lupus erythematosus. Ann Rheum Dis 35:398, 1976.

336. Isenberg DA, Snaith ML: Muscle disease in systemic lupus erythematosus: A study of its nature, frequency, and cause. J Rheumatol 8:917, 1981.
337. Williams TJ, O'Hehir RE, Czarny D, et al: Acute myopathy in severe acute asthma treated with intravenously administered corticosteroids. Am Rev Respir Dis 137:460, 1988.
338. Borman JB, Davidson JT, Blondheim SH: Idiopathic rhabdomyolysis (myoglobinuria) as an acute respiratory problem. Br Med J 2:726, 1963.
339. Berenson M, Yarvote P, Grace WJ: Idiopathic myoglobinuria with respiratory paralysis. Am Rev Respir Dis 94:956, 1966.
340. Taverner D, Zardawi IM, Walls J: Acute ventilatory failure and myoglobinuria. Neurology 34:369, 1984.
341. Prockop LD, Engel WK, Shug AL: Nearly fatal muscle carnitine deficiency with full recovery after replacement therapy. Neurology 33:1629, 1983.
342. Newman JH, Neff TA, Ziporin P: Acute respiratory failure associated with hypophosphatemia. N Engl J Med 296:1101, 1977.
343. Aubier M, Murcino D, Legocquic Y, et al: Effect of hypophosphatemia on diaphragmatic contractility in patients with acute respiratory failure. N Engl J Med 31:420, 1985.
344. Varsano S, Shapiro M, Taragan R, et al: Hypophosphatemia as a reversible cause of refractory ventilatory failure. Crit Care Med 11:908, 1983.
345. Fisher J, Magid N, Kallman C, et al: Respiratory illness and hypophosphatemia. Chest 83:504, 1983.
346. Lewis JF, Hodsman AB, Driedger AA, et al: Hypophosphatemia and respiratory failure: Prolonged abnormal energy metabolism demonstrated by nuclear magnetic resonance spectroscopy. Am J Med 83:1139, 1987.
347. Fischer DS, Nichol BA: Intraventricular conduction defect and respiratory tract paralysis in diabetic ketoacidosis. Am J Med 35:123, 1963.
348. Dorin RI, Crapo LM: Hypokalemic respiratory arrest in diabetic ketoacidosis. JAMA 257:1517, 1987.
349. Hermann RA, Mead AW, Spritz N, et al: Hypopotassemia with respiratory paralysis. Case due to renal tubular acidosis. Arch Intern Med 108:925, 1961.
350. Jenny DB, Goris GB, Urwiller RD, et al: Hypermagnesemia following irrigation of renal pelvis. Cause of respiratory depression. JAMA 240:1378, 1978.
351. Ferdinandus J, Pederson JA, Whang R: Hypermagnesemia as a cause of refractory hypotension, respiratory depression, and coma. Arch Intern Med 141:669, 1981.
352. Rodman T, Sobel M, Close HP: Arterial oxygen unsaturation and the ventilation-perfusion defect of Laënnec's cirrhosis. N Engl J Med 263:73, 1960.
353. Heinemann HO, Emirgil C, Mijnssen JP: Hyperventilation and arterial hypoxemia in cirrhosis of the liver. Am J Med 28:239, 1960.
354. Abelmann WH, Kramer GE, Verstraeten JM, et al: Cirrhosis of the liver and decreased arterial oxygen saturation. Arch Intern Med 108:34, 1961.
355. Rodman T, Hurwitz JK, Paston BH, et al: Cyanosis clubbing and arterial oxygen unsaturation associated with Laënnec's cirrhosis. Am J Med Sci 238:534, 1959.
356. Shaldon S, Ceasar J, Chiandussi L, et al: The demonstration of porta-pulmonary anastomoses in portal cirrhosis with the use of radioactive krypton (Kr-85). N Engl J Med 265:410, 1961.
357. Berthelot P, Walker JG, Sherlocks S, et al: Arterial changes in the lungs in cirrhosis of the liver—Lung spider nevi. N Engl J Med 274:291, 1966.
358. Freeman LJ, Nixon PG: Are coronary artery spasm and progressive damage to the heart associated with the hyperventilation syndrome? Br Med J 291:851, 1985.
359. Furukawa T, Hara N, Yasumoto K, et al: Arterial hypoxemia in patients with hepatic cirrhosis. Am J Med Sci 287:10, 1984.
360. Ruff F, Hughes JMB, Stanley N, et al: Regional lung function in patients with hepatic cirrhosis. J Clin Invest 50:2403, 1971.
361. Krowka MJ, Cortese DA: Pulmonary aspects of chronic liver disease and liver transplantation. Mayo Clin Proc 60:407, 1985.
362. Sherlock S: The liver-lung interface. Semin Respir Med 9:247, 1988.
363. Mélot C, Naeije R, Dechamps P, et al: Pulmonary and extrapulmonary contributors to hypoxemia in liver cirrhosis. Am Rev Respir Dis 139:632, 1989.
364. Schaefer JW, Reeves JT: The lung and the liver. Chest 80:526, 1981.
365. Picklemann JR, Evans LS, Kane JM, et al: Tuberculosis after jejunoileal bypass for obesity. JAMA 234:744, 1975.
366. Wolfe JD, Taskin DP, Holly FE, et al: Hypoxemia of cirrhosis. Detection of abnormal small pulmonary vascular channels by a quantitative radionuclide method. Am J Med 63:746, 1977.
367. Chen NS, Barnett CA, Farrer PA: Reversibility of intrapulmonary arteriovenous shunts in liver cirrhosis documented by serial radionuclide perfusion lung scans. Clin Nucl Med 9:279, 1984.
368. Shub C, Tajik AJ, Seward JB, et al: Detecting intrapulmonary right to left shunt with contrast echocardiography: Observations in a patient with diffuse pulmonary arteriovenous fistulas. Mayo Clin Proc 51:81, 1976.
369. Krowka MJ, Cortese DA: Severe hypoxemia associated with liver disease: Mayo Clinic experience and the experimental use of almitrine bismesylate. Mayo Clin Proc 62:164, 1987.
370. Stanley MN, Woodgate DJ: Mottled chest radiograph and gas transfer defect in chronic liver disease. Thorax 27:315, 1972.
371. Robin ED, Horn B, Goris ML, et al: Detection, quantitation and pathophysiology of lung "spiders." Trans Assoc Am Physicians 88:202, 1975.
372. Robin ED, Laman D, Horn BR, et al: Platypnea related to orthodeoxia caused by true vascular shunts. N Engl J Med 294:941, 1976.
373. Kennedy TC, Knudson RJ: Exercise-aggravated hypoxemia and orthodeoxia in cirrhosis. Chest 72:305, 1977.
374. Brownstein MH, Ballard HS: Hepatoma associated with erythrocytosis. Report of eleven new cases. Am J Med 40:204, 1966.
375. Palmer KNV, Gardiner AJS, McGregor MH: Hypoxaemia after partial gastrectomy. Thorax 20:73, 1965.
376. Diament ML, Palmer KNV: Postoperative changes in gas tensions of arterial blood and in ventilatory function. Lancet 2:180, 1966.
377. Diament ML, Palmer KNV: Venous/arterial pulmonary shunting as the principal cause of postoperative hypoxemia. Lancet 1:15, 1967.
378. Harris JC, Rumack BH, Peterson RG, et al: Methemoglobinemia resulting from absorption of nitrates. JAMA 242:2869, 1979.
379. Jaffé ER: Hereditary methemoglobinemias associated with abnormalities in the metabolism of erythrocytes. Am J Med 41:786, 1966.
380. Wetherhold JM, Linch AL, Charsha RC: Chemical cyanosis—Causes, effects, prevention. Arch Environ Health 1:353, 1960.
381. Simmel ER: Methemoglobinemia due to aminosalicylic acid (PAS). Am Rev Respir Dis 85:105, 1962.
382. Comly HH: Cyanosis in infants caused by nitrates in well water. JAMA 129:112, 1945.
383. Carlson DJ, Shapiro FL: Methemoglobinemia from well water nitrates: A complication of home dialysis. Ann Intern Med 73:757, 1970.
384. Ternberg JL, Luce E: Methemoglobinemia: A complication of the silver nitrate treatment of burns. Surgery 63:328, 1968.
385. Strauch B, Buch W, Grey W, et al: Successful treatment of methemoglobinemia secondary to silver nitrate therapy. N Engl J Med 281:257, 1969.
386. Finch CA: Methemoglobinemia and sulfhemoglobinemia. N Engl J Med 239:470, 1948.
387. Douglas WW, Fairbanks VF: Methemoglobinemia induced by a topical anesthetic spray (Cetacaine). Chest 71:587, 1977.
388. O'Donohue WJ, Moss LM, Angelillo VA: Acute methemoglobinemia induced by topical benzocaine and lidocaine. Arch Intern Med 140:1508, 1980.
389. Editorial: Carbon monoxide poisoning—A timely warning. N Engl J Med 278:849, 1968.
390. Jackson DL, Menges H: Accidental carbon monoxide poisoning. JAMA 243:772, 1980.
391. Fisher J, Rubin KP: Occult carbon monoxide poisoning. Arch Intern Med 142:1270, 1982.
392. Swada Y, Takahashi M, Ohashi N, et al: Computerized tomography as an indication of long-term outcome after acute carbon monoxide poisoning. Lancet 1:783, 1980.
393. Fein A, Grossman RF, Gareth Jones J, et al: Carbon monoxide effect on alveolar epithelial permeability. Chest 78:726, 1980.
394. Hopkinson JM, Pearce PJ, Oliver JS: Carbon monoxide poisoning mimicking gastroenteritis. Br Med J 281:214, 1980.
395. Goldman AL: Carboxyhemoglobin levels in primary and secondary cigar and pipe smokers. Chest 72:33, 1977.
396. Turner JAM, Sillett RW, McNicol MW: Effect of cigar smoking on carboxyhaemoglobin and plasma nicotine concentration in primary pipe and cigar smokers and ex-cigarette smokers. Br Med J 2:1387, 1977.
397. Jabara JW, Keefe TJ, Beaulieu HJ, et al: Carbon monoxide—Dosimetry in occupational exposures in Denver, Colorado. Arch Environ Health 35:198, 1980.
398. Froman C, Smith AC: Hyperventilation associated with low pH of cerebrospinal fluid after intracranial haemorrhage. Lancet 1:780, 1966.
399. Morse SR, Chandrasekhar AJ, Cugell DW: Cheyne-Stokes respiration redefined. Chest 66:345, 1974.
400. Cherniack NS, Longobardo GS: Cheyne-Stokes breathing: An instability in physiologic control. N Engl J Med 288:952, 1973.
401. Cherniack NS: Commentary: Abnormal breathing patterns, their mechanisms and clinical significance. JAMA 230:57, 1974.
402. Gotoh F, Meyer JS, Takagi Y: Cerebral venous and arterial blood gases during Cheyne-Stokes respiration. Am J Med 47:534, 1969.
403. Findley LJ, Zwillich CW, Ancoli-Israel S, et al: Cheyne-Stokes breathing during sleep in patients with left ventricular heart failure. South Med J 78:11, 1985.

21

404. Brown HW, Plum F: The neurologic basis of Cheyne-Stokes respiration. Am J Med *30*:849, 1961.
405. Karp HR, Sieker HO, Heyman A: Cerebral circulation and function in Cheyne-Stokes respiration. Am J Med *30*:861, 1961.
406. Findley LJ, Blackburn MR, Goldberger AL, et al: Apneas and oscillation of cardiac ectopy in Cheyne-Stokes breathing during sleep. Am Rev Respir Dis *130*:937, 1984.
407. Lewis RA, Howell JBL: Definition of the hyperventilation syndrome. Bull Eur Physiopathol Respir *22*:201, 1986.
408. Moss PD, McEvedy CP: An epidemic of overbreathing among schoolgirls. Br Med J *2*:1295, 1966.
409. Ley R: Panic disorder and agoraphobia: Fear of fear or fear of the symptoms produced by hyperventilation? J Behav Ther Exp Psychiat *18*:305, 1987.
410. Rice RL: Symptom patterns of the hyperventilation syndrome. Am J Med *8*:691, 1950.
411. Bass C, Gardner WN: Respiratory and psychiatric abormalities in chronic symptomatic hyperventilation. Br Med J *290*:1387, 1985.
412. Nisam M, Albertson TE, Panacek E, et al: Effects of hyperventilation on conjunctival oxygen tension in humans. Crit Care Med *14*:12, 1986.
413. Coyle PK, Sternman AP: Focal neurologic symptoms in panic attacks. Am J Psychiatry *143*:648, 1986.
414. Blau JN, Dexter SL: Hyperventilation in migraine attacks. Br Med J *280*:1254, 1980.
415. Magarian GJ, Olney RK: Absence spells. Hyperventilation syndrome as a previously unrecognized cause. Am J Med *76*:905, 1984.
416. Tavel ME: Hyperventilation syndrome with unilateral somatic symptoms. JAMA *187*:301, 1964.
417. Aronson PR: Hyperventilation syndrome. A comparative study of the effects of tranquilizers and a sedative upon the electrocardiogram. Clin Pharmacol Ther *5*:553, 1964.
418. Heckerling PS, Hanashiro PK: ST segment elevation in hyperventilation syndrome. Ann Emerg Med *14*:1122, 1985.
419. Motoyama EK, Rivard G, Acheson F, et al: Adverse effect of maternal hyperventilation on the foetus. Lancet *1*:286, 1966.
420. Annotations: Hyperventilation and foetal acidosis. Lancet *2*:1401, 1966.
421. Eichenholz A: Respiratory alkalosis. Arch Intern Med *116*:699, 1965.
422. Huckabee WE: Abnormal resting blood lactate. II. Lactate acidosis. Am J Med *30*:840, 1961.
423. Dossetor JB, Zborowski D, Dixon HB, et al: Hyperlactatemia due to hyperventilation: Use of CO inhalation. Ann NY Acad Sci *119*:1153, 1965.
424. Papadopoulos CN, Keats AS: The metabolic acidosis of hyperventilation produced by controlled respiration. Anesthesiology *20*:156, 1959.
425. Bates JH, Adamson JS, Pierce JA: Death after voluntary hyperventilation. N Engl J Med *274*:1371, 1966.
426. Anderson RJ, Potts DE, Gabow PA, et al: Unrecognized adult salicylate intoxication. Ann Intern Med *85*:745, 1976.
427. Alexander JK, Spalter HF, West JR: Modification of the respiratory response to carbon dioxide by salicylates. J Clin Invest *34*:533, 1955.
428. Rossing TH, Boixeda D, Maffeo N, et al: Hyperventilation with hypoproteinemia. J Lab Clin Med *112*:553, 1988.

Appendix

TABLE A–1

HOMOGENEOUS OPACITIES WITHOUT RECOGNIZABLE SEGMENTAL DISTRIBUTION

This pattern is epitomized by acute airspace pneumonia caused by *Streptococcus pneumoniae*. Typically the inflammation begins in the subpleural parenchyma and spreads centrifugally through pores of Kohn; since segmental boundaries do not impede such spread, consolidation tends to be nonsegmental. An air bronchogram is almost invariable and should not be misinterpreted as evidence of inhomogeneity. If the distribution of the disease is roughly segmental (for example, when acute airspace pneumonia fills a whole lobe), the presence of an air bronchogram should take precedence over apparent segmental distribution in suggesting the pathogenesis and therefore the etiology of the disease.

The nonsegmental character of parenchymal consolidation relates largely to its pathogenesis. For example, the volume of lung affected by acute irradiation pneumonitis corresponds roughly to the area irradiated, with little tendency to segmental or lobar distribution.

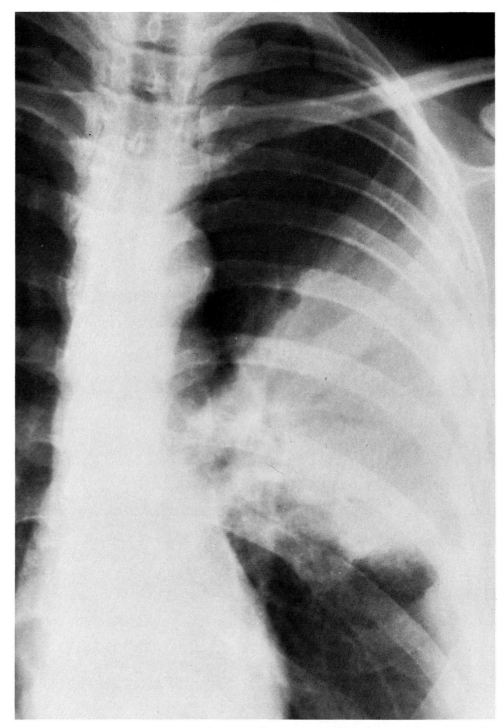

Figure 1. Homogeneous Nonsegmental Consolidation: Acute Pneumococcal Pneumonia. A view of the left hemithorax from a posteroanterior roentgenogram reveals consolidation of the axillary zone of the left upper lobe; the consolidation is homogeneous except for a well-defined air bronchogram. There is no loss of volume. The spreading margins are fairly sharply circumscribed despite the fact that they do not abut against a fissure. This pattern is virtually pathognomonic of acute airspace pneumonia, most commonly caused by *Streptococcus pneumoniae.*

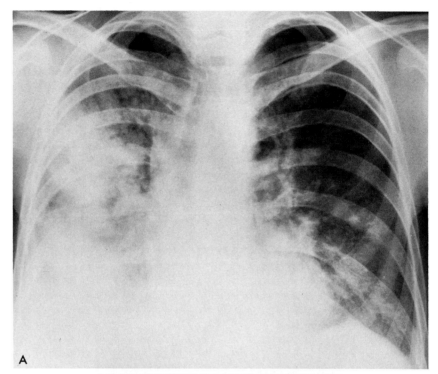

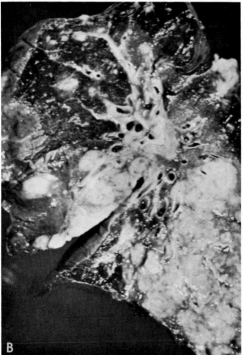

Figure 2. Homogeneous Nonsegmental Consolidation: Hodgkin's Disease. A posteroanterior roentgenogram *(A)* reveals extensive consolidation of much of the right lung, particularly its lower two thirds: the consolidation possesses no clear-cut segmental distribution. An air bronchogram is present. There is little, if any, loss of volume. Patchy shadows of a similar nature can be identified in the lower portion of the left lung. A photograph of a cut section of the right lung removed at necropsy *(B)* shows extensive replacement of the lower and middle lobes by Hodgkin's tissue; the nonsegmental distribution is indicated by the lack of involvement of portions of the superior and anterior segments of the lower lobe. The patient was a 27-year-old woman.

A–1
Homogeneous Opacities Without Recognizable Segmental Distribution

	ETIOLOGY	LOSS OF VOLUME	ANATOMIC DISTRIBUTION
DEVELOPMENTAL	Pulmonary arteriovenous fistula	0	Lower lobe predilection.
INFECTIOUS	**Bacteria**		
	Streptococcus pneumoniae.	0 to +	Influence of gravity; therefore dependent portions of upper and lower lobes. Usually unilobar.
	Klebsiella-Enterobacter-Serratia species.	Tendency to expansion of involved lung, although volume may be normal or even reduced.	Upper lobe predilection; often multilobar.
	Mycobacterium tuberculosis (primary).	0 to +	Slightly more frequent in upper lobes; no predilection for either anterior or posterior segments.
	Mycobacterium tuberculosis (postprimary).	0 to +	Upper lobe predilection, predominantly posterior (influence of gravity on endobronchial spread).
	Francisella tularensis (tularemia).	0	No lobar predilection; may be multilobar.
	Legionella pneumophila.	0 to +	Usually unilateral and unilobar when first seen, with tendency to multilobar and bilateral involvement with time. Lower lobe predilection.
	Pseudomonas aeruginosa.	0	Generalized or nonspecific.
	Pseudomonas pseudomallei.	0	Single or multiple lobes.
	Haemophilus influenzae.	0	No lobar predilection.
	Yersinia pestis (the Black Plague).	0	No lobar predilection.
	Anaerobic bacteria.	0	Posterior portion of upper or lower lobes.
	Escherichia coli.	0	Strong lower lobe anatomic bias, usually multilobar.
	Actinomyces israelii (actinomycosis). *Nocardia* species (nocardiosis).	0	Lower lobe predilection, often bilateral.

A–1
Homogeneous Opacities Without Recognizable Segmental Distribution *(Continued)*

ADDITIONAL FINDINGS	COMMENTS
Fairly extensive racemose opacity, ill-defined but homogeneous, occupying much of one bronchopulmonary segment (but not truly segmental).	Represents a complex angiomatous mass possessing one or more feeding and draining vessels. (*See* page 752.)
Air bronchogram almost invariable; fairly sharply circumscribed margins, even where not abutting against fissure; cavitation rare except with superimposed anaerobic infection.	Confluent airspace consolidation begins in subpleural parenchyma and spreads centrifugally via pores of Kohn; therefore no tendency to segmental involvement. (*See* page 831.)
Cavitation common; air bronchogram almost invariable; pleural effusion may be present.	Differs from pneumococcal pneumonia in propensity to cavitation and tendency to expand involved lung. (*See* page 846.)
Ipsilateral hilar or paratracheal lymph node enlargement almost invariable in children but in only about 50 per cent of adults. Pleural effusion in 10 per cent of affected children (almost always associated with parenchymal disease) and in approximately one third of adults (often as the sole manifestation). Cavitation and miliary spread rare.	(*See* page 891.)
Cavitation common. Individual acinar shadows frequently identifiable elsewhere in lungs due to endobronchial spread. Air bronchogram invariable.	Acute tuberculous pneumonia. Infection may transgress interlobar fissures from one lobe to another or occasionally may extend into chest wall and form abscesses (empyema necessitatis). (*See* page 915.)
Hilar lymph node enlargement and pleural effusion common; cavitation rare.	May be extensive involvement of both lungs; oval or spherical homogeneous consolidation. (*See* page 870.)
Abscess formation uncommon except in immunocompromised patients. Pleural effusion in 35 to 63 per cent of cases.	Consolidation may progress rapidly despite antibiotic therapy. Resolution is often prolonged. (*See* page 861.)
Pleural effusion common.	Less common method of presentation than homogeneous segmental consolidation (Table A–2). The majority of infections are acquired in hospital. (*See* page 855.)
———	Homogeneous consolidation due to confluence of multiple areas of airspace consolidation. Involvement may be extensive, resembling pulmonary edema. (*See* page 860.)
Effusion common.	Uncommon presentation. (*See* page 853.)
Pleural effusion in some cases.	May be overwhelming infection, with multilobar involvement and pulmonary edema pattern simulating ARDS. (*See* page 850.)
Tends to progress to lung abscess.	Acute airspace pneumonia tends to occur when aspirate is of watery consistency. (*See* page 895.)
Pleural effusion frequent; cavitation uncommon.	Affects chiefly debilitated patients. (*See* page 849.)
Cavitation common; pleural effusion and extension into chest wall characteristic (with or without rib destruction). Similarly, may transgress interlobar fissures from one lobe to another.	Roentgenographic patterns of these organisms are indistinguishable. (*See* pages 1024 and 1028.)

Table continued on following page

A–1
Homogeneous Opacities Without Recognizable Segmental Distribution *(Continued)*

	ETIOLOGY	LOSS OF VOLUME	ANATOMIC DISTRIBUTION
	Fungi		
	Blastomyces dermatitidis (blastomycosis).	0	Upper lobe predilection in ratio of 3:2.
	Histoplasma capsulatum (histoplasmosis).	0	No predilection.
	Coccidioides immitis (coccidioidomycosis).	0	Lower lobe predilection.
	Candida albicans (candidiasis).	0	No predilection.
	Geotrichum candidum (geotrichosis).	0	Upper lobe predilection.
	Aspergillus species (invasive aspergillosis).	0	No predilection.
INFECTIOUS *(Continued)*	*Cryptococcus neoformans* (cryptococcosis).	0	Lower lung zones.
	Parasites		
	Entamoeba histolytica (amebiasis).	0	Right lower lobe almost exclusively.
	Paragonimus westermani (paragonimiasis).	0	No predilection.
	Ascaris lumbricoides (ascariasis).	0	Multilobar.
	Strongyloides stercoralis.	0	Multilobar.
	Ancylostoma duodenale.	0	Multilobar.
	Pneumocystis carinii.	0	Generalized.
	Löffler's syndrome.	0	Peripherally situated without lobar predilection.
IMMUNOLOGIC	Chronic eosinophilic pneumonia.	0	Peripheral lung zones without lobar predilection.
	Polyarteritis nodosa (PAN).	0	Peripheral lung zones, without lobar predilection.
	Hodgkin's disease.	0	No predilection.
NEOPLASTIC	Non-Hodgkin's lymphoma.	0	No predilection.
	Bronchiolo-alveolar carcinoma.	0	No predilection.

A–1
Homogeneous Opacities Without Recognizable Segmental Distribution (*Continued*)

ADDITIONAL FINDINGS	COMMENTS
Cavitation uncommon (15 per cent); pleural effusion and lymph node enlargement rare, as is chest wall involvement.	Contrast with actinomycosis and nocardiosis in frequency of cavitation, pleural effusion, and chest wall involvement. (*See* page 970.)
Hilar lymph node enlargement common; cavitation may occur.	This pneumonic type is considerably less common than inhomogeneous primary histoplasmosis. (*See* page 947.)
Hilar and paratracheal lymph node enlargement may be present; cavitation common.	(*See* page 958.)
May cavitate.	Less common presentation than inhomogeneous segmental pattern (*see* Table A–4). (*See* page 987.)
Cavitation common, usually thin-walled.	(*See* page 1018.)
Cavitation uncommon.	Much less common form of disease than fungus ball or mucoid impaction. (*See* page 1007.)
Cavitation uncommon, as is node enlargement.	Less common roentgenographic presentation than a discrete mass. (*See* page 977.)
Right pleural effusion very common. Cavitation occurs in minority of cases.	Organisms enter thorax via diaphragm from liver abscesses. (*See* page 1081.)
Isolated nodular shadows, usually cavitary; may be pleural effusion.	Organisms enter thorax via diaphragm; spread via bronchial tree. (*See* page 1109.)
———	Löffler-type pattern suggested by fleeting nature of consolidation. (*See* page 1093.)
———	Löffler-type pattern. (*See* page 1094.)
———	Löffler-type pattern. (*See* page 1097.)
Pleural effusion very uncommon.	Massive airspace consolidation represents the terminal stage of pulmonary disease. (*See* page 1085.)
Foci of consolidation may be single or multiple, generally ill-defined and transitory or migratory in character. Cavitation, pleural effusion, lymph node enlargement, and cardiomegaly do not occur. Eosinophilia invariable.	Main differential diagnosis is allergic bronchopulmonary aspergillosis. (*See* page 1291.)
Blood eosinophilia common but not invariable.	In contrast to Löffler's syndrome, lesions tend to remain unchanged for days or weeks. Response to corticosteroid therapy characteristically dramatic. (*See* page 1292.)
Consolidation tends to be patchy and fleeting in nature and thus indistinguishable from Löffler's syndrome.	Whether pulmonary disease is caused by PAN *per se* is controversial; the majority of roentgenographic abnormalities are probably attributable to chronic renal disease, hypertension, or cardiac decompensation. (*See* page 1253.)
Almost invariably associated with hilar or mediastinal lymph node enlargement. Pleural effusion in 30 per cent of cases. Air bronchogram almost invariable.	Individual lesions may coalesce to form larger areas of homogeneous consolidation. (*See* page 1507.)
Often without associated hilar and mediastinal node enlargement. Pleural effusion in one third. Air bronchogram invariable.	(*See* page 1535.)
Air bronchogram invariable.	Malignant cells may be found in sputum, which is usually mucoid and sometimes copious. (*See* page 1414.)

Table continued on following page

A–1
Homogeneous Opacities Without Recognizable Segmental Distribution *(Continued)*

	ETIOLOGY	LOSS OF VOLUME	ANATOMIC DISTRIBUTION
	Pulmonary parenchymal contusion.	0 to +	Usually in lung directly deep to area traumatized, although it may develop as well or even predominantly on the side opposite from the trauma due to contracoup effect. No conformity to lobes or segments.
TRAUMATIC	Acute irradiation pneumonitis.	+ + to + + + +	The volume of lung affected generally but not always corresponds to the area irradiated; no tendency to segmental or lobar distribution.
	Lung torsion.	0 to +	A whole lobe or lung.

A–1
Homogeneous Opacities Without Recognizable Segmental Distribution (*Continued*)

ADDITIONAL FINDINGS	COMMENTS
Roentgenographic changes develop soon after trauma, almost invariably within six hours. Increase in size and loss of definition of vascular markings extending out from the hila indicate hemorrhage and edema in the major interstitial space.	The most common pulmonary complication of blunt chest trauma. The roentgenographic pattern varies from irregular patchy areas of airspace consolidation to diffuse and extensive homogeneous consolidation. Consolidation results from exudation of edema fluid and blood into the parenchyma of the lung in both its airspace and interstitial components. (*See* page 2481.)
Despite severe loss of volume, segmental bronchi tend to be unaffected so that an air bronchogram is almost invariable. Roentgenographically demonstrable pleural effusion is very uncommon although there may be fairly extensive thickening of the pleura.	The reaction of the lung to irradiation is affected by a number of variables including the dosage of radiation administered, the time over which it is given, the site to which the radiation is directed, and the condition of the lung prior to irradiation. (*See* page 2551.)
Torsion occurs through 180 degrees so that the base of the lung or lobe comes to lie at the apex of the hemithorax and the apex at the base: the pattern of pulmonary vascular markings is thus altered in a predictable manner.	If torsion is not relieved, vascular supply is compromised and the lung becomes opaque owing to exudation of blood into the airspaces and interstitial tissues. (*See* page 2494.)

TABLE A–2

HOMOGENEOUS OPACITIES OF RECOGNIZABLE SEGMENTAL DISTRIBUTION

The pattern is caused most often by endobronchial obstructing lesions—segmental atelectasis with or without obstructive pneumonitis. Since the pathogenesis involves bronchial obstruction, the resultant shadow necessarily is of specific bronchopulmonary segmental distribution. An air bronchogram should be absent except when the atelectasis is "adhesive" or "nonobstructive" in type or when therapy has relieved the obstruction, thereby permitting the entry of air into the involved segmental bronchi.

Acute confluent bronchopneumonia, commonly of staphylococcal etiology, also produces this pattern. The pathogenesis of bronchopneumonia implies a segmental distribution; the virulence of the infection results in confluence of consolidation and consequent homogeneity. As in obstructive pneumonitis, an air bronchogram seldom is present.

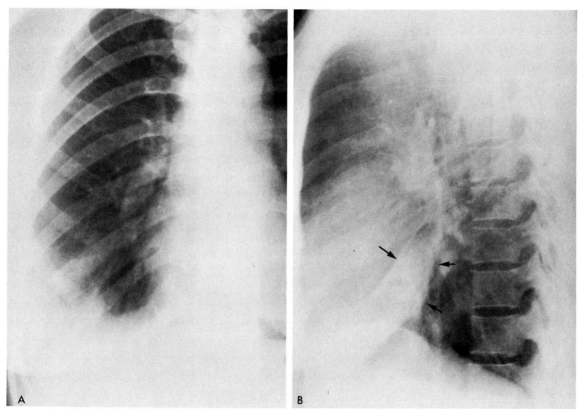

Figure 3. Homogeneous Segmental Consolidation: Acute Confluent Bronchopneumonia. Views of the right hemithorax from posteroanterior *(A)* and lateral *(B)* roentgenograms reveal homogeneous consolidation confined to the precise anatomic distribution of the anterior basal bronchopulmonary segment of the right lower lobe. The consolidation occupies a triangular segment of lung with its apex at the hilum and its base at the visceral pleura *(arrows in B)*. There is no evidence of an air bronchogram. Heavy growth of *Staphylococcus aureus* from the sputum; complete roentgenologic resolution in 10 days.

Figure 4. Homogeneous Segmental Consolidation Atelectasis: Bronchogenic Carcinoma. A triangular shadow of homogeneous density is situated in the anterior portion of the left upper lobe, its base continguous to the retrosternal pleura and its apex at the left hilum. The shadow is seen *en face* in posteroanterior projection *(A)* and in profile in lateral projection (standard roentgenogram [*B*] and tomogram [*C*]). The absence of an air bronchogram indicates bronchial obstruction; the relatively minor degree of loss of volume denotes obstructive pneumonitis. Squamous cell carcinoma of the anterior segmental bronchus of the left upper lobe. A lateral roentgenogram of the resected lung *(D)* shows the sharp definition and precise segmental distribution of the shadow to excellent advantage. (Courtesy Montreal Chest Hospital Center.)

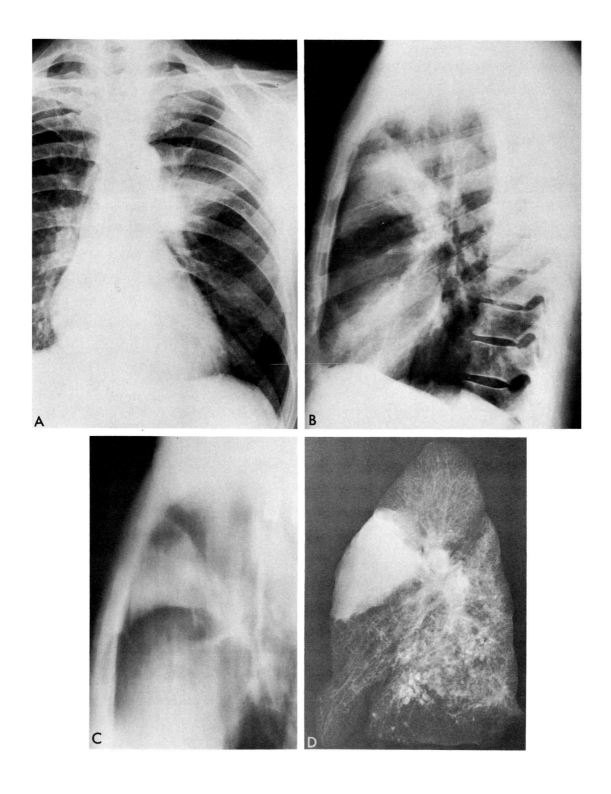

A–2
Homogeneous Opacities of Recognizable Segmental Distribution

	ETIOLOGY	LOSS OF VOLUME	ANATOMIC DISTRIBUTION
DEVELOPMENTAL	Pulmonary arteriovenous fistula	+ to + + + +	Predilection for lower lobes.
	Bacteria		
	Staphylococcus aureus.	0 to + +	No lobar predilection.
	Mycobacterium tuberculosis (primary).	0 to + + + +	2:1 predominance of right lung over left; predilection for anterior segment of upper lobe or medial segment of middle lobe.
	Streptococcus pneumoniae.	0 to +	Influence of gravity; therefore dependent portions of upper and lower lobes.
	Streptococcus pyogenes.	0 to + +	Predominantly lower lobes.
	Pseudomonas aeruginosa.	0 to + +	Predominantly lower lobes.
	Bordetella (Haemophilus) pertussis (whooping cough pneumonia).	+ to + +	Predominantly lower lobes.
INFECTIOUS	*Anaerobic organisms.*	0 to + +	*Reflects influence of gravity— posterior segments of upper lobes and superior segment of lower lobes.*
	All other bacteria listed in Table A–4.	0 to + +	*Predominantly lower lobes.*
	Fungi		
	Histoplasma capsulatum.	+ to + + + +	Predilection for right middle lobe.
	Mucorales order (mucormycosis).	0 to +	No predilection.
	Other fungi listed in Tables A–1 and A–4.	0 to +	Predominantly lower lobes.
	Viruses and Rickettsiae		
	Coxiella burnetii (Q fever).	0	Predominantly lower lobes.
	All viruses listed in Table A–4 (as well as *Mycoplasma*).	0 to + + +	Lower lobe predilection.

A–2
Homogeneous Opacities of Recognizable Segmental Distribution (*Continued*)

ADDITIONAL FINDINGS	COMMENTS
The feeding artery and draining vein may be partly or completely obscured by the shadow of the collapsed segment.	Bronchial compression with resultant atelectasis or obstructive pneumonitis is a rare complication. (*See* page 752.)
Abscess formation common; pleural effusion (empyema) common, particularly in children, with or without bronchopleural fistula (pyopneumothorax).	This is confluent bronchopneumonia; air bronchogram exceptional. Disease is bilateral in over 60 per cent of adults. (*See* page 836.)
Associated paratracheal or hilar lymph node enlargement in two thirds of patients.	Atelectasis results either from compression from enlarged lymph nodes or from endobronchial tuberculosis. In adults, tuberculous bronchostenosis tends to show a female sex predominance and a lower lobe predilection. (*See* page 891.)
Air bronchogram almost invariable; cavitation rare.	True segmental distribution very uncommon, and only when whole lobe involved. (*See* page 828.)
Pleural effusion almost invariable.	As confluent bronchopneumonia, this is a more common method of presentation than inhomogeneous involvement. (*See* page 835.)
Abscess formation with empyema common, with or without bronchopleural fistula (pyopneumothorax).	Confluent bronchopneumonia; a more common method of presentation than homogeneous nonsegmental consolidation. (*See* page 855.)
"Shaggy heart" sign. Hilar node enlargement in 30 per cent of patients.	Confluent bronchopneumonia, associated with some degree of atelectasis in at least 50 per cent of cases; pneumonia may be caused by secondary invader or by *Bordetella pertussis* itself. (*See* page 869.)
Abscess formation in the majority of cases. Empyema common.	Results from aspiration of anaerobically infected material in patients with poor oral hygiene. Tends to have a protracted, insidious course. (*See* page 875.)
———	These bacteria characteristically produce an inhomogeneous consolidation, but on occasion the densities may be confluent, thus leading to homogeneous consolidation.
Enlargement of bronchopulmonary lymph nodes an invariable accompaniment.	Compression from enlarged nodes results in obstructive pneumonitis or atelectasis. Calcification of compressing lymph nodes may be associated with erosion into the bronchial lumen (broncholithiasis.) (*See* page 949.)
———	Segmental consolidation may occur either from direct parenchymal invasion of the organism (confluent bronchopneumonia) or from pulmonary infarction secondary to pulmonary arterial invasion. (*See* page 1016.)
———	These fungi characteristically produce an inhomogeneous consolidation (bronchopneumonia), but on occasion the densities may be confluent, thus leading to homogeneous consolidation.
Pleural effusion is occasionally seen. Hilar lymph node enlargement rare.	Extent of consolidation may range from one segment to a complete lobe. (*See* page 1077.)
Pleural effusion and hilar node enlargement very uncommon.	These organisms characteristically cause inhomogeneous segmental consolidation, but on occasion the densities may be confluent. During the stage of resolution of adenoviral pneumonia, particularly in children, there may occur severe adhesive ("nonobstructive") atelectasis; despite the marked loss of volume, an air bronchogram usually is present.

Table continued on following page

A–2
Homogeneous Opacities of Recognizable Segmental Distribution *(Continued)*

	ETIOLOGY	LOSS OF VOLUME	ANATOMIC DISTRIBUTION
IMMUNOLOGIC	Hypersensitivity bronchopulmonary aspergillosis and mucoid impaction.	0 to + +	Predilection for upper lobes.
	Wegener's granulomatosis.	+ to + + +	No predilection.
	Pulmonary carcinoma.	+ to + + + +	The ratio of right to left lung is 6:4 and a similar ratio exists from upper to lower lobes. The neoplasm arises from the main or lobar bronchi in 20 to 40 per cent of cases and from segmental bronchi in 60 to 80 per cent.
	Carcinoid tumor.	+ to + + + +	Tends to arise from large or segmental bronchi. May occur in any lobe without clear-cut lobar predilection.
	Tracheobronchial gland neoplasms.	+ to + + + +	Lower lobe predilection.
	Tracheobronchial papillomas.	+ to + + + +	No predilection.
NEOPLASTIC	Neoplasms of muscle. Neoplasms of vascular tissue. Neoplasms of bone and cartilage. Neoplasms of neural tissue. Neoplasms of adipose tissue. Neoplasms of fibrohistiocytic tissue. Neoplasms of mixed mesenchymal appearance. Miscellaneous neoplasms of uncertain histogenesis. Miscellaneous tumors of non-neoplastic or uncertain nature.	+ to + + + +	No definite predilection.
	Hodgkin's disease.	+ to + + + +	No known predilection.
	Non-Hodgkin's lymphoma.	+ to + + + +	No known lobar predilection.

A–2
Homogeneous Opacities of Recognizable Segmental Distribution (*Continued*)

ADDITIONAL FINDINGS	COMMENTS
Round, oval, or elliptical masses seen in proximal bronchi. The pulmonary parenchyma distal to the mucous plug may be collapsed or show varying degrees of obstructive pneumonitis but commonly contains air due to collateral air drift from contiguous segments. Lungs are often overinflated as a result of associated spasmodic asthma.	Following disappearance of the mucous plugs, there remains a typical pattern of "proximal" bronchiectasis, which is diagnostic. (*See* page 993.)
Single or multiple masses, sometimes with cavitation.	Atelectasis caused by endobronchial involvement. (*See* page 1241.)
The neoplasm may be identified as a mass distinct from the obstructive pneumonitis. Enlarged lymph nodes may be present in the hilum and elsewhere. Pleural effusion in 10 to 15 per cent of cases.	Oligemia and air trapping distal to bronchial obstruction are uncommon manifestations. (*See* page 1368.)
Typical findings are those of "obstructive pneumonitis." The tumor may be identified on the plain roentgenograms or by CT. Enlarged lymph nodes occasionally may be identified in the hilum or elsewhere. Osseous metastases rare.	In 75 per cent of cases this is the method of presentation of this neoplasm. (*See* page 1477.)
Tend to arise in central airways.	Comprise less than 0.5 per cent of all pulmonary neoplasms. Several distinct histologic varieties have been described. (*See* page 1497).
Endobronchial papillomas are commonly multiple and are associated with similar lesions in the larynx and trachea. Tomography of the larynx, trachea, and lungs may be diagnostic. Bronchiectasis and abscess formation distal to the endobronchial lesions are frequent. Excavation of the lesions may occur.	(*See* page 1502.)
———	Rarely any of these neoplasms may arise from the bronchial wall and obstruct the bronchial lumen leading to obstructive pneumonitis. The more common method of presentation is as a solitary nodule. (*See* pages 1577 to 1608.)
Hilar and/or mediastinal lymph-node enlargement commonly associated. Other patterns of lung involvement also may be associated, particularly parenchymal consolidation presenting as a homogeneous density possessing no recognizable segmental distribution.	Atelectasis (with or without obstructive pneumonitis) results from bronchial obstruction, almost always due to endobronchial involvement by Hodgkin's tissue; rarely may be caused by compression from enlarged lymph nodes. Absence of air bronchogram of differential value. (*See* page 1507.)
Hilar and/or mediastinal lymph node enlargement commonly associated. Other patterns of lung involvement also may be associated, particularly parenchymal consolidation presenting as a homogeneous density possessing no recognizable segmental distribution.	Rarely presents as an endobronchial deposit leading to segmental atelectasis and pneumonitis, and only in the secondary form of the disease. (*See* page 1545.)

A–2
Homogeneous Opacities of Recognizable Segmental Distribution *(Continued)*

	ETIOLOGY	LOSS OF VOLUME	ANATOMIC DISTRIBUTION
THROMBOEMBOLIC	Thromboembolism with infarction.	0 to + +	Lower lobes, usually posteriorly but often nestled in the costophrenic sinus; less than 10 per cent in upper lobes. May be multiple.
INHALATIONAL	Aspiration of solid foreign bodies.	+ to + + + +	Lower lobes almost exclusively, ratio of right to left being 2:1.
	Lipoid pneumonia.	0 to +	Generally dependent portions of lower and upper lobes (occasionally right middle lobe or lingula).
TRAUMATIC	Bronchial fracture.	+ + to + + + +	One or more lobes or an entire lung.
	Postoperative adhesive atelectasis.	+ to + + +	Left lower lobe predilection.
METABOLIC	Bronchopulmonary amyloidosis.	+ to + + +	No predilection.
IDIOPATHIC	Sarcoidosis.	+ to + + + +	No predilection.

A–2
Homogeneous Opacities of Recognizable Segmental Distribution (*Continued*)

ADDITIONAL FINDINGS	COMMENTS
Ipsilateral hemidiaphragm frequently raised; increase in size and abrupt tapering of feeder artery is characteristic; pleural effusion is common. Signs of postcapillary hypertension due to associated cardiac disease may be present.	The size of the infarcted area is generally 3 to 5 cm in diameter but ranges from barely visible to 10 cm in diameter; occasionally shows truncated cone appearance ("Hampton's hump"). (*See* page 1724.)
The foreign body is opaque (e.g., a tooth) in approximately 10 per cent of patients.	Segmental collapse or consolidation occurs in only 25 per cent of cases, the remainder being categorized by "obstructive overinflation." (*See* page 2382.)
None.	The characteristic roentgenographic pattern is alveolar consolidation, commonly homogeneous but sometimes associated with isolated acinar shadows, particularly in the early stages of the disease. The segmental nature of the consolidation may be quite precise. (*See* page 2398.)
Pneumothorax, pneumomediastinum, and subcutaneous emphysema. Fractures of the first three ribs frequently associated, particularly in adults (53 per cent of cases).	Atelectasis develops as a result of displacement of fracture ends and is commonly a late development. The occurrence of atelectasis sometime after an accident should strongly suggest the diagnosis (additional confirmatory evidence provided by fractures of one or more of the first three ribs). (*See* page 2485.)
The usual findings associated with postoperative thoracotomy—pleural effusion, diaphragmatic elevation, and so forth.	Occurs predominantly following cardiac surgery, particularly with use of extracorporeal circulation. The degree of collapse varies considerably. Since the mechanism of atelectasis operates peripherally, an air bronchogram is invariable. (*See* page 2532.)
Sometimes associated with solitary or multiple pulmonary nodules or masses.	Atelectasis or obstructive pneumonitis is caused by intramural masses of amyloid. (*See* page 2578.)
Almost invariably associated with more characteristic changes such as hilar and mediastinal lymph node enlargement and a diffuse reticulonodular pattern.	A rare complication of endobronchial sarcoidosis that may be suspected from other roentgenographic findings and can be confirmed by bronchoscopy and bronchial biopsy. (*See* page 2611.)

TABLE A–3

INHOMOGENEOUS OPACITIES WITHOUT RECOGNIZABLE SEGMENTAL DISTRIBUTION

Postprimary tuberculosis undoubtedly is the most common cause of this pattern—focal areas of parenchymal consolidation separated by zones of air-containing lung. Although tuberculosis commonly is localized to the apical and posterior *regions* of an upper lobe, it seldom is truly segmental; in other words, it does not tend to affect a pyramidal section of lung of which the apex is at the hilum and base at the visceral pleura. It must be emphasized that the presence of cavitation *in itself* should not be interpreted as a cause of inhomogeneity. For example, acute confluent bronchopneumonia, which typically produces homogeneous segmental consolidation, may cavitate and thus create a shadow of relative inhomogeneity; such disease clearly is different pathogenetically from postprimary tuberculosis, in which cavitation accentuates an already inhomogeneous pattern.

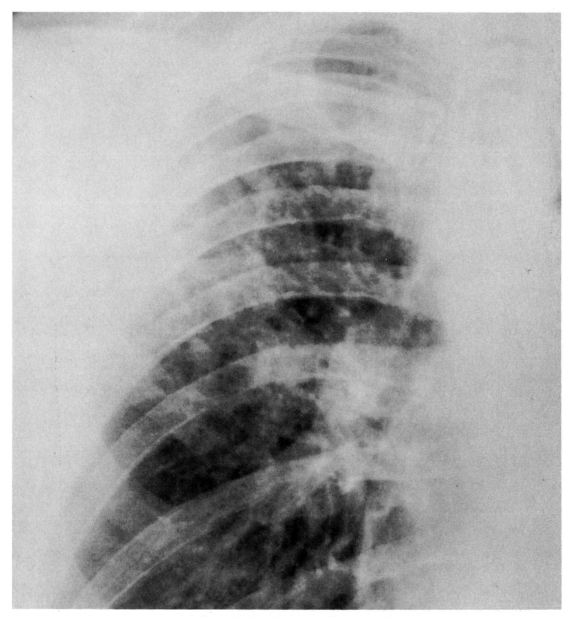

Figure 5. Inhomogeneous Nonsegmental Consolidation: Exudative Pulmonary Tuberculosis. A view of the upper half of the right lung from a posteroanterior roentgenogram demonstrates numerous patchy opacities separated by zones of air-containing lung. Both the posterior portion of the upper lobe and the superior portion of the lower lobe are affected, but involvement is not truly segmental. A moderate-sized cavity accentuates the inhomogeneity. The patient was a 40-year-old man. *Mycobacterium tuberculosis* was cultured from the sputum. (Courtesy Dr. J.F. Meakins, Montreal.)

Figure 6. Inhomogeneous Nonsegmental Consolidation: Acute Irradiation Pneumonitis. A posteroanterior roentgenogram reveals extensive disease throughout the right lung, possessing random distribution without confinement to specific segments; the central and mid-lung zones are affected more than the peripheral. An air bronchogram indicates that the process is chiefly one of airspace consolidation, although there is moderate loss of lung volume as evidenced by mediastinal shift and right hemidiaphragmatic elevation. The patient was a 68-year-old woman approximately 2 months following a course of cobalt therapy to anterior mediastinal lymph nodes for metastatic carcinoma of the breast; complete roentgenologic resolution occurred in 6 months.

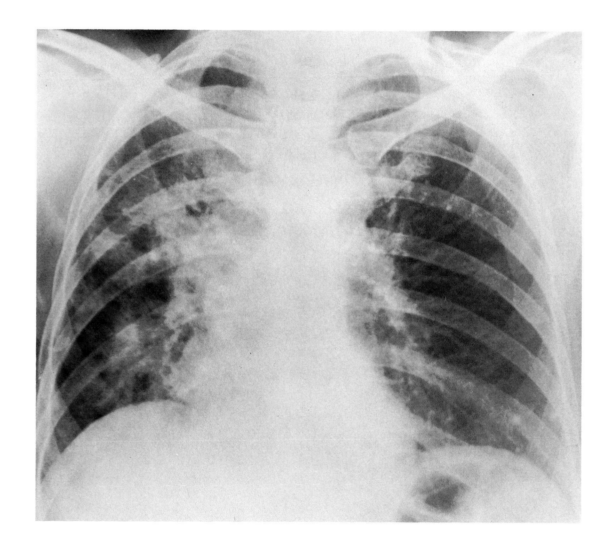

A–3
Inhomogeneous Opacities Without Recognizable Segmental Distribution

	ETIOLOGY	LOSS OF VOLUME	ANATOMIC DISTRIBUTION
DEVELOPMENTAL	Congenital cystic adenomatoid malformation	None	—
INFECTIOUS	**Bacteria** *Mycobacterium tuberculosis.*	0	Apical and posterior portion of upper lobes (rarely anterior alone); superior portion of lower lobes.
	Pseudomonas pseudomallei.	+ to + + +	Predominantly upper lobes.
	Klebsiella-Enterobacter-Serratia species.	+ to + + +	Predominantly upper lobes.
	Bacillus anthracis.	0	No known predilection.
	Fungi *Paracoccidioides (Blastomyces) brasiliensis.*	0	Lower lobe predominance.
	Histoplasma capsulatum.	0	Primary infection commonly in lower lobes; postprimary disease usually in upper lobes.
	Coccidioides immitis.	0	Upper lobes.
	Blastomyces dermatitidis.	0	Upper lobe predominance in ratio of 3:2.
	Viruses and Mycoplasma All viruses listed in Table A–4.	0	Predominantly lower lobes.
IMMUNOLOGIC	Löffler's syndrome.	0	Peripheral lung zones without upper or lower predilection.
TRAUMATIC	Chronic irradiation fibrosis; irradiation pneumonitis.	+ + + to + + + +	Generally corresponds to the area irradiated.
IDIOPATHIC	Ankylosing spondylitis and upper lobe pulmonary fibrosis.	+ + + to + + + +	Uniquely upper lobes.

A–3
Inhomogeneous Opacities Without Recognizable Segmental Distribution *(Continued)*

ADDITIONAL FINDINGS	COMMENTS
Tends to expand involved hemithorax. Mass contains numerous irregular air-containing cysts.	Seen predominantly in infants; mass communicates with bronchial tree and is supplied by the pulmonary circulation. *(See page 719.)*
Cavitation not infrequent; effusion and lymph node enlargement rare.	Postprimary tuberculosis. *(See pages 911 and 938.)*
Frequently associated with cavitation.	Resembles postprimary tuberculosis. Has been described as "unresolved pneumonia" and is the chronic form of the disease. *(See page 860.)*
May be associated with cavitation.	The chronic phase of the disease; closely simulates pulmonary tuberculosis. *(See page 846.)*
Mediastinal lymph node enlargement predominant finding.	Opacities due to pulmonary hemorrhage, not to pneumonia. *(See page 842.)*
Hilar node enlargement variable.	Progressive disease indistinguishable in pattern from postprimary tuberculosis except for lobar predominance. *(See page 975.)*
In primary disease, hilar lymph node enlargement frequent; pleural effusion may be present but is not common. In postprimary disease, cavitation may be present, but as with postprimary tuberculosis, hilar lymph node enlargement is uncommon. In postprimary disease, a calcified focus elsewhere in the lungs is frequently present, similar to Ranke's complex of primary tuberculosis.	There are no clear-cut distinguishing roentgenographic features from primary or postprimary tuberculosis. *(See page 853.)*
Densities may be "fleeting" in character and may leave behind thin-walled cavities.	This is the so-called benign form of the disease and generally does not produce symptoms. *(See page 962.)*
Cavitation in 15 per cent of cases; bone involvement in 25 per cent, either by direct extension across pleura or by bloodstream. Pleural effusion and lymph node enlargement rare.	*(See page 970.)*
None.	A specific segmental distribution may not be recognizable at certain stages of these acute pneumonias.
Consolidation generally ill-defined and transitory or migratory in character.	Consolidation more characteristically homogeneous. Eosinophilia invariable. *(See page 1291.)*
Characteristically there is obliteration of all architectural markings owing to replacement with fibrous tissue. Dense fibrotic strands frequently extend from the hilum to the periphery.	Differentiation from lymphangitic spread of carcinoma may be difficult if changes are bilateral although lack of progression over a period of time should permit differentiation. Acute irradiation pneumonitis characteristically produces a homogeneous nonsegmental pattern *(see Table A–1)* but in some cases it is inhomogeneous. *(See page 2551.)*
Bone and joint manifestations of ankylosing spondylitis.	Cavitation is fairly frequent and may be associated with mycetoma formation. *(See page 1208.)*

TABLE A–4

INHOMOGENEOUS OPACITIES OF
RECOGNIZABLE SEGMENTAL DISTRIBUTION

This pattern characterizes bronchopneumonia or "lobular" pneumonia. The infection is propagated distally in the bronchovascular bundles and thus invariably is of segmental distribution. The parenchymal changes consist of a combination of focal consolidation, atelectasis, and overinflation, resulting in an inhomogeneous roentgenographic pattern. Bronchiectasis produces the same appearance.

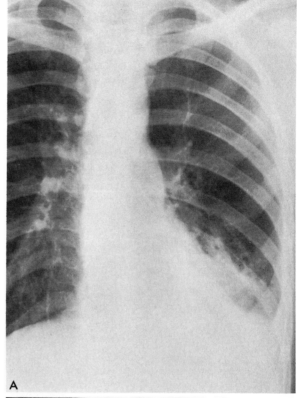

Figure 7. Inhomogeneous Segmental Consolidation: Acute Bronchopneumonia. Views of the left hemithorax from posteroanterior *(A)* and lateral *(B)* roentgenograms show patch inhomogeneous consolidation of the posterior and lateral bronchopulmonary segments of the left lower lobe. The affected lung is roughly conical in shape with its apex at the hilum and its base at the diaphragmatic visceral pleura. There is some loss of volume as evidenced by elevation of the left hemidiaphragm and shift of the mediastinum. Heavy growth of *Haemophilus influenzae* from the sputum.

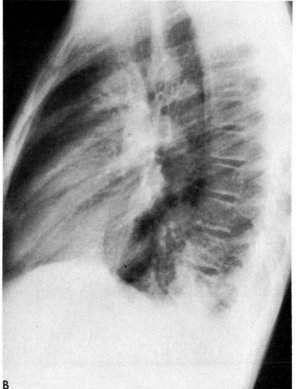

Figure 8. Inhomogeneous Segmental Consolidation: Cylindrical Bronchiectasis. Views of the left lung from posteroanterior *(A)* and lateral *(B)* roentgenograms demonstrate patchy shadows of increased density occupying all basal bronchopulmonary segments of the left lower lobe; in posteroanterior projection particularly, the shadows are oriented in the distribution of the bronchovascular bundles. There is little loss of volume. A bronchogram *(C)* shows cylindrical dilatation of all basal bronchi of the left lower lobe. The affected bronchi terminate abruptly, and there is no peripheral bronchiolar filling. The patient was a 14-year-old girl.

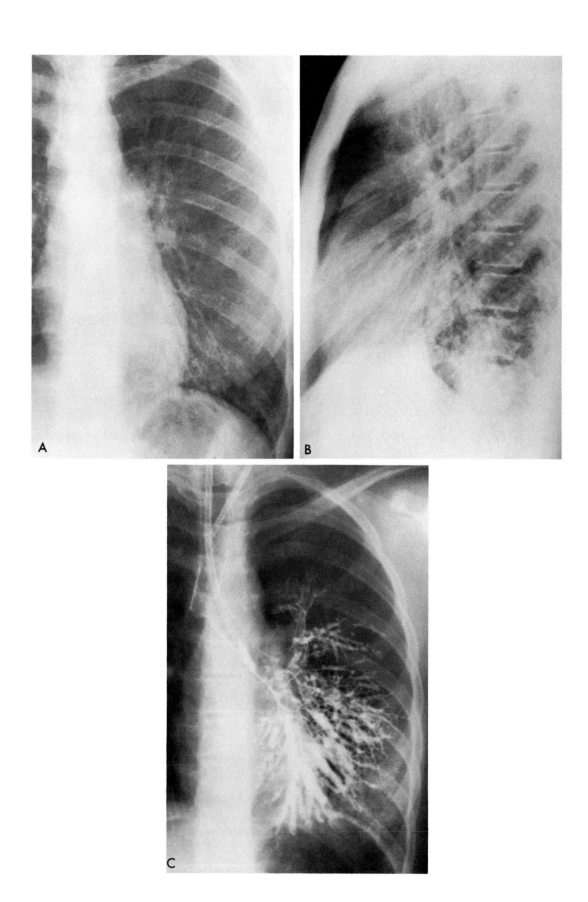

A–4
Inhomogeneous Opacities of Recognizable Segmental Distribution

	ETIOLOGY	LOSS OF VOLUME	ANATOMIC DISTRIBUTION
	Bacteria		
	Haemophilus influenzae.	+ to + +	Predominantly lower lobes.
	Streptococcus pneumoniae.	+ to + +	Dependent portions of upper or lower lobes.
	Mycobacterium tuberculosis (postprimary).	+ to + + +	Apical and posterior segments upper lobes; superior segment lower lobes.
	Salmonella species. *Brucella* species. *Staphylococcus aureus.* *Streptococcus pyogenes.* *Haemophilus pertussis.* *Klebsiella-Enterobacter-Serratia* genera.	+ to + +	Predominantly lower lobes.
	Fungi		
	Histoplasma capsulatum.	+ to + + +	Upper lobes.
	Candida albicans.	+ to + +	No predilection.
INFECTIOUS	*Mucorales* order (including *Mucor* species). *Sporothrix schenckii.*	+ to + +	No known predilection.
	All other fungi listed in Table A–4.	+ to + +	Variable.
	Viruses		
	Mycoplasma pneumoniae.	0	Predominantly lower lobes.
	Influenza. Adenoviruses. Psittacosis (ornithosis). Parainfluenza. Coxsackie.	0	Predominantly lower lobes.
	ECHO. Rubeola.	0	Predominantly lower lobes.
	Respiratory syncytial.	0	Predominantly lower lobes.
	Parasites		
	Toxoplasma gondii.	0	No predilection.

A–4
Inhomogeneous Opacities of Recognizable Segmental Distribution (*Continued*)

ADDITIONAL FINDINGS	COMMENTS
Pleural effusion common.	Typical roentgenographic pattern of bronchopneumonia. (*See* page 853.)
Often in disabled hospitalized patients with COPD.	Atypical presentation. Conforms to the usual pattern of acute bronchopneumonia. (*See* page 833.)
Frequently associated with tuberculous bronchiectasis and sometimes with cavitation.	Chronic stage of the disease, usually fibrotic (but not necessarily inactive). (*See* pages 911 and 938.)
Variable with specific organism.	On rare occasions, any of these organisms may give rise to an inhomogeneous segmental pattern.
———	Indistinguishable in appearance from chronic postprimary tuberculosis. (*See* page 953.)
May be associated with cavitation.	This pattern of bronchopneumonia is the usual method of presentation. (*See* page 987.)
———	Bronchopneumonia. (*See* pages 1016 and 1019.)
Variable with specific organism.	The chronic stage of the disease—usually fibrotic.
Pleural effusion and lymph node enlargement rare in adults. Hilar lymph node enlargement found in 25 per cent of children.	Characteristic reticular pattern with superimposed patchy areas of airspace consolidation. Generally indistinguishable from viral pneumonitis. (*See* page 1038.)
Hilar lymph node enlargement is seen in some patients with ornithosis.	Roentgenographic pattern indistinguishable within the group and indistinguishable from that of *Mycoplasma* pneumonia.
Hilar lymph node enlargement frequent.	In measles this pattern is probably due to superimposed bacterial bronchopneumonia. (*See* pages 1050 and 1056.)
Diffuse overinflation secondary to bronchitis and bronchiolitis.	Characteristically a disease of infants and young children, but may occur in adults. (*See* page 1049.)
Hilar lymph node enlargement common.	(*See* page 1081.)

Table continued on following page

A-4
Inhomogeneous Opacities of Recognizable Segmental Distribution *(Continued)*

	ETIOLOGY	LOSS OF VOLUME	ANATOMIC DISTRIBUTION
IMMUNOLOGIC	Systemic lupus erythematosus.	Progressive loss of lung volume may be characteristic but is unrelated to roentgenographic evidence of localized pulmonary disease.	Commonly peripherally situated in the lung bases.
NEOPLASTIC	Hodgkin's disease.	0	No predilection.
	All endobronchial neoplasms, either benign or malignant.	0 to + + + +	No predilection.
INHALATIONAL	Chronic aspiration.	+ to + + +	Posterior segments of lower or upper lobes; on serial roentgenographic examinations, anatomic distribution may vary considerably.
	Aspiration of solid foreign bodies.	+ to + +	Almost exclusively lower lobes, the ratio of right to left being 2:1.
	Lipoid pneumonia.	0 to +	Dependent portions of upper and lower lobes (occasionally right middle lobe or lingula).
AIRWAYS DISEASE	Bronchiectasis.	+ to + + +	More frequent in lower lobes and right middle lobe. Multiple segments or lobes may be involved.

A–4
Inhomogeneous Opacities of Recognizable Segmental Distribution *(Continued)*

ADDITIONAL FINDINGS	COMMENTS
Cardiac enlargement in 35 to 50 per cent of patients, commonly due to pericardial effusion. Bilateral pleural effusion common.	Pulmonary change is nonspecific, generally in form of basal pneumonitis or focal atelectasis. (*See* page 1189.)
Mediastinal and hilar lymph node enlargement almost invariable. Kerley lines in some cases. Pleural effusion in 30 per cent of cases.	The most common form of pulmonary parenchymal involvement. Results from direct extension from mediastinal and hilar nodes along interstitial tissues. (*See* page 1507.)
———	In any situation where a neoplasm has resulted in obstructive pneumonitis, the partial relief of the obstruction during therapy may permit visualization of air-containing distorted channels within the obstructed segment.
Almost always associated with underlying condition such as Zenker's diverticulum, esophageal stenosis, achalasia, or disturbances in swallowing of neuromuscular origin.	The roentgenographic picture suggests typical "bronchopneumonia." Multiple segments may be involved. Bronchiectasis may develop in involved segments. (*See* page 2387.)
The foreign body is radiopaque in approximately 10 per cent of cases.	The pattern is purely segmental and is produced by a combination of atelectasis and pneumonitis secondary to bronchial obstruction. May be associated with bronchiectasis. (*See* page 2382.)
CT can sometimes reveal the fatty nature of the opacity.	A reticular pattern may develop as a result of the movement of oil (in macrophages) from the airspaces into the interstitial tissues. (*See* page 2398.)
Saccular bronchiectasis may show fluid levels. Compensatory overinflation may be present in unaffected lung.	(*See* page 2186.)

TABLE A–5

CYSTIC AND CAVITARY DISEASE

This table includes all forms of pulmonary disease characterized by circumscribed air-containing spaces with distinct walls. This broad definition includes such entities as blebs, bullae, and cystic bronchiectasis. Air-fluid levels may be present or absent. Cavities may be single or multiple.

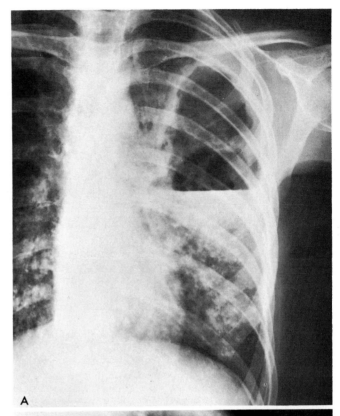

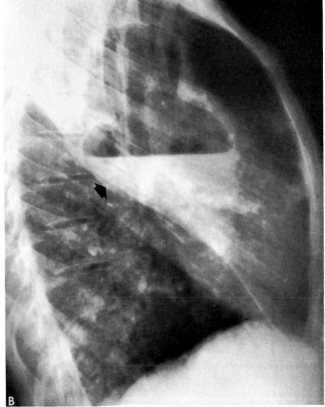

Figure 9. Cavitary Disease: Acute Lung Abscess. Posteroanterior *(A)* and lateral *(B)* roentgenograms show a large cavity in the posterior portion of the left upper lobe, possessing a prominent air-fluid level. The cavity wall is of moderate thickness and possesses an irregular, shaggy inner lining. The major fissure is bowed posteriorly *(arrow in B)*. The patchy shadows in both lungs represent contrast medium from previous bronchography. The patient was a 24-year-old woman with a long-standing history of spasmodic asthma. Heavy growth of *Staphylococcus aureus* from the sputum.

Figure 10. Cavitary Disease: Chronic Tuberculous Cavity Containing a Mycetoma. Views of the upper half of the right lung from a posteroanterior roentgenogram *(A)* and an anteroposterior tomogram *(B)* reveal a thin-walled, irregular cavity in the paramediastinal zone. Situated within it is a smooth, oblong shadow of homogeneous density whose relationships to the wall of the cavity change from the erect *(A)* to the supine *(B)* positions. A photomicrograph of the intracavitary mass revealed multiple mycelial threads characteristic of *Aspergillus*. The cavity was of tuberculous etiology.

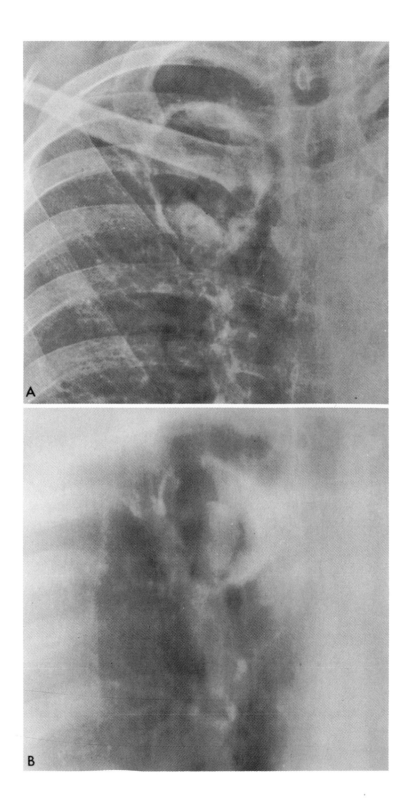

A–5
Cystic and Cavitary Disease

	ETIOLOGY	ANATOMIC DISTRIBUTION	CHARACTER OF WALL
DEVELOPMENTAL	Intralobar bronchopulmonary sequestration.	Two thirds of cases left lower lobe, one third right lower lobe. Almost invariably contiguous to diaphragm.	May be thin- or thick-walled.
	Bronchial cyst.	Medial third of lower lobes.	Thin-walled.
	Congenital adenomatoid malformation.	No definite predilection.	Multiple air-containing cysts scattered irregularly through a mass of unit density.
INFECTIOUS	**Bacteria**		
	Staphylococcus aureus.	No lobar predilection.	Tends to be thick with ragged inner lining.
	Klebsiella-Enterobacter-Serratia species.	Upper lobes predominate.	Tends to be thick with ragged inner lining.
	Mycobacterium species.	Apical and posterior regions of upper lobes and apical region of lower lobes.	Tends to be of moderate thickness. Inner lining generally smooth.
	Pseudomonas aeruginosa. *Escherichia coli.*	Predominantly lower lobes.	Highly variable.
	Streptococcus pneumoniae.	Upper lobe predilection.	Thick, with ragged inner lining.
	Pseudomonas pseudomallei.	Upper lobes predominate.	Moderately thick.
	Anaerobic organisms.	Posterior portion of both lungs.	Tends to be thick with ragged inner lining.
	Actinomyces israelii. *Nocardia* species.	Lower lobe predilection, bilateral.	Generally thick-walled.
	Fungi		
	Histoplasma capsulatum.	Predominantly upper lobes.	Variable.
	Coccidioides immitis.	Predominantly upper lobes.	Tends to be very thin-walled.
	Blastomyces dermatitidis.	No predilection.	Variable, but generally thick-walled.
	Cryptococcus neoformans.	Predominantly lower lobes.	Variable, but generally thick-walled.
	Geotrichum species. *Sporothrix schenckii.*	Upper lobe predilection.	Characteristically thin-walled.
	Mucorales order.	Not distinctive.	———
	Aspergillus species.	———	———

A–5
Cystic and Cavitary Disease *(Continued)*

ADDITIONAL FINDINGS	COMMENTS
Air-fluid levels may be present. The cyst volume may change on serial roentgenographic examinations. Cyst may be masked by pneumonia in surrounding parenchyma.	Cyst may be solitary but more commonly multilocular or multiple. (*See* page 702.)
An air-fluid level may be present. When pneumonitis leads to communication between cyst and the bronchial tree, the cavity may be masked by the surrounding pneumonia.	75 per cent of bronchial cysts eventually become air-containing as a result of communication with contiguous lung. (*See* page 712.)
An expanding process, causing enlargement of affected lung and hemithorax.	Volume of lung affected varies considerably. (*See* page 719.)
Pleural effusion (empyema) with or without bronchopleural fistula (pyopneumothorax) almost invariable in children and may occur in adults.	In adults, cavities result from tissue necrosis; in children, air-containing spaces commonly due to pneumatocele formation. Staphylococcal pyemia may lead to multiple small abscesses widely distributed throughout both lungs. (*See* page 836.)
Pleural effusion (empyema) may be present. Cavity rarely contains large masses of necrotic lung—acute lung gangrene.	Abscess formation in acute pneumonia. Cavities are usually single but tend to be multilocular. Multiple cavities may be present if pneumonia is multilobar. (*See* page 846.)
Cavities may be multiple.	Cavitation tends to be a more prominent feature of atypical mycobacterial disease than of *Mycobacterium tuberculosis* infection. (*See* pages 913 and 938.)
Empyema frequent.	Often the result of bacteremia from an extrathoracic focus (GU tract). Tends to occur in debilitated states (alcoholism or diabetes). (*See* page 855.)
The cavity may contain large irregular masses of necrotic lung—acute lung gangrene.	A rare complication of fulminating pneumococcal pneumonia. (*See* page 831.)
Effusions rare.	(*See* page 860.)
Cavities frequently multiple. Empyema common.	Tend to be associated with debilitation, alcoholism, and poor oral hygiene. (*See* page 875.)
Pleural effusion (empyema) is common as is extension into the chest wall with or without rib destruction.	Roentgenographic patterns in infections with these two organisms are indistinguishable. (*See* pages 1024 and 1028.)
Cavities may be multiple.	No clear-cut distinguishing roentgenographic features from postprimary tuberculosis. (*See* page 953.)
These thin-walled cavities tend to occur in the asymptomatic form of the disease following "fleeting" pneumonitis.	Not to be confused with cavitating nodules, which tend to be somewhat thicker-walled and frequently multiple. (*See* page 962.)
Cavitation occurs in about 15 per cent of cases. Pleural effusion and hilar lymph node enlargement very uncommon.	(*See* page 970.)
Cavitation occurs in about 15 per cent of cases. Pleural effusion and hilar lymph node enlargement very uncommon.	(*See* page 977.)
———	(*See* pages 1018 and 1019.)
———	(*See* page 1016.)
———	The invasive form of the disease is often associated with cavitation. (*See* page 1007.)

Table continued on following page

A–5
Cystic and Cavitary Disease *(Continued)*

	ETIOLOGY	ANATOMIC DISTRIBUTION	CHARACTER OF WALL
INFECTIOUS *(Continued)*	**Parasites**		
	Entamoeba histolytica (amebiasis).	Almost restricted to right lower lobe.	Generally thick-walled with irregular ragged inner lining.
	Paragonimus westermani.	No predilection.	Characteristically thin-walled, with local elevation or hump on inner lining.
	Echinococcus granulosus (hydatid cyst).	Lower lobe predilection.	Air may dissect between ectocyst and endocyst, creating a halo; or contents of cyst may be expelled into bronchial tree, leaving a thin-walled cystic space.
	Pneumocystis carinii.	Upper lobe predilection.	Thin-walled.
IMMUNOLOGIC	Wegener's granulomatosis.	Widely distributed and bilateral, with no predilection for upper or lower lung zones.	Usually thick, with irregular inner lining. In time, cavities may become thin-walled cystic spaces.
	Rheumatoid (necrobiotic) nodule.	Peripheral subpleural parenchyma, commonly in lower lobes.	Thick with smooth inner lining. With remission of the arthritis, cavities may become thin-walled and gradually disappear.
NEOPLASTIC	Pulmonary carcinoma.	Clear-cut predilection for upper lobes, both lungs being affected equally.	Tends to be thick, with an irregular, nodular inner lining (mural nodules). Thin-walled cavities simulating bronchial cysts occur occasionally.
	Hematogeneous metastases.	Cavitation occurs more frequently in upper than in lower lobe lesions.	May be thin- or thick-walled.
	Hodgkin's disease.	Lower lobe predilection.	Thin- or thick-walled.
THROMBOEMBOLIC	Septic embolism.	Lower lobe predilection, predominantly posterior and lateral segments.	Usually thin-walled but may be thick, with shaggy inner lining.
INHALATIONAL	Silicosis—large opacities (progressive massive fibrosis).	Strong predilection for upper lobes.	Tends to be thick with irregular inner lining.
	Coal workers' pneumoconiosis—large opacities (progressive massive fibrosis).	Strong predilection for upper lobes.	Tends to be thick with irregular inner lining.

A–5
Cystic and Cavitary Disease *(Continued)*

ADDITIONAL FINDINGS	COMMENTS
Right pleural effusion almost invariable.	Organisms enter thorax via right hemidiaphragm from liver abscess. *(See page 1081.)*
In addition to cavities, there may be isolated nodular shadows containing vacuoles. Pleural effusion rarely.	Organisms enter thorax via diaphragm from peritoneal space. *(See page 1109.)*
Irregularities of fluid layer caused by collapsed membranes (water-lily sign or sign of the camalote). Hydropneumothorax occasionally.	*(See page 1102.)*
Typical widespread interstitial/airspace disease; pneumothorax frequent.	This pattern is occurring with increasing frequency in patients with AIDS. *(See page 1085.)*
Cavities commonly multiple but all masses do not necessarily cavitate.	Cavitation occurs eventually in from one third to one half of patients. With treatment, cavitary lesions may disappear or heal with scar formation. *(See page 1241.)*
Pleural effusion or spontaneous pneumothorax.	Well-circumscribed masses are more frequently multiple than solitary and range in size from 3 mm to 7 cm. Cavitary nodules wax and wane in concert with frequently associated subcutaneous nodules. *(See page 1211.)*
Chunks of necrotic cancer occasionally may become detached and lie free within the cavity, simulating fungus ball.	Cavitation occurs in 2 to 10 per cent of pulmonary carcinomas, most commonly in lesions peripherally located. The majority are squamous-cell in type (adenocarcinomas and large cell carcinomas cavitate occasionally, small cell carcinomas rarely if ever). *(See page 1411.)*
Cavitation may involve only a few of multiple nodules throughout the lungs, such nodules characteristically showing considerable variation in size.	Cavitation in metastatic neoplasms less common (4 per cent) than in primary neoplasms (9 per cent). Occurs more frequently in squamous cell neoplasms but also in adenocarcinoma (particularly from the large bowel) and sarcoma. *(See page 1628.)*
Cavities are frequently multiple. Commonly associated with mediastinal and hilar lymph node enlargement.	Cavitation occurs characteristically in peripheral parenchymal consolidation. *(See page 1508.)*
Prominent feeding artery, associated pleural effusion, raised diaphragm, or multiple lesions may suggest the diagnosis. A mass of necrotic lung may separate and lie within the cavity, simulating fungus ball.	A rare manifestation which may be misdiagnosed unless clinical picture and associated roentgenographic findings suggest the possibility. Cavitation can also occur as a result of bacterial superinfection of a bland infarct. *(See page 1751.)*
Background of nodular or reticulonodular disease is inevitable although serial examinations may reveal diminution in the number of nodules due to incorporation into the massive consolidation. Hilar lymph node enlargement is the rule, with or without eggshell calcification.	Cavitation in conglomerate lesions can be the result of either superimposed tuberculosis or ischemic necrosis. *(See page 2289.)*
Background of simple coal workers' pneumoconiosis throughout the remainder of the lungs.	Cavitation in conglomerate shadows can be caused by either superimposed tuberculosis or ischemic necrosis. *(See page 2313.)*

Table continued on following page

A–5
Cystic and Cavitary Disease *(Continued)*

	ETIOLOGY	ANATOMIC DISTRIBUTION	CHARACTER OF WALL
AIRWAYS DISEASE	Blebs or bullae.	Predilection for upper lobes, particularly extreme apex.	Thin-walled.
	Cystic bronchiectasis.	Predilection for lower lobes.	Thin-walled.
TRAUMATIC	Pulmonary parenchymal laceration (traumatic lung cyst).	Characteristically in the peripheral subpleural parenchyma immediately underlying the point of maximum injury.	Typically thin-walled.
IDIOPATHIC	Sarcoidosis.	No predilection.	No typical characteristics.

A–5
Cystic and Cavitary Disease *(Continued)*

ADDITIONAL FINDINGS	COMMENTS
With infection, fluid levels may develop. In some cases, roentgenologic evidence of diffuse emphysema will be present.	The thinness of the wall is the main differentiating feature from true cavitation. *(See* page 2166.)
Usually considerable loss of volume of affected segment or segments.	"Cavities" represent severely dilated segmental bronchi. Usually multiple and commonly with air-fluid levels. *(See* page 2186.)
The presence of laceration may be masked by surrounding pulmonary contusion. In some cases of bullet wounds of the lung, a central radiolucency may be observed along the course of the bullet track, simulating a cavity when viewed in the same direction as the wound.	Approximately half these lesions present as thin-walled air-filled cavities (with or without air-fluid levels) and the remainder as pulmonary hematomas. They may be single or multiple, unilocular or multilocular; they are oval or spherical in shape and range from 2 to 14 cm in diameter. *(See* page 2481.)
Cavities may contain mycetomas.	True cavitation in sarcoidosis is rare. Important to exclude all other causes of cavitation before accepting the diagnosis. *(See* page 2611.)

TABLE A–6

SOLITARY PULMONARY NODULES LESS THAN 3 CM IN DIAMETER

For the purposes of this table, the criteria for inclusion in this category are as follows:

1. The presence of a solitary roentgenographic shadow not exceeding 3 cm in its largest diameter.

2. The lesion is fairly discrete but not necessarily sharply defined.

3. It may have any contour (smooth, lobulated, or umbilicated) or shape.

4. It may be calcified or cavitated.

5. Satellite lesions may be present.

6. The lesion is surrounded by air-containing lung; *or* if it is adjacent to the visceral pleural surface over the convexity of the thorax, at least two thirds of its circumference is contiguous to air-containing lung.

7. Symptoms may be present.

A logarithmic approach to the investigation of a solitary pulmonary nodule is given on page 1461.

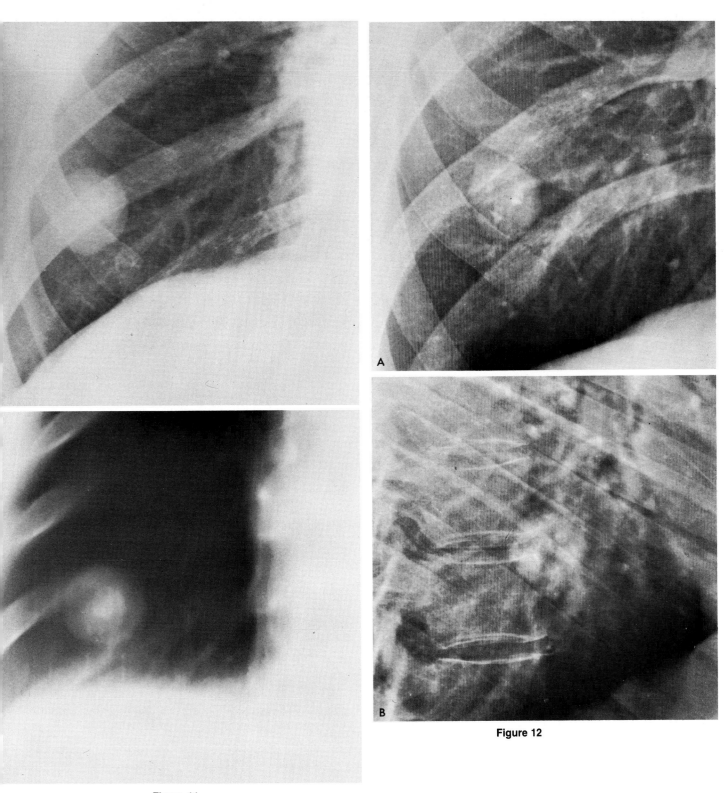

Figure 11

Figure 11. Solitary Nodule: Histoplasmoma. Views of the lower portion of the right lung from a posteroanterior roentgenogram *(A)* and an anteroposterior tomogram *(B)* reveal a solitary, sharply circumscribed nodule measuring 3.0 cm in diameter. The lesion is spherical and is homogeneous in density except for a central nidus of calcification seen to best advantage on the tomogram. Pathologically, the lesion was characterized by chronic granulomatous inflammation, probably due to histoplasmosis. This roentgenographic appearance is typical of histoplasmoma, particularly the central calcific focus that produces the so-called target appearance. (Courtesy Dr. Max Palayew, Jewish General Hospital, Montreal.)

Figure 12. Solitary Nodule: Hamartoma. Views of the lower portion of the right lung from posteroanterior *(A)* and lateral *(B)* roentgenograms show a solitary, sharply circumscribed nodule measuring 3 cm in diameter. Irregular calcium deposits throughout the lesion are suggestive of the descriptive designation "popcorn." This was a proved hamartoma. (Courtesy Dr. David Berger, Montreal Chest Hospital Center.)

A–6
Solitary Pulmonary Nodules Less Than 3 cm in Diameter

	ETIOLOGY	INCIDENCE	LOCATION
	Pulmonary bronchial cyst.	Peak incidence third decade; predilection for males and Yemenite Jews.	Lower lobe predilection, most commonly medial third.
	Pulmonary arteriovenous fistula.	0.6 per cent of Bateson's series. In two thirds of cases, lesions are single.	More common in lower lobes.
DEVELOPMENTAL			
	Varicosity of a pulmonary vein.	Very rare (47 cases reported by 1976).	Medial third of lung (lingular vein on left or medial basal pulmonary vein on right).
	Congenital bronchial atresia with mucoid impaction.	Very rare.	Strong predilection for the apicoposterior bronchus of the left upper lobe.
	Bacteria *Mycobacterium tuberculosis* (tuberculoma).	Common.	Predilection for upper lobes, the right more often than the left.
	Fungi *Histoplasma capsulatum* (histoplasmoma).	Common.	More frequently in the lower than in the upper lobes.
	Coccidioides immitis.	Rare.	Upper lobe predilection.
INFECTIOUS	*Aspergillus* species (mucoid impaction).	Very uncommon; largely restricted to patients with bronchospasm.	Upper lobe predilection.
	Aspergillus species (mycetoma)	Uncommon.	Upper lobe predilection.

A–6
Solitary Pulmonary Nodules Less than 3 cm in Diameter *(Continued)*

SHAPE	CALCIFICATION	CAVITATION	COMMENTS
Round or oval, smooth, well defined.	Rarely in wall; calcium has been reported in cyst contents.	Yes, when communication occurs with bronchial tree.	Cysts are homogeneous until communication established with contiguous lung, usually because of infection (occurs eventually in 75 per cent of cases). (*See* page 712.)
Round or oval, slightly lobulated, sharply defined.	Occasionally, probably due to phleboliths.	No.	Diagnosis by identification of feeding artery and draining vein. Angiography of *both lungs* imperative if surgery is contemplated in order to identify multiple fistulae not visible on plain roentgenograms. 40 to 65 per cent of cases have hereditary hemorrhagic telangiectasia. (*See* page 752.)
Round or oval, lobulated, well defined.	No.	No.	Change in size with Valsalva and Mueller procedures. Differential diagnosis from arteriovenous fistula by late filling and slow drainage on pulmonary angiography. (*See* page 742.)
Oval, smooth, sharply defined.	No.	No.	The mass consists of inspissated mucus which accumulates within the bronchus immediately distal to the point of obliteration; the lung parenchyma distal to the occlusion is overinflated owing to collateral air drift. (*See* page 721.)
Round or oval; 25 per cent are lobulated.	Frequent.	Uncommon.	"Satellite" lesions in 80 per cent; the draining bronchus may show irregular thickening of its wall or occasionally bronchostenosis. (*See* pages 923 and 938.)
Round or oval; typically sharply circumscribed.	Common, often central in location, thus producing the "target" appearance.	Rare.	"Satellite" lesions fairly common. Histoplasmomas may be multiple, varying considerably in size. Associated hilar lymph node calcification is common. (*See* page 949.)
Round or oval; typically sharply circumscribed.	In some cases.	Common; may be thin- or thick-walled.	(*See* page 962.)
Tends to be finger-like but may be Y-shaped or V-shaped in conformity with bronchial subdivision.	No.	Air-fluid levels may be visible within the markedly dilated bronchus, simulating cavitation.	The mass is caused by mucoid impaction within a proximal segmental bronchus. It tends to be transient in nature, although it may persist unchanged for weeks or even months, or may increase in size while under observation. When the lesion clears, it leaves as a residuum cylindrical or saccular dilatation of the affected bronchi. The impacted bronchus may or may not cause atelectasis of the involved segment; atelectasis frequently is prevented by collateral air drift. (*See* page 993.)
Round or oval.	No.	Invariably situated *within* a cavity.	This is only one of several fungi capable of forming an intracavitary "fungus ball." (*See* page 991.)

Table continued on following page

A–6
Solitary Pulmonary Nodules Less Than 3 cm in Diameter *(Continued)*

	ETIOLOGY	INCIDENCE	LOCATION
INFECTIOUS *(Continued)*	**Parasites** *Echinococcus* (hydatid cyst).	Common in endemic areas.	Lower lobe predilection, right more often than left.
	Dirofilaria immitis.	Rare.	No known predilection.
	Rheumatoid (necrobiotic) nodule.	Rare.	In the peripheral subpleural zone, usually lower lobes.
IMMUNOLOGIC	Wegener's granulomatosis.	Rare.	No predilection.
	Pulmonary carcinoma.	Varies widely; in patients referred for resection, approximately 40 per cent of solitary nodules will be malignant.	Predominantly upper lobes.
	Carcinoid tumor.	Incidence compared to pulmonary carcinoma 1:50. 20 to 25 per cent of all carcinoid tumors present as solitary nodules.	Predilection for right upper and middle lobes and lingula.
	Hamartoma.	Constitute approximately 5 per cent of solitary peripheral nodules.	No lobar predilection.
NEOPLASTIC	Neoplasms of muscle, vascular tissue, bone and cartilage, neural tissue, adipose tissues, fibrohistiocytic tissue, and mixed mesenchymal tissue. Miscellaneous neoplasms of uncertain histogenesis. Miscellaneous tumors of non-neoplastic or uncertain nature.	Very rare.	No definite predilection.
	Hematogenous metastasis.	3 to 5 per cent of asymptomatic nodules.	Predominantly lower lobes.

A–6
Solitary Pulmonary Nodules Less than 3 cm in Diameter (Continued)

SHAPE	CALCIFICATION	CAVITATION	COMMENTS
Almost always well circumscribed. Tendency to bizarre, irregular shape.	Very rare.	Common.	(See page 1102.)
Well defined.	No.	Sometimes.	Involvement of larger pulmonary arteries may result in a shadow simulating pulmonary infarction. (See page 1100.)
Well defined, smooth.	No.	Common. Cavities possess thick walls and smooth inner lining.	More commonly multiple than solitary. Pleural effusion may be present. Eosinophilia in some patients. Nodules wax and wane in concert with the frequently associated subcutaneous nodules and in proportion to the activity of the rheumatoid arthritis. (See page 1211.)
Tend to be well defined.	No.	In one third to one half of cases.	Much less common manifestation than multiple nodules, although solitary nodules were observed in 4 of 20 cases in one series. (See page 1241.)
Margins tend to be ill-defined, lobulated, or umbilicated.	Very rare.	2 to 10 per cent.	Satellite lesions very uncommon. (See pages 1383 and 1461.)
Round or oval, sharply defined, slightly lobulated.	Rare.	Rare.	The remaining 75 to 80 per cent of carcinoid tumors relate to a bronchial lumen and lead to segmental atelectasis or obstructive pneumonitis. (See page 1477.)
Well defined; more often lobulated than smooth in a ratio of 2:1.	Incidence varies widely in reported series, but certainly occurs in a minority of cases. "Popcorn" configuration virtually diagnostic.	No.	10 per cent arise endobronchially and then may cause bronchial obstruction, atelectasis, or obstructive pneumonitis. Serial examination may reveal slow growth. (See page 1608.)
Usually well defined.	Rarely.	No.	Rarely these neoplasms may arise within a bronchial wall and thus be manifested roentgenographically by bronchial obstruction and peripheral atelectasis or obstructive pneumonitis. (See pages 1577 to 1608.)
Smooth or slightly lobulated. Tend to be well defined.	Rarely and only in osteogenic sarcoma or chondrosarcoma.	Occasionally.	In 25 per cent of cases, metastatic lesions to the lungs are solitary. (See page 1628.)

Table continued on following page

A–6
Solitary Pulmonary Nodules Less Than 3 cm in Diameter *(Continued)*

	ETIOLOGY	INCIDENCE	LOCATION
	Bronchiolo-alveolar carcinoma.	The most common method of presentation of this neoplasm.	No predilection.
NEOPLASTIC *(Continued)*	Non-Hodgkin's lymphoma.	Rare.	No predilection.
	Multiple myeloma (plasmacytoma).	Rare.	No predilection.
	Pulmonary hematoma.	Uncommon.	Usually in a peripheral subpleural location.
TRAUMATIC			
METABOLIC	Bronchopulmonary amyloidosis.	Extremely rare.	No predilection.

A–6
Solitary Pulmonary Nodules Less than 3 cm in Diameter *(Continued)*

SHAPE	CALCIFICATION	CAVITATION	COMMENTS
Round, smooth, or lobulated; may be sharply or ill-defined.	No.	Rarely.	An air bronchogram or air bronchiologram is a common roentgenographic feature, except in the smaller lesions. Tends to be very slow growing. (*See* page 1414.)
Round, ovoid, triangular or polyhedral; tends to have fuzzy outline.	No.	In large cell lymphoma, "cyst-like" lesions may occur that resemble cavitation.	May be a manifestation of either primary or secondary disease. (*See* page 1535.)
Lobulated.	No.	No.	No distinguishing features from those of peripheral pulmonary carcinoma. (*See* page 1558.)
Oval or round, sharply defined, smooth.	No.	A hematoma occurs as a result of hemorrhage into a pulmonary parenchymal laceration or traumatic lung cyst—thus, an air-fluid level may be present as a result of communication with the bronchial tree.	Generally undergo slow but progressive decrease in size, although they may persist for long periods of time, sometimes up to 4 months. May be multiple. Not uncommonly result from segmental or wedge resection of lung parenchyma. The presence of a hematoma may be masked by surrounding pulmonary contusion. (*See* page 2481.)
	Occasionally in the periphery.	Occasionally.	(*See* page 2578.)

TABLE A–7

SOLITARY PULMONARY MASSES
3 CM OR MORE IN DIAMETER

The general characteristics of lesions included in this table are the same as for solitary nodules less than 3 cm in diameter.

The separation of a group of entities into this category on the basis of size alone is perhaps arbitrary but appears to be necessary in view of the restriction on size imposed by most authorities for inclusion of solitary nodules as so-called coin lesions.

Figure 13. Solitary Nodule: Squamous Cell Carcinoma.
Views of the lower half of the right lung from a posteroanterior
roentgenogram *(A)* and an anteroposterior tomogram *(B)* demonstrate a solitary mass that measures 5 cm in its greatest diameter.
The mass is situated within the right middle lobe (note the silhouette
sign). Its margins are fairly sharply circumscribed although somewhat irregular. The mass is perfectly homogeneous and shows no
evidence of calcification. The size of the mass and its nodular
contour suggest primary bronchogenic cancer. This was a 60-year-
old asymptomatic male.

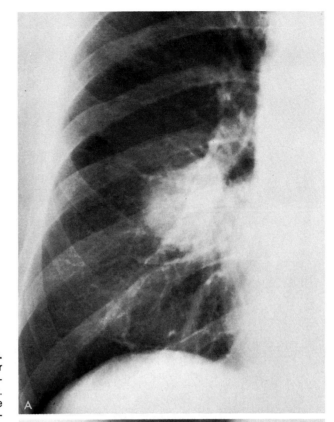

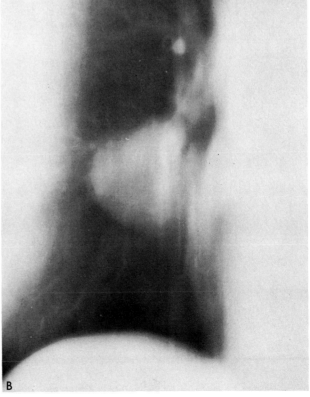

Figure 14. Masses Over 3 cm in Diameter: Echinococcus (Hydatid) Cyst. A posteroanterior roentgenogram of the chest of an 11-year-old girl *(A)* reveals a large, sharply defined mass situated in the lower portion of the right lung. Tomographic sections in anteroposterior *(B)* and lateral *(C)* projections show the mass to be located within the right lower lobe; it is homogeneous in density and contains no calcium. Its superior border shows a sharp indentation that gives the mass a rather bizarre shape reminiscent in lateral projection of a valentine heart. Such bizarre shapes are common in hydatid cyst and result from impingement by the soft, fluid-filled mass on comparatively rigid pulmonary structures such as bronchovascular bundles. The child was asymptomatic; an abnormality was known to have been present on her chest roentgenogram 2 years previously. At thoracotomy, the cyst was readily enucleated from the surrounding lung and was removed intact without the necessity for removal of normal lung tissue.

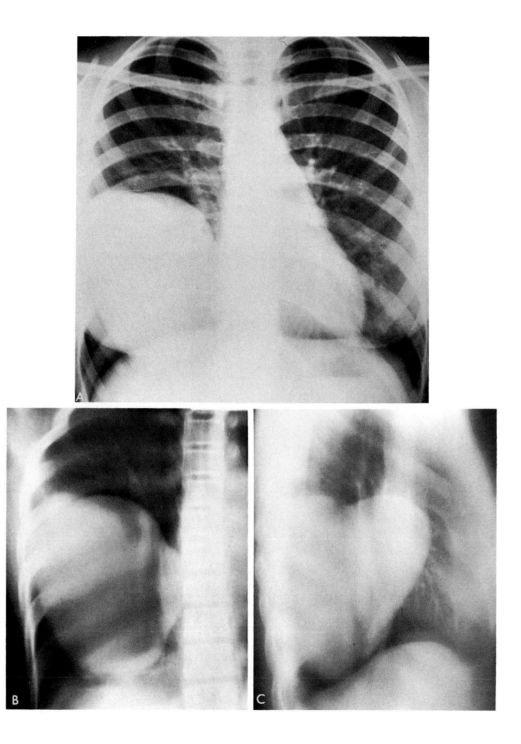

A–7
Solitary Pulmonary Masses 3 cm or More in Diameter

	ETIOLOGY	LOCATION
DEVELOPMENTAL	Intralobar bronchopulmonary sequestration.	Two thirds of cases left lower lobe; one third of cases right lower lobe; rare elsewhere. Almost invariably contiguous to diaphragm in posterior bronchopulmonary segment.
	Extralobar bronchopulmonary sequestration.	Related to left hemidiaphragm in 90 per cent of cases, lying immediately above, below, or within it.
	Pulmonary bronchial cyst.	Lower lobe predilection, usually in medial third.
	Congenital adenomatoid malformation.	No lobar predominance.
INFECTIOUS	Acute or chronic lung abscess.	Predilection for posterior portions of upper or lower lobes.
	Cryptococcus neoformans.	Lower lobe predominance, usually in the periphery.
	Blastomyces dermatitidis.	No lobar predominance.
	Nocardia asteroides.	Lower lobe predominance.
	Actinomyces israelii.	Lower lobe predominance.
	Coccidioides immitis.	Lower lobe predominance.
	Echinococcus granulosus (hydatid cyst).	Predilection for lower lobes, right more often than left.

A–7
Solitary Pulmonary Masses 3 cm or More in Diameter *(Continued)*

SHAPE	CALCIFICATION	CAVITATION	COMMENTS
Round, oval, or triangular in shape and typically well defined.	No.	Frequent.	Enclosed within visceral pleura of affected lung. Although cystic in nature, mass remains homogeneous until communication established with contiguous lung as a result of infection. Supplied by systemic artery and drains via pulmonary veins (*See* page 702.)
Well-defined homogeneous mass.	No.	Seldom.	Frequently associated with other anomalies and sometimes with diaphragmatic eventration. Enclosed within its own visceral pleural layer—therefore seldom infected or air-containing (*cf.* intralobar). Supplied by systemic artery (usually from abdominal aorta) and drains via systemic rather than pulmonary veins (IVC or azygos system). (*See* page 709.)
Round or oval.	Rarely in wall.	Only after they have become infected.	Incidence of mediastinal and pulmonary cysts varies, the former predominating in some series and the latter in others. Infection occurs eventually in 75 per cent of cases. (*See* page 712.)
Round or oval.	No.	See comments.	The solid form is much less common than the cystic. Manifested as a large, space-occupying homogeneous mass. (*See* page 719.)
Tends to be round; somewhat ill-defined when acute but sharply defined when chronic.	No.	Almost inevitable.	Usually of staphylococcal or anaerobic etiology. The mass may remain unchanged for many weeks without perforation into bronchial tree. (*See* pages 836 and 875.)
Tends to be well defined, homogeneous in density, and solitary.	No.	Reported in 16 per cent of cases.	Commonly pleural based. (*See* page 977.)
Margins tend to be ill-defined.	No.	Uncommon.	Frequency of this manifestation varies widely in reported series. May simulate pulmonary carcinoma. (*See* page 970.)
Indistinguishable from actinomycosis.	No.	Frequent.	The initial roentgenographic presentation in 4 of 12 cases in one series, with cavitation in all. (*See* page 1028.)
Somewhat ill-defined. Simulates pulmonary carcinoma.	No.	Frequent.	The initial roentgenographic presentation in 6 of 15 cases in one series. (*See* page 1024.)
Round or oval.	No.	Uncommon.	Can simulate a peripheral pulmonary carcinoma. (*See* page 958.)
Sharply defined; tends to possess bizarre, irregular shape.	Extremely rare.	Common.	Communication with bronchial tree may produce the "meniscus" sign or sign of the camalote. (*See* page 1102.)

Table continued on following page

A–7
Solitary Pulmonary Masses 3 cm or More in Diameter *(Continued)*

ETIOLOGY	LOCATION
Wegener's granulomatosis.	No predilection.

IMMUNOLOGIC

ETIOLOGY	LOCATION
Pulmonary carcinoma.	Predominantly upper lobes.
All neoplasms of soft tissue, bone, and cartilage listed in Table A–6.	No definite predilection.
Hematogenous metastasis.	Predominantly lower lobes.
Bronchiolo-alveolar carcinoma.	No predilection.

NEOPLASTIC

Hodgkin's disease.	No predilection.
Non-Hodgkin's lymphoma.	No clear-cut lobar predilection; tends to be more centrally than peripherally located.
Multiple myeloma (plasmacytoma).	Over the convexity of thorax contiguous to chest wall.

A–7
Solitary Pulmonary Masses 3 cm or More in Diameter (Continued)

SHAPE	CALCIFICATION	CAVITATION	COMMENTS
Well circumscribed.	No.	In one third to one half of cases.	Solitary nodules much less common than multiple. Range from a few millimeters to 9 cm in diameter. The lesion was solitary in 4 of 20 cases in one series. (See page 1241.)
Margins tend to be ill-defined, lobulated, or umbilicated.	No.	Fairly common.	Most common method of presentation of large cell carcinoma, somewhat less common in adenocarcinoma and squamous-cell carcinoma and very uncommon in small cell carcinoma. (See pages 1342 and 1367.)
Well defined, smooth.	Rarely.	No.	Any of these neoplasms may reach a large size.
Tend to be sharply defined, somewhat lobulated.	Rare—restricted to metastatic osteogenic sarcoma or chondrosarcoma.	Predominantly in upper lobe lesions but is uncommon.	(See page 1625.)
Tends to be ill-defined.	No.	No.	Tends to be very slow growing; may occupy most of the volume of a lobe, but there is no tendency to cross interlobar fissures. Air bronchogram frequent. (See page 1414.)
Shaggy and ill-defined.	No.	Sometimes.	Size ranges widely and may vary with time. An air bronchogram should be visible. (See page 1507.)
Smooth and fairly sharply defined.	No.	Rare.	May be a manifestation of either primary or secondary lymphoma. The primary form is often without associated hilar or mediastinal lymph node enlargement, and tends to grow slowly. Rarely obstructs the bronchial tree so that an air bronchogram is almost invariable. (See page 1535.)
Sharply defined, possessing an obtuse angle with the chest wall.	No.	No.	Due to protrusion into the thorax of a primary lesion originating in a rib—thus almost invariably associated with a destructive lesion of one or more ribs. May reach a very large size. (See page 1558.)

Table continued on following page

A–7
Solitary Pulmonary Masses 3 cm or More in Diameter *(Continued)*

	ETIOLOGY	LOCATION
	Lipoid pneumonia.	Dependent portions of upper and lower lobes (occasionally right middle lobe or lingula).
	Silicosis (progressive massive fibrosis).	Characteristically conglomerate shadows develop in the periphery of the mid or upper lung zones and in time tend to migrate toward the hilum.
INHALATIONAL	Coal workers' pneumoconiosis (progressive massive fibrosis).	Marked predilection for upper lobes; tends to originate in the periphery of the lung, migrating toward the hilum over a period of years.
	Asbestosis (large opacities).	Lower zonal predominance in contrast to similar lesions of silicosis and coal workers' pneumoconiosis.
	Talcosis (large opacities).	Lower zonal predominance.
TRAUMATIC	Pulmonary hematoma.	Usually deep to point of maximum trauma.
INCIDENTAL	Round atelectasis.	Lower zonal predominance.

A–7
Solitary Pulmonary Masses 3 cm or More in Diameter *(Continued)*

SHAPE	CALCIFICATION	CAVITATION	COMMENTS
Well defined, smooth or lobulated. Sometimes with very shaggy outer margin.	No.	No.	Usually homogeneous in density. Closely simulates peripheral pulmonary carcinoma. (*See* page 2402.)
Tend to be broader in the sagittal plane than in the coronal. Their margins may be irregular and somewhat ill-defined so as to simulate peripheral pulmonary carcinoma.	No.	Sometimes.	The background pattern of diffuse silicosis may be quite apparent, but the more extensive the progressive massive fibrosis, the less the nodularity apparent in the remainder of the lungs (due to incorporation of nodular lesions into the massive consolidation). Because of cicatrization atelectasis, compensatory overinflation or overt emphysema of remainder of lung is common. Cavitation may occur in conglomerate lesions. Hilar lymph node enlargement is usual and in an occasional case may be associated with "eggshell calcification." (*See* page 2282.)
Similar to large opacities of silicosis.	No.	Sometimes.	The background of diffuse nodular or reticulonodular shadows is usually evident, although incorporation of the individual foci into the conglomerate consolidation may render the nodular pattern inconspicuous. Compensatory overinflation or emphysema develops in lower lobes in response to cicatrization atelectasis. (*See* page 2282.)
Tend to be smaller than large opacities of silicosis. Round or oval; ill-defined.	No.	No.	Background pattern of diffuse pulmonary asbestosis, usually with pleural thickening, plaques, and calcification. (*See* pages 2316 and 2345.)
Variable	No.	No.	Background pattern of general haziness, nodulation, and reticulation. Pleural plaque formation common. (*See* page 2354.)
Sharply defined, round or oval.	No.	No.	Hematomas are usually less than 6 cm in diameter but occasionally are very large. Resolution may take several months. (*See* page 2481.)
Round or oval.	No.	No.	Invariably associated with pleural fibrosis and often with asbestos-related pleural disease. (*See* pages 489 and 2328.)

TABLE A–8

MULTIPLE PULMONARY NODULES, WITH OR WITHOUT CAVITATION

The individual lesions generally possess the same characteristics as those described in Tables A–6 and A–7.

Cavitation or calcification may be present or absent in some or all of the lesions.

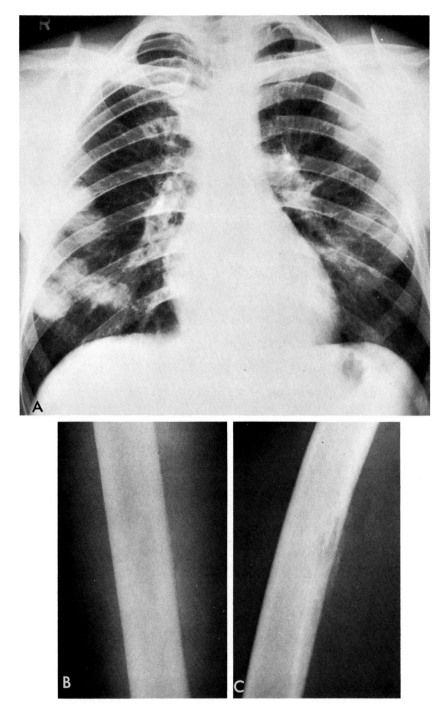

Figure 15. Multiple Nodules: Pyemic Abscesses. A posteroanterior roentgenogram *(A)* reveals several sharply circumscribed nodules ranging from 2 to 3 cm in diameter situated predominantly in the right lower lobe and the left upper lobe. The masses are homogeneous in density and show no evidence of cavitation (although cavitation eventually occurred in the majority). Anteroposterior *(B)* and lateral *(C)* views of the midshaft of the right femur show an irregular area of rarefaction in the cortex, associated with subperiosteal new bone formation along the posterior and medial aspects of the bone. This 24-year-old man first developed symptoms referable to his chest, consisting of a severe "chest cold" with retrosternal and bilateral axillary pain and cough productive of moderate quantities of yellow-brown sputum; approximately 10 days later swelling and throbbing pain developed in the thigh. The possibility of Ewing's sarcoma was entertained until the patient developed severe constitutional symptoms consisting of night sweats, chills, and high fever. *Staphylococcus aureus* was cultured from the sputum and from pus obtained from the thigh at incision and drainage. Acute osteomyelitis and metastatic pyemic abscesses.

Figure 16. Multiple Nodules: Hematogenous Metastases. A posteroanterior roentgenogram reveals multiple, sharply circumscribed nodules scattered widely throughout both lungs; they range in diameter from 1 to 6 cm and are homogeneous in density and roughly spherical. A photograph of a cross section of the lung removed at necropsy *(B)* shows the sharp definition and marked variation in size of the metastatic nodules; the large mass in the left lower lobe has undergone hemorrhagic necrosis. Primary fibrosarcoma of the ilium with hematogenous metastases. The patient was a 72-year-old man.

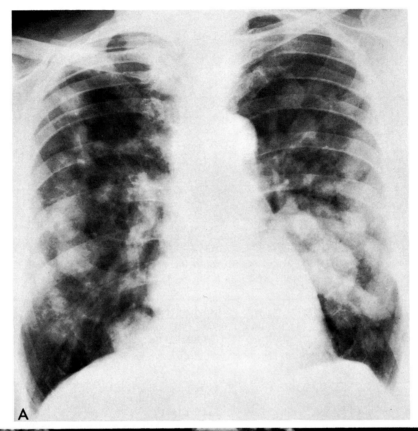

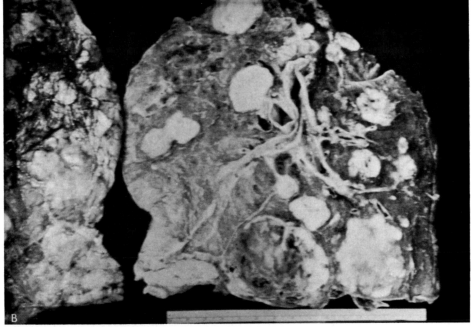

Multiple Pulmonary Nodules, With or Without Cavitation

	ETIOLOGY	LOCATION	SIZE AND SHAPE
DEVELOPMENTAL	Pulmonary arteriovenous fistula.	Lower lobe predilection.	One to several centimeters; round or oval, lobulated, well defined.
	Varicosities of the pulmonary veins.	Medially, close to left atrium.	1 to 3 cm; round or oval.
INFECTIOUS	Pyemic abscesses.	Generalized but more numerous in lower lobes.	Range from 0.5 to 4 cm; usually round and well defined.
	Pseudomonas pseudomallei.	No predilection.	4 to 11 mm; irregular and poorly defined.
	Coccidioides immitis.	Upper lobe predilection.	0.5 to 3.0 cm; round or oval, well defined.
	Histoplasma capsulatum.	No predilection.	0.5 to 3.0 cm; round and sharply defined.
	Paragonimus westermani.	Lower lobe predilection, usually in the periphery.	3 to 4 cm; well defined.
IMMUNOLOGIC	Wegener's granulomatosis.	Widely distributed, bilateral, no predilection for upper or lower lung zones.	5 mm to 9 cm; round, sharply defined.
	Rheumatoid (necrobiotic) nodules.	Peripheral subpleural parenchyma, more commonly lower lobes.	3 mm to 7 cm; round, well defined, smooth.
NEOPLASTIC	Tracheobronchial papillomas.	No predilection.	Up to several centimeters; round, sharply defined.
	Hematogenous metastases.	Predilection for lower lobes.	3 mm to 6 cm or more; typically round and sharply defined.
	Non-Hodgkin's lymphoma.	More numerous in lower lung zones.	3 mm to 7 cm; round, ovoid, triangular, or polyhedral, usually with fuzzy outlines.
	Multiple myeloma (plasmacytoma).	No predilection.	Lobulated.
THROMBOEMBOLIC	Septic emboli.	Lower lobe predilection.	Highly variable; commonly 2 to 6 cm. Round or wedge-shaped.
TRAUMATIC	Multiple pulmonary hematomas.	Unilateral or bilateral, generally in lung deep to maximum trauma.	Highly variable. Commonly 2 to 6 cm but may be very large. Sharply defined.
METABOLIC	Bronchopulmonary amyloidosis.	Widely distributed.	Highly variable.
IDIOPATHIC	Sarcoidosis.	Widely distributed.	Average diameter greater than 1 cm.

CALCIFICATION	CAVITATION	GENERAL COMMENTS
No.	No.	Multiple in one third of all cases. Diagnosis by identification of feeding artery and draining vein; lesions may change in size between Valsalva and Mueller procedures; angiography necessary to identify all fistulae. 40 to 65 per cent of cases associated with hereditary hemorrhagic telangiectasia. (*See* page 752.)
No.	No.	May be congenital or acquired. Consists of tortuosity and dilatation of pulmonary veins just before their entrance into the left atrium. Diagnosis by angiography or CT. (*See* page 742.)
No.	Common, usually thick-walled.	Commonly caused by *Staphylococcus aureus*. (*See* page 838.)
No.	Common.	Nodules tend to enlarge, coalesce, and cavitate as the disease progresses. (*See* page 860.)
Sometimes.	Common; may be thin- or thick-walled.	In approximately 2 per cent of affected patients, multiple cavities may be associated with pneumothorax and empyema. In contrast to tuberculosis, cavitary disease may occur in anterior segment of an upper lobe. (*See* page 962.)
Sometimes.	No.	May remain unchanged over many years or may undergo slow growth. Seldom exceed 4 or 5 in number. (*See* page 949.)
Occasionally.	Common.	Multiple ring opacities or thin-walled cysts are characteristic. (*See* page 1109.)
No.	In one third to one half of patients; characteristically thick-walled, with irregular, shaggy inner lining.	May be associated with focal areas of pneumonitis. Typically occur in patients who manifest no allergic background. Note related but somewhat different condition "allergic granulomatosis." (*See* page 1241.)
No.	Common, usually with thick walls and smooth inner lining.	Nodules tend to wax and wane in concert with subcutaneous nodules and in proportion to the activity of the rheumatoid arthritis. With remission of arthritis, cavities may become thin-walled and gradually disappear. In Caplan's syndrome, nodules tend to develop rapidly and appear in crops; both cavitation and calcification may occur in this variety of rheumatoid nodule. (*See* page 1211.)
No.	Frequent.	Obstruction of airways leads to peripheral atelectasis and obstructive pneumonitis. Diagnosis is suggested by a combination of multiple solid or cavitary lesions throughout the lungs associated with laryngeal or tracheal papillomas. (*See* page 1502.)
Rare, but if present, virtually diagnostic of osteogenic sarcoma or chondrosarcoma.	In approximately 4 per cent of cases, more frequently in upper lobes.	Wide range in size of multiple nodules is highly suggestive of the diagnosis. Seldom associated with mediastinal or bronchopulmonary lymph node enlargement. (*See* page 1625.)
No.	"Cyst-like" lesions may occur in large cell lymphoma, simulating cavitation.	Most often a manifestation of *secondary* lymphoma. Mediastinal and bronchopulmonary lymph node enlargement is associated in some cases. (*See* page 1535.)
No.	No.	(*See* page 1558.)
No.	Frequent, usually with thin walls.	Nodules tend to be peripherally located and ill-defined. May develop a central loose body (the "target sign") representing detached fragments of necrotic lung within a cavity. (*See* page 1751.)
No.	No.	Generally undergo slow but progressive decrease in size and may persist for weeks or even months. Initially, hematomas may be masked by surrounding pulmonary contusion. (*See* page 2481.)
Lesions may be calcified or ossified.	Sometimes.	This is the parenchymal form of the disease. (*See* page 2578.)
No.	No.	A rare pattern in sarcoidosis (in only 3 of 150 patients in one series). Simulates metastases. (*See* page 2611.)

TABLE A–9

DIFFUSE PULMONARY DISEASE WITH A PREDOMINANTLY ACINAR PATTERN

"Diffuse" implies involvement of all lobes of both lungs. Although the disease necessarily is widespread, it need not affect all lung regions uniformly. For example, the lower lung zones may be involved to a greater or lesser degree than the upper, or the central and mid portions of the lungs may be more severely affected than the peripheral ("bat's wing" distribution).

The term "acinar pattern" implies airspace consolidation, which may be confluent and thereby render individual acinar shadows unidentifiable.

Other abnormalities such as pleural effusion and cardiac enlargement may be present.

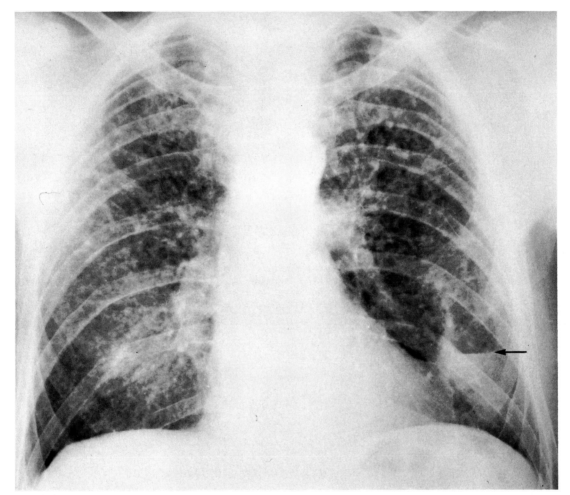

Figure 17. Diffuse Disease (Acinar): Bronchogenic Spread of *Mycobacterium tuberculosis*. A posteroanterior roentgenogram reveals a prominent air-fluid level in the lower portion of the left lung *(arrow)*; the wall of the abscess cavity is rather poorly visualized in this projection. Throughout the remainder of both lungs are multiple, rather ill-defined shadows ranging from 4 to 6 mm in diameter. Several of these densities are discrete and can be identified as individual acinar shadows; the upper two thirds of the lungs are involved to a greater extent than the lower. This is a characteristic picture of bronchogenic spread of *Mycobacterium tuberculosis*; the source of the organisms was the left lower lobe abscess.

Figure 18. Diffuse Disease (Acinar): Pulmonary Edema. A posteroanterior roentgenogram reveals extensive involvement of both lungs by shadows possessing the typical characteristics of airspace consolidation. In most areas, the shadows are confluent so as to produce homogeneous density; in other areas, individual acinar shadows can be identified. An air bronchogram is readily visualized, particularly in the right lung. This diffuse airspace edema had completely resolved roentgenologically 48 hours later. Pulmonary edema secondary to mitral stenosis.

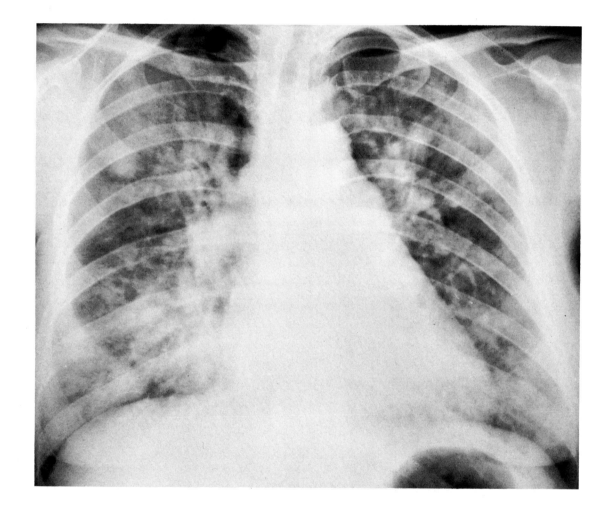

A–9
Diffuse Pulmonary Disease With a Predominantly Acinar Pattern

	ETIOLOGY	ANATOMIC DISTRIBUTION	VOLUME OF THORAX
INFECTIOUS	*Histoplasma capsulatum.*	Generalized.	Unaffected.
	Varicella-zoster virus (chickenpox pneumonia).	Widespread; acinar lesions may be confluent in central areas of lungs.	Unaffected.
	Influenza virus.	Uniform.	Unaffected.
	Ascaris lumbricoides or *Ascaris suum.*	Generalized.	Unaffected.
IMMUNOLOGIC	Goodpasture's syndrome and idiopathic pulmonary hemorrhage.	Widespread but more prominent in perihilar areas and in mid-lung and lower lung zones.	Unchanged.
	Leukocytoclastic vasculitis	Generalized	Unaffected.
NEOPLASTIC	Bronchiolo-alveolar carcinoma.	Diffuse.	Unaffected.
	Hematogenous metastases.	Widespread.	Unaffected.
THROMBOEMBOLIC	Fat embolism.	Diffuse, although predominantly peripheral.	Unaffected.
	Amniotic fluid embolism.	Generalized.	Unaffected.
CARDIOVASCULAR	Pulmonary edema, either hydrostatic or permeability in type.	Usually bilateral and symmetric. Cortex of lung may be relatively spared (the "butterfly" pattern).	Commonly reduced.
INHALATIONAL	Acute aspiration pulmonary edema (near-drowning).	Diffuse.	Unaffected.
	Acute berylliosis (fulminating variety).	Diffuse.	Unaffected.
	Acute berylliosis (insidious variety).	Diffuse.	Unaffected.
	Acute silicoproteinosis.	Diffuse.	May be severely reduced.

A–9
Diffuse Pulmonary Disease With a Predominantly Acinar Pattern (*Continued*)

ADDITIONAL FINDINGS	COMMENTS
Hilar lymph node enlargement frequent.	Acute widely disseminated histoplasmosis; symptoms may be disproportionately mild. Over a period of years, healing may result in multiple small calcific foci. (*See* page 947.)
Hilar lymph node enlargement in some cases.	Over a period of many years, healing may result in multiple small calcific foci throughout the lungs. (*See* page 1062.)
"Mitral configuration" of the heart may be present.	This pattern in acute influenza virus pneumonia occurs particularly in patients who have mitral stenosis or who are pregnant. (*See* page 1043.)
None.	Represents severe edema occasioned by allergic response to the passage of larvae through the pulmonary circulation. (*See* page 1093.)
Confluence of opacities may occur, in which circumstances an air bronchogram will be seen. Lymph node enlargement may be recognized occasionally.	An acinar pattern is seen in relatively pure form in the early stages of these diseases, but with the accumulation of hemosiderin in interstitial space, the pattern becomes reticular. (*See* page 1181.)
None.	Histologic term indicating small vessel vasculitis associated with more or less diffuse airspace hemorrhage. Occurs most frequently with Wegener's granulomatosis and SLE. (*See* page 1264.)
Pleural effusion in 8 to 10 per cent. Mediastinal lymph node enlargement uncommon.	Diffuse disease occurs more often in a mixed pattern. (*See* page 1414.)
———	A rare manifestation of hematogenous metastases. (*See* page 1625.)
Fracture of extremities, pelvis, or axial skeleton usually present. Heart size normal.	Lesions appear within 1 to 2 days after trauma and resolve within 1 to 4 weeks. Opacities tend to be peripheral rather than central. Absence of cardiac enlargement and of signs of postcapillary hypertension aid in differentiation from pulmonary edema of cardiac origin. (*See* page 1782.)
If vascular occlusion is severe enough, the heart may be enlarged as a result of cor pulmonale.	Airspace pulmonary edema indistinguishable from that of any other cause. (*See* page 1788.)
Associated findings depend largely on the etiology of the edema—for example, signs of interstitial pulmonary edema (septal lines, and so forth) in edema of cardiac origin.	(*See* pages 1899 and 1927.)
To be noted are the normal cardiac size and the absence of signs of pulmonary venous hypertension.	Roentgenographic pattern is one of diffuse patchy airspace consolidation typical of pulmonary edema. May occur with aspiration of fresh or sea water (in near-drowning), ethyl alcohol, kerosene, and, by far the most common, acid gastric juice (Mendelson's syndrome). (*See* pages 2387 and 2406.)
———	Morphologic changes consist of severe proteinaceous edema of the lungs. Roentgenologic changes characteristically develop rapidly following an overwhelming exposure. (*See* page 2363.)
None.	Roentgenographic changes consist of diffuse bilateral "haziness" with subsequent development of irregular patchy densities scattered widely throughout the lungs; develop 1 to 4 weeks after the onset of symptoms. Roentgenographic clearing may take two to three months. (*See* page 2363.)
Hilar lymph node enlargement.	Roentgenographic pattern is similar or identical to that of alveolar proteinosis. An acute, rapidly progressive course is characteristic. Most commonly seen in sandblasters. (*See* page 2300.)

Table continued on following page

A–9
Diffuse Pulmonary Disease With a Predominantly Acinar Pattern *(Continued)*

	ETIOLOGY	ANATOMIC DISTRIBUTION	VOLUME OF THORAX
	Drugs		
	Acetylsalicylic acid (aspirin).	Diffuse.	Unaffected.
	Heroin and other narcotics.	Diffuse.	Unaffected.
	Contrast media.	Diffuse.	Unaffected.
	Poisons (ingested or inhaled)		
	Flurocarbon/hydrocarbon ingestion.	Bilateral and predominantly basal.	Unaffected.
DRUGS AND POISONS	Paraquat ingestion.	Predominantly lower zones early, then diffuse.	Unaffected.
	Inhaled toxic gases and aerosols Nitrogen dioxide. Sulfur dioxide. Hydrogen sulfide. Ammonia. Chlorine. Phosgene. Cadmium. Associated with burns.	Diffuse.	Unaffected.
METABOLIC	Alveolar proteinosis.	Bilateral and symmetric, commonly in a "butterfly" distribution. Resolution tends to occur asymmetrically.	Unaffected.
IDIOPATHIC	Sarcoidosis.	Diffuse.	Unaffected.

A–9
Diffuse Pulmonary Disease With a Predominantly Acinar Pattern *(Continued)*

ADDITIONAL FINDINGS	COMMENTS
None.	Permeability pulmonary edema, usually following ingestion of large doses. (*See* page 2442.)
None.	Permeability pulmonary edema. Resolution often occurs in as brief a time as 24 to 48 hours. (*See* page 2444.)
None.	Permeability pulmonary edema. Responsible media include ethiodized oil and high osmolar water-soluble agents. (*See* page 2444.)
A pneumatocele can develop occasionally as a consequence of bronchiolar obstruction.	The roentgenographic pattern consists of patchy airspace consolidation caused by edema. The hila tend to be hazy and indistinct. (*See* page 2451.)
None.	Roentgenographic changes appear 3 to 7 days after ingestion and consist initially of fine granular opacities, predominantly basal in location. This is followed shortly by a pattern of diffuse pulmonary edema. (*See* page 2448.)
None.	Acute pulmonary edema develops within hours of exposure, and usually clears completely if the patient survives. (*See* pages 2453 to 2464.)
None.	Differentiated from pulmonary edema on the basis of absence of cardiac enlargement and of signs of pulmonary venous hypertension; Kerley B lines have been reported, however. (*See* page 2572.)
Hilar and mediastinal lymph node enlargement in many cases.	An uncommon pattern in this disease. May be the predominant pattern (in 20 per cent of patients) or associated with a reticulonodular pattern elsewhere in the lungs. (*See* page 2611.)

TABLE A–10

DIFFUSE PULMONARY DISEASE WITH A
PREDOMINANTLY NODULAR, RETICULAR, OR
RETICULONODULAR PATTERN

The large number of diseases capable of producing an "interstitial" pattern within the lungs has made this table the longest in the group. As with diseases characterized by an acinar pattern, "diffuse" involvement connotes affection of all lobes of both lungs, although the pattern may be more marked in some areas. Other abnormalities may be present, such as pleural effusion, hilar and mediastinal lymph node enlargement, and cardiac enlargement. The individual patterns may be described as follows.

NODULAR. The purely nodular interstitial diseases of the lungs perhaps are best epitomized by hematogenous infections such as miliary tuberculosis. Since the infecting organism arrives via the circulation and is trapped in the capillary sieve, it must be purely interstitial in location, at least early in its course. The pattern consists of discrete punctate opacities that range from tiny nodules 1 mm in diameter (barely visible roentgenographically) to 5 mm.

RETICULAR. This pattern consists of a network of linear opacities which may be regarded as a series of "rings" surrounding spaces of air density. It is useful to describe a reticular pattern according to the size of the "mesh": the terms fine, medium, and coarse are widely used and appear generally acceptable.

RETICULONODULAR. This pattern may be produced by a mixture of nodular deposits and diffuse linear thickening throughout the interstitial space. In addition, although a linear network throughout the interstitial tissue may appear roentgenographically as a purely reticular pattern, the orientation of some of the linear densities parallel to the x-ray beam may suggest a nodular component.

THE HONEYCOMB PATTERN. In this book, the term "honeycomb pattern" is restricted to a very coarse reticulation in which the airspaces in the "mesh" measure not less than 5 mm in diameter.

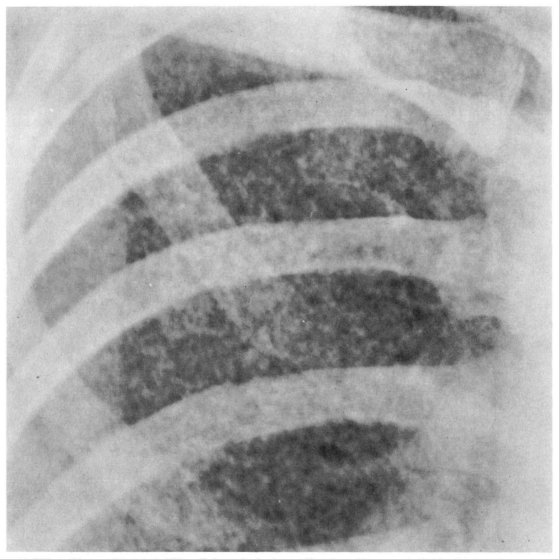

Figure 19. Diffuse Disease (Nodular): Miliary Tuberculosis. A magnified view of the upper half of the right lung from a posteroanterior roentgenogram shows multiple nodules of uniform size measuring approximately 2 mm in diameter. The shadows are quite discrete. This was proved miliary tuberculosis. (Courtesy Dr. Romeo Ethier, Montreal Neurological Hospital.)

Figure 20. Diffuse Disease (Reticular): Interstitial Pulmonary Fibrosis (Rheumatoid Lung Disease). A posteroanterior roentgenogram *(A)* reveals a duffuse reticular pattern throughout both lungs, more marked in the bases than elsewhere. The reticulation is "fine" in character. No other roentgenographic abnormalities are apparent. A magnified view of the lower portion of the left lung *(B)* reveals the pattern to better advantage. From a purely objective point of view, this pattern is not in any way diagnostic. This was a 68-year-old woman with established rheumatoid arthritis.

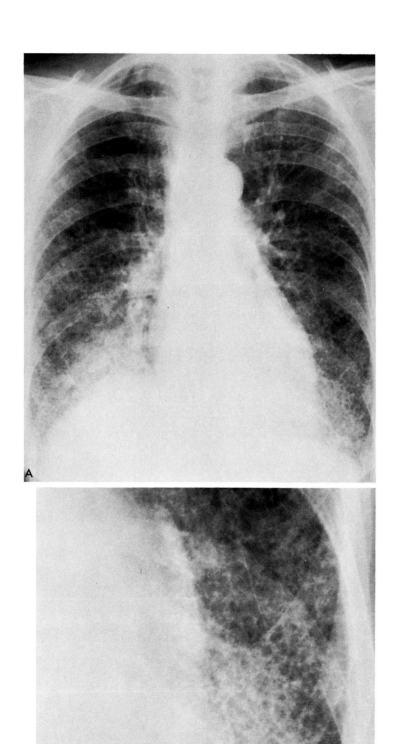

A–10
Diffuse Pulmonary Disease With a Predominantly Nodular, Reticular, or Reticulonodular Pattern

	ETIOLOGY	ANATOMIC DISTRIBUTION	VOLUME OF THORAX
	Bacteria *Mycobacterium tuberculosis.*	Generalized, uniform.	Unaffected.
	Staphylococcus aureus.	Generalized, uniform.	Unaffected.
	Salmonella species.	Generalized, uniform.	Unaffected.
	Fungi *Coccidioides immitis.*	Generalized, uniform.	Unaffected.
	Cryptococcus neoformans.	Generalized, uniform.	Unaffected.
	Paracoccidioides (Blastomyces) brasiliensis.	Generalized, uniform.	Unaffected.
	Blastomyces dermatitidis.	Generalized, uniform.	Unaffected.
	Histoplasma capsulatum.	Generalized, uniform.	Unaffected.
INFECTIOUS			
	Viruses *Mycoplasma pneumoniae.*	*Generalized, uniform.*	*Unaffected.*
	Rubeola.	*Generalized, uniform.*	*Unaffected.*
	Cytomegalovirus.	Generalized, uniform.	Unaffected.
	Parasites *Schistosoma* species (schistosomiasis).	Generalized, uniform.	Unaffected.
	Filaria species (filariasis).	Generalized, uniform.	Unaffected.
	Pneumocystis carinii.	Generalized, uniform.	Unaffected.
	Toxoplasma gondii.	Generalized, uniform.	Unaffected.

A–10
Diffuse Pulmonary Disease With a Predominantly Nodular, Reticular,
or Reticulonodular Pattern (*Continued*)

ADDITIONAL FINDINGS	COMMENTS
None.	Characteristic miliary pattern resulting from hematogenous dissemination. (*See* page 919.)
When of sufficient size, lesions may excavate to produce microabscesses.	Miliary pattern (hematogenous dissemination). (*See* page 836.)
There may be disseminated destructive lesions of bone.	Miliary pattern (hematogenous dissemination). (*See* page 850.)
Generalized, hematogenous spread may lead to destructive lesions of bone.	Miliary pattern (hematogenous dissemination). (*See* page 965.)
None.	Miliary pattern (hematogenous dissemination). (*See* page 977.)
None.	Hematogenous dissemination with production of miliary pattern is the only pulmonary manifestation of the disease. Seen only in South America. (*See* page 975.)
Thoracic or remote bone involvement.	Miliary pattern (hematogenous dissemination). *See* page 970.)
Hilar node enlargement in the majority of cases.	The "epidemic" form of the disease, typically developing in groups of people heavily exposed to organisms in caves or in locales of contaminated soil. Acute nodular opacities measuring 3 to 4 mm may heal to form multiple discrete calcifications many years later. (*See* page 947.)
Kerley B lines in some cases.	The presenting pattern in 28 of 100 cases in one series. Symptoms tend to be mild in contrast to the more common acute segmental disease. (*See* page 1038.)
Lymph node enlargement is common.	Reticulonodular. Primary measles infection of lungs may be associated with secondary bacterial pneumonia. (*See* page 1050.)
None.	Early stage manifestation, followed shortly by patchy acinar consolidation. (*See* page 1068.)
The central pulmonary arteries may be dilated secondary to vascular obstruction.	Hematogenous dissemination with production of a reticulonodular pattern. (*See* page 1111.)
Hilar lymph node enlargement in some cases.	Tropical pulmonary eosinophilia. Hematogenous dissemination with production of very fine reticulonodular pattern of low density. (*See* page 1097.)
No lymph node enlargement or pleural effusion.	Early manifestation. (*See* page 1085.)
Hilar lymph node enlargement common.	Represents the pattern seen in the early stages of diffuse disease. (*See* page 1081.)

Table continued on following page

A–10
Diffuse Pulmonary Disease With a Predominantly Nodular, Reticular, or Reticulonodular Pattern *(Continued)*

	ETIOLOGY	ANATOMIC DISTRIBUTION	VOLUME OF THORAX
	Idiopathic pulmonary hemorrhage. Goodpasture's syndrome.	Usually widespread but may be more prominent in the perihilar areas and the mid and lower lung zones.	May be a slight decrease in late stages of the disease.
	Progressive systemic sclerosis.	Generalized but more prominent in lung bases.	Serial roentgenographic studies may reveal progressive loss of lung volume.
	Rheumatoid disease.	Generalized but more prominent in lung bases.	Serial roentgenographic studies may reveal progressive loss of lung volume.
	Extrinsic allergic alveolitis.	Generalized.	Unaffected.
IMMUNOLOGIC	Dermatomyositis and polymyositis.	Generalized but more prominent in lung bases.	Serial studies may reveal progressive loss of lung volume, particularly if polymyositis involves the muscles of respiration.
	Sjögren's syndrome.	Generalized but more prominent in lung bases.	Unaffected.
	Systemic lupus erythematosus.	Generalized.	Serial studies may reveal progressive loss of lung volume.
	Necrotizing "sarcoidal" angiitis and granulomatosis.	Generalized.	Unaffected.
	Bronchiolo-alveolar carcinoma.	Diffuse.	Unaffected.
	Lymphangitic carcinomatosis.	Commonly generalized but more prominent in the lower lung zones.	Serial roentgenographic studies may reveal progressive reduction in volume.
NEOPLASTIC	Hodgkin's disease.	Generalized.	Unaffected.
	Non-Hodgkin's lymphoma.	Diffuse.	Unaffected.
	Leukemia.	Diffuse.	Unaffected.

A–10
Diffuse Pulmonary Disease With a Predominantly Nodular, Reticular, or Reticulonodular Pattern (*Continued*)

ADDITIONAL FINDINGS	COMMENTS
———	Early in the disease, the pattern represents a transition stage from acute hemorrhage into the airspaces to complete resolution, but in the later stages interstitial fibrosis is permanent. (*See* page 1181.)
Associated findings include esophageal dysperistalsis, terminal pulp calcinosis, absorption of distal phalanges, and widening of the periodontal membrane. Pleural effusion uncommon.	The roentgenographic pattern in the early stages consists of a fine reticulation which tends to coarsen and become reticulonodular as the disease progresses. Small cysts measuring up to 1 cm in diameter may be identified in the lung periphery, particularly in the bases. (*See* page 1220.)
Incidence of coexisting pleural effusion and pulmonary disease not clear, but the two are probably independent. Roentgenographic evidence of rheumatoid arthritis in most patients.	In the early stages the roentgenographic pattern is punctate or nodular in character; in the later or fibrotic stage the pattern consists of medium to coarse reticulation. (*See* page 1200.)
Vary somewhat depending on specific causative antigen, chiefly regarding hilar and mediastinal lymph node enlargement.	Considerable similarity exists in the roentgenographic pattern observed with different antigens, ranging from a diffuse nodular pattern through coarse reticulation characteristic of diffuse interstitial fibrosis. While the pattern is generally "interstitial" in type, involvement of airspaces in the form of acinar opacities may be observed in most if not all during the acute stage of the disease. Irreversible changes of fibrosis tend to occur with continuous or repeated exposure. (*See* pages 1273 and 1286.)
Additional findings may be those associated with progressive systemic sclerosis or rheumatoid disease. When polymyositis involves the muscles of respiration, small-volume lungs may be apparent.	In patients with diffuse lung involvement, the roentgenographic pattern is reticular or reticulonodular and may be indistinguishable from the changes of progressive systemic sclerosis or rheumatoid disease. These diseases sometimes occur in conjunction with primary malignancy elsewhere. (*See* page 1230.)
This syndrome consists of a triad of keratoconjunctivitis sicca, xerostomia, and recurrent swelling of the parotid gland. Occasionally appears in association with any of the connective tissue diseases.	One third of patients show a diffuse reticulonodular pattern similar to that of other collagen diseases characterized by vascular involvement. Joint changes resemble rheumatoid or psoriatic arthritis. Remarkable female sex predominance. (*See* page 1233.)
Pleural effusions common. Enlargement of cardiovascular silhouette usually due to pericardial effusion.	Etiology of reticular pattern varied. (*See* page 1189.)
———	Predominantly nodular pattern. Nodules may be well-defined or ill-defined. Pattern indistinguishable from sarcoidosis roentgenologically but associated with angiitis and necrosis pathologically. (*See* page 1258.)
Pleural effusion in 8 to 10 per cent, always in association with pulmonary involvement.	The roentgenographic pattern is basically nodular; less common than a mixed pattern. Metastatic carcinoma of the pancreas may produce a pattern indistinguishable roentgenologically or morphologically. (*See* page 1414.)
Hilar or mediastinal lymph node enlargement is frequent but is not necessary to the diagnosis. Kerley B lines frequent.	Although the basic change is linear or reticular, there may be a coarse nodular component as well. (*See* page 1632.)
Mediastinal and hilar lymph node enlargement almost invariably associated.	Differentiation from sarcoidosis or lymphangitic carcinomatosis may be difficult or impossible on purely roentgenologic grounds. (*See* page 1507.)
Pleural effusion in about one third of cases. Mediastinal and hilar lymph node enlargement may be inconspicuous or absent.	In some cases of large cell lymphoma, this diffuse pattern may be due to Sjögren's syndrome. The roentgenographic pattern may simulate lymphangitic carcinomatosis. (*See* page 1535.)
Mediastinal and hilar lymph node enlargement may be present but not necessarily. Pleural effusion in some cases.	This is the usual pattern of pulmonary parenchymal involvement, but tends to occur only in the terminal stages of the disease. Resembles lymphangitic carcinomatosis. (*See* page 1554.)

Table continued on following page

A–10
Diffuse Pulmonary Disease With a Predominantly Nodular, Reticular, or Reticulonodular Pattern (Continued)

	ETIOLOGY	ANATOMIC DISTRIBUTION	VOLUME OF THORAX
NEOPLASTIC (Continued)	Waldenström's macroglobulinemia.	Diffuse.	Unaffected.
	Embolism from oily contrast media.	Diffuse, uniform.	Unaffected.
THROMBOEMBOLIC	Talc granulomatosis of drug addicts.	Usually generalized.	May be reduced in the presence of severe fibrosis.
	Metaic mercury embolism.	Predominantly lower lung zones.	Unaffected.
	Schistosomiasis.	Generalized.	Unaffected.
CARDIOVASCULAR	Interstitial pulmonary edema.	Diffuse but predominantly lower lung zones.	May be reduced.
	Pulmonary fibrosis secondary to chronic postcapillary hypertension.	Predominantly mid and lower lung zones.	Unaffected.
INHALATIONAL	Silicosis (simple).	Generalized but often predominantly mid and upper lung zones.	Little affected.
	Coal workers' pneumoconiosis (simple).	Generalized.	Unaffected.
	Asbestosis.	In the early stages, predominantly lower lung zones; later generalized.	Normal or slightly reduced.
	Talcosis.	Identical to asbestosis.	As with asbestosis.
	Kaolin (china-clay) pneumoconiosis.	Generalized.	Unaffected.
	Chronic berylliosis.	Diffuse.	In advanced cases there may be marked loss of lung volume.
	Aluminum pneumoconiosis (aluminosis, bauxitosis, Shaver's disease).	Diffuse.	Considerable loss of lung volume may occur.

A–10
Diffuse Pulmonary Disease With a Predominantly Nodular, Reticular, or Reticulonodular Pattern (*Continued*)

ADDITIONAL FINDINGS	COMMENTS
Pleural effusion in about 50 per cent of cases.	This rare lymphoproliferative disorder is one of the plasma cell dyscrasias. (*See* page 1552.)
None.	The typical pattern is finely reticular; complete clearing usually occurs within 48 to 72 hours, although an abnormal pattern may persist for up to 11 days. In the early stages an arborizing pattern may be apparent owing due to filling of arterioles with contrast medium (similar to that seen on pulmonary arteriography). This complication usually occurs following lymphangiography with ultrafluid Lipiodol. (*See* page 1803.)
Pulmonary arterial hypertension and cor pulmonale in advanced cases.	Creates a pure micronodular pattern similar to alveolar microlithiasis. (*See* page 1794.)
A local collection of mercury may be present in the heart, usually near the apex of the right ventricle.	Roentgenographic appearance distinctive because of the very high density of the intravascular mercury. May be in the form of spherules or of short tubular opacities. (*See* page 1803.)
May be associated with signs of pulmonary arterial hypertension and cor pulmonale.	Presumably results from the passage of ova through vessel walls and the foreign body reaction to them. (*See* page 1111.)
Varies with the etiology of the edema, but usually those associated with pulmonary venous hypertension.	Roentgenographic pattern consists of loss of normal sharp definition of pulmonary vascular markings and thickening of the interlobular septa (Kerley B lines). (*See* page 1790.)
Typical cardiac configuration of chronic mitral valve disease. Almost invariably associated with signs of severe pulmonary venous and arterial hypertension. Ossific nodules may be present.	Roentgenographic pattern consists of a rather coarse but poorly defined reticulation. Probably related to recurrent episodes of airspace and interstitial edema and hemorrhage. (*See* page 1876.)
Hilar lymph node enlargement frequent, uncommonly associated with "eggshell calcification" (5 per cent). Pleural thickening in late stages. Kerley A and B lines are common and may be present without visible nodules.	The roentgenographic pattern ranges from well-defined nodular opacities of uniform density ranging from 1 to 10 mm in diameter to a reticular or reticulonodular appearance. (*See* page 2289.)
Enlargement of hilar lymph nodes is present in some cases but is seldom a predominant feature.	The roentgenographic pattern is typically nodular but may be predominantly reticular in the early stages. Nodules range from 1 to 10 mm in size and tend to be somewhat less well defined than in silicosis. (*See* page 2313.)
The pleural manifestations dominate the picture roentgenographically and consist of plaque formation and general thickening with or without calcification. Hilar lymph node enlargement is seldom if ever a notable feature.	The roentgenographic pattern may be divided into three stages: a fine reticulation occupying predominantly the lower lung zones and creating a ground-glass appearance of the lungs—the early changes; a stage in which the interstitial reticulation becomes more marked, producing the "shaggy heart" sign; and a late stage in which reticulation is generalized throughout the lungs. Note high incidence of associated neoplasia. (*See* page 2336.)
The hallmark in the roentgenologic diagnosis of talcosis is pleural plaque formation—often diaphragmatic in position and massive. Large opacities may develop identical to those seen in silicosis and coal workers' pneumoconiosis.	Pulmonary involvement similar to asbestosis. (*See* page 2354.)
Progressive massive fibrosis may occur as a late manifestation, as in silicosis and coal workers' pneumoconiosis.	The roentgenographic pattern ranges from no more than a generalized increase in lung markings to a diffuse nodular or "miliary" mottling. (*See* page 2356.)
Focal areas of emphysema may be identified in advanced cases, usually in the upper lobes. Spontaneous pneumothorax occurs in over 10 per cent of patients.	The roentgenographic pattern varies with degree of exposure: if minor, there is a diffuse granular "haziness"; with moderate exposure, the pattern is nodular, the nodules being ill-defined and of moderate size (calcification of nodules has been observed); in advanced cases, the pattern may be chiefly reticular. (*See* page 2363.)
Pleural thickening occasionally. Emphysematous bullae develop commonly and are associated with a high incidence of pneumothorax.	The roentgenographic pattern consists of a fine to coarse reticular pattern, sometimes with a nodular component. (*See* page 2366.)

Table continued on following page

A–10
Diffuse Pulmonary Disease With a Predominantly Nodular, Reticular, or Reticulonodular Pattern *(Continued)*

	ETIOLOGY	ANATOMIC DISTRIBUTION	VOLUME OF THORAX
INHALATIONAL *(Continued)*	Pneumoconiosis due to inert radiopaque dusts. Siderosis. Argyrosiderosis. Stannosis (tin oxide). Baritosis (barium sulfate). Antimony pneumoconiosis. Rare earth pneumoconiosis (cerium, etc.).	Generalized.	Unaffected.
	Thesaurosis.	Diffuse.	Unaffected.
AIRWAYS DISEASE	Chronic obstructive pulmonary disease (chronic bronchitic type).	Generalized, uniform.	Slight to moderate increase.
	Cystic fibrosis.	Generalized, uniform.	Considerable overinflation.
	Diffuse panbronchiolitis.	Generalized but predominantly lower lobes.	Overinflation, characteristically severe and generalized.
	Familial dysautonomia (Riley-Day syndrome).	Generalized.	Increased.
DRUGS AND POISONS	**Drug-induced** Nitrofurantoin.	Generalized.	Unaffected.
	Busulfan. Bleomycin. Mitomycin. Pepleomycin. Cyclophosphamide. Chlorambucil. Melphalan. BCNU. Amiodarone. Phenytoin.	Generalized.	Unaffected.
METABOLIC	Lipid storage disease Gaucher's disease. Niemann-Pick disease. Hermansky-Pudlak syndrome.	Generalized.	Unaffected.
	Bronchopulmonary amyloidosis.	Generalized.	Unaffected.
IDIOPATHIC	Sarcoidosis.	Usually generalized but in stages of development or resolution may show some lack of uniformity.	Usually unaffected although fibrosis may be associated with emphysema and overinflation.
	Cryptogenic fibrosing alveolitis; interstitial pulmonary fibrosis.	There is a predilection for the lower lung zones in the early stages, but becoming more generalized and uniform as the disease progresses.	Sequential studies will show progressive loss of lung volume.

A–10
Diffuse Pulmonary Disease With a Predominantly Nodular, Reticular, or Reticulonodular Pattern (*Continued*)

ADDITIONAL FINDINGS	COMMENTS
Lymph node enlargement is not a feature.	In siderosis, the roentgenographic pattern is reticulonodular in type, the deposits being of rather low density compared with the silicotic nodule. In the siderosis of silver polishers, a fine stippled pattern is created. If the free silica content of dust is high (siderosilicosis), the pattern is indistinguishable from that of silicosis. The roentgenographic pattern of the other dusts is basically nodular, the nodules being of very high density. None of these dusts is fibrogenic. (*See* page 2357.)
None.	A questionable entity. Pattern consists of a fine micronodulation which tends to clear with discontinuance of exposure to hair spray. (*See* page 2467.)
Signs of pulmonary arterial hypertension are inevitable, often associated with cor pulmonale.	The pattern is better described as a coarse increase in lung markings rather than reticular or reticulonodular. May be referred to as "increased markings (IM)" emphysema. (*See* page 2135.)
May be associated with segmental areas of consolidation or atelectasis due to bronchopneumonia or bronchiectasis.	The pattern is one of accentuation of the linear markings throughout the lungs giving a coarse reticular appearance. (*See* page 2208.)
Large cystic spaces may be evident on CT.	Unique to Japan. A nodular pattern is characteristic as is hyperinflation. (*See* page 2224.)
Local areas of segmental consolidation and atelectasis may be present, particularly in the right upper lobe and less frequently the right middle and left lower lobes.	The roentgenographic pattern is identical to that of cystic fibrosis. (*See* page 2219.)
Pleural effusion in some cases.	Disease occurs in two forms, acute and chronic. In both, the pattern consists of a diffuse reticulation. The acute form is invariably associated with peripheral blood eosinophilia, the chronic form sometimes. (*See* page 2434.)
None.	Each of these drugs causes a diffuse reticulonodular pattern initially; this may progress to patchy airspace disease. (*See* pages 2418 to 2438. *See* also Table 14–1, page 2419.)
Occasionally lytic bone lesions in Gaucher's disease.	Pattern is usually reticulonodular but may be miliary. (*See* pages 2590 to 2592.)
Hilar and mediastinal lymph node enlargement may be massive, and nodes can be densely calcified.	This is the diffuse alveolar septal form of the disease. (*See* page 2578.)
Hilar and mediastinal lymph node enlargement often constitutes the earliest roentgenologic finding, with diffuse lung involvement developing subsequently (with or without disappearance of the node enlargement). In approximately 25 per cent of cases, the pulmonary changes exist alone.	The pattern is usually reticulonodular in type, although ranging from purely nodular to purely reticular. In the approximately 20 per cent of cases that progress to fibrosis the pattern is coarsely reticular, somewhat uneven in distribution and associated with bulla formation and generalized overinflation. (*See* page 2611.)
Hilar lymph node enlargement and pleural effusion do not occur.	In the early stages the pattern is one of fine reticulation predominantly in the lung bases; the later stage is characterized by a generalized coarse reticular or reticulonodular pattern with "honeycombing" in some cases. (*See* page 2662.)

Table continued on following page

A–10
Diffuse Pulmonary Disease With a Predominantly Nodular, Reticular,
or Reticulonodular Pattern *(Continued)*

	ETIOLOGY	ANATOMIC DISTRIBUTION	VOLUME OF THORAX
IDIOPATHIC *(Continued)*	Eosinophilic granuloma.	Diffuse but with a tendency for predominance of lesions in the upper lung zones.	Usually normal or increased.
	Pulmonary lymphangioleiomyomatosis and tuberous sclerosis.	Usually generalized but predominantly basal.	Increased.
	Neurofibromatosis.	Generalized.	May be increased.
	Alveolar microlithiasis.	Diffuse.	Unaffected.
OTHER CAUSES	Spider angiomas in cirrhosis of the liver.	Predominantly basal.	Unaffected.

A–10
Diffuse Pulmonary Disease With a Predominantly Nodular, Reticular, or Reticulonodular Pattern (*Continued*)

ADDITIONAL FINDINGS	COMMENTS
Hilar and mediastinal lymph-node enlargement are exceedingly rare as is pleural effusion. Spontaneous pneumothorax in some cases.	The roentgenographic pattern varies with the stage of the disease, beginning with nodular and progressing to reticulonodular and finally to a typical honeycomb pattern. Probably the most common cause of a honeycomb pattern.
Chylous pleural effusion and pneumothorax common. Sclerotic (and sometimes lytic) lesions in bone.	The basic pattern is coarse reticulonodular in type and may progress to a typical "honeycomb" appearance. (*See* page 2672.)
Diffuse interstitial fibrosis usually associated with multiple bullae. Scoliosis and mediastinal neurofibromas.	Fibrosis is widespread with some basal predominance, whereas bullae are predominantly upper zonal. (*See* page 2679.)
Spontaneous pneumothorax is a rare complication.	The roentgenographic pattern is virtually pathognomonic, consisting of a myriad of tiny micronodular opacities. Conceivably could be confused with similar (although less numerous) opacities in talcosis of intravenous drug abuse. (*See* page 2693.)
None.	Pattern consists of ill-defined nodules of small size. Associated with hypoxemia due to veno-arterial shunting. (*See* page 2999.)

TABLE A–11

DIFFUSE PULMONARY DISEASE
WITH A MIXED ACINAR
AND RETICULONODULAR PATTERN

The pattern created by combined airspace consolidation and interstitial disease is best exemplified by pulmonary edema secondary to pulmonary venous hypertension. The roentgenographic manifestations of interstitial involvement consist of increased size and loss of definition of lung markings due to the presence of edema fluid within the bronchovascular sheath; airspace consolidation is manifested by discrete and confluent "fluffy" opacities characteristic of acinar-filling processes.

Another example of the mixed pattern is that produced by generalized bronchiolo-alveolar carcinoma: nodular and acinar components reflect the replacement of air spaces by malignant cells, and the linear or reticular component is due to the extension of carcinoma along the bronchovascular bundles, both within and around lymphatics (lymphangitic carcinoma).

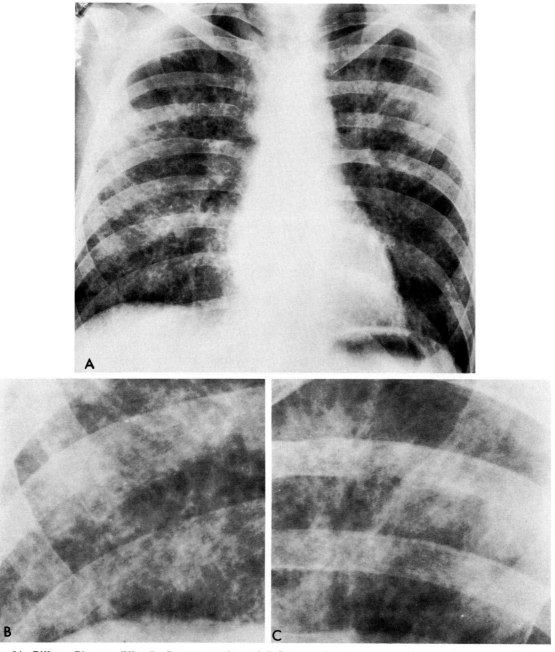

Figure 21. Diffuse Disease (Mixed): *Pneumocystis carinii* **Pneumonia.** A posteroanterior roentgenogram *(A)* demonstrates generalized involvement of both lungs by a process whose pattern is coarsely reticulonodular (seen to better advantage in a magnified view of the right lower lung [*B*]). Superimposed upon this pattern in the upper lung zones are confluent acinar shadows representing airspace consolidation (magnified view of left upper lung [*C*]). *Pneumocystis carinii* organisms were identified premortem in material obtained by needle aspiration and at necropsy throughout both lungs. This 32-year-old male had been the recipient of a renal transplant 2½ years previously and was receiving maintenance doses of corticosteroids and immunosuppressive drugs.

Figure 22. Diffuse Disease (Mixed): Idiopathic Pulmonary Hemosiderosis. A posteroanterior roentgenogram *(A)* shows extensive bilateral parenchymal disease, only the lung apices being spared. The patterns of disease are different in the two lungs, that in the right being finely reticulonodular (as revealed in a magnified view of the upper portion of the right lung [*B*]) and that in the left lung being chiefly acinar in type (magnified view of left upper lung [*C*]). Serial roentgenographic studies of this patient over the past several years had shown repeated episodes of acute pulmonary hemorrhage that, for some unknown reason, had affected chiefly the right lung. As a consequence, this lung had shown progressive deposition of hemosiderin in the interstitial space with a resultant reticular pattern; these changes had become irreversible. Just prior to this roentgenogram, the patient had suffered a fresh pulmonary hemorrhage that involved chiefly the left lung—thus the typical pattern of diffuse airspace consolidation on this side. While predominantly unilateral involvement is most unusual in this disease, idiopathic pulmonary hemosiderosis characteristically produces a mixed roentgenographic pattern—a predominant acinar pattern due to intra-alveolar hemorrhage followed by a reticular pattern due to passage of blood constituents into the interstitial space. In *A*, the longitudinal shadow visualized on the right side of the mediastinum is due to a markedly dilated esophagus secondary to achalasia.

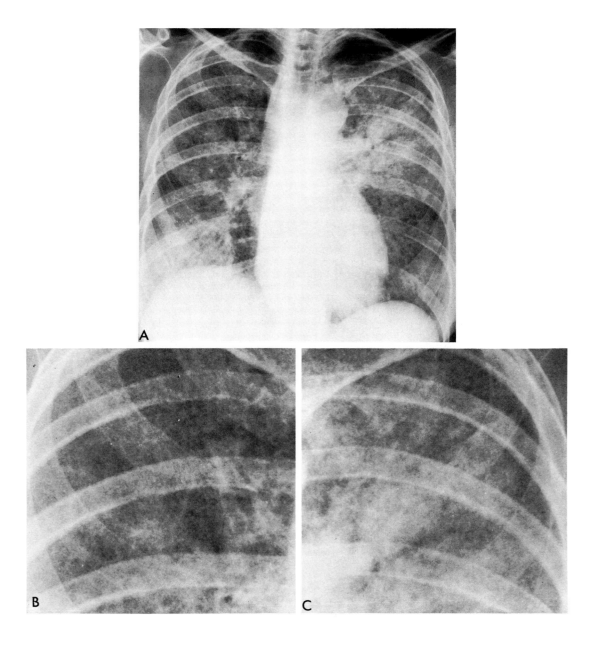

A–11
Diffuse Pulmonary Disease With a Mixed Acinar and Reticulonodular Pattern

	ETIOLOGY	ANATOMIC DISTRIBUTION	VOLUME OF THORAX
INFECTIOUS	Cytomegalovirus.	Generalized, uniform.	Usually unaffected.
	Pneumocystis carinii.	Usually generalized.	Unaffected.
	Mycoplasma pneumoniae and all viruses listed in Table A–4.	Generalized, uniform.	Unaffected or slightly decreased.
	Strongyloides stercoralis.	Generalized.	Unaffected.
IMMUNOLOGIC	Idiopathic pulmonary hemorrhage and Goodpasture's syndrome.	Usually widespread but may be more prominent in the perihilar areas and the mid and lower lung zones.	Usually unaffected.
	Extrinsic allergic alveolitis.	Generalized.	Unaffected.
NEOPLASTIC	Bronchiolo-alveolar carcinoma.	Generalized.	Unaffected.
CARDIOVASCULAR	Pulmonary edema.	Usually generalized.	May be reduced.
DRUGS AND POISONS	Bleomycin.	Diffuse.	Unaffected.
	Methotrexate.⎱ Azathioprine.⎰	Diffuse.	Unaffected.
	Busulfan.	Diffuse.	Unaffected.
	Mitomycin.	Lower zonal predominance.	Unaffected.
	Cyclophosphamide.	Diffuse.	Can be reduced in children.
	Amiodarone.	Diffuse with some lower zonal predominance.	Unaffected.
	Gold.	Diffuse.	Unaffected.
IDIOPATHIC	Sarcoidosis.	Generalized.	Unaffected.
	Diffuse fibrosing alveolitis (desquamative interstitial pneumonitis).	Generalized but with lower zone predominance	Progressive loss of lung volume common.

A–11
Diffuse Pulmonary Disease With a Mixed Acinar and Reticulonodular Pattern (Continued)

ADDITIONAL FINDINGS	COMMENTS
None.	Combined interstitial and airspace disease with production of mixed reticulonodular and acinar patterns. (*See* page 1068.)
None.	Pattern is combined reticulonodular and acinar. Sometimes occurs in combination with cytomegalovirus infection. (*See* page 1085.)
None.	Diffuse reticular pattern early, with superimposition of patchy airspace consolidation. (*See* page 1036.)
None.	Represents overwhelming infestation in a compromised host. (*See* page 1094.)
Rarely hilar lymph node enlargement. Coalescence of lesions may permit visualization of an air bronchogram.	The mixed pattern is caused by a combination of patchy airspace consolidation from hemorrhage and the presence of hemosiderin and fibrous tissue in the interstitium. It may clear completely or may leave a residuum of reticulation due to irreversible interstitial fibrosis. (*See* page 1181.)
Vary somewhat, depending on specific causative antigen, chiefly regarding hilar and mediastinal lymph node enlargement.	The majority of these cases are manifested by a relatively pure "interstitial" pattern which is either nodular or reticulonodular. However, in some cases acinar shadows representing airspace involvement are superimposed on the reticular pattern during the acute stage of the disease. (*See* page 1273.)
Prominent linear opacities extending along the bronchovascular bundles toward the hila usually represent lymphatic permeation. Pleural effusion in 8 to 10 per cent. Mediastinal lymph node enlargement uncommon.	The mixed pattern consists of acinar, nodular, and reticulonodular components. (*See* page 1414.)
Cardiomegaly common but not invariable.	Combined interstitial and airspace edema. (*See* page 1899.)
None.	Toxicity in 1 to 2 per cent caused by oxidants in most cases, hypersensitivity in a minority. As with other drugs in this column, the roentgenographic pattern is reticulonodular at the beginning, then becomes acinar. (*See* page 2418.)
Rarely enlargement of hilar lymph nodes.	Toxicity in 5 per cent of patients caused by a cellular immune response. Mortality rate about 1 per cent. (*See* page 2433.)
Pleural effusion very uncommon.	Clinically recognized toxicity occurs in only about 4 per cent of patients and only with long-term use. (*See* page 2427.)
Pleural effusion is a more common feature than in other cytotoxic drug reactions.	Mortality rate is said to be about 50 per cent. (*See* page 2426.)
Occasionally, severe airspace pulmonary edema.	Incidence of toxicity very low, probably less than 1 per cent. (*See* page 2428.)
Sometimes accompanied by peripheral consolidation resembling chronic eosinophilic pneumonia.	Incidence of toxicity ranges from 1 to 6 per cent. (*See* page 2438.)
None.	The mechanism is thought to be a hypersensitivity reaction, approximately one third of patients showing peripheral eosinophilia. (*See* page 2443.)
Hilar and mediastinal lymph node enlargement may coexist.	A mixed acinar and reticulonodular pattern is more common than a predominantly acinar pattern alone. (*See* page 2611.)
Hilar and mediastinal lymph node enlargement uncommon.	Early changes have been described as "ground-glass" opacification of both lungs. (*See* page 2662.)

TABLE A–12

GENERALIZED PULMONARY OLIGEMIA

This table includes all diseases in which there is reduction in the caliber of the pulmonary arterial tree throughout the lungs. As stressed previously, appreciation of such vascular change is a subjective process based on a thorough familiarity with the normal. Since reduction in the size of peripheral vessels constitutes the main criterion of diagnosis of all diseases in this category, differentiation depends upon secondary signs. The two ancillary signs of major importance are abnormal size and configuration of the central hilar vessels and general pulmonary overinflation. Three combinations of changes are possible:

1. Small peripheral vessels; no overinflation; normal or small hila. This combination indicates reduction in pulmonary blood flow from central causes and is virtually pathognomonic of cardiac disease, usually congenital.

2. Small peripheral vessels; no overinflation; enlarged hilar pulmonary arteries. This combination may result from peripheral or central causes (respectively, primary pulmonary arterial hypertension or massive pulmonary artery thrombosis without infarction).

3. Small peripheral vessels; general pulmonary overinflation; normal or enlarged hilar pulmonary arteries. This combination is virtually pathognomonic of pulmonary emphysema.

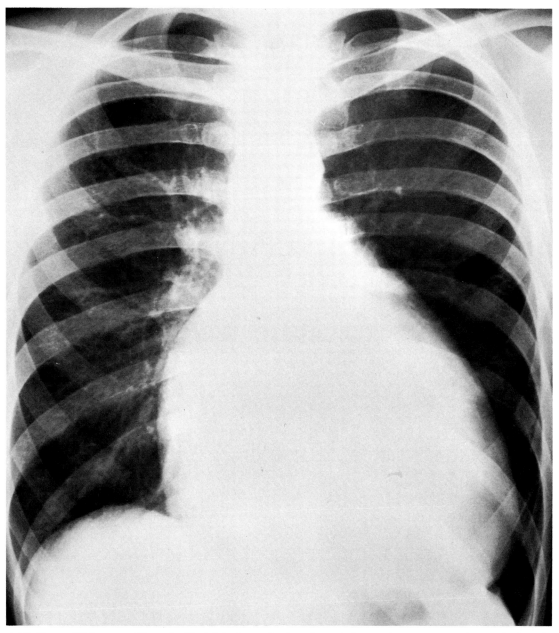

Figure 23. General Pulmonary Oligemia: Ebstein's Anomaly. A posteroanterior roentgenogram reveals a markedly enlarged heart whose right border strongly suggests dilatation of the right atrium. The hila are diminutive and the peripheral vessels narrow and attenuated. Pulmonary oligemia is uniform throughout both lungs. This 20-year-old man was relatively asymptomatic and was able to take part in sports; there was no cyanosis. The anomaly was surgically corrected.

Figure 24. General Pulmonary Oligemia: Emphysema. A posteroanterior roentgenogram *(A)* reveals generalized reduction in the caliber of peripheral vessels throughout the lungs, seen to better advantage on a tomogram of both lungs in anteroposterior projection *(B)*. There is severe generalized pulmonary overinflation (note the low flattened configuration of the diaphragm). There is no evidence of cardiomegaly, and the hilar pulmonary arteries are not enlarged; thus, despite the generalized oligemia, there is no evidence of pulmonary arterial hypertension.

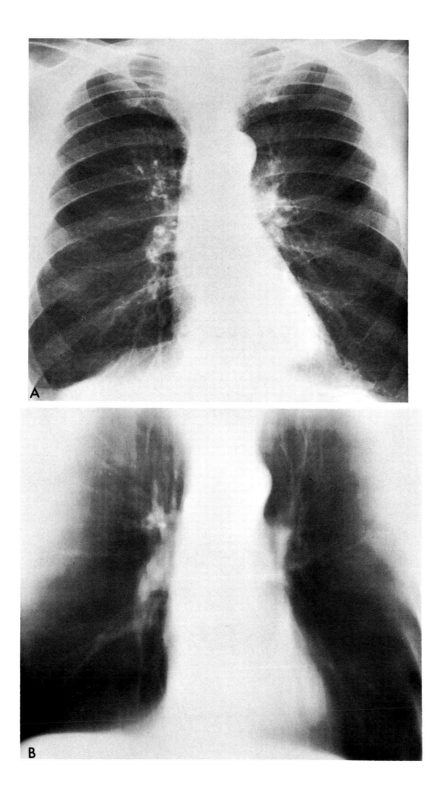

A–12
Generalized Pulmonary Oligemia

	ETIOLOGY
	Pulmonary artery stenosis or coarctation.

DEVELOPMENTAL	**Congenital cardiac anomalies**
	  Isolated pulmonic stenosis.
	  Tetralogy of Fallot with pulmonary atresia.
	  Persistent truncus arteriosus (type IV).
	  Ebstein's anomaly.

INFECTIOUS	*Schistosoma* species.
IMMUNOLOGIC	Pulmonary hypertension associated with connective tissue disease, notably SLE, progressive systemic sclerosis, and the CREST syndrome.
NEOPLASTIC	Metastases from trophoblastic neoplasms.
THROMBOEMBOLIC	Widespread embolic disease to small arteries.
CARDIOVASCULAR	Chronic postcapillary hypertension (mitral stenosis). Primary pulmonary hypertension.
AIRWAYS DISEASE	Emphysema. Bullous disease of the lung.

A–12
Generalized Pulmonary Oligemia (*Continued*)

DIFFERENTIAL CHARACTERISTICS	COMMENTS
Absence of overinflation and expiratory air trapping differentiates this from emphysema. Pulmonary arteriography essential to differentiate it from primary pulmonary hypertension or multiple peripheral embolization.	Diffuse pulmonary oligemia occurs when lesions are *multiple* and *peripheral*. Pulmonary arterial hypertension and cor pulmonale common. Associated cardiovascular anomalies frequent (60 per cent), particularly pulmonic stenosis. (*See* page 735.)
Cardiac enlargement present in some cases; no overinflation or air trapping. Hila diminutive as a rule, permitting differentiation from primary pulmonary hypertension and multiple peripheral embolization (exception is poststenotic dilatation of main or left pulmonary artery in valvular pulmonic stenosis).	Pulmonary vascular pattern formed partly or wholly by hypertrophied bronchial circulation (may be studied by selective bronchial arteriography or flood aortography). (*See* page 755.)
Indistinguishable from pattern of primary pulmonary hypertension. Central pulmonary arteries can be huge. Absence of overinflation.	More common method of presentation is a diffuse reticulonodular pattern. (*See* page 1111.)
Indistinguishable from primary pulmonary hypertension. No overinflation.	Often associated with Raynaud's phenomenon. (*See* page 1230.)
Indistinguishable from primary pulmonary hypertension. No overinflation.	Acute cor pulmonale responds to treatment in some cases. (*See* page 1651.)
Indistinguishable from primary pulmonary hypertension. No overinflation.	Multiple pulmonary emboli result in pulmonary artery hypertension; in contrast to emphysema, lung volume is either normal or decreased. (*See* pages 1718 and 1848.)
Characteristic configuration of enlarged heart, particularly left atrium. Diffuse oligemia represents late stage of chronic venous and arterial hypertension.	Commonly associated with episodes of interstitial or airspace edema. Roentgenographic evidence of hemosiderosis and ossific nodules in an occasional case. (*See* page 1861.)
Main and hilar pulmonary arteries are enlarged and show increased amplitude of pulsation fluoroscopically. Peripheral vessels diminutive. Absence of overinflation.	Preponderance in young women; familial tendency; dramatic response to intravenous injection of acetylcholine in some cases. (*See* page 1842.)
Generalized overinflation serves to differentiate this disease from others characterized by diffuse oligemia. Bullae may be present.	The oligemia may be predominant in the upper or lower lung zones or in one lung. (*See* page 2120.)
Margins of bullae may be identified as curved, hairline opacities. Hyperinflation as in diffuse emphysema.	A pattern of diffuse oligemia is rare in bullous disease of the lungs without emphysema, but may be seen when bullae are numerous and have enlarged maximally. (*See* page 2166.)

TABLE A–13

UNILATERAL, LOBAR, OR SEGMENTAL
PULMONARY OLIGEMIA

The same three combinations of changes apply in this pattern as in general pulmonary oligemia (the major difference between local and general oligemia is in its effect on pulmonary hemodynamics):

1. Small peripheral vessels, no overinflation; normal or small hilum. This is epitomized by lobar or unilateral hyperlucent lung (Swyer-James or Macleod's syndrome).

2. Small peripheral vessels; no overinflation; enlarged hilar pulmonary arteries (or an enlarged hilum). This combination is due almost invariably to unilateral pulmonary artery embolism without infarction.

3. Small peripheral vessels; overinflation; normal hilar pulmonary arteries. This combination is distinctive of obstructive emphysema.

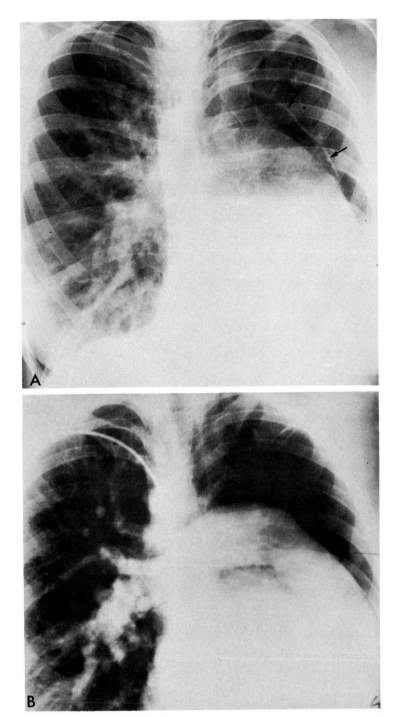

Figure 25. Local Pulmonary Oligemia: Agenesis of the Left Pulmonary Artery. On the posteroanterior roentgenogram *(A)*, there is evidence of marked shift of the mediastinum to the left. The visible portion of the left lung shows a severe diminution in the size of its vascular markings while those in the right lung are markedly increased in size; a left hilar complex cannot be identified. The overinflated right lung has extended across the anterior mediastinal septum into the left hemithorax, the vertical line shadow *(arrows)* representing four layers of pleura at the interface of the two lungs. A pulmonary angiogram *(B)* shows no evidence of a left pulmonary artery, the total right ventricular output passing into the right lung. As is so often the case in agenesis of the left pulmonary artery, this patient had a congenital intracardiac anomaly in the form of a ventricular septal defect.

Figure 26. Local Pulmonary Oligemia: Unilateral Emphysema (Swyer-James or Macleod's Syndrome). A posteroanterior roentgenogram of a 13-year-old asymptomatic boy *(A)* reveals considerable disparity in the density of the two lungs, the left being generally more radiolucent. The vascular markings throughout the left lung are diminutive, the disparity in blood flow to the two lungs being well illustrated in a pulmonary angiogram *(B)* and in a lung scan *(C)*. The left lung is of approximately normal volume compared to the right. (Courtesy Dr. William Beamish, Royal Alexandra Hospital, Edmonton.)

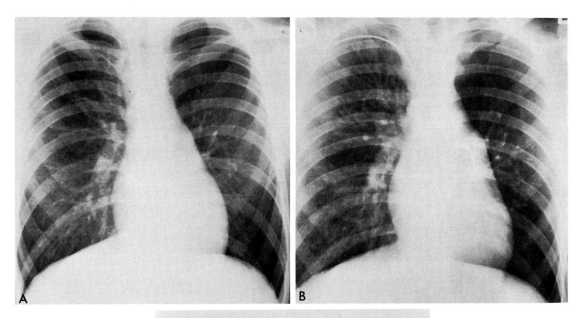

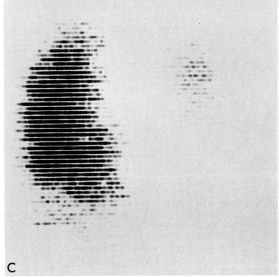

A–13
Unilateral, Lobar, or Segmental Pulmonary Oligemia

	ETIOLOGY
	Hypogenetic lung syndrome.
	Proximal interruption of the right or left pulmonary artery.
DEVELOPMENTAL	Anomalous origin of left pulmonary artery from the right.
	Congenital bronchial atresia.
	Neonatal lobar hyperinflation (congenital lobar emphysema).
INFECTIOUS	*Mycobacterium tuberculosis* (primary).
	Staphylococcus aureus.
IMMUNOLOGIC	Relapsing polychondritis.
	Pulmonary carcinoma.
NEOPLASTIC	Carcinoid tumor.
	Tracheobronchial gland tumors.
	All neoplasms of soft tissues, bone, and cartilage listed in Table A–2.
	Hodgkin's disease.
	Non-Hodgkin's lymphoma.
THROMBOEMBOLIC	Pulmonary thromboembolism without infarction.

A–13
Unilateral, Lobar, or Segmental Pulmonary Oligemia (*Continued*)

DIFFERENTIAL CHARACTERISTICS	COMMENTS
Anomalous vein forms "scimitar sign," which is diagnostic.	Partial hypoplasia of the right lung and right pulmonary artery; associated anomalies include dextrocardia, mirror-image bronchial tree, and anomalous venous drainage of right lung to inferior vena cava. Right lung supplied by systemic arteries, in part or wholly (*see* page 748.)
Absent or diminutive hilum. Differentiation from Swyer-James (Macleod's) syndrome by absence of air trapping on forced expiration. Confirmation of diagnosis by pulmonary arteriography.	Involved lung hypoplastic and of reduced volume; supplied by hypertrophied bronchial circulation. Anomalous artery usually on side opposite aortic arch: when on *left*, high incidence of associated cardiovascular anomalies. (*See* page 729.)
If right main bronchus is compressed, whole right lung may be radiolucent due to air trapping—thus, lung is *overinflated*. Confirmation by demonstration of posterior displacement of barium-filled esophagus due to interposition of anomalous artery between lower trachea and esophagus: arteriography diagnostic.	If anomalous artery compresses trachea rather than right main bronchus, both lungs will show overinflation and expiratory air trapping. Severe compression may result in atelectasis of right lung. (*See* page 731.)
Almost invariably associated with a smooth, lobulated soft tissue mass (due to inspissated mucus) distal to the point of atresia.	May involve a variety of segmental bronchi but most commonly affects the apicoposterior segment of the left upper lobe. Affected bronchopulmonary segments are air-containing owing to collateral air drift. (*See* page 721.)
Characterized by severe overinflation of a pulmonary lobe, most commonly the left upper or right middle lobe. Air trapping is severe and results in marked enlargement of the lobe and contralateral displacement of the mediastinum.	Only about a third of cases become manifest at birth, the remainder not being recognized until some weeks later. Cyanosis may develop in severe cases. (*See* page 722.)
Ipsilateral hilar lymph node enlargement is present in most cases of primary tuberculosis. There is a predilection for anterior segment of upper lobe and medial segment of middle lobe.	Overinflation and oligemia result from partial bronchial obstruction. Although the majority of cases with this pattern are consequent upon extrabronchial compression from lymph nodes, some may develop as a result of bronchostenosis from tuberculous granuloma. Atelectasis may replace localized oligemia at a later stage. (*See* page 895.)
Large pneumatoceles develop as a complication of acute staphylococcal pneumonia and may fill an entire hemithorax. Air-fluid levels are present in some cases. Characteristically undergo rapid change in size.	Common in infants and children, rare in adults. (*See* page 836.)
Oligemia is usually unilateral and involves a whole lung. It results from hypoxic vasoconstriction secondary to alveolar hypoventilation caused by narrowing of a major bronchus. Air trapping is present on expiration.	A rare cause of local oligemia. (*See* page 1238.)
A segment, lobe, or whole lung may be affected. A mass is almost invariably identifiable. Air trapping may be noted on forced expiration.	This is a rare manifestation of pulmonary carcinoma. It may progress to a pattern of homogeneous segmental consolidation and atelectasis as a result of obstructive pneumonitis. Lymphatic spread of neoplasm to hilar lymph nodes occasionally results in compression of a bronchus, with resultant oligemia. (*See* page 1369.)
Air trapping on expiration and oligemia may be followed by atelectasis or obstructive pneumonitis.	Volume of affected parenchyma usually smaller than normal at full inspiration. Air trapping and oligemia result from partial endobronchial obstruction and hypoxic vasoconstriction. (*See* pages 1477, 1497, and 1577.)
Asymmetric lymph node enlargement in paratracheal, retrosternal, and hilar areas is almost invariable.	Local oligemia is a rare manifestation of endobronchial Hodgkin's disease. (*See* page 1507.)
Usually in association with hilar and mediastinal lymph node enlargement. Indistinguishable from Hodgkin's disease.	A rare manifestation of the secondary form of non-Hodgkin's lymphoma; results from partial endobronchial obstruction. (*See* page 1535.)
Almost invariably associated with obstruction of a major pulmonary artery (*e.g.*, lobar). Affected artery is characteristically widened and of sharper than normal definition. The involved bronchopulmonary segments may show moderate loss of volume—of value in differentiation from other causes of local oligemia.	Local oligemia resulting from thromboembolism constitutes Westermark's sign. (*See* page 1718.)

Table continued on following page

A–13
Unilateral, Lobar, or Segmental Pulmonary Oligemia *(Continued)*

	ETIOLOGY
INHALATIONAL	Foreign body aspiration.
	Local obstructive emphysema.
	Unilateral or lobar emphysema (Swyer-James syndrome).
AIRWAYS DISEASE	
	Bullae.
METABOLIC	Bronchopulmonary amyloidosis.
	Sarcoidosis.
IDIOPATHIC	
	Neurofibromatosis.

A–13
Unilateral, Lobar, or Segmental Pulmonary Oligemia (*Continued*)

DIFFERENTIAL CHARACTERISTICS	COMMENTS
Lower lobe predominance, invariably segmental in distribution. Foreign body identifiable as an opaque shadow in some cases.	Air trapping and local oligemia are more common manifestations of foreign body inhalation than atelectasis or obstructive pneumonitis. (*See* page 2382.)
In addition to showing air trapping on expiration (as in Swyer-James syndrome), affected zones are overinflated at TLC.	Approximately 50 per cent of cases of emphysema have local rather than diffuse involvement of the lungs as assessed roentgenologically, although function tests usually indicate generalized disease. Affected areas may be upper zones or lower zones, more frequently the latter. (*See* page 2120.)
Oligemia characteristically involves a whole lung, producing unilateral radiolucency; however, single lobes may be similarly affected. Both the hilar and peripheral vessels are diminutive, although structurally normal. The volume of affected lung at TLC is normal or reduced, seldom if ever increased. Air trapping on expiration is a *sine qua non* to the diagnosis, and permits differentiation from agenesis of a pulmonary artery. Bronchiectasis is demonstrable in most cases.	There is convincing evidence that this abnormality results from acute pneumonia during infancy or childhood, frequently of viral etiology; infection of the peripheral airways leads to bronchiolitis obliterans and a morphologic picture virtually indistinguishable from emphysema. (*See* page 2177.)
Characterized by sharply defined, air-containing spaces bounded by curvilinear, hairline shadows; range in size from 1 cm to the volume of a hemithorax. Vascular markings are absent; adjacent lung parenchyma is compressed. Overinflation and air trapping are usual.	Predominantly unilateral in contrast to the bilateral disease described in Table A–12. Unlike unilateral emphysema, the vasculature is absent rather than attenuated. (*See* pages 2132 and 2166.)
A manifestation of endobronchial amyloid deposits producing partial bronchial obstruction. Parenchymal lesions may be present as well.	A rare cause of local oligemia. This is the tracheobronchial form of this disorder. (*See* page 2578.)
Oligemia results from partial bronchial obstruction and consequent air trapping and overinflation. Usually lobar or multilobar. Diagnosis may be suspected from symmetric hilar and paratracheal lymph node enlargement.	A rare cause of local oligemia. Although bronchial compression from enlarged nodes may be the cause, obstruction more often results from endobronchial sarcoid deposits. (*See* page 2611.)
Multiple bullae, usually with upper zonal predominance, often associated with diffuse interstitial fibrosis but can occur alone.	Usually associated with numerous cutaneous nodules and other stigmata. (*See* page 2679.)

TABLE A–14

PLEURAL EFFUSION UNASSOCIATED WITH OTHER ROENTGENOGRAPHIC EVIDENCE OF DISEASE IN THE THORAX

This title is self-explanatory. Effusion may be unilateral or bilateral. It must be emphasized that the lack of association with other abnormalities in the chest implies the absence of other *roentgenologically demonstrable* abnormality. Obviously, disease may be present but be roentgenographically invisible; for example, pulmonary involvement in rheu- matoid disease may have no definite roentgenographic manifestations, although a considerable degree of pulmonary interstitial fibrosis may be apparent histologically. Conversely, diseases in which pulmonary abnormality is obscured by an effusion (e.g., lobar collapse due to an obstructing endobronchial cancer) are *not* included in this table, since the presence of underlying pulmonary disease would be clearly demonstrable by CT or after thoracentesis.

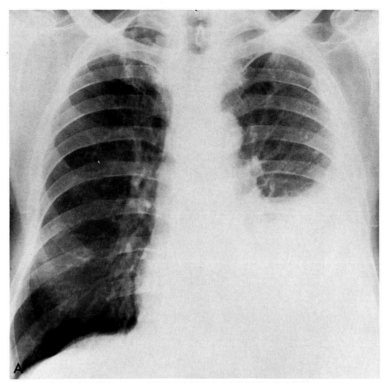

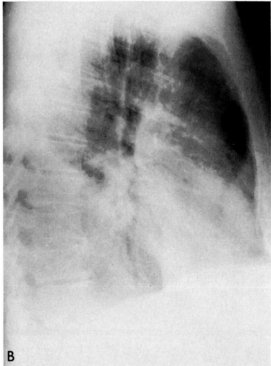

Figure 27. Pleural Effusion in Rheumatoid Pleuropulmonary Disease. Posteroanterior *(A)* and lateral *(B)* roentgenograms reveal the typical appearance of a moderate accumulation of fluid in the left pleural space. Following thoracentesis, the lungs were regarded as normal roentgenologically, although subsequent examination of the lungs at necropsy estalished the presence of extensive changes compatible with rheumatoid disease.

A–14
Pleural Effusion Unassociated With Other Roentgenographic Evidence of Disease in the Thorax

	ETIOLOGY	CHARACTER OF THE FLUID
INFECTIOUS	**Bacteria** *Mycobacterium tuberculosis.*	Serous exudate. Predominantly lymphocytic reaction; erythrocytes may be present but seldom in great numbers. Blood glucose levels below 25 mg/100 ml highly suggestive (N.B.: differentiate from effusions of rheumatoid disease).
	Viruses All viruses and *Mycoplasma.*	Serous exudate.
	Subphrenic abscess.	Serous exudate.
IMMUNOLOGIC	Systemic lupus erythematosus.	Serous exudate.
	Rheumatoid disease.	Serous exudate; tends to be turbid and greenish-yellow. Predominance of lymphocytes. Glucose concentration characteristically low, with failure to rise on IV glucose infusion (failure of glucose-transport mechanism).
NEOPLASTIC	Neoplasms arising within thorax: Lymphoma.	Usually serosanguineous exudate; may be chylous or chyliform.
	Neoplasms arising outside the thorax: Metastatic carcinoma.	Serous exudate; varies in blood content from none to grossly hemorrhagic. Glucose content greater than 80 mg/100 ml is common but not diagnostic.
	Ovarian neoplasms (Meigs-Salmon syndrome).	Usually serous exudate; occasionally serosanguineous.
	Carcinoma of the pancreas.	Serous exudate.
	Retroperitoneal lymphoma.	Serous exudate.
	Leukemia.	Serous exudate.

A–14
Pleural Effusion Unassociated with Other Roentgenographic Evidence of Disease in the Thorax (Continued)

CRITERIA FOR PRESUMPTIVE DIAGNOSIS	CRITERIA FOR POSITIVE DIAGNOSIS	COMMENTS
Combination of positive tuberculin reaction and predominantly lymphocytic pleural fluid.	Positive pleural biopsy. Culture of tubercle bacili from pleural fluid.	A negative tuberculin test may be found in early cases. Strong tendency to subsequent development of active pulmonary tuberculosis if effusion not treated. Effusions rarely bilateral. A manifestation of primary tuberculosis more common in the adult (approximately 40 per cent) than in children (10 per cent). (See page 2717.)
None.	Elevated agglutinin titer to offending organism.	May be bilateral. (See page 2722.)
Elevation and fixation of hemidiaphragm.	Gas and fluid in subphrenic space.	More commonly associated with basal pulmonary disease ("plate" atelectasis or pneumonitis). (See page 2736.)
Clinical findings of typical rash, renal disease, heart murmur, and so forth.	Positive antinuclear antibodies or LE-cell test in association with characteristic clinical findings.	Occurs as isolated abnormality in slightly more than 10 per cent of cases. Effusion usually small, but may be moderate or even massive; bilateral in about 50 per cent. Usually clears without residua. Often associated with pericardial effusion. (See page 2723.)
Clinical or roentgenologic changes of rheumatoid arthritis. High titer of rheumatoid factor in serum highly suggestive but not conclusive. Biopsy of pleura showing typical rheumatoid granulation tissue.	Pleural fluid glucose abnormalities associated with one or more presumptive criteria.	Almost exclusively in men. Usually unilateral, on right slightly more often than on left. May antedate signs and symptoms of rheumatoid arthritis, but usually follows. Effusion often persists for several months. (See page 2725.)
Peripheral lymph node enlargement, hepatosplenomegaly, and so forth.	Finding of typical cells in pleural fluid or biopsy of pleura or lymph node.	This broad heading includes both Hodgkin's disease and non-Hodgkin's lymphoma. Approximately 30 per cent of cases have pleural effusion, but seldom without associated pulmonary or mediastinal node involvement. (See page 2729.)
Identification of remote primary neoplasm.	Finding of characteristic tissue on needle biopsy or malignant cells in pleural fluid.	Most commonly from breast; also from pancreas, stomach, ovary, kidney. (See page 2730.)
Pleural fluid negative for malignant cells; pelvic mass.	Presence of ovarian neoplasm with ascites; disappearance of effusion following oophorectomy.	Ovarian neoplasm may be fibroma, thecoma, cystadenoma, adenocarcinoma, granulosa-cell tumor; occasionally leiomyoma of uterus. (See page 2737.)
Pleural fluid negative for malignant cells; clinical signs of intra-abdominal neoplasia.	Disappearance of fluid following removal of primary.	Effusion may occur without direct involvement of thorax by primary; probably related to transport of fluid into thorax via diaphragmatic lymphatics. (See page 2730.)
Pleural fluid negative for malignant cells; clinical signs of intra-abdominal neoplasia.	Disappearance of fluid following treatment of primary.	
Disappearance of effusion following treatment of leukemia.	Demonstration of leukemic cells in peripheral blood.	Second in frequency only to mediastinal node enlargement. (See page 2730.)

Table continued on following page

Pleural Effusion Unassociated With Other Roentgenographic Evidence of Disease in the Thorax (Continued)

	ETIOLOGY	CHARACTER OF THE FLUID
THROMBOEMBOLIC	Pulmonary embolism.	Almost invariably serosanguineous.
CARDIOVASCULAR	Cardiac decompensation.	Transudate.
INHALATIONAL	Asbestosis.	Sterile, serous or blood-tinged exudate.
TRAUMATIC	Closed-chest trauma.	Blood (hemothorax). Chyle (chylothorax). Contains ingested food (esophageal rupture).
	Following abdominal surgery.	Serous exudate.
DRUG-INDUCED	Bromcriptine. Methysergide. Dantrolene sodium. Nitrofurantoin.	Serous exudate.
MISCELLANEOUS CAUSES	Pancreatitis.	Usually serous exudate but may be serosanguineous. Pleural fluid amylase higher than serum amylase.
	Nephrotic syndrome and other causes of diminished plasma osmotic pressure.	Transudate.
	Acute glomerulonephritis.	Transudate.
	Myxedema.	Serous exudate.
	Cirrhosis with ascites.	Transudate.
	Hydronephrosis and urinothorax.	Serous exudate.
	Uremic pleuritis.	Serous exudate. Sometimes fibrinous.
	Dialysis.	Serous exudate, sometimes sanguineous as a result of anticoagulation.
	Lymphedema.	High protein content.
	Familial recurring polyserositis.	Serofibrinous exudate.
	Dressler's syndrome.	Serosanguineous exudate.

A–14
Pleural Effusion Unassociated with Other Roentgenographic Evidence of
Disease in the Thorax (*Continued*)

CRITERIA FOR PRESUMPTIVE DIAGNOSIS	CRITERIA FOR POSITIVE DIAGNOSIS	COMMENTS
History of sudden onset of pleural pain with or without peripheral thrombophlebitis. Rarely may observe relative diminution of peripheral vasculature roentgenologically.	Lung scan or pulmonary angiogram or both.	Frequency of effusion as sole manifestation of pulmonary embolism not precisely known, but probably very uncommon. (*See* page 2731.)
Clinical signs of cardiac decompensation.	Disappearance of the fluid on treatment of the failure.	Frequently unilateral on the right, seldom on the left. (*See* page 2731.)
History of asbestos exposure.	Only following exclusion of other diagnostic possibilities, particularly tuberculosis and mesothelioma.	Diagnosis should be made with caution. Effusions frequently recurrent, usually bilateral, and often associated with chest pain. (*See* page 2727.)
History.	Thoracentesis and history.	May originate from chest wall, diaphragm, mediastinum, or lung. (*See* page 2732.)
History. Time lag between trauma and development of effusion.	Thoracentesis; lymphangiography.	Side of chylothorax depends on site of thoracic duct rupture. (*See* page 2735.)
History.	Thoracentesis; esophagogram.	Almost always left-sided. Generally due to surgical procedure. (*See* page 2732.)
History of recent abdominal surgery.	Unnecessary. Almost always self-limited.	Usually requires lateral decubitus roentgenograms for identification. Present in 49 per cent of patients in one series. (*See* page 2736.)
History of specific drug therapy.	Resolution following withdrawal of the drug.	(*See* Chapter 14, page 2417.)
Clinical picture of acute abdomen.	Elevated level of pleural fluid anylase.	May occur in acute, chronic or relapsing pancreatitis. Majority of effusions are left-sided. (*See* page 2736.)
General edema.	Thoracentesis; biochemical assay of serum and urine.	Effusion commonly infrapulmonary. (*See* page 2738.)
Usual findings of acute glomerulonephritis.	———	(*See* page 2738.)
Studies of thyroid activity.	———	Effusion occurs more often in pericardium. (*See* page 2738.)
Demonstration of cirrhosis and ascites. (N.B.: exclude carcinoma of liver.)	———	Ascitic fluid enters pleural space via diaphragmatic lymphatics (as in Meigs-Salmon syndrome). (*See* page 2738.)
Demonstration of hydronephrosis.	Disappearance of effusion following removal of urinary obstruction.	Mechanism not clear; possibly related to transport of fluid via diaphragmatic lymphatics. (*See* page 2737.)
Clinical findings of uremia.	———	May not be possible to distinguish from effusion associated with dialysis. (*See* page 2738.)
History of peritoneal or hemodialysis.	———	May not be possible to distinguish from effusion associated with uremia itself. (*See* page 2737.)
Associated clinical findings of lymphedema elsewhere.	———	Results from hypoplasia of the lymphatic system. May be associated with Milroy's disease. (*See* page 2738.)
Combination of symptoms and signs in specific racial groups.	———	Heredofamilial; limited to Armenians, Arabs, and Jews. Episodic acute attacks of abdominal and chest pain. Most episodes of pleurisy associated with arthritis and arthralgia. (*See* page 2739.)
History of myocardial infarction or surgical procedure on the pericardium.	———	Syndrome can occur years after the causative episode. (*See* page 2739.)

TABLE A–15

PLEURAL EFFUSION ASSOCIATED WITH
OTHER ROENTGENOGRAPHIC EVIDENCE OF
DISEASE IN THE THORAX

This table includes all diseases in which unilateral or bilateral pleural effusion is associated with roentgenologic evidence of another abnormality in the thorax—local or general pulmonary disease, hilar or mediastinal lymph node enlargement, cardiomegaly, diaphragmatic abnormality, disease of the pleura, bony thorax, or chest wall, or any combination of these. This widely ranging list makes a long and rather cumbersome table; however, it seemed preferable to create a single, all-inclusive table than to subdivide diseases into separate categories according to the anatomic structures involved.

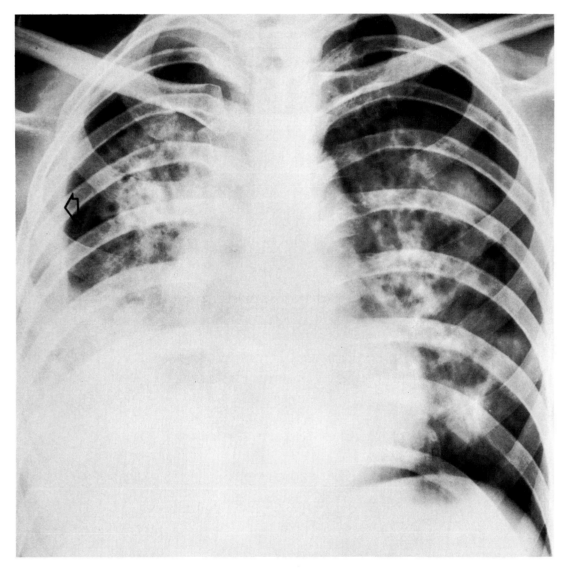

Figure 28. Pleural Effusion Associated with Pulmonary Consolidation and Mediastinal Lymph Node Enlargement: Hodgkin's Disease. A posteroanterior roentgenogram reveals a moderate accumulation of fluid in the right pleural space, possessing a somewhat atypical configuration *(arrow)* due to the presence of extensive underlying pulmonary disease. Bilateral hilar and right paratracheal lymph node enlargement is also present. This was proved Hodgkin's granuloma. (Courtesy Montreal Chest Hospital Center.)

Figure 29. Pleural Effusion Associated with Diaphragmatic Abnormality: Subphrenic Abscess. A posteroanterior roentgenogram demonstrates a small right pleural effusion obliterating the right costophrenic sulcus. The right hemidiaphragm is moderately elevated and immediately beneath it there is a small accumulation of gas containing an air-fluid level *(arrow)*. Subphrenic abscess two weeks following subtotal gastrectomy.

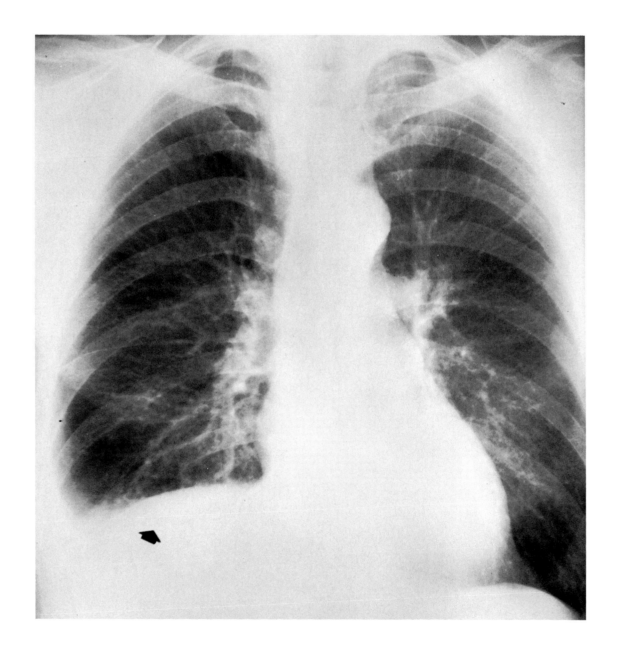

A–15
Pleural Effusion Associated With Other Roentgenographic Evidence of Disease in the Thorax

	ETIOLOGY	CHARACTER OF THE FLUID
	Bacteria	
	Klebsiella-Enterobacter-Serratia genera.	Purulent; predominant polymorphonuclear response.
	Francisella tularensis (tularemia).	Serous.
	Staphylococcus aureus.	Usually purulent but may be serous or serosanguineous.
	Streptococcus pneumoniae.	Serous.
	Mycobacterium tuberculosis.	Serous or purulent.
INFECTIOUS	*Yersinia pestis* (the plague).	Serous.
	Streptococcus pyogenes.	Varies from serous effusion to frank pus.
	Pseudomonas aeruginosa.	
	Escherichia coli.	
	Salmonella species.	Purulent.
	Acinetobacter calcoaceticus.	
	Haemophilus influenzae.	

A-15
Pleural Effusion Associated With Other Roentgenographic Evidence of Disease in the Thorax (*Continued*)

CRITERIA FOR PRESUMPTIVE DIAGNOSIS	CRITERIA FOR POSITIVE DIAGNOSIS	COMMENTS
Cavitating airspace pneumonia, often in upper lobes.	Culture of organism from sputum or pleural fluid.	Acute airspace pneumonia; cavitation frequent. Involved lobe may be expanded. (*See* page 2720.)
Combination of spherical or oval pulmonary densities with enlarged hilar nodes. History of animal exposure.	Rising serum agglutinin titers against *F. tularensis*. Isolation of the organism from sputum or pleural fluid.	Pleural effusion in 25 to 50 per cent of pneumonias. Hilar lymph node enlargement frequent. Pulmonary and pleural involvement much more frequent in typhoidal form (50 to 77 per cent) than in nontyphoidal (8 to 26 per cent). (*See* page 2721.)
In infants and children, pneumonia and empyema almost pathognomonic, particularly with abscess and pneumatocele formation.	Identification of organism by smear or culture from sputum or pleural fluid.	Rapidly progressive pneumonia—typically confluent segmental bronchopneumonia. Empyema more common in children (90 per cent) than in adults (50 per cent). (*See* page 2720.)
Typical roentgen characteristics of acute airspace pneumonia.	Isolation of organism.	Demonstrable effusion very uncommon on standard roentgenograms in erect position. (*See* page 2720.)
Positive PPD reaction	Granulomas on pleural biopsy; acid-fast organisms on smear of sputum or pleural fluid. Culture of organism from sputum or pleural fluid.	Combined pleural effusion and roentgenographically demonstrable parenchymal disease an uncommon manifestation of either primary or postprimary tuberculosis. Effusion may occur as a manifestation of widely disseminated hematogenous disease or disease of the thoracic skeleton. (*See* page 2717.)
Combination of confluent pneumonia, enlarged peripheral lymph nodes, and history of animal exposure.	Isolation of organism from sputum, blood, or aspirate of lymph node.	Pulmonary disease may simulate acute pulmonary edema. (*See* page 850.)
———	Smear or culture of organism from pleural fluid (may be very difficult to identify).	Inhomogeneous or homogeneous segmental bronchopneumonia; abscess formation variable. In children, commonly preceded by viral disease, especially exanthems. (*See* page 2720.)
Characteristically in patients with low resistance—e.g., chronic diseases, alcoholism.	Isolation of organism.	Homogeneous segmental bronchopneumonia. (*See* page 855.) Acute airspace pneumonia, commonly multilobar. (*See* page 849.) Segmental bronchopneumonia; abscess formation variable. Involvement of GI tract may not be obvious. (*See* page 850.) Pneumonia, commonly with abscesses. Pyopneumothorax usual owing to bronchopleural fistula. (*See* page 868.) Inhomogeneous segmental bronchopneumonia. In children, associated with acute upper respiratory tract symptoms. (*See* page 853.)

Table continued on following page

A–15
Pleural Effusion Associated With Other Roentgenographic Evidence of Disease in the Thorax (*Continued*)

ETIOLOGY	CHARACTER OF THE FLUID
Anaerobic organisms.	Purulent
Actinomyces israelii (actinomycosis). *Nocardia* species.	Purulent.
Fungi *Blastomyces dermatitidis.* *Cryptococcus neoformans.*	Serous exudate.
Aspergillus species.	Nonpurulent serous exudate.
Viruses All viruses and *Mycoplasma pneumoniae.*	Serous exudate.
Parasites *Entamoeba histolytica* (amebiasis).	Usually serofibrinous but may become frankly purulent when secondarily infected. Occasionally fluid contains bile and necrotic liver tissue and then possesses characteristic "chocolate-sauce" appearance.
Paragonimus westermani.	Serous exudate.
Echinococcus granulosus (hydatid disease).	Cloudy serous fluid.
Extrathoracic infection Subphrenic abscess.	Serous exudate.
Systemic lupus erythematosus.	Serous exudate.
Rheumatoid disease.	Exudate (*see* Table A–14); low serum glucose values.

INFECTIOUS *(Continued)*

IMMUNOLOGIC

A–15
Pleural Effusion Associated With Other Roentgenographic Evidence of Disease in the Thorax
(Continued)

CRITERIA FOR PRESUMPTIVE DIAGNOSIS	CRITERIA FOR POSITIVE DIAGNOSIS	COMMENTS
Characteristically in patients with low resistance—e.g., chronic diseases, alcoholism, and poor oral hygiene.	Isolation of organisms.	Segmental bronchopneumonia; incidence of infection higher than generally believed; organism requires anaerobic culture; may be intrapleural gas production. (*See* page 875.)
Combination of cavitary pneumonia, pleural effusion (empyema), and chest wall involvement should strongly suggest these etiologies.	Isolation of organism from sputum, pleural fluid, or chest wall abscess.	Homogeneous nonsegmental airspace pneumonia almost invariable; abscess formation and chest wall involvement common, sometimes with rib destruction. Empyema necessitatis. (*See* pages 1022 and 1028.)
None.	Isolation of organism.	Effusion very uncommon in blastomycosis and rare in cryptococcosis. Associated with homogeneous nonsegmental airspace pneumonia; cavitation uncommon (15 per cent). Chest-wall involvement rare. (*See* pages 968 and 975.)
None.	Isolation of organism.	Usually an opportunistic invader in postoperative empyema cavity; does not form pus. (*See* page 988.)
May be suggested by acute segmental pneumonia with combined interstitial and airspace elements. Clinical picture helpful.	Positive serologic tests. Isolation of organism.	Combined interstitial and airspace pneumonia (segmental). Effusion uncommon. (*See* page 1035.)
Combination of lower lobe consolidation, pleural effusion, and enlarged liver, especially in a patient with diarrhea.	Recovery of cysts or trophozoites from sputum, pleural fluid, or stool.	Elevation and fixation of right hemidiaphragm; homogeneous consolidation of right lower lobe, with or without abscess formation. Organisms infiltrate from liver abscess through diaphragm into pleura and lung. May form bronchohepatic fistula. (*See* page 1081.)
Thin-walled cystic spaces in lower lobes in a patient from an endemic area.	Recovery of ova from sputum or feces.	Isolated nodular opacities, usually in lower lobes, commonly with cavitation. Metacercariae migrate from free peritoneal space through diaphragm into the pleura and lung. (*See* page 1109.)
Commonly hydropneumothorax; floating scolices and daughter cysts producing "water lily" sign.	Positive Casoni skin test or complement fixation test. Recovery of hooklets from sputum or pleural fluid.	Pleural effusion develops as a result of rupture of a pulmonary hydatid cyst; a collapsed cystic space may be observed in the lungs; other solid hydatid cysts may be present. Rupture more commonly occurs into bronchus. (*See* page 1102.)
Elevated fixed hemidiaphragm with basal atelectasis and effusion (usually small).	Gas and fluid in subphrenic space.	Hemidiaphragm elevated and fixed; usually basal atelectasis, with or without pneumonia. (*See* page 2736.)
Combination of bilateral pleural effusion, nonspecific cardiac enlargement, and basal atelectasis or pneumonia should suggest the diagnosis.	Positive antinuclear antibodies in association with characteristic clinical findings.	Pulmonary changes nonspecific—generally in form of basal "pneumonitis" or atelectasis; cardiac enlargement in 30 to 50 per cent of all cases, commonly due to pericardial effusion. Progressive loss of lung volume may be a characteristic. (*See* page 2723.)
Pleuropulmonary disease in patients with rheumatoid arthritis.	High titer of rheumatoid factor in blood suggestive but not conclusive.	Diffuse reticulonodular pattern, predominantly basal in distribution. Pleural effusion most commonly an isolated finding; incidence of coexistent pleural effusion and pulmonary disease not clear but probably independent. (*See* page 2725.)

Table continued on following page

A–15
Pleural Effusion Associated With Other Roentgenographic Evidence of Disease in the Thorax (*Continued*)

	ETIOLOGY	CHARACTER OF THE FLUID
IMMUNOLOGIC (*Continued*)	Wegener's granulomatosis.	Exudate.
	Pulmonary carcinoma.	Serous exudate; may be sanguineous.
	Lymphoma.	Serosanguineous or chylous.
	Metastatic carcinoma.	Serous or serosanguineous.
	Mesothelioma.	Almost invariably bloody; hyaluronic acid levels may be elevated.
NEOPLASTIC	Bronchioloalveolar carcinoma.	Serous or serosanguineous.
	Multiple myeloma.	Commonly serosanguineous.
	Primary neoplasms of chest wall.	Serosanguineous.
	Neoplastic involvement of pleura by direct invasion of a nonpulmonary carcinoma.	Serosanguineous.
	Waldenström's macroglobulinemia.	Serous.
THROMBOEMBOLIC	Pulmonary embolism and infarction.	Serosanguineous.

A–15
Pleural Effusion Associated With Other Roentgenographic Evidence of Disease in the Thorax (*Continued*)

CRITERIA FOR PRESUMPTIVE DIAGNOSIS	CRITERIA FOR POSITIVE DIAGNOSIS	COMMENTS
Combination of pleural effusion and single or multiple pulmonary nodules (with or without cavitation), especially if associated with renal disease.	Biopsy of pulmonary or renal lesions.	Effusion was present in 6 of 11 cases in one series. (*See* page 1241.)
Obstructive pneumonitis with pleural effusion very strong presumptive evidence *per se*.	Recovery of cells from pleural fluid or sputum; positive pleural, bronchoscopic, or mediastinal node biopsy.	Commonly associated with obstructive pneumonitis. May or may not be associated with hilar or mediastinal node enlargement. Although the effusion may not contain cells, its presence is ominous. (*See* page 2729.)
Combination of zones of consolidation (commonly separate from hilum) and pleural effusion, especially with enlargement of hilar and mediastinal nodes, constitutes strong presumptive evidence.	Biopsy of pleura, lung, or lymph node. Recovery of cells from pleural fluid.	Includes Hodgkin's disease and non-Hodgkin's lymphoma. Single or multiple areas of consolidated lung of varying size—may be massive; usually homogeneous. Hilar and mediastinal nodes also may be enlarged. Parenchymal involvement seldom if ever the presenting feature. (*See* page 2729.)
Combination of diffuse pulmonary densities and pleural effusion highly suggestive, particularly if heart size is normal; differentiation from bronchioloalveolar carcinoma may be difficult.	Identification of primary lesion; positive pleural biopsy or malignant cells in pleural fluid; cells occasionally identified in sputum.	Hematogenous: generally nodular. Lymphangitic: often predominantly linear but may have nodular component. Hilar and mediastinal nodes may be involved but this is seldom a prominent roentgenographic feature. (*See* page 2730.)
In local variety, peripherally situated mass usually having obtuse angles with chest wall. In diffuse type, history of exposure to asbestos. Volume of ipsilateral hemithorax may be reduced despite massive opacification.	Recovery of cells from pleural fluid. Positive pleural biopsy.	Effusion uncommon in local variety but almost invariable in diffuse malignant type. Either local or diffuse variety may be obscured by pleural fluid. (*See* page 2770.)
High index of suspicion. Difficult to differentiate from metastatic neoplasm or widely disseminated lymphoma.	Malignant cells in pleural fluid or sputum. Biopsy.	Widely disseminated nodular densities of variable size, generally discrete but may be confluent in areas. Lymph nodes enlarged pathologically in 25 per cent of cases but may not be apparent roentgenologically. (*See* page 2729.)
Single or multiple soft-tissue masses arising from chest wall and protruding into thoracic space. Expansion of ribs almost pathognomonic.	Rib or chest wall biopsy; characteristic changes in bone marrow; electrophoretic pattern of serum proteins. Plasma cells may be numerous in pleural fluid.	Pleural effusion uncommon. Destructive lesions of one or more ribs with or without expansion. Soft-tissue masses commonly protrude into thorax. Also destructive lesions in shoulder girdle or thoracic spine. Lungs may be involved. (*See* page 2730.)
Combination of expanding lesion of chest wall and pleural effusion highly suggestive. May be indistinguishable from myeloma unless the latter is multiple.	Malignant cells in pleural fluid or biopsy.	Osteolytic, osteoblastic, or mixed neoplasms of ribs (or occasionally thoracic vertebrae) may extend into thoracic cavity. Primary mesenchymal neoplasms of intercostal spaces may act similarly. (*See* page 2955.)
In breast carcinoma, absence of breast shadow or history of mastectomy suggestive but not conclusive.	Typical cells in pleural fluid; pleural biopsy.	May occur occasionally from breast carcinoma, and rarely from liver or pancreas neoplasm. (*See* page 2730.)
Diffuse reticulonodular pattern in the lungs of a patient with anemia, lymphocytic or plasmacytoid infiltration of the bone marrow, and monoclonal IgM gammopathy.	Lung biopsy. IgM gammopathy in blood and pleural fluid.	Effusion occurs in roughly 50 per cent of cases with lung involvement. (*See* page 2730.)
Any basal shadow associated with diaphragmatic elevation and pleural effusion should suggest the possibility. Clinical picture usually distinctive. Positive ventilation-perfusion scan highly suggestive.	Pulmonary angiogram.	Pulmonary changes vary from major segmental area of consolidation to line shadows of varying extent. Hemidiaphragm commonly elevated. Pleural effusion almost always small. (*See* page 2731.)

Table continued on following page

A–15
Pleural Effusion Associated With Other Roentgenographic Evidence of Disease
in the Thorax (*Continued*)

	ETIOLOGY	CHARACTER OF THE FLUID
	Cardiac decompensation.	Transudate.
CARDIOVASCULAR	Constrictive pericarditis.	Transudate.
	Obstruction of superior vena cava or azygos vein.	Transudate.
INHALATIONAL	Asbestos-related disease.	Sterile, serous, or blood-tinged exudate.
TRAUMATIC	Open- or closed-chest trauma.	Blood (hemothorax). Chyle (chylothorax). Ingested food (esophageal rupture).
IDIOPATHIC	Sarcoidosis.	Exudate containing a predominance of lymphocytes.
	Lymphangioleiomyomatosis. Tuberous sclerosis.	Chylous.

A–15
Pleural Effusion Associated With Other Roentgenographic Evidence of Disease
in the Thorax (*Continued*)

CRITERIA FOR PRESUMPTIVE DIAGNOSIS	CRITERIA FOR POSITIVE DIAGNOSIS	COMMENTS
Cardiac enlargement, usually general and "nonspecific." Clinical signs of cardiac decompensation.	Nature of the fluid on thoracentesis; its disappearance with treatment of cardiac decompensation.	Most commonly with failure of both sides of the heart. Frequently unilateral on the right, seldom on the left, but may be bilateral. (*See* page 2731.)
Signs of systemic venous hypertension.	Pericardial calcification with reduced amplitude of pulsation.	Effusion present in approximately 50 per cent of cases. (*See* page 2731.)
Clinical signs of superior vena cava syndrome.	Angiography or CT.	(*See* page 2879.)
History of asbestos exposure plus background of pulmonary asbestosis.	Only following exclusion of other diagnostic possibilities, particularly tuberculosis and mesothelioma.	Effusions frequently recurrent, usually bilateral and often associated with chest pain. Association with asbestosis is more common than pleural effusion alone. (*See* page 2727.)
Associated findings should allow precise diagnosis in majority of cases.	Thoracentesis always diagnostic with positive history.	Wide variety of changes, including fractured ribs, pulmonary hemorrhage or hematoma, mediastinal hematoma, aortic aneurysm, pneumothorax, pneumomediastinum. (*See* page 2732.)
Association with biopsy-proved pulmonary sarcoidosis.	Identification of nonnecrotizing granulomas on pleural biopsy.	Invariably associated with pulmonary sarcoidosis, often of moderately advanced form. Incidence ranges from 0.7 to 7 per cent. (*See* page 2611.)
Presence of numerous sclerotic lesions in the skeleton, renal angiomyolipomas, and intracranial calcifications in tuberous sclerosis.	Typical changes on lung biopsy. Diffuse reticulonodular pattern in a young woman in lymphangioleiomyomatosis.	Effusion can occur rarely in the absence of pulmonary disease and is rare in tuberous sclerosis. (*See* page 2673.)

TABLE A–16

HILAR AND MEDIASTINAL LYMPH NODE ENLARGEMENT

This table includes all conditions producing lymph node enlargement within the thorax, either alone or in combination with other roentgenographic abnormalities. It is to be noted that a number of diseases are included in which node enlargement is a common manifestation in infants and children but uncommon in adults; since we have excluded much reference to pediatric diseases of the chest in the text, their inclusion here is a compromise to space limitation.

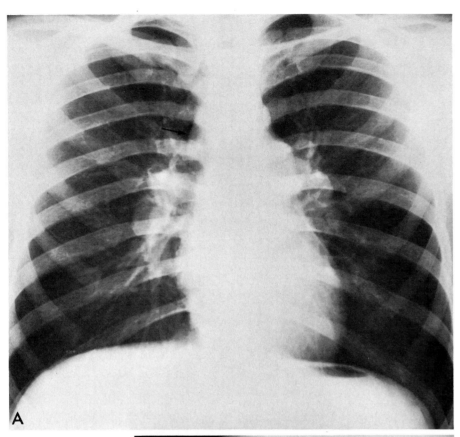

Figure 30. Hilar and Mediastinal Lymph Node Enlargement: Sarcoidosis. Posteroanterior *(A)* and lateral *(B)* roentgenograms reveal marked enlargement of both hilar shadows due to enlarged lymph nodes; the lobulated contour is particularly well demonstrated in lateral projection. Bilateral paratracheal and tracheobronchial lymph node enlargement is also present, the azygos lymph node being clearly visible in posteroanterior projection *(arrow)*. The lungs are clear.

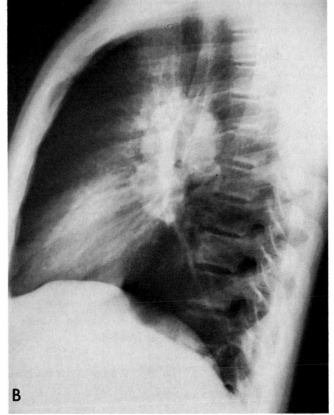

Figure 31. Hilar and Mediastinal Lymph Node Enlargement: Chronic Lymphatic Leukemia. Posteroanterior *(A)* and lateral *(B)* roentgenograms demonstrate enlarged lymph nodes in both hila and in the anterior mediastinal (prevascular) compartment *(arrows* on both illustrations). Such enlargement of the anterior mediastinal chain is highly suggestive of lymphoma.

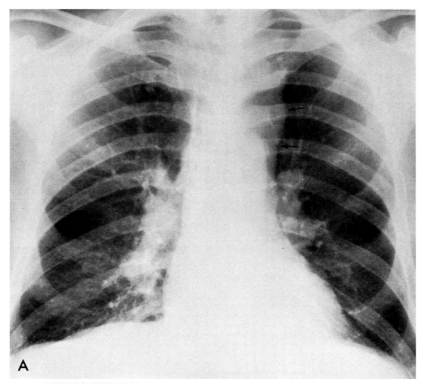

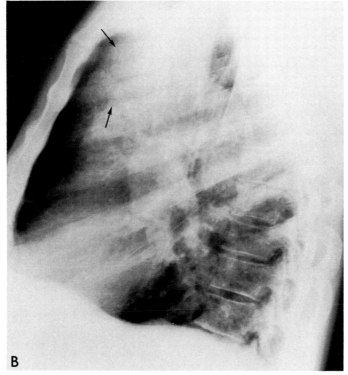

A–16
Hilar and Mediastinal Lymph Node Enlargement

	ETIOLOGY	SYMMETRY	NODE GROUPS INVOLVED
INFECTIOUS	**Bacteria**		
	Mycobacterium tuberculosis (primary).	Unilateral in 80 per cent of cases.	Approximately 60 per cent hilar and 40 per cent combined hilar and paratracheal.
	Francisella tularensis.	Unilateral.	Hilar.
	Bordetella pertussis.	Unilateral.	Hilar.
	Bacillus anthracis.	Symmetric.	All.
	Yersinia pestis (the plague).	Symmetric.	Hilar and paratracheal.
	Fungi		
	Histoplasma capsulatum.	May be unilateral or bilateral.	Hilar or paratracheal or both.
	Coccidioides immitis.	Unilateral or bilateral.	Hilar or paratracheal or both.
	Sporothrix schenkii.	Unilateral.	Hilar.
	Mycoplasma and viruses		
	Mycoplasma pneumoniae.	Unilateral or bilateral.	Hilar.
	Rubeola.	Bilateral.	Hilar.
	ECHO virus.	Bilateral.	Hilar.
	Varicella-zoster.	Bilateral.	Hilar.
	Chlamydia psittaci (ornithosis).	Unilateral or bilateral.	Hilar.
	Epstein-Barr mononucleosis.	Bilateral symmetric.	Predominantly hilar.
	Parasites		
	Tropical eosinophilia.	Bilateral.	Hilar.

A–16
Hilar and Mediastinal Lymph Node Enlargement (*Continued*)

ADDITIONAL FINDINGS	COMMENTS
Almost always associated with ipsilateral parenchymal disease.	Rarely the presentation may be bilateral, symmetric hilar node enlargement as sole manifestation. (*See* page 894.)
Oval areas of parenchymal consolidation; pleural effusion common.	Ipsilateral hilar node enlargement in 25 to 50 per cent of pneumonic tularemia. (*See* page 870.)
Ipsilateral segmental pneumonia.	Pneumonia is the result of secondary infection in some cases. (*See* page 869.)
Occasionally patchy nonsegmental opacities throughout lungs due to pulmonary hemorrhage; pleural effusion is common.	Node enlargement due to hemorrhage and edema; extension of inflammatory reaction into adjacent mediastinal tissues may obscure typical nodal configuration. (*See* page 842.)
———	Rarely, roentgenographic changes may be restricted to node enlargement, without associated pulmonary manifestations. (*See* page 850.)
Enlarged nodes may obstruct airways through extrinsic pressure, resulting in obstructive pneumonitis and atelectasis.	Node enlargement is usually associated with parenchymal disease but may occur without, particularly in children. (*See* page 949.)
Node enlargement may occur with or without associated parenchymal disease.	Involvement of paratracheal lymph nodes should raise suspicion of imminent dissemination. (*See* page 957.)
Associated with parenchymal disease in some cases.	A rare form of mycotic infection. (*See* page 1019.)
Always with segmental inhomogeneous or homogeneous pneumonia.	Lymph node enlargement is rare in adults but common in children. (*See* page 1036.)
Diffuse interstitial pattern throughout the lungs.	This pattern results from infection with rubeola virus itself and not from secondary infection. (*See* page 1050.)
Accompanied by increase in bronchovascular markings.	Lymph node enlargement rare in adults and pneumonia extremely rare in infants. (*See* page 1056.)
Diffuse airspace pneumonia may mask hilar node enlargement.	(*See* page 1062.)
Parenchymal involvement may be homogeneous consolidation or a diffuse reticular pattern.	Hilar node enlargement has not been reported as sole manifestation of the disease. (*See* page 1074.)
Splenomegaly.	Rarely associated with roentgenographic changes in the lungs. (*See* page 1071.)
A widespread micronodular pattern throughout the lungs.	Diffuse parenchymal disease is usually not accompanied by node enlargement. (*See* page 1097.)

Table continued on following page

A–16
Hilar and Mediastinal Lymph Node Enlargement *(Continued)*

	ETIOLOGY	SYMMETRY	NODE GROUPS INVOLVED
IMMUNOLOGIC	Extrinsic allergic alveolitis.	Symmetric.	Bronchopulmonary.
NEOPLASTIC	Pulmonary carcinoma.	Unilateral almost invariably.	Hilar nodes usually; paratracheal and posterior mediastinal nodes in some cases.
	Hodgkin's disease.	Typically bilateral but asymmetric; unilateral node enlargement is very unusual.	Paratracheal and bifurcation group involved as often as or more often than bronchopulmonary group. Involvement of anterior mediastinal and retrosternal nodes frequent.
	Non-Hodgkin's lymphoma.	Bilateral but asymmetric.	Similar to Hodgkin's disease.
	Leukemia.	Usually symmetric.	Mediastinal and hilar.
	Lymphangitic carcinomatosis.	Unilateral or bilateral.	Hilar or mediastinal or both.
	Bronchioloalveolar carcinoma.	Unilateral or bilateral.	Hilar or mediastinal or both.
	Angioimmunoblastic lymphadenopathy.	Bilateral but asymmetric.	Similar to Hodgkin's disease.
INHALATIONAL	Silicosis.	Symmetric.	Predominantly hilar.
	Chronic berylliosis.	Symmetric.	Hilar.
IDIOPATHIC	Sarcoidosis.	Almost invariably symmetric, unilateral node enlargement occurring in 1 to 3 per cent of cases only. The outer borders of the enlarged hila are usually lobulated.	Paratracheal, tracheobronchial, and bronchopulmonary groups. Paratracheal enlargement seldom if ever occurs without concomitant enlargement of hilar nodes.
	Histiocytosis X (eosinophilic granuloma).	Symmetric.	Hilar and mediastinal.
	Idiopathic pulmonary hemorrhage.	Symmetric.	Hilar.
AIRWAYS	Cystic fibrosis.	Unilateral or bilateral.	Hilar.
METABOLIC	Bronchopulmonary amyloidosis.	Symmetric.	Hilar and mediastinal.

A–16
Hilar and Mediastinal Lymph Node Enlargement (*Continued*)

ADDITIONAL FINDINGS	COMMENTS
Diffuse reticulonodular (sometimes acinar) pattern invariably associated.	Hilar node enlargement fairly common in mushroom-workers' lung but rare in other varieties. (*See* page 1273.)
Involvement of the bifurcation or posterior mediastinal groups of nodes may displace the barium-filled esophagus.	Enlargement of mediastinal lymph nodes may be the sole abnormality roentgenographically and almost always indicates spread from a small cell carcinoma. (*See* page 1415.)
Pulmonary involvement occurs in less than 30 per cent of patients and is almost invariably associated with mediastinal node enlargement. Pleural effusion in approximately 30 per cent of cases, usually in association with other intrathoracic manifestations. The sternum may be destroyed by direct extension from retrosternal nodes.	Intrathoracic involvement occurs in 90 per cent of patients at some stage of the disease, most commonly in the form of mediastinal lymph node enlargement; the latter is seen on the initial chest roentgenogram in approximately 50 per cent of patients. (*See* page 1507.)
Sometimes associated with pleuropulmonary involvement.	The most common intrathoracic manifestation of the disease; however, large cell lymphoma tends to be manifested by parenchymal consolidation without associated node enlargement. (*See* page 1535.)
Both pleural effusion and parenchymal involvement may be associated.	The most common roentgenographic manifestation of leukemia within the thorax (25 per cent of patients). A much more common manifestation of lymphocytic than of myelocytic leukemia. (*See* page 1554.)
Usually associated with a diffuse reticular or reticulonodular pattern throughout the lungs, predominantly basal in distribution.	Septal (Kerley B) lines are frequently present. (*See* page 1632.)
Node enlargement may occur in association with either local or diffuse pulmonary disease.	A rare finding in this neoplasm. (*See* page 1414.)
The lungs are occasionally affected in a pattern similar to that in Hodgkin's disease.	A hyperimmune disorder, most probably of B lymphocytes. Lymph node enlargement predominates and is identical to that of Hodgkin's disease. (*See* page 1570.)
Diffuse nodular or reticulonodular disease throughout both lungs. Pleural thickening in late stages. Eggshell calcification of lymph nodes occurs in approximately 5 per cent of cases and may also be observed in lymph nodes in the anterior and posterior mediastinum, the thoracic wall, and occasionally the retroperitoneal and intraperitoneal nodes.	Enlargement of hilar nodes may occur without roentgenographic evidence of pulmonary disease, although this is a rare presenting picture. (*See* page 2289.)
Diffuse micronodular pattern invariably associated.	Hilar node enlargement occurs in a minority of cases. (*See* page 2363.)
75 to 90 per cent of patients with sarcoid show mediastinal and hilar lymph node enlargement and approximately 40 per cent of these show diffuse parenchymal disease as well.	75 per cent of patients with hilar lymph node enlargement show complete resolution of the enlarged nodes. Symmetric appearance, lack of involvement of retrosternal nodes, and diminution of lymph node size with onset of diffuse lung disease aid in differentiating sarcoidosis from lymphoma and tuberculosis. (*See* page 2611.)
Early diffuse micronodular pattern which may become coarse in later stages.	Intrathoracic lymph node enlargement is rarely a manifestation of this disease. (*See* page 2682.)
Diffuse alveolar and interstitial disease.	Predominantly in acute stage. (*See* page 1183.)
Diffuse increase in markings with hyperinflation and areas of atelectasis and bronchiectasis.	Hilar node enlargement is an uncommon finding in this disease. (*See* page 2213.)
Enlarged nodes may be densely calcified.	Usually associated with diffuse pulmonary involvement. (*See* page 2578.)

TABLE A–17

MEDIASTINAL WIDENING

The conditions listed in this table include all those responsible for increase in the width or mass of the mediastinum. Of necessity, there is considerable overlap of diseases in Tables A–16 and A–17; since enlargement of lymph nodes causes mediastinal widening, it is clear that all diseases listed in Table A–16 could be included in this category. However, in Table A–17, emphasis is placed on those diseases that cause widening of the mediastinal silhouette in which contour does *not* suggest node enlargement.

The headings in this table include *anatomic location* of the various disease processes within the mediastinal compartments: the designation +++ indicates that the process is almost invariably within that compartment, ++ that it predominates in that compartment, and + that it sometimes is located in that compartment. Thus, those diseases indicated by a single + in all compartments show no definite anatomic predilection. Where possible, the order in which the diseases are listed has been arranged to comply with predominant anatomic location; thus, under *Neoplastic,* tumors that tend to occupy the anterior compartment are listed first, the middle compartment second, and the posterior compartment last.

No attempt has been made to include diseases of the heart, since such clearly is outside the scope of this book. Similarly, abnormalities of mediastinal contour that relate directly or indirectly to cardiac anomalies have been excluded (e.g., the "snowman" configuration of anomalous pulmonary venous return).

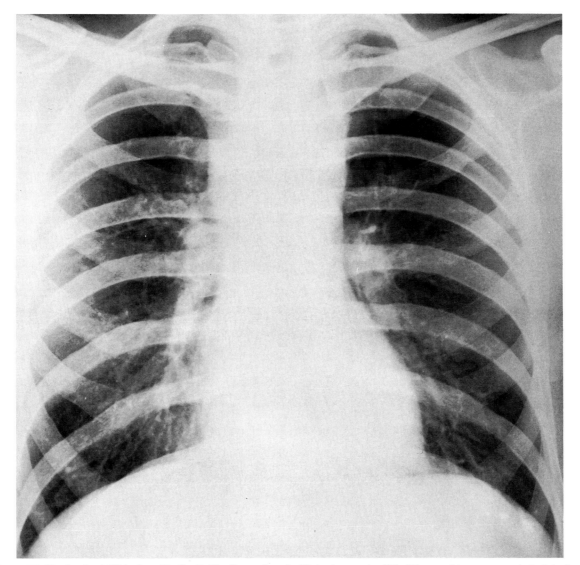

Figure 32. Mediastinal Widening: Mediastinitis Secondary to Histoplasmosis. This 30-year-old man presented clinically with a superior vena caval syndrome. A posteroanterior roentgenogram reveals moderate widening of the superior mediastinum, the contour being smooth rather than nodular as might be expected from lymph node enlargement. Multiple tiny punctate calcifications that were present throughout the spleen (not visualized on this illustration) lent support to other evidence for a diagnosis of histoplasmosis.

Figure 33. Mediastinal Widening: Malignant Thymoma. Posteroanterior *(A)* and lateral *(B)* roentgenograms reveal a marked widening of the upper mediastinum by a smooth, sharply circumscribed soft-tissue mass of homogeneous density situated predominantly in the anterior mediastinal compartment (note the poorly defined increase in density in the anterior portion of the thorax in lateral projection). The elevation of the left hemidiaphragm was unexplained. This was proved malignant thymoma.

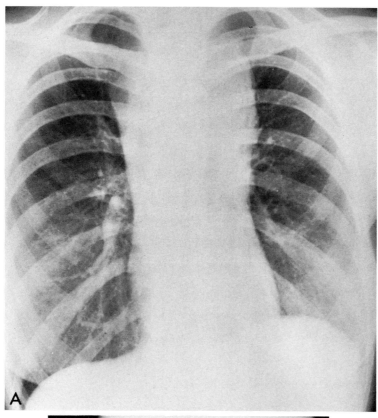

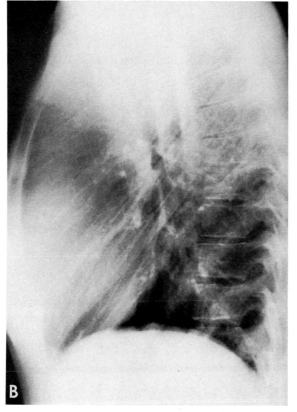

A–17
Mediastinal Widening

		LOCATION		
	ETIOLOGY	ANTERIOR	MIDDLE	POSTERIOR
DEVELOPMENTAL	Bronchial cyst.	+	+ +	+ +
	Mesothelial cyst (pericardial and pleuropericardial cysts).	+	+ +	
	Diverticula of the pharynx or esophagus.			+ + +
	Gastroenteric (neurenteric) cyst.			+ + +
	Meningocele and meningomyelocele.			+ + +
INFECTIOUS	Chronic sclerosing mediastinitis.	+	+	+
	Acute mediastinitis.	+	+	+
	Anthrax.	+	+	
	Suppurative spondylitis.			+ + +

A–17
Mediastinal Widening *(Continued)*

CONTOUR	ADDITIONAL FINDINGS	COMMENTS
Round or oval, well defined. Contour may be affected by contact with more solid structures.	May compress tracheobronchial tree or esophagus. Calcification rare (however, *see* Figure 5–10, page 718.)	Cyst may be multilocular. Seldom communicates with tracheobronchial tree. May look like a solid mass on CT because of high attenuation of contents. (*See* page 714.)
Usually round, oval, or "tear-drop" in appearance, with smooth margin.	Variation in shape of cyst may occur on changing position of patient.	Almost always do not cause symptoms. (*See* page 2867.)
Cyst-like structure in superior (pharyngeal) or inferior (esophageal) regions.	Invariably communicate with pharynx or esophagus. May displace contiguous esophagus.	Aspiration pneumonia may develop from pharyngeal (Zenker's) diverticulum. (*See* page 2903.)
Oval or lobulated, sharply defined, homogeneous.	Spinal anomalies in many cases. Rarely air is found in cyst.	Often discovered in infancy. May reach large size, and may be unilateral or bilateral. (*See* page 2902.)
Sharply circumscribed, solitary or multiple, unilateral or bilateral.	Frequently spine and rib deformities. No calcification.	Usually communicate with spinal subarachnoid space. (*See* page 2901.)
Lobulated, usually in right paramediastinal area.	May show calcification. Compression of SVC or other vessel or major airway in some cases.	The cause of approximately 10 per cent of mediastinal widening. (*See* page 2796.)
Symmetric widening due to diffuse involvement or localized due to abscess formation.	May be air in mediastinum.	Most cases due to esophageal rupture. (*See* page 2796.)
Symmetric widening resulting from hemorrhagic edema of lymph nodes.	Patchy nonsegmental opacities may be present in lungs, owing to hemorrhagic edema. Pleural effusion common.	Disease commonest in sorters and combers in the wool industry. Organism (*B. anthracis*) is extremely virulent. (*See* page 842.)
Widening of lower mediastinum with fusiform mass.	Erosion or destruction of vertebrae at level of paravertebral mass.	(*See* page 2908.)

Table continued on following page

ETIOLOGY	LOCATION		
	ANTERIOR	MIDDLE	POSTERIOR
Tumors and tumor-like conditions of the thymus: Thymic hyperplasia.	+ + +		
Thymolipoma.	+ + +		
Thymic cysts.	+ + +		
Thymoma.	+ + +		
Thymic neuroendocrine neoplasms.	+ + +		
Thymic carcinoma.	+ + +		
Thymic lymphoma.	+ + +		

Germ cell neoplasms:
    Teratoma.
    Seminoma.
    Choriocarcinoma.
    Endodermal sinus tumor.
		+ + +	+

Thyroid tumors.	+ +		+
Parathyroid tumors.	+ + +		
Soft-tissue tumors and tumor-like conditions: Lipomatosis.	+ +	+	+
Lipoma. Liposarcoma. Hemangioma. Angiosarcoma. Hemangiopericytoma. Lymphangioma. Leiomyoma. Leiomyosarcoma. Fibroma. Fibrosarcoma.	+ +	+	+
Lymphoma and leukemia.	+ +	+ + +	
Metastatic lymph node enlargement.	+	+ + +	+

NEOPLASTIC

CONTOUR	ADDITIONAL FINDINGS	COMMENTS
Smooth or lobulated.	None.	Defined as an increase in the size of the gland associated with an intact gross architecture and normal histologic appearance. (*See* page 2815.)
Smooth or lobulated.	None.	These tumors can grow very large, and because of their fat content and soft pliable consistency tend to slump toward the diaphragm, leaving the upper mediastinum relatively clear. (*See* page 2818.)
Smooth.	None.	Cystic nature should be readily apparent on CT. (*See* page 2820.)
Smooth or lobulated; well defined.	Contains calcium in some cases.	Close relationship to myasthenia gravis. CT is the examination of choice. (*See* page 2820.)
Lobulated.	Contain calcium in some cases.	Derived from neuroendocrine cells; the most common histologic type is carcinoid tumor. (*See* page 2831.)
Irregular, poorly defined.	Invasion of adjacent structures common at the time of diagnosis.	Bulky masses ranging from 5 to 15 cm in diameter. Prognosis poor. (*See* page 2834.)
Smooth or lobulated.	Mediastinal lymph node enlargement in some cases.	Hodgkin's disease and lymphoblastic lymphoma most common types. (*See* page 2835.)
Smooth or lobulated, oval or round. May protrude to either side or bilaterally.	Calcification, bone, teeth, or fat may be identified in teratomas.	CT or MRI is the examination of choice. (*See* page 2835.)
Smooth or lobulated.	Anterior tumors displace the trachea posteriorly and laterally; posterior tumors displace trachea anteriorly and esophagus posteriorly. Calcification fairly common.	Typically a nodular goiter. Radioactive isotopic studies are usually diagnostic although CT may be required. (*See* page 2844.)
Smooth or lobulated.	Evidence of hyperparathyroidism in the thoracic skeleton. Mass may displace esophagus.	Arteriography or CT may reveal smaller lesions. Hypercalcemia and hypophosphatemia. (*See* page 2846.)
Smooth and symmetric; sometimes lobulated.	Enlargement of pleuropericardial fat pads.	Usually associated with Cushing's syndrome or long-term corticosteroid therapy, occasionally with simple obesity. If necessary, CT diagnostic. (*See* page 2848.)
Commonly smooth and well defined.	Variable.	Each of these tumors can occur in any mediastimal compartment but are usually located anteriorly. (*See* pages 2846 to 2858.)
Symmetrically widened mediastinum or solitary or multiple lobulated masses.	Pulmonary consolidation and pleural effusion in some cases.	Most common mediastinal "mass." (*See* page 2858.)
Commonly unilateral with pulmonary carcinoma. Predominant involvement may occur in paratracheal or hilar groups.	Phrenic nerve involvement may result in diaphragmatic paralysis.	Primary usually pulmonary carcinoma. May originate from GI tract, breast, kidney, and so forth. (*See* page 1415.)

Table continued on following page

A–17
Mediastinal Widening *(Continued)*

ETIOLOGY	LOCATION		
	ANTERIOR	MIDDLE	POSTERIOR
Giant lymph node hyperplasia.	+	+ + +	+
Tumors and tumor-like conditions of neural tissue: Aorticopulmonary paraganglioma (chemodectoma).		+ + +	
Aorticosympathetic (paravertebral) paraganglioma.			+ + +
Tumors of peripheral nerves (neurofibroma, neurilemoma, neurogenic sarcoma). Tumors of sympathetic ganglia (ganglioneuroma, ganglioneuroblastoma, neuroblastoma).			+ + +
Esophageal neoplasms.			+ + +
Bone and cartilage neoplasms.	+		+ + +
Aortic aneurysm.	+	+	+
Buckling or aneurysm of the innominate artery.		+ + +	
Superior vena caval dilatation.		+ + +	
Azygos and hemiazygos dilatation.		+	+ +
Dilatation of pulmonary artery.		+ + +	
Aortic vascular ring.		+	+

NEOPLASTIC *(Continued)* — rows: Giant lymph node hyperplasia through Bone and cartilage neoplasms.

CARDIOVASCULAR — rows: Aortic aneurysm through Aortic vascular ring.

A–17
Mediastinal Widening (Continued)

CONTOUR	ADDITIONAL FINDINGS	COMMENTS
Usually solitary and sharply circumscribed.	No calcification.	In anterior mediastinum a multilobulated appearance may suggest thymic or teratoid tumors. (*See* page 2861.)
Smooth or lobulated.	None.	A neoplasm of the extra-adrenal paraganglionic system, arising from aorticopulmonary paraganglia. (*See* page 2866.)
Smooth or lobulated.	None.	Arises from segmental ganglia of the sympathetic chain in the pasterior mediastinum. (*See* page 2901.)
Round or oval, well defined. Rarely dumbbell-shaped.	Majority are paravertebral in location, usually unilateral. Rib or vertebral erosion variable. Rarely calcification in tumor.	CT, with or without myelography, usually required for diagnosis. (*See* page 2898.)
Smooth, rounded margin; usually unilateral.	Smooth compression of esophageal lumen on barium swallow.	Usually carcinoma or leiomyoma. (*See* page 2903.)
Rounded, paravertebral mass.	Destruction of affected bone, often associated with soft tissue mass protruding into and compressing lung.	(*See* page 2908.)
Fusiform or saccular.	Erosion of bony thoracic cage where pulsatile aneurysm is contiguous. Calcification may be present in wall.	Aortography or CT may be needed for definitive diagnosis. (*See* page 2885.)
Smooth, lateral bulging, convex laterally from level of aortic arch upwards.	Tortuous thoracic aorta due to atherosclerosis may also be noted.	Angiography or CT may be required for definitive diagnosis but is seldom indicated. (*See* page 2888.)
Smooth, extending from hilum along right paramediastinal border.	Signs of etiology—e.g., cardiac dilatation, mediastinal mass, and so forth.	Secondary to central pressure rise or to compression and obstruction. (*See* page 2879.)
Smooth, round or oval mass at tracheobronchial angle.	Change in size with Valsalva and Mueller procedures and with change in body position.	Azygography or CT may be required for definitive diagnosis. (*See* page 2879.)
Smooth.	Stenotic pulmonary valve or peripheral vascular attenuation in secondary types.	Angiography or CT may be required to differentiate this from mediastinal tumors. (*See* page 2869.)
A vessel situated between trachea and esophagus.	Compression of esophagus or trachea.	Usually detected in first year of life. (*See* page 731.)

Tale continued on following page

A–17
Mediastinal Widening *(Continued)*

ETIOLOGY	LOCATION		
	ANTERIOR	MIDDLE	POSTERIOR
Pneumomediastinum.	+	+	+
TRAUMATIC Mediastinal hemorrhage or hematoma.	+	+	+
Fracture of vertebra with hematoma.			+ + +
Herniation through foramen of Morgagni.	+ + +		
Esophageal hiatus hernia.			+ + +
MISCELLANEOUS CAUSES Herniation through foramen of Bochdalek.			+ + +
Megaesophagus.			+ + +
Extramedullary hematopoiesis.			+ + +

A–17
Mediastinal Widening *(Continued)*

CONTOUR	ADDITIONAL FINDINGS	COMMENTS
Smooth; unilateral or bilateral.	Unilateral or bilateral pneumothorax. Subcutaneous and interstitial emphysema.	Much more commonly spontaneous. Readily diagnosed by presence of mediastinal air. (*See* page 2498.)
May be local or diffuse, commonly in upper mediastinum.	Rarely SVC compression.	History of trauma (including surgery) or dissecting aneurysm. (*See* page 2499.)
Smooth paravertebral swelling, usually bilateral.	Vertebral and rib fractures.	(*See* page 2908.)
Round or oval; usually to right of pericardium.	If completely radiopaque, CT may differentiate this from epicardial fat or pericardial cyst.	Often in asymptomatic individuals. Examination of the colon may be diagnostic. (*See* page 2867.)
Retrocardiac mass of variable size containing air and fluid; usually smooth.	May contain several fluid levels; rarely completely opaque. Barium usually outlines contents.	Contains stomach, rarely bowel, omentum, liver, or spleen. (*See* page 2906.)
Round or oval retrocardiac density. Unilateral and rarely bilateral.	———	Occasionally contains bowel loops, more often omentum or solid abdominal viscera. (*See* page 2908.)
Broad vertical opacity on the right side of the mediastinum.	Air in lumen with fluid level at varying distance from diaphragm.	Usually the result of progressive systemic sclerosis or achalasia. (*See* page 2906.)
Smooth or lobulated, usually bilateral.	Spleen may be enlarged.	Anemia and hepatosplenomegaly. (*See* page 2908.)

NAME INDEX

CUMULATIVE SUBJECT INDEX

Note: Page numbers in *italics* refer to illustrations;
page numbers followed by a t refer to tables.